Health Care Careers
Directory 2008-2009

36th Edition

Indispensable information on
8,000 programs in 77 professions

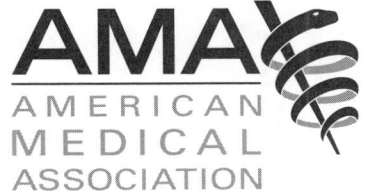

AMERICAN
MEDICAL
ASSOCIATION

Health Care Careers Directory 2008-2009

Copyright 2008 by the American Medical Association
All rights reserved
Printed in the United States of America

No part of this publication may be reproduced, stored in a retrieval system, or transmitted in any form or by any means—electronic, mechanical, photocopying, recording, or otherwise—without the prior written permission of the American Medical Association.

Internet address: www.ama-assn.org

The American Medical Association and its authors and editors have checked with sources believed to be reliable to confirm that the information presented herein is accurate and complete and in accordance with current accepted practices. However, the AMA does not warrant that the information is in every respect accurate and complete, and is not responsible for any errors or omissions or for any consequences from application of the information in this book. This book is intended for information purposes only. It is not intended to constitute legal advice. If legal advice is desired or needed, a licensed attorney should be consulted.

Order Information

To order additional copies of the *Health Care Careers Directory*, call the American Medical Association toll free at 800 621-8335. Mention product number OP417508

For other correspondence address inquiries to:
Fred Donini-Lenhoff
Medical Education Products
American Medical Association
515 N State St
Chicago, IL 60610
312 464-5333
312 464-5830 Fax
E-mail: fred.lenhoff@ama-assn.org

ISBN 978-1-60359-005-1
BP19:08-P-017

Contents

 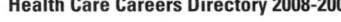

Contents

Preface

The *2008-2009 Health Care Careers Directory* now encompasses
- 8,000 programs
- 2,600 sponsoring institutions
- 77 health care careers

Organization of the Directory

The *Health Care Careers Directory* contains information on more than 8,000 educational programs in 77 health care careers.

Section I: Health Care Careers and Educational Programs includes career descriptions, employment characteristics, and information about educational programs, such as length, curriculum, and educational standards, for the majority of the health care fields listed. Section I also provides sources for information on careers, certification, licensure, and registration.

This information is followed by a complete list of accredited/approved educational programs in alphabetical order by state, for each occupation. Most program listings include the educational program name and address and Web site address.

The list of programs is followed by a data chart showing class capacity (per start date or session), month(s) classes begin, program length(s), yearly tuition cost (resident and nonresident), yearly stipend (if any), academic award(s) granted, availability of evening/weekend courses, whether a program offers education/courses in medical/ health care terms in non-English languages, availability of distance education, and whether the program offers education in cultural competence or in patient communication. These data are shown only for those programs that completed the 2007 AMA Survey of Health Professions Education Programs.

Section II: Institutions Sponsoring Accredited Programs lists 2,600 institutions sponsoring the educational programs listed in Section I. Sponsoring institutions are listed by state and city in alphabetical order. The majority of entries for each institution include the name, address, telephone number, and e-mail address of the chief executive officer and a list of the accredited health education programs for which the institution is a sponsor.

Section III: Additional Health Professions Information provides information on health care careers not included in Section I, as well as information on leading national organizations involved in promoting health care careers and providing workforce data.

Section IV: Health Professions Education Data offers data tables and sources for additional information on the health professions.

Annual Survey of Health Professions Education Programs

In 2007, the AMA used an online survey to collect data on health professions education programs for the 2006-2007 academic year. The Internet-based survey, available at www.ama-assn.org/go/hpsurvey, helps reduce survey mailing costs and allowed for the collection of racial/ethnic program data, which had been discontinued in 1996 due to the costs and difficulty of obtaining accurate data. Aggregate survey data are published in Section IV and in the *Health Professions Education Data Book* (see below).

Health Care Careers e-Letter

This monthly electronic newsletter covers educational trends and career-related issues in the professions included in the *Directory*. The *e-Letter* is distributed free of charge via e-mail to all program and institution personnel listed in the *Directory* who opt in to receive it. To view the current issue, click on www.ama-assn.org/go/hpe-letter; to subscribe, see www.ama-assn.org/go/enews or e-mail alliedhealth@ama-assn.org.

Health Professions Education Data Book

Data collected on the annual survey are available in the *Health Professions Education Data Book*. For more information or to order, call 312 464-5333 or e-mail enza.perrone@ama-assn.org, or access www.ama-assn.org/go/hpdatabook.

Health Professions Data Service/Mailing Labels

The AMA's Health Professions Data Service offers a wide range of custom data and mailing labels for the health professions. These data, both current and historical, are collected on the Annual Survey of Health Professions Education Programs. Available data variables include:

Student data
- data on program enrollments, attrition, and graduates by gender

Program data
- tuition cost(s) (total for first-year student)
- class capacity (per start date or session)
- availability of evening/weekend classes
- program length(s), in months
- program start date(s)
- credential(s) awarded
- data on percentages of recent graduates (within last 6 months) finding employment or seeking additional education
- name, address, telephone/fax numbers, and e-mail addresses of program officials.

For more information, contact Medical Education Products at 312 464-5333 or enza.perrone@ama-assn.org.

Disclaimer

The AMA does not certify or register health personnel and does not recognize or approve certifying agencies or the professions listed in the *Directory*. The certifying agencies listed in Section I do not represent an inclusive listing. For more information on certifying agencies, contact the National Organization for Competency Assurance at www.noca.org.

Acknowledgments

The AMA gratefully acknowledges the cooperative relationships with the participating health professions accrediting agencies, listed on the inside front cover; these relationships and the hard work of accrediting agency staff throughout the year are essential for establishing the survey population and for providing information about and updates to accredited programs. The AMA also expresses its deep appreciation for the continued cooperation of program directors, the majority of whom respond to the Annual Survey of Health Professions Education Programs.

Acknowledgments are also due to Enza Perrone and Arecia Washington for survey and data assistance; Rod Hill for production support; and AMA customer service staff for handling the questions generated by this product. In addition, thanks are due to the AMA Book Group staff listed on page ii.

Fred Donini-Lenhoff, MA, Editor
Dorothy Grant-Bryant, Survey and Database Coordinator
Paul H Rockey, MD, MPH, Director, Division of Graduate Medical
  Education

Health Care Careers QuickConsult

American Medical Association

515 N State St, Chicago, IL 60610   312 464-5000
www.ama-assn.org

Membership information	*800 621-8335*
Council on Ethical and Judicial Affairs	312 464-4823
www.ama-assn.org/go/ceja	
Council on Medical Education	312 464-4515
www.ama-assn.org/go/councilmeded	
Council on Science and Public Health	312 464-5046
www.ama-assn.org/go/csa	
Allied Health	312 464-5333
www.ama-assn.org/go/alliedhealth	
Adolescent Health	312 464-5315
www.ama-assn.org/go/adolescenthealth	
Domestic Violence	312 464-5437
www.ama-assn.org/go/violence	
Genetics and Molecular Medicine	312 464-4964
www.ama-assn.org/go/genetics	
Health Disparities	312 464-4452
www.ama-assn.org/go/healthdisparities	
Health Literacy	312 464-5357
www.amafoundation.org	
Medical Education	312 464-5333
www.ama-assn.org/go/meded	
Minority Affairs Consortium	312 464-5622
www.ama-assn.org/go/mac	
Section on Medical Schools	312 464-4655
www.ama-assn.org/go/sms	
Virtual Mentor	312 464-5260
www.virtualmentor.org	

Health Care Careers Information

Anesthesiologist Assisting
American Academy of Anesthesiologists' Assistants
804 565-6353   www.anesthetist.org

Art Therapy
American Art Therapy Association
888 290-0878 or 703 212-2238   www.arttherapy.org

Subscribe to our free e-mail newsletter!

The *Health Care Careers e-Letter* is a monthly electronic newsletter that covers educational trends and career-related issues in the professions included in the *Directory*. The *e-Letter* is distributed free of charge via e-mail to all program and institution personnel listed in the *Directory*.

    To view the current issue, click on
        www.ama-assn.org/go/hpe-letter
    To subscribe, see:
        www.ama-assn.org/go/enews

Athletic Training
National Athletic Trainers' Association
800 TRY-NATA or 214 637-6282   www.nata.org

Audiology
American Speech-Language-Hearing Association
800 638-8255   www.asha.org

Blindness and Visual Impairment Professions
Association for Education and Rehabilitation of the Blind and Visually Impaired
703 671-4500 or 877 492-2708   www.aerbvi.org

Blood Bank Technology, Specialist in
American Society for Clinical Pathology
312 541-4999   www.ascp.org

Cardiovascular Technology
Society for Vascular Ultrasound
301 459-7550   www.svunet.org

American Society of Echocardiography
919 861-5574   www.asecho.org

Clinical Laboratory Science/Medical Technology
American Society for Clinical Laboratory Science
301 657-2768   www.ascls.org

American Society of Clinical Pathologists
312 541-4999   www.ascp.org

Counseling
American Counseling Association
800 347-6647   www.counseling.org

Cytotechnology
American Society of Cytopathology
302 429-8802   www.cytopathology.org

Dance Therapy
American Dance Therapy Association
410 997-4040   www.adta.org

Dentistry
American Dental Association
312 440-2500   www.ada.org

Dental Assisting
American Dental Assistants Association
312 541-1550   www.dentalassistant.org

Dental Hygiene
American Dental Hygienists' Association
312 440-8900   www.adha.org

Dental Laboratory Technician
National Association of Dental Laboratories
800 950-1150 or 850 205-5626   www.nadl.org

Diagnostic Medical Sonography
Society of Diagnostic Medical Sonographers
800 229-9506 or 214 473-8057   www.sdms.org

Dietetics
American Dietetic Association
800 877-1600   www.eatright.org

Electroneurodiagnostic Technology
American Society of Electroneurodiagnostic Technologists
816 931-1120   www.aset.org

Emergency Medical Technician-Paramedic
National Association of Emergency Medical Technicians
800 34-NAEMT   www.naemt.org

Exercise Science
American Alliance for Health, Physical Education,
Recreation, and Dance
800 213-7193   www.aahperd.org

Genetic Counseling
National Society of Genetic Counselors
312 321-6834   www.nsgc.org

Health Information Management
American Health Information Management Association
312 233-1100   www.ahima.org

Histotechnology
National Society for Histotechnology
301 262-6221   www.nsh.org

Kinesiotherapy
American Kinesiotherapy Association
800 296-2582   www.akta.org

Massage Therapy
American Massage Therapy Association
877 905-2700   www.amtamassage.org

Medical Assisting
American Association of Medical Assistants
312 899-1500   www.aama-ntl.org

Medical Librarian
Medical Library Association
312 419-9094   www.mlanet.org/career

Music Therapy
American Music Therapy Association
301 589-3300   www.musictherapy.org

Nuclear Medicine Technology
Society of Nuclear Medicine—Technologist Section
703 708-9000   www.snm.org

Nursing
National League for Nursing
800 669-1656   www.nln.org

American Nurses Association
800-274-4ANA   http://nursingworld.org

Occupational Therapy
American Occupational Therapy Association
301 652-2682   www.aota.org

Ophthalmic Dispensing Optician
Opticians Association of America
847 202-1411   www.opticians.org

Ophthalmic Medical Technology
Joint Comm. on Allied Health Personnel in Ophthalmology
800 284-3937   www.jcahpo.org/newsite

Optometrist
American Optometric Association
800 365-2219   www.aoa.org

Orthoptist
American Orthoptic Council
608 233-5383   www.orthoptics.org

Orthotist and Prosthetist
American Orthotic and Prosthetic Association
571 431-0876   www.aopanet.org

Pathologists' Assisting
American Association of Pathologists' Assistants
800 532-AAPA   www.pathologistsassistants.org

Perfusionist
American Society of Extra-Corporeal Technologists
804 565-6363   www.amsect.org

Pharmacist
American Pharmacists Association
202 628-4410   www.aphanet.org

Pharmacy Technician
American Association of Pharmacy Technicians
919 686-3800   www.pharmacytechnician.com

Physical Therapy
American Physical Therapy Association
800 999-2782 or 703 684-2782   www.apta.org

Physician (allopathic)
American Medical Association
312 464-5000   www.ama-assn.org/go/becominganmd

Physician (osteopathic)
American Osteopathic Association
800 621-1773 or 312 202-8000   www.osteopathic.org

Physician Assistant
American Academy of Physician Assistants
703 836-2272   www.aapa.org

Podiatrist
American Podiatric Medical Association
301 581-9200   www.apma.org/careers

Polysomnographic Technology
Association of Polysomnographic Technologists
708 492-0796   www.aptweb.org

Psychologist
American Psychological Association
800 374-2721 or 202 336-5500   www.apa.org/students

Radiologic Technology
American Society of Radiologic Technologists
800 444-2778 or 505 298-4500   www.asrt.org

Rehabilitation Counseling
National Council on Rehabilitation Education
618 549-3267   www.rehabeducators.org

Respiratory Therapy
American Association for Respiratory Care
972 243-2272   www.aarc.org

Speech-language Pathology
American Speech-Language-Hearing Association
800 638-8255   www.asha.org

Surgical Technology
Association of Surgical Technologists
303 694-9130   www.ast.org

Therapeutic Recreation Specialist
American Therapeutic Recreation Association
703 683-9420   www.atra-tr.org/atra.htm

Veterinary Medicine, Veterinary Technology
American Veterinary Medical Association
847 925-8070   www.avma.org

Accrediting Agencies

Accreditation Council for Occupational Therapy Education

www.aota.org
- Occupational therapist
- Occupational therapy assistant

Accreditation Council for Pharmacy Education

www.acpe-accredit.org
- Pharmacist

Accreditation Council on Optometric Education

www.aoa.org
- Optometrist, Optometric Technician

Accreditation Review Commission on Education for the Physician Assistant

www.arc-pa.org
- Physician assistant

American Art Therapy Association

www.arttherapy.org
- Art therapist

American Board of Genetic Counseling

www.abgc.net
- Genetic counselor

American Dance Therapy Association

www.adta.org
- Dance therapist

American Orthoptic Council

www.orthoptics.org
- Orthoptist

American Psychological Association Committee on Accreditation

www.apa.org
- Psychologist

American Society of Health System-Pharmacists

www.ashp.org
- Pharmacy technician

American Veterinary Medical Association, Committee on Veterinary Technician Education and Activities

www.avma.org/education/cvea/
- Veterinary Technologist

American Veterinary Medical Association, Council on Education

www.avma.org/education/cvea/
- Veterinarian

Association for Education and Rehabilitation of the Blind and Visually Impaired

www.aerbvi.org
- Orientation and mobility specialist
- Teacher of the visually impaired
- Rehabilitation teacher
- Low vision therapist

Commission on Accreditation for Dietetics Education of the American Dietetic Association

www.eatright.org/cade
- Dietitian/nutritionist
- Dietetic technician

Commission on Accreditation for Health Informatics and Information Management Education

www.cahiim.org
- Health information administrator
- Health information technician

Commission on Accreditation in Physical Therapy Education

www.apta.org
- Physical therapist
- Physical therapist assistant

Commission on Accreditation of Athletic Training Education

www.jrc-at.org
- Athletic trainer

Commission on Accreditation of Ophthalmic Medical Programs

www.jcahpo.org
- Ophthalmic medical technical/technologist
- Ophthalmic Assistant

Commission on Accreditation of Allied Health Education Programs

www.caahep.org
- Anesthesiologist assistant
- Cardiovascular technologist
- Cytotechnologist
- Diagnostic medical sonographer
- Electroneurodiagnostic technologist
- Emergency medical technician-paramedic
- Exercise physiologist (applied and clinical)
- Exercise science professional
- Kinesiotherapist
- Medical assistant
- Medical illustrator
- Orthotist/prosthetist
- Perfusionist
- Polysomnographic technologist
- Respiratory therapist advanced
- Respiratory therapy entry level
- Specialist in blood bank technology
- Surgical assistant
- Surgical technologist

Commission on Collegiate Nursing Education

www.aacn.nche.edu/accreditation
- Nurse

Commission on Dental Accreditation of the American Dental Association

www.ada.org
- Dentist
- Dental assistant
- Dental hygienist
- Dental laboratory technologist

Commission on Massage Therapy Accreditation

www.comta.org
- Therapeutic Massage and Bodywork

Commission on Opticianry Accreditation

www.COAccreditation.com
- Ophthalmic laboratory technician
- Ophthalmic Dispensing Optician

Commission on Osteopathic College Accreditation

www.osteopathic.org
- Physician (osteopathic)

Council for Accreditation of Counseling and Related Educational Programs

www.cacrep.org
- Community counselor
- Marriage, couple, and family counselor/therapist
- Mental health counselor
- Student affairs practitioner
- School counselor

Council on Academic Accreditation in Audiology and Speech-Language Pathology

www.asha.org
- Audiologist
- Speech-language pathologist

Council on Accreditation of the National Recreation and Park Association

www.councilonaccreditation.org
- Therapeutic recreation specialist

Council on Podiatric Medical Education

www.cpme.org
- Podiatrist

Council on Rehabilitation Education

http://core-rehab.org
- Rehabilitation counselor

Joint Review Committee on Education in Radiologic Technology

www.jrcert.org
- Medical Dosimetrist
- Magnetic Resonance Technologist
- Radiation therapist
- Radiographer

Joint Review Committee on Educational Programs in Nuclear Medicine Technology

www.jrcnmt.org
- Nuclear medicine technologist

Liaison Committee on Medical Education

www.lcme.org
- Physician (allopathic)

Medical Library Association

www.mlanet.org
- Medical librarian

National Accrediting Agency for Clinical Laboratory Sciences

www.naacls.org
- Clinical assistant
- Clinical laboratory scientist/medical technologist
- Clinical laboratory technician/medical lab technician
- Cytogenetic technologist
- Diagnostic molecular scientist
- Histotechnologist
- Pathologists' assistant
- Phlebotomist

National Association of Schools of Music

www.arts-accredit.org
- Music therapist

Section I: *Health Care Careers and Educational Programs* offers descriptions and general information for 77 health care careers and includes listings for 8,000 accredited educational programs in all 50 states, Puerto Rico, Canadian provinces, and some other countries.

Each profession description contains many if not all of the following elements, identified by an icon:

History describes the development of the profession over time, from the origin and evolution of each profession's key duties and responsibilities, and the establishment of the first sponsoring institutions and programs, to important convocations of decision-makers, accrediting bodies, and market forces that have shaped and defined the current state of the profession.

Career Description details the general duties of the profession within the context of the health care environment in which it exists. Background information on the area of medical care that the profession supports (eg, laboratory testing, physical rehabilitation, surgery, administration, diet and nutrition) is also included. Also included is a more in-depth depiction of the day-to-day activities of each profession, including the duties and responsibilities that could be expected or assigned, depending on the facility, physical location, staff needs, and work environment.

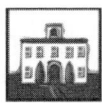

Employment Characteristics describes the workplace, facility, or physical location where the profession's duties are typically performed. Lengths of shifts, typical work weeks, and on-call status are also included, if available.

Salary ranges, from a variety of government, professional association, and industry survey sources, are provided if available. (*Note:* Salary data are also shown, by profession, in Table 5, Section IV.)

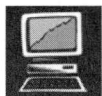

Employment Outlook, if available, gives statistics or trend summaries from government, professional associations, and industry surveys about overall projections for demand, growth, and staffing needs within each profession's field of activity.

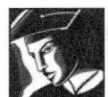

Educational Programs offers general information regarding the length, prerequisites, typical coursework, and specific subjects of study for accredited educational programs in the chosen profession. This section also describes the various levels of educational attainment (eg, certificate, associate's degree, bachelor's degree, master's level) that are offered, as well as those that are required, to work in the selected profession.

Licensure, Certification, and Registration specifies the legal and/or professional requirements, if any, for practicing in a chosen profession. Renewal cycles for certification and continuing education standards, as well as information on national and local accrediting bodies, may also be included.

Inquiries lists names, addresses, and other contact information for national professional associations, accrediting bodies, and related information resources.

The lists of accredited educational programs are in alphabetical order by state, then city, for each occupation. Most program listings include the name and address of the educational program and Web site address.

At the end of each profession's section is a data chart showing class capacity (per start date or session), month(s) classes begin, program length(s), yearly tuition cost (resident and nonresident), yearly stipend (if any), academic award(s) granted, availability of evening/weekend courses, whether a program offers education/courses in medical/health care terms in non-English languages, availability of distance education, and whether the program offers education in cultural competence or in patient communication. These data are shown only for those programs that completed the 2007 AMA Survey of Health Professions Programs.

For more information about a specific educational program, contact the program officials directly.

Data Sources; Updates to Listings

The data in each of the program listings (Section I) and institution listings (Section II) are the product of two processes: The cooperative relationships between the AMA and the applicable health professions accrediting agencies, and the cooperation of program directors and institutional officials in responding to the Annual Survey of Health Professions Education Programs.

Program directors or institutional officials wishing to update the listings in Sections I or II should make the required changes on the annual survey, available online at www.ama-assn.org/go/hpsurvey. Updates can also be sent to the AMA at the following address:

Medical Education Products
American Medical Association
attn: Dorothy Grant-Bryant
515 N State Street
Chicago, IL 60610
312 464-4936
312 464-5830 Fax
E-mail: dorothy.grant-bryant@ama-assn.org

Anesthesiologist Assistant

The anesthesiologist assistant (AA) functions as a specialty physician assistant under the direction of a licensed and qualified anesthesiologist, principally in medical centers. The AA assists the anesthesiologist in developing and implementing the anesthesia care plan. This may include:

- Collecting preoperative data, such as taking an appropriate health history
- Performing various preoperative tasks, such as the insertion of intravenous and arterial catheters and special catheters for central venous pressure monitoring, if necessary
- Performing airway management and drug administration for induction and maintenance of anesthesia
- Assisting in the administering and monitoring of regional and peripheral nerve blockade
- Administering supportive therapy, for example, with intravenous fluids and cardiovascular drugs
- Adjusting anesthetic levels on a minute-to-minute basis
- Performing intraoperative monitoring
- Providing recovery room care
- Functioning in the intensive care unit

The AA may also be used in pain clinics or may participate in administrative and educational activities.

Career Description
In addition to the duties described in the occupational description above, anesthesiologist assistants provide other support according to established protocols. Such activities may include pretesting anesthesia delivery systems and patient monitors and operating special monitors and support devices for critical cardiac, pulmonary, and neurological systems. AAs may be involved in the operation of bedside electronic computer-based monitors and have supervisory responsibilities for laboratory functions associated with anesthesia and operating room care. They provide cardiopulmonary resuscitation in association with other anesthesia care team members and in accordance with approved emergency protocols.

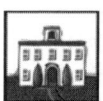
Employment Characteristics
Anesthesiologist assistants work as members of the anesthesia care team in any locale where they may be appropriately directed by legally responsible anesthesiologists. The AAs most often work within organizations that also employ nurse anesthetists, and their responsibilities are identical. Experience to date has been that AAs are most commonly employed in larger facilities that perform procedures such as cardiac surgery, neurosurgery, transplant surgery, and trauma care, given the training in extensive patient monitoring devices and complex patients and procedures emphasized in AA educational programs. However, AAs are used in hospitals of all sizes and assist anesthesiologists in a variety of settings and for a wide range of procedures.

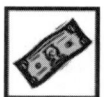
Salary
Starting salaries for 2006 graduates are $95,000 up to $120,000 for the 40-hour work week plus benefits and consideration of on-call activity. The high end of the salary range is around $160,000 to $180,000 for experienced anesthetists (including overtime). Refer to Section IV, Table 5 of this *Directory* for more information, or see www.ama-assn.org/go/hpsalary.

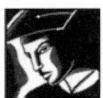
Educational Programs
Length. These postbaccalaureate programs are essentially 24 to 28 months.
Prerequisites. The programs require an undergraduate premedical background (premedical courses in biology, chemistry, physics, and math) and a baccalaureate degree. Although any baccalaureate major is acceptable (if premedical requirements are met), majors typically are biology, chemistry, physics, mathematics, computer science, or one of the allied health professions, such as respiratory therapy, medical technology, or nursing.

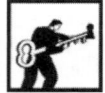
Certification
The National Commission for Certification of Anesthesiologist Assistants (NCCAA), which was founded in 1989, provides the certification process for AAs in the United States. The Commission includes anesthesiologists and anesthesiologist assistants. NCCAA contracts with the National Board of Medical Examiners to assist with the certification process, including task analyses, development of content grids, item writing and editing, and administration of examinations. The certification process incorporates a 6-year cycle of certifying examination, examination for continued demonstration of qualifications, and registration of continuing medical education.

Inquiries
Careers. Curriculum inquiries should be directed to the individual programs. Inquiries regarding AA careers should be directed to

American Academy of Anesthesiologist Assistants
PO Box 13978
Tallahassee, FL 32317
866 328-5858
850 656-3038 Fax
www.anesthetist.org

Certification
National Commission for Certification of Anesthesiologist Assistants
PO Box 15519
Atlanta, GA 30333-0519
404 687-9978 Fax

Program Accreditation
Commission on Accreditation of Allied Health Education Programs (CAAHEP) in collaboration with:
Accreditation Review Committee for the Anesthesiologist Assistant
Brad Maxwell
c/o CAAHEP
1361 Park Street
Clearwater, FL 33756
727 210-2350

Anesthesiologist Assistant

Florida

Nova Southeastern University
Anesthesiologist Asst Prgm
3200 S University Dr
Fort Lauderdale, FL 33328-2018
Prgm Dir: Robert Wagner, MMSc AA-C
Tel: 954 262-1166   *Fax:* 954 262-1181
E-mail: rwagner@nsu.nova.edu

Georgia

Emory University
Anesthesiologist Asst Prgm
57 Executive Park South, Ste 300
Atlanta, GA 30329
www.emoryaaprogram.org
Prgm Dir: Richard Brouillard, ScD
Tel: 404 727-3188   *Fax:* 404 727-3021
E-mail: rick_brouillard@emoryhealthcare.org

South University
Cosponsor: Mercer University School of Medicine
Anesthesiologist Asst Prgm
709 Mall Blvd
Savannah, GA 31406
www.southuniversity.edu
Prgm Dir: A William Paulsen, MMSc PhD CCE AAC
Tel: 912 201-8000   *Fax:* 912 201-8070
E-mail: bpaulsen@southuniversity.edu

Ohio

Case Western Reserve University
Anesthesiologist Asst Prgm
11100 Euclid Ave
Lakeside Hospital Rm 2532
Cleveland, OH 44106-5007
Prgm Dir: Joseph Rifici, AA-C MEd
Tel: 216 844-3161   *Fax:* 216 844-7349
E-mail: joseph.rifici@uhhs.com

Anesthesiologist Assistant

Programs*	Class Capacity	Begins	Length (months)	Award	Res. Tuition	Non-res. Tuition	Stipend	Offers:‡ 1	2	3	4
Georgia											
Emory University (Atlanta)	50	Aug	24	MMSc	$27,720	$27,720					
South University (Savannah)	25	Jun	28	MMSc	$27,180	$27,180				•	

*Data are shown only for programs that completed the 2007 AMA Survey of Health Professions Education Programs.
‡Key to Offers: 1: Evening or weekend classes; 2: Non-English instruction; 3: Cultural competence instruction; 4: Distance education component.

History

Art therapy emerged as a distinct profession in the 1940s when hospitals and rehabilitation facilities increasingly began to include art therapy programs along with traditional "talk therapies," underscoring the recognition that art making enhanced recovery, health, and wellness. Since that time, the profession of art therapy has grown into an effective and important method of treatment and assessment with children, adults, families, and groups in a variety of settings. Currently, the field of art therapy has gained attention in health care facilities throughout the United States and within psychiatry, medicine, psychology, counseling, education, and the arts.

The American Art Therapy Association (AATA), the official member organization for professionals and students, was founded in 1969 to develop and promote educational, professional, and ethical standards for the field of art therapy. The AATA sponsors annual conferences, approves educational programs, and publishes *Art Therapy: Journal of the American Art Therapy Association* (first published in 1983), the quarterly *AATA Newsletter,* the *AATA E-Newsletter,* books, and monographs. In the 1970s, the first master's degrees in art therapy were awarded. Today, there are 34 AATA-approved master's degree programs, and university and college curricula across the US include undergraduate introductory courses and preparatory programs in art therapy.

Career Description

Art therapy is a mental health profession that uses the creative process of art making to improve and enhance the physical, mental, and emotional well being of individuals of all ages. It is based on the belief that the creative process of artistic self-expression helps people to resolve conflicts and problems, develop interpersonal skills, manage behavior, reduce stress, increase self-esteem and self-awareness, and achieve insight.

Art therapy integrates the fields of human development, visual art (drawing, painting, sculpture, and other art forms), and the creative process with models of counseling and psychotherapy. Art therapy is used with children, adolescents, adults, older adults, groups, and families to assess and treat the following:

- Anxiety, depression, and other mental and emotional problems and disorders
- Substance abuse and other addictions
- Family and relationship issues
- Abuse and domestic violence
- Social and emotional difficulties related to disability and illness
- Trauma and loss
- Physical, cognitive, and neurological problems
- Psychosocial difficulties related to medical illness

Art therapy programs and art therapists are found in a variety of settings including hospitals, clinics, public, social service, and community agencies, wellness centers, educational institutions, businesses, and private practices.

Art therapists use drawing, painting, and other art processes to assess and treat clients with emotional, cognitive, physical, and/or developmental needs and disorders. Using their skills in evaluation and psychotherapy, they choose materials and interventions appropriate to their clients' needs and design sessions to achieve therapeutic goals and objectives. Art therapists also maintain

appropriate charts, records, and periodic reports on client progress as required by agency guidelines and professional standards; participate in professional staff meetings and conferences; and provide information and consultation regarding the client's clinical progress. They also may function as supervisors, administrators, consultants, and expert witnesses.

With the growing acceptance of complementary therapies and recent research findings on art therapy with medical populations, there is an increase in the application of art therapy to a variety of patient groups. For example, art therapists work with cancer, burn, pain, post-surgery, HIV-positive, asthma, and substance abuse patients, among others, and with pediatric, geriatric, and other medical populations. In hospitals, art therapists may be part of psychiatric departments, child life programs, arts in hospital programs, or creative arts therapies or activity therapies departments. Many art therapists also hold credentials in mental health counseling or marriage and family therapy because of their training and experience.

An understanding of the application of various art media and art processes to treatment is central to the practice of art therapy. In general, an art therapist must be sensitive to a variety of human needs and possess emotional stability, patience, interpersonal skills, and a capacity for insight into psychological processes. An art therapist also must be an attentive listener and keen observer and be able to develop a rapport with people. Flexibility and a sense of humor are important in adapting to work with people with a wide range of mental health and healthcare needs and in a variety of settings.

Employment Characteristics

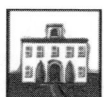

Art therapists work in a many different healthcare environments, including, but not limited to, the following: hospitals and clinics (medical and psychiatric); outpatient mental health agencies and day treatment facilities; residential treatment centers; domestic violence and homeless shelters; community agencies and nonprofit settings; sheltered workshops; correctional facilities; elder care facilities; art studios; private practice; and schools, colleges, and universities.

An art therapist may work as part of a team that includes physicians, psychologists, nurses, mental health counselors, marriage and family therapists, rehabilitation counselors, social workers, and/or teachers. Together, they determine each client's therapeutic goals and objectives and implement a treatment plan. Other art therapists work independently and maintain private practices with children, adolescents, adults, groups, and/or families.

Salary

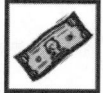

Earnings for art therapists vary depending on type of practice, job responsibilities, and practice location. The average entry-level income (2006 data) is approximately $32,000, median income is between $38,000 and $48,000, and top earning potential for salaried administrators is between $50,000 and $80,000. Art therapists who possess doctoral degrees and/or licensure or who qualify in their state to conduct a private practice can earn an average of $85 to $120 per hour as an independent practitioner. Refer to Section IV, Table 5 of this *Directory* for more information, or see www.ama-assn.org/go/hpsalary.

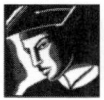

Educational Programs

Length. Art therapy master's degree programs are no less than 2 years and must include a minimum of 24 graduate credit hours in the art therapy core curriculum.

Prerequisites. Applicants to master's degree programs must hold a baccalaureate degree from an accredited US institution or have equivalent academic preparation from an institution outside the United States. In addition, prospective students must submit a portfolio of original artwork and must document 15 semester hours in studio art and 12 semester hours in psychology.

Curriculum. Educational requirements include theories of art therapy, counseling, and psychotherapy; psychopathology; ethics and standards of practice; assessment and evaluation; individual, group, and family techniques; human and creative development; multicultural issues; research methods; and practicum experiences in clinical, community, and/or other settings.

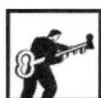

Registration and Certification

The Art Therapy Credentials Board (ATCB) Inc, an independent organization, grants a credential, Art Therapist Registered (ATR), after reviewing documentation of completion of graduate education and supervised postgraduate experience. Registered art therapists who successfully complete a written examination administered by the ATCB are qualified as Board Certified (ATR-BC). Recertification is required every 5 years by documentation of continuing education credits (CECs).

Inquiries

Education, Program Approval, Careers, Resources
American Art Therapy Association (AATA), Inc
5999 Stevenson Avenue
Alexandria, VA 22304
888 290-0878
703 212-2238
E-mail: info@arttherapy.org
www.arttherapy.org

Art Therapist

California

Notre Dame de Namur University
Art Therapy Prgm
1500 Ralston Ave
Belmont, CA 94002
Prgm Dir: Richard Carolan, EdD ATR-BC
Tel: 650 508-3556   *Fax:* 650 508-3426
E-mail: rcarolan@ndnu.edu

Phillips Graduate Institute
Art Therapy Prgm
5445 Balboa Blvd
Encino, CA 91316-1509
www.pgi.edu
Prgm Dir: Noah Hass-Cohen, MA ATR-BC LMFT
Tel: 818 386-5611
E-mail: noah@pgi.edu

Loyola Marymount University
Art Therapy Prgm
Grad Dept of Marital and Family Therapy
1 LMU Dr
Los Angeles, CA 90045-2659
Prgm Dir: Debra Linesch, PhD MFT ATR-BC
Tel: 310 338-4562   *Fax:* 310 338-4518
E-mail: dlinesch@lmu.edu

Colorado

Naropa University
Art Therapy Prgm
2130 Arapahoe Ave
Boulder, CO 80302
Prgm Dir: Michael Franklin, MA ATR-BC
Tel: 303 546-3545
E-mail: michaelf@naropa.edu

Connecticut

Albertus Magnus College
Art Therapy Prgm
700 Prospect St
New Haven, CT 06511
Prgm Dir: Donna Kaiser, PhD ATR-BC LPC
Tel: 203 773-8903   *Fax:* 203 773-3117
E-mail: dkaiser@albertus.edu

District of Columbia

George Washington University
Art Therapy Prgm
2129 G St NW, Bldg L, Rear
Washington, DC 20052
Prgm Dir: Heidi Bardot, MA ATR-BC
Tel: 202 994-6285   *Fax:* 202 994-1404
E-mail: hbardot@gwu.edu

Florida

Florida State University
Art Therapy Prgm
028 William Johnston Building
Tallahassee, FL 32306-1232
www.fsu.edu/~are
Prgm Dir: Marcia Rosal, PhD
Tel: 850 644-5473   *Fax:* 850 644-5067
E-mail: mrosal@fsu.edu

Illinois

Adler School of Professional Psychology
Art Therapy Prgm
65 E Wacker Pl, Ste 2100
Chicago, IL 60601-7298
www.adler.edu
Prgm Dir: Nancy Slater, PhD ATR-BC
Tel: 312 201-5900, Ext 220   *Fax:* 312 201-5917
E-mail: nslater@adler.edu

School of the Art Institute of Chicago
Art Therapy Prgm
Dept of Art Therapy
37 S Wabash
Chicago, IL 60603-3103
www.saic.edu
Prgm Dir: Catherine Moon, MA ATR-BC
Tel: 312 899-7481   *Fax:* 312 899-1477
E-mail: arttherapy@saic.edu

Southern Illinois University
Art Therapy Prgm
Dept of Art and Design
Box 1764
Edwardsville, IL 62026-1764
www.siue.edu/art/areas/art_therapy/
Prgm Dir: P Gussie Klorer, PhD ATR-BC LCSW LCPC
Tel: 618 650-3183   *Fax:* 618 650-3106
E-mail: pklorer@siue.edu

Kansas

Emporia State University
Art Therapy Prgm
1200 Commercial St, Campus Box 4031
Emporia, KS 66801
Prgm Dir: Gaelynn Wolf Bordonaro, PhD ATR
Tel: 620 341-5809
E-mail: gwolf@emporia.edu

Kentucky

University of Louisville
Art Therapy Prgm
Coll of Education and Human Dev Expressive Therapies
Louisville, KY 40292
Prgm Dir: John Begley
Tel: 502 852-8796   *Fax:* 502 852-4598
E-mail: john.begley@louisville.edu

Massachusetts

Lesley University
Art Therapy Prgm
Expressive Therapies
29 Everett St
Cambridge, MA 02138
Prgm Dir: Michaela Kirby, PhD ATR-BC CGP
Tel: 617 349-8433   *Fax:* 617 349-8431
E-mail: mkirby@lesley.edu

Springfield College
Art Therapy Prgm
Springfield Coll Visual and Performing Arts
263 Alden St
Springfield, MA 01109-3797
Prgm Dir: Simone Alter-Muri, EdD
Tel: 413 748-3752   *Fax:* 413 748-3580
E-mail: simone_alter-muri@spfldcol.edu

Michigan

Wayne State University
Art Therapy Prgm
163 Community Arts Bldg
Detroit, MI 48202
Prgm Dir: Holly Feen, PhD ATR-BC
Tel: 313 577-1823   *Fax:* 313 993-7558
E-mail: hfeen@wayne.edu

New Jersey

Caldwell College
Art Therapy Prgm
9 Ryerson Ave
Caldwell, NJ 07006
Prgm Dir: Marie Wilson, MA ATR-BC LPC
Tel: 973 618-3511
E-mail: mwilson@caldwell.edu

New Mexico

Southwestern College
Art Therapy Prgm
PO Box 4788
Santa Fe, NM 87502-4788
www.swc.edu
Prgm Dir: Deborah Schroder, MS ATR-BC LPAT LPAT
Tel: 505 471-5756, Ext 22   *Fax:* 505 471-4071
E-mail: info@swc.edu

New York

Pratt Institute
Art Therapy Prgm
200 Willoughby Ave
East 3
Brooklyn, NY 11205
Prgm Dir: Laurel Thompson, MPS ADTR ATR-BC LCAT
Tel: 718 636-3428   *Fax:* 718 636-3597
E-mail: lthompso@pratt.edu

Long Island University - C W Post Campus
Art Therapy Prgm
720 Northern Blvd
Brookville, NY 11548
Prgm Dir: Christine Kerr, PhD ATR-BC CGP
Tel: 516 299-2935, Ext 2944   *Fax:* 516 299-2858
E-mail: christine.kerr@liu.edu

Hofstra University
Art Therapy Prgm
124 Hofstra University
Hempstead, NY 11549-1240
Prgm Dir: Joan Bloomgarden, PhD ATR-BC CGP
Tel: 516 463-5752   *Fax:* 516 463-6184
E-mail: Joan.S.Bloomgarden@hofstra.edu

College of New Rochelle
Art Therapy Prgm
29 Castle Pl
Chapel Hall G 15
New Rochelle, NY 10805
Prgm Dir: Patricia St John, EdD ATR-BC
Tel: 914 654-5280   *Fax:* 914 654-5593
E-mail: pstjohn@cnr.edu

New York University
Art Therapy Prgm
34 Stuyvesant St
New York, NY 10003
Prgm Dir: Ikuko Acosta, MA ATR-BC
Tel: 212 998-5726   *Fax:* 212 995-4320
E-mail: ia4@nyu.edu

School of Visual Arts
Art Therapy Prgm
209 E 23rd St
New York, NY 10010
www.sva.edu
Prgm Dir: Deborah Farber, MPS ATR-BC LCAT
Tel: 212 592-2610   *Fax:* 917 606-0461
E-mail: arttherapy@sva.edu

Nazareth College of Rochester
Art Therapy Prgm
4245 East Ave
Rochester, NY 14618-3790
Prgm Dir: Ellen G Horovitz, PhD ATR-BC
Tel: 585 389-2535   *Fax:* 585 586-2452
E-mail: ehorovi4@naz.edu

Ohio

Ursuline College
Art Therapy Prgm
2550 Lander Rd
Pepper Pike, OH 44124
Prgm Dir: Gail Rule-Hoffman, MEd ATR-BC
Tel: 440 646-8139   *Fax:* 440 684-6135
E-mail: grulehof@ursuline.edu

Oregon

Marylhurst University
Art Therapy Prgm
Dept of Graduate Studies in Art Therapy Counseling
17600 Pacific Hwy, PO Box 261
Marylhurst, OR 97036
www.marylhurst.edu
Prgm Dir: Christine Turner, ATR-BC LPC NCC ACS
Tel: 503 699-6244   *Fax:* 503 534-4062
E-mail: cturner@marylhurst.edu

Pennsylvania

Seton Hill University
Art Therapy Prgm
PO Box 467F Seton Hill Dr
Greensburg, PA 15601
Prgm Dir: Nina Denninger, MA ATR-BC
Tel: 724 830-1047, Ext 4368   *Fax:* 724 830-1295
E-mail: denninger@setonhill.edu

Drexel University
Art Therapy Prgm
Hahnemann Creative Arts in Therapy Program
245 N 15th St
Philadelphia, PA 19102-1192
www.drexel.edu/cnhp/creativearts/
Prgm Dir: Nancy Gerber, PhD ATR-BC LPC
Tel: 215 762-6928   *Fax:* 215 762-6933
E-mail: ng27@drexel.edu

Marywood University
Art Therapy Prgm
Art Dept
2300 Adams Ave
Scranton, PA 18509
Prgm Dir: Stephanie Wise, ATR-BC LCAT
Tel: 570 348-6278, Ext 2525   *Fax:* 570 340-6023
E-mail: swise@marywood.edu

Quebec, Canada

Concordia University
Art Therapy Prgm
1455 de Maisonneuve Blvd W
Montreal, QC H3G 1M8
Prgm Dir: Josee Leclerc, PhD ATR ATPQ
Tel: 514 848-2424, Ext 4795   *Fax:* 514 848-4969
E-mail: cats@vax2.concordia.ca

Virginia

Eastern Virginia Medical School
Art Therapy Prgm
PO Box 1980
Norfolk, VA 23501
www.evms.edu/hlthprof/art-therapy.html
Prgm Dir: Kay Stovall, ATR-BC MFT
Tel: 757 446-5895   *Fax:* 757 446-6179
E-mail: ARTthrpy@evms.edu

Washington

Antioch University - Seattle
Art Therapy Prgm
2326 Sixth Ave
Seattle, WA 98121-1814
Prgm Dir: Janice Hoshino, PhD
Tel: 206 268-4818
E-mail: jhoshino@antiochsea.edu

Wisconsin

Mount Mary College
Art Therapy Prgm
2900 N Menomonee River Pkwy
Milwaukee, WI 53222-4545
Prgm Dir: Bruce Moon, PhD ATR-BC
Tel: 414 256-1215, Ext 302   *Fax:* 414 256-1205
E-mail: moonb@mtmary.edu

Art Therapist

Programs*	Class Capacity	Begins	Length (months)	Award	Res. Tuition	Non-res. Tuition	Stipend	Offers:‡ 1	2	3	4
California											
Phillips Graduate Institute (Encino)	50	Sep Jan	24, 36	MA	$675	$675		•		•	
Florida											
Florida State University (Tallahassee)	14	Fall	24, 36	MS, PhD	$7,080	$26,040	$3,200	•		•	
Illinois											
Adler School of Professional Psychology (Chicago)	15	Fall Winter	24	Dipl, Cert, MA, PM CAT				•		•	
School of the Art Institute of Chicago	30	Sep	24	MAAT	$30,000	$30,000				•	
Southern Illinois University (Edwardsville)	10	Aug	36	Dipl, MA	$3,216	$6,432				•	
Massachusetts											
Springfield College	20	Sep	20	MS	$43,000	$0		•		•	
New Mexico											
Southwestern College (Santa Fe)	65	Fall (FT) Winter	24, 30	Dipl, Cert, MA	$16,758	$16,758		•		•	
New York											
School of Visual Arts (New York)	25	Fall semester	24	MPS	$13,060	$13,060		•			
Oregon											
Marylhurst University	20	Sep	21	Cert, MA	$17,752	$17,752		•		•	
Pennsylvania											
Drexel University (Philadelphia)	22	Sep	24	MA	$16,875	$0				•	
Marywood University (Scranton)	12	Sep Jan	27	Cert, MA	$20,160	$20,160		•		•	
Virginia											
Eastern Virginia Medical School (Norfolk)	15	Aug	24	MS	$19,800	$19,800				•	

*Data are shown only for programs that completed the 2007 AMA Survey of Health Professions Education Programs.
‡Key to Offers: 1: Evening or weekend classes; 2: Non-English instruction; 3: Cultural competence instruction; 4: Distance education component.

PROGRAMS

The athletic trainer, with the consultation and direction of attending and/or consulting physicians, is an integral part of the health care system associated with physical activity and sports. Through preparation in both academic education and clinical experience, the athletic trainer provides a variety of services, including injury prevention, assessment, immediate care, treatment, and rehabilitation after physical injury or trauma.

Career Description

Past role delineation studies have concluded that the role of an athletic trainer includes, but may not be limited to:

- Prevention
- Recognition, evaluation, and assessment
- Immediate care
- Treatment, rehabilitation, and reconditioning
- Organization and administration
- Professional development

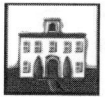

Employment Characteristics

Athletic trainers typically provide their services in one or more of the following settings: secondary schools, colleges and universities, professional athletic organizations, physician offices, hospital-based clinics, private sports medicine and rehabilitation clinics, industrial/occupational, military, and performing arts.

Salary

Entry-level salaries in 2005 averaged $35,000. The average overall salary is $45,000, with the upper ranges from $55,000 to $75,000. Refer to Section IV, Table 5 of this *Directory* for more information, or see www.ama-assn.org/go/hpsalary.

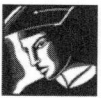

Educational Programs

Length. Baccalaureate degree programs require 4 years of study. Postbaccalaureate programs are generally 2 years.

Prerequisites. Applicants for the 4-year baccalaureate degree programs must have a high school diploma or equivalent and meet institutional entrance requirements. Applicants for postbaccalaureate programs should have a baccalaureate degree that includes appropriate course work and clinical experience, as specified by the institution.

Curriculum. The professional curriculum includes formal instruction in risk management and injury/illness prevention, pathology of injury/illness, assessment of injury/illness, general medical conditions and disabilities, therapeutic modalities, therapeutic exercise, rehabilitative techniques, health care administration, weight management and body composition, psychosocial intervention and referral, medical ethics and legal issues, pharmacology, and professional development and responsibilities. The didactic curriculum is augmented by a series of structured laboratory and clinical experiences.

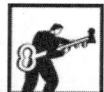

Certification

Almost all states require that athletic trainers hold the ATC® (Athletic Trainer, Certified) credential, which is issued by the Board of Certification Inc. The ATC credential is supported by three pillars: the BOC certification examination, BOC Standards of Practice and Disciplinary Process, and continuing competence requirements. The 1-day, three-part examination verifies that the knowledge, skills, and abilities required for competent performance as an entry-level athletic trainer have been met.

Inquiries

Careers
National Athletic Trainers' Association, Inc
2952 Stemmons Freeway, Suite 200
Dallas, TX 75247
214 637-6282
800 TRY-NATA
214 637-2206 Fax
www.NATA.org

Certification
Board of Certification Inc
BOC Administrative Offices
4223 S 143rd Circle
Omaha, NE 68137
402 559-0091
402 561-0598 Fax
www.bocatc.org

Program Accreditation
Commission on Accreditation of Athletic Training Education (CAATE)
2201 Double Creek Drive, Suite 5006
Round Rock, TX 78664
512 733-9700
512 733-9700 Fax
E-mail: caate@sbcglobal.net
www.caate.net

Athletic Trainer
Alabama

Samford University
Athletic Training Prgm
800 Lakeshore Dr
PO Box 292448
Birmingham, AL 35229
Prgm Dir: Chris A Gillespie, MEd ATC LAT
Tel: 205 726-2379 *Fax:* 205 726-2607
E-mail: cagilles@samford.edu

University of West Alabama
Athletic Training Prgm
Station 14
Livingston, AL 35470
http://at.uwa.edu
Prgm Dir: R T Floyd, EdD ATC LAT CSCS
Tel: 205 652-3714 *Fax:* 205 652-3799
E-mail: rtf@uwa.edu

University of Mobile
Athletic Training Prgm
5735 College Pkwy
Mobile, AL 36663-0220
Prgm Dir: William Carroll, EdD JD ATC
Tel: 251 442-2324 *Fax:* 251 442-2519
E-mail: bcarroll@mail.umobile.edu

Huntingdon College
Athletic Training Prgm
1500 E Fairview Ave
Montgomery, AL 36106
Prgm Dir: Shelby Searcy, EdD
Tel: 334 833-4267 *Fax:* 334 833-4206
E-mail: ssearcy@huntingdon.edu

Troy University
Athletic Training Prgm
3212 Veterans Stadium Dr, 2nd Fl
Dept of Athletic Training Education
Troy, AL 36082
Prgm Dir: John Anderson, MS BS ATC
Tel: 334 670-3722, Ext 3722 *Fax:* 334 670-3870
E-mail: athtrain@troy.edu

University of Alabama - Tuscaloosa
Athletic Training Prgm
Dept of Health Science
Box 870311
Tuscaloosa, AL 35487-0311
Prgm Dir: Deidre Leaver-Dunn, PhD ATC
Tel: 205 348-9176 *Fax:* 205 348-7568
E-mail: dleaver@bama.ua.edu

Arizona

Northern Arizona University
Athletic Training Prgm
PO Box 15094
Flagstaff, AZ 86011-5094
www.nau.edu/hp/at
Prgm Dir: Debbie Craig, PhD ATC LAT
Tel: 928 523-0704 *Fax:* 928 523-4315
E-mail: debbie.craig@nau.edu

Grand Canyon University
Athletic Training Prgm
3300 W Camelback Rd
Phoenix, AZ 85017
Prgm Dir: Cindy Seminoff, MS ATC CSCS
Tel: 602 589-2741 *Fax:* 602 589-2716
E-mail: cseminoff@gcu.edu

Arkansas

Henderson State University
Athletic Training Prgm
HSU Box 7552
Arkadelphia, AR 71999-0001
Prgm Dir: John K Miller, MSE ATC
Tel: 870 230-5360 *Fax:* 870 230-5073
E-mail: millerj@hsu.edu

Ouachita Baptist University
Athletic Training Prgm
Box 3700
Arkadelphia, AR 71998
www.obu.edu/atep
Prgm Dir: Terry DeWitt, PhD ATC
Tel: 870 245-5264 *Fax:* 870 245-5241
E-mail: dewittt@obu.edu

University of Central Arkansas
Athletic Training Prgm
Prince Center 133E
201 Donaghey Ave
Conway, AR 72035-0001
www.uca.edu/divisions/academic/kped/
Prgm Dir: Ellen Epping
Tel: 501 450-5112 *Fax:* 501 450-5087
E-mail: eepping@uca.edu

University of Arkansas
Athletic Training Prgm
HPER 308h
Fayetteville, AR 72701
Prgm Dir: Jeffrey A Bonacci, DA ATC
Tel: 479 575-4112 *Fax:* 479 575-3119
E-mail: bonacci@uark.edu

Southern Arkansas University
Athletic Training Prgm
100 E University
PO Box 9299
Magnolia, AR 71754
Prgm Dir: Jan Kiilsgaard, MS LAT ATC
Tel: 870 235-4248 *Fax:* 870 235-4988
E-mail: jmkiilsgaard@saumag.edu

Harding University
Athletic Training Prgm
HU Box 12281
Searcy, AR 72148
Prgm Dir: Randy Lambeth, EdD
Tel: 501 279-4308
E-mail: rlambeth@harding.edu

Arkansas State University
Athletic Training Prgm
PO Box 240
State University, AR 72467
www.clt.astate.edu/hpess/AthleticTrainingProgram/atho
me.html
Prgm Dir: Matthew Comeau, PhD LAT ATC CSCS
Tel: 870 972-3066 *Fax:* 870 972-3096
E-mail: mcomeau@astate.edu

California

Humboldt State University
Athletic Training Prgm
1 Harpst St
Arcata, CA 95521
www.humboldt.edu
Prgm Dir: Thomas "T K" Koesterer, PhD ATC
Tel: 707 826-5967 *Fax:* 707 826-5480
E-mail: tk@humboldt.edu

Azusa Pacific University
Athletic Training Prgm
Dept of Exercise and Sport Science
701 E Foothill Blvd
Azusa, CA 91702
www.apu.edu/bas/exercisesport/atep/
Prgm Dir: Christopher Schmidt, PhD ATC
Tel: 626 815-6000, Ext 5194 *Fax:* 626 815-5084
E-mail: cschmidt@apu.edu

Vanguard University
Athletic Training Prgm
55 Fair Dr
Costa Mesa, CA 92626
Prgm Dir: Terry Zeigler, EdD ATC
Tel: 714 556-3610, Ext 280 *Fax:* 714 668-6144
E-mail: tzeigler@vanguard.edu

California State University - Fresno
Athletic Training Prgm
5275 N Campus Dr
Fresno, CA 93740-8018
Prgm Dir: Robert Pettitt, PhD
Tel: 209 278-3178 *Fax:* 209 278-7010
E-mail: rpettitt@csufresno.edu

California State University - Fullerton
Athletic Training Prgm
PO Box 6870
Fullerton, CA 92834-6870
http://hdcs.fullerton.edu/at/
Prgm Dir: Robert Kersey, PhD ATC CSCS
Tel: 714 278-3430 *Fax:* 714 278-5317
E-mail: rkersey@fullerton.edu

Concordia Univesity - Irvine
Athletic Training Prgm
1530 Concordia West
Irvine, CA 92612
Prgm Dir: Christopher S Teich, MS ATC
Tel: 949 854-8002, Ext 1445 *Fax:* 949 854-6771
E-mail: chris.teich@cui.edu

University of La Verne
Athletic Training Prgm
1950 Third St
La Verne, CA 91750
www.ulv.edu/athletictraining
Prgm Dir: Marilyn Oliver, MS ATC
Tel: 909 593-3511, Ext 4270 *Fax:* 909 392-2760
E-mail: oliverm@ulv.edu

California State University - Long Beach
Athletic Training Prgm
Department of Kinesiology
1250 Bellflower Blvd
Long Beach, CA 90840
Prgm Dir: Keith Freesemann, EdD
Tel: 562 985-4669
E-mail: kfreesemn@csulb.edu

California State University - Northridge
Athletic Training Prgm
18111 Nordhoff St
Department of Kinesiology
Northridge, CA 91330-8287
www.csun.edu
Prgm Dir: Shane Stecyk, PhD ATC CSCS
Tel: 818 677-3205, Ext 4738 *Fax:* 818 677-3207
E-mail: shane.stecyk@csun.edu

Chapman University
Athletic Training Prgm
One University Dr
Orange, CA 92866
www.chapman.edu/educ/atep
Prgm Dir: Ky Kugler, EdD ATC
Tel: 714 997-6642 *Fax:* 714 997-6991
E-mail: kekugler@chapman.edu

California State University - Sacramento
Athletic Training Prgm
CSUS 6000 J St
Sacramento, CA 95819
www.hhs.csus.edu/KHS/AthleticTraining
Prgm Dir: Doris E Fennessy Flores, MS
Tel: 916 278-6401   *Fax:* 916 278-7664
E-mail: floresde@csus.edu

Point Loma Nazarene University
Athletic Training Prgm
3900 Lomaland Dr
San Diego, CA 92106
Prgm Dir: Jeff Sullivan, PhD
Tel: 619 849-2629   *Fax:* 619 849-2553
E-mail: jeffsullivan@pointloma.edu

San Diego State University
Athletic Training Prgm
5500 Campanile Dr
Exercise and Nutrition Science Department
San Diego, CA 92182
Prgm Dir: Marcia Klaiber, MA ATC
Tel: 619 594-4094   *Fax:* 619 594-6553
E-mail: mklaiber@mail.sdsu.edu

San Jose State University
Athletic Training Prgm
One Washington Square
Department of Kinesiology
San Jose, CA 95192-0054
www.sjsu.edu/at
Prgm Dir: KyungMo Han, PhD ATC CSCS
Tel: 408 924-3041   *Fax:* 408 924-3053
E-mail: han@kin.sjsu.edu

University of the Pacific
Athletic Training Prgm
Dept of Sport Sciences
3601 Pacific Ave
Stockton, CA 95211
Prgm Dir: Jolene Baker, MA
Tel: 209 946-3182   *Fax:* 209 946-3225
E-mail: jbaker@pacific.edu

California Lutheran University
Athletic Training Prgm
60 W Olsen Rd, MC 3400
Thousand Oaks, CA 91360
Prgm Dir: Kavin Tsang, PhD
Tel: 805 493-3547   *Fax:* 805 493-3860
E-mail: ktsang@callutheran.edu

Colorado

Metropolitan State College of Denver
Athletic Training Prgm
Campus Box 25
PO Box 173362
Denver, CO 80217-3362
Prgm Dir: Christine Odell, MA
Tel: 303 556-3148   *Fax:* 303 556-8301
E-mail: codell6@mscd.edu

Fort Lewis College
Athletic Training Prgm
1000 Rim Dr
Durango, CO 81301-3999
Prgm Dir: Carrie Meyer, EdD
Tel: 970 247-7581   *Fax:* 970 247-7568
E-mail: meyer_c@fortlewis.edu

Mesa State College
Athletic Training Prgm
1100 North Ave
Grand Junction, CO 81501
Prgm Dir: Robert Ryan, MA
Tel: 970 845-1985
E-mail: rryan@mesastate.edu

University of Northern Colorado
Athletic Training Prgm
Sch of Kinesiology and Phys Ed
Butler-Hancock 124
Greeley, CO 80639
Prgm Dir: Shannon Courtney, ATC
Tel: 970 351-1860   *Fax:* 970 351-4310
E-mail: shannon.courtney@unco.edu

Colorado State University - Pueblo
Athletic Training Prgm
T250 - 2200 Bonforte Blvd
Pueblo, CO 81001
www.colostate-pueblo.edu
Prgm Dir: Roger Clark, PhD ATC
Tel: 719 549-2530   *Fax:* 719 549-2519
E-mail: roger.clark@colostate-pueblo.edu

Connecticut

Sacred Heart University
Athletic Training Prgm
5151 Park Ave
Fairfield, CT 06432
Prgm Dir: Timothy Speicher, MS
Tel: 203 396-8012
E-mail: speichert@sacredheart.edu

Quinnipiac University
Athletic Training Prgm
275 Mount Carmel Ave
Hamden, CT 06518
www.quinnipiac.edu
Prgm Dir: Lennart D Johns, PhD ATC
Tel: 203 582-8557
E-mail: lenn.johns@quinnipiac.edu

Central Connecticut State University
Athletic Training Prgm
1615 Stanley St
New Britain, CT 06050-4010
Prgm Dir: Peter Morano, BS
Tel: 860 832-2609   *Fax:* 860 832-2159
E-mail: moranop@ccsu.edu

Southern Connecticut State University
Athletic Training Prgm
Pelz Gymnasium
501 Crescent St
New Haven, CT 06515
Prgm Dir: Gary E Morin, PhD ATC
Tel: 203 392-6089   *Fax:* 203 392-6093
E-mail: moring1@southernct.edu

University of Connecticut
Athletic Training Prgm
Dept of Kinesiology
2095 Hillside Rd, U-1110
Storrs, CT 06269-1110
Prgm Dir: Stephanie M Mazerolle, PhD ATC
Tel: 860 486-4536   *Fax:* 860 486-1123
E-mail: stephanie.mazerolle@uconn.edu

Delaware

University of Delaware
Athletic Training Prgm
Human Performance Laboratory, Fred Rust Ice Arena
541 S College Ave
Newark, DE 19716
Prgm Dir: Thomas Kaminski, PhD ATC FACSM
Tel: 302 831-6402   *Fax:* 302 831-3693
E-mail: kaminski@udel.edu

District of Columbia

George Washington University
Athletic Training Prgm
Department of Exercise Science
817 23rd St NW
Washington, DC 20052
Prgm Dir: Beverly J Westerman, EdD ATC
Tel: 202 994-3862   *Fax:* 202 994-1420
E-mail: bev@gwu.edu

Florida

University of Miami
Athletic Training Prgm
PO Box 248065
Coral Gables, FL 33124
www.education.miami.edu/AthleticTraining/
Prgm Dir: Kysha Harriell, MS ATC LAT
Tel: 305 284-3201   *Fax:* 305 284-5168
E-mail: kharriell@miami.edu

Nova Southeastern University
Athletic Training Prgm
3301 College Ave
Fort Lauderdale, FL 33314
Prgm Dir: Elizabeth Swann, PhD
Tel: 954 262-8334
E-mail: swann@nsu.nova.edu

Florida Gulf Coast University
Athletic Training Prgm
10501 FGCU Blvd South
Fort Myers, FL 33965
Prgm Dir: Jason Craddock, MS
Tel: 239 482-5399   *Fax:* 239 482-4353
E-mail: jcraddoc@fgcu.edu

University of Florida
Athletic Training Prgm
Dept of Applied Physiology and Kinesiology
160 FL Gym, Box 118205
Gainesville, FL 32611-8205
www.hhp.ufl.edu/apk/undergrad/2006atweb/
  athletictraining.htm
Prgm Dir: Erik Wikstrom, MS ATC LAT
Tel: 352 392-0584, Ext 1402   *Fax:* 352 392-5262
E-mail: ewikstrom@hhp.ufl.edu

University of North Florida
Athletic Training Prgm
1 UNF Drive
Brooks College of Health
Jacksonville, FL 32224-2673
www.unf.edu/brooks/cohatweb.htm
Prgm Dir: Joel Beam, EdD ATC LAT
Tel: 904 620-1424   *Fax:* 904 620-2848
E-mail: jbeam@unf.edu

Florida Southern College
Athletic Training Prgm
111 Lake Hollingsworth Dr
Lakeland, FL 33801-5698
www.flsouthern.edu
Prgm Dir: Sue Stanley-Green, MS ATC LAT
Tel: 863 680-4262   *Fax:* 863 680-4251
E-mail: sstanleygreen@flsouthern.edu

Barry University
Athletic Training Prgm
11300 NE 2nd Ave
Miami Shores, FL 33161-6695
www.barry.edu/hpls
Prgm Dir: Carl R Cramer, EdD RKT ATC LAT
Tel: 305 899-3497   *Fax:* 305 899-4809
E-mail: ccramer@mail.barry.edu

University of Central Florida
Athletic Training Prgm
4000 Central Florida Blvd, HPA II Rm 121
Orlando, FL 32816-2200
Prgm Dir: Kristen Schellhase, MEd ATC CSCS
Tel: 407 823-3463
E-mail: kschellh@mail.ucf.edu

University of West Florida
Athletic Training Prgm
11000 University Pkwy
Pensacola, FL 32524
www.uwf.edu
Prgm Dir: Richard Frazee
Tel: 850 473-7245   *Fax:* 850 474-2106
E-mail: rfrazee@uwf.edu

Florida State University
Athletic Training Prgm
422 Sandels Bldg - NFES
Tallahassee, FL 320306
Prgm Dir: Angela Sehgal, EdD
Tel: 850 644-1899   *Fax:* 850 645-5000
E-mail: asehgal@fsu.edu

University of South Florida
Athletic Training Prgm
3500 E Fletcher Ave, Ste 511, MDC 106
Tampa, FL 33613
www.health.usf.edu/nocms/medicine/orthopaedic/atep/
Prgm Dir: Jeff Konin, PhD
Tel: 813 396-9627   *Fax:* 813 396-9195
E-mail: jkonin@health.usf.edu

University of Tampa
Athletic Training Prgm
401 W Kennedy Blvd, Box 30F
Tampa, FL 33606
www.ut.edu
Prgm Dir: J C Andersen, PhD ATC PT SCS
Tel: 813 253-3333, Ext 3127   *Fax:* 813 258-7497
E-mail: jcandersen@ut.edu

Palm Beach Atlantic University
Athletic Training Prgm
PO Box 24708
West Palm Beach, FL 33416-4708
www.pba.edu
Prgm Dir: Tyler Hamilton, MS ATC LAT
Tel: 561 803-2378   *Fax:* 561 803-2370
E-mail: Tyler_Hamilton@pba.edu

Georgia

University of Georgia
Athletic Training Prgm
Ramsey Center, 330 River Rd
Department of Kinesiology
Athens, GA 30602
www.coe.uga.edu/kinesiology/exs/athletictraining/
Prgm Dir: Michael S Ferrara, PhD ATC
Tel: 706 542-4801   *Fax:* 706 542-3148
E-mail: mferrara@uga.edu

North Georgia College & State University
Athletic Training Prgm
Memorial Hall
Dahlonega, GA 30597
Prgm Dir: Derek Suranie, MEd ATC
Tel: 706 867-2770   *Fax:* 706 867-2865
E-mail: djsuranie@ngcsu.edu

Georgia College & State University
Athletic Training Prgm
Campus Box 65
Milledgeville, GA 31061
Prgm Dir: Earl R Cooper, Jr, EdD ATC CSCS
Tel: 478 445-4072, Ext 1786   *Fax:* 478 445-1790
E-mail: bud.cooper@gcsu.edu

Georgia Southern University
Athletic Training Prgm
PO Box 8076
Hollis Bldg
Statesboro, GA 30460-8076
Prgm Dir: Thomas Buckley, EdD ATC
Tel: 912 681-5268   *Fax:* 912 681-0381
E-mail: tbuckley@georgiasouthern.edu

Valdosta State University
Athletic Training Prgm
Dept KSPE
Valdosta, GA 31698
www.valdosta.edu/coe/
Prgm Dir: Chuck Conner, MA LAT ATC
Tel: 229 333-5354   *Fax:* 229 333-5972
E-mail: cconner@valdosta.edu

Hawaii

University of Hawaii
Athletic Training Prgm
Dept of KLS
1337 Lower Campus Rd PE, A Rm 231
Honolulu, HI 96822
Prgm Dir: Michelle Cleary, PhD
Tel: 808 956-3804   *Fax:* 808 956-3106
E-mail: mcleary@hawaii.edu

Idaho

Boise State University
Athletic Training Prgm
Dept of Kinesiology, K209
1910 University Dr
Boise, ID 83725
Prgm Dir: John W McChesney, PhD ATC
Tel: 208 426-1481   *Fax:* 208 426-1894
E-mail: johnmcchesney@boisestate.edu

University of Idaho
Athletic Training Prgm
Department of HPERD
PO Box 442401
Moscow, ID 83844-2401
www.uidaho.edu
Prgm Dir: Jacqueline M Williams, MS LAT ATC
Tel: 208 885-2185   *Fax:* 208 885-5929
E-mail: jwilli@uidaho.edu

Illinois

Aurora University
Athletic Training Prgm
347 S Gladstone Ave
Aurora, IL 60506
Prgm Dir: Oscar H Krieger, MS ATC CIE
Tel: 630 844-4224   *Fax:* 630 844-7809
E-mail: okrieger@aurora.edu

Olivet Nazarene University
Athletic Training Prgm
1 University Ave
Bourbonnais, IL 60914-2345
Prgm Dir: Brian Hyma, MA
Tel: 815 939-5115   *Fax:* 815 939-7933
E-mail: bhyma@olivet.edu

Southern Illinois University Carbondale
Athletic Training Prgm
Department of Kinesiology
1075 S Normal Ave
Carbondale, IL 62901
www.siu.edu/~athtrain
Prgm Dir: Toby Brooks, PhD
Tel: 618 453-3116   *Fax:* 618 453-3329
E-mail: tbrooks@siu.edu

Eastern Illinois University
Athletic Training Prgm
Department of Kinesiology and Sport Studies
600 Lincoln Ave, 2220 Lantz Gymnasium
Charleston, IL 61920
www.eiu.edu/~athtrain
Prgm Dir: Lee Ann Price, ABD LAT ATC
Tel: 217 581-7615   *Fax:* 217 581-7973
E-mail: lprice@eiu.edu

North Park University
Athletic Training Prgm
3225 W Foster Ave
Chicago, IL 60625
Prgm Dir: Andrew Lundgren, MA Ed
Tel: 773 244-6293   *Fax:* 773 244-4952
E-mail: alundgren@northpark.edu

Millikin University
Athletic Training Prgm
1184 W Main
Decatur, IL 62522
Prgm Dir: Tisha Hess, MS ATC/L
Tel: 217 420-6624   *Fax:* 217 363-6414
E-mail: thess@mail.millikin.edu

Trinity International University
Athletic Training Prgm
2065 Half Day Rd
Deerfield, IL 60015
Prgm Dir: Karl Glass, MS
Tel: 847 317-7066   *Fax:* 847 317-8056
E-mail: kglass@tiu.edu

Northern Illinois University
Athletic Training Prgm
Dept of Kinesiology and Physical Education
DeKalb, IL 60115
Prgm Dir: Gretchen A Schlabach, PhD ATC/L
Tel: 815 753-1424   *Fax:* 815 753-1413
E-mail: gas@niu.edu

McKendree University
Athletic Training Prgm
701 College Rd
Lebanon, IL 62254-1299
www.mckendree.edu/athletictraining
Prgm Dir: Dawn M Hankins, PhD ATC LAT
Tel: 618 537-6917   *Fax:* 618 537-6876
E-mail: dhankins@mckendree.edu

Western Illinois University
Athletic Training Prgm
Brophy Hall 220B
One University Circle
Macomb, IL 61455
www.wiu.edu/kinesiology/atraining.html
Prgm Dir: Renee Polubinsky, EdD ATC CSCS
Tel: 309 298-2050   *Fax:* 309 298-2981
E-mail: RL-Polubinsky@wiu.edu

North Central College
Athletic Training Prgm
30 N Brainard
Naperville, IL 60540
Prgm Dir: Heidi M Matthews, MS ATC/L
Tel: 630 637-5511   *Fax:* 630 637-5360
E-mail: hmmatthews@noctrl.edu

Illinois State University
Athletic Training Prgm
208 Horton
Normal, IL 61790-5120
www.kinrec.ilstu.edu/at
Prgm Dir: Todd A McLoda, PhD ATC LAT
Tel: 309 438-2605   *Fax:* 309 438-5559
E-mail: tamcloda@ilstu.edu

Lewis University
Athletic Training Prgm
One University Parkway, Box 10
Romeoville, IL 60446
Prgm Dir: Cathy Oczkowski, MA
Tel: 815 836-5921
E-mail: oczkowca@lewisu.edu

Univ of Illinois at Urbana-Champaign
Athletic Training Prgm
331 Freer Hall
906 S Goodwin Ave
Urbana, IL 61801-3841
Prgm Dir: Steven Broglio, PhD
Tel: 217 244-7322   *Fax:* 217 244-7322
E-mail: broglio@uiuc.edu

Indiana

Anderson University
Athletic Training Prgm
1100 E 5th St
Anderson, IN 46012-1362
www.anderson.edu
Prgm Dir: Jennifer Popp, EdD ATC LAT
Tel: 765 641-4494   *Fax:* 765 641-3841
E-mail: jkpopp@anderson.edu

Indiana University - Bloomington
Athletic Training Prgm
Sportsmedicine Dept, Assembly Hall
1001 E 17th St
Bloomington, IN 47408-1590
Prgm Dir: Katie Grove, PhD
Tel: 812 856-3640   *Fax:* 812 855-1810
E-mail: kagrove@indiana.edu

University of Evansville
Athletic Training Prgm
1800 Lincoln Ave, Wallace Graves Hall 217
Evansville, IN 47722
Prgm Dir: Jeffrey Tilly, MS ATC LAT
Tel: 812 488-1054   *Fax:* 812 479-2717
E-mail: jt3@evansville.edu

Franklin College
Athletic Training Prgm
Franklin College
Spurlock Center
Franklin, IN 46131
www.franklincollege.edu/athweb/training/
Prgm Dir: Kathy Taylor Remsburg, MS
Tel: 317 738-8135   *Fax:* 317 738-8248
E-mail: kremsburg@franklincollege.edu

DePauw University
Athletic Training Prgm
Kinesiology Department
702 S College St
Greencastle, IN 46135
Prgm Dir: Marie Pickerill, PhD
Tel: 765 658-6689   *Fax:* 765 658-4964
E-mail: mariapickerill@depauw.edu

University of Indianapolis
Athletic Training Prgm
1400 E Hanna Ave
Indianapolis, IN 46227
www.athtrg.uindy.edu
Prgm Dir: Connie Pumpelly, MS LAT ATC
Tel: 317 788-6143   *Fax:* 317 788-3472
E-mail: cpumpelly@uindy.edu

Indiana Wesleyan University
Athletic Training Prgm
4201 S Washington St
Marion, IN 46953
http://cas.indwes.edu/hkrss/athletictraining/
Prgm Dir: Adam Thompson, PhD ATC LAT
Tel: 765 677-2335, Ext 2335   *Fax:* 765 677-2328
E-mail: adam.thompson@indwes.edu

Ball State University
Athletic Training Prgm
HP 209
Muncie, IN 47306
Prgm Dir: Thomas Weidner, PhD
Tel: 765 285-5039   *Fax:* 765 285-8254
E-mail: tweidner@bsu.edu

Manchester College
Athletic Training Prgm
Box PERC
North Manchester, IN 46962
Prgm Dir: Mark W Huntington, PED ATC PT
Tel: 260 982-5033   *Fax:* 260 982-5405
E-mail: mwhuntington@manchester.edu

Indiana State University
Athletic Training Prgm
Arena Rm C-09
Terre Haute, IN 47809
www.indstate.edu/athtrn
Prgm Dir: Catherine L Stemmans, PhD ATC/L
Tel: 812 237-8336   *Fax:* 812 237-4368
E-mail: cstemmmans@isugw.indstate.edu

Purdue University
Athletic Training Prgm
Dept of Health and Kinesiology
800 W Stadium Ave
West Lafayette, IN 47907
www.cla.purdue.edu/hk/sportsmed
Prgm Dir: Larry J Leverenz, PhD ATC
Tel: 765 494-3167   *Fax:* 765 496-1239
E-mail: llevere@purdue.edu

Iowa

Iowa State University
Athletic Training Prgm
225 Forker Bldg
Ames, IA 50011
Prgm Dir: Mary Meier, MS ATC LAT
Tel: 515 294-3587   *Fax:* 515 294-8740
E-mail: mkmeier@iastate.edu

University of Northern Iowa
Athletic Training Prgm
203 Wellness Recreation Center
Cedar Falls, IA 50614-0241
Prgm Dir: Kelli Snyder, MS
Tel: 319 273-7264   *Fax:* 319 273-5958
E-mail: kelli.snyder@uni.edu

Coe College
Athletic Training Prgm
1220 First Ave NE
Cedar Rapids, IA 52402
Prgm Dir: Chad Libby, MS
Tel: 319 399-8014   *Fax:* 319 399-8721
E-mail: clibby@coe.edu

Luther College
Athletic Training Prgm
700 College Dr
Decorah, IA 52101
Prgm Dir: Brian Solberg
Tel: 563 387-1246
E-mail: solberbr@luther.edu

Clarke College
Athletic Training Prgm
1550 Clarke Dr, MS 1757
Dubuque, IA 52001
www.clarke.edu
Prgm Dir: Melody "Dee" Higgins
Tel: 563 588-6549
E-mail: dee.higgins@clarke.edu

Loras College
Athletic Training Prgm
1450 Alta Vista
Dubuque, IA 52004-0178
Prgm Dir: Susan P Wehring
Tel: 563 588-7020
E-mail: susie.wehring@loras.edu

Upper Iowa University
Athletic Training Prgm
605 Washington St
PO Box 1857
Fayette, IA 52142
www.uiu.edu
Prgm Dir: Angela Leete, MS ATC LAT
Tel: 563 425-5782   *Fax:* 563 425-5379
E-mail: leetea@uiu.edu

Simpson College
Athletic Training Prgm
701 North C St
Indianola, IA 50125
Prgm Dir: Mike Hadden, MS
Tel: 515 961-1751   *Fax:* 515 961-1279
E-mail: hadden@simpson.edu

University of Iowa
Athletic Training Prgm
414 FH
Iowa City, IA 52242-1020
www.hawkeyehealthcare.com/Education/venue05.htm
Prgm Dir: Danny T Foster, PhD ATC LAT
Tel: 319 335-9393   *Fax:* 319 335-9398
E-mail: danny-foster@uiowa.edu

Graceland University
Athletic Training Prgm
1 University Place
Lamoni, IA 50140
Prgm Dir: Diane Bartholomew, DHSc ATC
Tel: 641 784-5043   *Fax:* 641 784-5472
E-mail: batholo@graceland.edu

Northwestern College
Athletic Training Prgm
101 7th St SW
Orange City, IA 51041-1998
www.nwciowa.edu
Prgm Dir: Jennifer J Rogers, MEd ATC
Tel: 712 707-7307   *Fax:* 712 707-7290
E-mail: jjaacks@nwciowa.edu

Central College
Athletic Training Prgm
812 University Box 6600
Pella, IA 50219
www.central.edu
Prgm Dir: John Roslien, MS
Tel: 641 628-5132   *Fax:* 641 628-5356
E-mail: roslienj@central.edu

Buena Vista University
Athletic Training Prgm
610 W Fourth St
Storm Lake, IA 50588
www.bvu.edu
Prgm Dir: Christopher Todden, MS ATC LAT
Tel: 712 749-2022   *Fax:* 712 749-1460
E-mail: todden@bvu.edu

Kansas

Benedictine College
Athletic Training Prgm
1020 N Second St
Atchison, KS 66002
Prgm Dir: Lanny Leroy
Tel: 913 367-5340, Ext 2541
E-mail: lannyl@benedictine.edu

Emporia State University
Athletic Training Prgm
1200 Commerical St, Box 4013
Emporia, KS 66801
www.emporia.edu/hper
Prgm Dir: Leslie Kenney, MS ATC LAT
Tel: 620 341-5955   *Fax:* 620 341-6953
E-mail: lkenney@emporia.edu

Fort Hays State University
Athletic Training Prgm
600 Park St
Hays, KS 67601
Prgm Dir: David Fitzhugh, PhD
Tel: 785 628-4354   *Fax:* 785 628-4126
E-mail: dkfitzhugh@fhsu.edu

Tabor College
Athletic Training Prgm
400 S Jefferson
Hillsboro, KS 67063
www.tabor.edu
Prgm Dir: James Moore, MS ATC CSCS
Tel: 620 947-3121, Ext 1306   *Fax:* 620 947-2607
E-mail: jimm@tabor.edu

University of Kansas
Athletic Training Prgm
1301 Sunnyside Ave
ROB 161-C
Lawrence, KS 66045
Prgm Dir: W David Carr, PhD ATC
Tel: 785 864-0799   *Fax:* 785 864-3343
E-mail: wdcarr@ku.edu

Kansas State University
Athletic Training Prgm
241 Justin Hall
Department of Human Nutrition
Manhattan, KS 66506-1407
https://www.k-state.edu/humec/hn/athleticcover.htm
Prgm Dir: Shawna Jordan, PhD ATC LAT
Tel: 785 532-0151   *Fax:* 785 532-3132
E-mail: jordan@ksu.edu

Bethel College
Athletic Training Prgm
300 E 27th St
North Newton, KS 67117
www.bethelks.edu
Prgm Dir: Doug Maury, MEd ATC LAT CSCS
Tel: 316 284-5298   *Fax:* 316 284-5286
E-mail: dmaury@bethelks.edu

Mid-America Nazarene University
Athletic Training Prgm
2030 E College Way
Olathe, KS 66062-1899
www.mnu.edu
Prgm Dir: Chad Keller
Tel: 913 971-3755   *Fax:* 913 971-3404
E-mail: cjkeller@mnu.edu

Kansas Wesleyan University
Athletic Training Prgm
100 E Claflin Ave
Salina, KS 67401-6196
Prgm Dir: Matthew Williams, ATC DSM
Tel: 785 827-5541, Ext 3194   *Fax:* 785 827-0927
E-mail: mjw@kwu.edu

Sterling College
Athletic Training Prgm
125 W Cooper
Sterling, KS 67579
Prgm Dir: Ryan Manely, MS
Tel: 620 278-4338   *Fax:* 620 278-4319
E-mail: pmanely@sterling.edu

Washburn University
Athletic Training Prgm
1700 SW College
Topeka, KS 66621
Prgm Dir: Bryan Dorrel, MS ATC LAT
Tel: 785 670-1965   *Fax:* 785 670-1059
E-mail: bryan.dorrel@washburn.edu

Southwestern College
Athletic Training Prgm
100 College St
Winfield, KS 67156
Prgm Dir: Lisa Braun, MEd LAT ATC
Tel: 620 229-6226   *Fax:* 620 229-6112
E-mail: lisa.braun@sckans.edu

Kentucky

Northern Kentucky University
Athletic Training Prgm
109 Albright Health Center
Highland Heights, KY 41099
Prgm Dir: Trey Morgan, MS ATC
Tel: 859 572-1399   *Fax:* 859 572-6090
E-mail: morgant@nku.edu

Murray State University
Athletic Training Prgm
Dept of Wellness and Therapeutic Sciences
102A Carr Health Bldg
Murray, KY 42071
www.murraystate.edu/academics/hshs/wts/
   athletictraining.htm
Prgm Dir: Jeremy Erdmann, MA ATC
Tel: 270 809-4517   *Fax:* 270 809-6803
E-mail: jeremy.erdmann@murraystate.edu

Eastern Kentucky University
Athletic Training Prgm
Moberly 224
521 Lancaster Ave
Richmond, KY 40475
Prgm Dir: Joseph Beckett, EdD ATC
Tel: 859 622-2134   *Fax:* 859 622-1254
E-mail: Joe.Beckett@eku.edu

Louisiana

Louisiana State University
Athletic Training Prgm
Department of Kinesiology
112 H P Long Fieldhouse
Baton Rouge, LA 70803
www.lsu.edu/kinesiology
Prgm Dir: Ray Castle, PhD ATC LAT
Tel: 225 578-7175   *Fax:* 225 578-3680
E-mail: rcastl1@lsu.edu

Southeastern Louisiana University
Athletic Training Prgm
SLU 10845
Hammond, LA 70402
Prgm Dir: Karen Lew, MEd
Tel: 985 549-2350   *Fax:* 985 549-5119
E-mail: klew@selu.edu

University of Louisiana at Lafayette
Athletic Training Prgm
225 Cajundome Blvd
Lafayette, LA 70506
http://kinesiology.louisiana.edu/Programs/ATEP/
Prgm Dir: Toby Dore, PhD ATC LAT
Tel: 337 482-6283   *Fax:* 337 482-6278
E-mail: tldore@louisiana.edu

Louisiana College
Athletic Training Prgm
1140 College Dr, Box 563
Pineville, LA 71359
Prgm Dir: Mike Brunet, PhD
Tel: 318 487-7519   *Fax:* 318 487-7174
E-mail: mbrunet@lacollege.edu

Nicholls State University
Athletic Training Prgm
PO Box 2090
Thibodaux, LA 70310
www.nicholls.edu/ahs/health/athletic
Prgm Dir: Celest Weuve, MS ATC CSCS LAT
Tel: 985 493-2613   *Fax:* 985 493-2614
E-mail: celest.weuve@nicholls.edu

Maine

University of New England
Athletic Training Prgm
11 Hills Beach Rd
Biddeford, ME 04005
Prgm Dir: Wayne Lamarre, MEd
Tel: 207 602-2412   *Fax:* 207 282-6379
E-mail: wlamarre@une.edu

University of Southern Maine
Athletic Training Prgm
105A Warren Hill Gymnasium
37 College Ave
Gorham, ME 04038
Prgm Dir: Ben Towne, MA
Tel: 207 228-8104   *Fax:* 207 780-4745
E-mail: btowne@usm.maine.edu

University of Maine - Orono
Athletic Training Prgm
108 Lengyel Hall
Orono, ME 04469
www.umaine.edu
Prgm Dir: Sherrie L Weeks, ATC
Tel: 207 581-2466   *Fax:* 207 581-1206
E-mail: Sherrie_Weeks@umit.maine.edu

University of Maine - Presque Isle
Athletic Training Prgm
181 Main St, 209 South Hal
Presque Isle, ME 04769
www.umpi.maine.edu/cms/academics/atep/index-200506
   22327/
Prgm Dir: Barbara Blackstone, MSS
Tel: 207 768-9415   *Fax:* 207 768-9553
E-mail: blackstb@umpi.maine.edu

Maryland

Frostburg State University
Athletic Training Prgm
Cordts Physical Education Center
Frostburg, MD 21532
Prgm Dir: John Wright, MS
Tel: 301 687-4477   *Fax:* 301 687-7961
E-mail: jwright@frostburg.edu

Salisbury University
Athletic Training Prgm
1101 Camden Ave
Department of Health, Physical Education & Human
   Performance
Salisbury, MD 21801
www.salisbury.edu
Prgm Dir: Donna Ritenour, EdD
Tel: 410 543-6348   *Fax:* 410 543-6434
E-mail: dmritenour@salisbury.edu

Towson University
Athletic Training Prgm
8000 York Rd
Kinesiology Department
Towson, MD 21252
www.towson.edu
Prgm Dir: Michael Higgins, PhD ATC/PT CSCS
Tel: 410 704-3166   *Fax:* 410 704-3912
E-mail: mhiggins@towson.edu

Massachusetts

Endicott College
Athletic Training Prgm
376 Hale St
Beverly, MA 01915
Prgm Dir: Deborah Swanton, EdD ATC
Tel: 978 232-2433 *Fax:* 978 232-2600
E-mail: dswanton@endicott.edu

Boston University
Athletic Training Prgm
635 Commonwealth Ave
Boston, MA 02215
www.bu.edu/sargent
Prgm Dir: Sara Brown, MS ATC
Tel: 617 353-7507 *Fax:* 617 353-9463
E-mail: sara@bu.edu

Northeastern University
Athletic Training Prgm
304 Dockser Hall
Boston, MA 02115
www.neu.edu
Prgm Dir: Jamie L Musler, MS Ed ATC
Tel: 617 373-5355 *Fax:* 617 373-5920
E-mail: j.musler@neu.edu

Bridgewater State College
Athletic Training Prgm
Dept of MAHPLS
Tinsley Center
Bridgewater, MA 02325
Prgm Dir: Marcia Anderson, PhD
Tel: 508 531-2072 *Fax:* 508 531-1717
E-mail: mkanderson@bridgew.edu

Lasell College
Athletic Training Prgm
1844 Commonwealth Ave
Newton, MA 02466
Prgm Dir: Christina Haverty, MEd
Tel: 617 243-2131 *Fax:* 617 243-2309
E-mail: chaverty@lasell.edu

Merrimack College
Athletic Training Prgm
315 Turnpike St
North Andover, MA 01845
Prgm Dir: Birgid Hopkins, MS ATC
Tel: 978 837-5332 *Fax:* 978 837-5032
E-mail: birgid.hopkins@merrimack.edu

Salem State College
Athletic Training Prgm
352 Lafayette St
Salem, MA 01970-5353
Prgm Dir: Joe Gallo, DSc
Tel: 978 542-6585 *Fax:* 978 542-6554
E-mail: jgallo@salemstate.edu

Springfield College
Athletic Training Prgm
Physical Education Complex
Springfield, MA 01109
http://catalog.spfldcol.edu/preview_program.php?catoid
=26&poid=877
Prgm Dir: Mary G Barnum, EdD ATC LAT
Tel: 413 748-3763 *Fax:* 413 748-3052
E-mail: mary_barnum@spfldcol.edu

Westfield State College
Athletic Training Prgm
Department of Movement Science
577 Western Ave
Westfield, MA 01086-1630
www.wsc.ma.edu/dept/mssls/atraining/
Prgm Dir: William Miller, DPE ATC LAT
Tel: 413 572-5450 *Fax:* 413 572-8214
E-mail: wmiller@wsc.ma.edu

Michigan

Albion College
Athletic Training Prgm
Box 4830
Albion, MI 49224
Prgm Dir: Robert Moss, PhD ATC
Tel: 517 629-0548 *Fax:* 517 629-0619
E-mail: rmoss@albion.edu

Grand Valley State University
Athletic Training Prgm
Movement Science Dept
192 Field House
Allendale, MI 49401
Prgm Dir: Shari Bartz-Smith, PhD ATC CSCS
Tel: 616 331-3044 *Fax:* 616 331-3232
E-mail: bartzs@gvsu.edu

Alma College
Athletic Training Prgm
614 W Superior St
Alma, MI 48801
www.alma.edu
Prgm Dir: Denny Griffin, MA ATC
Tel: 989 463-7988, Ext 989 *Fax:* 989 463-7018
E-mail: griffin@alma.edu

University of Michigan
Athletic Training Prgm
401 Washtenaw Ave
Kinesiology Bldg
Ann Arbor, MI 48109-2214
Prgm Dir: Brian Czajika, MS
Tel: 734 647-2702 *Fax:* 734 936-1925
E-mail: baczajka@umich.edu

Michigan State University
Athletic Training Prgm
105 IM Circle
East Lansing, MI 48824
Prgm Dir: Tracey Covassin, PhD
Tel: 517 353-2010 *Fax:* 517 432-2944
E-mail: covassin@msu.edu

Aquinas College
Athletic Training Prgm
1607 Robinson Rd SE
Hruby Hall 42
Grand Rapids, MI 49506-1799
Prgm Dir: JoAnne Gorant, MS
Tel: 616 632-2899 *Fax:* 616 732-4487
E-mail: goranjoa@aquinas.edu

Hope College
Athletic Training Prgm
PO Box 9000
Holland, MI 49423
www.hope.edu/academic/kinesiology/athtrain
Prgm Dir: Richard Ray, EdD ATC
Tel: 616 395-7708 *Fax:* 616 395-7175
E-mail: ray@hope.edu

Western Michigan University
Athletic Training Prgm
Health, Physical Education and Recreation
1903 W Michigan Ave #5426
Kalamazoo, MI 49008
www.wmich.edu
Prgm Dir: Jennifer O'Donoghue, MA ATC CSCS
Tel: 269 387-2703
E-mail: ODonoghueJ@groupwise.wmich.edu

Northern Michigan University
Athletic Training Prgm
Dept of HPER
1401 Presque Isle Ave
Marquette, MI 49855
Prgm Dir: Julie A Rochester, MS ATC
Tel: 906 227-2026 *Fax:* 906 227-2181
E-mail: jrochest@nmu.edu

Central Michigan University
Athletic Training Prgm
HPB 1171
Mount Pleasant, MI 48859
www.chp.cmich.edu/atep
Prgm Dir: Rene Shingles, PhD ATC
Tel: 989 774-2378 *Fax:* 989 774-2923
E-mail: shing1rr@cmich.edu

Lake Superior State University
Athletic Training Prgm
650 W Easterday Ave
Sault Ste Marie, MI 49783
www.lssu.edu
Prgm Dir: Joseph D Susi II, MS ATC
Tel: 906 635-2161 *Fax:* 906 635-2753
E-mail: jsusi@lssu.edu

Saginaw Valley State University
Athletic Training Prgm
7400 Bay Rd
University Center, MI 48710
www.svsu.edu
Prgm Dir: Paul Ballard, EdD
Tel: 989 964-7269 *Fax:* 989 964-4564
E-mail: pballard@svsu.edu

Eastern Michigan University
Athletic Training Prgm
310 Porter Bldg
Ypsilanti, MI 48197
Prgm Dir: Jodi Johnson, MS ATC
Tel: 734 487-7120, Ext 2722 *Fax:* 734 487-2024
E-mail: jjohnson@emich.edu

Minnesota

University of Minnesota - Duluth
Athletic Training Prgm
110 Sports and Health Center
1216 Ordean Court
Duluth, MN 55812
www.d.umn.edu/hper/undergraduate/majors/
   athletic_training/
Prgm Dir: William Gear, PhD
Tel: 218 726-8654 *Fax:* 218 726-6243
E-mail: wgear@d.umn.edu

Minnesota State University - Mankato
Athletic Training Prgm
1400 Highland Center
Mankato, MN 56001
Prgm Dir: Patrick Sexton, EdD ATC/R CSCS
Tel: 507 389-2092 *Fax:* 507 389-5618
E-mail: patrick.sexton@mnsu.edu

Minnesota State University - Moorhead
Athletic Training Prgm
106 D Alex Namzek Hall
Moorhead, MN 56563
Prgm Dir: Dawn Hammerschmidt, MEd
Tel: 218 477-2318 *Fax:* 218 477-2363
E-mail: hammerda@mnstate.edu

St Cloud State University
Athletic Training Prgm
720 4th Ave South, Halenbeck Hall 339
St Cloud, MN 56301
Prgm Dir: William Picconatto, PhD
Tel: 320 308-3079 *Fax:* 320 308-5399
E-mail: wjpicconatto@stcloudstate.edu

Bethel University
Athletic Training Prgm
3900 Bethel Dr
St Paul, MN 55112
Prgm Dir: Neal S Dutton
Tel: 651 638-6255
E-mail: dutnea@bethel.edu

Gustavus Adolphus College
Athletic Training Prgm
800 W College Ave
St Peter, MN 56082
Prgm Dir: John Mattson, PhD ATC
Tel: 507 933-7674   *Fax:* 507 933-8412
E-mail: jmattson@gac.edu

Winona State University
Athletic Training Prgm
Memorial Hall 117
Winona, MN 55987-5838
www.winona.edu/athletictraining
Prgm Dir: Shellie F Nelson, EdD ATC
Tel: 507 457-5214   *Fax:* 507 457-5606
E-mail: snelson@winona.edu

Mississippi

Delta State University
Athletic Training Prgm
PO Box B-2
Cleveland, MS 38733
Prgm Dir: Timothy Colbert, MS
Tel: 662 846-4562   *Fax:* 662 846-4571
E-mail: tcolbert@deltastate.edu

University of Southern Mississippi
Athletic Training Prgm
Dept of Human Performance and Recreation
118 College Dr, Box 5142
Hattiesburg, MS 39405-0001
www.usm.edu/athletictraining/
Prgm Dir: Benito Velasquez, DA
Tel: 601 266-6058   *Fax:* 601 266-4445
E-mail: benito.velasquez@usm.edu

Missouri

Southwest Baptist University
Athletic Training Prgm
1600 University Ave
Bolivar, MO 65613
Prgm Dir: Todd A John
Tel: 417 328-1988
E-mail: tjohn@sbuniv.edu

Culver-Stockton College
Athletic Training Prgm
1 College Hill
Canton, MO 63435
Prgm Dir: Robert W Carmichael
Tel: 573 288-6304   *Fax:* 573 288-6442
E-mail: rcarmichael@culver.edu

Southeast Missouri State University
Athletic Training Prgm
One University Plaza MS7650
Cape Girardeau, MO 63701
Prgm Dir: Craig Elder, PhD ATC CSCS
Tel: 573 651-5193   *Fax:* 573 651-5150
E-mail: celder@semo.edu

Central Methodist University
Athletic Training Prgm
411 CMC Square
Fayette, MO 65248
Prgm Dir: Wade Welton, MS ATC/L
Tel: 660 248-6217   *Fax:* 660 248-6381
E-mail: wwelton@centralmethodist.edu

William Woods University
Athletic Training Prgm
One University Ave
Fulton, MO 65251
Prgm Dir: Anthony Lungstrum, MS
Tel: 573 592-1638   *Fax:* 573 592-1641
E-mail: anthony.lungstrum@williamwoods.edu

Truman State University
Athletic Training Prgm
Pershing Bldg
Kirksville, MO 63501
http://hes.truman.edu/atmaj
Prgm Dir: Michelle Boyd, MS
Tel: 660 785-7364   *Fax:* 660 785-4166
E-mail: mboyd@truman.edu

Missouri Valley College
Athletic Training Prgm
500 E College St
Marshall, MO 65340
Prgm Dir: Karla Bruntzel, PhD ATC
Tel: 660 831-4103   *Fax:* 660 831-4030
E-mail: bruntzelk@moval.edu

Park University
Athletic Training Prgm
8700 NW Riverpark Dr
Parkville, MO 64152
Prgm Dir: Thomas Bertoncino, MS ATC
Tel: 816 584-6864   *Fax:* 816 587-8907
E-mail: thomas.bertoncino@park.edu

Missouri State University
Athletic Training Prgm
Professional Bldg 160
901 S National Ave
Springfield, MO 65897
Prgm Dir: Gary Ward, MS ATC LAT PT
Tel: 417 836-8553   *Fax:* 417 836-8554
E-mail: GaryWard@MissouriState.edu

Lindenwood University
Athletic Training Prgm
209 S Kings Hwy
St Charles, MO 63301
Prgm Dir: Randy Biggerstaff, MS
Tel: 636 949-4683   *Fax:* 636 949-4636
E-mail: rbiggerstaff@lindenwood.edu

University of Central Missouri
Athletic Training Prgm
Humphreys 204
Warrensburg, MO 64093
Prgm Dir: Brian Hughes, EdD
Tel: 660 543-8062
E-mail: bhughes@ucmo.edu

Montana

Montana State University - Billings
Athletic Training Prgm
PE 119
1500 University Dr
Billings, MT 59101
Prgm Dir: Mike Diede, PhD ATC
Tel: 406 657-2351
E-mail: mdiede@msubillings.edu

University of Montana
Athletic Training Prgm
Health and Human Performance Dept
McGill Hall 101
Missoula, MT 59812-1055
www.soe.umt.edu/hhp/athletic_training/
Prgm Dir: Scott T Richter, EdM
Tel: 406 243-5246   *Fax:* 406 243-6252
E-mail: scott.richter@mso.umt.edu

Nebraska

University of Nebraska - Kearney
Athletic Training Prgm
905 W 25th St
Cushing Bldg Rm 158
Kearney, NE 68849
Prgm Dir: Scott Unruh
Tel: 308 865-8627   *Fax:* 308 865-8073
E-mail: unruhsa@unk.edu

Nebraska Wesleyan University
Athletic Training Prgm
5000 St Paul Ave
Lincoln, NE 68504
Prgm Dir: Dana Bates, MS
Tel: 402 465-7545   *Fax:* 402 465-2170
E-mail: dbates@nebrwesleyan.edu

University of Nebraska - Lincoln
Athletic Training Prgm
231 Mabel Lee Hall
Lincoln, NE 68588-0234
Prgm Dir: Jeffrey P Rudy
Tel: 402 472-5978
E-mail: jrudy2@unl.edu

Creighton University
Athletic Training Prgm
2500 California Plaza, KFC 234
Omaha, NE 68178
Prgm Dir: Charles Pfeifer, MS
Tel: 402 280-2402   *Fax:* 402 280-4732
E-mail: pcp@creighton.edu

University of Nebraska - Omaha
Athletic Training Prgm
HPER 207
6001 Dodge St
Omaha, NE 68182-0216
http://coe.unomaha.edu/hper/at/at_index.php
Prgm Dir: Joshua Nichter, MS ATC CSCS
Tel: 402 554-3224   *Fax:* 402 554-3693
E-mail: jnichter@mail.unomaha.edu

Nevada

University of Nevada - Las Vegas
Athletic Training Prgm
4505 Maryland Pkwy
PO Box 453034
Las Vegas, NV 89154-3034
Prgm Dir: Mack Rubley, PhD LAT ATC CSCS
Tel: 702 895-2457   *Fax:* 702 895-1500
E-mail: mack.rubley@unlv.edu

New Hampshire

University of New Hampshire
Athletic Training Prgm
Dept of Kinesiology
145 Main St, Field House
Durham, NH 03824
www.shhs.unh.edu/kin_at/
Prgm Dir: Daniel R Sedory, MS ATC NHLAT
Tel: 603 862-1831   *Fax:* 603 862-4198
E-mail: dan.sedory@unh.edu

Keene State College
Athletic Training Prgm
229 Main St
Keene, NH 03435-2301
Prgm Dir: Wanda Swiger, EdD
Tel: 603 358-2783   *Fax:* 603 358-2075
E-mail: wswiger@keene.edu

Colby-Sawyer College
Athletic Training Prgm
541 Main St
New London, NH 03257
Prgm Dir: Jennifer Austin, PhD
Tel: 603 526-3619   *Fax:* 603 526-3872
E-mail: jaustin@colby-sawyer.edu

Plymouth State University
Athletic Training Prgm
MSC 22
Plymouth, NH 03264
www.plymouth.edu
Prgm Dir: Linda S Levy, EdD ATC
Tel: 603 535-2577   *Fax:* 603 535-2395
E-mail: levy@plymouth.edu

New Jersey

Rowan University
Athletic Training Prgm
201 Mullica Hill Rd
Glassboro, NJ 08028
Prgm Dir: Robert Sterner, PhD
Tel: 856 256-4500, Ext 376　*Fax:* 856 256-5613
E-mail: sterner@rowan.edu

Seton Hall University
Athletic Training Prgm
400 S Orange Ave
South Orange, NJ 07079
Prgm Dir: Carolyn Goeckel, MA ATC
Tel: 973 275-2826
E-mail: goeckeca@shu.edu

Kean University
Athletic Training Prgm
D'Angola Gym, Morris Ave
Union, NJ 07083
Prgm Dir: Gary Ball, EdD MEd BS ATC
Tel: 908 737-0659　*Fax:* 908 353-7199
E-mail: gball@kean.edu

Montclair State University
Athletic Training Prgm
1 Normal Ave
Upper Montclair, NJ 07043
Prgm Dir: David Middlemas, EdD
Tel: 973 655-7090　*Fax:* 973 655-5461
E-mail: middlemasd@mail.montclair.edu

William Paterson Univ of New Jersey
Athletic Training Prgm
Dept of Exercise and Movement Science
300 Pompton Rd
Wayne, NJ 07470
www.wpunj.edu/cos/ex-movsci/atep.htm
Prgm Dir: Robb Rehberg, PhD ATC CSCS NREMT
Tel: 973 720-2267　*Fax:* 973 720-2034
E-mail: rehbergr@wpunj.edu

New Mexico

University of New Mexico
Athletic Training Prgm
South Athletic Complex
Albuquerque, NM 87131
Prgm Dir: Susan McGowen
Tel: 505 277-5151　*Fax:* 505 277-6227
E-mail: yorex@unm.edu

New Mexico State University
Athletic Training Prgm
Box 30001, MSC 3FAC
Las Cruces, NM 88003-0001
www.nmsu.edu
Prgm Dir: Karen Hostetter, PhD ATC
Tel: 505 646-5038　*Fax:* 505 646-3564
E-mail: khosttet@nmsu.edu

New York

Alfred University
Athletic Training Prgm
1 Saxon Dr
Alfred, NY 14802
www.las.alfred.edu
Prgm Dir: Timothy Howell, EdD ATC CSCS
Tel: 607 871-2784　*Fax:* 607 871-2712
E-mail: howellt@alfred.edu

SUNY Brockport
Athletic Training Prgm
260 Tuttle South
Brockport, NY 14420
Prgm Dir: Timothy J Henry, PhD ATC
Tel: 585 395-5357　*Fax:* 585 395-2771
E-mail: thenry@brockport.edu

Long Island University - Brooklyn Campus
Athletic Training Prgm
1 University Plaza
HS 312
Brooklyn, NY 11201-8423
www.brooklyn.liu.edu/athletictraining
Prgm Dir: Tracye Rawls-Martin, MS ATC
Tel: 718 780-4081　*Fax:* 718 488-1432
E-mail: tmartin@liu.edu

Canisius College
Athletic Training Prgm
2001 Main St
Buffalo, NY 14208-1098
www.canisius.edu/sportsmed/
Prgm Dir: Peter Koehneke, MS ATC
Tel: 716 888-2954　*Fax:* 716 888-3216
E-mail: koehneke@canisius.edu

University at Buffalo - SUNY
Athletic Training Prgm
405 Kimball Tower
3435 Main St
Buffalo, NY 14214
Prgm Dir: Karl Kozlowski, EdM
Tel: 716 829-2941, Ext 282　*Fax:* 716 829-2428
E-mail: kfk@buffalo.edu

SUNY College at Cortland
Athletic Training Prgm
PO Box 2000
Cortland, NY 13045
www.cortland.edu/kin
Prgm Dir: John Cottone, EdD ATC
Tel: 607 753-4962　*Fax:* 607 753-5975
E-mail: cottoneJ@cortland.edu

Hofstra University
Athletic Training Prgm
220 Hofstra University
The Dome
Hempstead, NY 11550
Prgm Dir: Jayne Kitsos-Ciarlante, MA ATC
Tel: 516 463-6952　*Fax:* 516 463-6275
E-mail: hprjmk@Hofstra.edu

Ithaca College
Athletic Training Prgm
48 Hill Center
Ithaca College
Ithaca, NY 14850
www.ithaca.edu/hshp/clinics/atclinic/
Prgm Dir: Paul Geisler, EdD ATC
Tel: 607 274-3006　*Fax:* 607 274-1943
E-mail: pgeisler@Ithaca.edu

Dominican College
Athletic Training Prgm
470 Western Hwy
Orangeburg, NY 10962
Prgm Dir: James T Crawley, MEd ATC PT
Tel: 845 848-6004, Ext 6004　*Fax:* 845 398-4895
E-mail: jim.crawley@dc.edu

Marist College
Athletic Training Prgm
3399 North Rd
McCann Center Rm 212
Poughkeepsie, NY 12601
www.marist.edu/science/athtrain
Prgm Dir: Sally Perkins, ATC
Tel: 845 575-3912　*Fax:* 845 575-3282
E-mail: sally.perkins@marist.edu

Stony Brook University
Athletic Training Prgm
School of Health Technology and Management
100 Nicolls Rd, Indoor Sports Complex
Stony Brook, NY 11794-3504
www.hsc.stonybrook.edu/shtm/at/
Prgm Dir: Kathryn A Koshansky, MS ATC
Tel: 631 632-2837　*Fax:* 631 632-7210
E-mail: kathryn.koshansky@stonybrook.edu

North Carolina

Lees-McRae College
Athletic Training Prgm
PO Box 128
375 College Dr
Banner Elk, NC 28604
Prgm Dir: Rita A Smith
Tel: 828 898-8768　*Fax:* 828 898-8742
E-mail: smithr@lmc.edu

Gardner-Webb University
Athletic Training Prgm
Department of Physical Edu, Wellness and Sport Studies
Campus 7257
Boiling Springs, NC 28017
www.gardner-webb.edu
Prgm Dir: Ashley White, MS LAT ATC
Tel: 704 406-3810　*Fax:* 704 406-3503
E-mail: awhite@gardner-webb.edu

Appalachian State University
Athletic Training Prgm
Hlth Leisure and Exercise Science
Boone, NC 28608
Prgm Dir: Jamie Moul, EdD ATC
Tel: 828 262-7630　*Fax:* 828 262-3138
E-mail: mouljl@appstate.edu

Campbell University
Athletic Training Prgm
PO Box 10
89 Pope St
Buies Creek, NC 27506
Prgm Dir: Mary Jones, PhD
Tel: 910 893-1362　*Fax:* 910 893-1424
E-mail: jonesm@campbell.edu

University of North Carolina - Chapel Hill
Athletic Training Prgm
211 Fetzer, CB 8700
Chapel Hill, NC 27599-8700
Prgm Dir: Darin Padua
Tel: 919 843-5117　*Fax:* 919 962-0489
E-mail: dpadua@email.unc.edu

Univ of North Carolina at Charlotte
Athletic Training Prgm
226 Belk Gymnasium
Dept of Kinesiology
Charlotte, NC 28223
www.health.uncc.edu/academic_programs.cfm?pname=
　bsat
Prgm Dir: Tricia J Hubbard, PhD ATC
Tel: 704 687-6202　*Fax:* 704 687-3350
E-mail: thubbar1@uncc.edu

Western Carolina University
Athletic Training Prgm
135 Moore Hall
Cullowhee, NC 28723
Prgm Dir: James Scifers, DScPT
Tel: 828 227-2147
E-mail: jscifers@email.wcu.edu

North Carolina Central University
Athletic Training Prgm
1801 Fayetteville St
PO Box 19542
Durham, NC 27707
www.nccu.edu
Prgm Dir: Dawn Maffucci, MA ATC LAT
Tel: 919 530-7239　*Fax:* 919 530-6156
E-mail: dmaffucci@nccu.edu

Elon University
Athletic Training Prgm
Campus Box 2525
Elon, NC 27244
Prgm Dir: Gregory Calone, MS
Tel: 336 278-6715　*Fax:* 336 278-5918
E-mail: gcalone@elon.edu

Methodist University
Athletic Training Prgm
5400 Ramsey St
Fayetteville, NC 28311
Prgm Dir: Hugh Harling, EdD
Tel: 910 630-7418   *Fax:* 910 630-7676
E-mail: hharling@methodist.edu

Greensboro College
Athletic Training Prgm
815 W Market St
Greensboro, NC 27401
www.gborocollege.edu
Prgm Dir: Michelle Lesperance, MS ATC LAT
Tel: 336 272-7102, Ext 629   *Fax:* 336 217-7237
E-mail: mlesperance@gborocollege.edu

University of North Carolina - Greensboro
Athletic Training Prgm
Dept of Exercise and Sport Science
250 HHP
Greensboro, NC 27412
www.uncg.edu/ess/atep
Prgm Dir: Jolene Henning, EdD ATC
Tel: 336 334-3694   *Fax:* 336 334-3238
E-mail: jmhenni2@uncg.edu

East Carolina University
Athletic Training Prgm
245 Ward Sports Medicine Bldg
Greenville, NC 27858
Prgm Dir: Katie Walsh, EdD ATC-L
Tel: 252 328-4560   *Fax:* 252 328-4565
E-mail: walshk@ecu.edu

Lenoir-Rhyne College
Athletic Training Prgm
PO Box 7356
Hickory, NC 28603
www.lrc.edu/hlss
Prgm Dir: Michael R McGee, EdD LAT ATC
Tel: 828 328-7127   *Fax:* 828 267-3445
E-mail: mcgee@lrc.edu

High Point University
Athletic Training Prgm
833 Montlieu Ave
High Point, NC 27262
Prgm Dir: Rick Proctor, EdD LAT ATC
Tel: 336 841-9267   *Fax:* 336 841-9182
E-mail: rproctor@highpoint.edu

Mars Hill College
Athletic Training Prgm
PO Box 6668
Mars Hill, NC 28754
Prgm Dir: Kelly Ottie, MA
Tel: 828 689-1217   *Fax:* 828 689-1313
E-mail: kottie@mhc.edu

University of North Carolina
Athletic Training Prgm
PO Box 1510
Pembroke, NC 28372
Prgm Dir: Susan Edkins, MS
Tel: 910 521-6480
E-mail: edkins@uncp.edu

Catawba College
Athletic Training Prgm
2300 W Innes St
Salisbury, NC 28144
www.catawba.edu
Prgm Dir: Robert Dingle, HSD LAT ATC
Tel: 704 637-4455   *Fax:* 704 637-5705
E-mail: rdingle@catawba.edu

University of North Carolina - Wilmington
Athletic Training Prgm
601 S College Rd
Wilmington, NC 28403-5956
http://people.uncw.edu/brownk/UNCAThomepage.htm
Prgm Dir: Kirk Brown, PhD LAT ATC
Tel: 910 962-7184   *Fax:* 910 962-7073
E-mail: brownk@uncw.edu

Barton College
Athletic Training Prgm
PO Box 5000
Wilson, NC 27893
www.barton.edu
Prgm Dir: Carla Stoddard, MS ATC LAT
Tel: 252 399-6377   *Fax:* 252 399-6516
E-mail: cstoddard@barton.edu

Wingate University
Athletic Training Prgm
Campus Box 3079
Wingate, NC 28174
www.wingate.edu/academics/sport_sciences/
   athletic_training/
Prgm Dir: Traci N Gearhart, PhD
Tel: 704 233-8179   *Fax:* 704 233-8365
E-mail: tgearhar@wingate.edu

North Dakota

University of Mary
Athletic Training Prgm
7500 University Dr
Bismarck, ND 58504-9652
www.umary.edu/UM/AcademicInformation/
   Undergraduate/hps/AthleticTraining/
Prgm Dir: Blaine Steiner, MS ATC LAT
Tel: 701 355-8188   *Fax:* 701 255-7687
E-mail: bsteiner@umary.edu

North Dakota State University
Athletic Training Prgm
Bentson Bunker Fieldhouse 9C
PO Box 5576
Fargo, ND 58105-5576
Prgm Dir: Pamela Hansen, EdD ATC
Tel: 701 231-8093   *Fax:* 701 231-8872
E-mail: pamela.j.hansen@ndsu.edu

University of North Dakota
Athletic Training Prgm
Div of Sports Medicine
2751 2nd Ave N, Stop 9013
Grand Forks, ND 58202-9013
www.und.nodak.edu
Prgm Dir: Steven Westereng, LATC MA ATC
Tel: 701 777-3886   *Fax:* 701 777-2536
E-mail: Wester@medicine.nodak.edu

Ohio

Ohio Northern University
Athletic Training Prgm
Dept of HPSS
243 Sports Center
Ada, OH 45810
Prgm Dir: Michelle Glon, MS ATC
Tel: 419 772-2443   *Fax:* 419 772-2437
E-mail: m-glon@onu.edu

University of Akron
Athletic Training Prgm
Memorial Hall 77D
Akron, OH 44325-5103
Prgm Dir: Stacey Buser, MS ATC LAT
Tel: 330 972-7475   *Fax:* 330 972-5293
E-mail: buser@uakron.edu

Mount Union College
Athletic Training Prgm
1972 Clark Ave
Alliance, OH 44601
Prgm Dir: Daniel M Gorman, MS ATC/L
Tel: 330 823-4882   *Fax:* 330 823-2399
E-mail: gormandm@muc.edu

Ashland University
Athletic Training Prgm
916 King Rd
Arthur L & Maxine Sheets Rybolt Sport Sciences Center
Ashland, OH 44805
www.ashland.edu
Prgm Dir: Dennis M Gruber, EdD ATC
Tel: 419 289-5446   *Fax:* 419 289-5460
E-mail: dgruber@ashland.edu

Ohio University
Athletic Training Prgm
Grover Center E-188
Athens, OH 45701-2979
Prgm Dir: Kristi White, PhD LAT
Tel: 740 597-1876   *Fax:* 740 593-0284
E-mail: whitek2@ohio.edu

Baldwin-Wallace College
Athletic Training Prgm
275 Eastland Rd
Berea, OH 44017
Prgm Dir: Karyn A Gentile, ATC/L
Tel: 440 826-3463   *Fax:* 440 826-6980
E-mail: kgentile@bw.edu

Bowling Green State University
Athletic Training Prgm
Eppler Complex N217
Bowling Green, OH 43403
Prgm Dir: Chris Schommer, MEd ATC
Tel: 419 372-6810   *Fax:* 419 372-0383
E-mail: schomme@bgnet.bgsu.edu

Cedarville University
Athletic Training Prgm
251 N Main St
Cedarville, OH 45314
www.cedarville.edu
Prgm Dir: Evan Hellwig, PhD PT ATC
Tel: 937 766-7691   *Fax:* 937 766-2795
E-mail: hellwige@cedarville.edu

College of Mt St Joseph
Athletic Training Prgm
Dept of Health Sciences
5701 Delhi Rd
Cincinnati, OH 45233-1870
www.msj.edu
Prgm Dir: Malissa Martin, EdD ATC CSCS
Tel: 513 244-4542   *Fax:* 513 244-4654
E-mail: Malissa_martin@mail.msj.edu

University of Cincinnati
Athletic Training Prgm
PO Box 210002
Cincinnati, OH 45221-0002
www.uc.edu/athletictraining
Prgm Dir: Pat Graman, MA ATC
Tel: 513 556-0576   *Fax:* 513 556-3898
E-mail: pat.graman@uc.edu

Xavier University
Athletic Training Prgm
3800 Victory Pkwy
Cincinnati, OH 45207-6312
Prgm Dir: Tina Davlin, PhD
Tel: 513 745-3430   *Fax:* 513 745-4291
E-mail: davlin@xavier.edu

Capital University
Athletic Training Prgm
Capital Center
1 College and Main
Columbus, OH 43209
Prgm Dir: Bonnie Goodwin, MESS ATC
Tel: 614 236-6667   *Fax:* 614 236-6178
E-mail: bgoodwin@capital.edu

Ohio State University
Athletic Training Prgm
Athletic Training Division
453 W 10th Ave
Columbus, OH 43210
http://amp.osu.edu/at
Prgm Dir: Mark Merrick, PhD ATC
Tel: 614 247-6231   *Fax:* 614 292-0210
E-mail: merrick.29@osu.edu

Wright State University
Athletic Training Prgm
Health and Physical Education Dept
Rm 303 Nutter Center
Dayton, OH 45435
Prgm Dir: L Tony Ortiz, ATC
Tel: 937 775-3827   *Fax:* 937 775-4252
E-mail: tony.ortiz@wright.edu

Defiance College
Athletic Training Prgm
701 N Clinton St
Defiance, OH 43512
www.defiance.edu/pages/edu_AT_home.html
Prgm Dir: Myra Stockdale, DHSc ATC LAT
Tel: 419 783-2393   *Fax:* 419 783-2369
E-mail: mstockdale@defiance.edu

University of Findlay
Athletic Training Prgm
1000 N Main St
Findlay, OH 45840
Prgm Dir: Keith Beck, MEd
Tel: 419 434-6962
E-mail: kbeck@findlay.edu

Denison University
Athletic Training Prgm
Dept of Physical Education
Granville, OH 43023
Prgm Dir: Eric R Winters, PhD ATC
Tel: 740 587-6311   *Fax:* 740 587-5742
E-mail: winterse@denison.edu

Kent State University
Athletic Training Prgm
School of Exercise Leisure and Sport
Rm 161D MACC Gym Annex
Kent, OH 44242
www.kent.edu/athletictraining
Prgm Dir: Kimberly S Peer, EdD ATC LAT
Tel: 330 672-0231   *Fax:* 330 672-4106
E-mail: kpeer@kent.edu

Marietta College
Athletic Training Prgm
Dept of Sports Medicine
215 Fifth St
Marietta, OH 45750-4031
www.marietta.edu
Prgm Dir: Richard Crowther, MS ATC
Tel: 740 376-4774   *Fax:* 740 376-4405
E-mail: crowthers@marietta.edu

Miami University
Athletic Training Prgm
KNH Dept
Oxford, OH 45056
Prgm Dir: J Brett Massie, EdD ATC
Tel: 513 529-8105   *Fax:* 513 529-5006
E-mail: massiejb@muohio.edu

Shawnee State University
Athletic Training Prgm
940 Second St
Portsmouth, OH 45662
www.shawnee.edu
Prgm Dir: Tony Ward, MS ATC LAT
Tel: 740 351-3348   *Fax:* 740 351-3172
E-mail: tward@shawnee.edu

University of Toledo
Athletic Training Prgm
College of Health Science and Human Service
Dept of Kinesiology, 2801 W Bancroft St
Toledo, OH 43606
http://homepages.utoledo.edu/sportsmed/
Prgm Dir: James M Rankin, PhD ATC
Tel: 419 530-2752   *Fax:* 419 530-2477
E-mail: james.rankin@utoledo.edu

Urbana University
Athletic Training Prgm
579 College Way
Urbana, OH 43078
Prgm Dir: Bradley K Adams, MEd
Tel: 937 652-1225   *Fax:* 937 484-1223
E-mail: badams@urbana.edu

Otterbein College
Athletic Training Prgm
160 Center St, Rike Center
Westerville, OH 43081
Prgm Dir: Joan E Rocks, MS LATC
Tel: 614 823-3505   *Fax:* 614 823-1966
E-mail: jrocks@otterbein.edu

Wilmington College
Athletic Training Prgm
1870 Quaker Way
Pyle Center Box 1246
Wilmington, OH 45177
http://www2.wilmington.edu/athletic-training/
Prgm Dir: Larry Howard, MA ATC LAT
Tel: 937 382-6661, Ext 257   *Fax:* 937 383-8566
E-mail: larry_howard@wilmington.edu

Oklahoma

East Central University
Athletic Training Prgm
1100 East 14th
Ada, OK 74820
Prgm Dir: Jeff Williams, ATC
Tel: 580 559-5357   *Fax:* 580 332-8361
E-mail: jwillims@ecok.edu

Southern Nazarene University
Athletic Training Prgm
6729 NW 39th Expressway
Bethany, OK 73008
Prgm Dir: Sylvia M Goodman, EdD LAT C
Tel: 405 717-6263   *Fax:* 405 717-6257
E-mail: sgoodman@snu.edu

Oklahoma State University
Athletic Training Prgm
191 Colvin Center
Stillwater, OK 74078
Prgm Dir: Aric Warren, EdD
Tel: 405 744-4060   *Fax:* 405 744-6507
E-mail: aric.warren@okstate.edu

University of Tulsa
Athletic Training Prgm
Chapman Hall 355
600 S College Ave
Tulsa, OK 74104-3189
Prgm Dir: Robin Ploeger, EdD ATC/L
Tel: 918 631-3170   *Fax:* 918 631-2068
E-mail: robin-ploeger@utulsa.edu

Southwestern Oklahoma State University
Athletic Training Prgm
100 Campus Dr
Weatherford, OK 73096
Prgm Dir: Michael Catterson, MS
Tel: 580 774-3073   *Fax:* 580 774-3749
E-mail: michael.catterson@swosu.edu

Oregon

Oregon State University
Athletic Training Prgm
226 Langton Hall
Corvallis, OR 97331-3302
Prgm Dir: Mark Hoffman, PhD
Tel: 541 737-6801   *Fax:* 541 737-2788
E-mail: Mark.hoffman@oregonstate.edu

Linfield College
Athletic Training Prgm
900 SE Baker St
McMinnville, OR 97128
www.linfield.edu
Prgm Dir: Gregor Hill, MS
Tel: 503 883-2386   *Fax:* 503 883-2453
E-mail: ghill@linfield.edu

George Fox University
Athletic Training Prgm
414 N Meridian St #6188
Newberg, OR 97132
www.georgefox.edu
Prgm Dir: Bethany Goldman, MS
Tel: 503 554-2922   *Fax:* 503 554-3864
E-mail: bgoldman@georgefox.edu

Pennsylvania

Neumann College
Athletic Training Prgm
One Neumann Dr
Aston, PA 19014
www.neumann.edu
Prgm Dir: Hurbert Lee, MA ATC CSCS
Tel: 610 361-2499   *Fax:* 610 361-2494
E-mail: leeh@neumann.edu

University of Pittsburgh - Bradford
Athletic Training Prgm
300 Campus Dr
Bradford, PA 16701
www.upb.pitt.edu
Prgm Dir: Jason Honeck, MSEd ATC
Tel: 814 362-7536   *Fax:* 814 362-7503
E-mail: honeck@exchange.upb.pitt.edu

California University of Pennsylvania
Athletic Training Prgm
250 University Ave
California, PA 15419
Prgm Dir: Amanda Allen, PhD ATC
Tel: 724 938-4562   *Fax:* 724 938-4342
E-mail: allen_a@cup.edu

East Stroudsburg University
Athletic Training Prgm
200 Prospect St
East Stroudsburg, PA 18301
Prgm Dir: John R Hauth, EdD
Tel: 570 422-3006   *Fax:* 570 422-3616
E-mail: jhauth@po-box.esu.edu

Mercyhurst College
Athletic Training Prgm
501 E 38th St
Erie, PA 16546-0001
Prgm Dir: Suzanne Gusuie, MA ATC
Tel: 814 824-2526, Ext 3012   *Fax:* 814 824-2204
E-mail: sgushie@mercyhurst.edu

Messiah College
Athletic Training Prgm
One College Ave
Grantham, PA 17027
Prgm Dir: Edwin A Bush, MS ATC
Tel: 717 691-6037, Ext 6037   *Fax:* 717 691-6044
E-mail: sbush@messiah.edu

Indiana University of Pennsylvania
Athletic Training Prgm
228 Zink Hall
1190 Maple St
Indiana, PA 15705
www.hhs.iup.edu/hped
Prgm Dir: Jose E Rivera, MS Ed ATC
Tel: 724 357-5507   *Fax:* 724 357-3777
E-mail: jose.rivera@iup.edu

Lock Haven University
Athletic Training Prgm
140 Health Professions Building
Lock Haven, PA 17745
www.lhup.edu/athletictraining
Prgm Dir: Eric L Lippincott, PT ATC
Tel: 570 484-2781   *Fax:* 570 484-2220
E-mail: elippinc@lhup.edu

Temple University
Athletic Training Prgm
Dept of Kinesiology
116 Pearson Hall
Philadelphia, PA 19122
www.temple.edu/chp/departments/kinesiology/Kine_BS.
  htm
Prgm Dir: Dani Moffit, MA
Tel: 215 204-8836   *Fax:* 215 214-4414
E-mail: moffitd@temple.edu

Duquesne University
Athletic Training Prgm
John G Rangos, Sr School of Health Sciences
122 Health Sciences Building
Pittsburgh, PA 15282
www.healthsciences.duq.edu/at/athome.html
Prgm Dir: Paula S Turocy, EdD ATC
Tel: 412 396-5695   *Fax:* 412 396-4160
E-mail: turocyp@duq.edu

University of Pittsburgh
Athletic Training Prgm
4049 Forbes Tower
Pittsburgh, PA 15260
www.shrs.pitt.edu
Prgm Dir: Kevin M Conley, PhD ATC
Tel: 412 383-6737   *Fax:* 412 383-6636
E-mail: kconley@pitt.edu

Alvernia College
Athletic Training Prgm
400 St Bernardine St
Reading, PA 19607
Prgm Dir: Thomas Porrazzo, PhD
Tel: 610 796-8311   *Fax:* 610 796-8349
E-mail: tom.porrazzo@alvernia.edu

Marywood University
Athletic Training Prgm
2300 Adams Ave
Mellow Center
Scranton, PA 18509-1598
Prgm Dir: Mary J Barron, PhD ATC
Tel: 570 348-6259, Ext 2692   *Fax:* 570 961-4743
E-mail: mjbarron@marywood.edu

Slippery Rock University of Pennsylvania
Athletic Training Prgm
Department of Exercise and Rehabilitative Sciences
114 West Gym
Slippery Rock, PA 16057
Prgm Dir: Bonnie Siple, MS ATC
Tel: 724 738-2930   *Fax:* 724 738-4890
E-mail: bonnie.siple@sru.edu

Eastern University
Athletic Training Prgm
1300 Eagle Rd
St David, PA 19087
Prgm Dir: Michele Monaco, MS
Tel: 610 225-5169   *Fax:* 610 341-1460
E-mail: mmonaco@eastern.edu

Penn State University
Athletic Training Prgm
275 Recreation Bldg
University Park, PA 16802
Prgm Dir: Lauren Kramer, PhD ATC
Tel: 814 863-1758   *Fax:* 814 865-1275
E-mail: lco100@psu.edu

Waynesburg College
Athletic Training Prgm
51 W College St
Waynesburg, PA 15370
Prgm Dir: Michele Kabay, MEd
Tel: 724 852-3309, Ext 309   *Fax:* 724 852-3295
E-mail: mkabay@waynesburg.edu

West Chester University
Athletic Training Prgm
Department of Sports Medicine
West Chester, PA 19383
http://health-sciences.wcupa.edu/sportsmed/
Prgm Dir: Neil Curtis, EdD ATC
Tel: 610 436-2969   *Fax:* 610 436-2803
E-mail: ncurtis@wcupa.edu

King's College
Athletic Training Prgm
133 N River St
Wilkes-Barre, PA 18711
www.kings.edu
Prgm Dir: Jeremy Simington, MS ATC
Tel: 570 208-5900, Ext 5636   *Fax:* 570 208-5988
E-mail: jeremysimington@kings.edu

South Carolina

Charleston Southern University
Athletic Training Prgm
9200 University Blvd
Charleston, SC 29406
www.charlestonsouthern.edu/ATEP
Prgm Dir: Kelly Harkins, MS
Tel: 843 863-7399   *Fax:* 843 863-7394
E-mail: kharkins@csuniv.edu

College of Charleston
Athletic Training Prgm
66 George St
Charleston, SC 29424
Prgm Dir: Susan L Rozzi, PhD ATC
Tel: 843 953-7163   *Fax:* 843 953-6757
E-mail: rozzis@cofc.edu

University of South Carolina
Athletic Training Prgm
212 Blatt PE Center
Columbia, SC 29208
Prgm Dir: Toni Torres-McGehee, PhD
Tel: 803 777-0636   *Fax:* 803 777-6250
E-mail: torresmc@gwm.sc.edu

Erskine College
Athletic Training Prgm
PO Box 338
Due West, SC 29639
www.erskine.edu
Prgm Dir: Scott DeGiantis, MS ATR
Tel: 864 379-8899   *Fax:* 864 379-2197
E-mail: deciantis@erskine.edu

Limestone College
Athletic Training Prgm
1115 College Dr
Gaffney, SC 29340
Prgm Dir: Vanessa B Fulbright, MA ATC
Tel: 864 488-8243   *Fax:* 864 488-8211
E-mail: vfulbright@llimestone.edu

Lander University
Athletic Training Prgm
PO Box 6026
Greenwood, SC 29649
Prgm Dir: Robert Bradley, MS ATC SCAT
Tel: 864 388-8170   *Fax:* 864 388-8660
E-mail: rbradley@lander.edu

Winthrop University
Athletic Training Prgm
117 Peabody Gymnasium
Rock Hill, SC 29733
www.winthrop.edu
Prgm Dir: Alice J McLaine, PhD ATC
Tel: 803 323-2123   *Fax:* 803 323-2124
E-mail: mclainea@winthrop.edu

South Dakota

South Dakota State University
Athletic Training Prgm
Health PE and Recreation
Box 2820
Brookings, SD 57007-1497
http://sdstate.edu
Prgm Dir: Jim Booher, PhD PT ATC
Tel: 605 688-5824   *Fax:* 605 688-5999
E-mail: jim.booher@sdstate.edu

Dakota Wesleyan University
Athletic Training Prgm
1200 W University, Box 912
Mitchell, SD 57301
www.dwu.edu/catalog/courses/athletic_training.htm
Prgm Dir: Dan Wagner, EdD ATC CSCS
Tel: 605 995-2145   *Fax:* 605 995-2143
E-mail: dnwagner@dwu.edu

National American University
Athletic Training Prgm
321 Kansas City St
Rapid City, SD 57701
Prgm Dir: Joshua Ellis, MSEd
Tel: 605 394-4860   *Fax:* 605 394-4871
E-mail: jellis@national.edu

Augustana College
Athletic Training Prgm
2001 S Summit Ave
Sioux Falls, SD 57197
www.augie.edu
Prgm Dir: Brian Gerry, MS ATC
Tel: 605 274-5534   *Fax:* 605 274-5298
E-mail: brian.gerry@augie.edu

Tennessee

University of Tennessee - Chattanooga
Athletic Training Prgm
615 McCallie Ave, Dept 6606
Chattanooga, TN 37403-2598
Prgm Dir: Marisa A Colston, PhD
Tel: 423 425-4743   *Fax:* 423 425-5395
E-mail: marisa-colston@utc.edu

Lee University
Athletic Training Prgm
1120 N Ocoee St
Cleveland, TN 37320-3450
Prgm Dir: Kelly Lumpkin, MS
Tel: 423 614-8474   *Fax:* 423 614-8438
E-mail: klumpkin@leeuniversity.edu

Bryan College
Athletic Training Prgm
721 Bryan Dr, Box 7814
Dayton, TN 37321
Prgm Dir: Christy Rodenbeck, MS
Tel: 423 775-7254   *Fax:* 423 775-7330
E-mail: rodenbch@bryan.edu

Tusculum College
Athletic Training Prgm
60 Shiloh Rd
Greeneville, TN 37743
www.tusculum.edu
Prgm Dir: Jane C Sandusky, MS ATC/L
Tel: 800 729-0256, Ext 5731   *Fax:* 423 636-7404
E-mail: jsandusk@tusculum.edu

Lincoln Memorial University
Athletic Training Prgm
6965 Cumberland Gap Pkwy
Harrogate, TN 37752
www.lmunet.edu
Prgm Dir: Jack Mansfield, EdD
Tel: 423 869-6322   *Fax:* 423 869-6382
E-mail: jack.mansfield@lmunet.edu

Union University
Athletic Training Prgm
1050 Union University Dr
PO Box 1824
Jackson, TN 38305
Prgm Dir: Cliff Pawley, MEd ATC
Tel: 731 661-5529   *Fax:* 731 661-5182
E-mail: cpawley@uu.edu

Carson-Newman College
Athletic Training Prgm
Box 71897
MSAC Rm 1013
Jefferson City, TN 37760
Prgm Dir: Eugene Dupas Jr, MS ATC
Tel: 865 471-4650   *Fax:* 865 471-2037
E-mail: edupas@cn.edu

Cumberland University
Athletic Training Prgm
One Cumberland Sq
Lebanon, TN 37087
www.cumberland.edu
Prgm Dir: Daniel Rogers, MS ATC
Tel: 615 547-1335   *Fax:* 615 444-2569
E-mail: drogers@cumberland.edu

University of Tennessee - Martin
Athletic Training Prgm
3006 Elam Center
Martin, TN 38238
www.utm.edu/departments/cebs/hhp/
    AthleticTraining.php
Prgm Dir: Janet Wilbert, EdD ATC
Tel: 731 881-7310   *Fax:* 731 881-7319
E-mail: jwilbert@utm.edu

Middle Tennessee State University
Athletic Training Prgm
PO Box 96
Murfreesboro, TN 37132
Prgm Dir: Helen Binkley, PhD
Tel: 615 904-8129   *Fax:* 615 904-8469
E-mail: hbinkley@mtsu.edu

Texas

Hardin-Simmons University
Athletic Training Prgm
2200 Hickory St
Box 16180
Abilene, TX 79698
www.hsutx.edu
Prgm Dir: David Stuckey, MS ATC LAT EMT-I
Tel: 325 670-1378   *Fax:* 325 670-5852
E-mail: dstuckey@hsutx.edu

University of Texas at Arlington
Athletic Training Prgm
Box 19259
Arlington, TX 76019
Prgm Dir: Louise Fincher, EdD ATC LAT
Tel: 817 272-3107   *Fax:* 817 272-3233
E-mail: lfincher@uta.edu

University of Texas at Austin
Athletic Training Prgm
1 University Station Stop D3700
Austin, TX 78712
www.edb.utexas.edu/atep
Prgm Dir: Brian Farr, MA ATC LAT CSCS
Tel: 512 471-9885   *Fax:* 512 471-0946
E-mail: bfarr@mail.utexas.edu

University of Mary Hardin-Baylor
Athletic Training Prgm
900 College St, Box 8010
Belton, TX 76513
www.umhb.edu
Prgm Dir: Courtney Burken, ATC LAT PhD
Tel: 254 295-5514   *Fax:* 254 295-4614
E-mail: cburken@umhb.edu

West Texas A&M University
Athletic Training Prgm
WTAMU Box 60216
Canyon, TX 79016
www.wtamu.edu/athletictraining
Prgm Dir: Lorna Strong, MS ATC LAT
Tel: 806 651-2370
E-mail: lstrong@mail.wtamu.edu

Texas A&M University - Commerce
Athletic Training Prgm
ATEP Dept of Health
Kinesiology and Sports Studies
Commerce, TX 75429-3011
Prgm Dir: Robert Conlin, MS
Tel: 903 886-5553   *Fax:* 903 886-5365
E-mail: Bob_Conlin@tamu-commerce.edu

Texas Christian University
Athletic Training Prgm
PO Box 297730
3005 Stadium Dr
Fort Worth, TX 76129
www.tcuathletictraining.com
Prgm Dir: Sean Willeford, MS ATC LAT
Tel: 817 257-6737   *Fax:* 817 257-7702
E-mail: s.willeford@tcu.edu

Texas Wesleyan University
Athletic Training Prgm
1201 Wesleyan St
Fort Worth, TX 76105
Prgm Dir: Pamela Rast, PhD
Tel: 817 531-4876
E-mail: prast@txwes.edu

Southwestern University
Athletic Training Prgm
PO Box 770
Georgetown, TX 78627-0770
Prgm Dir: Miguel A Benavides, MEd ATC LAT
Tel: 512 863-1385   *Fax:* 512 863-1393
E-mail: benavidm@southwestern.edu

Texas Tech Univ Health Sciences Center
Athletic Training Prgm
3601 4th St, Stop 6226
Lubbock, TX 79430-6226
www.ttuhsc.edu
Prgm Dir: LesLee Taylor, PhD ATC LAT
Tel: 806 743-1032   *Fax:* 806 743-3518
E-mail: leslee.taylor@ttuhsc.edu

East Texas Baptist University
Athletic Training Prgm
1209 N Grove
Marshall, TX 75670
Prgm Dir: Dawn Johnston, MSE ATC LAT
Tel: 903 923-2237   *Fax:* 903 935-0162
E-mail: djohnston@etbu.edu

Stephen F Austin State University
Athletic Training Prgm
PO Box 13015-SFA Station
Nacogdoches, TX 75962
www.kin.sfasu.edu
Prgm Dir: Linda Bobo, PhD ATC LAT
Tel: 936 468-1599   *Fax:* 936 468-1850
E-mail: lbobo@sfasu.edu

Angelo State University
Athletic Training Prgm
ASU Station #10899
2601 West Ave N
San Angelo, TX 76909
www.angelo.edu/org/sportmed
Prgm Dir: Troy Hill, MS ATC LAT
Tel: 325 942-2264, Ext 247   *Fax:* 325 942-2272
E-mail: troy.hill@angelo.edu

University of the Incarnate Word
Athletic Training Prgm
4301 Broadway, CPO 472
San Antonio, TX 78209
Prgm Dir: Brad Robinson, MS ATC LAT
Tel: 210 829-2787   *Fax:* 210 829-3174
E-mail: brad.robinson@uiwtx.edu

Texas State University - San Marcos
Athletic Training Prgm
Dept of Health, Physical Education and Recreation
Jowers Center 601 University Dr
San Marcos, TX 78666
http://uweb.txstate.edu/~jr41/
Prgm Dir: Matt Kutz, PhD ATC
Tel: 512 245-2956   *Fax:* 512 245-8678
E-mail: mk22@txstate.edu

Texas Lutheran University
Athletic Training Prgm
1000 W Court St
Seguin, TX 78155
Prgm Dir: Brian Coulombe, MS
Tel: 830 372-6952   *Fax:* 830 372-8135
E-mail: bcoulombe@tlu.edu

Baylor University
Athletic Training Prgm
One Bear Place #97313
HHPR Dept
Waco, TX 76798-7313
http://www3.baylor.edu/HHPR/Undergraduate/Programs/
    ATSM/
Prgm Dir: Lori Greenwood, PhD
Tel: 254 710-4026   *Fax:* 254 710-3527
E-mail: Lori_Greenwood@baylor.edu

Midwestern State University
Athletic Training Prgm
3410 Taft Blvd
Wichita Falls, TX 76308
Prgm Dir: Jennifer Lancaster, MS ATC LAT
Tel: 940 397-6229
E-mail: jennifer.lancaster@mwsu.edu

Utah

Southern Utah University
Athletic Training Prgm
351 W University Blvd
Cedar City, UT 84720
www.suu.edu
Prgm Dir: Ben Davidson, MS
Tel: 435 586-7823   *Fax:* 435 865-8057
E-mail: davidson@suu.edu

Weber State University
Athletic Training Prgm
2801 University Circle
Ogden, UT 84408-2801
http://programs.weber.edu/athletictraining
Prgm Dir: Valerie Herzog, EdD
Tel: 801 626-7656   *Fax:* 801 626-6228
E-mail: valerieherzog@weber.edu

Brigham Young University
Athletic Training Prgm
Dept of Exercise Sciences
267 SFH
Provo, UT 84602-2111
Prgm Dir: Mike Diede, PhD
Tel: 801 422-2145   *Fax:* 801 422-0555
E-mail: Mike_Diede@byu.edu

University of Utah
Athletic Training Prgm
1850 East 250 South, Rm 241
Salt Lake City, UT 84112-0920
Prgm Dir: Bradley Hayes, PhD
Tel: 801 581-7362   *Fax:* 801 585-3992
E-mail: bradley.hayes@hsc.utah.edu

Vermont

University of Vermont
Athletic Training Prgm
305 Rowell Building
106 Carrigan Dr
Burlington, VT 05405
www.uvm.edu
Prgm Dir: Alan Maynard, MEd LAT ATC
Tel: 802 656-7678   *Fax:* 802 656-3492
E-mail: alan.maynard@uvm.edu

Castleton State College
Athletic Training Prgm
Glenbrook Gym
Castleton, VT 05735
Prgm Dir: Reese Barber, MS
Tel: 802 468-1435   *Fax:* 802 468-2189
E-mail: reese.barber@castleton.edu

Norwich University
Athletic Training Prgm
158 Harmon Dr
Northfield, VT 05663
www.norwich.edu
Prgm Dir: Todd Neuharth, ATC LAT MA
Tel: 802 485-2231   *Fax:* 802 485-2333
E-mail: tneuhart@norwich.edu

Virginia

Bridgewater College
Athletic Training Prgm
402 E College St, Box 66
Bridgewater, VA 22812
Prgm Dir: Barbara Long, MS VATL ATC
Tel: 540 828-5771   *Fax:* 540 828-5734
E-mail: bhlong@bridgewater.edu

Averett University
Athletic Training Prgm
420 W Main St
Danville, VA 24541
Prgm Dir: Lee Burton, PhD
Tel: 434 791-5821   *Fax:* 434 791-5740
E-mail: lburton@averett.edu

Emory & Henry College
Athletic Training Prgm
PO Box 947
Emory, VA 24327-0947
www.ehc.edu
Prgm Dir: Dennis Cobler, MA ATC CSCS
Tel: 276 944-6589   *Fax:* 276 944-6738
E-mail: dcobler@ehc.edu

Longwood University
Athletic Training Prgm
201 High St
Farmville, VA 23909
www.longwood.edu/hrk/athletic_training/
Prgm Dir: Sharon Menegoni, MS ATC
Tel: 434 395-2845   *Fax:* 434 395-2380
E-mail: menegonism@longwood.edu

James Madison University
Athletic Training Prgm
Department of Health Sciences
MSC 4301
Harrisonburg, VA 22807
Prgm Dir: Paula Maxwell, PhD
Tel: 540 568-8872   *Fax:* 540 568-3336
E-mail: maxwelpj@jmu.edu

Liberty University
Athletic Training Prgm
Department of Health Sciences and Kinesiology
1971 University Blvd
Lynchburg, VA 24502
Prgm Dir: Vance Pickard, EdD
Tel: 434 592-3762   *Fax:* 434 582-2412
E-mail: vpickard@liberty.edu

Lynchburg College
Athletic Training Prgm
1501 Lakeside Dr
Lynchburg, VA 24501
www.lynchburg.edu
Prgm Dir: Debbie Bradney, DPE
Tel: 434 544-8522   *Fax:* 434 544-8365
E-mail: bradney@lynchburg.edu

George Mason University
Athletic Training Prgm
10900 University Blvd, MSN 4E5
Manassas, VA 20110-2203
Prgm Dir: Shane Caswell, PhD
Tel: 703 993-4638   *Fax:* 703 993-2025
E-mail: scaswell@gmu.edu

Radford University
Athletic Training Prgm
Dept of Exercise, Sport and Health Education
PO Box 6957
Radford, VA 24142
Prgm Dir: Angela Mickle, PhD ATC
Tel: 540 831-5330   *Fax:* 540 831-6053
E-mail: ammickle@radford.edu

Roanoke College
Athletic Training Prgm
221 College Lane
Salem, VA 24153
Prgm Dir: James Buriak, MS ATC
Tel: 540 375-2343   *Fax:* 540 375-2031
E-mail: buriak@roanoke.edu

Shenandoah University
Athletic Training Prgm
1460 University Dr
Winchester, VA 22601
Prgm Dir: Rose Schmieg, DHSc
Tel: 540 665-5534   *Fax:* 540 545-7387
E-mail: Rschmieg@SU.edu

Washington

Eastern Washington University
Athletic Training Prgm
200 Physical Eductation Building, PEHR Dept
Cheney, WA 99004-2476
www.ewu.edu/x3356.xml
Prgm Dir: Garth Babcock, PhD ATC
Tel: 509 359-2427   *Fax:* 509 359-4833
E-mail: gbabcock@mail.ewu.edu

Washington State University
Athletic Training Prgm
Dept of Educational Leadership and Counseling
   Psycholgy
PEB 122
Pullman, WA 99164-1410
Prgm Dir: Kasee Hildenbrand, PhD
Tel: 509 335-8834   *Fax:* 509 335-6961
E-mail: khildenbrand@wsu.edu

Whitworth College
Athletic Training Prgm
300 W Hawthorne Rd
Spokane, WA 99251-2501
Prgm Dir: Russell J Richardson, MA ATC
Tel: 509 777-3244   *Fax:* 509 777-3720
E-mail: rrichardson@whitworth.edu

West Virginia

Concord University
Athletic Training Prgm
PO Box 1000
Campus Box 77
Athens, WV 24712
Prgm Dir: Steven Rathbone, DA ATC
Tel: 304 384-6063   *Fax:* 304 384-5117
E-mail: srathbone@concord.edu

West Virginia Wesleyan College
Athletic Training Prgm
59 College Ave
Buckhannon, WV 26201-2995
www.wvwc.edu
Prgm Dir: Rae Emrick, MS
Tel: 304 473-8002   *Fax:* 304 473-8349
E-mail: emrick_r@wvwc.edu

University of Charleston
Athletic Training Prgm
2300 MacCorkle Ave SE
Charleston, WV 25304
Prgm Dir: Ericka Zimmerman, MS ATC
Tel: 304 357-4828   *Fax:* 304 357-4965
E-mail: erickazimmerman@ucwv.edu

Marshall University
Athletic Training Prgm
College of Education and Human Services
400 Hal Greer Blvd
Huntington, WV 25755-2450
www.marshall.edu/coehs/essr/athletic.training/
Prgm Dir: R Daniel Martin, EdD ATC
Tel: 304 696-2412   *Fax:* 304 696-2928
E-mail: martind@marshall.edu

West Virginia University
Athletic Training Prgm
PO Box 6116 Coliseum
Morgantown, WV 26506-6116
Prgm Dir: Vincent Stilger, HSD ATC
Tel: 304 293-3295, Ext 5148   *Fax:* 304 293-4641
E-mail: vstilger@mail.wvu.edu

Alderson-Broaddus College
Athletic Training Prgm
Box 2062
101 College Hill Rd
Philippi, WV 26416
www.ab.edu
Prgm Dir: Eric Shor, MS ATC
Tel: 304 457-6276   *Fax:* 304 457-6291
E-mail: shorem@mail.ab.edu

Wisconsin

University of Wisconsin - Eau Claire
Athletic Training Prgm
Dept of Kinesiology
213 McPhee Center
Eau Claire, WI 54702-4004
www.uwec.edu/kin
Prgm Dir: Robert Stow, PhD
Tel: 715 836-2022   *Fax:* 715 836-4074
E-mail: stowrc@uwec.edu

Carthage College
Athletic Training Prgm
2001 Alford Park Dr
Kenosha, WI 53140
Prgm Dir: Daniel Ruffner, MS
Tel: 262 551-5741   *Fax:* 262 551-5951
E-mail: druffner@carthage.edu

University of Wisconsin - La Crosse
Athletic Training Prgm
135 Mitchell Hall
La Crosse, WI 54601
Prgm Dir: Mark H Gibson, MS LAT PT
Tel: 608 785-8190   *Fax:* 608 785-8172
E-mail: gibson.mark@uwlax.edu

University of Wisconsin - Madison
Athletic Training Prgm
2000 Observatory Dr, Rm 1037
Madison, WI 53706
Prgm Dir: Andrew Winterstein, PhD
Tel: 608 265-2503   *Fax:* 608 262-1656
E-mail: winterstein@education.wisc.edu

Concordia University Wisconsin
Athletic Training Prgm
12800 N Lake Shore Dr
Mequon, WI 53097
Prgm Dir: Russell DeLap, MBA ATC CSCS
Tel: 262 243-4323, Ext 4323   *Fax:* 262 243-2969
E-mail: russell.delap@cuw.edu

Marquette University
Athletic Training Prgm
PO Box 1881
Milwaukee, WI 53201-1881
Prgm Dir: Christopher F Geiser, MS
Tel: 414 288-6210   *Fax:* 414 288-6079
E-mail: christopher.geiser@marquette.edu

University of Wisconsin - Milwaukee
Athletic Training Prgm
Dept of Human Movement Sciences
Enderis 413
Milwaukee, WI 53201-0413
Prgm Dir: Jennifer Earl, PhD
Tel: 414 229-3227   *Fax:* 414 229-2619
E-mail: jearl@uwm.edu

University of Wisconsin - Oshkosh
Athletic Training Prgm
169H Kolf Center
Oshkosh, WI 54901
Prgm Dir: Hal Strough, PhD LAT ATC
Tel: 920 424-1298   *Fax:* 920 424-1068
E-mail: strough@uwosh.edu

University of Wisconsin - Stevens Point
Athletic Training Prgm
129 HEC
Stevens Point, WI 54481
Prgm Dir: Holly Schmies, MS
Tel: 715 346-2922   *Fax:* 715 346-4655
E-mail: hschmies@uwsp.edu

Carroll College
Athletic Training Prgm
100 N East Ave
Physical Therapy Building
Waukesha, WI 53186
www.cc.edu
Prgm Dir: John Lichosik, MS MA ATC LAT
Tel: 262 524-7701   *Fax:* 262 524-7690
E-mail: jlichosi@cc.edu

Wyoming

University of Wyoming
Athletic Training Prgm
Div of Kinesiology and Health Dept 3196
1000 E University Ave
Laramie, WY 82071
http://uwadmnweb.uwyo.edu/athtrn/
Prgm Dir: William T Lyons, MS ATC
Tel: 307 766-5285   *Fax:* 307 766-4090
E-mail: iceit@uwyo.edu

Athletic Trainer

Programs*	Class Capacity	Begins	Length (months)	Award	Res. Tuition	Non-res. Tuition	Stipend	Offers:‡ 1	2	3	4
Alabama											
Troy University	33	Aug	12	BS	$2,082	$4,164					
University of West Alabama (Livingston)	40	Aug	48	Dipl, BS	$3,838	$7,676					
Arizona											
Northern Arizona University (Flagstaff)	45	Aug	24	BS	$4,076	$12,596					
Arkansas											
Arkansas State University	12	Jan	36	Dipl, BS	$2,607	$5,787					
Ouachita Baptist University (Arkadelphia)	12	Aug	18	Dipl, BA	$18,900	$18,900					•
Southern Arkansas University (Magnolia)	8	Aug	36	BS	$2,130	$3,225		•			
University of Central Arkansas (Conway)	12	Jan	25	BS	$2,347	$2,347		•		•	
California											
Azusa Pacific University	15	Jan	20	BA	$31,580	$31,580					
California State University - Fullerton	10	Aug	30	Cert, BS	$1,260	$8,136					
California State University - Northridge	15	Jun	24	BS	$1,389	$5,643					
California State University - Sacramento	40	Sep	48	BS	$3,558	$17,989		•			
Chapman University (Orange)	60	Aug	36	BS	$35,000	$35,000					
Humboldt State University (Arcata)	10	Aug	36	Dipl, BS	$1,034	$1,156					•
Point Loma Nazarene University (San Diego)	16	Aug	36	Dipl, BA	$22,000	$22,000					
San Jose State University	40	Aug Jan	48	BS	$2,500	$9,700					
University of La Verne	30	Fall	27	Dipl, BS	$25,590	$25,590				•	
University of the Pacific (Stockton)	30	Aug	16	Dipl, BA	$28,480	$28,480					
Colorado											
Colorado State University - Pueblo	32	Aug	20	Dipl, BS	$1,973	$7,257					
Fort Lewis College (Durango)	24	Aug	24	BA	$5,318	$13,848					
Connecticut											
Quinnipiac University (Hamden)	22	Sep	48	Dipl, BS	$26,280	$26,280					

*Data are shown only for programs that completed the 2007 AMA Survey of Health Professions Education Programs.
‡Key to Offers: 1: Evening or weekend classes; 2: Non-English instruction; 3: Cultural competence instruction; 4: Distance education component.

Athletic Trainer

Programs*	Class Capacity	Begins	Length (months)	Award	Res. Tuition	Non-res. Tuition	Stipend	Offers:‡ 1	2	3	4
Florida											
Barry University (Miami Shores)	20	Sep	48	BS	$22,430	$22,430		•		•	
Florida Southern College (Lakeland)	48	Aug		Dipl, BS	$18,500	$19,700					
Palm Beach Atlantic University (West Palm Beach)	24	Aug	30	BS	$18,740	$18,740					
University of Florida (Gainesville)	20	Aug	24	BS	$3,206	$17,791		•			
University of Miami (Coral Gables)	60	Aug		Dipl, BS Ed	$31,288	$31,288					
University of North Florida (Jacksonville)	55	Aug	22	Dipl, BS	$3,101	$6,959					
University of South Florida (Tampa)	30	Summer	24	Dipl, BS	$3,460	$16,170				•	
University of Tampa	24	Aug	36	Dipl, BS	$20,882	$0					
University of West Florida (Pensacola)	24	Aug	24	BS/HLE	$3,000	$9,500		•			
Georgia											
Georgia Southern University (Statesboro)	45	Aug	36	Dipl, BSK	$2,714	$10,856				•	
North Georgia College & State University (Dahlonega)	12	Aug	20	Dipl, BS	$2,560	$10,242					
University of Georgia (Athens)	45	Aug	24	BSEd	$4,964	$18,040					
Valdosta State University	16	Aug	36	BS	$1,733	$5,537		•			
Idaho											
University of Idaho (Moscow)	30	Aug	48	BS	$4,410	$14,490					
Illinois											
Eastern Illinois University (Charleston)	18	Aug	28	Dipl, BS	$3,996	$9,202		•			
Illinois State University (Normal)	22	Jan	36	BS	$7,689	$15,741					
McKendree University (Lebanon)	40	Aug	48	BS	$27,000	$27,000					
Southern Illinois University Carbondale	40	Aug	30	Dipl, BS	$3,102	$6,204					
Western Illinois University (Macomb)	33	Aug Jan	35, 28	BS	$5,538	$7,714		•			
Indiana											
Anderson University	32	Aug Sep	36	BA	$19,990	$19,990					
DePauw University (Greencastle)	8	Jan	30	BA	$27,000	$0		•			
Franklin College	26	Aug	27	Dipl, BA	$21,000	$21,000		•			
Indiana State University (Terre Haute)	17	Aug	48, 12	Dipl, BS, MS	$6,102	$13,518				•	
Indiana Wesleyan University (Marion)	40	Sep	32	BS	$24,652	$24,652					
Purdue University (West Lafayette)	15	Aug	27	BS	$7,750	$23,224					
University of Evansville	16	Sep	48	Dipl, BS	$27,000	$27,000					
University of Indianapolis	14	Aug	48	Dipl, BS	$19,540	$19,540				•	
Iowa											
Buena Vista University (Storm Lake)	27	Aug	36	Dipl, BA	$22,556	$22,556		•			
Central College (Pella)	32	Aug	30	BA	$23,898	$23,898		•			
Clarke College (Dubuque)	12	Aug	30	Dipl, BS						•	
Northwestern College (Orange City)	28	Aug	32	BS	$21,648	$21,648				•	
University of Iowa (Iowa City)	16	Aug	29	BS/BA	$5,376	$18,548		•	•	•	
Upper Iowa University (Fayette)	12	Aug	36	BS	$19,625	$19,625					
Kansas											
Bethel College (North Newton)	12	Sep	27	BS	$13,000	$13,000					
Emporia State University	24	Aug	36	Dipl, BS	$1,431	$5,199					
Fort Hays State University	12	Aug	36	BS	$3,355	$10,543		•		•	
Kansas State University (Manhattan)	20	Aug	30	Dipl, BS	$1,572	$6,543		•			
Mid-America Nazarene University (Olathe)	23	Fall	12	Cert, BA	$8,045	$8,045					
Southwestern College (Winfield)	24	Aug	36	BS	$15,350	$15,350					
Sterling College	8	Aug	30	Dipl, BS	$15,500	$15,500					
Tabor College (Hillsboro)	16	Sep	27	BA	$15,574	$15,574					
University of Kansas (Lawrence)	20	Fall	18	Dipl, BSE	$2,266	$9,034		•		•	•
Washburn University (Topeka)	12	Aug	36	BS	$3,936	$8,904		•			
Kentucky											
Murray State University	36	Jan	30	BS	$4,998	$13,566			•	•	
Louisiana											
Louisiana State University (Baton Rouge)	24	Aug	28	BS	$4,286	$11,086		•			•
Nicholls State University (Thibodaux)	15	Aug	48	BS	$3,555	$9,002					
University of Louisiana at Lafayette	60	Aug	25	Dipl, Cert, BA	$2,589	$8,769					
Maine											
University of Maine - Orono	60	Sep Jan	36	Dipl, BS	$4,710	$13,410		•			
University of Maine - Presque Isle	10	Fall		BS						•	
Maryland											
Salisbury University	48	Jan	30	Dipl, BS	$6,412	$14,500				•	
Towson University	60	Aug	42	BS	$7,100	$16,000					
Massachusetts											
Boston University	80	Sep	36	BS	$33,330	$33,330				•	
Endicott College (Beverly)	25	Sep Jan	32	BS	$19,690	$19,690					

*Data are shown only for programs that completed the 2007 AMA Survey of Health Professions Education Programs.
‡Key to Offers: 1: Evening or weekend classes; 2: Non-English instruction; 3: Cultural competence instruction; 4: Distance education component.

Athletic Trainer

Programs*	Class Capacity	Begins	Length (months)	Award	Res. Tuition	Non-res. Tuition	Stipend	Offers:‡ 1	2	3	4
Merrimack College (North Andover)	18	Sep	48	BS	$29,310	$29,310		•			
Northeastern University (Boston)	28	Sep Jan	54	Dipl, BS	$13,375	$13,375				•	
Springfield College	30	Sep	48	BS	$22,715	$22,715					
Westfield State College	24	Sep	36	BS	$970	$7,050					
Michigan											
Alma College	24	Sep	36	Dipl, BA, BS	$19,786	$19,786		•			
Central Michigan University (Mount Pleasant)	14	Aug Jan	36	BS	$6,024	$14,016				•	
Hope College (Holland)	24	Aug	36	BA	$23,660	$23,660				•	
Lake Superior State University (Sault Ste Marie)	16	Junior year	24	BS	$6,558	$13,116				•	
Saginaw Valley State University (University Center)	10	Fall, Winter semesters	27	Dipl, BS	$171	$404		•		•	
Western Michigan University (Kalamazoo)	45	Aug	36	BS	$6,478	$9,378				•	
Minnesota											
Minnesota State University - Moorhead											
St Cloud State University	12	Spring semester		Dipl, BA							
University of Minnesota - Duluth	16	Sep	36	Dipl, BASc	$7,605	$18,712					
Winona State University	26	Aug-Dec Jan-May	28	BS	$2,470	$4,443					
Mississippi											
Delta State University (Cleveland)	12	Fall	10, 11	Dipl, BS	$3,762	$8,950		•	•		
University of Southern Mississippi (Hattiesburg)	25	Jun 27	20	Dipl, BS	$2,053	$2,585		•			
Missouri											
Lindenwood University (St Charles)	32	Aug	36	BS	$12,000	$12,000					
Missouri State University (Springfield)	100	Aug	46	BS	$179	$349					
Truman State University (Kirksville)	20	Aug	24	BS	$6,210	$10,820					
William Woods University (Fulton)	48	Aug	48	BS	$15,150	$15,150					
Montana											
Montana State University - Billings	10	Jul 24	21	Dipl, MS	$4,300	$10,400		•			
University of Montana (Missoula)	20	Sep	36	Dipl, BS	$11,846	$21,052		•			
Nebraska											
Nebraska Wesleyan University (Lincoln)	28	Aug	12	BS	$19,930	$0					
University of Nebraska - Omaha	40	Jul Aug	24, 36	BS Ed, MA	$3,937	$11,602		•			
Nevada											
University of Nevada - Las Vegas	15	Jan	29	BS	$3,660	$6,563					
New Hampshire											
Colby-Sawyer College (New London)	14	Sep	27	BS	$24,700	$24,700				•	
Plymouth State University	32	Aug	48	BS, MEd	$6,040	$13,640		•			•
University of New Hampshire (Durham)	20	Sep	36	BS	$9,778	$21,498					
New Jersey											
Rowan University (Glassboro)	24	Sep	48	BA	$9,566	$12,696					
William Paterson Univ of New Jersey (Wayne)	40	Jan	20	Dipl, BS	$9,996	$16,242		•		•	
New Mexico											
New Mexico State University (Las Cruces)	40	Aug	32	BS	$3,936	$13,206		•			
New York											
Alfred University	40	Sep	48	BS	$18,498	$18,498					
Canisius College (Buffalo)	16	Sep	45	Dipl, BS	$24,000	$24,000					
Ithaca College	45	Aug	48	Dipl, BS	$28,670	$0				•	
Long Island University - Brooklyn Campus	20	Sep	36	BS/MS	$24,000	$24,000		•			
Marist College (Poughkeepsie)	60	Sep	27, 18	Dipl, BS	$23,560	$23,560		•		•	
Stony Brook University	24	Jun	23	Dipl, BS	$6,578	$12,838				•	
SUNY College at Cortland	40	Sep	30	BS	$4,350	$10,610					
University at Buffalo - SUNY	15	May	36	BS/MS	$6,900	$10,920				•	
North Carolina											
Appalachian State University (Boone)	42	Jan	30	BS	$4,241	$13,983					
Barton College (Wilson)	10	Third semester	20	Dipl, BS	$17,490	$17,490					
Catawba College (Salisbury)	12	Aug	27	BS	$28,000	$28,000					
Elon University	36	Aug	36	Dipl, BS	$20,171	$20,171					
Gardner-Webb University (Boiling Springs)	10	Jan	35	Dipl, BS	$18	$18				•	
Greensboro College	10		30	Dipl, BS	$20,544	$20,544		•	•	•	
High Point University	15	Aug	24	BS	$15,280	$15,280					
Lenoir-Rhyne College (Hickory)	30	Aug	18	BS	$29,000	$29,000					
North Carolina Central University (Durham)	36	Jan	20	Dipl, BS	$8,152	$17,896				•	
Univ of North Carolina at Charlotte	16	Junior year	24	Dipl, BS							
University of North Carolina - Greensboro	10	Jun	24	Dipl, MS	$3,119	$13,683					
University of North Carolina - Wilmington	50	Aug	48	Dipl, BA	$2,050	$7,017					
Wingate University	45	Aug	36	BS	$24,500	$24,500					

*Data are shown only for programs that completed the 2007 AMA Survey of Health Professions Education Programs.
‡Key to Offers: 1: Evening or weekend classes; 2: Non-English instruction; 3: Cultural competence instruction; 4: Distance education component.

Athletic Trainer

Programs*	Class Capacity	Begins	Length (months)	Award	Res. Tuition	Non-res. Tuition	Stipend	Offers:‡ 1	2	3	4
North Dakota											
North Dakota State University (Fargo)	20	Aug	36	Dipl, BS, MS	$2,800	$7,000					
University of Mary (Bismarck)	30	Aug	30	BS, BA	$9,990	$9,990		•			
University of North Dakota (Grand Forks)	15	Aug	34	BS	$5,792	$13,786					
Ohio											
Ashland University	40	Aug	36	BS	$31,380	$31,380		•			
Capital University (Columbus)	30	Aug	18, 27	BA	$24,100	$24,100					
Cedarville University	12	Aug	36	BA	$18,400	$18,400					
College of Mt St Joseph (Cincinnati)	60	Aug	36	BS	$19,500	$0					
Defiance College	36	Aug	36	BS	$20,120	$20,120					
Kent State University	60	Aug	20	BS	$7,504	$14,516		•		•	
Marietta College		Aug	48	Dipl, BS	$23,200	$23,200		•			
Miami University (Oxford)	60	Aug	24	BS	$11,538	$22,618					
Ohio State University (Columbus)	66	Sep	27	BS	$8,667	$20,562					
Shawnee State University (Portsmouth)		Fall Spring		BS	$5,830	$9,970		•			
University of Cincinnati	35	Sep	27	BS	$8,329	$21,351					
University of Toledo	32	Aug	33	BS	$6,815	$15,627					
Wilmington College	60	Aug	36	BS	$21,578	$21,578	$1,500				
Wright State University (Dayton)	20	Sep	28	BS	$4,335	$8,670					
Oklahoma											
East Central University (Ada)	10	Fall semester	36	Dipl, BS	$3,457	$8,437					
Southwestern Oklahoma State University (Weatherford)	16	Aug	24	Dipl, BS	$3,300	$7,800		•			
Oregon											
George Fox University (Newberg)	10	Aug	36	Dipl, BS	$21,720	$21,720					
Linfield College (McMinnville)	12	Aug	27	Dipl, BS, BA	$24,500	$0					
Pennsylvania											
Alvernia College (Reading)	10	Fall semester	36	BS	$20,000	$20,000					
California University of Pennsylvania	60	Sep	27	Dipl, BS AT	$1,684	$4,283					•
Duquesne University (Pittsburgh)	30	Sep	32	BS	$24,462	$24,462					•
Indiana University of Pennsylvania	28	Aug	18	Dipl, BS	$5,177	$12,944		•		•	
King's College (Wilkes-Barre)	15	Aug	36	Dipl, BS	$23,450	$23,450					
Lock Haven University	17	Jan	30	Dipl, BS	$5,178	$12,944					
Marywood University (Scranton)	25	Aug	48	BS	$23,040	$23,040		•		•	
Neumann College (Aston)	44	Aug	48	Dipl, BS	$17,992	$17,992		•			
Penn State University (University Park)	36	Jan	40, 45	Dipl, BS	$21,000	$31,000					•
Temple University (Philadelphia)	16	Sep	24, 48	Dipl, BA, MEd	$9,680	$17,724					
University of Pittsburgh	20	Aug	24	BS	$14,308	$26,290					
University of Pittsburgh - Bradford	24	Aug	48	BS	$11,000	$21,000					
West Chester University	24	Aug	48	BS	$5,038	$12,598					
South Carolina											
Charleston Southern University	15	Aug	24	Dipl, BS	$17,620	$17,620					
Erskine College (Due West)	24	Sep Feb	36	BS	$23,954	$23,954					
Lander University (Greenwood)	10		27	Dipl, BS	$5,000	$8,000		•			
Winthrop University (Rock Hill)	26	Aug	28	BS	$10,210	$19,034					
South Dakota											
Augustana College (Sioux Falls)	24	Sep	27	Dipl, BA	$20,743	$20,743					
Dakota Wesleyan University (Mitchell)	26	Aug	54	BA	$17,500	$17,500		•			
South Dakota State University (Brookings)	36	Aug	24	BS, MA	$1,221	$3,881					
Tennessee											
Cumberland University (Lebanon)	10	Aug	30	BS	$14,710	$14,710	$4,000				
Lincoln Memorial University (Harrogate)	45	Aug	48	BS	$16,400	$16,400					
Tusculum College (Greeneville)	32	Aug	36	BA	$17,385	$0					
University of Tennessee - Chattanooga	16	Early Jul	23	DiplMS	$5,854	$15,816					•
University of Tennessee - Martin	20	Aug	48	Dipl, BSHHP	$2,441	$7,177					
Texas											
Angelo State University (San Angelo)	32	Aug	48	Dipl, BS	$4,577	$12,827					
Baylor University (Waco)	48	Aug	36	BS Ed	$18,900	$18,900					
Hardin-Simmons University (Abilene)	22	Aug	45	Dipl, BBS	$535	$535	$500			•	
Stephen F Austin State University (Nacogdoches)	10	Summer II semester	22	Dipl, Cert, MS	$48	$282				•	•
Texas Christian University (Fort Worth)	12	Aug	48	BS	$24,820	$24,820		•			
Texas Lutheran University (Seguin)	16	Aug	36	BS	$18,720	$18,720					
Texas State University - San Marcos	16	Aug	36	Dipl, BS	$4,016	$12,026					
Texas Tech Univ Health Sciences Center (Lubbock)	28	Late May, Early Jun	24	MAT	$8,100	$18,500					
University of Mary Hardin-Baylor (Belton)	42	Aug	45	BS	$15,750	$15,750		•			
University of Texas at Austin	45	Fall semester	36	BS	$4,000	$8,500		•			
West Texas A&M University (Canyon)		Fall semester	36	BS	$5,200	$13,260					

*Data are shown only for programs that completed the 2007 AMA Survey of Health Professions Education Programs.

‡Key to Offers: 1: Evening or weekend classes; 2: Non-English instruction; 3: Cultural competence instruction; 4: Distance education component.

Athletic Trainer

Programs*	Class Capacity	Begins	Length (months)	Award	Res. Tuition	Non-res. Tuition	Stipend	Offers:‡ 1	2	3	4
Utah											
Brigham Young University (Provo)	20	Sep Jan	32	BS	$3,620	$7,240		•			
Southern Utah University (Cedar City)	24	Aug	48	BS, BA	$3,060	$10,098				•	
Weber State University (Ogden)	18	Fall	30, 42	BS	$2,988	$10,459		•		•	
Vermont											
Norwich University (Northfield)	12	Aug	15	BS	$18,000	$18,000		•		•	
University of Vermont (Burlington)	60	Sep	48	Dipl, BS	$5,211	$13,153				•	
Virginia											
Bridgewater College	40	Jan	22	BS, BA	$30,800	$30,800				•	
Emory & Henry College	36	Aug	32	BS, BA	$28,220	$28,220					
George Mason University (Manassas)	80	Aug	32	BS	$2,724	$7,908		•			
Liberty University (Lynchburg)	40	Aug	48	BS	$20,750	$20,750					
Longwood University (Farmville)	32	Aug	30	BS	$9,100	$16,350				•	
Lynchburg College	15	Fall semester		Dipl, BS							
Radford University	16	Aug	48	BS	$4,140	$11,202					
Roanoke College (Salem)	24	Jan	30	BS	$30,143	$30,143					
Washington											
Eastern Washington University (Cheney)	15	Sep	27	BS	$4,485	$13,350				•	
Washington State University (Pullman)	18	Aug	48	BS	$5,506	$14,514					
West Virginia											
Alderson-Broaddus College (Philippi)	24	Aug	18	BS	$25,000	$0					
Concord University (Athens)	24	Aug	48	BS	$8,136	$12,216					
Marshall University (Huntington)	24	Sep Jan	48	BA	$2,575	$5,076		•		•	•
University of Charleston	35	Aug	30	BS	$20,200	$20,200					
West Virginia Wesleyan College (Buckhannon)	32	Aug	36	Dipl, BS	$27,105	$27,105					
Wisconsin											
Carroll College (Waukesha)	15			Dipl AT							
University of Wisconsin - Eau Claire	45	Sep	27	BS	$4,864	$19,040		•		•	
University of Wisconsin - La Crosse	13	Sep	33	BS	$5,820	$13,300					
University of Wisconsin - Stevens Point	35	Sep	36	BS	$3,932	$14,782					
Wyoming											
University of Wyoming (Laramie)	64	Aug	48	BS	$3,554	$10,394					

*Data are shown only for programs that completed the 2007 AMA Survey of Health Professions Education Programs.
‡Key to Offers: 1: Evening or weekend classes; 2: Non-English instruction; 3: Cultural competence instruction; 4: Distance education component.

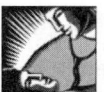

Career Description

Audiologists are professionals who work with people that exhibit hearing, balance, and related ear problems. They examine individuals of all ages and identify those with the symptoms of hearing loss and other auditory, balance, and related neural problems. They then assess the nature and extent of the problems and help the individuals manage them. Using audiometers, computers, and other testing devices, they measure the loudness at which a person begins to hear sounds, the ability to distinguish between sounds, and the impact of hearing loss or balance problems on an individual's daily life. Audiologists interpret these results and may coordinate them with medical, educational, and psychological information to make a diagnosis and determine a course of treatment. Audiologists must effectively communicate diagnostic test results, interpretation, and proposed treatment in a manner easily understood to patients/clients and their families/care givers.

Hearing disorders can result from a variety of causes, including trauma at birth, viral infections, genetic disorders, exposure to loud noise, certain medications, or aging. Treatment may include examining and cleaning the ear canal, fitting and dispensing hearing aids, fitting and tuning cochlear implants, and providing aural rehabilitation. Aural rehabilitation emphasizes counseling on adjusting to hearing loss, training on the use of hearing instruments, and teaching communication strategies for use in a variety of listening environments. Audiologists also may recommend, fit, and dispense personal or large area amplification systems and alerting devices.

Some audiologists specialize in work with the elderly, children, or hearing-impaired individuals who need special therapy programs. Others develop and implement ways to protect workers' ears from on-the-job injuries. They measure noise levels in workplaces and conduct hearing protection programs in factories, as well as in schools and communities.

A graduate degree is necessary to practice as an audiologist in most states. A doctoral degree (PhD) is required for work in some areas.

Audiologists specialize in the study of:

- Normal and impaired hearing
- Prevention of hearing loss
- Identification and assessment of hearing and balance problems
- Rehabilitation of persons with hearing and balance disorders
- In addition, audiologists may:
- Prepare future professionals in colleges and universities
- Manage agencies, clinics, or private practices
- Engage in research to enhance knowledge about normal hearing, and the evaluation and treatment of hearing disorders
- Design hearing instruments and testing equipment

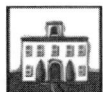

Employment Characteristics

Audiologists may work in a wide range of settings, including schools, hospitals, rehabilitation centers, skilled nursing facilities, government health facilities, community clinics, geriatric facilities, health maintenance organizations (HMOs), public health departments, research laboratories, private practice, or industrial corporations.

Salary

Salaries of audiologists depend on educational background, specialty, and experience, along with the geographical location and type of setting in which they work. The median salary range in 2006 for audiologists certified by the American Speech-Language-Hearing Association (ASHA) was $65,000. Persons in supervisory positions—for example, in administration and management—may earn well over $78,000 per year. While the 2004 median starting salary for certified audiologists with 1 to 3 years' experience was $52,000, the median salary for certified audiologists with clinical doctorate degrees was $68,000 and $90,000 for those with research doctorate degrees. Good benefits packages, such as insurance programs and leave, are usually available to audiologists. Refer to Section IV, Table 5 of this *Directory* for more information, or see www.ama-assn.org/go/hpsalary.

Employment Outlook

Employment of audiologists is expected to grow about as fast as the average for all occupations through the year 2014 (www.bls.gov/oco/ocos085.htm#outlook). Because hearing loss is strongly associated with aging, rapid growth in the population age 55 and older will cause the number of persons with hearing impairment to increase markedly. Members of the baby boom generation are now entering middle age, when the possibility of neurological disorders and associated hearing impairments increases. Medical advances are also improving the survival rate of premature infants and trauma and stroke victims, who then need assessment and possible treatment. Many states now require that all newborns be screened for hearing loss and receive appropriate early intervention services. Opportunities in research and higher education are expected to increase as baby boomers currently in these positions retire and a clinical doctoral degree is required as the minimum educational requirement for new clinicians. Greater awareness of the importance of early identification and diagnosis of speech, language, and hearing disorders also will increase employment.

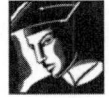

Educational Programs

Approximately 80 universities in the United States offer graduate education programs in audiology at the clinical doctoral level that prepare students for entry into practice. Although master's degree programs had been the prominent degree programs for preparation for professional practice since 1965, clinical doctoral degree programs have replaced these master's programs in the US. Most programs can be identified as Doctor of Audiology programs or AuD programs; some clinical doctoral programs have chosen to use other degree designations such as Clinical PhD or Doctor of Science (ScD). Some advanced degree programs are available for further study with an emphasis on clinical issues or in research. *Note:* As of January 1, 2007, the Council on Academic Accreditation in Audiology and Speech-Language Pathology and Audiology (CAA) no longer accredits master's level programs in audiology. Few master's programs in audiology are available.

Length. Most clinical doctoral programs are designed to be completed in 4 years, including summers, for full-time study and include intensive clinical training designed to meet requirements for licensure and certification; most master's degree programs in audiology usually take at least 2 years, including summers.

Prerequisites. Coursework in the biological sciences, physical sciences, mathematics, and behavioral or social sciences is required for graduate study. Undergraduate programs in communication sciences and disorders will provide a background in linguistics, phonetics, psychology, normal speech, and language development, and introductory course work in audiology. Excellent oral and written communication skills are expected.

Curriculum. Graduate programs should offer a curriculum to allow a student to meet the knowledge and skills necessary to enter independent practice in audiology. A typical graduate program of study includes courses in genetics; normal and abnormal communication development; auditory, balance, and neural systems assessment and treatment; diagnosis and treatment; pharmacology; and ethics. Opportunities to work in a variety of different clinical settings and with a broad range of clients should be provided during the graduate program of study. Most clinical doctoral programs will expect the completion of a 9- to 12-month clinical externship as part of the degree program.

Licensure and Certification

In most states, audiologists must comply with state regulatory (licensure) standards and/or have state teacher certification to practice in specific settings. Earning a graduate degree, completion of a 9- to 12-month clinical experience, and passage of a national examination are typically required to achieve the credentials. Individuals should contact the appropriate state licensure board or teacher certification agency for more information about requirements. ASHA offers the Certificate of Clinical Competence in Audiology (CCC-A), a nationally recognized credential that offers certificate holders ease in qualifying for state credentials because those requirements are similar or identical to ASHA's CCC requirements, recognition as a "highest qualified provider" of audiology services for reimbursement, and increased opportunities for employment or promotion, as certain positions in hospitals, educational programs, or private practices may require ASHA certification. In 2012, a doctoral degree will be required by ASHA to award certification in audiology; further, some states also will require a doctoral degree for licensure.

Inquiries

For information about a specific program, write to the director of the audiology program in care of the institution listed.

For additional information about the professions or program accreditation, contact:

American Speech-Language-Hearing Association (ASHA)
2200 Research Blvd
Rockville, MD 20850
800 498-2071
www.asha.org

Audiologist

Alabama

Auburn University
Audiologist Prgm
Dept of Comm Disorders
1199 Haley Center
Auburn University, AL 36849-5232
Prgm Dir: Lawrence F Molt, PhD
Tel: 334 844-9613   *Fax:* 334 844-4585
E-mail: moltlaw@auburn.edu

University of South Alabama
Audiologist Prgm
Dept of Speech Pathology and Audiology
2000 University Commons
Mobile, AL 36688-0002
Prgm Dir: Paul Dagenais, PhD CCC-SLP
Tel: 334 380-2600, Ext 4-2608   *Fax:* 334 380-2699
E-mail: pdagenais@usouthal.edu

Arizona

Arizona State University
Audiologist Prgm
Dept of Speech and Hearing
PO Box 870102
Tempe, AZ 85287-0102
www.asu.edu/clas/shs/pg-aud.html
Prgm Dir: William A Yost, PhD
Tel: 480 965-2905   *Fax:* 480 965-8516
E-mail: William.yost@asu.edu

University of Arizona
Audiologist Prgm
Speech, Language, and Hearing Sciences
PO Box 210071
Tucson, AZ 85721
Prgm Dir: Elena Plante, PhD
Tel: 520 621-1644   *Fax:* 520 651-9901
E-mail: eplante@email.arizona.edu

Arkansas

University of Arkansas for Medical Sciences
Cosponsor: University of Arkansas at Little Rock
Audiologist Prgm
Dept of Audiology and Speech Pathology
UP 600
Little Rock, AR 72204-1099
www.uams.edu/chrp/audiospeech/
Prgm Dir: Laura Smith-Olinde, PhD
Tel: 501 569-3155   *Fax:* 501 569-3157
E-mail: lso@uams.edu

California

California State University - Los Angeles
Audiologist Prgm
Dept of Communication Disorders
5151 State University Dr
Los Angeles, CA 90032
Prgm Dir: Edward S Klein, PhD
Tel: 323 343-4690   *Fax:* 323 343-4698
E-mail: eklein@cslanet.calstatela.edu

California State University - Northridge
Audiologist Prgm
Dept of Communicative Disorders
18111 Nordhoff St
Northridge, CA 91330-8279
Prgm Dir: J Stephen Sinclair, PhD
Tel: 818 677-2852   *Fax:* 818 677-2632
E-mail: steve.sinclair@csun.edu

California State University - Sacramento
Audiologist Prgm
Dept of Speech Pathology and Audiology
6000 J St
Sacramento, CA 95819-6071
www.csus.edu
Prgm Dir: Laureen O'Hanlon, PhD
Tel: 916 278-6601   *Fax:* 916 278-7730
E-mail: ohanlon@csus.edu

San Diego State University
Cosponsor: University of California San Diego
Audiologist Prgm
School of Speech, Language, and Hearing Sciences
5500 Campanile Dr MC-1518
San Diego, CA 92182-1518
http://chhs.sdsu.edu/slhs/audmain.php
Prgm Dir: Steven Kramer, PhD
Tel: 619 594-6140   *Fax:* 619 594-7109
E-mail: skramer@mail.sdsu.edu

San Francisco State University
Audiologist Prgm
College of Health and Human Services
1600 Holloway Ave, Gym 105
San Francisco, CA 94132-4158
Prgm Dir: Marcia Raggio, PhD
Tel: 415 338-7653   *Fax:* 415 338-0907
E-mail: mraggio@sfsu.edu

Colorado

University of Colorado at Boulder
Audiologist Prgm
2501 Kittredge Loop Rd
UCB 409
Boulder, CO 80309-0409
www.colorado.edu/slhs
Prgm Dir: Susan M Moore
Tel: 303 492-5284   *Fax:* 303 492-3274
E-mail: susan.moore@colorado.edu

University of Northern Colorado
Audiologist Prgm
Audiology and Speech Language Sciences
Gunter 1400, Box 140
Greeley, CO 80639-0030
www.unco.edu/nhs/asls
Prgm Dir: Ellen Meyer Gregg, PhD CCC-SLP
Tel: 970 351-1597   *Fax:* 970 351-2974
E-mail: ellen.gregg@unco.edu

Connecticut

Southern Connecticut State University
Audiologist Prgm
Communication Disorders
501 Crescent St
New Haven, CT 06515
Prgm Dir: James Dempsey, PhD
Tel: 203 392-5954   *Fax:* 203 392-5968
E-mail: dempseyj1@southernct.edu

University of Connecticut
Audiologist Prgm
Communication Sciences
850 Bolton Rd, Unit 1085
Storrs, CT 06268-1085
Prgm Dir: Harvey R Gilbert
Tel: 860 486-2817   *Fax:* 860 486-5422
E-mail: harvey.gilbert@uconn.edu

District of Columbia

Gallaudet University
Audiologist Prgm
Audiology and Speech-Lang Path
800 Florida Ave NE
Washington, DC 20002-3695
Prgm Dir: James J Mahshie, PhD
Tel: 202 651-5329   *Fax:* 202 651-5324
E-mail: james.mahshie@gallaudet.edu

Howard University
Audiologist Prgm
Comm Sciences and Disorders
525 Bryant St NW
Washington, DC 20059
Prgm Dir: Ovetta Harris
Tel: 202 806-6990   *Fax:* 202 806-4046
E-mail: oharris@howard.edu

Florida

Nova Southeastern University
Audiologist Prgm
3200 S University Dr
Fort Lauderdale, FL 33328
Prgm Dir: Barry A Freeman, PhD
Tel: 954 262-7745   *Fax:* 954 262-1181
E-mail: freemanb@nova.edu

University of Florida
Audiologist Prgm
Comm Processes and Disorders
335 Dauer Hall, PO Box 117420
Gainesville, FL 32611-7420
Prgm Dir: Kenneth J Logan, PhD
Tel: 352 392-2113   *Fax:* 352 846-0243
E-mail: logan@csd.ufl.edu

University of South Florida
Audiologist Prgm
Communication Sciences and Disorders
4202 E Fowler Ave PCD 1017
Tampa, FL 33620-8150
www.usf.edu
Prgm Dir: Theresa Chisolm, PhD
Tel: 813 974-2006   *Fax:* 813 974-0822
E-mail: chisolm@cas.usf.edu

Idaho

Idaho State University
Audiologist Prgm
Communication Sciences & Disorders and Education of
   the Deaf
Box 8116
Pocatello, ID 83209-0009
Prgm Dir: Jeff Brockett, EdD CCC-A
Tel: 208 282-2556   *Fax:* 208 236-4571
E-mail: brocjeff@isu.edu

Illinois

Univ of Illinois at Urbana-Champaign
Audiologist Prgm
220 Speech and Hearing Sci Bldg
901 S 6th St
Champaign, IL 61820
Prgm Dir: Ron D Chambers, PhD
Tel: 217 333-2230   *Fax:* 217 244-2235
E-mail: rdc@uiuc.edu

Rush University Medical Center
Audiologist Prgm
Comm Disorders and Sciences
1653 W Congress Pkwy
Chicago, IL 60612
Prgm Dir: Dianne Meyer, PhD
Tel: 312 942-3289   *Fax:* 312 942-7211
E-mail: dianne_h_meyer@rush.edu

Northern Illinois University
Audiologist Prgm
Communicative Disorders
DeKalb, IL 60115-2899
Prgm Dir: Pamela Jackson, PhD
Tel: 815 753-6510   *Fax:* 815 753-9123
E-mail: plj@niu.edu

Northwestern University
Audiologist Prgm
Comm Sciences and Disorders
2240 Campus Dr
Evanston, IL 60208-3540
Prgm Dir: Dean C Garstecki, PhD
Tel: 847 491-3066   *Fax:* 847 491-4975
E-mail: d-garstecki@northwestern.edu

Illinois State University
Audiologist Prgm
Speech Pathology and Audiology
Fairchild Hall #204
Normal, IL 61790-4720
www.ilstu.edu
Prgm Dir: Joe Smaldino, PhD
Tel: 309 438-8643   *Fax:* 309 438-5221
E-mail: wsmoski@ilstu.edu

Indiana

Indiana University - Bloomington
Audiologist Prgm
Speech and Hearing Sciences
200 S Jordan Ave
Bloomington, IN 47405-7002
Prgm Dir: Phil Connell, PhD
Tel: 812 855-4156   *Fax:* 812 855-5531
E-mail: pconnell@indiana.edu

Ball State University
Audiologist Prgm
Speech Pathology and Audiology
2000 University Ave
Muncie, IN 47306
www.bsu.edu/spaa
Prgm Dir: David Coffin, AuD
Tel: 765 285-8160   *Fax:* 765 285-5623
E-mail: dcoffin@bsu.edu

Purdue University
Audiologist Prgm
Speech, Language, and Hearing Sciences
500 Oval Dr
West Lafayette, IN 47907-2038
Prgm Dir: Robert Novak, PhD CCC-A
Tel: 765 494-3788   *Fax:* 765 494-9771
E-mail: novakr@purdue.edu

Iowa

University of Iowa
Audiologist Prgm
Speech Pathology and Audiology
119 SHC
Iowa City, IA 52242
www.shc.uiowa.edu
Prgm Dir: Paul Abbas
Tel: 319 335-8718   *Fax:* 319 335-8851
E-mail: paul-abbas@uiowa.edu

Kansas

University of Kansas
Audiologist Prgm
Intercampus Program in Communicative Disorders
3901 Rainbow Blvd
Kansas City, KS 66160-7605
www.ukans.edu/~splh/
Prgm Dir: John Ferraro, PhD
Tel: 913 588-5937   *Fax:* 913 588-5923
E-mail: jferraro@kumc.edu

Wichita State University
Audiologist Prgm
Communication Sciences and Disorders
1845 N Fairmount
Wichita, KS 67260-0075
Prgm Dir: Kathy Coufal, PhD
Tel: 316 978-3171   *Fax:* 316 978-3291
E-mail: kathy.coufal@wichita.edu

Kentucky

University of Louisville
Audiologist Prgm
Surgery/Graduate Program in Communicative Disorders
Health Sciences Center, Myers Hall
Louisville, KY 40292
Prgm Dir: Barbara M Baker, PhD
Tel: 502 852-5274   *Fax:* 502 852-0865
E-mail: barbara.baker@louisville.edu

Louisiana

Louisiana State Univ and A&M College
Audiologist Prgm
Communication Disorders
Music & Dramatic Arts Bldg, Rm 163
Baton Rouge, LA 70803-2606
Prgm Dir: Paul R Hoffman
Tel: 225 578-2545   *Fax:* 225 578-2528
E-mail: cdhoff@lsu.edu

Louisiana Tech University
Audiologist Prgm
Dept of Speech
PO Box 3165
Ruston, LA 71272
www.latech.edu/slp-aud
Prgm Dir: Sheryl Shoemaker, AuD
Tel: 318 257-4764   *Fax:* 318 257-4492
E-mail: sshoemaker@latech.edu

Maryland

Univ of Maryland at College Park
Audiologist Prgm
Hearing and Speech Science
Le Frak Hall
College Park, MD 20742
www.bsos.umd.edu/hesp/
Prgm Dir: Nan Ratner
Tel: 301 405-4214   *Fax:* 301 314-2023
E-mail: Nratner@hesp.umd.edu

Towson University
Audiologist Prgm
Audiology, Speech Language Pathology and Deaf Studies
8000 York Rd
Towson, MD 21252
Prgm Dir: Sharon Glennen, PhD
Tel: 410 704-4153   *Fax:* 410 704-4131
E-mail: sglennen@towson.edu

Massachusetts

University of Massachusetts - Amherst
Audiologist Prgm
Communication Disorders
715 N Pleasant St
Amherst, MA 01003-9304
Prgm Dir: Jane Baran, PhD
Tel: 413 545-0131   *Fax:* 413 545-0803
E-mail: baran@comdis.umass.edu

Northeastern University
Audiologist Prgm
Speech-Language Pathology and Audiology
106 Forsyth Bldg, 360 Huntington Ave
Boston, MA 02115
Prgm Dir: Linda J Ferrier, PhD
Tel: 617 373-3698   *Fax:* 617 373-2239
E-mail: l.ferrier@neu.edu

Michigan

Wayne State University
Audiologist Prgm
Communication Sciences and Disorders
207 Rackham Building
Detroit, MI 48202
www.clas.wayne.edu/CSD
Prgm Dir: Alex Johnson, PhD
Tel: 313 577-3339   *Fax:* 313 577-8885
E-mail: ajohnson@wayne.edu

Michigan State University
Audiologist Prgm
378 Comm Arts and Sciences Bldg
East Lansing, MI 48824-1220
Prgm Dir: Michael W Casby, PhD
Tel: 517 353-8780   *Fax:* 517 353-3176
E-mail: casby@msu.edu

Western Michigan University
Audiologist Prgm
Speech Pathology and Audiology
Kalamazoo, MI 49008-5355
Prgm Dir: John M Hanley, PhD
Tel: 616 387-8045   *Fax:* 616 381-8044
E-mail: john.hanley@wmich.edu

Central Michigan University
Audiologist Prgm
Communication Disorders
Health Professions Bldg 1183
Mount Pleasant, MI 48859
Prgm Dir: Gerald Church, PhD CCC-A
Tel: 989 774-7301   *Fax:* 989 774-2799
E-mail: churc1g@cmich.edu

Minnesota

University of Minnesota - Minneapolis
Audiologist Prgm
115 Shevlin Hall
164 Pillsbury Dr SE
Minneapolis, MN 55455
www.slhs.umn.edu
Prgm Dir: Jennifer Windsor, PhD
Tel: 612 624-3322   *Fax:* 612 624-7586
E-mail: windsor@umn.edu

Mississippi

University of Southern Mississippi
Audiologist Prgm
Dept of Speech and Hearing Sciences
PO Box 5092
Hattiesburg, MS 39406-5092
Prgm Dir: Stephen E Oshrin, PhD
Tel: 601 266-5216   *Fax:* 601 266-5224
E-mail: steve.oshrin@usm.edu

Missouri

Missouri State University
Audiologist Prgm
Communication Disorders
901 S National Ave
Springfield, MO 65897-0095
www.missouristate.edu/csd/
Prgm Dir: Neil J DiSarno, PhD
Tel: 417 836-5368, Ext 66511   *Fax:* 417 836-4242
E-mail: neildisarno@missouristate.edu

Washington University
Audiologist Prgm
Program in Audiology and Communication Sciences
660 S Euclid Ave, Campus Box 8042
St Louis, MO 63110
http://pacs.wustl.edu
Prgm Dir: William W Clark, PhD
Tel: 314 747-0103   *Fax:* 314 747-0105
E-mail: clarkw@msnotes.wustl.edu

University of Central Missouri
Audiologist Prgm
Speech Pathology and Audiology
Martin Bldg 41
Warrensburg, MO 64093
Prgm Dir: Carl Harlan, PhD CCC-SP
Tel: 660 543-4606, Ext 660   *Fax:* 660 543-8234
E-mail: harlan@ucmo.edu

Nebraska

University of Nebraska - Lincoln
Audiologist Prgm
Dept of Special Education and Communication
   Disorders
301 Barkley Center
Lincoln, NE 68583-0234
www.unl.edu/Barkley/audiology
Prgm Dir: John Bernthal, PhD
Tel: 402 472-2145   *Fax:* 402 472-7697
E-mail: jbernthal1@unl.edu

New York

University at Buffalo - SUNY
Audiologist Prgm
Dept of Communicative Disorders and Sciences
122 Cary Hall
Buffalo, NY 14214-3005
http://cdswebserver.med.buffalo.edu/drupal/
Prgm Dir: Elaine Stathopoulos, PhD
Tel: 716 829-2797, Ext 625   *Fax:* 716 829-3979
E-mail: stathop@buffalo.edu

Adelphi University
Cosponsor: Hofstra University, St. John's University
Audiologist Prgm
Comm Sciences and Disorders
Hy Weinberg Center, Rm 001
Garden City, NY 11530
www.adelphi.edu
Prgm Dir: Janet Schoepflin, PhD
Tel: 516 877-4770   *Fax:* 516 877-4783
E-mail: schoepfl@adelphi.edu

Hofstra University
Audiologist Prgm
Dept of Speech-Language-Hearing Sciences
110 Hofstra University
Hempstead, NY 11549
Prgm Dir: Carole Ferrand, PhD
Tel: 516 463-5511   *Fax:* 516 463-5260
E-mail: Carole.T.Ferrand@hofstra.edu

St John's University
Audiologist Prgm
Speech and Hearing Ctr
8000 Utopia Pkwy
Jamaica, NY 11439
http://new.stjohns.edu
Prgm Dir: Donna Geffner, PhD
Tel: 718 990-6480   *Fax:* 718 990-1917
E-mail: geffnerd@stjohns.edu

CUNY Hunter College
Cosponsor: Hunter College, Brooklyn College
Audiologist Prgm
Clinical Doctoral Programs
365 Fifth Ave
New York, NY 10016
www.gc.cuny.edu
Prgm Dir: Barabara Weinstein, PhD
Tel: 212 817-7981   *Fax:* 212 817-1680
E-mail: bweinstein@gc.cuny.edu

Syracuse University
Audiologist Prgm
Dept of Communication Sciences and Disorders
805 S Crouse Ave
Syracuse, NY 13244-2280
Prgm Dir: Raymond H Colton, PhD
Tel: 315 443-9637   *Fax:* 315 443-1113
E-mail: rhcolton@syr.edu

North Carolina

University of North Carolina - Chapel Hill
Audiologist Prgm
Division of Speech and Hearing Sciences
CB 7190 Wing D Medical School
Chapel Hill, NC 27599-7190
Prgm Dir: Jackson Roush, PhD
Tel: 919 966-1006   *Fax:* 919 966-0100
E-mail: jroush@med.unc.edu

East Carolina University
Audiologist Prgm
Dept of Communication Sciences and Disorders
College of Allied Health Sciences
Greenville, NC 27858-4353
www.ecu.edu/csd/
Prgm Dir: Gregg D Givens, PhD
Tel: 252 744-6080   *Fax:* 252 744-6081
E-mail: givensg@ecu.edu

Ohio

University of Akron
Cosponsor: Northeast Ohio Audiology Consortium
Audiologist Prgm
School of Speech-Language and Audiology
Polsky Building, Rm 184B
Akron, OH 44325-3001
www.uakron.edu/sslpa
Prgm Dir: Sharon Lesner, PhD
Tel: 330 972-6118   *Fax:* 330 972-7884
E-mail: lesner@uakron.edu

Ohio University
Audiologist Prgm
School of Hearing, Speech and Language Sciences
Grover Center W218
Athens, OH 45701-2979
Prgm Dir: Brooke Hallowell, PhD
Tel: 740 593-1356   *Fax:* 740 593-0287
E-mail: hsls@ohio.edu

University of Cincinnati
Audiologist Prgm
Communication Sciences and Disorders
Mail Station 379
Cincinnati, OH 45221-0379
Prgm Dir: Nancy Creaghead, PhD
Tel: 513 558-8501   *Fax:* 513 558-8500
E-mail: nancy.creaghead@uc.edu

Ohio State University
Audiologist Prgm
Dept of Speech and Hearing Sciences
110 Pressey Hall, 1070 Carmack Rd
Columbus, OH 43210-1002
Prgm Dir: Robert Allen Fox, PhD
Tel: 614 292-8207   *Fax:* 614 292-7504
E-mail: fox.2@osu.edu

Oklahoma

Univ of Oklahoma Health Sciences Center
Audiologist Prgm
Communication Sciences and Disorders
825 NE 14th, PO Box 26901
Oklahoma City, OK 73190
Prgm Dir: Stephen Painton, PhD
Tel: 405 271-4214, Ext 46054   *Fax:* 405 271-3360
E-mail: stephen-painton@ouhsc.edu

Oregon

Portland State University
Audiologist Prgm
Speech and Hearing Sciences
PO Box 751
Portland, OR 97207-0751
Prgm Dir: Thomas Dolan, PhD
Tel: 503 725-3533   *Fax:* 503 725-9171
E-mail: dolant@pdx.edu

Pennsylvania

Bloomsburg University
Audiologist Prgm
Dept of Audiology and Speech Pathology
400 E 2nd St, Centennial Hall
Bloomsburg, PA 17815-1301
Prgm Dir: Dianne Angelo, PhD
Tel: 570 389-4436   *Fax:* 570 389-5022
E-mail: dangelo@bloomu.edu

University of Pittsburgh
Audiologist Prgm
Communication Science and Disorders
4033 Fobes Tower, Atwood St
Pittsburgh, PA 15260
www.shrs.pitt.edu/csd/
Prgm Dir: Malcolm McNeil, PhD
Tel: 412 383-6540   *Fax:* 412 383-6555
E-mail: mcneil@pitt.edu

Penn State University
Audiologist Prgm
Dept of Communication Sciences and Disorders
110 Moore Bldg
University Park, PA 16802-3100
Prgm Dir: Gordon Blood, PhD
Tel: 814 865-3177   *Fax:* 814 863-3759
E-mail: F2X@psu.edu

Rhode Island

University of Rhode Island
Audiologist Prgm
Dept of Communicative Disorders
Independence Sq, Ste 1
Kingston, RI 02881-0821
Prgm Dir: Jay Singer, PhD
Tel: 401 874-5969   *Fax:* 401 874-4404
E-mail: DrJay@uri.edu

South Dakota

University of South Dakota
Audiologist Prgm
Dept of Communication Disorders
414 E Clark St
Vermillion, SD 57069-2390
www.usd.edu/dcom
Prgm Dir: Teri J Bellis, PhD
Tel: 605 677-5474   *Fax:* 605 677-5767
E-mail: tbellis@usd.edu

Tennessee

East Tennessee State University
Audiologist Prgm
Dept of Communicative Disorders
PO Box 70643
Johnson City, TN 37614-0643
Prgm Dir: Marc Fagelson, PhD
Tel: 423 439-4583   *Fax:* 423 439-4607
E-mail: fagelson@etsu.edu

University of Tennessee - Knoxville
Audiologist Prgm
Audiology and Speech Pathology
578 S Stadium Hall
Knoxville, TN 37996-0740
Prgm Dir: Patricia M Visser
Tel: 865 974-5019   *Fax:* 865 974-1539
E-mail: pvisser@utk.edu

University of Memphis
Audiologist Prgm
School of Audiology and Speech-Language Pathology
807 Jefferson Ave
Memphis, TN 38105
www.ausp.memphis.edu
Prgm Dir: Maurice I Mendel, PhD
Tel: 901 678-5800   *Fax:* 901 525-1282
E-mail: mmendel@memphis.edu

Vanderbilt University Medical Center
Audiologist Prgm
Hearing and Speech Sciences
1215 21st Ave S, Rm 8310
Nashville, TN 37232-8718
http://vanderbiltbillwilkersoncenter.com/dhss.html
Prgm Dir: Fred H Bess, PhD
Tel: 615 936-5000   *Fax:* 615 936-5014
E-mail: fred.h.bess@vanderbilt.edu

Texas

University of Texas at Austin
Audiologist Prgm
Communication Sciences and Disorders
1 University Station, A1100
Austin, TX 78712-1089
Prgm Dir: Craig Champlin, PhD
Tel: 512 471-4119   *Fax:* 512 471-2957
E-mail: champlin@austin.utexas.edu

Lamar University
Audiologist Prgm
Dept of Communication
Box 10076, Lamar Station
Beaumont, TX 77710
Prgm Dir: Sumalai Maroonroge, PhD
Tel: 409 880-8177   *Fax:* 409 880-2265
E-mail: maroonroge@aol.com

University of Texas at Dallas
Audiologist Prgm
Program in Communication Disorders
1966 Inwood Rd
Dallas, TX 75235-7298
Prgm Dir: Robert D Stillman, PhD
Tel: 214 905-3060   *Fax:* 214 905-3006
E-mail: stillman@utdallas.edu

University of North Texas
Audiologist Prgm
Dept of Speech and Hearing Sciences
PO Box 305010
Denton, TX 76203-5010
Prgm Dir: Jeffrey Cokely
Tel: 940 565-2481   *Fax:* 940 565-4058
E-mail: cokely@unt.edu

Texas Tech Univ Health Sciences Center
Audiologist Prgm
Dept of Speech, Language, and Hearing Sciences
STOP 6073 - 3601 4th St
Lubbock, TX 79430
www.ttuhsc.edu/SAH
Prgm Dir: Candace Hicks, PhD
Tel: 806 743-5660, Ext 230   *Fax:* 806 743-5670
E-mail: candace.hicks@ttuhsc.edu

Utah

Utah State University
Audiologist Prgm
Comm Disorders and Deaf Educ
1000 Old Main Hill
Logan, UT 84322-1000
www.usu.edu
Prgm Dir: James C Blair, PhD
Tel: 435 797-1375   *Fax:* 435 797-0221
E-mail: jimb@cc.usu.edu

University of Utah
Audiologist Prgm
390 South 1530 East
Rm 1201 BEH S
Salt Lake City, UT 84322-1000
Prgm Dir: Bruce L Smith, PhD
Tel: 801 581-6725   *Fax:* 801 581-7955
E-mail: angelina.harder@hsc.utah.edu

University of Utah Health Science Center
Audiologist Prgm
Communication Sciences and Disorders
1201 Behavioral Science Bldg
Salt Lake City, UT 84112
Prgm Dir: Lisa Hunter, PhD
Tel: 801 581-6725   *Fax:* 801 571-7955
E-mail: lisa.hunter@hsc.utah.edu

Virginia

James Madison University
Audiologist Prgm
Communication Sciences and Disorders
MSC 4304
Harrisonburg, VA 22807
Prgm Dir: Vicki Reed, EdD
Tel: 540 568-6440   *Fax:* 540 568-8077
E-mail: reedva@jmu.edu

Washington

Washington State University
Audiologist Prgm
Speech and Hearing Sciences
201 Daggy Hall, PO Box 642420
Pullman, WA 99164-2420
Prgm Dir: Gail Chermak
Tel: 509 335-4526   *Fax:* 509 335-8357
E-mail: chermak@wsu.edu

University of Washington
Audiologist Prgm
Speech and Hearing Sciences
1417 NE 42nd St
Seattle, WA 98105-6246
Prgm Dir: Christopher Moore
Tel: 206 685-7402   *Fax:* 206 543-1093
E-mail: camoore@u.washington.edu

West Virginia

West Virginia University
Audiologist Prgm
Speech Pathology and Audiology
805 Allen Hall, Box 6122
Morgantown, WV 26506-6122
Prgm Dir: Lynn R Cartwright, EdD
Tel: 304 293-4241   *Fax:* 304 293-7565
E-mail: lcartwri@wvu.edu

Wisconsin

University of Wisconsin - Madison
Cosponsor: University of Wisconsin - Stevens Point
Audiologist Prgm
Communicative Disorders
1975 Willow Dr - Goodnight Hall
Madison, WI 53706
www.comdis.wisc.edu
Prgm Dir: Cynthia Fowler, PhD
Tel: 608 262-3951   *Fax:* 608 262-6466
E-mail: cgfowler@wisc.edu

University of Wisconsin - Stevens Point
Cosponsor: UW - Madison
Audiologist Prgm
Communicative Disorders
1901 4th Ave
Stevens Point, WI 54481-3897
http://http:/www.uwsp.edu/commD/
Prgm Dir: Gary Cumley, PhD
Tel: 715 346-4699   *Fax:* 715 346-2157
E-mail: gcumley@uwsp.edu

Audiologist

Programs*	Class Capacity	Begins	Length (months)	Award	Res. Tuition	Non-res. Tuition	Stipend	Offers:‡ 1	2	3	4
Arizona											
Arizona State University (Tempe)	12	Aug	48	Dipl, AuD						•	
Arkansas											
University of Arkansas for Medical Sciences (Little Rock)	9	Fall semester	48, 21	Dipl, AuD	$257	$555		•		•	
California											
California State University - Sacramento	50	Fall	24	BS						•	
San Diego State University	10	Fall	46	Dipl, AuD	$3,200	$0	$2,000			•	
Colorado											
University of Colorado at Boulder	8	Fall	48	Dipl, AuD, PhD						•	
University of Northern Colorado (Greeley)	8	Aug	48	AuD	$5,118	$14,832		•		•	
Florida											
University of South Florida (Tampa)	14	Aug	48	AuD	$7,000	$27,000	$10,000				
Illinois											
Illinois State University (Normal)	10		48	AuD	$3,000	$6,000		•			
Indiana											
Ball State University (Muncie)	10	Aug	48	Dipl, AuD	$12,416	$27,983				•	
Iowa											
University of Iowa (Iowa City)	8	Fall semester	48	AuD	$7,158	$19,158					
Kansas											
University of Kansas (Kansas City)	10	Jun Aug Jan	48	Dipl, AuD, PhD	$6,000	$12,000		•		•	
Louisiana											
Louisiana Tech University (Ruston)	16	Fall	48	Dipl, AuD	$3,600	$12,000	$8,000	•			
Maryland											
Univ of Maryland at College Park	15	Aug	48	AuD, PhD	$10,250	$17,500	$8,000				
Michigan											
Central Michigan University (Mount Pleasant)	40	Aug	48	Dipl, AuD	$416	$753				•	
Wayne State University (Detroit)	12	Fall term	45	AuD	$15,600	$32,650					
Minnesota											
University of Minnesota - Minneapolis	20	Fall	44	Dipl	$8,748	$15,848				•	
Missouri											
Missouri State University (Springfield)	60	Aug	44	AuD	$5,860	$11,718				•	
Washington University (St Louis)	12	Aug	48	Dipl, Cert, AuD	$21,100	$21,100					
Nebraska											
University of Nebraska - Lincoln	24	Aug	48	AuD, PhD	$211	$569				•	
New York											
Adelphi University (Garden City)	25	Sep Jan		AuD	$22,000	$22,000			•	•	
CUNY Hunter College (New York)	12	Fall	4	Dipl, AuD					•	•	
St John's University (Jamaica)		Sep	24, 48	AUD	$860	$0			•	•	
University at Buffalo - SUNY	30	Aug	36	PhD							
North Carolina											
East Carolina University (Greenville)	10	Fall	60	Dipl, PhD	$2,912	$13,228	$14,000			•	
Ohio											
University of Akron	20	Aug	48	Dipl, AuD	$11,132	$20,892				•	
Pennsylvania											
University of Pittsburgh	41	Aug 28	45, 60	Dipl, AuD, PhD	$24,576	$31,920	$17,234	•		•	
South Dakota											
University of South Dakota (Vermillion)	10	Aug Sep	48	AuD	$3,006	$5,448				•	

*Data are shown only for programs that completed the 2007 AMA Survey of Health Professions Education Programs.
‡Key to Offers: 1: Evening or weekend classes; 2: Non-English instruction; 3: Cultural competence instruction; 4: Distance education component.

Audiologist

Programs*	Class Capacity	Begins	Length (months)	Award	Res. Tuition	Non-res. Tuition	Stipend	Offers:‡ 1	2	3	4
Tennessee											
University of Memphis	35	Fall semester	48, 24	AuD, MA	$9,434	$23,868	$4,500	•			
Vanderbilt University Medical Center (Nashville)	15	Aug 27	48	Dipl, Cert, AuD, PhD	$26,500	$34,248			•	•	
Texas											
Texas Tech Univ Health Sciences Center (Lubbock)	10	Fall	45	Dipl, AuD	$8,039	$19,638				•	
Utah											
Utah State University (Logan)	6	Aug	36	AuD	$4,558	$14,488	$5,000				
Wisconsin											
University of Wisconsin - Madison	15	Fall	48	Dipl, AuD, PhD	$12,000	$36,000				•	•
University of Wisconsin - Stevens Point	5	Fall	48	Dipl, Cert, AuD	$13,258	$21,798	$4,000	•			

*Data are shown only for programs that completed the 2007 AMA Survey of Health Professions Education Programs.
‡Key to Offers: 1: Evening or weekend classes; 2: Non-English instruction; 3: Cultural competence instruction; 4: Distance education component.

PROGRAMS

Includes:
- Low Vision Therapist
- Orientation and mobility specialist
- Teacher of the visually impaired
- Vision rehabilitation therapist (formerly Rehabilitation teacher)

Orientation and Mobility Specialist

Career Description
Orientation and mobility specialists teach people who are blind or visually impaired the skills and concepts they need to travel independently and safely at home, in the classroom, in their communities, and wherever they may want to go.

Orientation and Mobility Instruction is a sequential process in which visually impaired individuals are taught to utilize their remaining senses to determine their position within their environment and to negotiate safe movement from one place to another. The skills involved in this teaching include but are not limited to:
- Concept development, which includes body image, spatial, temporal, positional, directional. and environmental concepts
- Motor development, including motor skills needed for balance, posture, and gait, as well as the use of adaptive devices and techniques to assist those with multiple disabilities
- Sensory development, which includes visual, auditory, vestibular, kinesthetic, tactile, olfactory, and proprioceptive senses, and the interrelationships of these systems
- Residual vision stimulation and training
- Human guide technique
- Upper and lower protective techniques
- Locating dropped objects
- Trailing
- Squaring-off
- Cane techniques
- Soliciting/declining assistance
- Following directions
- Utilizing landmarks
- Search patterns
- Compass directions
- Route planning
- Analysis and identification of intersections and traffic patterns
- Use of traffic control devices
- Techniques for crossing streets
- Techniques for travel in indoor environments, outdoor residential, small and large business districts, mall travel, and rural areas
- Problem solving
- Use of public transportation
- Evaluation with sun filters for the reduction of glare
- Instructional use of low vision devices

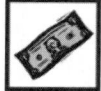

Salary
According the 2002 Salary Survey of the AER, the average full-time salary for orientation and mobility specialists is $46,564. Refer to Section IV, Table 5 of this

Directory for more information, or see www.ama-assn.org/go/salary.

Teacher of the Visually Impaired

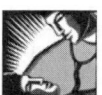

Career Description
Teachers of the visually impaired (or VI teachers) are specialized teachers with unique competencies to meet the diverse needs of the visually impaired.

VI teachers work within the special education system but address the unique needs of children with visual impairments. In addition to working with the children (usually in a one-to-one relationship), VI teachers work closely with other teachers, parents, and other people and organizations in the community. VI teachers are specialists at translating medical information into educational practices.

VI teachers understand basic diagnostic information about vision and visual impairments. They take information on a student's visual diagnosis and conduct a functional vision evaluation and a learning media assessment. Based on those sources of information, VI teachers develop a plan to best teach the student and work with others to address instructional needs, including basic core curriculum and student-specific needs.

Specific duties of a VI teacher might include:
- Teaching a toddler to enjoy playing with a variety of toys
- Teaching a young child how to read and write Braille
- Teaching students how to make a favorite snack
- Working with other educators and paraprofessionals to modify materials to address the impact of the visual impairment

VI teachers are certified by states thought the educator certification systems. Depending on the state, VI teachers can be certified with a bachelors degree, a post-bachelors certification, and/or a masters degree. Teachers must have a degree in education or special education.

Vision Rehabilitation Therapist

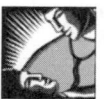

Career Description
- Vision rehabilitation therapists (formerly rehabilitation teachers) instruct persons with vision impairment in the use of compensatory skills and assistive technology that will enable them to live safe, productive, and independent lives. Specific responsibilities include
- Assessing and evaluating learners' needs in home, work, and community environments
- Developing and implementing instructional programs, case management, and record keeping
- Helping persons with visual impairment identify and use local and national resources
- Facilitate psychosocial adjustment to blindness and vision loss

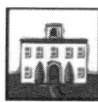

Employment Characteristics
Vision rehabilitation therapists work in organizations that enhance vocational opportunities, independent

living, and educational development of persons with vision loss. This may include working in center-based or itinerant settings, including clients' homes and workplaces. Vision rehabilitation therapists provide individualized programs of instruction that accommodate the unique needs of specialized groups, including persons who are aging, deaf-blind, or disabled.

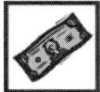

Salary
According to the 2002 Salary Survey of the AER, the average full-time salary for vision rehabilitation therapists is $37,055. Refer to Section IV, Table 5 of this *Directory* for more information, or see www.ama-assn.org/go/salary.

Inquiries
Careers/Curriculum
Association for Education and Rehabilitation of the Blind and Visually Impaired
1703 N Beauregard Street, Suite 440
Alexandria, VA 22311-1744
703 671-4500
703 671-6391 Fax
www.aerbvi.org

Certification
Academy for Certification of Vision Rehabilitation and Education Professionals
300 N Commerce Park Loop, #200
Tucson, AZ 85745
520 887-6816
520 887-6826 Fax
E-mail: info@acvrep.org
www.acvrep.org

Program Accreditation
Association for Education and Rehabilitation of the Blind and Visually Impaired
1703 N Beauregard Street, Suite 440
Alexandria, VA 22311-1744
703 671-4500
703 671-6391 Fax
www.aerbvi.org

Low Vision Therapist

Pennsylvania

Pennsylvania College of Optometry
Low Vision Therapy Prgm
Vision Rehabilitation Therapy & O&M Therapy
Dept of Graduate Studies in Vision Impairment
Elkins Park, PA 19027-1598
Prgm Dir: Maureen A Duffy, CVRT
Tel: 215 780-1362   *Fax:* 215 780-1357
E-mail: mduffy@pco.edu

Orientation and Mobility Specialist

Arizona

University of Arizona
Orientation and Mobility Specialist Prgm
PO Box 210069
Tucson, AZ 85721
Prgm Dir: Jane Erin, PhD
Tel: 520 621-0945
E-mail: Jerin@u.arizona.edu

Arkansas

University of Arkansas at Little Rock
Orientation and Mobility Specialist Prgm
2801 S University Ave
Little Rock, AR 72204
Prgm Dir: William H Jacobson, EdD
Tel: 501 569-8505   *Fax:* 501 224-3170
E-mail: WHJacobson@UALR.Edu

California

California State University - Los Angeles
Orientation and Mobility Specialist Prgm
5151 State University Dr
Los Angeles, CA 90032
Prgm Dir: Diane Fazzi, PhD COMS
Tel: 323 343-4411   *Fax:* 323 343-5605
E-mail: dfazzi@calstatela.edu

San Francisco State University
Orientation and Mobility Specialist Prgm
1600 Holloway Ave
San Francisco, CA 94132
www.sfsu.edu/~mobility
Prgm Dir: Sandra Rosen, PhD COMS
Tel: 415 338-1245   *Fax:* 415 338-0566
E-mail: srosen@sfsu.edu

Colorado

University of Northern Colorado
Orientation and Mobility Specialist Prgm
NCLID, McKee Hall Campus Box 146
Greeley, CO 80639
Prgm Dir: Paula Conroy, EdD TVI COMS
Tel: 970 351-1651   *Fax:* 970 351-1061
E-mail: paula.conroy@unco.edu

Florida

Florida State University
Orientation and Mobility Specialist Prgm
205 Stone Bldg
Tallahassee, FL 32306-4459
www.careersinblindness.com
Prgm Dir: Eileen Bischof, COMS
Tel: 850 644-8407   *Fax:* 850 644-8715
E-mail: epace@mailer.fsu.edu

Illinois

Northern Illinois University
Orientation and Mobility Specialist Prgm
Dept of Teaching and Learning
DeKalb, IL 60115
Prgm Dir: Jodi Sticken, MSEd COMS
Tel: 815 753-8456   *Fax:* 815 753-8594
E-mail: jsticken@niu.edu

Michigan

Western Michigan University
Orientation and Mobility Specialist Prgm
Dept of Blindness and Low Vision Studies
Mail Stop 5218
Kalamazoo, MI 49008
Prgm Dir: Marvin Weessies
Tel: 269 387-3447
E-mail: marvin.weessies@wmich.edu

New York

CUNY Hunter College
Cosponsor: The Lavelle Fund for the Blind, Inc
Orientation and Mobility Specialist Prgm
695 Park Ave, 916 W
New York, NY 10021
www.hunter.cuny.edu/education/deptsprograms/
    chart.shtml
Prgm Dir: Rosanne K Silberman, EdD
Tel: 212 772-4740   *Fax:* 212 650-3542
E-mail: rsilberm@hunter.cuny.edu

New Zealand

Massey University
Orientation and Mobility Specialist Prgm
School of Health Sciences
Private Bag 11222
Palmerston North, NZ
Prgm Dir: Steven La Grow
Tel: 646 350-9099   *Fax:* 646 350-5688
E-mail: S.J.Lagrow@massey.ac.nz

North Carolina

North Carolina Central University
Orientation and Mobility Specialist Prgm
712 Cecil St
Durham, NC 27707
Prgm Dir: Brad R Walker, PhD
Tel: 919 715-5172   *Fax:* 919 530-7291
E-mail: Brad.Walker@ncmail.net

Ontario, Canada

Mohawk College
Orientation and Mobility Specialist Prgm
411 Elgin St
Brantford, ON N3T 5V2
Prgm Dir: Mary-Maureen Snook-Hill, EdD
Tel: 519 758-6029
E-mail: mary-maureen.atkin@mohawkcollege.ca

Pennsylvania

Pennsylvania College of Optometry
Orientation and Mobility Specialist Prgm
Dept of Graduate Studies
8360 Old York Rd
Elkins Park, PA 19027
Prgm Dir: Laurel Leigh
Tel: 215 780-1360   *Fax:* 215 780-1357
E-mail: lleigh@pco.edu

University of Pittsburgh
Orientation and Mobility Specialist Prgm
Vision Studies Specialization
5316 WWPH
Pittsburgh, PA 15260
Prgm Dir: George J Zimmerman, PhD
Tel: 412 624-7247   *Fax:* 412 648-7081
E-mail: gjz@pitt.edu

South Carolina

South Carolina State University
Orientation and Mobility Specialist Prgm
Dept of Human Services
PO Box 7417, 300 College St
Orangeburg, SC 29117
Prgm Dir: Shirley Madison, MA COMS CRC
Tel: 803 533-3956   *Fax:* 803 533-3636
E-mail: smadison@scsu.edu

Texas

Texas Tech University
Orientation and Mobility Specialist Prgm
Personnel Preparation/Visual Impairment
Box 41071
Lubbock, TX 79409-1071
Prgm Dir: Nora Griffin-Shirley
Tel: 806 742-1997, Ext 247   *Fax:* 806 742-2326
E-mail: n.griffin-shirley@ttu.edu

Stephen F Austin State University
Orientation and Mobility Specialist Prgm
13019 SFA Station
Nacogdoches, TX 75962
Prgm Dir: Bill Bryan
Tel: 936 468-2906   *Fax:* 936 468-1342
E-mail: bbryan@sfasu.edu

Teacher of the Visually Impaired

Arizona

University of Arizona
Teacher of the Visually Impaired Prgm
Education Bldg, Rm 412
PO Box 210069
Tucson, AZ 85721
Prgm Dir: Jane Erin
Tel: 520 621-0945
E-mail: Jerin@u.arizona.edu

Florida

Florida State University
Teacher of the Visually Impaired Prgm
205 Stone Bldg
Tallahassee, FL 32306
Prgm Dir: Sandra Lewis
Tel: 850 644-4880
E-mail: lewis@coe.fsu.edu

Illinois

Northern Illinois University
Teacher of the Visually Impaired Prgm
Department of Teaching and Learning
DeKalb, IL 60115
Prgm Dir: Toni Heinze
Tel: 815 753-8452
E-mail: theinze@niu.edu

Michigan

Michigan State University
Teacher of the Visually Impaired Prgm
313 Erickson Hall
East Lansing, MI 48824
Prgm Dir: Rosario Garcia
Tel: 517 353-5901
E-mail: Mact@msu.edu

Missouri

Missouri State University
Teacher of the Visually Impaired Prgm
901 S National Ave
Springfield, MO 65897
Prgm Dir: Paris DePaepe
Tel: 417 836-4761
E-mail: parisdepaepe@missouristate.edu

Orientation and Mobility Specialist

Programs*	Class Capacity	Begins	Length (months)	Award	Res. Tuition	Non-res. Tuition	Stipend	Offers:‡ 1	2	3	4
California											
San Francisco State University	12	Fall Spring Summer	16	Cert, MA	$4,098	$14,268	$6,000	•		•	
Florida											
Florida State University (Tallahassee)	12	Aug	17	MS	$4,720	$17,360	$2,500			•	
New York											
CUNY Hunter College (New York)	12	Fall semester	12	Dipl, Cert, MSEd	$1,135	$1,635	$2,500	•		•	•
North Carolina											
North Carolina Central University (Durham)			12	MA							
South Carolina											
South Carolina State University (Orangeburg)	8	Fall Spring	18	Cert, MA	$2,600	$4,000		•			•

*Data are shown only for programs that completed the 2007 AMA Survey of Health Professions Education Programs.
‡Key to Offers: 1: Evening or weekend classes; 2: Non-English instruction; 3: Cultural competence instruction; 4: Distance education component.

New Mexico

New Mexico State University
Teacher of the Visually Impaired Prgm
MSC 3SPE
PO Box 30001
Las Cruces, NM 88003
Prgm Dir: Janice Duseau
Tel: 505 646-4234
E-mail: jduseau@nmsu.edu

Pennsylvania

Pennsylvania College of Optometry
Teacher of the Visually Impaired Prgm
Elkins Park Campus
8360 Old York Rd
Elkins Park, PA 19027
Prgm Dir: Diane P Wormsley
Tel: 215 780-1366
E-mail: dwormsley@pco.edu

Tennessee

Vanderbilt University
Cosponsor: Peabody College of Optometry
Teacher of the Visually Impaired Prgm
Box 328
Nashville, TN 37203
Prgm Dir: Anne Corn
Tel: 615 322-2249
E-mail: Anne.Corn@Vanderbilt.edu

Vision Rehabilitation Therapist

Arkansas

University of Arkansas at Little Rock
Vision Rehabilitation Therapy Prgm
Dept of CARE
2801 S University Ave
Little Rock, AR 72204-1099
www.ualr.edu/rehdept
Prgm Dir: Patricia Smith, EdD CVRT
Tel: 501 569-3169   *Fax:* 501 569-8129
E-mail: pbsmith@ualr.edu

Florida

Florida State University
Vision Rehabilitation Therapy Prgm
205 Stone Bldg
Tallahassee, FL 32306-4489
www.careersinblindness.com
Prgm Dir: Lynda Jones, RTC
Tel: 850 644-5610   *Fax:* 850 644-8715
E-mail: jonesl@coe.fsu.edu

Illinois

Northern Illinois University
Vision Rehabilitation Therapy Prgm
Dept of Teaching and Learning
DeKalb, IL 60115
Prgm Dir: Jodi Sticken, MSEd COMS
Tel: 815 753-8456   *Fax:* 815 753-8594
E-mail: jsticken@niu.edu

Michigan

Western Michigan University
Vision Rehabilitation Therapy Prgm
Dept of Blindness and Low Vision Studies
3413 Sangren Hall
Kalamazoo, MI 49008-5218
Prgm Dir: Susan Ponchillia, EdD MA CVRT
Tel: 269 387-3450   *Fax:* 269 387-3567
E-mail: susan.ponchillia@wmich.edu

New York

CUNY Hunter College
Vision Rehabilitation Therapy Prgm
Dept of Special Education
695 Park Ave
New York, NY 10065
www.hunter.cuny.edu/education/programs/bvi_rehab/
Prgm Dir: Rosanne Silberman, EdD
Tel: 212 772-4740   *Fax:* 212 650-3542
E-mail: rsilberm@hunter.cuny.edu

Ontario, Canada

Mohawk College
Vision Rehabilitation Therapy Prgm
11 Elgin St
Brantford, ON N3T 5V2
Prgm Dir: Mary-Maureen Snook-Hill
Tel: 519 758-6029   *Fax:* 519 758-6043
E-mail: mary-maureen.atkin@mohawkcollege.ca

Pennsylvania

Pennsylvania College of Optometry
Vision Rehabilitation Therapy Prgm
Dept of Graduate Studies in Vision Impairment
8360 Old York Rd
Elkins Park, PA 19027-1598
Prgm Dir: Maureen A Duffy, RTC
Tel: 215 780-1362   *Fax:* 215 780-1357
E-mail: mduffy@pco.edu

Vision Rehabilitation Therapist

Programs*	Class Capacity	Begins	Length (months)	Award	Res. Tuition	Non-res. Tuition	Stipend	Offers:‡ 1	2	3	4
Arkansas											
University of Arkansas at Little Rock	Var	Every semester		MA	$280	$280	$5,700	•		•	•
Florida											
Florida State University (Tallahassee)	12	Aug	17	MS	$4,720	$34,720	$7,500			•	
New York											
CUNY Hunter College (New York)	12	Fall semester	30, 12	Dipl, Cert, MSEd, COMS	$270	$500	$1,100	•		•	•

*Data are shown only for programs that completed the 2007 AMA Survey of Health Professions Education Programs.
‡Key to Offers: 1: Evening or weekend classes; 2: Non-English instruction; 3: Cultural competence instruction; 4: Distance education component.

Specialists in blood bank technology (SBBs) perform both routine and specialized tests in blood donor centers, transfusion services, reference laboratories, and research facilities. SBBs use methodology that conforms to the Standards for Blood Centers and Transfusion Services of the American Association of Blood Banks (AABB).

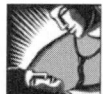

Career Description

Specialists in blood bank technology demonstrate a superior level of technical proficiency and problem-solving ability in such areas as

- Testing for blood group antigens, compatibility, and antibody identification
- Investigating abnormalities such as hemolytic diseases of the newborn, hemolytic anemias, and adverse reactions to transfusion
- Supporting physicians in transfusion therapy for patients with coagulopathies (diseases affecting blood clotting) or candidates for organ and cellular transplantation/therapy
- Performing blood collection and processing, including selecting donors, collecting blood, typing blood, molecular testing, and performing viral marker testing to ensure the safety of the patient.

Accordingly, supervision, management, and/or teaching make up a considerable part of the responsibilities of the specialist in blood bank technology educational program.

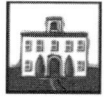

Employment Characteristics

Specialists in blood bank technology work in many types of facilities, including community blood centers, private hospital blood banks, university-affiliated blood banks, transfusion services, and independent laboratories. They also may be part of a university faculty. Specialists may have some weekend and night duty, including emergency calls. Qualified specialists may advance to supervisory or administrative positions or move into teaching or research activities. The criteria for advancement in this field are experience, technical expertise, and completion of advanced education courses.

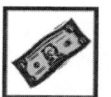

Salary

Salaries for specialists in blood banking range from a national average of $50,000 for bench techs and $60,000 for supervisors to $70,000 for managers. Salaries may be higher in certain regions of the country. Refer to Section IV, Table 5 of this Directory for more information, or see www.ama-assn.org/go/hpsalary.

Educational Programs

Length. Most of the educational programs are approximately 12 months. Some programs offer a master's degree and are approximately 24 months.

Prerequisites. Applicants must be certified in medical technology by the Board of Registry and possess a baccalaureate degree from a regionally accredited college or university. If applicants are not certified in medical technology by the Board of Registry, they must possess both a baccalaureate degree from a regionally accredited college or university with a major in any of the biological or physical sciences and have work experience in a blood bank.

Curriculum. Each specific educational program defines its own criteria for measurement of student achievement, and the sequence of instruction is at the discretion of the medical director and the program director and/or educational coordinator of the program. The clinical material available in the educational program provides the student with a full range of experiences. The educational design and environment are conducive to the development of competence in all technical areas of the modern blood bank. The didactic experience covers all theoretical concepts of blood bank immunohematology and transfusion medicine.

Inquiries

Careers/Curriculum

American Association of Blood Banks (AABB)
8101 Glenbrook Road
Bethesda, MD 20814-2749
301 215-6482   301 951-3729 Fax

Certification/Registration

Board of Registry
PO Box 12277
Chicago, IL 60612-0277
312 738-1336
E-mail: bor@ascp.org

Program Accreditation

Commission on Accreditation of Allied Health Education Programs (CAAHEP) in collaboration with:
Committee on Accreditation of SBB Schools
American Association of Blood Banks (AABB)
8101 Glenbrook Road
Bethesda, MD 20814-2749
301 215-6482 Education Department
301 907-6895 Fax
E-mail: education@aabb.org Website: www.aabb.org

Specialist in Blood Bank Technology

District of Columbia

Walter Reed Army Medical Center
Specialist in BB Tech Prgm
US Army Blood Bank Fellowship
Dept of Pathology, 6900 Georgia Ave NW
Washington, DC 20307-5001
Prgm Dir: William Turcan, MT(ASCP)SBB
Tel: 202 782-6210   *Fax:* 202 782-4502
E-mail: william.turcan@na.amedd.army.mil

Florida

Transfusion Med Acad Ctr FL Blood Svcs
Specialist in BB Tech Prgm
10100 Dr Martin Luther King Jr St N
St Petersburg, FL 33716-3806
Prgm Dir: Marjorie Doty, MT(ASCP)SBB
Tel: 727 568-5433, Ext 1514   *Fax:* 727 568-1177
E-mail: mdoty@fbsblood.org

Illinois

Rush University
Specialist in BB Tech Prgm
Department of Clinical Laboratory Sciences
600 S Paulina St, 1014 A-AAC
Chicago, IL 60612
www.rushu.rush.edu/cls/
Prgm Dir: Veronica N Lewis, MS MT(ASCP)SBB
Tel: 312 942-2402   *Fax:* 312 942-6464
E-mail: Veronica_Lewis@rush.edu

Indiana

Indiana Blood Center
Specialist in BB Tech Prgm
3450 N Meridian St
Indianapolis, IN 46208
Prgm Dir: Jayanna Slayten, MS MT(ASCP)SBB
Tel: 317 916-5186

Louisiana

Medical Center of Louisiana
Specialist in BB Tech Prgm
Blood Bank
2021 Perdido St
New Orleans, LA 70112
Prgm Dir: Cindy A Eicher, MHS MT(ASCP) SBB
Tel: 504 903-4851   *Fax:* 504 903-3437
E-mail: ceiche@lsuhsc.edu

Maryland

Johns Hopkins Hospital
Specialist in BB Tech Prgm
Carnegie Bldg #667
600 N Wolfe St
Baltimore, MD 21287-6667
Prgm Dir: Jan Light, MAS MT(ASCP)SBB
Tel: 410 955-6580   *Fax:* 410 955-0618
E-mail: jlight5@jhmi.edu

NIH Clinical Center Blood Bank
Specialist in BB Tech Prgm
Department of Transfusion Medicine, Bldg 10,
   Rm 1C 711
10 Center Dr MSC 1184
Bethesda, MD 20892
www.cc.nih.gov/dtm/dtm_training_&_education_sbb_
   program.htm
Prgm Dir: Sherry Sheldon, MT(ASCP)SBB
Tel: 301 451-8654   *Fax:* 301 496-9990
E-mail: SSheldon@cc.nih.gov

Ohio

University of Cincinnati Medical Center
Cosponsor: Hoxworth Blood Center
Specialist in BB Tech Prgm
3130 Highland Ave, PO Box 670055
Cincinnati, OH 45267-0055
Prgm Dir: Susan L Wilkinson, EdD MT(ASCP)SBB
Tel: 513 558-1271   *Fax:* 513 558-1279
E-mail: pamela.inglish@uc.edu

ARC Blood Svcs - Central Ohio Region
Cosponsor: OSU Transfusion Service
Specialist in BB Tech Prgm
995 E Broad
Columbus, OH 43205
Prgm Dir: Joanne Kosanke, MT(ASCP)SBB
Tel: 614 253-2740, Ext 2270   *Fax:* 614 253-2487
E-mail: kosankej@usa.redcross.org

Texas

Univ of Texas Southwestern Med Ctr
Specialist in BB Tech Prgm
5323 Harry Hines Blvd
Dallas, TX 75390-8878
http://www8.utsouthwestern.edu/utsw/cda/dept48940/
   files/210758.html
Prgm Dir: Lynn M Little, PhD MT (ASCP)
Tel: 214 648-1780   *Fax:* 214 648-1029
E-mail: barbara.fryer@utsouthwestern.edu

University of Texas Medical Branch
Specialist in BB Tech Prgm
301 University Blvd
Galveston, TX 77555-1140
http://http:www.utmb.edu/sbb
Prgm Dir: Janet L Vincent, MS SBB(ASCP)
Tel: 409 772-9476   *Fax:* 409 772-9470
E-mail: jvincent@utmb.edu

Gulf Coast School of Blood Bank Technology
Specialist in BB Tech Prgm
1400 La Concha Ln
Houston, TX 77054-1802
Prgm Dir: Clare Wong, MT(ASCP)SBB SLS
Tel: 713 791-6201   *Fax:* 713 791-6610
E-mail: cwong@giveblood.org

Univ of Texas Hlth Sci Ctr at San Antonio
Cosponsor: University Hospital Health System
Specialist in BB Tech Prgm
Dept of Clinical Laboratory Sci, 6246
7703 Floyd Curl Dr
San Antonio, TX 78229-3900
Prgm Dir: Linda A Smith, PhD Bonnie Fodermaier,
   SBB(ASCP)
Tel: 210 567-8869   *Fax:* 210 567-8875
E-mail: smithla@uthscsa.edu

Wisconsin

Blood Center of Southeast Wisconsin
Specialist in BB Tech Prgm
638 N 18th St
Milwaukee, WI 53233
Prgm Dir: Susan T Johnson, MT(ASCP) SBB
Tel: 414 937-6403   *Fax:* 414 937-6202
E-mail: stjohnson@bcsew.edu

Specialist in Blood Bank Technology

Programs*	Class Capacity	Begins	Length (months)	Award	Res. Tuition	Non-res. Tuition	Stipend	Offers:‡ 1	2	3	4
Alabama											
Univ of Alabama at Birmingham/Amer Red Cross	2	Jan	12, 14	Cert, SBB	$17,000	$0					•
District of Columbia											
Walter Reed Army Medical Center (Washington)	6	Jul	18	Dipl, Cert, SBB, MSHS							
Illinois											
Rush University (Chicago)	10	Sep	12, 16	Cert, MS	$13,000	$13,000					•
Indiana											
Indiana Blood Center (Indianapolis)	4	Nov	12	Cert	$2,400	$2,400					•

*Data are shown only for programs that completed the 2007 AMA Survey of Health Professions Education Programs.
‡Key to Offers: 1: Evening or weekend classes; 2: Non-English instruction; 3: Cultural competence instruction; 4: Distance education component.

Specialist in Blood Bank Technology

Programs*	Class Capacity	Begins	Length (months)	Award	Res. Tuition	Non-res. Tuition	Stipend	Offers:‡ 1	2	3	4
Louisiana											
Medical Center of Louisiana (New Orleans)	4	Jan	12, 24	Cert							
Maryland											
Johns Hopkins Hospital (Baltimore)	6	Jul	12	Cert, SBB							
NIH Clinical Center Blood Bank (Bethesda)	3	Jul	12	Cert							
Ohio											
ARC Blood Svcs - Central Ohio Region (Columbus)	4	Jan	24	Cert	$1,000	$0					
University of Cincinnati Medical Center	2	Sep	15	MS	$12,111	$21,945	$15,000				
Texas											
Gulf Coast School of Blood Bank Technology (Houston)	6	May	12	Cert	$2,400	$2,400					•
Univ of Texas Southwestern Med Ctr (Dallas)	8	Aug	24	Cert	$1,944	$6,948					•
University of Texas Medical Branch (Galveston)	30	Mar	12	Cert	$2,400	$2,400					•

*Data are shown only for programs that completed the 2007 AMA Survey of Health Professions Education Programs.
‡Key to Offers: 1: Evening or weekend classes; 2: Non-English instruction; 3: Cultural competence instruction; 4: Distance education component.

Cardiovascular Technologist

The cardiovascular technologist performs diagnostic examinations and therapeutic interventions of the heart and/or blood vessels at the request or direction of a physician in one or more of the following:

- Invasive cardiology—Cardiac catheterization
- Noninvasive cardiology—Echocardiography
- Noninvasive peripheral vascular study—Vascular ultrasound

Through subjective sampling and/or recording, the technologist creates an easily definable foundation of data from which a correct anatomic and physiologic diagnosis may be established for each patient.

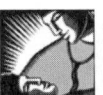

Career Description

The cardiovascular technologist is qualified by specific didactic, laboratory, and clinical technological education to perform various cardiovascular/peripheral vascular diagnostic and therapeutic procedures. The role of the cardiovascular technologist may include but is not limited to:

- Reviewing and/or recording pertinent patient history and supporting clinical data
- Performing appropriate clinical procedures and obtaining a record of anatomical, pathological, and/or physiological data for interpretation by a physician
- Exercising discretion and judgment in the performance of cardiovascular diagnostic and therapeutic services

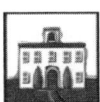

Employment Characteristics

Cardiovascular technologists may provide their services to patients in any medical setting under the supervision of a doctor of medicine or osteopathy (MD or DO). The procedures performed by the cardiovascular technologist may be found in, but are not limited to, one of the following general settings:

- Invasive cardiovascular laboratories, including cardiac catheterization, blood gas, and electrophysiology laboratories
- Noninvasive cardiovascular laboratories, including echocardiography, exercise stress test, and electrocardiography laboratories
- Noninvasive peripheral vascular studies laboratories, including Doppler ultrasound, thermography, and plethysmography laboratories.

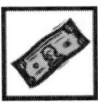

Salary

In 2006, entry-level salaries ranged from $36,000 to $45,000. The overall average was $50,000 to $65,000, with the upper ranges at $75,000 plus. Refer to Section IV, Table 5 of this *Directory* for more information, or see www.ama-assn.org/go/hpsalary.

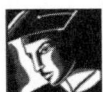

Educational Programs

Length. Programs may be from 1 to 4 years, depending on student qualifications and number of areas of diagnostic evaluation selected: invasive cardiology, noninvasive cardiology, or noninvasive peripheral vascular study.

Prerequisites. High school diploma or equivalent or qualifications in a clinically related allied health profession.

Curriculum. Curricula of accredited programs include didactic instruction, formal laboratory experiences, and patient-based clinical instruction. Suggested areas of instruction in the core curriculum include an introduction to the field of cardiovascular technology, general and/or applied sciences, human anatomy and physiology, basic pharmacology, and basic medical electronics and medical instrumentation. Emphasis, following the core curriculum, is given in the specialty area(s) selected: invasive cardiology, noninvasive cardiology, and noninvasive peripheral vascular study. Both didactic instruction and clinical experiences are provided in these areas.

Inquiries

Careers/Curriculum

Society for Vascular Ultrasound
4601 Presidents Drive, Suite 260
Lanham, MD 20706-4365
301 459-7550 or 800 SVT-VEIN
301 459-5651 Fax

American Society of Echocardiography
1500 Sunday Drive, Suite 102
Raleigh, NC 27607
919 861-5574
919 787-4916 Fax
www.asecho.org

Society of Invasive Cardiovascular Professionals
1500 Sunday Drive, Suite 102
Raleigh, NC 27607
919 861-4546
www.sicp.com

Certification/Registration

Cardiovascular Credentialing International
1500 Sunday Drive, Suite 102
Raleigh, NC 27607
800 326-0268
919 787-4916 Fax
www.cci-online.org

American Registry of Diagnostic Medical Sonographers
51 Monroe Street, Plaza East One
Rockville, MD 20850-2400
301 738-8401
301 738-0312 Fax
www.ardms.org

Program Accreditation

Commission on Accreditation of Allied Health Education Programs (CAAHEP) in collaboration with:
Joint Review Committee on Education in Cardiovascular Technology
1248 Harwood Road
Bedford, TX 76021-4244
214 206-3117
817 354-8519
E-mail: jrccvt@heasc.org

Cardiovascular Technologist

California

Orange Coast College
Cardiovascular Technology Prgm
2701 Fairview Rd
Costa Mesa, CA 92628-5005
Prgm Dir: Darryl Isaac
Tel: 714 432-5549   *Fax:* 714 432-5535
E-mail: disaac@mail.occ.cccd.edu

Grossmont College
Cardiovascular Technology Prgm
Invasive/Noninvasive/Vascular Tracks
8800 Grossmont College Dr
El Cajon, CA 92020-1799
www.grossmont.edu
Prgm Dir: Rick D Kirby, RICS RCS MA
Tel: 619 644-7302   *Fax:* 619 644-7961
E-mail: rick.kirby@gcccd.net

Naval School of Health Sciences, San Diego
Cardiovascular Technology Prgm
Invasive Track
34101 Farenholt Ave
San Diego, CA 92134
Prgm Dir: Trevor E Smith, AAS RCIS CCT MTS
Tel: 619 532-5223   *Fax:* 619 532-6750
E-mail: trevor.smith@med.navy.mil

Florida

Edison College
Cardiovascular Technology Prgm
Invasive Track
8099 College Pkwy SW
Fort Myers, FL 33906
www.edison.edu
Prgm Dir: Robert Jeff Davis, RRT RCIS
Tel: 239 489-9430   *Fax:* 239 985-8352
E-mail: jdavis@edison.edu

Santa Fe Community College
Cardiovascular Technology Prgm
Invasive/Noninvasive/Vascular Tracks
3000 NW 83rd St
Gainesville, FL 32653
Prgm Dir: Reeda Fullington
Tel: 352 395-5707   *Fax:* 352 395-5711
E-mail: reeda.fullington@sfc.edu

Central Florida Institute
Cardiovascular Technology Prgm
Invasive/Noninvasive/Cardiovascular Ultrasound Tracks
30522 US Hwy 19 N
Palm Harbor, FL 34684
Prgm Dir: Thomas O'Brien, MBA BBA AS CCT
Tel: 727 786-4707   *Fax:* 727 781-9421
E-mail: tobrien@cfinstitute.com

Georgia

Harry T Harper Jr Sch of Cardiac & Vas Tech
Cosponsor: Augusta Technical College & USC Columbia
Cardiovascular Technology Prgm
University Hospital
1350 Walton Way
Augusta, GA 30901
Prgm Dir: Patricia L Thomas, MBA RCIS BSRT
Tel: 706 774-5044   *Fax:* 706 774-8644
E-mail: pthomas@uh.org

Kentucky

Norton Healthcare
Cardiovascular Technology Prgm
Invasive Cardiology and Cardiac Sonography
1 Audubon Plaza Dr
Louisville, KY 40217
Prgm Dir: Steve Janto, RCVT
Tel: 502 636-7124   *Fax:* 502 636-7146
E-mail: steve.janto@nortonhealthcare.org

Spencerian College
Cardiovascular Technology Prgm
Invasive Cardiovascular Technologist Program
4627 Dixie Hwy
Louisville, KY 40216
www.spencerian.edu
Prgm Dir: Vicki Lemaster
Tel: 502 447-1000, Ext 7876   *Fax:* 502 449-7866
E-mail: vlemaster@spencerian.edu

Louisiana

Louisiana State Univ Health Sciences Center
Cardiovascular Technology Prgm
1900 Gravier St
New Orleans, LA 70112
www.lsuhsc.edu
Prgm Dir: Andy Pellett, PhD
Tel: 504 568-4230   *Fax:* 504 568-4249
E-mail: apelle@lsuhsc.edu

Maryland

Howard Community College
Cardiovascular Technology Prgm
Invasive Track
10901 Little Patuxent Pkwy
Columbia, MD 21044
Prgm Dir: Mary Patricia English, RTR(CV) MS RLIS
Tel: 410 772-4466   *Fax:* 410 772-4494
E-mail: penglish@howardcc.edu

Michigan

Carnegie Institute
Cardiovascular Technology Prgm
Noninvasive Peripheral Vascular, Invasive CVT & Noninv Echo
550 Stephenson Hwy Ste 100
Troy, MI 48083
Prgm Dir: Bonnie M Normile, RN CCVT
Tel: 248 589-1078   *Fax:* 248 589-1631
E-mail: info@Carnegie-Institute.edu

Minnesota

Northland Community & Technical College
Cardiovascular Technology Prgm
Invasive Track
2022 Central Ave NE
East Grand Forks, MN 56721
Prgm Dir: Connie Schimke, BS RCIS
Tel: 218 773-3441, Ext 4797   *Fax:* 218 773-4502
E-mail: connie.schimke@northlandcollege.edu

St Cloud Technical College
Cardiovascular Technology Prgm
Invasive and Echocardiography
1540 Northway Dr
St Cloud, MN 56303
Prgm Dir: Patrick McGuire
Tel: 320 308-6010
E-mail: pmcguire@sctc.edu

Nebraska

BryanLGH College of Health Sciences
Cosponsor: BryanLGH Medical Center
Cardiovascular Technology Prgm
5035 Everett St
Lincoln, NE 68506-1398
www.bryanlghcollege.org
Prgm Dir: Diane Kathol, MSN MEd
Tel: 402 481-8847   *Fax:* 402 481-8421
E-mail: dkathol@bryanlgh.org

New Jersey

Morristown Memorial Hospital
Cardiovascular Technology Prgm
Invasive/Noninvasive/Vascular Tracks
100 Madison Ave
Morristown, NJ 07962-1956
http://atlantichealth.org
Prgm Dir: Susan Smith, BA RDCS RVS
Tel: 973 971-6336   *Fax:* 973 290-7310
E-mail: susan.smith@atlantichealth.org

Univ of Medicine & Dent of New Jersey
Cardiovascular Technology Prgm
Vascular Technology Program
1776 Raritan Rd
Scotch Plains, NJ 07076
Prgm Dir: Clifford T Araki, PhD RVT
Tel: 908 889-2468   *Fax:* 908 889-0417
E-mail: arakict@umdnj.edu

New York

Molloy College
Cardiovascular Technology Prgm
1000 Hempstead Ave
PO Box 5002
Rockville Centre, NY 11571-5002
www.molloy.edu
Prgm Dir: Michael Hartman, MS RDMS RVT RT(R)
Tel: 516 678-5000, Ext 6958   *Fax:* 516 256-2252
E-mail: mhartman@molloy.edu

Ohio

University of Toledo
Cardiovascular Technology Prgm
Noninvasive Cardiovascular (Echo) Track
2801 W Bancroft St, Mail Stop 119
Toledo, OH 43606-3390
www.utoledo.edu
Prgm Dir: Suzanne Wambold, PhD RN RDCS FASE
Tel: 419 530-4688   *Fax:* 419 530-4780
E-mail: suzanne.wambold@utoledo.edu

Pennsylvania

Geisinger Medical Center
Cardiovascular Technology Prgm
Invasive Track
100 N Academy Ave
Danville, PA 17822-2011
www.geisinger.org
Prgm Dir: Stephanie Ranck, BA RCIS
Tel: 570 271-6638   *Fax:* 570 214-5088
E-mail: sranck@geisinger.edu

Gwynedd-Mercy College
Cardiovascular Technology Prgm
Invasive/Noninvasive Tracks
1325 Sumneytown Pike, PO Box 901
Gwynedd Valley, PA 19437
Prgm Dir: Andrea Reiley-Helzner, MS RCIS
Tel: 215 542-4659   *Fax:* 215 641-5559
E-mail: reiley.a@gmc.edu

Lancaster Gen Coll of Nursing & Hlth Sciences
Cardiovascular Technology Prgm
410 N Lime St
Lancaster, PA 17602
Prgm Dir: William L Fisher, RCIS MEd
Tel: 717 290-5511, Ext 44700   *Fax:* 717 290-5970
E-mail: wlfisher@LancasterGeneral.org

South Carolina

Sister of Charity Providence Hospital
Cardiovascular Technology Prgm
School of Cardiovascular Diagnostics
Department 7195
Columbia, SC 29204
Prgm Dir: Eric Walker, RDCS RVT
Tel: 803 256-5636   *Fax:* 803 256-5913
E-mail: eric.walker@providencehospitals.com

South Dakota

Southeast Technical Institute
Cardiovascular Technology Prgm
Invasive/Noninvasive/Vascular Tracks
2320 N Career Ave
Sioux Falls, SD 57107
Prgm Dir: Catherine J Miller, BS LPN RVT
Tel: 605 367-4634   *Fax:* 605 367-6108
E-mail: cathy.miller@southeasttech.com

Tennessee

Northeast State Technical Comm College
Cardiovascular Technology Prgm
Invasive Track
PO Box 246, 2425 Hwy 75
Blountville, TN 37617-0246
Prgm Dir: Connie Marshall, RT(R) RCIS
Tel: 423 279-3680   *Fax:* 423 477-4859
E-mail: cmarshall@NortheastState.edu

Texas

El Centro College
Cardiovascular Technology Prgm
Echocardiology Technology Program
Main and Lamar
Dallas, TX 75202
Prgm Dir: Catherine Carolan, RDMS RDCS RVT
Tel: 214 860-2310   *Fax:* 214 860-2268
E-mail: cmc5540@dcccd.edu

US Army Medical Dept Center & School
Cardiovascular Technology Prgm
Invasive/Noninvasive Tracks
MCCS-HMD, 2250 Stanley Rd, Bldg 2398
Fort Sam Houston, TX 78234-6170
www.cs.amedd.army.mil/300y6/
Prgm Dir: Harrell Carmichael
Tel: 210 221-3472   *Fax:* 210 221-1197
E-mail: harrell.carmichael@cen.amedd.army.mil

Virginia

Sentara Norfolk General Hospital
Cardiovascular Technology Prgm
Invasive/Noninvasive/Vascular Tracks
600 Gresham Dr
Norfolk, VA 23507
Prgm Dir: Kathy Butterbaugh
Tel: 757 668-2900   *Fax:* 757 668-2905
E-mail: klbutter@sentara.com

Washington

Spokane Community College
Cardiovascular Technology Prgm
Invasive/Noninvasive Tracks
N 1810 Greene St MS 2090
Spokane, WA 99217-5499
Prgm Dir: Darren Powell, RCIS FSICP
Tel: 509 533-7306   *Fax:* 509 533-8621
E-mail: dpowell@scc.spokane.edu

Wisconsin

Milwaukee Area Technical College
Cardiovascular Technology Prgm
Invasive Track
700 W State St
Milwaukee, WI 53233-1443
www.matc.edu
Prgm Dir: Erwin Wuehr, CP
Tel: 414 297-8517   *Fax:* 414 297-8955
E-mail: wuehre@matc.edu

Cardiovascular Technologist

Programs*	Class Capacity	Begins	Length (months)	Award	Res. Tuition	Non-res. Tuition	Stipend	Offers:‡ 1	2	3	4
California											
Grossmont College (El Cajon)	54	Aug	24	Cert, AS	$580	$5,307				•	
Naval School of Health Sciences, San Diego	16	Feb Aug	13	Cert						•	
Florida											
Edison College (Fort Myers)	20	Aug	22	AS	$2,628	$9,796					
Kentucky											
Norton Healthcare (Louisville)	10	Sep	18	Cert	$12,500	$12,500					
Spencerian College (Louisville)	10	Jan Mar Jun Sep	21	AASD	$12,120	$12,120				•	
Louisiana											
Louisiana State Univ Health Sciences Center (New Orleans)	15	May	24	BS	$5,035	$8,160				•	
Michigan											
Carnegie Institute (Troy)	48	Mar Sep	18, 24	Dipl	$12,630	$12,630		•			
Nebraska											
BryanLGH College of Health Sciences (Lincoln)	24	Aug	21	AS	$10,500	$10,500				•	
New Jersey											
Morristown Memorial Hospital	15	Sep	18	Dipl	$18,000	$18,000					
Univ of Medicine & Dent of New Jersey (Scotch Plains)	12	Sep	15	Cert, BS	$9,000	$13,500				•	
New York											
Molloy College (Rockville Centre)	18	Sep	24	AAS	$18,000	$18,000		•			
Ohio											
University of Toledo	10	Aug	24	AAS, BS	$15,000	$28,000					
Pennsylvania											
Geisinger Medical Center (Danville)	5	Aug	12	Dipl	$8,500	$8,500					
Gwynedd-Mercy College (Gwynedd Valley)	16	Aug	24	Cert, AS	$19,720	$19,720				•	
Texas											
El Centro College (Dallas)	15	Jun	12, 24	Cert, AAS	$3,068	$5,588				•	•
US Army Medical Dept Center & School (Fort Sam Houston)	15	Apr	21, 36	Dipl, Cert						•	
Washington											
Spokane Community College	30	Sep	20	AAS	$2,864	$5,348				•	•
Wisconsin											
Milwaukee Area Technical College	12	Aug	19	AAS	$3,100	$17,500		•			

*Data are shown only for programs that completed the 2007 AMA Survey of Health Professions Education Programs.
‡Key to Offers: 1: Evening or weekend classes; 2: Non-English instruction; 3: Cultural competence instruction; 4: Distance education component.

Includes:
- Clinical assistant
- Clinical laboratory scientist/medical technologist
- Clinical laboratory technician/medical laboratory technician
- Cytogenetic technologist
- Diagnostic molecular scientist
- Histologic technician/histotechnologist
- Pathologists' assistant
- Phlebotomist

Clinical Assistant

Laboratory tests play an important role in the detection, diagnosis, and treatment of diseases. Clinical assistants are formally prepared multiskilled health care providers with a laboratory focus. Clinical assistants are trained to work under the supervision of an appropriately qualified person in chemistry, donor room collection screening, component processing, hematology, immunology, microbiology, phlebotomy, and/or urinalysis.

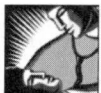

Career Description

Clinical assistants follow standard operating procedures to collect specimens; prepare blood and body fluid specimens for analysis according to standard operating procedures; prepare/reconstitute reagents, standards, and controls according to standard operating procedure; perform appropriate tests at the clinical assistant level; perform and record vital sign measurements; and follow established quality control protocols. Clinical assistants follow infection control and safety practices and use information systems necessary to accomplish job functions.

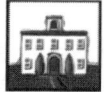

Employment Characteristics

Many clinical assistants are employed in hospital laboratories. Others are employed in physicians' private laboratories and clinics; by the armed forces; or by city, state, and federal health agencies.

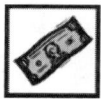

Salary

Salaries vary depending on the employer and geographic location. Refer to Section IV, Table 5 of this *Directory* for more information, or see www.ama-assn.org/go/hpsalary.

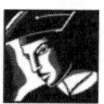

Educational Programs

Length. Approved programs culminate in a postsecondary certificate.

Prerequisites. High school diploma or equivalent. The applicant must also meet the admission requirements of the sponsoring institution.

Curriculum. Clinical assistant programs are conducted in junior or community colleges, hospitals, medical laboratories, proprietary schools, and other equivalent postsecondary educational institutions.

Clinical Laboratory Scientist/ Medical Technologist

Laboratory tests play an important role in the detection, diagnosis, and treatment of many diseases. Clinical laboratory scientists/medical technologists perform these tests in conjunction with pathologists (physicians who diagnose the causes and nature of disease) and other physicians or scientists who specialize in clinical chemistry, microbiology, or the other biological sciences. Clinical laboratory scientists/medical technologists develop data on the blood, tissues, and fluids of the human body by using a variety of precise methodologies and technologies.

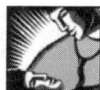

Career Description

In addition to possessing the skills of clinical laboratory technicians/medical laboratory technicians, clinical laboratory scientists/medical technologists perform complex analyses, fine-line discrimination, and error correction. They are able to recognize the interdependency of tests and have knowledge of physiological conditions affecting test results so that they can confirm these results and develop data that may be used by a physician in determining the presence, extent, and, as far as possible, cause of a disease.

Clinical laboratory scientists/medical technologists assume responsibility and are held accountable for accurate results. They establish and monitor quality assurance and quality improvement programs and design or modify procedures as necessary. Tests and procedures performed or supervised by clinical laboratory scientists/medical technologists in the clinical laboratory focus on major areas of hematology, microbiology, immunohematology, immunology, clinical chemistry, and urinalysis.

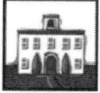

Employment Characteristics

Most clinical laboratory scientists/medical technologists are employed in hospital laboratories. Others are employed in physicians' private laboratories and clinics; by the armed forces; by city, state, and federal health agencies; in industrial medical laboratories; in pharmaceutical houses; in numerous public and private research programs dedicated to the study of specific diseases; and as faculty of accredited programs preparing medical laboratory personnel. While many graduates are employed in the clinical laboratory setting, career options are abundant, with opportunities in all areas of health care. As a clinical laboratory scientist/medical technologist, one may decide to specialize in:
- Biomedical research and development
- Andrology and assisted reproductive technology laboratories
- Organ transplantation
- Genetic testing
- Infection control
- Health information management
- Health care industry
- Consultative and entrepreneurial opportunities
- Forensic testing

Salary
Salaries vary depending on the employer and geographic location. Based on a 2005 survey published in *Laboratory Medicine*, median salaries ranged from $44,500 to $52,000, and median manager salaries ranged from $69,500 to $72,000. Refer to Section IV, Table 5 of this *Directory* for more information, or see www.ama-assn.org/go/hpsalary.

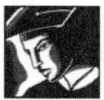

Educational Programs
Length. Programs are at least 1 year of professional/clinical education in conjunction with either a baccalaureate or a master's degree.

Prerequisites. College courses and number of required credits are those necessary to ensure admission of a student who is prepared for the clinical educational program. Content areas should include general chemistry, general biological sciences, organic and/or biochemistry, microbiology, immunology, and mathematics. Survey courses do not qualify as fulfillment of chemistry and biological science prerequisites, and remedial mathematics courses will not satisfy the mathematics requirement.

College/university programs that integrate preprofessional and professional coursework are structured with professional courses in the junior and senior years or at the graduate level.

Curriculum. There must be a structured laboratory program, including instruction pertaining to theory and practice in hematology, clinical chemistry, microbiology, immunology, and immunohematology. The program must culminate in a baccalaureate degree for those students not already possessing the degree but may also culminate in a master's degree.

Clinical Laboratory Technician/ Medical Laboratory Technician

Laboratory tests play an important role in the detection, diagnosis, and treatment of many diseases and in the promotion of health. Clinical laboratory technicians/medical laboratory technicians perform these tests under the supervision or direction of pathologists (physicians who diagnose the causes and nature of disease) and other physicians, clinical laboratory scientists/medical technologists, or other scientists who specialize in clinical chemistry, microbiology, or the other biological sciences. Clinical laboratory technicians/medical laboratory technicians develop data on the blood, tissues, and fluids of the human body by using a variety of precise methodologies and technologies.

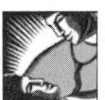

Career Description
Associate degree clinical laboratory technicians/medical laboratory technicians perform all the routine tests in an up-to-date medical laboratory and can demonstrate discrimination between closely similar items and correction of errors by the use of preset strategies. The technician has knowledge of specific techniques and instruments and is able to recognize factors that directly affect procedures and results. The technician also monitors quality assurance procedures.

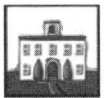

Employment Characteristics
Most clinical laboratory technicians/medical laboratory technicians work in hospital, clinic, or physician office laboratories.

Salary
Salaries vary, depending upon the employer and geographic location. Based on a 2005 survey published in *Laboratory Medicine,* median salaries ranged from $37,100 to $41,000. Refer to Section IV, Table 5 of this *Directory* for more information, or see www.ama-assn.org/go/hpsalary.

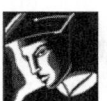

Educational Programs
Length. The period of education is usually 2 academic years and culminates in an associate degree.

Prerequisites. High school diploma or equivalent. The applicant also must meet the admission requirements of the sponsoring educational institution.

Curriculum. Associate degree programs are conducted in junior or community colleges, in 2-year divisions of universities and colleges, or in other recognized institutions granting associate degrees. Courses are taught on campus and usually in affiliated hospitals. Classroom and laboratory classes focus on general knowledge and basic skills; understanding principles and master procedures of laboratory testing; and basic laboratory mathematics, computer technology, communication skills, and interpersonal relationships and responsibilities. The clinical courses include application of basic principles commonly used in the diagnostic laboratory. Clinical instruction includes procedures in hematology, microbiology, immunohematology, immunology, clinical chemistry, and urinalysis.

Cytogenetic Technologist

Laboratory tests play an important role in the detection, diagnosis, and treatment of diseases. Cytogenetic technologists study the morphology of chromosomes and their relationship to disease. Cytogenetic analysis provides important data for the diagnosis, prognosis, and treatment of genetic disorders and malignant diseases.

Career Description
Cytogenetic technologists evaluate the correct method of collection, transport, and handling of various specimen types for cytogenetic analysis; identify culture techniques based on tissue type and reason for referral; and perform chromosomal staining, microscopic analysis, and karyotyping (organizing chromosomes according to a standardized ideogram). In addition to practicing good general laboratory skills, quality assurance principles, and safety protocols, cytogenetic technologists understand the legal implications of their work environment and exhibit appropriate ethical and professional health care standards while demonstrating professional conduct, stress management, and interpersonal and communication skills with patients, peers, other health care personnel, and the public.

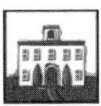

Employment Characteristics
Cytogenetic technologists are employed in hospital laboratories, private medical laboratories, and research facilities. They may also serve as faculty in cytogenetic education programs.

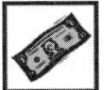

Salary
Salaries vary depending upon the employer and geographic location. Refer to Section IV, Table 5 of this *Directory* for more information, or see www.ama-assn.org/go/hpsalary.

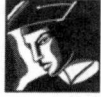

Educational Programs

Length. Programs are at least 1 year. Cytogenetic technologists attend a baccalaureate or postbaccalaureate program that includes professional and clinical education. Certification is desired by most employers.

Prerequisites. College courses and a number of required credits necessary to ensure admission of a student who is prepared for the clinical education program. College and university programs that integrate preprofessional and professional coursework are structured with professional courses in the junior and senior years or at the graduate level.

Curriculum. Cytogenetic technology programs are conducted in colleges and universities, hospitals, private medical laboratories, and other equivalent postsecondary educational institutions. The areas of study that must be included in either the professional program or as prerequisites are biology, chemistry, biochemistry or cellular biology, genetics, cytogenetics, hematology, microbiology, immunology, laboratory information systems, laboratory safety, and quality control.

Diagnostic Molecular Scientist

The diagnostic molecular scientist performs diagnostic assay or testing using a variety of manual techniques and precision instruments. The results of these tests are used to detect and diagnose disease and other abnormalities. The main responsibilities of the diagnostic molecular scientist are all aspects of genetic testing, including DNA and RNA isolation, amplification and detection, infectious disease testing, and viral load analysis.

Career Description

Diagnostic molecular scientists provide service in the molecular diagnosis of acquired, inherited, and infectious diseases. This includes researching, evaluating, implementing, and monitoring methods of collection, transport, and handling of various specimen types for molecular analysis; researching and developing principles, practices, and applications of molecular-based testing for laboratory utilization and clinical decisions for client outcomes; and performing appropriate techniques utilizing instrumentation and information management systems for molecular analysis and correlating results with acquired, inherited, and infectious diseases. Finally, diagnostic molecular scientists apply the principles of management and supervision when they function as section supervisors and of educational methodology when they teach students.

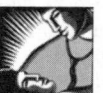

Employment Characteristics

Most diagnostic molecular scientists work in hospital laboratories.

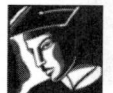

Educational Programs

Length. Programs for the diagnostic molecular scientist usually lead to a master's degree.

Prerequisites. College level courses as required by the sponsoring institution.

Curriculum. The curriculum includes both didactic instruction and practical demonstration in the areas of organic and/or biochemistry, genetics, cell biology, microbiology, immunology, diagnostic molecular biology, principles and methodologies for all major areas commonly practiced by a modern diagnostic molecular laboratory, and clinical significance of laboratory procedures in

diagnosis and treatment. It also includes principles and practices of

- Laboratory administration, supervision, safety, and problem solving
- Quality management
- Computer science (including acquisition and evaluation of laboratory information systems)
- Professional conduct

Histotechnician

Physicians (usually pathologists) and other scientists specializing in biological sciences or related clinical areas such as chemistry work in partnership with medical laboratory workers to analyze blood, tissues, and fluids from humans (and sometimes animals), using a variety of precision instruments. The results of these tests are used to detect and diagnose disease and other abnormalities.

The main responsibility of the histotechnician in the clinical laboratory is preparing sections of body tissue for examination by a pathologist. This includes the preparation of tissue specimens of human and animal origin for diagnostic, research, or teaching purposes. Tissue sections prepared by the histotechnician for a variety of disease entities enable the pathologist to diagnose body dysfunction and malignancy.

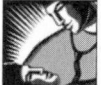

Career Description

Histotechnicians process sections of body tissue by fixation, dehydration, embedding, sectioning, decalcification, microincineration, mounting, and routine and special staining. They identify tissue structures, cell components, and their staining characteristics and relate them to physiological functions; and institute proper procedures to maintain accuracy and precision.

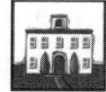

Employment Characteristics

Most histotechnicians work in hospital or reference laboratories.

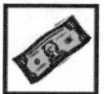

Salary

Based on a 2005 survey published in *Laboratory Medicine,* median salaries ranged from $40,250 to $40,580. Refer to Section IV, Table 5 of this *Directory* for more information, or see www.ama-assn.org/go/hpsalary.

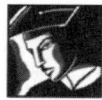

Educational Programs

Length. Programs for the histotechnician are 12 months, unless the curriculum is an integral part of a college program.

Prerequisites. High school diploma or equivalent.

Curriculum. The curriculum includes both didactic instruction and practical demonstration in the areas of medical ethics, medical terminology, chemistry, laboratory mathematics, computer technology, organic and/or biochemistry, immunology, electron microscopy, management, anatomy, histology, histochemistry, quality control, instrumentation, microscopy, processing techniques, preparation of museum specimens, and record and administration procedures. It is recommended that the curriculum be an integral part of a junior or community college program culminating in an associate degree and that the course of study include chemistry, biology, and mathematics.

Histotechnologist

Physicians (usually pathologists) and other scientists specializing in biological sciences or related clinical areas such as chemistry work in partnership with medical laboratory workers to analyze blood, tissues, and fluids from humans (and sometimes animals), using a variety of precision instruments. The results of these tests are used to detect and diagnose disease and other abnormalities.

The main responsibility of the histotechnologist in the clinical laboratory is preparing sections of body tissue for examination by a pathologist. This includes the preparation of tissue specimens of human and animal origin for diagnostic, research, or teaching purposes. Tissue sections prepared by the histotechnologist for a variety of disease entities enable the pathologist to diagnose body dysfunction and malignancy.

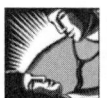

Career Description

Histotechnologists process sections of body tissue by fixation, dehydration, embedding, sectioning, decalcification, microincineration, mounting, and routine and special staining. In addition, histotechnologists perform the more complex procedures for processing tissues. They identify tissue structures, cell components, and their staining characteristics and relate them to physiological functions; implement and test new techniques and procedures; make judgments concerning the results of quality control measures; and institute proper procedures to maintain accuracy and precision. Histotechnologists apply the principles of management and supervision when they function as section supervisors and of educational methodology when they teach students.

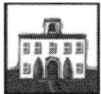

Employment Characteristics

Most histotechnologists work in hospital, reference, or research laboratories.

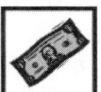

Salary

Based on a 2005 survey published in *Laboratory Medicine,* median salaries ranged from $44,970 to $49,360. Refer to Section IV, Table 5 of this *Directory* for more information, or see www.ama-assn.org/go/hpsalary.

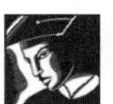

Educational Programs

Length. Programs for the histotechnologist are 4 years and lead to a baccalaureate degree.

Prerequisites. High school diploma or equivalent.

Curriculum. The curriculum includes both didactic instruction and practical demonstration in the areas of medical ethics, medical terminology, chemistry, laboratory mathematics, computer technology, organic and/or biochemistry, immunology, electron microscopy, management, anatomy, histology, histochemistry, quality control, instrumentation, microscopy, processing techniques, preparation of museum specimens, and record and administration procedures. The baccalaureate-level program includes coursework designed to provide supervisors and teachers with advanced capabilities.

Pathologists' Assistant

Anatomic pathologists are physicians who examine tissue specimens from patients and perform autopsies to diagnose the disease processes involved. Pathologists' assistants participate in autopsies and in the examination, dissection, and processing of tissue specimens. They function as physician extenders.

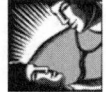

Career Description

The following services are provided under the direct supervision of a licensed and board-certified pathologist and should include, but not be limited to, the following:

Surgical pathology. Assisting in the preparation and performance of surgical specimen dissection by ensuring appropriate specimen accessioning, obtaining pertinent clinical information and studies, describing gross anatomic features, dissecting surgical specimens, preparing and submitting tissue for histologic processing, obtaining and submitting specimens for additional analytic procedures (immunostaining, flow cytometry, image analysis, bacterial and viral cultures, toxicology, etc), and assisting in photographing gross and microscopic specimens.

Autopsy pathology. Assisting in the performance of postmortem examination by ascertaining proper legal authorization; obtaining and reviewing the patient's chart and other pertinent clinical data and studies; notifying involved personnel of all special procedures and techniques required; coordinating special requests for specimens; notifying involved clinicians and appropriate authorities and individuals; assisting in the postmortem examination; selecting and preparing tissue for histologic processing and special studies; obtaining specimens for biological and toxicologic analysis; assisting in photographing gross and microscopic specimens and photomicrography; and participating in the completion of the autopsy report.

Additional duties. Assuming duties as may be assigned relative to teaching, administrative, supervisory, and budgetary functions in anatomic pathology.

Employment Characteristics

Pathologists' assistants are employed in a variety of settings, including community and regional hospitals, university medical centers, private pathology laboratories, and medical examiners/coroners' offices.

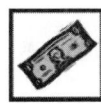

Salary

Salaries vary with geographic location and type of employing institution. Entry-level salaries average $55,000-$75,000. Refer to Section IV, Table 5 of this *Directory* for more information, or see www.ama-assn.org/go/hpsalary.

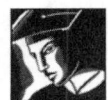

Educational Programs

Length. Minimum of 22 months.

Degree. Most programs are at the master's level.

Prerequisites. Variable among programs and dependent on the degree offered. Baccalaureate programs require a minimum of 60 hours of acceptable credits, with variable specific requirements.

Curriculum. The curriculum includes both didactic and practical training to provide a sound background in the basic medical sciences and the necessary skills to work in an anatomic pathology laboratory. Coursework includes anatomy, physiology, and medical terminology, as well as general, systemic, pediatric, and forensic pathology. Clinical training includes autopsy pathology, surgical pathology, forensic pathology, and medical photography.

Phlebotomist

Laboratory tests play an important role in the detection, diagnosis, and treatment of diseases. Phlebotomists collect blood specimens for many of these tests. Phlebotomists practice safe blood collection and handling techniques that protect patients from injury, safeguard themselves from accidents, and produce high-quality specimens while demonstrating compassion for the patient.

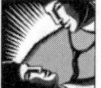

Career Description

Phlebotomists collect, transport, handle, and process blood specimens for analysis; identify and select equipment, supplies, and additives used in blood collection; and understand factors that affect specimen collection procedures and test results. Recognizing the importance of specimen collection in the overall patient care system, phlebotomists adhere to infection control and safety policies and procedures. They monitor quality control within predetermined limits while demonstrating professional conduct, stress management, and communication skills with patients, peers, and other health care personnel as well as with the public.

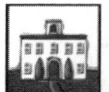

Employment Characteristics

Many phlebotomists are employed in hospital laboratories. Others are employed in physicians' private laboratories and clinics; by the armed forces; by city, state, and federal health agencies; in industrial medical laboratories; in pharmaceutical houses; in numerous public and private research programs; and as faculty of approved programs preparing medical laboratory personnel.

Salary

Salaries vary depending on the employer and geographic location. Based on a 2005 survey published in *Laboratory Medicine,* median salaries ranged from $24,315 to $29,120. Refer to Section IV, Table 5 of this *Directory* for more information, or see www.ama-assn.org/go/hpsalary.

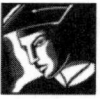

Educational Programs

Length. Approved programs contain at least 100 hours of clinical practicum and culminate in a postsecondary certificate.

Prerequisites. High school diploma or equivalent. The applicant must also meet the admission requirements of the sponsoring institution.

Curriculum. Phlebotomy programs are conducted in junior or community colleges, hospitals, medical laboratories, proprietary schools, and other equivalent postsecondary educational institutions. The curriculum includes didactic instruction and 100 hours of applied experiences, performance of a minimum of 100 successful unaided collections, and instruction in a variety of collection techniques, including vacuum collection devices, syringe, and capillary/skin-puncture methods.

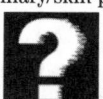

Inquiries

Careers/Curriculum

American Society for Clinical Laboratory Science
7910 Woodmont Avenue, Suite 530
Bethesda, MD 20814

301 657-2768
301 657-2909 Fax
E-mail: ascls@ascls.org
www.ascls.org

American Society for Clinical Pathology
33 West Monroe, Suite 1600
Chicago, IL 60603
312 541-4999
E-mail: info@ascp.org
www.ascp.org

Association of Genetic Technologists
Executive Office
PO Box 15945-288
Lenexa, KS 66285
913 541-9077

National Society for Histotechnology
4201 Northview Drive, Suite 502
Bowie, MD 20716-2604
301 262-6221
301 262-9188 Fax
E-mail: histo@nsh.org
www.nsh.org

American Association of Pathologists' Assistants
8030 Old Cedar Avenue, Suite 225
Bloomington, MN 55425-1215
800 532-AAPA
E-mail: mspindler@mn.state.net
www.pathologistsassistants.org

Certification/Registration

American Society for Clinical Pathology
Board of Registry
PO Box 12270
Chicago, IL 60612
312 738-1336, Ext 1341
E-mail: bor@ascp.org
www.ascp.org

National Certification Agency for Medical Laboratory Personnel
PO Box 15945-289
Lenexa, KS 66285
913 438-5110
E-mail: nca-info@goamp.com
www.nca-info.org

American Association of Bioanalysts
Board of Registry
906 Olive Street, Suite 1200
St. Louis, MO 63101-1434
www.aab.org

American Medical Technologists
710 Higgins Road
Park Ridge, IL 60068-5765
847 823-5169
E-mail: amtmail@aol.com
www.amt1.com

Program Accreditation
Dianne M Cearlock, PhD
Chief Executive Officer (CEO)
National Accrediting Agency for Clinical Laboratory Sciences
8410 W Bryn Mawr Avenue, Suite 670
Chicago, IL 60631-3415
773 714-8880
773 714-8886 Fax
E-mail: dcearlock@naacls.org
www.naacls.org

Clinical Assistant

Massachusetts

Springfield Technical Community College
Clinical Assisting Prgm
Clinical Laboratory Assistant Program
One Amory Square
Springfield, MA 01105-1204
Prgm Dir: Susan A Schneider, MEd MT(ASCP) CLS(NCA)
Tel: 413 755-4846   *Fax:* 413 755-6312
E-mail: SASchneider@stcc.edu

Oregon

Clackamas Community College
Clinical Assisting Prgm
19600 S Molalla Ave
Oregon City, OR 97045-7998
Prgm Dir: Helen Wand, MT(ASCP)
Tel: 503 657-6958, Ext 5505   *Fax:* 503 722-5878
E-mail: helenw@clackamas.edu

Clinical Laboratory Scientist/Medical Technologist

Alabama

University of Alabama at Birmingham
Clin Lab Scientist/Med Technologist Prgm
RMSB 446
1705 University Blvd
Birmingham, AL 35294-1212
http://main.uab.edu/Shrp/default.aspx?pid=78012
Prgm Dir: Janelle M Chiasera, PhD MT(ASCP)
Tel: 205 934-7384   *Fax:* 205 975-7302
E-mail: chiasera@uab.edu

University of South Alabama
Clin Lab Scientist/Med Technologist Prgm
Dept of Clinical Laboratory Sciences
1504 Springhill Ave, Rm 2309
Mobile, AL 36604
www.southalabama.edu/alliedhealth/cls/
Prgm Dir: George A Harwell, EdD MT(ASCP)SC CLS(NCA)
Tel: 251 434-3468   *Fax:* 251 434-3403
E-mail: gharwell@usouthal.edu

Auburn University Montgomery
Clin Lab Scientist/Med Technologist Prgm
PO Box 244023
Montgomery, AL 36124-4023
www.aum.edu/cls/
Prgm Dir: Virginia C Hughes, MS MT(ASCP)SBB
Tel: 334 244-3606   *Fax:* 334 244-3146
E-mail: vhughes@mail.aum.edu

Baptist Medical Center South
Clin Lab Scientist/Med Technologist Prgm
2105 E South Blvd
PO Box 11010
Montgomery, AL 36111-0100
Prgm Dir: Jeanne Whitney, MS MT(ASCP)CM
Tel: 334 286-2899   *Fax:* 334 286-3351
E-mail: jwhitney@baptistfirst.org

Tuskegee University
Clin Lab Scientist/Med Technologist Prgm
BIOE 71-271
Booker T Washington Blvd
Tuskegee, AL 36088
www.tuskegee.edu
Prgm Dir: Floyd C Raven, MS MT(ASCP)
Tel: 334 727-8335   *Fax:* 334 727-8259
E-mail: fraven@tuskegee.edu

Alaska

University of Alaska Anchorage
Clin Lab Scientist/Med Technologist Prgm
3211 Providence Dr
Anchorage, AK 99508
Prgm Dir: Heidi Mannion, MS MT(ASCP)
Tel: 907 786-6923   *Fax:* 907 786-6938
E-mail: afham@uaa.alaska.edu

Arizona

Arizona State University
Clin Lab Scientist/Med Technologist Prgm
School of Life Sciences
PO Box 874501
Tempe, AZ 85287-4501
http://sols.asu.edu/cls/
Prgm Dir: Diana Mass, MA MT(ASCP)CLS
Tel: 480 965-7090   *Fax:* 480 965-8126
E-mail: Diana.Mass@asu.edu

Arkansas

Baptist Health Schools Little Rock
Clin Lab Scientist/Med Technologist Prgm
11900 Colonel Glenn Rd, Ste 1000
Little Rock, AR 72210-2820
Prgm Dir: Sandra G Ackerman, MT(ASCP)SH
Tel: 501 202-7409   *Fax:* 501 202-6220
E-mail: sgackerm@baptist-health.org

University of Arkansas for Medical Sciences
Clin Lab Scientist/Med Technologist Prgm
4301 W Markham St, Slot 597
Little Rock, AR 72205
www.uams.edu/chrp/medtech.htm
Prgm Dir: Karen K Hunter, MS MT(ASCP)
Tel: 501 686-5776   *Fax:* 501 526-6563
E-mail: hunterkarenk@uams.edu

Clinical Assistant

Programs*	Class Capacity	Begins	Length (months)	Award	Res. Tuition	Non-res. Tuition	Stipend	Offers:‡ 1	2	3	4
Massachusetts											
Springfield Technical Community College	18	Sep-May	9	Cert	$1,408	$6,016				•	

*Data are shown only for programs that completed the 2007 AMA Survey of Health Professions Education Programs.
‡Key to Offers: 1: Evening or weekend classes; 2: Non-English instruction; 3: Cultural competence instruction; 4: Distance education component.

Arkansas State University
Clin Lab Scientist/Med Technologist Prgm
PO Box 910
State University, AR 72467
www.astate.edu
Prgm Dir: R Whitney Williams, PhD MT(ASCP)SC
Tel: 870 972-3073   *Fax:* 870 972-2004
E-mail: wwilliam@astate.edu

California

California State University - Dominguez Hills
Clin Lab Scientist/Med Technologist Prgm
1000 E Victoria Blvd
Carson, CA 90747-9960
www.csudh.edu
Prgm Dir: Cheryl Jackson-Harris, MS MT(ASCP)SH
Tel: 310 243-3748, Ext 3899   *Fax:* 310 516-3542
E-mail: charris@csudh.edu

Loma Linda University
Clin Lab Scientist/Med Technologist Prgm
School of Allied Health Professions, Dept of CLS
Nichol Hall, Rm A918
Loma Linda, CA 92350
www.llu.edu
Prgm Dir: Katherine Davis, MS MT(ASCP) CLS(NCA)
Tel: 909 558-4966   *Fax:* 909 558-0458
E-mail: kdavis@llu.edu

Univ of California Irvine Med Ctr
Clin Lab Scientist/Med Technologist Prgm
101 City Dr S, Rte 38
Orange, CA 92868
www.ucihs.uci.edu/com/pathology/medtechprog.html
Prgm Dir: Laura S Ogata, MA MT(ASCP)
Tel: 714 456-6305   *Fax:* 714 456-6090
E-mail: logata@uci.edu

Eisenhower Medical Center
Clin Lab Scientist/Med Technologist Prgm
39000 Bob Hope Dr
Rancho Mirage, CA 92270
Prgm Dir: Joan M Steiner-Adler, EdD MA MS MT(ASCP)
Tel: 760 773-4525   *Fax:* 760 773-4363
E-mail: jsteiner@emc.org

Univ of California Davis Health System
Clin Lab Scientist/Med Technologist Prgm
Specialty Testing Center
3740 Business Dr
Sacramento, CA 95820
www.ucdmc.ucdavis.edu/pathology/education/
    cls_training_program/
Prgm Dir: Jiunn Huang, PhD MT(ASCP)
Tel: 916 734-0231   *Fax:* 916 734-0320
E-mail: jiunn.huang@ucdmc.ucdavis.edu

San Francisco State University
Clin Lab Scientist/Med Technologist Prgm
Ctr for Biomedical Laboratory Sci 211
San Francisco, CA 94132
Prgm Dir: Geraldine M Albee, MA CLS(NCA) CNMT
Tel: 415 405-3779   *Fax:* 415 338-7747
E-mail: galbee@sfsu.edu

San Jose State University
Clin Lab Scientist/Med Technologist Prgm
One Washington Square
San Jose, CA 95192-0100
www.sjsu.edu/cls
Prgm Dir: Mara Williams, MS MT(ASCP)
Tel: 408 924-4851   *Fax:* 408 924-4840
E-mail: cls@science.sjsu.edu

Santa Barbara Cottage Hospital
Clin Lab Scientist/Med Technologist Prgm
Pueblo at Bath Sts
PO Box 689
Santa Barbara, CA 93102
www.cottagehealthsystem.org
Prgm Dir: Lynette Hansen, MHA MT(ASCP)EdD CLS
Tel: 805 569-7378   *Fax:* 805 569-8223
E-mail: lhansen@cottagehealthsystem.org

Colorado

Centura Health/Penrose-St Francis Hlth Serv
Clin Lab Scientist/Med Technologist Prgm
2222 N Nevada Ave
Colorado Springs, CO 80907-7021
www.penrosestfrancis.org
Prgm Dir: Sr Rose V Brown, MEd MT(ASCP) CLS(NCA)
Tel: 719 776-5221   *Fax:* 719 776-5584
E-mail: rosebrown@centura.org

Colorado Center for Med Laboratory Science
Clin Lab Scientist/Med Technologist Prgm
1719 E 19th Ave
Denver, CO 80218
Prgm Dir: Karen E Myers, MA MT(ASCP)SC
Tel: 303 839-6485   *Fax:* 303 869-1720
E-mail: kmyers@coloradohealth.org

Parkview Medical Center
Clin Lab Scientist/Med Technologist Prgm
400 W 16th St
Pueblo, CO 81003
www.parkviewmc.com
Prgm Dir: Mary Chasteen, MA MT(ASCP)SBB
    CLS(NCA)
Tel: 719 584-4429   *Fax:* 719 584-4658
E-mail: mary_chasteen@parkviewmc.com

Connecticut

Danbury Hospital
Clin Lab Scientist/Med Technologist Prgm
School of Medical Technology
24 Hospital Ave
Danbury, CT 06810
www.danburyhospital.org/educationandresidencies/
    medical_technology.htm
Prgm Dir: Ana H Vicente, MHA MT(ASCP)
Tel: 203 739-7804   *Fax:* 203 739-8900
E-mail: Ana.Vicente@danhosp.org

Hartford Hospital
Clin Lab Scientist/Med Technologist Prgm
School of Allied Health
80 Seymour St
Hartford, CT 06115
Prgm Dir: Wayne A Aguiar, MS MT(ASCP)
Tel: 860 545-5632   *Fax:* 860 545-5066
E-mail: waguiar@harthosp.org

University of Hartford
Clin Lab Scientist/Med Technologist Prgm
Dana Hall/Rm 429
200 Bloomfield Ave
West Hartford, CT 06117-1599
www.hartford.edu
Prgm Dir: Karen Barrett, MS MT(ASCP)
Tel: 860 768-4489   *Fax:* 860 768-4558
E-mail: barrett@hartford.edu

Delaware

University of Delaware
Clin Lab Scientist/Med Technologist Prgm
Dept of Medical Technology
305 Willard Hall Education Building
Newark, DE 19716
www.udel.edu/medtech
Prgm Dir: Anna P Ciulla, MCC MT(ASCP)SC CC(NRCC)
    CLS(NCA)
Tel: 302 831-2849   *Fax:* 302 831-4180
E-mail: aciulla@udel.edu

District of Columbia

George Washington University
Clin Lab Scientist/Med Technologist Prgm
2300 I St NW, Ste 503
Washington, DC 20037
www.gwumc.edu/healthsci/programs/cls/
Prgm Dir: Sylvia Silver, DA MT(ASCP)
Tel: 202 994-2945   *Fax:* 202 994-5056
E-mail: ssilver@gwu.edu

Howard University
Clin Lab Scientist/Med Technologist Prgm
6th and Bryant Sts NW
Coll of Phar, Nursing & Allied Hlth Sciences
Washington, DC 20059
Prgm Dir: Marguerite E Neita, PhD MT(ASCP)
Tel: 202 806-5632   *Fax:* 202 806-7918
E-mail: mneita@howard.edu

Walter Reed Army Medical Center
Clin Lab Scientist/Med Technologist Prgm
Clinical Lab Officer Course
6900 Georgia Ave NW, DPALS
Washington, DC 20307-5001
Prgm Dir: Patricia Fishback, MA MT(ASCP)
Tel: 202 782-8353   *Fax:* 202 782-4502
E-mail: patricia.fishback@us.army.mil

Washington Hospital Center
Clin Lab Scientist/Med Technologist Prgm
110 Irving St NW
Department of Pathology and Laboratory Medicine
Washington, DC 20010
www.whcenter.org/departments/pathology
Prgm Dir: John C Rees, PhD MS MT(ASCP)
Tel: 202 877-3346   *Fax:* 202 877-5263
E-mail: john.c.rees@medstar.net

Florida

Shands Jacksonville
Clin Lab Scientist/Med Technologist Prgm
655 W Eighth St
Jacksonville, FL 32209
http://jax.shands.org/education/medtech/
Prgm Dir: James D Sigler, MT(ASCP) CLSup(NCA) CLS
Tel: 904 244-9520   *Fax:* 904 244-2899
E-mail: jim.sigler@jax.ufl.edu

St Vincent's Medical Center
Clin Lab Scientist/Med Technologist Prgm
1800 Barrs St
Jacksonville, FL 32204
www.jaxhealth.com/medicalscience
Prgm Dir: Lynnette Chakkaphak, MS MT(ASCP)
Tel: 904 308-3817   *Fax:* 904 308-2970
E-mail: Lchak001@stvincentshealth.com

University of Central Florida
Clin Lab Scientist/Med Technologist Prgm
4000 Central Florida Blvd, HPA II 335A
Orlando, FL 32816-2360
www.biomed.ucf.edu
Prgm Dir: Dorilyn J Hitchcock, MS MT(ASCP)
Tel: 407 823-5220   *Fax:* 407 823-3095
E-mail: hitchcod@mail.ucf.edu

University of West Florida
Clin Lab Scientist/Med Technologist Prgm
11000 University Pkwy
Pensacola, FL 32514-5751
http://uwf.edu/clinicallabsciences
Prgm Dir: Swarna Krothapalli, MS MT(ASCP)
Tel: 850 474-2988   *Fax:* 850 474-2749
E-mail: skrothap@uwf.edu

Bayfront Medical Center
Clin Lab Scientist/Med Technologist Prgm
701 Sixth St S
St Petersburg, FL 33701
www.bayfront.org
Prgm Dir: Dawn Tripolino, MBA MT(ASCP)
Tel: 727 893-6604   *Fax:* 727 893-6861
E-mail: dawn.tripolino@bayfront.org

Tampa General Hospital
Clin Lab Scientist/Med Technologist Prgm
PO Box 1289
Tampa, FL 33601
Prgm Dir: Donald W Vendrone, MPH MT(ASCP)
Tel: 813 844-7284   *Fax:* 813 844-4160
E-mail: dvendron@tgh.org

Georgia

Medical College of Georgia
Clin Lab Scientist/Med Technologist Prgm
EC-3422
1120 15th St
Augusta, GA 30912-0500
www.mcg.edu/SAH/brt/MT.htm
Prgm Dir: Barbara L Russell, EdD MT(ASCP)SH
Tel: 706 721-3046   *Fax:* 706 721-7631
E-mail: brussell@mcg.edu

Armstrong Atlantic State University
Clin Lab Scientist/Med Technologist Prgm
11935 Abercorn St
Savannah, GA 31419-1997
www.medtech.armstrong.edu
Prgm Dir: Hassan Aziz, PhD CLS/NCA
Tel: 912 927-5204   *Fax:* 912 921-5585
E-mail: azizhass@mail.armstrong.edu

Thomas University
Clin Lab Scientist/Med Technologist Prgm
1501 Millpond Rd
Thomasville, GA 31792
www.thomasu.edu
Prgm Dir: Jill Dennis, MEd MT(ASCP) CLS(NCA)
Tel: 229 226-1621, Ext 146   *Fax:* 229 227-6947
E-mail: jdennis@thomasu.edu

Hawaii

University of Hawaii
Clin Lab Scientist/Med Technologist Prgm
1960 East-West Rd/Bio C206
Honolulu, HI 96822
www.hawaii.edu/medtech/Medtech.html
Prgm Dir: Andre Theriault, PhD CLS(C)
Tel: 808 956-8557   *Fax:* 808 956-5457
E-mail: andret@hawaii.edu

Idaho

Idaho State University
Clin Lab Scientist/Med Technologist Prgm
Dept of Biological Sciences
741 S Seventh, Box 8007
Pocatello, ID 83209
http://isu.edu/cls
Prgm Dir: Kathleen Spiegel, PhD MT(ASCP), Acting PD
Tel: 208 236-4378
E-mail: spiekath@isu.edu

Illinois

Rush University
Clin Lab Scientist/Med Technologist Prgm
600 S Paulina St, Ste 1019 AAC
Chicago, IL 60612
www.rushu.rush.edu/cls
Prgm Dir: Herbert J Miller, PhD MT(ASCP) CLS(NCA)
Tel: 312 942-7251   *Fax:* 312 942-6464
E-mail: herb_j_miller@rush.edu

Northern Illinois University
Clin Lab Scientist/Med Technologist Prgm
1425 W Lincoln Hwy
DeKalb, IL 60115-2825
Prgm Dir: Jeanne M Isabel, MSEd
Tel: 815 753-1382   *Fax:* 815 753-1653
E-mail: jisabel@niu.edu

Evanston Northwestern Healthcare - Evanston
Clin Lab Scientist/Med Technologist Prgm
2650 Ridge Ave, Rm 1927D
Department of Pathology and Laboratory Medicine
Evanston, IL 60201
www.enh.org/academicprograms
Prgm Dir: Marcia Hicks, MAdEd MT(ASCP)
Tel: 847 570-2737   *Fax:* 847 570-1938
E-mail: mhicks@enh.org

Edward Hines Jr VA Hospital
Clin Lab Scientist/Med Technologist Prgm
PO Box 5000/113/School
Hines, IL 60141-5113
www.hines.med.va.gov/edu/mt.htm
Prgm Dir: Donna M Wray, MT(ASCP)
Tel: 708 202-8387, Ext 23212   *Fax:* 708 202-2588
E-mail: Donna.Wray@va.gov

Illinois State University
Clin Lab Scientist/Med Technologist Prgm
5220 Health Sciences
Normal, IL 61790-5220
www.healthsciences.ilstu.edu
Prgm Dir: Meridee Van Draska, MS MT(ASCP)
    CLS(NCA)
Tel: 309 438-8269   *Fax:* 309 438-2450
E-mail: mrust@ilstu.edu

Rosalind Franklin Univ of Medicine & Science
Clin Lab Scientist/Med Technologist Prgm
Dept of Clinical Laboratory Sciences
3333 Green Bay Rd
North Chicago, IL 60064
Prgm Dir: Lillian Mundt, MHS CLS(NCA) SpH
Tel: 847 578-8636   *Fax:* 847 578-8651
E-mail: Lillian.Mundt@rosalindfranklin.edu

OSF St Francis Medical Center
Clin Lab Scientist/Med Technologist Prgm
530 NE Glen Oak Ave
Peoria, IL 61637
www.osfhealthcare.org
Prgm Dir: Carol E Becker, MS MT(ASCP) CLS(NCA)
Tel: 309 624-9021   *Fax:* 309 624-9150
E-mail: carol.e.becker@osfhealthcare.org

OSF St Anthony Medical Center
Clin Lab Scientist/Med Technologist Prgm
5666 E State St
Rockford, IL 61108
Prgm Dir: James F Beam, MT(ASCP) CLS(NCA)
Tel: 815 395-5119   *Fax:* 815 395-5364
E-mail: jim.beam@osfhealthcare.org

St John's Hospital
Clin Lab Scientist/Med Technologist Prgm
800 E Carpenter St
Springfield, IL 62769
www.st-johns.org
Prgm Dir: Gilma Roncancio-Weemer, MS CLS(NCA)
    MT(ASCP)
Tel: 217 757-6788   *Fax:* 217 535-3775
E-mail: gilma.roncancio-weemer@st-johns.org

University of Illinois at Springfield
Clin Lab Scientist/Med Technologist Prgm
One University Plaza
MS HSB 314
Springfield, IL 62703
Prgm Dir: Linda J McCown, MS CLS(NCA) MT(ASCP)
Tel: 217 206-7550   *Fax:* 217 206-6162
E-mail: lmcco2@uis.edu

Indiana

St Francis Hospital & Health Centers
Clin Lab Scientist/Med Technologist Prgm
1600 Albany St
Beech Grove, IN 46107
www.stfrancishospitals.org
Prgm Dir: DeAnne S Maxwell, MT(ASCP)
Tel: 317 783-8195   *Fax:* 317 783-8801
E-mail: deanne.maxwell@ssfhs.org

Parkview Hospital
Clin Lab Scientist/Med Technologist Prgm
328 Ley Rd
Fort Wayne, IN 46825
Prgm Dir: Brian Goff, MA MT(ASCP)
Tel: 219 373-9406   *Fax:* 219 373-9418
E-mail: brian.goff@parkview.com

St Margaret Mercy Healthcare Centers
Clin Lab Scientist/Med Technologist Prgm
5454 Hohman Ave
Hammond, IN 46320
www.ssfhs.org
Prgm Dir: Rosemary Ann Duda, MS MT(ASCP)I SM
Tel: 219 932-2300, Ext 34199   *Fax:* 219 852-2508
E-mail: rose.butkiewicz@ssfhs.org

Clarian Health Partners Inc
Clin Lab Scientist/Med Technologist Prgm
3501 W 11th St
Indianapolis, IN 46206
Prgm Dir: Carla B Clem, MS MT(ASCP)
Tel: 317 491-6217   *Fax:* 317 962-2102
E-mail: cclem@clarian.org

Indiana University
Clin Lab Scientist/Med Technologist Prgm
School of Medicine
350 W 11th St
Indianapolis, IN 46202
http://http:www.pathology.iupui.edu/htm/
    clinical_sci.htm
Prgm Dir: Diane S Leland, PhD MT(ASCP)SM
Tel: 317 491-6646   *Fax:* 317 491-6649
E-mail: dleland@iupui.edu

Ball Memorial Hospital
Cosponsor: PA LABS
Clin Lab Scientist/Med Technologist Prgm
2401 University Ave
Muncie, IN 47303
Prgm Dir: Shirley A Replogle, MT(ASCP)
Tel: 765 254-6289, Ext 2289   *Fax:* 765 747-3133
E-mail: replogles@palab.com

Good Samaritan Hospital
Clin Lab Scientist/Med Technologist Prgm
520 S Seventh St
Vincennes, IN 47591
Prgm Dir: Michaele R McDonald, MS MT(ASCP)
Tel: 812 885-3361   *Fax:* 812 885-3135
E-mail: mmcdonald@gshvin.org

Iowa

St Luke's Hospital
Clin Lab Scientist/Med Technologist Prgm
1026 A Ave NE
Cedar Rapids, IA 52402
www.stlukescr.org
Prgm Dir: Nadine Sojka, MS MT(ASCP)SH
Tel: 319 369-7309   *Fax:* 319 369-8095
E-mail: sojkan@crstlukes.com

Mercy Medical Center
Clin Lab Scientist/Med Technologist Prgm
1111 6th Ave
Des Moines, IA 50314
Prgm Dir: Kyla Deibler, MS MT(ASCP) CLS(NCA)
Tel: 515 247-4469   *Fax:* 515 643-8810
E-mail: kdeibler@mercydesmoines.org

Mercy Medical Center - Sioux City
Clin Lab Scientist/Med Technologist Prgm
801 5th St
Sioux City, IA 51101
www.mercysiouxcity.com/services/clinical/
Prgm Dir: Mary K Smith, MS BS MT(ASCP)
Tel: 712 279-2371   *Fax:* 712 279-2372
E-mail: smithmk@mercyhealth.com

St Luke's College
Clin Lab Scientist/Med Technologist Prgm
2720 Stone Park Blvd
Sioux City, IA 51104
www.stlukes.org
Prgm Dir: Pamela G Briese, MS MT(ASCP)SC
Tel: 712 279-3967   *Fax:* 712 233-8017
E-mail: briesepg@stlukes.org

Kansas

University of Kansas Medical Center
Clin Lab Scientist/Med Technologist Prgm
3901 Rainbow Blvd, MS 4048
G014 Eaton
Kansas City, KS 66160
www.cls.kumc.edu
Prgm Dir: Venus J Ward, PhD MT(ASCP) CLS(NCA)
Tel: 913 588-0154   *Fax:* 913 588-5222
E-mail: vward@kumc.edu

Wichita State University
Clin Lab Scientist/Med Technologist Prgm
1845 Fairmount Box 43
Wichita, KS 67260
www.wsu.edu
Prgm Dir: Mary E Conrad, PhD MT(ASCP)
Tel: 316 978-5655, Ext 5655   *Fax:* 316 978-3025
E-mail: mary.conrad@wichita.edu

Kentucky

St Elizabeth Medical Center
Clin Lab Scientist/Med Technologist Prgm
One Medical Village Dr
Edgewood, KY 41017
www.stelizabeth.com
Prgm Dir: Beth Warning, MS MT(ASCP) CLS(NCA)
Tel: 859 301-2417   *Fax:* 859 301-5560
E-mail: bwarning@stelizabeth.com

University of Kentucky
Clin Lab Scientist/Med Technologist Prgm
Div of Clinical Lab Sci
CHS Bldg, 900 S Limestone, Rm 209
Lexington, KY 40536-0200
Prgm Dir: Linda Gorman, PhD MT(ASCP)
Tel: 859 323-1100, Ext 80855   *Fax:* 859 257-2454
E-mail: Linda.Gorman@uky.edu

Bellarmine University
Clin Lab Scientist/Med Technologist Prgm
Lansing Sch of Nursing and Hlth Sci, 108 Pasteur Hall
2001 Newburg Rd
Louisville, KY 40205-0671
http://lansing.bellarmine.edu/cls/
Prgm Dir: Karen Golemboski, MT(ASCP) PhD
Tel: 502 452-8387   *Fax:* 502 452-8389
E-mail: kgolemboski@bellarmine.edu

Owensboro Medical Health System
Clin Lab Scientist/Med Technologist Prgm
PO Box 20007
Owensboro, KY 42304-0007
Prgm Dir: Lisa Sellars Cecil, MS MT(ASCP)
Tel: 270 688-2934   *Fax:* 270 688-2938
E-mail: Lcecil@omhs.org

Eastern Kentucky University
Clin Lab Scientist/Med Technologist Prgm
Dizney 220
521 Lancaster Ave
Richmond, KY 40475-3102
Prgm Dir: David C Hufford, PhD MT(ASCP)
Tel: 859 622-3078   *Fax:* 859 622-1939
E-mail: david.hufford@eku.edu

Louisiana

Rapides Regional Medical Center
Clin Lab Scientist/Med Technologist Prgm
211 Fourth St, PO Box 30101
Alexandria, LA 71301
Prgm Dir: Laine O Reeder, MT(ASCP) SC
Tel: 318 473-3175, Ext 3809   *Fax:* 318 473-3079
E-mail: laine.poe@hcahealthcare.com

Our Lady of the Lake College
Clin Lab Scientist/Med Technologist Prgm
7434 Perkins Rd
Baton Rouge, LA 70808
www.ololcollege.edu
Prgm Dir: Todd Casanova, PhD MT(ASCP)
Tel: 225 768-1745   *Fax:* 225 768-0819
E-mail: tcasanov@ololcollege.edu

Lake Charles Mem Hosp Sch of Med Tech
Clin Lab Scientist/Med Technologist Prgm
1701 Oak Park Blvd
Lake Charles, LA 70601
Prgm Dir: Dianne D Malveaux, MEd MT(ASCP)
Tel: 337 494-3000, Ext 3366   *Fax:* 337 494-2464
E-mail: DMalveaux@LCMH.com

McNeese State University
Clin Lab Scientist/Med Technologist Prgm
4205 Ryan St
Lake Charles, LA 70609-2000
Prgm Dir: Donna Calvert, MEd MT(ASCP)
Tel: 337 475-5655   *Fax:* 337 475-5677
E-mail: dcalvert@mail.mcneese.edu

St Francis Medical Center
Clin Lab Scientist/Med Technologist Prgm
309 Jackson St
PO Box 1901
Monroe, LA 71201-1901
Prgm Dir: Melanie S Chapman, MEd MT(ASCP)
Tel: 318 327-4359   *Fax:* 318 327-4857
E-mail: chapmam@stfran.com

Louisiana State Univ Health Sciences Center
Clin Lab Scientist/Med Technologist Prgm
1900 Gravier St
New Orleans, LA 70112
www.alliedhealth.lsuhsc.edu/ClinicalLaboratory
Prgm Dir: Louann Lawrence, DrPH CLS(NCA) MT(ASCP)SH
Tel: 504 568-4276   *Fax:* 504 568-6761
E-mail: llawre@lsuhsc.edu

Louisiana State U Hlth Sci Ctr - Shreveport
Clin Lab Scientist/Med Technologist Prgm
PO Box 33932
1501 Kings Hwy
Shreveport, LA 71130-3932
www.sh.lsuhsc.edu/ah
Prgm Dir: Lynda A Britton, PhD CLS(NCA)
Tel: 318 675-6609   *Fax:* 318 675-6937
E-mail: lbritt1@lsuhsc.edu

Overton Brooks VA Medical Center
Clin Lab Scientist/Med Technologist Prgm
510 E Stoner Ave
Shreveport, LA 71101-4295
Prgm Dir: Vanessa Jones Johnson, MBA MT(ASC) CLS(NCA)
Tel: 318 424-6169   *Fax:* 318 424-6093
E-mail: vanessa.johnson@med.va.gov

Maine

Eastern Maine Medical Center
Clin Lab Scientist/Med Technologist Prgm
489 State St
Bangor, ME 04401
www.medtech.emmc.org
Prgm Dir: Ellen M Libby, MS MT(ASCP) CLS(NCA)
Tel: 207 973-7616   *Fax:* 207 973-5823
E-mail: elibby@emh.org

Maryland

Morgan State University
Clin Lab Scientist/Med Technologist Prgm
Cold Spring Ln and Hillen Rd
Baltimore, MD 21251
Prgm Dir: Diane Wilson, PhD MT(ASCP)
Tel: 443 885-3611   *Fax:* 443 885-8285
E-mail: dwilson1@jewel.morgan.edu

University of Maryland
Clin Lab Scientist/Med Technologist Prgm
Clin Lab Scientist/Med & Research Technology Prgm
100 Penn St, AHB
Baltimore, MD 21201-1082
http://medschool.umaryland.edu/dmrt
Prgm Dir: Deirdre D Parsons, MS MT(ASCP)SBB
Tel: 410 706-1829   *Fax:* 410 706-0073
E-mail: dparsons@som.umaryland.edu

Salisbury University
Clin Lab Scientist/Med Technologist Prgm
1101 Camden Ave
Salisbury, MD 21801
www.salisbury.edu/healthsci/MDTC1.htm
Prgm Dir: Johanna W Laird, MS MT(ASCP)CM CLS(NCA)
Tel: 410 543-6364   *Fax:* 410 548-9185
E-mail: jwlaird@salisbury.edu

Massachusetts

Northeastern University
Clin Lab Scientist/Med Technologist Prgm
360 Huntington Ave
312 Robinson Hall
Boston, MA 02215
www.neu.edu
Prgm Dir: Mary Louise Turgeon, EdD CLS(NCA)
Tel: 617 373-4192   *Fax:* 617 373-3665
E-mail: m.turgeon@neu.edu

University of Massachusetts - Lowell
Clin Lab Scientist/Med Technologist Prgm
Department of Clinical Laboratory and Nutritional
Sciences
3 Solomont Way, Ste 4, Weed Hall
Lowell, MA 01854
www.uml.edu/college/she/
Prgm Dir: Kathleen (Kay) Doyle, PhD MT(ASCP)
Tel: 978 934-4425, Ext 4425 *Fax:* 978 934-3006
E-mail: Kathleen_Doyle@uml.edu

University of Massachusetts - Dartmouth
Clin Lab Scientist/Med Technologist Prgm
Dept of Med Lab Science
285 Old Westport Rd
North Dartmouth, MA 02747-2300
www.umassd.edu/cas/medlabscience/welcome.cfm
Prgm Dir: Dorothy A Bergeron, MS CLS(NCA)
Tel: 508 999-8584 *Fax:* 508 999-8418
E-mail: dbergeron@umassd.edu

Berkshire Medical Center
Clin Lab Scientist/Med Technologist Prgm
725 North St
Pittsfield, MA 01201
www.berkshirehealth.com
Prgm Dir: Lori Moore, MEd MT(ASCP)
Tel: 413 447-2580 *Fax:* 413 447-2097
E-mail: Lmoore@bhs1.org

Michigan

Andrews University
Clin Lab Scientist/Med Technologist Prgm
Department of Clinical and Laboratory Sciences
Halenz Hall 326
Berrien Springs, MI 49104
www.andrews.edu/cls
Prgm Dir: Marcia Kilsby, PhD MT(ASCP)SBB CLS(NCA)
Tel: 269 471-6294 *Fax:* 269 471-6218
E-mail: kilsby@andrews.edu

Ferris State University
Clin Lab Scientist/Med Technologist Prgm
VFS210A
200 Ferris Dr
Big Rapids, MI 49307-2740
www.ferris.edu/cls
Prgm Dir: Barbara Ross, MS MT(ASCP)
Tel: 231 591-2317 *Fax:* 231 591-3788
E-mail: rossb@ferris.edu

DMC University Laboratories
Clin Lab Scientist/Med Technologist Prgm
4201 St Antoine
Detroit, MI 48201
www.dmc.org/univ
Prgm Dir: Joyce Salancy, MS MT(ASCP)
Tel: 313 993-0482 *Fax:* 313 993-2900
E-mail: jsalancy@dmc.org

Wayne State University
Clin Lab Scientist/Med Technologist Prgm
Eugene Applebaum College of Pharmacy and Health
Sciences
Ste 4690
Detroit, MI 48201
Prgm Dir: Janet M Brown, MS MT(ASCP) CLS(NCA)
Tel: 313 577-1384 *Fax:* 313 577-5497
E-mail: aa3663@wayne.edu

Michigan State University
Clin Lab Scientist/Med Technologist Prgm
322 N Kedzie Hall
East Lansing, MI 48824
www.medtech.cls.msu.edu
Prgm Dir: Kathryn M Doig, PhD CLS(NCA)
Tel: 517 353-7800, Ext 8 *Fax:* 517 432-2006
E-mail: doig@msu.edu

Hurley Medical Center
Clin Lab Scientist/Med Technologist Prgm
One Hurley Plaza
Flint, MI 48503
Prgm Dir: Sheila Moore, MSA MT(ASCP)SH
Tel: 810 762-7092 *Fax:* 810 762-7082
E-mail: smoore3@hurleymc.com

Grand Valley State University
Clin Lab Scientist/Med Technologist Prgm
301 Michigan St NE, Ste 200
Grand Rapids, MI 49503-3314
www.gvsu.edu/cls/
Prgm Dir: Linda Goossen, PhD MT(ASCP)
Tel: 616 331-8540 *Fax:* 616 331-5999
E-mail: goossenl@gvsu.edu

St John Health
Cosponsor: St John Health Laboratories
Clin Lab Scientist/Med Technologist Prgm
19251 Mack Ave, Ste 460
Grosse Pointe Woods, MI 48236
www.stjohn.org/labcareers
Prgm Dir: Marilyn Held, SpM MT(ASCP)DLM
Tel: 313 343-3508 *Fax:* 313 881-4727
E-mail: marilyn.held@stjohn.org

Northern Michigan University
Clin Lab Scientist/Med Technologist Prgm
1401 Presque Isle Ave
3513 West Science
Marquette, MI 49855
Prgm Dir: Lucille A Contois, MA MT(ASCP)
Tel: 906 227-1660 *Fax:* 906 227-1309
E-mail: lcontois@nmu.edu

William Beaumont Hospital
Clin Lab Scientist/Med Technologist Prgm
3601 W 13 Mile Rd
Department of Clinical Pathology - RI 105
Royal Oak, MI 48073-6769
www.beaumont.edu/alliedhealth
Prgm Dir: Nancy E Ramirez, MS MT(ASCP) SH
CLS(NCA)
Tel: 248 551-8023, Ext 15135 *Fax:* 248 551-3694
E-mail: nramirez@beaumont.edu

Eastern Michigan University
Clin Lab Scientist/Med Technologist Prgm
342 Marshall Building
Ypsilanti, MI 48197
Prgm Dir: Gary Hammerberg, EdD MT(ASCP)
Tel: 734 487-3223 *Fax:* 734 487-4095
E-mail: gary.hammerberg@emich.edu

Minnesota

Fairview Health Services
Clin Lab Scientist/Med Technologist Prgm
2450 Riverside Ave, F180-56
Minneapolis, MN 55454
www.fairview.org/cls
Prgm Dir: Carol T McCoy, PhD MT(ASCP) CLS(NCA)
Tel: 612 672-4298 *Fax:* 612 672-4280
E-mail: cmccoy1@fairview.org

Hennepin County Medical Center
Clin Lab Scientist/Med Technologist Prgm
701 Park Ave S, Lab P4
Minneapolis, MN 55415
www.hcmc.org
Prgm Dir: Roberta J Montgomery, MLS MT(ASCP)SI
CLS(NCA)
Tel: 612 873-3022 *Fax:* 612 904-4229
E-mail: robbi.montgomery@co.hennepin.mn.us

University of Minnesota - Minneapolis
Clin Lab Scientist/Med Technologist Prgm
420 Delaware St SE, MMC 711
Minneapolis, MN 55455
Prgm Dir: Carol L Wells, PhD MT(ASCP)
Tel: 612 625-5951 *Fax:* 612 625-5901
E-mail: wells002@umn.edu

Mississippi

University of Southern Mississippi
Clin Lab Scientist/Med Technologist Prgm
118 College Dr #5134
Hattiesburg, MS 39406-0001
www.usm.edu/medtech
Prgm Dir: M Jane Hudson, PhD MT(ASCP)SM
CLS(NCA)
Tel: 601 266-4908 *Fax:* 601 266-4913
E-mail: jane.hudson@usm.edu

Mississippi Baptist Medical Center
Clin Lab Scientist/Med Technologist Prgm
1225 N State St
Jackson, MS 39202
www.mbhs.org
Prgm Dir: Jennifer Knight, MHS CLS (NCA) MT(ASCP)
Tel: 601 968-3070, Ext 7376 *Fax:* 601 974-6286
E-mail: jknight@mbhs.org

University of Mississippi Medical Center
Clin Lab Scientist/Med Technologist Prgm
2500 N State St
Jackson, MS 39216
Prgm Dir: LaToya Richards, PhD MT(ASCP)
Tel: 601 984-6321 *Fax:* 601 815-1717
E-mail: lrichards@shrp.umsmed.edu

North Mississippi Medical Center
Clin Lab Scientist/Med Technologist Prgm
830 S Gloster
Tupelo, MS 38801
www.nmhs.net/medtech
Prgm Dir: Lee H Montgomery, MT(ASCP)
Tel: 662 377-3066 *Fax:* 662 377-3109
E-mail: Lmontgomery@nmhs.net

Missouri

**Southeast Missouri Hospital College of
Nursing and Health Sciences**
Clin Lab Scientist/Med Technologist Prgm
2001 William St
Cape Girardeau, MO 63703
www.southeastmissourihospital.com/college
Prgm Dir: Ann Green, MS MAEd MT(ASCP)
Tel: 573 334-6825, Ext 31 *Fax:* 573 339-7805
E-mail: agreen@sehosp.org

St John's Regional Medical Center
Clin Lab Scientist/Med Technologist Prgm
2727 McClelland Blvd
Joplin, MO 64804-1695
Prgm Dir: Connie Wilkins, MS MT(ASCP)
Tel: 417 625-2135 *Fax:* 417 659-6429
E-mail: cjwilkin@stj.com

Saint Luke's Hospital
Clin Lab Scientist/Med Technologist Prgm
4401 Wornall Rd
Kansas City, MO 64111
www.saintlukeshealthsystem.org
Prgm Dir: Jane M Rachel, MA MT(ASCP)
Tel: 816 932-2413 *Fax:* 816 932-3822
E-mail: jrachel@saint-lukes.org

North Kansas City Hospital
Clin Lab Scientist/Med Technologist Prgm
2800 Clay Edwards Dr
North Kansas City, MO 64116-3220
www.nkch.org/lab
Prgm Dir: Marisa James, MA MT(ASCP)
Tel: 816 691-1321 *Fax:* 816 346-7304
E-mail: marisa.james@nkch.org

CoxHealth
Clin Lab Scientist/Med Technologist Prgm
3801 S National Ave
Springfield, MO 65807
www.coxhealth.com
Prgm Dir: Douglas D Hubbard, MT(ASCP)
Tel: 417 269-6633   *Fax:* 417 269-4600
E-mail: doug.hubbard@coxhealth.com

Saint Louis University
Clin Lab Scientist/Med Technologist Prgm
3437 Caroline St
St Louis, MO 63104-1111
http://cls.slu.edu
Prgm Dir: Mary Lou Vehige, MA MT(ASCP) CLS (NCA)
Tel: 314 977-8518   *Fax:* 314 977-8503
E-mail: vehigeml@slu.edu

St John's Mercy Medical Center
Clin Lab Scientist/Med Technologist Prgm
615 S New Ballas Rd
St Louis, MO 63141
www.stjohnsmercy.org/sjmmc/departmentservices/scls/
Prgm Dir: Teresa A Taff, MA MT(ASCP)SM
Tel: 314 251-6855   *Fax:* 314 251-4580
E-mail: taffta@stlo.mercy.net

Nebraska

Nebraska Methodist Hospital
Clin Lab Scientist/Med Technologist Prgm
Pathology Center
8303 Dodge St
Omaha, NE 68114
www.unmc.edu/AlliedHealth/medtech
Prgm Dir: Julie Richards, MPA MT(ASCP) BB
Tel: 402 354-4563   *Fax:* 402 354-4535
E-mail: Julie.Richards@nmhs.org

University of Nebraska Medical Center
Clin Lab Scientist/Med Technologist Prgm
987549 Nebraska Medical Center
Omaha, NE 68198-7549
www.unmc.edu/AlliedHealth/medtech
Prgm Dir: Linda L Fell, MS MT(ASCP)SH
Tel: 402 559-7739   *Fax:* 402 559-9044
E-mail: lfell@unmc.edu

Nevada

University of Nevada - Las Vegas
Clin Lab Scientist/Med Technologist Prgm
4505 Maryland Pkwy
Mail Box 453021
Las Vegas, NV 89154-3021
http://alliedhealth.unlv.edu/cls/
Prgm Dir: Janice M Conway-Klaassen, MT(ASCP)SM
CLS(NCA)
Tel: 702 895-3788   *Fax:* 702 895-3872
E-mail: janice.klaassen@unlv.edu

New Hampshire

University of New Hampshire
Clin Lab Scientist/Med Technologist Prgm
210 Kendall Hall
129 Main St
Durham, NH 03824
Prgm Dir: Adele Marone, MS MT(ASCP)
Tel: 603 862-1376   *Fax:* 603 862-3758
E-mail: amarone@cisunix.unh.edu

New Jersey

Monmouth Medical Center
Clin Lab Scientist/Med Technologist Prgm
300 2nd Ave
Long Branch, NJ 07740
Prgm Dir: John A Mihok, MS Ed MT SM(ASCP) CLS
Tel: 732 923-7367   *Fax:* 732 923-7355
E-mail: jmihok@sbhcs.com

Morristown Memorial Hospital
Clin Lab Scientist/Med Technologist Prgm
Atlantic Health System
100 Madison Ave
Morristown, NJ 07960
Prgm Dir: Phyllis R Vail, EdM MT(ASCP)
Tel: 973 971-5282   *Fax:* 973 290-7370
E-mail: phyllis.vail@atlantichealth.org

Jersey Shore University Medical Center
Clin Lab Scientist/Med Technologist Prgm
Florence M Cook School of Medical Laboratory Science
3rd Floor Mehandru Pavilion
Neptune, NJ 07753
www.meridianhealth.com
Prgm Dir: Perla L Simmons, MPA MT(ASCP)SH
Tel: 732 776-4603   *Fax:* 732 776-4592
E-mail: psimmons@meridianhealth.com

Univ of Medicine & Dent of New Jersey
Clin Lab Scientist/Med Technologist Prgm
School of Health Related Professions
65 Bergen St
Newark, NJ 07107-3006
http://shrp.umdnj.edu/programs/cls/medic.htm
Prgm Dir: Elaine M Keohane, PhD CLS(NCA)
Tel: 973 972-5510   *Fax:* 973 972-8527
E-mail: keohanem@umdnj.edu

The Valley Hospital
Clin Lab Scientist/Med Technologist Prgm
223 N Van Dien Ave
Ridgewood, NJ 07450
Prgm Dir: Jacqueline M Opera, MT(ASCP)BB
Tel: 201 447-8234   *Fax:* 201 447-8657
E-mail: jopera@valleyhealth.com

New Mexico

University of New Mexico
Clin Lab Scientist/Med Technologist Prgm
MSC09 5250
1 University of New Mexico
Albuquerque, NM 87131-0001
http://hsc.unm.edu/pathology/medlab/
Prgm Dir: Leslie Danielson, PhD MT(ASCP)
Tel: 505 272-5434   *Fax:* 505 272-8079
E-mail: Ldanielson@salud.unm.edu

New York

New York Methodist Hospital
Clin Lab Scientist/Med Technologist Prgm
506 Sixth St
Brooklyn, NY 11215
Prgm Dir: Lori A Burkard, MS MT(ASCP)
Tel: 718 780-3706   *Fax:* 718 780-3673
E-mail: lab9026@nyp.org

Long Island University - C W Post Campus
Clin Lab Scientist/Med Technologist Prgm
720 Northern Blvd
Brookville, NY 11548
www.liu.edu/health
Prgm Dir: Angela L Meisse, MPA MT(ASCP) SBB
CLS(NCA)
Tel: 516 299-3039   *Fax:* 516 299-3106
E-mail: angela.meisse@liu.edu

University at Buffalo - SUNY
Clin Lab Scientist/Med Technologist Prgm
26 Cary Hall
3435 Main St
Buffalo, NY 14214-3005
www.smbs.buffalo.edu/cls/
Prgm Dir: Robert Klick, MS MT(ASCP)
Tel: 716 829-3630, Ext 109   *Fax:* 716 829-3601
E-mail: klick@buffalo.edu

St John's University
Clin Lab Scientist/Med Technologist Prgm
Dr Andrew J Bartilucci Center
175-07 Horace Harding Exp
Fresh Meadows, NY 11365
Prgm Dir: Ann Paula Zero, MS MT(ASCP) CLS
Tel: 718 990-8421   *Fax:* 718 990-8445
E-mail: zeroa@stjohns.edu

Woman's Christian Association Hospital
Clin Lab Scientist/Med Technologist Prgm
PO Box 840
207 Foote Ave
Jamestown, NY 14702
www.wcahospital.org/mtschool
Prgm Dir: Michele G Harms, MS MT(ASCP)
Tel: 716 664-8484   *Fax:* 716 664-8306
E-mail: michele.harms@wcahospital.org

St Vincent's Hospital Manhattan SVCMC
Clin Lab Scientist/Med Technologist Prgm
153 W 11th St
New York, NY 10011
Prgm Dir: Sr Catherine Sherry, MS MT(ASCP)
Tel: 212 604-8385   *Fax:* 212 604-8426
E-mail: csherry@svcmcny.org

Marist College
Clin Lab Scientist/Med Technologist Prgm
Dept of Medical Laboratory Sciences, DN 228,
  3399 North Rd
Donnelly Hall, Rm 109
Poughkeepsie, NY 12601-1387
http://Marist.edu
Prgm Dir: Robert Sullivan, PhD MT(ASCP)
Tel: 845 575-3000, Ext 2501   *Fax:* 845 575-3184
E-mail: Robert.Sullivan@Marist.edu

Rochester General Hospital
Clin Lab Scientist/Med Technologist Prgm
1425 Portland Ave
Rochester, NY 14621
Prgm Dir: Nancy C Mitchell, MS MT(ASCP)DLM
Tel: 585 922-4274   *Fax:* 585 922-2088
E-mail: nancy.mitchell@viahealth.org

Stony Brook University
Clin Lab Scientist/Med Technologist Prgm
Sch of Hlth Tech and Management
Stony Brook, NY 11794-8205
www.hsc.sunysb.edu/shtm
Prgm Dir: Kathleen Finnegan, MS MT(ASCP)SH
Tel: 631 444-3224   *Fax:* 631 444-8821
E-mail: kathleen.finnegan@stonybrook.edu

SUNY Upstate Medical University
Clin Lab Scientist/Med Technologist Prgm
750 E Adams St
Syracuse, NY 13210
Prgm Dir: Susan Graham, MS MT(ASCP)SH
Tel: 315 464-4608   *Fax:* 315 464-4609
E-mail: grahams@upstate.edu

North Carolina

University of North Carolina - Chapel Hill
Clin Lab Scientist/Med Technologist Prgm
4100 Bondurant Hall, CB # 7145
Division of Clinical Laboratory Science
Chapel Hill, NC 27599-7145
www.med.unc.edu/ahs/clinical
Prgm Dir: Susan J Beck, PhD CLS(NCA)
Tel: 919 966-3033 *Fax:* 919 966-5200
E-mail: sbeck@med.unc.edu

Carolinas College of Health Sciences
Clin Lab Scientist/Med Technologist Prgm
PO Box 32861
Charlotte, NC 28232
Prgm Dir: Elizabeth T Anderson, MHDL MT(ASCP)
CLS(NCA)
Tel: 704 355-4275 *Fax:* 704 355-5967
E-mail: banderson@carolinas.org

Western Carolina University
Clin Lab Scientist/Med Technologist Prgm
120 Moore Hall
Cullowhee, NC 28723
www.wcu.edu/aps/healths/HS_UG-CLS.htm
Prgm Dir: Russell Cheadle, MS MT(ASCP)
Tel: 704 227-3515 *Fax:* 704 227-7446
E-mail: cheadle@email.wcu.edu

East Carolina University
Clin Lab Scientist/Med Technologist Prgm
Department of Clinical Laboratory Science
School of Allied Hlth Sciences
Greenville, NC 27858-4353
www.edu.edu/clsc
Prgm Dir: Richard Bamberg, PhD MT(ASCP)SH
CLDir(NCA) CHES
Tel: 252 744-6064 *Fax:* 252 744-6018
E-mail: bambergw@ecu.edu

Wake Forest University Baptist Medical Center
Clin Lab Scientist/Med Technologist Prgm
Medical Center Blvd
Winston-Salem, NC 27157
http://www1.wfubmc.edu/pathology/medtech
Prgm Dir: Elizabeth Skillman Gaither, MBA MT(ASCP)
SM
Tel: 336 716-4727 *Fax:* 336 716-6359
E-mail: bgaither@wfubmc.edu

Winston-Salem State University
Clin Lab Scientist/Med Technologist Prgm
CLS Dept FL Atkins Ste 401
601 Martin Luther King Jr Dr
Winston-Salem, NC 27110
Prgm Dir: Denny Ryman, EdD MT(ASCP)
Tel: 336 750-2510 *Fax:* 336 750-2517
E-mail: rymand@wssu.edu

North Dakota

MeritCare Medical Center
Clin Lab Scientist/Med Technologist Prgm
737 Broadway
PO Box MC
Fargo, ND 58122-0041
https://www.meritcare.com/jobs
Prgm Dir: Sandra Matthey, MS BS MT(ASCP)
Tel: 701 234-2481 *Fax:* 701 234-2403
E-mail: sandra.matthey@meritcare.com

University of North Dakota
Clin Lab Scientist/Med Technologist Prgm
University of North Dakota
Dept of Pathology/CLS
Grand Forks, ND 58202-9037
http://pathology.med.und.nodak.edu/cls/
Prgm Dir: Ruth Paur, MS CLS(NCA) MT(ASCP)
Tel: 701 777-2651 *Fax:* 701 777-2404
E-mail: ruthpaur@medicine.nodak.edu

Ohio

Ohio Northern University
Clin Lab Scientist/Med Technologist Prgm
525 S Main St
Ada, OH 45810
www.onu.edu
Prgm Dir: Cara L Calvo, MS MT(ASCP)SH CLS(NCA)
Tel: 419 772-3084 *Fax:* 419 772-2330
E-mail: c-calvo@onu.edu

Children's Hospital Medical Ctr of Akron
Clin Lab Scientist/Med Technologist Prgm
One Perkins Square
Akron, OH 44308
www.akronchildrens.org
Prgm Dir: Sharon K Shriber, MBA MT(ASCP)SH
Tel: 330 543-8676 *Fax:* 330 543-6303
E-mail: sshriber@chmca.org

Bowling Green State University
Clin Lab Scientist/Med Technologist Prgm
504 Life Science Bldg
Bowling Green, OH 43403
www.bgsu.edu/departments/medt.html
Prgm Dir: Robert Harr, MS MT(ASCP)
Tel: 419 372-8109 *Fax:* 419 372-0332
E-mail: rharr@bgnet.bgsu.edu

University of Cincinnati Medical Center
Clin Lab Scientist/Med Technologist Prgm
3202 Eden Ave
Rm 371 French East, ML 0394
Cincinnati, OH 45267-0394
www.cahs.uc.edu
Prgm Dir: Linda J Graeter, PhD MT(ASCP)
Tel: 513 558-2018 *Fax:* 513 558-6002
E-mail: graetel@email.uc.edu

Ohio State University
Clin Lab Scientist/Med Technologist Prgm
453 W 10th Ave
535 Atwell Hall
Columbus, OH 43210
www.amp.osu.edu/mt/
Prgm Dir: Sally V Rudmann, PhD MT(ASCP)SBB
Tel: 614 292-7303, Ext 5 *Fax:* 614 292-0210
E-mail: rudmann.1@osu.edu

Wright State University
Clin Lab Scientist/Med Technologist Prgm
235A Biological Sciences Bldg
3640 Colonel Glenn Hwy
Dayton, OH 45435
Prgm Dir: Cheryl Conley, PhD MT(ASCP)
Tel: 937 775-2306 *Fax:* 937 775-3320
E-mail: cheryl.conley@wright.edu

Southwest General Health Center
Clin Lab Scientist/Med Technologist Prgm
18697 E Bagley Rd
Middleburg Heights, OH 44130
www.swgeneral.com
Prgm Dir: Corinne Hartwell, MS MT(ASCP)
Tel: 440 816-8879 *Fax:* 440 816-8690
E-mail: chartwell@swgeneral.com

St Vincent Mercy Medical Center
Clin Lab Scientist/Med Technologist Prgm
2222 Cherry St
Toledo, OH 43608
www.ehealthconnection.com/regions/toledo/content/
Integrated_CLS_Mercy_Program.asp
Prgm Dir: Karlyn Lange
Tel: 419 251-8252 *Fax:* 419 251-7816
E-mail: Karlyn_Lange@mhsnr.org

Oklahoma

Valley View Regional Hospital
Clin Lab Scientist/Med Technologist Prgm
430 N Monta Vista
Ada, OK 74820
www.valeyviewregional.com/medicalservices/laboratory
Prgm Dir: Leah Babcock, MSHR MT(ASCP)
Tel: 405 421-1596 *Fax:* 405 421-1525
E-mail: lbabcock@vvrh.com

Comanche County Memorial Hospital
Clin Lab Scientist/Med Technologist Prgm
PO Box 129
Lawton, OK 73502
Prgm Dir: Gary Jackson, SH(ASCP)
Tel: 405 355-8699, Ext 3362 *Fax:* 405 585-5462
E-mail: jacksong@memorialhealthsource.com

Muskogee Regional Medical Center
Clin Lab Scientist/Med Technologist Prgm
300 Rockefeller Dr
Muskogee, OK 74401
Prgm Dir: Tamme A Garrison, BS MT(ASCP)
Tel: 918 684-2139 *Fax:* 918 684-2223
E-mail: tamme.garrison@capellahealth.com

Saint Francis Hospital
Clin Lab Scientist/Med Technologist Prgm
6161 S Yale Ave
Tulsa, OK 74136
Prgm Dir: Theresa D Foster, MPH MT(ASCP)SH
Tel: 918 494-6342 *Fax:* 918 494-1497
E-mail: tdfoster@saintfrancis.com

Oregon

Oregon Health & Science University
Cosponsor: Oregon Insitute of Technology
Clin Lab Scientist/Med Technologist Prgm
3181 SW Sam Jackson Park Rd, MTGH
Portland, OR 97239-3098
www.oit.edu/cls
Prgm Dir: Marian Ewell, MT(ASCP)SBB
Tel: 503 494-8589 *Fax:* 503 494-2730
E-mail: ewellm@ohsu.edu

Pennsylvania

Altoona Regional Health System
Clin Lab Scientist/Med Technologist Prgm
Altoona Hospital Campus
620 Howard Ave
Altoona, PA 16601-4899
Prgm Dir: Joseph R Noel, CLS(NCA) MT(ASCP)
Tel: 814 889-2835 *Fax:* 814 889-6001
E-mail: jnoel@altoonaregional.org

Neumann College
Clin Lab Scientist/Med Technologist Prgm
One Neumann Dr
Aston, PA 19014
Prgm Dir: Sandra M Weiss, EdD MT (ASCP) CLS (NCA)
Tel: 610 558-5607 *Fax:* 610 361-5314
E-mail: sweiss@neumann.edu

Saint Vincent Health Center
Clin Lab Scientist/Med Technologist Prgm
232 W 25th St
Erie, PA 16544-0002
www.saintvincenthealth.com/medicalprofessionals/
medical_technology.htm
Prgm Dir: Stephen M Johnson, MS MT(ASCP)
Tel: 814 452-5365 *Fax:* 814 456-4784
E-mail: sjohnson@svhs.org

Conemaugh Memorial Medical Center
Clin Lab Scientist/Med Technologist Prgm
1086 Franklin St
Johnstown, PA 15905-4398
Prgm Dir: Abra Elkins, MA MT(ASCP)
Tel: 814 534-5578   *Fax:* 814 534-3253
E-mail: aelkins@conemaugh.org

Lancaster Gen Coll of Nursing & Hlth Sciences
Clin Lab Scientist/Med Technologist Prgm
410 N Lime St
Lancaster, PA 17602
www.lancastergeneral.org
Prgm Dir: Wendy S Gayle, MS MT(ASCP) CLS(NCA)
Tel: 717 544-7208   *Fax:* 717 544-5970
E-mail: wsgayle@lancastergeneral.org

Pennsylvania Hospital
Clin Lab Scientist/Med Technologist Prgm
800 Spruce St
Rm 756 Preston Building
Philadelphia, PA 19107
www.uphs.upenn.edu/pahedu/med_tech
Prgm Dir: Jean Buchenhorst, MS MT(ASCP)
Tel: 215 829-7634   *Fax:* 215 829-7564
E-mail: Jean.Buchenhorst@uphs.upenn.edu

St Christopher's Hospital for Children
Clin Lab Scientist/Med Technologist Prgm
Dept of Pathology and Laboratory Medicine
E Erie Ave at N Front St
Philadelphia, PA 19134
Prgm Dir: Richard Vandell, MS MT(ASCP) SC SH
Tel: 215 427-5050
E-mail: Richard.Vandell@Tenethealth.com

Thomas Jefferson University
Clin Lab Scientist/Med Technologist Prgm
130 S 9th St, Ste 1924
Philadelphia, PA 19107
Prgm Dir: Janet Devine, EdD MT(ASCP)
Tel: 215 503-8187   *Fax:* 215 503-2189
E-mail: Janet.Devine@jefferson.edu

Reading Hospital & Medical Center
Clin Lab Scientist/Med Technologist Prgm
PO Box 16052
Reading, PA 19612-6052
www.readinghospital.org
Prgm Dir: Sharon Kay Strauss, MS CLS(NCA)
   MT(ASCP)SM CLSp(NCA)
Tel: 610 988-8273   *Fax:* 610 988-5964
E-mail: strausss@readinghospital.org

Robert Packer Hospital
Cosponsor: Guthrie Health Systems
Clin Lab Scientist/Med Technologist Prgm
Guthrie Square
Sayre, PA 18840
www.guthrie.org/medtech
Prgm Dir: Brian D Spezialetti, MS MT(ASCP)
Tel: 570 882-4736   *Fax:* 570 882-6509
E-mail: spezialetti_brian@ghs.guthrie.org

Mount Nittany Medical Center
Clin Lab Scientist/Med Technologist Prgm
1800 E Park Ave
State College, PA 16803
www.mountnittany.org
Prgm Dir: Michael W Archer, MEd MT(ASCP)
Tel: 814 231-7279   *Fax:* 814 231-7390
E-mail: marcher@mountnittany.org

Williamsport Hosp & Medical Center
Clin Lab Scientist/Med Technologist Prgm
777 Rural Ave
Williamsport, PA 17701
www.shscares.edu
Prgm Dir: Loretta A Moffatt, MHA MT(ASCP)
Tel: 570 321-2326   *Fax:* 570 321-2727
E-mail: lmoffatt@susquehannahealth.org

York Hospital/WellSpan Health
Clin Lab Scientist/Med Technologist Prgm
1001 S George St
York, PA 17405-7198
www.wellspan.org/EducationResearch/AlliedHealthEduc
   ation_YHLabScience.htm
Prgm Dir: Carolyn Darr, MA MT(ASCP)
Tel: 717 851-2473   *Fax:* 717 851-2934
E-mail: cdarr@wellspan.org

Puerto Rico

Pontifical Catholic University
Clin Lab Scientist/Med Technologist Prgm
2250 Las Americas Ave, Ste 588
Ponce, PR 00717-9997
Prgm Dir: Maribel Figueroa Pena, MS MT(ASCP)
Tel: 787 841-2000, Ext 1585   *Fax:* 787 651-2000
E-mail: tecmed@email.pucpr.edu

Inter American University of Puerto Rico
Clin Lab Scientist/Med Technologist Prgm
Call Box 5100
San German, PR 00683-9801
www.sg.inter.edu
Prgm Dir: Irma Mendez, MS MT(ASCP)
Tel: 787 264-1912, Ext 7711   *Fax:* 787 892-6350
E-mail: imendez@sg.inter.edu

**Inter American University of Puerto Rico -
   Metro Campus**
Clin Lab Scientist/Med Technologist Prgm
Sein St, Road 1
Francisco Sein State Rd 1
San Juan, PR 00926
Prgm Dir: Ida Mejias, PhD MT(ASCP)
Tel: 787 250-1912, Ext 2406   *Fax:* 787 767-5081
E-mail: iamejias@metro.inter.edu

University of Puerto Rico
Clin Lab Scientist/Med Technologist Prgm
Med Sciences Campus, School of Health Professions
PO Box 365067
San Juan, PR 00936-5067
http://cprsweb.rcm.upr.edu
Prgm Dir: Carmen Ofelia Melendez, EdD MT(ASCP)
Tel: 787 758-2525, Ext 2106   *Fax:* 787 756-7220
E-mail: ofeliamelendez@cprs.rcm.upr.edu

Rhode Island

Our Lady of Fatima Hospital
Clin Lab Scientist/Med Technologist Prgm
200 High Service Ave
North Providence, RI 02904
Prgm Dir: Frances Ingersoll, MS MT(ASCP) CLS(NCA)
Tel: 401 456-3416   *Fax:* 401 456-3695
E-mail: fingersoll@saintjosephri.com

Rhode Island Hospital
Clin Lab Scientist/Med Technologist Prgm
593 Eddy St
PO Building, Rm 034
Providence, RI 02903
Prgm Dir: David J Mello, MS MT(ASCP) CLS(NCA)
Tel: 401 444-5724   *Fax:* 401 444-0151
E-mail: djmello@lifespan.org

South Carolina

Palmetto Health Baptist
Clin Lab Scientist/Med Technologist Prgm
Taylor at Marion Sts
Columbia, SC 29220
Prgm Dir: Jennifer R Gray, MPH MT(ASCP) HT(ASCP)
Tel: 803 296-5014
E-mail: jennifer.gray@palmettohealth.org

McLeod Regional Medical Center
Clin Lab Scientist/Med Technologist Prgm
555 E Cheves St
PO Box 100551
Florence, SC 29506
www.peedeeahec.net
Prgm Dir: Vicki Anderson, MT(ASCP)
Tel: 843 777-2497   *Fax:* 843 777-2071
E-mail: vanderson@mcleodhealth.org

Lexington Medical Center
Clin Lab Scientist/Med Technologist Prgm
2720 Sunset Blvd
West Columbia, SC 29169
www.lexmed.com
Prgm Dir: Ann Beaman, MSW BS MT(ASCP)
Tel: 803 936-8126   *Fax:* 803 936-8910
E-mail: ajbeaman@lexhealth.org

South Dakota

Rapid City Regional Hospital
Clin Lab Scientist/Med Technologist Prgm
353 Fairmont Blvd
Rapid City, SD 57701
www.rcrh.org/clsp
Prgm Dir: Pam Kieffer, MS CLS(NCA) MT(ASCP)
Tel: 605 719-8092   *Fax:* 605 719-2205
E-mail: pkieffer@rcrh.org

Sanford Medical Center
Cosponsor: Sanford Health
Clin Lab Scientist/Med Technologist Prgm
1305 W 18th St
Sioux Falls, SD 57117-5039
www.sanfordhealth.org
Prgm Dir: Renee Rydell, MBA MS MT(ASCP)
Tel: 605 333-7104   *Fax:* 605 333-1532
E-mail: rydellr@sanfordhealth.org

Tennessee

Austin Peay State University
Clin Lab Scientist/Med Technologist Prgm
PO Box 4718
Clarksville, TN 37044
www.apsu.edu/medtech
Prgm Dir: Robert D Robison, PhD MT(ASCP)
Tel: 931 221-7018   *Fax:* 931 221-6323
E-mail: RobisonR@apsu.edu

Lincoln Memorial University
Clin Lab Scientist/Med Technologist Prgm
6965 Cumberland Gap Pkwy
Harrogate, TN 37752
www.lmunet.edu
Prgm Dir: Bill Engle, DD ThD MS(CLS) MT(ASCP)
Tel: 423 869-6471   *Fax:* 423 869-6244
E-mail: bengle@lmunet.edu

Univ of Tennessee Medical Ctr at Knoxville
Clin Lab Scientist/Med Technologist Prgm
1924 Alcoa Hwy SW
Knoxville, TN 37920
www.utmedicalcenter.org/health_professionals/
   educational_services/medical_technology_program
Prgm Dir: Betty M White, MAT MT(ASCP)
Tel: 865 544-9087   *Fax:* 865 525-5762
E-mail: BMWhite@mc.utmck.edu

University of Tennessee Health Science Ctr
Clin Lab Scientist/Med Technologist Prgm
930 Madison Ave, #664
Memphis, TN 38163
www.utmem.edu/allied/mthome.html
Prgm Dir: Linda Ross, MS BS MT(ASCP) CLS(NCA)
Tel: 901 448-6304   *Fax:* 901 448-7545
E-mail: lross@utmem.edu

Tennessee State University
Clin Lab Scientist/Med Technologist Prgm
3500 John A Merritt Blvd
Nashville, TN 37203
www.tnstate.edu
Prgm Dir: Theola Copeland, MS MT(ASCP)
Tel: 615 963-5062   *Fax:* 615 963-2538
E-mail: tcopeland@tnstate.edu

Vanderbilt University Medical Center
Clin Lab Scientist/Med Technologist Prgm
4605D The Vanderbilt Clinic
1165 21st Ave S
Nashville, TN 37232-5310
Prgm Dir: Maralie Gaffron Exton, MT(ASCP)SH
Tel: 615 322-6940   *Fax:* 615 343-8420
E-mail: maralie.exton@vanderbilt.edu

Texas

Austin State Hospital
Clin Lab Scientist/Med Technologist Prgm
4110 Guadalupe St
Austin, TX 78751-4296
Prgm Dir: Judith D Larsen, MT(ASCP)SH
Tel: 512 419-2038   *Fax:* 512 419-2039
E-mail: judy.larsen@mhmr.state.tx.us

CHRISTUS Hospital - St Elizabeth
Clin Lab Scientist/Med Technologist Prgm
2830 Calder St, PO Box 5405
Beaumont, TX 77726-5405
www.christusste.org
Prgm Dir: Deborah R Zink, MBA MT(ASCP)
Tel: 409 899-7150, Ext 4002   *Fax:* 409 899-7991
E-mail: debbi.zink@christushealth.org

Texas A&M University - Corpus Christi
Clin Lab Scientist/Med Technologist Prgm
College of Science and Technology
6300 Ocean Dr
Corpus Christi, TX 78412
Prgm Dir: Christina Thompson, EdD MT(ASCP)SBB
Tel: 361 825-2473   *Fax:* 361 825-3719
E-mail: cthomp@falcon.tamucc.edu

Univ of Texas Southwestern Med Ctr
Clin Lab Scientist/Med Technologist Prgm
5323 Harry Hines Blvd
Dallas, TX 75390-8878
www.utsouthwestern.edu/utsw/medlabsci
Prgm Dir: Lynn M Little, PhD MBA CLS(NCA)
MT(ASCP)M
Tel: 214 648-1780   *Fax:* 214 648-1029
E-mail: lynn.little@utsouthwestern.edu

Univ of Texas - Pan American
Clin Lab Scientist/Med Technologist Prgm
1201 W University Dr
Edinburg, TX 78541
www.panam.edu/dept/clinlab/
Prgm Dir: Karen Chandler, MA MT(ASCP) CLS (NCA)
Tel: 956 381-2296   *Fax:* 956 318-5253
E-mail: kchandler@utpa.edu

University of Texas at El Paso
Clin Lab Scientist/Med Technologist Prgm
1101 N Campbell, Rm 714
El Paso, TX 79902
http://academics.utep.edu/cls
Prgm Dir: M Lorraine Torres, MS MT(ASCP) ABD
Tel: 915 747-7282   *Fax:* 915 747-7207
E-mail: lorit@utep.edu

Tarleton State University
Clin Lab Scientist/Med Technologist Prgm
1501 Enderly Place
Fort Worth, TX 76104
Prgm Dir: Sally S Lewis, MS MT(ASCP) HTL (ASCP)
Tel: 817 926-1101   *Fax:* 817 922-8103
E-mail: slewis@tarleton.edu

University of Texas Medical Branch
Clin Lab Scientist/Med Technologist Prgm
School of Allied Health Sciences
301 University Blvd
Galveston, TX 77555-1140
www.sahs.utmb.edu/cls/
Prgm Dir: Vicki S Freeman, PhD MT(ASCP)SC
Tel: 409 772-3056   *Fax:* 409 772-9470
E-mail: vfreeman@utmb.edu

Methodist Hospital
Clin Lab Scientist/Med Technologist Prgm
6565 Fannin, B154
Houston, TX 77030
Prgm Dir: Judy Jobe, MT(ASCP)
Tel: 713 441-2599   *Fax:* 713 793-7408
E-mail: jjobe@tmhs.org

Texas Southern University
Clin Lab Scientist/Med Technologist Prgm
3100 Cleburne Ave
Houston, TX 77004
www.tsu.edu
Prgm Dir: Dorothy J Quiller, MEd BS MT(ASCP)
Tel: 713 313-7248   *Fax:* 713 313-1094
E-mail: quiller_dj@tsu.edu

Univ of Texas M D Anderson Cancer Ctr
Clin Lab Scientist/Med Technologist Prgm
1100 Holcombe Blvd, Unit 0204
Houston, TX 77030
www.mdanderson.org/healthsciences
Prgm Dir: Karen McClure, MS CLS(NCA)
MT(ASCP)SBB
Tel: 713 745-1648   *Fax:* 713 745-3337
E-mail: kmcclure@mdanderson.org

Texas Tech Univ Health Sciences Center
Clin Lab Scientist/Med Technologist Prgm
School of Allied Health Sciences
3601 4th St
Lubbock, TX 79430
Prgm Dir: Lori Rice-Spearman, MS MT(ASCP)
Tel: 806 743-3252   *Fax:* 806 743-3249
E-mail: lori.ricespearman@ttuhsc.edu

Univ of Texas Hlth Sci Ctr at San Antonio
Clin Lab Scientist/Med Technologist Prgm
7703 Floyd Curl Dr
San Antonio, TX 78229-3900
www.uthscsa.edu/sah/cls/cls.html
Prgm Dir: Shirlyn B McKenzie, PhD
Tel: 210 567-8860, Ext 7-8868   *Fax:* 210 567-8875
E-mail: mckenzie@uthscsa.edu

Texas State University - San Marcos
Clin Lab Scientist/Med Technologist Prgm
601 University Dr
San Marcos, TX 78666-4616
www.txstate.edu/cls
Prgm Dir: David M Falleur, MEd MT(ASCP) CLS(NCA)
Tel: 512 245-3500   *Fax:* 512 245-7860
E-mail: dfalleur@txstate.edu

Scott & White Hospital
Clin Lab Scientist/Med Technologist Prgm
2401 S 31st St
Temple, TX 76508
www.sw.org
Prgm Dir: Mary Ruth Beckham, MEd MT(ASCP
Tel: 254 724-5970   *Fax:* 254 724-8395
E-mail: mbeckham@swmail.sw.org

Hillcrest Baptist Medical Center
Clin Lab Scientist/Med Technologist Prgm
3000 Herring Ave
Waco, TX 76708
Prgm Dir: Kele D Johnson, MHSM MT(ASCP)
Tel: 254 202-8133   *Fax:* 254 202-5675
E-mail: kjohnson@hillcrest.net

United Regional Health Care Systems
Clin Lab Scientist/Med Technologist Prgm
1600 Eleventh St
Wichita Falls, TX 76301
Prgm Dir: Gwendolyn Morman, MS MA MT(ASCP)
Tel: 940 764-3187   *Fax:* 940 764-3328
E-mail: gmorman@urhcs.org

Utah

Weber State University
Clin Lab Scientist/Med Technologist Prgm
3905 University Circle
Ogden, UT 84408-3905
Prgm Dir: Yasmen Simonian, PhD MT(ASCP) CLS(NCA)
Tel: 801 626-7080   *Fax:* 801 626-7508
E-mail: ysimonian@weber.edu

Brigham Young University
Clin Lab Scientist/Med Technologist Prgm
375 WIDB
Provo, UT 84602
http://mmbio.byu.edu/home/page/About_the_Program.
aspx
Prgm Dir: Shauna C Anderson, PhD CLS (NCA)
MT(ASCP)
Tel: 801 422-8757   *Fax:* 801 422-0014
E-mail: shauna_anderson@byu.edu

University of Utah Health Science Center
Clin Lab Scientist/Med Technologist Prgm
Dept of Pathology
30 North 1900 East
Salt Lake City, UT 84132
http://path.utah.edu/mls
Prgm Dir: Larry Schoeff, MS MT(ASCP)
Tel: 801 585-6989   *Fax:* 801 585-2463
E-mail: lschoeff@path.utah.edu

Vermont

University of Vermont
Clin Lab Scientist/Med Technologist Prgm
Medical Laboratory and Radiation Sciences
302 Rowell Hall
Burlington, VT 05405
www.uvm.edu/mlrs
Prgm Dir: Paula Deming, PhD MT(ASCP)
Tel: 802 656-3811   *Fax:* 802 656-2191
E-mail: paula.deming@uvm.edu

Virginia

Inova Fairfax Hospital
Clin Lab Scientist/Med Technologist Prgm
3300 Gallows Rd
Falls Church, VA 22046
Prgm Dir: Amy Shoemaker, MT(ASCP)DLM
Tel: 703 698-2891   *Fax:* 703 698-2407
E-mail: amy.shoemaker@inova.org

Augusta Medical Center
Clin Lab Scientist/Med Technologist Prgm
PO Box 1000
78 Medical Center Dr
Fishersville, VA 22939
www.augustamed.com/cls
Prgm Dir: Bernadette Bekken, CLS(NCA)MT(ASCP)BB
Tel: 540 332-4539   *Fax:* 540 332-4543
E-mail: bbekken@augustamed.com

Rockingham Memorial Hospital
Clin Lab Scientist/Med Technologist Prgm
235 Cantrell Ave
Harrisonburg, VA 22801
Prgm Dir: Sue W Lawton, MS MA MT(ASCP)
Tel: 540 564-5407   *Fax:* 540 433-4284
E-mail: slawton@rhcc.com

Norfolk State University
Clin Lab Scientist/Med Technologist Prgm
700 Park Ave
Norfolk, VA 23504
www.nsu.edu
Prgm Dir: Mildred Fuller, PhD MT(ASCP) CLS(NCA)
Tel: 757 823-2366 *Fax:* 757 823-2909
E-mail: mkfuller@nsu.edu

Old Dominion University
Clin Lab Scientist/Med Technologist Prgm
School of Med Laboratory and Radiation Sciences
2118 Health Sciences Bldg
Norfolk, VA 23529
http://hs.odu.edu/medlab/academics/medtech/
Prgm Dir: Faye E Coleman, MS MT(ASCP) CLS
Tel: 757 683-3588 *Fax:* 757 683-5028
E-mail: fcoleman@odu.edu

Virginia Commonwealth University
Cosponsor: VCU Medical Center
Clin Lab Scientist/Med Technologist Prgm
PO Box 980583, Medical Center Campus
301 College St
Richmond, VA 23298-0583
Prgm Dir: Teresa Nadder, PhD CLS(NCA) MT(ASCP)
Tel: 804 828-9469 *Fax:* 804 828-1911
E-mail: tsnadder@vcu.edu

Carilion Medical Center
Clin Lab Scientist/Med Technologist Prgm
Carilion Roanoke Community Hospital
101 Elm Ave SW
Roanoke, VA 24013
Prgm Dir: Maribeth Greenway, MEd MT (ASCP)SH
Tel: 540 985-8109 *Fax:* 540 224-4457
E-mail: mgreenway@carilion.com

Washington

University of Washington
Clin Lab Scientist/Med Technologist Prgm
School of Medicine
Dept of Laboratory Medicine, Box 357110
Seattle, WA 98195-7110
Prgm Dir: Mary F Lampe, PhD
Tel: 206 598-2135 *Fax:* 206 598-6189
E-mail: lampe@u.washington.edu

Sacred Heart Medical Center
Clin Lab Scientist/Med Technologist Prgm
101 W Eighth Ave
Spokane, WA 99220-2555
www.shmclab.org
Prgm Dir: Cynthia Hamby, MEd MT(ASCP)
Tel: 509 474-3339 *Fax:* 509 474-5056
E-mail: hambyc@shmc.org

Yakima Regional CLS Program
Cosponsor: Heritage University
Clin Lab Scientist/Med Technologist Prgm
1120 W Spruce St
Yakima, WA 98902
Prgm Dir: Claudia R Steen, MS MT(ASCP)
Tel: 509 454-6100 *Fax:* 509 454-6117
E-mail: yakimacls@yakima.hma-corp.com

West Virginia

Marshall University
Clin Lab Scientist/Med Technologist Prgm
One John Marshall Dr
Huntington, WV 25755
www.marshall.edu/clinical
Prgm Dir: Dorothy J Fike, MS MT(ASCP)
Tel: 304 969-3165 *Fax:* 304 696-3243
E-mail: fike@marshall.edu

West Virginia University
Clin Lab Scientist/Med Technologist Prgm
2163E Health Sciences Ctr N, PO Box 9211
Morgantown, WV 26506-9211
www.hsc.wvu.edu/som/medtech
Prgm Dir: Martha J Lake, EdD CLS(NCA) MT(ASCP)
Tel: 304 293-2069 *Fax:* 304 293-6249
E-mail: mlake@hsc.wvu.edu

West Liberty State College
Clin Lab Scientist/Med Technologist Prgm
Dept of Health Sciences
West Liberty, WV 26074
https://www.westliberty.edu
Prgm Dir: William C Wagener, PhD MT(ASCP)
Tel: 304 336-8177 *Fax:* 304 336-5104
E-mail: wagenerw@westliberty.edu

Wisconsin

Affinity Health System
Clin Lab Scientist/Med Technologist Prgm
St Elizabeth Hospital
1506 S Oneida St
Appleton, WI 54915
Prgm Dir: Cecelia W Landin, MS MT(ASCP)
Tel: 920 738-2132 *Fax:* 920 831-8518
E-mail: clandin@affinityhealth.org

Sacred Heart Hospital
Clin Lab Scientist/Med Technologist Prgm
900 W Clairemont Ave
Eau Claire, WI 54701
Prgm Dir: James R Sorenson, MT(ASCP)
Tel: 715 839-4232 *Fax:* 715 833-4941
E-mail: jsorenson@shec.hshs.org

University of Wisconsin - Madison
Clin Lab Scientist/Med Technologist Prgm
1300 University Ave, 6175 MSC
Madison, WI 53706
www.clsmedtech.wisc.edu
Prgm Dir: Sharon Ehrmeyer, PhD MT(ASCP)
Tel: 608 262-2085 *Fax:* 608 262-9520
E-mail: ehrmeyer@wisc.edu

St Joseph's Hospital
Cosponsor: Marshfield Clinic
Clin Lab Scientist/Med Technologist Prgm
Marshfield Laboratories
611 St Joseph Ave
Marshfield, WI 54449
https://my.marshfieldclinic.org/reference/
Prgm Dir: Julie J Seehafer, MS MT(ASCP)SH
Tel: 715 387-7202 *Fax:* 715 387-7121
E-mail: seehafer.julie@marshfieldclinic.org

Clement J Zablocki VA Medical Center
Clin Lab Scientist/Med Technologist Prgm
5000 W National Ave
Milwaukee, WI 53295
Prgm Dir: Mark J Maticek, MT(ASCP)
Tel: 414 384-2000, Ext 41332 *Fax:* 414 389-4187
E-mail: mark.maticek@med.va.gov

Marquette University
Clin Lab Scientist/Med Technologist Prgm
PO Box 1881
Milwaukee, WI 53201-1881
www.marquette.edu/chs/clls/
Prgm Dir: Linda Milson, MS MT(ASCP)
Tel: 414 288-7566 *Fax:* 414 288-5847
E-mail: linda.milson@marquette.edu

University of Wisconsin - Milwaukee
Clin Lab Scientist/Med Technologist Prgm
Department of Health Sciences
PO Box 413
Milwaukee, WI 53201
http://cfprod.imt.uwm.edu/chs/academics/
    undergraduate/healthsciences/medicaltechnology/
Prgm Dir: Cindy Brown, MA(Ed) CLS(NCA) MT(ASCP)
Tel: 414 229-5299 *Fax:* 414 229-2619
E-mail: cbrown@uwm.edu

University of Wisconsin - Stevens Point
Clin Lab Scientist/Med Technologist Prgm
D127 Science Bldg
Stevens Point, WI 54481-3897
www.uwsp.edu/hlthsci/
Prgm Dir: Susan L Raab, EdD MT(ASCP)
Tel: 715 346-3777 *Fax:* 715 346-2640
E-mail: sraab@uwsp.edu

Aspirus Wausau Hospital
Clin Lab Scientist/Med Technologist Prgm
333 Pine Ridge Blvd
Wausau, WI 54401
www.aspirus.org
Prgm Dir: Susan Flaker Johnson, MEd MT(ASCP)
Tel: 715 847-2000, Ext 53210 *Fax:* 715 847-2930
E-mail: susanj@aspirus.org

Clinical Laboratory Scientist/Medical Technologist

Programs*	Class Capacity	Begins	Length (months)	Award	Res. Tuition	Non-res. Tuition	Stipend	Offers:‡ 1	2	3	4
Alabama											
Auburn University Montgomery	50	Aug	24	Cert	$6,132	$18,096					
Baptist Medical Center South (Montgomery)	8	Jan Jul	12	Cert							
Tuskegee University	10	Aug	24	BSCLS	$11,290	$11,290					
University of Alabama at Birmingham	24	Aug	21	Cert, BS, MS	$6,080	$8,512					
University of South Alabama (Mobile)	14	Aug	21	Dipl, BSCLS	$4,445	$8,890					
Arizona											
Arizona State University (Tempe)	24	Jan	16	Cert, BS	$4,686	$15,846				•	

*Data are shown only for programs that completed the 2007 AMA Survey of Health Professions Education Programs.
‡Key to Offers: 1: Evening or weekend classes; 2: Non-English instruction; 3: Cultural competence instruction; 4: Distance education component.

Clinical Laboratory Scientist/Medical Technologist

Programs*	Class Capacity	Begins	Length (months)	Award	Res. Tuition	Non-res. Tuition	Stipend	Offers:‡ 1	2	3	4
Arkansas											
Arkansas State University	20	Jun	24	BS	$149	$389					•
Baptist Health Schools Little Rock	8	Jul	12	Cert	$4,835	$4,835					
University of Arkansas for Medical Sciences (Little Rock)	30	Aug	18, 12	Dipl, BSMT	$5,100	$12,330					
California											
California State University - Dominguez Hills (Carson)	24	Jul	12	Cert, BS	$3,382	$9,715	$6,000		•		
Eisenhower Medical Center (Rancho Mirage)	4	Oct	12	Cert, MT-CLS	$0	$0	$12,000				
Loma Linda University	22	Mid-Aug	20	Dipl, BS	$23,000	$23,000				•	
San Jose State University	20	Mar Sep	12	Cert	$5,000	$12,000	$14,000				•
Santa Barbara Cottage Hospital	4	Sep	12	Cert, MT	$0	$0	$12,000				
Univ of California Davis Health System (Sacramento)	20	Sep	12	Cert	$0	$0	$1,000				
Univ of California Irvine Med Ctr (Orange)	6	Sep	12	Cert	$0	$0	$6,000				
Colorado											
Centura Health/Penrose-St Francis Hlth Serv (Colorado Springs)	4	Aug	12	Cert	$1,000	$1,000	$900				
Colorado Center for Med Laboratory Science (Denver)	21	Aug	12	Cert, BS	$6,840	$6,840					
Parkview Medical Center (Pueblo)	4	Jul	12	Cert						•	
Connecticut											
Danbury Hospital	6	Mid-Jun	12	Cert						•	
University of Hartford (West Hartford)	8	Jan Jun Sep	12, 48	Cert, MT, BS	$25,806	$25,806				•	
Delaware											
University of Delaware (Newark)	26	Sep	18	BS	$6,980	$17,690					
District of Columbia											
George Washington University	30	Aug	24, 12	Cert, BS	$15,244	$15,244		•		•	•
Walter Reed Army Medical Center (Washington)	6	Aug	12	Cert						•	
Washington Hospital Center	14	Aug	12	Cert, BS	$5,000	$5,000	$9,000				
Florida											
Bayfront Medical Center (St Petersburg)	6	Aug	12	Cert	$1,000	$2,000					
Shands Jacksonville	6	Jul Jan	12	Cert							
St Vincent's Medical Center (Jacksonville)	10	Jan Jul	12	Cert, BS							
Tampa General Hospital	6	Aug	12	Cert	$1,500	$1,500					
University of Central Florida (Orlando)	20	Aug	24	BS	$3,282	$12,868					
University of West Florida (Pensacola)	20	Jan	15	BS	$2,782	$13,520					
Georgia											
Armstrong Atlantic State University (Savannah)	25	Aug	16	Cert, BS	$2,864	$10,180				•	•
Medical College of Georgia (Augusta)	50	Aug Jan May	12, 24	Cert, BS, BS Web	$5,730	$22,900		•		•	•
Thomas University (Thomasville)	12	Jan	24	BS	$12,000	$12,000		•			•
Hawaii											
University of Hawaii (Honolulu)	16	Aug	30	Cert, BS	$5,390	$14,654					
Idaho											
Idaho State University (Pocatello)	32	Sep	12, 24	BS, MS	$4,050	$8,400					•
Illinois											
Edward Hines Jr VA Hospital	8	Aug	11	Cert							
Evanston Northwestern Healthcare - Evanston	8	Sep	10	Cert	$8,000	$8,000					
Illinois State University (Normal)	32	Fall	24	BS	$6,495	$11,847					
Northern Illinois University (DeKalb)	32	Aug	18	BS	$6,652	$11,713				•	•
OSF St Anthony Medical Center (Rockford)	4	Aug	9	Cert, CLS/MT							
OSF St Francis Medical Center (Peoria)	6	Aug	11	BS	$1,000	$2,000				•	
Rush University (Chicago)	30	Sep Jan	20	BS, MS	$16,250	$0				•	
St John's Hospital (Springfield)	6	Jun	11	Cert	$800	$800					
University of Illinois at Springfield	20	Aug	21	BS	$5,580	$14,730				•	
Indiana											
Ball Memorial Hospital (Muncie)	6-8	Jul	12	Cert, BS	$3,000	$3,000	$1,000				
Clarian Health Partners Inc (Indianapolis)	24	Aug	11	Cert, BS	$3,000	$3,000					
Good Samaritan Hospital (Vincennes)	6	Aug	12	Cert, BS	$0	$0	$3,000				
Indiana University (Indianapolis)	12	Aug	11	BS	$7,900	$23,200					
Parkview Hospital (Fort Wayne)	4	Jul	11	Cert	$3,000	$3,000					
St Francis Hospital & Health Centers (Beech Grove)	8	Jul	11	Cert, BA/BS	$3,000	$3,000				•	
St Margaret Mercy Healthcare Centers (Hammond)	9	Aug	12	Cert	$1,500	$1,500					
Iowa											
Mercy Medical Center (Des Moines)	6	Aug	12	Cert, BS	$3,000	$3,000					
Mercy Medical Center - Sioux City	4	Aug	12	Cert, BS	$3,000	$3,000				•	
St Luke's College (Sioux City)	6	Aug	12	Cert	$4,000	$4,000					
St Luke's Hospital (Cedar Rapids)	5	Jul	12	Cert	$3,000	$3,000					
Kansas											
University of Kansas Medical Center (Kansas City)	30	Aug	24	BS	$6,522	$18,984					•
Wichita State University	45	Jan Jun Aug	17	BS	$9,638	$24,297			•	•	

*Data are shown only for programs that completed the 2007 AMA Survey of Health Professions Education Programs.
‡Key to Offers: 1: Evening or weekend classes; 2: Non-English instruction; 3: Cultural competence instruction; 4: Distance education component.

PROGRAMS

Clinical Laboratory Scientist/Medical Technologist

Programs*	Class Capacity	Begins	Length (months)	Award	Res. Tuition	Non-res. Tuition	Stipend	Offers:‡ 1	2	3	4
Kentucky											
Bellarmine University (Louisville)	16	Fall Spring	20, 16	Cert, BHS	$25,200	$25,200				•	
Eastern Kentucky University (Richmond)	24	Jan Aug	17	BS	$2,597	$7,269					
Owensboro Medical Health System	6	Jul	12	Cert, BS	$1,200	$1,200					
St Elizabeth Medical Center (Edgewood)	4	Jun	12	Cert	$3,500	$3,500				•	
Louisiana											
Lake Charles Mem Hosp Sch of Med Tech	10	Jan Aug	12	Cert	$50	$0					
Louisiana State U Hlth Sci Ctr - Shreveport	20	Spring Summer Fall	16	BS	$5,181	$8,306					
Louisiana State Univ Health Sciences Center (New Orleans)	28	Jan	16	Dipl, BS	$5,285	$8,410				•	
McNeese State University (Lake Charles)	10	Aug Jan	12	BS	$4,500	$9,000					
Our Lady of the Lake College (Baton Rouge)	14	Jun	18	BS	$226	$226				•	
Overton Brooks VA Medical Center (Shreveport)	8	Jan Jul	12	Cert	$1,500	$1,500					
Rapides Regional Medical Center (Alexandria)	8	Jan Jul	12	Cert, BS, BA							
Maine											
Eastern Maine Medical Center (Bangor)	6	Aug	11	Cert	$6,368	$6,368				•	
Maryland											
Morgan State University (Baltimore)	10	Sep	24	Dipl, BS	$2,120	$5,750					
Salisbury University	12	Aug	18	BS	$4,814	$12,902					
University of Maryland (Baltimore)	60	Aug Jan	18	Cert, BSMRT, MSMRT	$6,981	$13,962				•	
Massachusetts											
Berkshire Medical Center (Pittsfield)	6	Jul	12	Cert, BS	$2,000	$2,000					
Northeastern University (Boston)	32	Sep	60, 24	BS	$31,500	$31,500					
University of Massachusetts - Dartmouth (North Dartmouth)	24	Sep	48	BS	$8,036	$17,536					
University of Massachusetts - Lowell	24	Sep	36	BS	$1,454	$8,567					
Michigan											
Andrews University (Berrien Springs)	24	Aug	11	Cert, BSCLS, MSCLS	$25,728	$25,728				•	
DMC University Laboratories (Detroit)	10	Aug Jan	10	Cert	$0	$0	$3,600				
Eastern Michigan University (Ypsilanti)	100	Sep	34	BS	$2,450	$6,500			•		
Ferris State University (Big Rapids)	32	May	24	Dipl, BS	$8,700	$15,900				•	
Grand Valley State University (Grand Rapids)	20	Jan	17	BS i	$7,240	$12,510					
Hurley Medical Center (Flint)	10	Sep	10	Cert							
Michigan State University (East Lansing)	18	Aug	30	Cert, BS	$8,603	$22,543					
St John Health (Grosse Pointe Woods)	12	Jul Aug	11	Cert	$0	$0	$5,500			•	
Wayne State University (Detroit)	30	Sep	16, 6	BS	$4,500	$8,000				•	
William Beaumont Hospital (Royal Oak)	12	Jul Jan	11	Cert, MT						•	
Minnesota											
Fairview Health Services (Minneapolis)	10	Jun 1	12	Cert	$5,000	$0				•	
Hennepin County Medical Center (Minneapolis)	8	Sep	9	Cert	$4,400	$4,400				•	
University of Minnesota - Minneapolis	42	Sep	15	BS, MS	$10,508	$26,608				•	
Mississippi											
Mississippi Baptist Medical Center (Jackson)	12	Sep	12	Cert	$1,000	$1,000					
North Mississippi Medical Center (Tupelo)	12	Aug	12	Cert, BS							
University of Mississippi Medical Center (Jackson)	25	Aug	18	BS	$3,232	$6,904					•
University of Southern Mississippi (Hattiesburg)	18	Aug Jan	15	Dipl, Cert, BS, MS	$4,594	$10,622					
Missouri											
CoxHealth (Springfield)	6	Jan Jun	12	CertCLS	$3,000	$3,000					
North Kansas City Hospital	6	Jun	11	Cert	$2,000	$2,000					
Saint Louis University (St Louis)	25	Aug Jan	36	BS	$26,250	$26,250					
Saint Luke's Hospital (Kansas City)	8	Jul	11	Cert	$3,000	$3,000				•	
Southeast Missouri Hospital College of Nursing and Health Sciences (Cape Girardeau)	9	Jul	11	Cert	$10,791	$10,791				•	
St John's Mercy Medical Center (St Louis)	8	Last wk of Jun	12	Cert, BSMT, MT/CLS	$4,800	$4,800					
St John's Regional Medical Center (Joplin)	8	Jan Jun	12	Cert, BS	$2,000	$2,000					
Nebraska											
Nebraska Methodist Hospital (Omaha)	10	Jun	11	Cert, BS	$6,610	$19,636				•	
University of Nebraska Medical Center (Omaha)	48	May 29	12	BS	$6,240	$20,500				•	•
Nevada											
University of Nevada - Las Vegas	24	Aug	24	Dipl, Cert, BS	$2,868	$12,334				•	
New Hampshire											
University of New Hampshire (Durham)	25	Sep	49	BS	$8,720	$21,770					
New Jersey											
Jersey Shore University Medical Center (Neptune)	6	Aug	11	Cert, BS	$3,000	$3,000					
Monmouth Medical Center (Long Branch)	8	Aug	11	Cert, BS	$2,600	$2,600				•	
Morristown Memorial Hospital	8	Sep	11	Cert, BS	$2,000	$2,000					
The Valley Hospital (Ridgewood)	4	Jun	12	Cert, BS	$2,000	$2,000					
Univ of Medicine & Dent of New Jersey (Newark)	24	Jun	15	Cert, BS	$11,176	$16,764				•	•

*Data are shown only for programs that completed the 2007 AMA Survey of Health Professions Education Programs.

‡Key to Offers: 1: Evening or weekend classes; 2: Non-English instruction; 3: Cultural competence instruction; 4: Distance education component.

Clinical Laboratory Scientist/Medical Technologist

Programs*	Class Capacity	Begins	Length (months)	Award	Res. Tuition	Non-res. Tuition	Stipend	Offers:‡ 1	2	3	4
New Mexico											
University of New Mexico (Albuquerque)	25	Jun Jan Sep	18	Cert, BS MLS	$4,800	$16,000				•	
New York											
Long Island University - C W Post Campus (Brookville)	20	Sep	24	Dipl, Cert, BS	$22,100	$22,100		•			
Marist College (Poughkeepsie)	30	Sep Jan	35	BS	$22,066	$22,066					
New York Methodist Hospital (Brooklyn)	10	Aug	12	Cert, BS	$7,500	$7,500					
Rochester General Hospital	18	Aug	12	Cert, BS	$5,800	$5,800					
St John's University (Fresh Meadows)	15	Jun	12	Dipl, Cert, BSMT	$26,000	$26,000					
St Vincent's Hospital Manhattan SVCMC (New York)	10	Jun	12	Cert, BS	$7,200	$7,200					
Stony Brook University	25	Aug	20	BS	$4,350	$10,610					
SUNY Upstate Medical University (Syracuse)	40	Aug	21	BS	$4,350	$10,610					
University at Buffalo - SUNY	35	Aug	21	BS	$4,655	$9,555					
Woman's Christian Association Hospital (Jamestown)	10	Aug	11	Cert	$5,800	$5,800				•	
North Carolina											
Carolinas College of Health Sciences (Charlotte)	12	Aug Jan	12	Cert	$5,000	$5,000					
East Carolina University (Greenville)	16	Aug 20	21	BS	$2,979	$12,635					•
University of North Carolina - Chapel Hill	24	Aug	16, 20	Cert, BS	$5,032	$19,680					
Wake Forest University Baptist Medical Center (Winston-Salem)	12	Jul Jan	12	Cert	$3,000	$3,000					
Western Carolina University (Cullowhee)	14	Aug	18	BS	$3,945	$13,528					
North Dakota											
MeritCare Medical Center (Fargo)	10	Jun	12	Cert, BS	$2,468	$2,886				•	
University of North Dakota (Grand Forks)	75	May	24, 12	Dipl, Cert, BS	$7,000	$0		•		•	•
Ohio											
Bowling Green State University	14	May	14	Cert, BS	$13,590	$24,552					
Children's Hospital Medical Ctr of Akron	9	Jul	12	Cert	$4,500	$4,500					
Ohio Northern University (Ada)	8	Jun	12	Cert, BS	$9,200	$9,200					
Ohio State University (Columbus)	70	Sep	22	Cert, BS	$8,667	$20,562					
Southwest General Health Center (Middleburg Heights)	6	Jul	12	Cert	$2,500	$2,500					
St Vincent Mercy Medical Center (Toledo)	4	Jul	12	Cert	$500	$500					
University of Cincinnati Medical Center	18*	Sep Jan Mar Jun	12, 26	Dipl, Cert, BS	$12,532	$31,896		•		•	•
Wright State University (Dayton)	12	Jun	12	Cert, BSCLS	$7,278	$14,004				•	
Oklahoma											
Comanche County Memorial Hospital (Lawton)	6	Aug	12	Cert	$1,250	$0					
Muskogee Regional Medical Center	5	Jun	12	Cert							
Valley View Regional Hospital (Ada)	6	Late May	12	Cert, BS						•	
Oregon											
Oregon Health & Science University (Portland)	26	Sep	15	BS	$14,728	$23,872					
Pennsylvania											
Conemaugh Memorial Medical Center (Johnstown)	8	Jul	12	Cert	$6,200	$6,200					
Lancaster Gen Coll of Nursing & Hlth Sciences	8	Aug	12	Cert	$10,500	$10,500				•	
Mount Nittany Medical Center (State College)	4	End of Jul	11	Cert	$8,000	$0					
Pennsylvania Hospital (Philadelphia)	6	Sep	11	Cert	$7,000	$7,000				•	
Reading Hospital & Medical Center	4	Jul	11	Cert	$4,000	$4,000				•	
Robert Packer Hospital (Sayre)	10	Aug	11	Cert	$5,900	$5,900					
Saint Vincent Health Center (Erie)	12	Jul	12	Cert, BS	$7,092	$7,092					
Williamsport Hosp & Medical Center	4	Aug	12	Cert	$3,500	$3,500					
York Hospital/WellSpan Health	6	Jul	12	Cert	$6,800	$6,800				•	
Puerto Rico											
Inter American University of Puerto Rico (San German)	18	Aug Feb	12	DiplCLS, BSMT	$6,000	$6,000					
University of Puerto Rico (San Juan)	40	Aug	17	Dipl, Cert, BSMT	$2,550	$0			•	•	
Rhode Island											
Our Lady of Fatima Hospital (North Providence)	6	Jul	11	Cert	$5,650	$5,650					
Rhode Island Hospital (Providence)	9	Jul	11	BS							
South Carolina											
Lexington Medical Center (West Columbia)	4	Aug	12	Cert	$0	$0	$2,000				
McLeod Regional Medical Center (Florence)	8	Aug	12	Cert	$2,000	$2,000					
Palmetto Health Baptist (Columbia)	4	Jan Jul	12	Cert							
South Dakota											
Rapid City Regional Hospital	10	Jun	12	Cert, BS	$4,000	$4,000					
Sanford Medical Center (Sioux Falls)	10	Jun	11	Cert, BA/BS	$4,000	$4,000				•	
Tennessee											
Austin Peay State University (Clarksville)	18	Jun	12	Cert, BS	$5,884	$17,316					
Lincoln Memorial University (Harrogate)	12	Aug	24	BS	$13,104	$13,104		•			
Tennessee State University (Nashville)	14	Aug	12	Cert, BS	$6,846	$21,387					
Univ of Tennessee Medical Ctr at Knoxville	8	Jan	12	Cert, BS	$8,000	$23,000					
University of Tennessee Health Science Ctr (Memphis)	20	Sep	21, 48	BS, MS	$6,830	$22,420					

*Data are shown only for programs that completed the 2007 AMA Survey of Health Professions Education Programs.
‡Key to Offers: 1: Evening or weekend classes; 2: Non-English instruction; 3: Cultural competence instruction; 4: Distance education component.

Clinical Laboratory Scientist/Medical Technologist

Clinical Laboratory Scientist/Medical Technologist

Programs*	Class Capacity	Begins	Length (months)	Award	Res. Tuition	Non-res. Tuition	Stipend	Offers:‡ 1	2	3	4
Texas											
CHRISTUS Hospital - St Elizabeth (Beaumont)	6	Aug	12	Cert	$300	$300					
Hillcrest Baptist Medical Center (Waco)	5	Jan Jul	12	Cert							
Methodist Hospital (Houston)	4	Aug	12	Cert, BSMT	$0	$0	$2,400				
Scott & White Hospital (Temple)	8	Aug	12	Cert	$500	$500					
Texas Southern University (Houston)	18	Aug	24	Cert, BS	$3,098	$8,760				•	
Texas State University - San Marcos	20	Sep	24	BS	$7,875	$17,488					
United Regional Health Care Systems (Wichita Falls)	6	Jul	12	Cert, BS	$0	$0	$1,500				
Univ of Texas - Pan American (Edinburg)	18	Sep	15	Cert, BS	$6,733	$19,189				•	
Univ of Texas Hlth Sci Ctr at San Antonio	30	Aug Jan	19	Cert, BS, MS	$3,480	$11,730				•	•
Univ of Texas M D Anderson Cancer Ctr (Houston)	20	Aug	12	Dipl, Cert, BS, CLS	$4,250	$16,500				•	
Univ of Texas Southwestern Med Ctr (Dallas)	24	Aug	16, 28	Cert, BSMT	$1,200	$7,824					
University of Texas at El Paso	20	Jun	22	BS	$6,600	$13,050					•
University of Texas Medical Branch (Galveston)	40	Aug	24	Cert, BS	$3,280	$12,000		•	•	•	•
Utah											
Brigham Young University (Provo)	14	Sep Jan	12	Dipl, BS	$3,840	$7,680					
University of Utah Health Science Center (Salt Lake City)	40	Aug	21	BS	$1,800	$4,000					
Weber State University (Ogden)	40	Aug	36	Cert, BS	$2,772	$8,612				•	
Vermont											
University of Vermont (Burlington)	20	Aug	48, 24	Cert, BS	$10,422	$26,306					
Virginia											
Augusta Medical Center (Fishersville)	5	Jul	12	Cert	$1,000	$1,000					
Norfolk State University	11	Aug	18	BS	$5,862	$18,966				•	
Old Dominion University (Norfolk)	Var	Aug	22	BSMT	$7,385	$20,475		•			•
Rockingham Memorial Hospital (Harrisonburg)	8	Jun	12	Cert, BS	$635	$635					
Virginia Commonwealth University (Richmond)	35	Aug	20	BS	$6,142	$18,686				•	
Washington											
Sacred Heart Medical Center (Spokane)	12	Jul	12	Cert						•	
Yakima Regional CLS Program	8	Sep	12	Cert, BS	$6,000	$6,000					
West Virginia											
Marshall University (Huntington)	6	Aug	18	BS	$3,360	$9,144		•		•	
West Liberty State College	16	Aug	24	BS	$3,686	$9,054					
West Virginia University (Morgantown)	29	Aug	21	BS	$5,650	$17,690					
Wisconsin											
Affinity Health System (Appleton)	6	Sep	9	Cert	$3,500	$3,500				•	
Aspirus Wausau Hospital	6	Aug	9	Cert	$1,000	$1,000				•	
Clement J Zablocki VA Medical Center (Milwaukee)	10	Jul	10	Cert							
Marquette University (Milwaukee)	96	Fall semester	37	BS	$26,270	$26,270					
Sacred Heart Hospital (Eau Claire)	4	Sep	9	Cert	$850	$1,200					
St Joseph's Hospital (Marshfield)	12	Aug	9	Cert, BS/MT	$850	$850				•	
University of Wisconsin - Madison	24	Sep	18	BS	$6,730	$20,730					
University of Wisconsin - Milwaukee	20	Sep	35	BS, MS	$6,630	$16,230				•	
University of Wisconsin - Stevens Point	30	Fall	6	BSCLS							•

*Data are shown only for programs that completed the 2007 AMA Survey of Health Professions Education Programs.

‡Key to Offers: 1: Evening or weekend classes; 2: Non-English instruction; 3: Cultural competence instruction; 4: Distance education component.

Clinical Laboratory Technician/Medical Laboratory Technician

Alabama

Jefferson State Community College
Clin Lab Technician/Med Lab Technician
2601 Carson Rd
Birmingham, AL 35215
www.jeffstateonline.com
Prgm Dir: Candy Hill, MA Ed MT(ASCP) CLS(NCA)
Tel: 205 856-6031 *Fax:* 205 856-7725
E-mail: chill@jeffstateonline.com

Gadsden State Community College
Clin Lab Technician/Med Lab Technician
PO Box 227
1001 George Wallace Dr
Gadsden, AL 35902-0227
www.gadsdenstate.edu
Prgm Dir: Sunita M Graves, MS MT(ASCP)
Tel: 256 549-8470 *Fax:* 256 549-8272
E-mail: sgraves@gadsdenstate.edu

Wallace State Community College
Clin Lab Technician/Med Lab Technician
801 Main St
PO Box 2000
Hanceville, AL 35077-2000
www.wallacestate.edu
Prgm Dir: Julie Welch, MS MT(ASCP)
Tel: 256 352-8347 *Fax:* 256 352-8320
E-mail: julie.welch@wallacestate.edu

Alaska

University of Alaska Anchorage
Clin Lab Technician/Med Lab Technician
3211 Providence Dr
Anchorage, AK 99508-4610
Prgm Dir: Heidi Mannion, PhD MT(ASCP)
Tel: 907 786-6924, Ext 102 *Fax:* 907 786-6938
E-mail: afham@uaa.alaska.edu

Arkansas

Arkansas State University - Beebe
Clin Lab Technician/Med Lab Technician
PO Box 1000
Beebe, AR 72012
www.asub.edu
Prgm Dir: Jimmy L Boyd, MS MHS CLS(NCA)
Tel: 501 882-8214 *Fax:* 501 882-8387
E-mail: jlboyd@asub.edu

South Arkansas Community College
Clin Lab Technician/Med Lab Technician
300 S West Ave
PO Box 7010
El Dorado, AR 71730
Prgm Dir: George H Roberts, EdD CLS(NCA)
Tel: 870 864-7102 *Fax:* 870 864-7140
E-mail: groberts@southark.edu

North Arkansas College
Clin Lab Technician/Med Lab Technician
1515 Pioneer Dr
Harrison, AR 72601-5599
www.northark.edu
Prgm Dir: Sherry Gibbany, MA MT(ASCP)
Tel: 870 391-3288 *Fax:* 870 743-5326
E-mail: sgibbany@northark.edu

Phillips Community College/U of Arkansas
Clin Lab Technician/Med Lab Technician
PO Box 785
1000 Campus Dr
Helena, AR 72342
Prgm Dir: Julie Byrd, MS MT(ASCP)
Tel: 870 338-6474, Ext 1109 *Fax:* 870 338-7542
E-mail: jbyrd@pccua.edu

National Park Community College
Clin Lab Technician/Med Lab Technician
101 College Dr
Hot Springs, AR 71913-9174
Prgm Dir: Carol A Spargo, BS MEd MT(ASCP)
Tel: 501 760-4130 *Fax:* 501 760-4141
E-mail: cspargo@npcc.edu

Arkansas State University
Clin Lab Technician/Med Lab Technician
PO Box 910
State University, AR 72467
www.clt.astate.edu/cls/
Prgm Dir: R Whitney Williams, PhD MT(ASCP)
Tel: 870 972-3073 *Fax:* 870 972-2004
E-mail: wwilliam@astate.edu

California

De Anza College
Clin Lab Technician/Med Lab Technician
21250 Stevens Creek Blvd
Cupertino, CA 95014
Prgm Dir: Debbie Wagner, MT(ASCP) CLS(NCA)
Tel: 408 864-8790
E-mail: wagnerdebbie@deanza.edu

Hartnell College
Clin Lab Technician/Med Lab Technician
156 Homestead Ave
Salinas, CA 93901-1697
Prgm Dir: Susan A McQuiston, MS JD MT(ASCP)
Tel: 831 770-6152 *Fax:* 831 770-6144
E-mail: smcquist@hartnell.edu

Naval School of Health Sciences, San Diego
Clin Lab Technician/Med Lab Technician
34101 Farenholt Ave
San Diego, CA 92134-5291
Prgm Dir: Luis A Nunez Jr, LT MSC USN MA MT(ASCP)
Tel: 619 532-7330 *Fax:* 619 532-7145
E-mail: lanunez@nshs-sd.med.navy.mil

Colorado

Arapahoe Community College
Clin Lab Technician/Med Lab Technician
5900 S Santa Fe Dr
PO Box 9002
Littleton, CO 80160-9002
Prgm Dir: Jennifer Wolff, MT(ASCP)
Tel: 303 797-5796 *Fax:* 303 797-5935
E-mail: jennifer.wolff@arapahoe.edu

Delaware

Delaware Technical & Community College - Owens Campus
Clin Lab Technician/Med Lab Technician
PO Box 610
Georgetown, DE 19947
Prgm Dir: Sheridan A Shupe, MEd MT(ASCP)
Tel: 302 855-5974 *Fax:* 302 858-5470
E-mail: sshupe@college.dtcc.edu

Florida

Brevard Community College
Clin Lab Technician/Med Lab Technician
1519 Clearlake Rd
Cocoa, FL 32922
www.brevardcc.edu
Prgm Dir: Celine Marilyn Hulme, MEd MT(ASCP)
Tel: 321 433-7543 *Fax:* 321 433-7599
E-mail: hulmem@brevardcc.edu

Keiser University
Clin Lab Technician/Med Lab Technician
1500 NW 49th St
Fort Lauderdale, FL 33309
www.keiseruniversity.edu
Prgm Dir: Lureen Samuel, MS BS BS MT(ASCP)
Tel: 954 776-4456, Ext 431 *Fax:* 954 776-5157
E-mail: lureens@keiseruniversity.edu

Indian River Community College
Clin Lab Technician/Med Lab Technician
3209 Virginia Ave
Fort Pierce, FL 34981
Prgm Dir: Marilyn Barbour, MEd MT(ASCP) CLS(NCA)
Tel: 772 462-7534 *Fax:* 772 462-7816
E-mail: mbarbour@ircc.edu

Florida Community College - Jacksonville
Clin Lab Technician/Med Lab Technician
North Campus, 4501 Capper Rd
Jacksonville, FL 32218
www.fccj.org
Prgm Dir: Rhoda S Jost, MS MT(ASCP)
Tel: 904 766-6580 *Fax:* 904 766-6654
E-mail: rjost@fccj.edu

Miami Dade College
Clin Lab Technician/Med Lab Technician
Medical Center Campus
950 NW 20th St
Miami, FL 33127
www.mdc.edu
Prgm Dir: Nilia Madan, MBA MT(ASCP)SH
Tel: 305 237-4041 *Fax:* 305 237-4278
E-mail: nilia.madan@mdc.edu

St Petersburg College
Clin Lab Technician/Med Lab Technician
PO Box 13489
St Petersburg, FL 33733-3489
www.spcollege.edu/hec/medlab
Prgm Dir: Valerie Polansky, MEd MT(ASCP)
Tel: 727 341-3714 *Fax:* 727 341-3740
E-mail: polansky.valerie@spcollege.edu

Erwin Technical Center
Clin Lab Technician/Med Lab Technician
2010 E Hillsborough Ave
Tampa, FL 33610-8299
Prgm Dir: Linda J Dickson, MT(ASCP) MSPH
Tel: 813 231-1800, Ext 1326 *Fax:* 813 231-1820
E-mail: linda.dickson@sdhc.k12.fl.us

Georgia

Darton College
Clin Lab Technician/Med Lab Technician
2400 Gillionville Rd
Albany, GA 31707
Prgm Dir: Nancy T Beamon, MS MT(ASCP)
Tel: 912 430-6846 *Fax:* 912 430-6910
E-mail: nancy.beamon@darton.edu

Coastal Georgia Community College
Clin Lab Technician/Med Lab Technician
3700 Altama Ave
Brunswick, GA 31520
www.cgcc.edu
Prgm Dir: Katherine Nisi Zell, EdS MT(ASCP) SH
 CLS/NCA
Tel: 912 264-7382 *Fax:* 912 262-3283
E-mail: nzell@cgcc.edu

North Georgia Technical College
Clin Lab Technician/Med Lab Technician
1500 Hwy 197 N, PO Box 65
Clarkesville, GA 30523
https://www.northgatech.edu
Prgm Dir: Lauren Strader, MEd MT(ASCP)
Tel: 706 754-7757 *Fax:* 706 754-7777
E-mail: lstrader@northgatech.edu

DeKalb Technical College
Clin Lab Technician/Med Lab Technician
495 N Indian Creek Dr
Clarkston, GA 30021-2397
Prgm Dir: Virginia D Roberts, MEd MT(AMT)
Tel: 404 297-9522, Ext 1160 *Fax:* 404 294-4234
E-mail: robertsg@dekalbtech.org

Dalton State College
Clin Lab Technician/Med Lab Technician
650 College Dr
Dalton, GA 30720-3778
Prgm Dir: Tyra D Stalling, MSHS CLS(NCA) MT(ASCP)
Tel: 706 272-2508 *Fax:* 706 272-2517
E-mail: tstalling@daltonstate.edu

Central Georgia Technical College
Clin Lab Technician/Med Lab Technician
3300 Macon Tech Dr
Macon, GA 31206
Prgm Dir: Tony Dugan, MS MT(ASCP)DLM
Tel: 478 757-3571 *Fax:* 478 757-3575
E-mail: tdugan@centralgatech.edu

Lanier Technical College
Clin Lab Technician/Med Lab Technician
2990 Landrum Education Dr
Oakwood, GA 30566
Prgm Dir: Kimberly A Randolph, MT(ASCP) MS
Tel: 770 531-6367 *Fax:* 770 531-6306
E-mail: krandolph@laniertech.edu

Southwest Georgia Technical College
Clin Lab Technician/Med Lab Technician
15689 US Hwy 19 N
Thomasville, GA 31792
www.swgtc.net
Prgm Dir: Richard Miller, PhD MBA MT(ASCP)CM
 CLS(NCA)
Tel: 229 225-5203 *Fax:* 229 225-5289
E-mail: rmiller@southwestgatech.edu

Valdosta Technical College
Clin Lab Technician/Med Lab Technician
4089 Val Tech Rd
Valdosta, GA 31602-0929
Prgm Dir: Angela Robinson, MEd MT(AMT) MLT(ASCP)
Tel: 229 249-4855
E-mail: arobinson@valdostatech.edu

Southeastern Technical College
Clin Lab Technician/Med Lab Technician
3001 E First St
Vidalia, GA 30474
Prgm Dir: Charlotte Bates, MEd MT(ASCP)
Tel: 912 538-3183
E-mail: cbates@southeasterntech.edu

West Central Technical College
Clin Lab Technician/Med Lab Technician
178 Murphy Campus Blvd
Waco, GA 30182
Prgm Dir: John W Ridley, PhD MT(ASCP)
Tel: 770 537-6043 *Fax:* 770 537-7992
E-mail: jridley@westcentraltech.edu

Okefenokee Technical College
Clin Lab Technician/Med Lab Technician
1701 Carswell Ave
Waycross, GA 31501
www.okefenokeetech.edu
Prgm Dir: Mary Ann Hursey, BS MT(ASCP)
Tel: 912 285-6166 *Fax:* 912 287-4865
E-mail: mhursey@okefenokeetech.edu

Hawaii

Kapi'olani Community College
Clin Lab Technician/Med Lab Technician
4303 Diamond Head Rd
Honolulu, HI 96816
Prgm Dir: Marcia A Armstrong, MS CLS(NCA)
 MT(ASCP)
Tel: 808 734-9231 *Fax:* 808 734-9126
E-mail: marciaa@hawaii.edu

Illinois

Southwestern Illinois College
Clin Lab Technician/Med Lab Technician
2500 Carlyle Rd
Belleville, IL 62221-5899
www.southwestern.cc.il.us
Prgm Dir: Jean M Deitz, MS MT(ASCP)
Tel: 618 235-2700, Ext 5386 *Fax:* 618 235-2052
E-mail: Jean.Deitz@swic.edu

Oakton Community College
Clin Lab Technician/Med Lab Technician
1600 E Golf Rd
Des Plaines, IL 60016
Prgm Dir: Lynne Steele, MS MT(ASCP)
Tel: 847 635-1889 *Fax:* 847 635-1987
E-mail: lynne@oakton.edu

Elgin Community College
Clin Lab Technician/Med Lab Technician
1700 Spartan Dr
Elgin, IL 60123-7193
www.elgin.edu
Prgm Dir: Wendy Miller, MS CLS(NCA) MT(ASCP)SI
Tel: 847 214-7308 *Fax:* 847 214-7527
E-mail: wmiller@elgin.edu

Southern Illinois Collegiate Common Market
Clin Lab Technician/Med Lab Technician
3213 S Park Ave
Herrin, IL 62948
Prgm Dir: Paula Ann Berry, MS Ed MT(ASCP)
Tel: 618 942-6902 *Fax:* 618 942-6658
E-mail: pberry@siccm.com

Kankakee Community College
Clin Lab Technician/Med Lab Technician
100 College Dr
Kankakee, IL 60901
www.kcc.edu
Prgm Dir: Manuela Sawalha, MHS MT(ASCP)
Tel: 815 802-8835 *Fax:* 815 802-8101
E-mail: nsawalha@kankakee.edu

Illinois Central College
Clin Lab Technician/Med Lab Technician
Thomas K Thomas Bldg
201 SW Adams St
Peoria, IL 61635-0001
www.icc.edu/hcps/hc_medicalLabTech.asp
Prgm Dir: Anh Strow, MPH MT(ASCP) CLS(NCA)
Tel: 309 999-4661 *Fax:* 309 673-9626
E-mail: astrow@icc.edu

Blessing Hospital
Clin Lab Technician/Med Lab Technician
School of MLT
Broadway at 11th St
Quincy, IL 62301
www.blessinghospital.com
Prgm Dir: Heather Ator, MT(ASCP)SM
Tel: 217 223-8400, Ext 6205 *Fax:* 217 223-7032
E-mail: hator@blessinghospital.org

Indiana

Indiana University Northwest
Clin Lab Technician/Med Lab Technician
3400 Broadway St
Gary, IN 46408
Prgm Dir: Susan A K Higgins, MS MT(ASCP)SC
Tel: 219 980-6923 *Fax:* 219 980-6649
E-mail: sahiggin@iun.edu

Ivy Tech Community College - South Bend
Clin Lab Technician/Med Lab Technician
220 Dean Johnson Blvd
South Bend, IN 46601-3415
Prgm Dir: Pamela B Primrose, ABD MLFSC MT(ASCP)
Tel: 574 289-7001, Ext 5401 *Fax:* 574 236-7166
E-mail: pprimros@ivytech.edu

Ivy Tech Community College - Terre Haute
Clin Lab Technician/Med Lab Technician
7999 US Hwy 41 S
Terre Haute, IN 47802-4898
www.goivytech.net
Prgm Dir: Janee Gambill, MS MT(ASCP)
Tel: 812 298-2243 *Fax:* 812 298-2392
E-mail: Jgambill@ivytech.edu

Iowa

Des Moines Area Community College
Clin Lab Technician/Med Lab Technician
2006 Ankeny Blvd, Bldg 9
Ankeny, IA 50023
www.dmacc.edu/programs/medlabtech/
Prgm Dir: Karen Campbell, MAT MT(ASCP) CLS(NCA)
Tel: 515 964-6296 *Fax:* 515 964-6440
E-mail: kjcampbell@dmacc.edu

Iowa Central Community College
Clin Lab Technician/Med Lab Technician
330 Ave M
Fort Dodge, IA 50501
Prgm Dir: Diane C Edwards, BS MT(ASCP)
Tel: 515 576-0099, Ext 2394 *Fax:* 515 576-5656
E-mail: edwards@triton.iccc.cc.ia.us

Hawkeye Community College
Clin Lab Technician/Med Lab Technician
1501 E Orange Rd
PO Box 8015
Waterloo, IA 50704
www.hawkeye.cc.ia.us
Prgm Dir: Amy R Kapanka, MS MT(ASCP)
Tel: 319 296-2329, Ext 1357 *Fax:* 319 296-2874
E-mail: akapanka@hawkeyecollege.edu

Kansas

Barton County Community College
Clin Lab Technician/Med Lab Technician
245 NE 30th Rd
Great Bend, KS 67530-9283
www.bartonccc.edu/mlt/home
Prgm Dir: Leonard Bunselmeyer, Jr, MS MT(ASCP)
Tel: 316 792-2701, Ext 393 *Fax:* 316 786-1164
E-mail: bunselmeyerl@bartonccc.edu

Seward County Community College
Clin Lab Technician/Med Lab Technician
PO Box 1137
Liberal, KS 67905
www.sccc.edu
Prgm Dir: Suzanne Campbell, PhD MS BS MT(ASCP)
Tel: 620 626-3077   *Fax:* 620 626-3040
E-mail: suzanne.campbell@sccc.edu

Wichita Area Technical College
Clin Lab Technician/Med Lab Technician
324 N Emporia St
Wichita, KS 67202-2512
www.watc.edu
Prgm Dir: Barbara C Wenger, MS MT(ASCP)
Tel: 316 677-1378   *Fax:* 316 677-1310
E-mail: bwenger@watc.edu

Kentucky

HCC/MCC Consortium
Cosponsor: Madisonville Community College
Clin Lab Technician/Med Lab Technician
2000 College Dr
Madisonville, KY 42431
www.madisonville.kctcs.edu
Prgm Dir: Karol Conrad, MS MT(ASCP)
Tel: 270 824-1741   *Fax:* 270 824-1879
E-mail: karol.conrad@kctcs.edu

Southeast Kentucky Comm & Tech College
Clin Lab Technician/Med Lab Technician
3300 US Highway 25E S
Pineville, KY 40977
Prgm Dir: Sheila Gibbs Miracle, MEd CLS(NCA)
   H(ASCP)cm
Tel: 606 248-0946   *Fax:* 606 248-3361
E-mail: sheila.miracle@kctcs.edu

Eastern Kentucky University
Clin Lab Technician/Med Lab Technician
Dizney 220
521 Lancaster Ave
Richmond, KY 40475-3102
Prgm Dir: David C Hufford, PhD MT(ASCP)
Tel: 859 622-3078   *Fax:* 859 622-1939
E-mail: david.hufford@eku.edu

Somerset Community College
Clin Lab Technician/Med Lab Technician
808 Monticello St
Somerset, KY 42501
Prgm Dir: Nancy W Powell, MAEd MT(ASCP)
Tel: 606 451-6842, Ext 16842   *Fax:* 606 679-3684
E-mail: nancy.powell@kctcs.edu

Louisiana

Louisiana State University - Alexandria
Clin Lab Technician/Med Lab Technician
8100 Hwy 71 S
Alexandria, LA 71302-9121
Prgm Dir: Sheryl B Herring, MSA MT(ASCP)
Tel: 318 473-6464   *Fax:* 318 473-6588
E-mail: slienhop@lsua.edu

MedVance Institute
Clin Lab Technician/Med Lab Technician
9255 Interline Ave
Baton Rouge, LA 70809
Prgm Dir: Laverne Floyd, MA MT(ASCP)
Tel: 225 248-1015   *Fax:* 225 248-9517
E-mail: laverne@frontiernet.net

Our Lady of the Lake College
Clin Lab Technician/Med Lab Technician
7434 Perkins Rd
Baton Rouge, LA 70808
www.ololcollege.edu
Prgm Dir: Todd Casanova, PhD MT(ASCP)
Tel: 225 768-1745   *Fax:* 225 768-0819
E-mail: tcasanov@ololcollege.edu

Louisiana Tech College - Lafayette Campus
Clin Lab Technician/Med Lab Technician
PO Box 4909
Lafayette, LA 70502
Prgm Dir: Karon E Hebert, MS MT(ASCP)
Tel: 337 262-5962, Ext 249   *Fax:* 337 262-5122
E-mail: ehebert@theltc.net

Delgado Community College
Clin Lab Technician/Med Lab Technician
615 City Park Ave
New Orleans, LA 70119
www.dcc.edu
Prgm Dir: Sheila M Hickman, MEd MT(ASCP)SBB
Tel: 504 671-6224   *Fax:* 504 483-4609
E-mail: shickm@dcc.edu

Southern Univ at Shreveport
Clin Lab Technician/Med Lab Technician
3050 Martin Luther King Jr Dr
Shreveport, LA 71107
www.susla.edu
Prgm Dir: Patricia Raphiel-Brown, MA CLS(AMT)
Tel: 318 674-3350   *Fax:* 318 676-5495
E-mail: pbrown@susla.edu

Maine

Central Maine Community College
Clin Lab Technician/Med Lab Technician
1250 Turner St
Auburn, ME 04210
Prgm Dir: Valerie V Ferrante, MS MT(ASCP)
Tel: 207 755-5420   *Fax:* 207 755-5496
E-mail: vferrante@cmcc.edu

University of Maine - Presque Isle
Cosponsor: University of Maine at Augusta
Clin Lab Technician/Med Lab Technician
Medical Laboratory Technology Program of Maine
181 Main
Presque Isle, ME 04769
Prgm Dir: Linda Graves, EdD MT(ASCP)
Tel: 207 768-9451   *Fax:* 207 768-9553
E-mail: graves@umpi.maine.edu

Maryland

Allegany College of Maryland
Clin Lab Technician/Med Lab Technician
12401 Willowbrook Rd SE
Cumberland, MD 21502-2596
Prgm Dir: Mary H Saunders-Bloom, MEd MT(ASCP)
Tel: 301 784-5548   *Fax:* 301 784-5015
E-mail: msaunders@allegany.edu

Massachusetts

Bristol Community College
Clin Lab Technician/Med Lab Technician
777 Elsbree St
Fall River, MA 02720
Prgm Dir: Paula Baptista, MS MT(ASCP)
Tel: 508 678-2811, Ext 2629   *Fax:* 508 730-3281
E-mail: Paula.Baptista@bristolcc.edu

Springfield Technical Community College
Clin Lab Technician/Med Lab Technician
One Armory Sq
PO Box 9000
Springfield, MA 01105-1204
Prgm Dir: Susan Schneider, MEd MT(ASCP) CLS(NCA)
Tel: 413 755-4846   *Fax:* 413 755-6312
E-mail: saschneider@stcc.edu

Michigan

Kellogg Community College
Clin Lab Technician/Med Lab Technician
450 North Ave
Battle Creek, MI 49017
www.kellogg.edu/alliedhealth/mlt/mltmain.html
Prgm Dir: Kathleen T Paff, MA CLS(NCA) MT(ASCP)
Tel: 269 965-3931, Ext 2316   *Fax:* 269 565-2059
E-mail: paffk@kellogg.edu

Ferris State University
Clin Lab Technician/Med Lab Technician
VFS210A
200 Ferris Dr
Big Rapids, MI 49307-2740
www.ferris.edu/cls
Prgm Dir: Barbara A Ross, MS MT(ASCP)
Tel: 231 591-2317   *Fax:* 231 591-3788
E-mail: rossb@ferris.edu

Northern Michigan University
Clin Lab Technician/Med Lab Technician
3513 West Science Bldg
Marquette, MI 49855
Prgm Dir: Lucille A Contois, MA MT(ASCP)
Tel: 906 227-1660   *Fax:* 906 227-1309
E-mail: lcontois@nmu.edu

Baker College of Owosso
Clin Lab Technician/Med Lab Technician
1020 S Washington St
Owosso, MI 48867
www.baker.edu
Prgm Dir: Mary Vuckovich, MBA MT(ASCP)
Tel: 789 729-3416   *Fax:* 789 729-3411
E-mail: mary.vuckovich@baker.edu

Minnesota

Alexandria Technical College
Clin Lab Technician/Med Lab Technician
1601 Jefferson St
Alexandria, MN 56308
Prgm Dir: Wanda Haberer, MS MT(ASCP) CLS(NCA)
Tel: 320 762-0221   *Fax:* 320 762-4501
E-mail: wandah@alx.tec.mn.us

North Hennepin Community College
Clin Lab Technician/Med Lab Technician
7411 85th Ave N
Brooklyn Park, MN 55445
Prgm Dir: Nancy C Denny, MAEd MT(ASCP)
Tel: 763 424-0768   *Fax:* 763 493-0571
E-mail: nancy.denny@nhcc.edu

Lake Superior College
Clin Lab Technician/Med Lab Technician
2101 Trinity Rd
Duluth, MN 55811
Prgm Dir: Mary Grace Werner, MSEd MT(ASCP)
   CLS(NCA)
Tel: 218 733-7679   *Fax:* 218 723-4921
E-mail: m.werner@lsc.edu

Argosy University - Twin Cities
Clin Lab Technician/Med Lab Technician
Twin Cities Campus
1515 Central Parkway
Eagan, MN 55121
www.argosyu.edu
Prgm Dir: Kevin Swanson, DC MT(ASCP)
Tel: 651 846-3555   *Fax:* 651 994-0144
E-mail: kswanson@argosyu.edu

Northland Community & Technical College
Clin Lab Technician/Med Lab Technician
2022 Central Ave NE
East Grand Forks, MN 56721
Prgm Dir: Paula Bowman, MS MT(ASCP)
Tel: 218 773-2149   *Fax:* 218 773-4502
E-mail: paula.bowman@northlandcollege.edu

South Central College
Clin Lab Technician/Med Lab Technician
1225 3rd St SW
Faribault, MN 55021
Prgm Dir: Darla Petersen, MA BS
Tel: 507 332-5852   *Fax:* 507 332-5888
E-mail: darla.petersen@southcentral.edu

Minnesota State Community and Technical Coll
Clin Lab Technician/Med Lab Technician
1414 College Way
Fergus Falls, MN 56537
www.minnesota.edu
Prgm Dir: Patricia Sjolie, AS BS MS MT(ASCP)
Tel: 218 736-1594   *Fax:* 218 736-1510
E-mail: pat.sjolie@minnesota.edu

Hibbing Community College
Clin Lab Technician/Med Lab Technician
1515 E 25th St
Hibbing, MN 55746
Prgm Dir: Mitzi Morris, MT(ASCP)
Tel: 218 262-7254   *Fax:* 218 262-6717
E-mail: mitzimorris@hibbing.edu

Saint Paul College
Clin Lab Technician/Med Lab Technician
235 Marshall Ave
St Paul, MN 55102-1807
www.saintpaul.edu
Prgm Dir: Michelle Briski, MEd MT(ASCP) CLS(NCA)
Tel: 651 846-1421
E-mail: michelle.briski@saintpaul.edu

Minnesota West Comm & Tech College
Clin Lab Technician/Med Lab Technician
1450 Collegeway Dr
Worthington, MN 56187
Prgm Dir: Rita MIller, MS (CLS) MT(ASCP)
Tel: 507 372-3422   *Fax:* 507 825-4656
E-mail: rmiller@wr.mnwest.mnscu.edu

Mississippi

Northeast Mississippi Community College
Clin Lab Technician/Med Lab Technician
101 Cunningham Blvd
Booneville, MS 38829
www.nemcc.edu
Prgm Dir: Rita Murry, MA MT(ASCP)
Tel: 601 720-7403   *Fax:* 601 728-1165
E-mail: rjmurry@nemcc.edu

Mississippi Gulf Coast Community College
Clin Lab Technician/Med Lab Technician
2300 Hwy 90, PO Box 100
Gautier, MS 39553
www.mgccc.edu
Prgm Dir: Peggy Caldwell, MA MT(ASCP)
Tel: 228 497-7846   *Fax:* 228 497-7676
E-mail: peggy.caldwell@mgccc.edu

Pearl River Community College
Clin Lab Technician/Med Lab Technician
5448 US Hwy 49 S
Hattiesburg, MS 39401
www.prcc.edu
Prgm Dir: Evelyn Wallace, BS MT(ASCP)
Tel: 601 554-5523   *Fax:* 601 554-5511
E-mail: ewallace@prcc.edu

Hinds Community College
Clin Lab Technician/Med Lab Technician
Nursing/Allied Hlth Ctr
1750 Chadwick Dr
Jackson, MS 39204-3402
www.hindscc.edu
Prgm Dir: Timothy Henry, MS MT(ASCP)
Tel: 601 371-3515   *Fax:* 601 371-3529
E-mail: Tghenry@hindscc.edu

Meridian Community College
Clin Lab Technician/Med Lab Technician
910 Hwy 19 N
Meridian, MS 39307
Prgm Dir: Cassandra Johnson, MHS MT(ASCP)
Tel: 601 484-8754   *Fax:* 601 484-8743
E-mail: cjohnson@meridiancc.edu

Mississippi Delta Community College
Clin Lab Technician/Med Lab Technician
PO Box 668
Moorhead, MS 38761
www.msdelta.edu
Prgm Dir: Patricia Kelly, MT(AMT)(ASCP)BB MBA
Tel: 662 246-6500   *Fax:* 662 246-6507
E-mail: pkelly@msdelta.edu

Copiah-Lincoln Community College
Clin Lab Technician/Med Lab Technician
PO Box 457
Wesson, MS 39191-0457
https://www.colin.edu/careertech/MedicalLab
Prgm Dir: Mary E Shivers, MT(ASCP)
Tel: 601 643-8391   *Fax:* 601 643-8214
E-mail: mary.shivers@colin.edu

Missouri

Three Rivers Community College
Clin Lab Technician/Med Lab Technician
2080 Three Rivers Blvd
Poplar Bluff, MO 63901
www.trcc.edu
Prgm Dir: Dionne M Thompson, MSE MT(ASCP)
Tel: 573 840-9677, Ext 677   *Fax:* 573 840-9657
E-mail: deethomp@trcc.edu

St Louis Community College - Forest Park
Clin Lab Technician/Med Lab Technician
5600 Oakland Ave
St Louis, MO 63110
www.stlcc.edu
Prgm Dir: Karen M Kiser, MA MT(ASCP) PBT
Tel: 314 644-9645   *Fax:* 314 644-9752
E-mail: kkiser@stlcc.edu

Nebraska

Central Community College
Clin Lab Technician/Med Lab Technician
PO Box 1024
E Hwy 6
Hastings, NE 68902-1024
http://cccneb.edu
Prgm Dir: Lori Van Boening, MT(ASCP)
Tel: 402 461-2451   *Fax:* 402 460-2138
E-mail: lvanboening@cccneb.edu

Southeast Community College
Clin Lab Technician/Med Lab Technician
8800 O St
Lincoln, NE 68520
www.southeast.edu
Prgm Dir: Janis K Bible, BA MT(ASCP)
Tel: 402 437-2760   *Fax:* 402 437-2404
E-mail: jbible@southeast.edu

Mid-Plains Community College
Clin Lab Technician/Med Lab Technician
North Campus
1101 Halligan Dr
North Platte, NE 69101
www.mpcc.edu/page.cfm?action=show_section&
pg_id=73#
Prgm Dir: Martin D Steinbeck, MT(ASCP)
Tel: 308 535-3754   *Fax:* 308 535-3794
E-mail: steinbeckm@mpcc.edu

Nevada

College of Southern Nevada
Clin Lab Technician/Med Lab Technician
6375 W Charleston Blvd
Las Vegas, NV 89146
www.ccsn.nevada.edu
Prgm Dir: Patricia R Castro, EdD MS MT(ASCP)BB
Tel: 702 651-5819   *Fax:* 702 651-5762
E-mail: patricia.castro@csn.edu

New Hampshire

New Hampshire Comm Tech Coll - Claremont
Clin Lab Technician/Med Lab Technician
1 College Dr
Claremont, NH 03743
www.claremont.nhctc.edu
Prgm Dir: Andrea Gordon, MEd MT(ASCP)SH
Tel: 603 542-7744, Ext 317   *Fax:* 603 543-1844
E-mail: agordon@nhctc.edu

New Jersey

Camden County College
Clin Lab Technician/Med Lab Technician
PO Box 200
College Dr
Blackwood, NJ 08012
www.camdencc.edu
Prgm Dir: Patricia A Chappell, MA MT(ASCP)
Tel: 856 227-7200, Ext 4330   *Fax:* 856 374-4891
E-mail: pchappell@camdencc.edu

Middlesex County College
Clin Lab Technician/Med Lab Technician
2600 Woodbridge Ave
Edison, NJ 08818-3050
www.middlesexcc.edu
Prgm Dir: Stephen P Larkin III, MHSA MT(ASCP)SH
Tel: 732 906-2581
E-mail: slarkin@middlesexcc.edu

Mercer County Community College
Clin Lab Technician/Med Lab Technician
PO Box B
1200 Old Trenton Rd
Trenton, NJ 08690
www.mccc.edu
Prgm Dir: Jane O'Reilly, MEd MT(ASCP)
Tel: 609 570-3387   *Fax:* 609 689-0762
E-mail: oreilly@mccc.edu

New Mexico

New Mexico State U at Alamogordo
Clin Lab Technician/Med Lab Technician
2400 N Scenic Dr
Alamogordo, NM 88310
http://alamo.nmsu.edu
Prgm Dir: Judith J O'Brien, BS MT(ASCP) MM
Tel: 505 439-3761   *Fax:* 505 439-3759
E-mail: jjobrien@nmsua.nmsu.edu

Central New Mexico Community College
Clin Lab Technician/Med Lab Technician
525 Buena Vista SE
Albuquerque, NM 87106
www.cnm.edu
Prgm Dir: Monya Kmetz, MA MT(ASCP)
Tel: 505 224-5021   *Fax:* 505 224-5033
E-mail: monya@cnm.edu

University of New Mexico - Gallup
Clin Lab Technician/Med Lab Technician
200 College Rd
Gallup, NM 87301
Prgm Dir: Michael Nye, MT(ASCP) MSM
Tel: 505 863-7598   *Fax:* 505 863-7513
E-mail: mnye@gallup.unm.edu

New York

Broome Community College
Clin Lab Technician/Med Lab Technician
PO Box 1017
Binghamton, NY 13902
Prgm Dir: Andrea C Wade, PhD MT(ASCP)
Tel: 607 778-5211
E-mail: wade_a@sunybroome.edu

Farmingdale State College, SUNY
Clin Lab Technician/Med Lab Technician
2350 Broadhollow Rd, Gleeson Hall, Rm 304
Farmingdale, NY 11735
Prgm Dir: Karen M Escolas, EdD MT(ASCP)
Tel: 631 420-2257   *Fax:* 631 420-2784
E-mail: Karen.Escolas@Farmingdale.edu

Nassau Community College
Clin Lab Technician/Med Lab Technician
One Education Dr
Garden City, NY 11530
Prgm Dir: Lois Lucca, MS MT(ASCP
Tel: 516 572-7072
E-mail: luccal@ncc.edu

Orange County Community College
Clin Lab Technician/Med Lab Technician
115 South St
Middletown, NY 10940
www.sunyorange.edu
Prgm Dir: Rosamaria B Contarino, MS MT(ASCP)
CLS(NCA)
Tel: 845 341-4136   *Fax:* 845 341-4122
E-mail: rcontari@sunyorange.edu

Clinton Community College
Clin Lab Technician/Med Lab Technician
Lake Shore Rd, Rte 9 S
136 Clinton Point Dr
Plattsburgh, NY 12901
Prgm Dir: Sharon T Columbus, MEd MT(ASCP)
Tel: 518 562-4273   *Fax:* 518 562-4158
E-mail: Sharon.Columbus@clinton.edu

Dutchess Community College
Clin Lab Technician/Med Lab Technician
53 Pendell Rd
Poughkeepsie, NY 12601
www.sunydutchess.edu
Prgm Dir: Karen Ann Ingham, MT(ASCP)
Tel: 845 431-8321   *Fax:* 845 431-8329
E-mail: ingham@sunydutchess.edu

Erie Community College - North Campus
Clin Lab Technician/Med Lab Technician
6205 Main St
Williamsville, NY 14221
www.ecc.edu
Prgm Dir: Marcia T Bermel, MS MT(ASCP)
Tel: 716 851-1553   *Fax:* 716 851-1550
E-mail: bermel@ecc.edu

North Carolina

Asheville-Buncombe Technical Comm College
Clin Lab Technician/Med Lab Technician
340 Victoria Rd
Asheville, NC 28801
www.abtech.edu
Prgm Dir: Melissa Hyatt, BS MT(ASCP) MHS
Tel: 828 254-1921, Ext 266   *Fax:* 828 281-9734
E-mail: Mhyatt@abtech.edu

Central Piedmont Community College
Clin Lab Technician/Med Lab Technician
PO Box 35009
Charlotte, NC 28235-5009
www.cpcc.edu
Prgm Dir: Rebecca C Sanders, MSA MT(ASCP)SM
Tel: 704 330-5028   *Fax:* 704 330-6131
E-mail: becky.sanders@cpcc.edu

Alamance Community College
Clin Lab Technician/Med Lab Technician
PO Box 8000
Graham, NC 27253-8000
www.alamancecc.edu
Prgm Dir: Pamela E Hall, MA MT(ASCP)SBB
Tel: 336 506-4196   *Fax:* 336 578-1987
E-mail: hallpm@alamancecc.edu

Coastal Carolina Community College
Clin Lab Technician/Med Lab Technician
444 Western Blvd
Jacksonville, NC 28546-6877
www.coastal.cc.nc.us
Prgm Dir: Christine N Weaver, MS MT(ASCP)
CLS(NCA)
Tel: 910 938-6275   *Fax:* 910 938-6806
E-mail: weaverc@coastal.cc.nc.us

Davidson County Community College
Clin Lab Technician/Med Lab Technician
PO Box 1287
297 DCCC Rd
Lexington, NC 27293-1287
www.davidsonccc.edu
Prgm Dir: Suzanne Rohrbaugh, MA MT(ASCP)
Tel: 336 249-8186, Ext 6721   *Fax:* 336 249-9060
E-mail: srohr@davidsonccc.edu

Western Piedmont Community College
Clin Lab Technician/Med Lab Technician
1001 Burkemont Ave
Morganton, NC 28655-0680
Prgm Dir: Nancy Shoaf, MA MT(ASCP)
Tel: 828 438-6128   *Fax:* 828 430-7183
E-mail: nshoaf@wpcc.edu

Sandhills Community College
Clin Lab Technician/Med Lab Technician
3395 Airport Rd
Pinehurst, NC 28374
www.sandhills.edu
Prgm Dir: Cheryl P McCormick, PhD MT(ASCP)
Tel: 910 695-3839   *Fax:* 910 693-2060
E-mail: mccormickc@sandhills.edu

Wake Technical Community College
Clin Lab Technician/Med Lab Technician
9101 Fayetteville Rd
2901 Holston Lane
Raleigh, NC 27610
www.waketech.edu
Prgm Dir: Pamela Horton, MEd BS MT(ASCP)
Tel: 919 212-3818   *Fax:* 919 250-4329
E-mail: pbhorton@waketech.edu

Southwestern Community College
Clin Lab Technician/Med Lab Technician
447 College Dr
Sylva, NC 28779
www.southwesterncc.edu/mlt
Prgm Dir: Andrea Kennedy, MBA MT(ASCP)
Tel: 828 586-4091, Ext 312   *Fax:* 828 586-3129
E-mail: andrea@southwesterncc.edu

Beaufort County Community College
Clin Lab Technician/Med Lab Technician
PO Box 1069
Highway 264 East
Washington, NC 27889
www.beaufort.cc.nc.us
Prgm Dir: Arthur S Keehnle, MS MT(ASCP)
Tel: 252 940-6207   *Fax:* 252 946-0271
E-mail: artk@email.beaufort.cc.nc.us

Halifax Community College
Clin Lab Technician/Med Lab Technician
PO Box 809
Weldon, NC 27890
Prgm Dir: Randy C Harris, PhD MT(ASCP)
Tel: 804 786-4370   *Fax:* 804 536-4144
E-mail: rcharris@hanover.k12.va.us

Southeastern Community College
Clin Lab Technician/Med Lab Technician
PO Box 151
Whiteville, NC 28472
www.sccnc.edu
Prgm Dir: Patricia Wright, MT(ASCP)
Tel: 910 642-7141, Ext 312   *Fax:* 910 642-3257
E-mail: pwright@sccnc.edu

North Dakota

Bismarck State College
Clin Lab Technician/Med Lab Technician
1500 Edwards Ave
PO Box 5587
Bismarck, ND 58506-5587
www.bismarckstate.edu
Prgm Dir: Angela Uhlich, MS MT(ASCP)SBB
Tel: 701 323-5482   *Fax:* 701 323-5831
E-mail: Angela.Uhlich@bsc.nodak.edu

Ohio

Cincinnati State Tech & Comm College
Clin Lab Technician/Med Lab Technician
3520 Central Pkwy
Cincinnati, OH 45223
www.cincinnatistate.edu
Prgm Dir: A Janelle Gohn, PhD MT(ASCP)SM
Tel: 513 569-1688   *Fax:* 513 487-1688
E-mail: janelle.gohn@cincinnatistate.edu

Cuyahoga Community College
Clin Lab Technician/Med Lab Technician
Metro Campus Health Careers and Science Bldg, 126I
2900 Community College Ave
Cleveland, OH 44115-3196
www.tri-c.edu/MLT/docs/contact.htm
Prgm Dir: Amy Gatautis, MT(ASCP)SC MBA
Tel: 216 987-4438, Ext 4438   *Fax:* 216 987-4386
E-mail: amy.gatautis@tri-c.edu

Columbus State Community College
Clin Lab Technician/Med Lab Technician
550 E Spring St
Columbus, OH 43216-1609
Prgm Dir: Sandra Arrighi, MEd MT(ASCP)SBB
Tel: 614 287-2518   *Fax:* 614 287-5144
E-mail: sarrighi@cscc.edu

Lorain County Community College
Clin Lab Technician/Med Lab Technician
1005 N Abbe Rd
Elyria, OH 44035
Prgm Dir: James E Daly, MEd MT(ASCP)
Tel: 440 366-7194, Ext 7194   *Fax:* 440 366-4116
E-mail: jdaly@lorainccc.edu

Lakeland Community College
Clin Lab Technician/Med Lab Technician
7700 Clocktower Dr
Kirtland, OH 44094-5198
Prgm Dir: Kathryn G Ertter, MSHS MT(ASCP)
Tel: 440 525-7169   *Fax:* 440 975-4733
E-mail: kertter@lakelandcc.edu

Washington State Community College
Clin Lab Technician/Med Lab Technician
710 Colegate Dr
Marietta, OH 45750
www.wscc.edu
Prgm Dir: Heather Kincaid, MEd MT(ASCP)
Tel: 740 374-8716, Ext 1674   *Fax:* 740 373-7496
E-mail: hkincaid@wscc.edu

Marion Technical College
Clin Lab Technician/Med Lab Technician
1467 Mt Vernon Ave
Marion, OH 43302
www.mtc.edu
Prgm Dir: Deborah L Bates, MBA MT(ASCP)SBB
Tel: 740 389-4636, Ext 254   *Fax:* 740 725-4018
E-mail: batesd@mtc.edu

Stark State College of Technology
Clin Lab Technician/Med Lab Technician
6200 Frank Ave NW
North Canton, OH 44720
www.starkstate.edu
Prgm Dir: Kozy Corsaut, MS Ed MT(ASCP)
Tel: 330 494-6170, Ext 4221   *Fax:* 330 966-6586
E-mail: kcorsaut@starkstate.edu

Shawnee State University
Clin Lab Technician/Med Lab Technician
940 Second St
Portsmouth, OH 45662
Prgm Dir: Marla H Thoroughman, MS MA MT(ASCP)
Tel: 740 351-3388 *Fax:* 740 351-3354
E-mail: mthoroughman@shawnee.edu

University of Rio Grande
Clin Lab Technician/Med Lab Technician
218 N College Ave, F-39
Rio Grande, OH 45674-0500
Prgm Dir: Keith Searls, BS MT(ASCP)
Tel: 740 245-7319   *Fax:* 740 245-7440
E-mail: keith.searls@med.va.gov
• Currently inactive

Clark State Community College
Clin Lab Technician/Med Lab Technician
570 E Leffel Ln
Springfield, OH 45501-0570
www.clarkstate.edu
Prgm Dir: Sandra Jean Horn, MS MT(ASCP)
Tel: 937 328-8077   *Fax:* 937 328-6138
E-mail: horns@clarkstate.edu

Jefferson Community College
Clin Lab Technician/Med Lab Technician
4000 Sunset Blvd
Steubenville, OH 43952
www.jcc.edu
Prgm Dir: Sondra Sutherland, MEd MT(ASCP)
CLS(NCA)
Tel: 740 264-5591, Ext 165   *Fax:* 740 264-9504
E-mail: ssutherlan@jcc.edu

Youngstown State University
Clin Lab Technician/Med Lab Technician
Dept of Health Professions
One University Plaza
Youngstown, OH 44555
www.ysu.edu
Prgm Dir: Maria E Delost, PhD MT(ASCP) CLS(NCA)
Tel: 330 941-1761   *Fax:* 330 941-2921
E-mail: medelost@ysu.edu

Zane State College
Clin Lab Technician/Med Lab Technician
1555 Newark Rd
Zanesville, OH 43701
www.zanestate.edu
Prgm Dir: Vicki Huntsman, MS MT(ASCP)
Tel: 740 588-1311, Ext 1311   *Fax:* 740 454-0035
E-mail: vhunstman@zanestate.edu

Oklahoma

Northeastern Oklahoma A&M College
Clin Lab Technician/Med Lab Technician
Second and I Sts NE
Miami, OK 74354
www.neoam.edu
Prgm Dir: Rita Kay Harris, MS MT(ASCP)NM
Tel: 918 540-6315   *Fax:* 918 540-6471
E-mail: kharris@neoam.edu

Rose State College
Clin Lab Technician/Med Lab Technician
6420 SE 15th St
Midwest City, OK 73110
www.rose.edu
Prgm Dir: Evelyn Paxton, MS MT(ASCP)
Tel: 405 733-7577   *Fax:* 405 736-0338
E-mail: epaxton@rose.edu

Seminole State College
Clin Lab Technician/Med Lab Technician
PO Box 351
2701 Boren Blvd
Seminole, OK 74818-0351
http://sscok.edu
Prgm Dir: Perthena Latchaw, MS MT(ASCP)
Tel: 405 382-9214   *Fax:* 405 382-3122
E-mail: p.latchaw@sscok.edu

Tulsa Community College
Clin Lab Technician/Med Lab Technician
909 S Boston Ave
10300 E 81st St, 74133
Tulsa, OK 74119
www.tulsacc.edu
Prgm Dir: Karen L Holmes, MA MT(ASCP)
Tel: 918 595-8666   *Fax:* 918 595-7091
E-mail: kholmes@tulsacc.edu

Oregon

Portland Community College
Clin Lab Technician/Med Lab Technician
PO Box 19000
Portland, OR 97280-0990
Prgm Dir: Jeffrey Josifek, MS CLS(NCA)
Tel: 503 978-5679   *Fax:* 503 978-5257
E-mail: jjosifek@pcc.edu

Pennsylvania

Montgomery County Community College
Clin Lab Technician/Med Lab Technician
340 DeKalb Pike
PO Box 400
Blue Bell, PA 19422
www.mc3.edu
Prgm Dir: Debra Lynn Eckman, MS MT(ASCP)
Tel: 215 641-6487   *Fax:* 215 619-7178
E-mail: deckman@mc3.edu

Harcum College
Clin Lab Technician/Med Lab Technician
750 Montgomery Ave
Bryn Mawr, PA 19010
Prgm Dir: Donna M Broderick, MS MT(ASCP)
CLS(NCA)
Tel: 610 526-6662   *Fax:* 610 526-6031
E-mail: dbroderick@harcum.edu

Harrisburg Area Community College
Clin Lab Technician/Med Lab Technician
One HACC Dr
Harrisburg, PA 17110-2999
Prgm Dir: Ruth A Negley, MEd MT(ASCP)SM CLS(NCA)
Tel: 717 337-3855   *Fax:* 717 780-2551
E-mail: ranegley@hacc.edu

Penn State University - Hazleton
Clin Lab Technician/Med Lab Technician
76 University Dr
Hazleton, PA 18202
www.hn.psu.edu/Academics/MLTassoc.htm?cn21
Prgm Dir: Patricia D Ferry, MS MT(ASCP)
Tel: 570 450-3090   *Fax:* 570 450-3182
E-mail: pdf1@psu.edu

Community College of Philadelphia
Clin Lab Technician/Med Lab Technician
1700 Spring Garden St
Philadelphia, PA 19130
Prgm Dir: Robin G Krefetz, MEd MT(ASCP) CLS(NCA)
Tel: 215 751-8511   *Fax:* 215 751-8937
E-mail: rkrefetz@ccp.edu

Reading Area Community College
Clin Lab Technician/Med Lab Technician
Ten S Second St, PO Box 1706
Reading, PA 19603
Prgm Dir: Sandra A Neiman, MA MT(ASCP) CLS(NCA)
Tel: 610 372-4721, Ext 5428   *Fax:* 610 607-6254
E-mail: sneiman@racc.edu

Comm College of Allegheny County
Clin Lab Technician/Med Lab Technician
1750 Clairton Rd, Rte 885
West Mifflin, PA 15122
www.ccac.edu
Prgm Dir: Jane Coughanour, MEd MT(ASCP)
Tel: 412 469-6280, Ext 6280   *Fax:* 412 469-6371
E-mail: jcoughanour@ccac.edu

Rhode Island

Community College of Rhode Island
Clin Lab Technician/Med Lab Technician
1762 Louisquisset Pike
Lincoln, RI 02865
Prgm Dir: Maggie Joseph
Tel: 401 333-7148   *Fax:* 401 333-7441
E-mail: mjosephs@ccri.edu

South Carolina

Trident Technical College
Clin Lab Technician/Med Lab Technician
PO Box 118067
7000 Rivers Ave
Charleston, SC 29423-8067
http://tridenttech.edu
Prgm Dir: Donna J Donaldson, MCLT MT(ASCP)
Tel: 843 574-6476   *Fax:* 843 574-6585
E-mail: donna.donaldson@tridenttech.edu

Midlands Technical College
Clin Lab Technician/Med Lab Technician
PO Box 2408
Columbia, SC 29202
www.midlandstech.edu
Prgm Dir: Mary Breci, MAT BSMT(ASCP)
Tel: 803 822-3557   *Fax:* 803 822-3417
E-mail: brecim@midlandstech.edu

Florence-Darlington Technical College
Clin Lab Technician/Med Lab Technician
PO Box 100548
Florence, SC 29501-0548
Prgm Dir: Kathleen Hanrahan, MHA MT PBT (ASCP)
Tel: 843 661-8105   *Fax:* 843 292-0851
E-mail: hanrahank@fdtc.edu

Greenville Technical College
Clin Lab Technician/Med Lab Technician
PO Box 5616/Station B
Greenville, SC 29606
www.greenvilletech.com
Prgm Dir: Tommie H Whitt, MHSA MT(ASCP)
Tel: 864 250-8292   *Fax:* 864 250-8462
E-mail: Tommie.Whitt@gvltec.edu

Orangeburg Calhoun Technical College
Clin Lab Technician/Med Lab Technician
3250 St Matthews Rd
Orangeburg, SC 29118
Prgm Dir: Bonnie D Fanning, MS MT(ASCP)
Tel: 803 535-1349   *Fax:* 803 535-1350
E-mail: fanningb@octech.edu

Tri-County Technical College
Clin Lab Technician/Med Lab Technician
PO Box 587
Pendleton, SC 29670-0587
Prgm Dir: Polly Kay, MHS MT(ASCP)
Tel: 864 646-1349 *Fax:* 864 646-1892
E-mail: pkay@tctc.edu

York Technical College
Clin Lab Technician/Med Lab Technician
452 S Anderson Rd
Rock Hill, SC 29730
www.yorktech.com
Prgm Dir: R Lynne Fantry, MLA MT(ASCP)
Tel: 803 981-7082 *Fax:* 803 981-7216
E-mail: lfantry@yorktech.com

Spartanburg Community College
Clin Lab Technician/Med Lab Technician
PO Drawer 4386
Spartanburg, SC 29305
Prgm Dir: Ellen F Romani, MHSA MT(ASCP) BBDLM
Tel: 864 592-4866 *Fax:* 864 592-4881
E-mail: romanie@stcsc.edu

South Dakota

Presentation College
Clin Lab Technician/Med Lab Technician
1500 N Main St
Aberdeen, SD 57401
Prgm Dir: Terry Piatz, MS MT(ASCP)
Tel: 605 229-8526 *Fax:* 605 229-8518
E-mail: Terry.Piatz@presentation.edu

Mitchell Technical Institute
Clin Lab Technician/Med Lab Technician
821 N Capital
Mitchell, SD 57301
www.mitchelltech.edu
Prgm Dir: Lynne M Smith, MT(ASCP) MEd
Tel: 605 995-3032 *Fax:* 605 996-3299
E-mail: lynne.smith@mitchelltech.edu

Lake Area Technical Institute
Clin Lab Technician/Med Lab Technician
200 NE 9th St
Watertown, SD 57201
Prgm Dir: Mona Gleysteen, MS CLS(NCA)
Tel: 605 882-5284, Ext 324 *Fax:* 605 882-6347
E-mail: mgleyste@lakeareatech.edu

Tennessee

MedVance Institute
Clin Lab Technician/Med Lab Technician
1025 Highway 111
Cookeville, TN 38501
www.medvance.org
Prgm Dir: LaVerne Floyd, MA MT(ASCP)
Tel: 931 528-8589 *Fax:* 931 528-5327
E-mail: laverne@multipro.com

Northeast State Technical Comm College
Clin Lab Technician/Med Lab Technician
Nave Center/1000 Jason Witten Way
Elizabethton, TN 37643
Prgm Dir: Linda S Lahr, MS MT(ASCP)
Tel: 423 547-4907 *Fax:* 423 543-2266
E-mail: lslahr@northeaststate.edu

Volunteer State Community College
Clin Lab Technician/Med Lab Technician
1480 Nashville Pike
Gallatin, TN 37066
Prgm Dir: Lisa Lee-Biggs, MS MT(ASCP)
Tel: 615 230-3363
E-mail: Lisa.Lee-Biggs@volstate.edu

Jackson State Community College
Clin Lab Technician/Med Lab Technician
Allied Health Department
2046 N Parkway
Jackson, TN 38301-3797
Prgm Dir: Peter P O'Brien, MBA MT(ASCP) CLS(NCA)
Tel: 731 425-2612, Ext 226 *Fax:* 731 425-9551
E-mail: pobrien@jscc.edu

Southwest Tennessee Community College
Clin Lab Technician/Med Lab Technician
PO Box 780
761 Linden Ave
Memphis, TN 38101
Prgm Dir: Darius Y Wilson, EdD MAT MT(ASCP)
Tel: 901 333-5407 *Fax:* 901 333-5391
E-mail: dwilson@southwest.tn.edu

Texas

Amarillo College
Clin Lab Technician/Med Lab Technician
PO Box 447
Amarillo, TX 79178
www.actx.edu/medical_lab or
    http://www.actx.edu/mltonline
Prgm Dir: Jan Martin, BA MEd-MLT/MT(ASCP)
    CLT/CLS(NCA)
Tel: 806 354-6059 *Fax:* 806 354-6076
E-mail: martin-jm@actx.edu

Austin Community College
Clin Lab Technician/Med Lab Technician
Eastview Campus
3401 Webberville Rd
Austin, TX 78702
Prgm Dir: Terry Kotrla, MS MT(ASCP)BB
Tel: 512 223-5932 *Fax:* 512 223-5898
E-mail: kotrla@austincc.edu

Univ Tx at Brownsville/Tx Southmost Coll
Clin Lab Technician/Med Lab Technician
80 Ft Brown
Brownsville, TX 78520
Prgm Dir: Consuelo Villalon, MPH MT(AMT)
Tel: 956 882-5010 *Fax:* 956 554-5012
E-mail: consuelo.villalon@utb.edu

Del Mar College
Clin Lab Technician/Med Lab Technician
101 Baldwin Blvd
Corpus Christi, TX 78404
www.delmar.edu
Prgm Dir: Duncan F Samo, MEd MT(ASCP) CLS(NCA)
Tel: 361 698-2824 *Fax:* 361 698-2811
E-mail: dsamo@delmar.edu

Navarro College
Clin Lab Technician/Med Lab Technician
3200 W Seventh Ave
Corsicana, TX 75110-4899
www.navarrocollege.edu
Prgm Dir: Evelyn Glass, MS MT(ASCP)
Tel: 903 875-7516 *Fax:* 903 875-7525
E-mail: evelyn.glass@navarrocollege.edu

El Centro College
Clin Lab Technician/Med Lab Technician
801 Main St
Dallas, TX 75202-3604
Prgm Dir: Lisa Lock, MBA BSMT MT(ASCP)BB
    CLS(NCA)
Tel: 214 860-2304, Ext 2304 *Fax:* 214 860-2268
E-mail: lal5630@dcccd.edu

Grayson County College
Clin Lab Technician/Med Lab Technician
6101 Grayson Dr
Denison, TX 75020
Prgm Dir: Alan Jackson, MS MT(ASCP)
Tel: 903 463-8779 *Fax:* 903 463-5284
E-mail: jacksona@grayson.edu

El Paso Community College
Clin Lab Technician/Med Lab Technician
PO Box 20500
El Paso, TX 79998
www.epcc.edu
Prgm Dir: Veronica Dominguez, MEd CLS(NCA)
Tel: 915 831-4085 *Fax:* 915 831-4114
E-mail: vdoming6@epcc.edu

US Army Medical Dept Center & School
Clin Lab Technician/Med Lab Technician
Academy of Health Sciences
3151 Scott Rd
Fort Sam Houston, TX 78234-6137
Prgm Dir: Donna S Whitlaker, PhD MT(ASCP)SBB
Tel: 210 221-7709 *Fax:* 210 221-7679
E-mail: donna.whitlaker@amedd.army.mil

Tarleton State University
Clin Lab Technician/Med Lab Technician
1501 Enderly Place
Fort Worth, TX 76104
Prgm Dir: Lynda Gunter, PhD MT(ASCP)
Tel: 817 926-1101, Ext 228
E-mail: gunter@tarleton.edu

Houston Community College
Clin Lab Technician/Med Lab Technician
1900 Pressler
Houston, TX 77030
www.hccs.edu
Prgm Dir: Theresa Spain, MEd MT(ASCP) CLS(NCA)
Tel: 713 718-5518 *Fax:* 713 718-7653
E-mail: theresa.spain@hccs.edu

Central Texas College
Clin Lab Technician/Med Lab Technician
6200 W Central TX Expressway
PO Box 1800
Killeen, TX 76541-9990
www.ctcd.edu
Prgm Dir: Donna E Poteet, MA CLS(NCA)
Tel: 254 526-1187 *Fax:* 254 526-1765
E-mail: donna.poteet@ctcd.edu

Laredo Community College
Clin Lab Technician/Med Lab Technician
West End Washington St
Laredo, TX 78040
www.laredo.edu
Prgm Dir: Bill Branim, Jr, MS Chem MPA MT(ASCP)
    DLM
Tel: 956 796-2155 *Fax:* 956 721-5421
E-mail: bill_branim@chs.net

Lamar State College - Orange
Clin Lab Technician/Med Lab Technician
410 Front St
Orange, TX 77630
Prgm Dir: Kathleen Ann Park, MEd MT(ASCP)
Tel: 409 882-3914 *Fax:* 409 882-3374
E-mail: Kathy.Park@lsco.edu

San Jacinto College Central
Clin Lab Technician/Med Lab Technician
8060 Spencer Hwy, PO Box 2007
Pasadena, TX 77501-2007
Prgm Dir: Terri C Simon, MS
Tel: 281 478-2730 *Fax:* 281 478-2754
E-mail: terri.simon@sjcd.edu

St Philip's College
Clin Lab Technician/Med Lab Technician
1801 Martin Luther King Dr
San Antonio, TX 78203-2098
www.accd.edu/spc
Prgm Dir: Jerri Lee Reynolds, PhD MT(ASCP)
Tel: 210 531-3449 *Fax:* 210 531-3459
E-mail: jreynolds@mail.accd.edu

882d Training Group
Clin Lab Technician/Med Lab Technician
382 Training Squadron/XYAC
917 Missile Rd, Ste 3
Sheppard AFB, TX 76311-2263
Prgm Dir: Barry T White, MS MT(ASCP)
Tel: 940 676-3869   *Fax:* 940 676-3850
E-mail: Barry.White@sheppard.af.mil

Tyler Junior College
Clin Lab Technician/Med Lab Technician
PO Box 9020
Tyler, TX 75711-9020
www.tjc.edu/medlab/home.asp
Prgm Dir: Daniel L Spencer, EdD MT(ASCP) CLS(NCA)
Tel: 903 510-2240   *Fax:* 903 510-2880
E-mail: dspe@tjc.edu

Victoria College
Clin Lab Technician/Med Lab Technician
2200 E Red River
Victoria, TX 77901
www.victoriacollege.edu/dept/mlt/
Prgm Dir: Larry S Dunn, MS MT(ASCP)
Tel: 361 572-6455   *Fax:* 361 572-6441
E-mail: larry.dunn@victoriacollege.edu

McLennan Community College
Clin Lab Technician/Med Lab Technician
1400 College Dr
Waco, TX 76708
www.mclennan.edu
Prgm Dir: Diane L Schmaus, MA MT(ASCP)
Tel: 254 299-8417   *Fax:* 254 299-8435
E-mail: dschmaus@mclennan.edu

Utah

Weber State University
Clin Lab Technician/Med Lab Technician
3905 University Cirlce
Ogden, UT 84408-3905
http://weber.edu/cls
Prgm Dir: Yasmen Simonian, PhD MT(ASCP) CLS(NCA)
Tel: 801 626-7080   *Fax:* 801 626-7508
E-mail: ysimonian@weber.edu

Salt Lake Community College
Clin Lab Technician/Med Lab Technician
PO Box 30808
Salt Lake City, UT 84130
Prgm Dir: Karen A Brown, MS MT(ASCP) CLS
Tel: 801 581-3544   *Fax:* 801 585-2463
E-mail: karen.brown@path.utah.edu

Virginia

Thomas Nelson Community College
Clin Lab Technician/Med Lab Technician
PO Box 9407
99 Thomas Nelson Dr
Hampton, VA 23670
http://tncc.edu
Prgm Dir: Linda A Dezern, MS MT(ASCP)
Tel: 757 825-2783   *Fax:* 757 825-3831
E-mail: dezernl@tncc.edu

Centra Health Systems of Lynchburg
Clin Lab Technician/Med Lab Technician
3300 Rivermont Ave
Lynchburg, VA 24501
Prgm Dir: Robin L Levandoski, MEd BS MT(ASCP) SC
Tel: 434 947-4551   *Fax:* 434 947-4035
E-mail: levandoskir@cvcc.vccs.edu

J Sargeant Reynolds Community College
Clin Lab Technician/Med Lab Technician
PO Box 85622
Richmond, VA 23285-5622
www.reynolds.edu
Prgm Dir: Becky Clark, MEd MT(ASCP)
Tel: 804 523-5772   *Fax:* 804 786-5298
E-mail: bclark@reynolds.edu

Northern Virginia Community College
Clin Lab Technician/Med Lab Technician
6699 Springfield Center Dr
Springfield, VA 22150
www.nvcc.edu
Prgm Dir: Glenn Flodstrom, MS MT(ASCP)
Tel: 703 822-6367   *Fax:* 703 822-6619
E-mail: gflodstrom@nvcc.edu

Wytheville Community College
Clin Lab Technician/Med Lab Technician
1000 E Main St
Wytheville, VA 24382
Prgm Dir: Lorri Huffard, MS MT(ASCP)SBB
Tel: 276 223-4828   *Fax:* 276 223-4778
E-mail: wchuffl@wcc.vccs.edu

Washington

Clover Park Technical College
Clin Lab Technician/Med Lab Technician
4500 Steilacoom Blvd SW
Lakewood, WA 98499-4098
www.cptc.ctc.edu
Prgm Dir: Anne G O'Neil, MT(ASCP) MEd
Tel: 253 589-5625   *Fax:* 253 589-5866
E-mail: anne.oneil@cptc.edu

Shoreline Community College
Clin Lab Technician/Med Lab Technician
16101 Greenwood Ave N
Seattle, WA 98133
Prgm Dir: Molly Morse, MS CLS(NCA) MT(ASCP)
Tel: 206 546-6947   *Fax:* 206 533-5103
E-mail: mmorse@shoreline.edu

Wenatchee Valley College
Clin Lab Technician/Med Lab Technician
1300 Fifth St
Wenatchee, WA 98801
Prgm Dir: David C Abbott, MSA MT(ASCP)
Tel: 509 682-6668   *Fax:* 509 682-6541
E-mail: dabbott@wvc.edu

West Virginia

Bluefield Regional Medical Center
Cosponsor: New River Technical and Community College
Clin Lab Technician/Med Lab Technician
500 Cherry St
Bluefield, WV 24701-3306
Prgm Dir: Mary Boysaw, MHE MT(ASCP)
Tel: 304 327-1596   *Fax:* 304 327-1591
E-mail: mboysaw@brmcwv.org

Fairmont State Univ
Cosponsor: Pierpont Comm & Tech College
Clin Lab Technician/Med Lab Technician
1201 Locust Ave
Fairmont, WV 26554
www.fairmontstate.edu
Prgm Dir: Rosemarie R Romesburg, PhD MT(ASCP)
Tel: 304 367-4284   *Fax:* 304 367-4268
E-mail: rromesburg@fairmontstate.edu

Marshall University
Clin Lab Technician/Med Lab Technician
Clinical Lab Science Dept
One John Marshall Dr
Huntington, WV 25755
Prgm Dir: Dorothy J Fike, MS MT(ASCP)
Tel: 304 696-3165   *Fax:* 304 696-3243
E-mail: fike@marshall.edu

Southern West Virginia Comm & Tech College
Clin Lab Technician/Med Lab Technician
Logan Campus/PO Box 2900
Mount Gay, WV 25637
http://southernwv.edu
Prgm Dir: Vernon R Elkins, MA BS MT(ASCP)
Tel: 304 792-7098, Ext 243   *Fax:* 304 792-7053
E-mail: vernone@southern.wvnet.edu

Wisconsin

Chippewa Valley Technical College
Clin Lab Technician/Med Lab Technician
620 W Clairemont Ave
Eau Claire, WI 54701
www.cvtc.edu/Programs/DeptPages/CLT/
   MLTHomePage.html
Prgm Dir: Patricia Griffin, MS MT(ASCP)
Tel: 715 833-6420   *Fax:* 715 833-6470
E-mail: pgriffin@cvtc.edu

Moraine Park Technical College
Clin Lab Technician/Med Lab Technician
235 N National Ave
PO Box 1940
Fond du Lac, WI 54936-1940
Prgm Dir: Linda Bau, MPA BS MT(ASCP)
Tel: 920 924-6373
E-mail: lbau@morainepark.edu

Northeast Wisconsin Technical College
Clin Lab Technician/Med Lab Technician
2740 W Mason St, PO Box 19042
Green Bay, WI 54307-9042
www.nwtc.edu
Prgm Dir: Patricia Moore-Cribb, MT(ASCP) MS
Tel: 920 498-6374   *Fax:* 920 498-2660
E-mail: patricia.cribb@nwtc.edu

Western Technical College
Clin Lab Technician/Med Lab Technician
304 N Sixth St, PO Box C-908
La Crosse, WI 54601
Prgm Dir: Carolyn Byom, MS MT(ASCP)
Tel: 608 789-6284   *Fax:* 608 785-9299
E-mail: byomc@wwtc.edu

Madison Area Technical College
Clin Lab Technician/Med Lab Technician
3550 Anderson St
Madison, WI 53704-2599
Prgm Dir: Sue Ellen S Beglinger, MS MT(ASCP)
   CLS(NCA)
Tel: 608 246-6459   *Fax:* 608 246-6013
E-mail: beglinger@matcmadison.edu

Milwaukee Area Technical College
Clin Lab Technician/Med Lab Technician
700 W State St
Milwaukee, WI 53233
www.matc.edu
Prgm Dir: Dennis Schmidt, MS MT(ASCP)
Tel: 414 297-7142   *Fax:* 414 297-6851
E-mail: SchmidtD@matc.edu

PROGRAMS

Clinical Laboratory Technician/Medical Laboratory Technician

Programs*	Class Capacity	Begins	Length (months)	Award	Res. Tuition	Non-res. Tuition	Stipend	Offers:‡ 1	2	3	4
Alabama											
Gadsden State Community College	17	Aug Jan	24	AAS	$3,780	$7,560					
Jefferson State Community College (Birmingham)	18	May Aug	24	Dipl, AAS	$7,548	$12,802					•
Wallace State Community College (Hanceville)	30	May Aug	19	Dipl, AAS	$3,420	$6,840					
Alaska											
University of Alaska Anchorage	13	Open enrollment	20	AAS	$2,574	$8,580				•	•
Arkansas											
Arkansas State University	20	Aug	24	AAS	$149	$384					
Arkansas State University - Beebe	15	Jul	12	AAS	$1,200	$1,824				•	
North Arkansas College (Harrison)	12	Jul	10	AAS	$2,040	$4,366					
South Arkansas Community College (El Dorado)	10	Aug	12	AAS	$3,500	$6,498		•			
Colorado											
Arapahoe Community College (Littleton)	30	Aug	24	AAS	$3,300	$12,030		•			•
Florida											
Brevard Community College (Cocoa)	16	Open entry	22	Dipl AS, ATD	$5,149	$18,772					
Erwin Technical Center (Tampa)	18	Jan	15	Dipl	$2,757	$10,998				•	
Florida Community College - Jacksonville	20	Aug Jan May	24	AS	$2,290	$9,158		•			•
Indian River Community College (Fort Pierce)	17	Aug	23	AS	$2,584	$9,310		•			•
Keiser University (Fort Lauderdale)	20	Jan Apr Aug	22	AS	$17,460	$17,460					
Miami Dade College	45	Aug Jan	22	AS	$5,200	$17,380		•		•	
St Petersburg College	40	Aug	24	AS	$2,648	$9,952					•
Georgia											
Central Georgia Technical College (Macon)	12	Oct	21	AAT	$1,812	$1,812					
Coastal Georgia Community College (Brunswick)	15	Aug	21	AS	$2,700	$9,843					
Dalton State College	12	Aug Jan	24	AAS	$1,872	$7,951				•	
Darton College (Albany)	36	Aug	17	AS	$2,406	$9,618		•			•
DeKalb Technical College (Clarkston)	28	Oct	24	AAS	$5,652	$14,324	$2,500			•	
Lanier Technical College (Oakwood)	12	Oct	24	AAS	$1,860	$3,720				•	
North Georgia Technical College (Clarkesville)	15	Oct	21	AAS	$1,868	$3,736		•			•
Okefenokee Technical College (Waycross)	14	Apr	24	AAT	$1,750	$0				•	
Southwest Georgia Technical College (Thomasville)	12	Apr	24	AAT	$2,554	$3,554					
Hawaii											
Kapi'olani Community College (Honolulu)	16	Jan	17	AS	$2,218	$9,070					
Illinois											
Blessing Hospital (Quincy)	8	Aug	12	Assoc	$1,000	$1,000				•	
Elgin Community College	15	Aug	22	AAS	$4,000	$15,000		•		•	•
Illinois Central College (Peoria)	16	Aug	20	AAS	$5,100	$10,540		•			•
Kankakee Community College	17	Aug	18, 12	AAS	$2,483	$6,484					
Oakton Community College (Des Plaines)	20	Aug	21	Dipl AAS	$3,500	$7,500				•	
Southwestern Illinois College (Belleville)	14	Aug	20	AAS	$3,500	$5,000					
Indiana											
Indiana University Northwest (Gary)	18	Aug	21	AS	$5,320	$13,875				•	
Ivy Tech Community College - South Bend	15	Aug	22	AAS	$3,200	$6,400		•			
Ivy Tech Community College - Terre Haute	24	Aug	21	AAS	$6,143	$12,495					
Iowa											
Des Moines Area Community College (Ankeny)	24	Aug	22	AAS	$3,492	$6,984					•
Hawkeye Community College (Waterloo)	24	Aug	21	AAS	$2,465	$4,930					
Kansas											
Barton County Community College (Great Bend)	25	Aug	24	Dipl, AAS	$2,700	$3,330					
Seward County Community College (Liberal)	15	Aug Jan	24	AAS	$3,300	$3,300					•
Wichita Area Technical College	18	Aug	24, 12	AAS	$7,016	$22,541				•	•
Kentucky											
Eastern Kentucky University (Richmond)	36	Aug Jan	22	AS	$2,597	$7,269					
HCC/MCC Consortium (Madisonville)	26	Aug	24	AAS	$3,706	$11,118					
Somerset Community College	15	Aug	21	AAS	$4,025	$12,075					
Southeast Kentucky Comm & Tech College (Pineville)	14	Aug	24	AAS	$115	$345					
Louisiana											
Delgado Community College (New Orleans)	12	Jan	24	AAS	$768	$2,258					
MedVance Institute (Baton Rouge)	40	Jan Apr Jul Oct	18	AOS	$16,663	$16,663					
Our Lady of the Lake College (Baton Rouge)	14	Jun	12	AS CLT	$7,700	$7,700				•	
Southern Univ at Shreveport	24	Aug	24	AS	$2,000	$3,700					
Maine											
University of Maine - Presque Isle	30	Sep	20	AS	$5,005	$12,460					
Massachusetts											
Springfield Technical Community College	18	Sep	22	Dipl, AS	$1,408	$6,016				•	

*Data are shown only for programs that completed the 2007 AMA Survey of Health Professions Education Programs.
‡Key to Offers: 1: Evening or weekend classes; 2: Non-English instruction; 3: Cultural competence instruction; 4: Distance education component.

Clinical Laboratory Technician/Medical Laboratory Technician

Programs*	Class Capacity	Begins	Length (months)	Award	Res. Tuition	Non-res. Tuition	Stipend	Offers:‡ 1	2	3	4
Michigan											
Baker College of Owosso	20	Mar	13	AAS	$20,720	$20,720		•		•	•
Ferris State University (Big Rapids)	32	May	13	Dipl, AAS	$8,700	$15,900				•	
Kellogg Community College (Battle Creek)	16	Aug	22	AAS	$2,624	$4,131					
Minnesota											
Argosy University - Twin Cities (Eagan)	12	Sep Jan May	24	AS	$18,000	$18,000		•		•	
Lake Superior College (Duluth)	30	Aug	20	AAS	$4,140	$6,401		•		•	
Minnesota State Community and Technical Coll (Fergus Falls)	15	Aug	19	AS	$153	$153		•		•	•
Saint Paul College (St Paul)	24	Aug	20	AAS	$144	$277		•		•	•
South Central College (Faribault)	50	Aug	22	AAS	$5,400	$8,100					•
Mississippi											
Copiah-Lincoln Community College (Wesson)	30	Aug Jan	24	AAS	$1,800	$3,500					
Hinds Community College (Jackson)	20	Aug	24	AAS	$2,490	$5,799					
Mississippi Delta Community College (Moorhead)	18	Jun	24	AAS	$1,800	$3,408				•	
Mississippi Gulf Coast Community College (Gautier)	16	Aug Jan	24	AS	$1,596	$3,192					
Northeast Mississippi Community College (Booneville)	15	Aug	22	AAS	$915	$1,830					
Pearl River Community College (Hattiesburg)	20	Aug	24	Dipl, AS	$1,620	$2,398		•			
Missouri											
St Louis Community College - Forest Park	20	Aug	20	AAS	$3,645	$6,660				•	•
Three Rivers Community College (Poplar Bluff)	20	Aug	22	Dipl, AAS	$2,100	$4,100					
Nebraska											
Central Community College (Hastings)	16	Aug	24	AAS	$2,176	$3,298					
Mid-Plains Community College (North Platte)	20	Aug	24	AAS	$2,622	$3,306		•			
Southeast Community College (Lincoln)	26	Jul	24	AAS	$2,887	$3,514		•	•		
Nevada											
College of Southern Nevada (Las Vegas)	12	Jan Aug	24	AAS	$1,880	$4,572		•	•		
New Hampshire											
New Hampshire Comm Tech Coll - Claremont	12	Sep	20	AS	$6,400	$14,664		•	•		
New Jersey											
Camden County College (Blackwood)	16	May	24	AAS	$3,564	$3,894		•	•		
Mercer County Community College (Trenton)	12	May	14	AAS	$3,038	$4,076				•	
Middlesex County College (Edison)	21	Sep	21	AAS	$4,000	$8,000		•			
New Mexico											
Central New Mexico Community College (Albuquerque)	20	Aug	20, 24	AS	$1,607	$1,897				•	•
New Mexico State U at Alamogordo	10	Aug	20	Assoc	$1,600	$5,310					
University of New Mexico - Gallup	12	Aug Jan	24, 30	AS	$1,438	$3,190				•	
New York											
Broome Community College (Binghamton)	24	Aug Jan	20	AAS	$3,058	$6,116				•	
Dutchess Community College (Poughkeepsie)	30	Aug	20	AAS	$2,700	$5,400		•			
Erie Community College - North Campus (Williamsville)	45	Sep	21	AAS	$2,987	$5,974				•	
Farmingdale State College, SUNY	40	Sep	24	AS	$4,350	$10,610					
Orange County Community College (Middletown)	18	Sep	18	AAS	$3,000	$6,000					
North Carolina											
Alamance Community College (Graham)	40	Aug Jan May	24	AAS	$1,500	$5,600			•	•	
Asheville-Buncombe Technical Comm College	16	Aug	21	AAS	$1,748	$9,706					
Beaufort County Community College (Washington)	13	Aug	22	AAS	$1,824	$10,128		•			
Central Piedmont Community College (Charlotte)	16	Aug	21	AAS	$2,000	$8,000					
Coastal Carolina Community College (Jacksonville)	20	Aug	22	AAS	$1,126	$6,134					
Davidson County Community College (Lexington)	24	Aug	21	AAS	$1,800	$10,500					•
Sandhills Community College (Pinehurst)	18	Aug	21	AAS	$836	$4,642				•	
Southeastern Community College (Whiteville)	20	Aug	23	AAS	$1,323	$7,353		•			•
Southwestern Community College (Sylva)	20	Aug	22	AAS	$1,264	$7,024		•			•
Wake Technical Community College (Raleigh)	24	Aug	21	AAS	$1,896	$10,536				•	
Western Piedmont Community College (Morganton)	16	Aug 20	21	AAS	$2,055	$11,240					•
North Dakota											
Bismarck State College	10	Aug	22	AS	$3,500	$8,950		•	•	•	
Ohio											
Cincinnati State Tech & Comm College	30	Sep	24	AAS	$5,100	$10,200				•	
Clark State Community College (Springfield)	28+	Sep Jan	18	AAS	$5,499	$8,687					•
Columbus State Community College	50	Mar Fall	21	AAS	$3,504	$7,728					
Cuyahoga Community College (Cleveland)	24	Aug	21	AAS	$2,275	$5,975				•	•
Jefferson Community College (Steubenville)	16	Aug	24	AAS	$3,017	$4,082					
Lorain County Community College (Elyria)	20	Aug	20	AAS	$2,769	$3,334					
Marion Technical College	15	Sep	21	AAS	$6,037	$8,263					
Stark State College of Technology (North Canton)	20	Aug	21	AAS	$4,500	$6,545					
Washington State Community College (Marietta)	16	Sep	21	AAS	$3,420	$6,840					•

*Data are shown only for programs that completed the 2007 AMA Survey of Health Professions Education Programs.
‡Key to Offers: 1: Evening or weekend classes; 2: Non-English instruction; 3: Cultural competence instruction; 4: Distance education component.

Clinical Laboratory Technician/Medical Laboratory Technician

Programs*	Class Capacity	Begins	Length (months)	Award	Res. Tuition	Non-res. Tuition	Stipend	Offers:‡ 1	2	3	4
Youngstown State University	15	Aug	24	AAS	$6,468	$11,974		•			•
Zane State College (Zanesville)	20	Sep	22	AAS	$85	$170		•		•	•
Oklahoma											
Northeastern Oklahoma A&M College (Miami)	12	Aug	18	AAS	$1,890	$4,690					
Rose State College (Midwest City)	20	Aug	24	AAS	$1,943	$6,438		•			
Seminole State College	20	Aug Jan	12, 24	AAS	$2,448	$5,667				•	
Tulsa Community College	16	Aug	24	AAS	$3,000	$6,000		•			
Oregon											
Portland Community College	78	Sep	21	Dipl, AAS	$3,672	$10,530					•
Pennsylvania											
Comm College of Allegheny County (West Mifflin)	20	Aug	20	AS	$96	$110				•	
Montgomery County Community College (Blue Bell)	16	Sep	21	AAS	$3,232	$6,304					
Penn State University - Hazleton	10	Aug	24	AS	$13,248	$20,380		•			•
Reading Area Community College	24	Sep	20	AAS	$2,436	$4,872		•		•	
South Carolina											
Greenville Technical College	22	Aug	24	AAS	$4,530	$9,480				•	
Midlands Technical College (Columbia)	18	May	24	AS	$4,601	$12,183					
Orangeburg Calhoun Technical College	24	Aug	21	AAS	$4,104	$5,148				•	
Tri-County Technical College (Pendleton)	20	Aug	21	AS	$2,736	$6,228				•	
Trident Technical College (Charleston)	20	Aug	24	AHS	$4,425	$8,379		•		•	
York Technical College (Rock Hill)	16	Aug	21	AHS	$2,988	$6,864				•	•
South Dakota											
Lake Area Technical Institute (Watertown)	20	Aug Jan	22	AAS	$3,145	$0		•			•
Mitchell Technical Institute	18	Aug	18	AAS	$2,340	$2,340					
Tennessee											
MedVance Institute (Cookeville)	20	Jan Apr Jul Oct	18, 21	AAS	$10,033	$10,033		•			
Northeast State Technical Comm College (Elizabethton)	15	Aug	24	AAS	$2,418	$8,860					
Southwest Tennessee Community College (Memphis)	20	Aug Jan	24	AAS	$1,324	$4,862		•			
Texas											
882d Training Group (Sheppard AFB)	30	6-7x/yr	13	Cert						•	
Amarillo College	20	Aug	23	AAS	$2,100	$2,800		•	•	•	•
Central Texas College (Killeen)	20	Aug Jan	24	Dipl, AAS	$1,200	$2,800					
Del Mar College (Corpus Christi)	24	Sep	21	AAS	$1,000	$1,900					
El Paso Community College	12	Aug	24	AAS	$2,576	$3,468					
Grayson County College (Denison)	24	Aug	24	AAS	$1,640	$1,886					
Houston Community College	24	Aug	24	AAS	$2,203	$4,417				•	
Laredo Community College	12	Aug	21	Dipl, AAS	$1,520	$2,454		•			
McLennan Community College (Waco)	24	Aug	24	AAS	$1,488	$2,928				•	
Navarro College (Corsicana)	25	Aug	21, 24	Dipl, AAS	$2,200	$4,500					
San Jacinto College Central (Pasadena)	25	Aug	23	AAS	$2,942	$4,598					
St Philip's College (San Antonio)	15	Aug	24	AAS	$1,800	$4,900					
Tyler Junior College	15	Aug	22	AAS	$4,849	$6,617				•	•
Victoria College	14	Aug	20	AAS	$1,617	$2,343					
Utah											
Salt Lake Community College (Salt Lake City)	15	Aug	24	AAS	$3,000	$9,000					
Weber State University (Ogden)	40	Aug Jan	18	AAS	$2,772	$8,612				•	
Virginia											
Centra Health Systems of Lynchburg	10	Aug	12	Cert	$2,900	$8,900					•
J Sargeant Reynolds Community College (Richmond)	80	Aug Jan May	22	AAS	$2,672	$7,836		•			•
Northern Virginia Community College (Springfield)	25	Aug	21	AAS	$2,459	$7,411		•		•	
Thomas Nelson Community College (Hampton)	63	Jan Jul	12, 24	Cert, AAS	$2,886	$91,908					
Washington											
Clover Park Technical College (Lakewood)	13	Mar	12	AAT	$4,801	$4,801					
West Virginia											
Bluefield Regional Medical Center	6	Aug	12	Cert, AAS	$1,500	$1,500					
Fairmont State Univ	13	Aug	22	AAS	$3,982	$8,860					
Southern West Virginia Comm & Tech College (Mount Gay)	20	Aug	21	AAS	$1,776	$6,744					
Wisconsin											
Chippewa Valley Technical College (Eau Claire)	28	Sep	21	AS	$3,200	$17,372					
Madison Area Technical College	14	Aug	21	AAS	$5,044	$17,591					
Milwaukee Area Technical College	16	Aug Jan	19	AAS	$94	$543		•	•	•	•
Northeast Wisconsin Technical College (Green Bay)	16	Aug	21	AS	$2,589	$14,275		•		•	

*Data are shown only for programs that completed the 2007 AMA Survey of Health Professions Education Programs.
‡Key to Offers: 1: Evening or weekend classes; 2: Non-English instruction; 3: Cultural competence instruction; 4: Distance education component.

Cytogenetic Technologist

Connecticut

University of Connecticut
Cytogenetic Technology Prgm
School of Allied Health, 222 Koons Halls
358 Mansfield Rd, Unit 2101
Storrs, CT 06269
www.uconn.edu
Prgm Dir: Martha Keagle, MEd CT(ASCP) CLSp(CG)
Tel: 860 486-0036   *Fax:* 860 486-5375
E-mail: martha.keagle@uconn.edu

Georgia

Kennesaw State University
Cytogenetic Technology Prgm
1000 Chastain Rd
Bldg 12
Kennesaw, GA 30144-5591
Prgm Dir: Xueya Hauge, PhD FABMG
Tel: 770 423-6163   *Fax:* 770 423-6625
E-mail: xhauge@kennesaw.edu

Michigan

Northern Michigan University
Cytogenetic Technology Prgm
1401 Presque Isle Ave
3513 W Science Bldg
Marquette, MI 49855-5346
Prgm Dir: Lucille A Contois, MA MT(ASCP)
Tel: 906 227-1660   *Fax:* 906 227-1309
E-mail: lcontois@nmu.edu

Minnesota

Mayo Clinic
Cytogenetic Technology Prgm
Hilton 512
200 1st St SW
Rocester, MN 55905
Prgm Dir: Peggy Stupca, MS CLSp(CG) CLSup
Tel: 507 284-3040
E-mail: pstupca@mayo.edu

Texas

Univ of Texas M D Anderson Cancer Ctr
Cytogenetic Technology Prgm
Unit 146, 1515 Holcombe Blvd
Houston, TX 77030-4095
www.mdanderson.org/healthsciences
Prgm Dir: Vicki Hopwood, MS CLSp(CG)
Tel: 713 563-3093   *Fax:* 713 745-3337
E-mail: vhopwood@mdanderson.org

Univ of Texas Hlth Sci Ctr at San Antonio
Cytogenetic Technology Prgm
Dept of Clin Lab Sci
7703 Floyd Curl Dr
San Antonio, TX 78284-7772
Prgm Dir: Betty Dunn, MS CLSp(CG)
Tel: 210 567-8865, Ext 1   *Fax:* 210 567-8875
E-mail: dunnb0@uthscsa.edu

Diagnostic Molecular Scientist

Kansas

University of Kansas Medical Center
Diagnostic Molecular Scientist Prgm
G014 Eaton
3901 Rainbow Blvd, MS 4048
Kansas City, KS 66160
www.cls.kumc.edu
Prgm Dir: Venus J Ward, PhD MT(ASCP) CLS(NCA)
Tel: 913 588-0154   *Fax:* 913 588-5222
E-mail: vward@kumc.edu

Michigan

Northern Michigan University
Diagnostic Molecular Scientist Prgm
1401 Presque Isle Ave
3513 W Science Bldg
Marquette, MI 49855-5346
Prgm Dir: Lucille A Contois, MA MT(ASCP)
Tel: 906 227-1660   *Fax:* 906 227-1309
E-mail: lcontois@nmu.edu

Texas

Univ of Texas M D Anderson Cancer Ctr
Diagnostic Molecular Scientist Prgm
Program in Molecular Genetic Technology
1515 Holcombe Blvd, Unit 146
Houston, TX 77030
Prgm Dir: Peter Hu, MS CLS(NCA) MP(ASCP)
    MT(ASCP)
Tel: 713 563-3095   *Fax:* 713 745-3337
E-mail: pchu@mdanderson.org

Texas Tech Univ Health Sciences Center
Diagnostic Molecular Scientist Prgm
Dept of Laboratory Sciences and Primary Care
3601 Fourth St, 2-B-181, MS 6281
Lubbock, TX 79430
Prgm Dir: Lori Rice-Spearman, MS MT(ASCP)
Tel: 806 743-3255   *Fax:* 806 743-3249
E-mail: lori.ricespearman@ttuhsc.edu

Cytogenetic Technologist

Programs*	Class Capacity	Begins	Length (months)	Award	Res. Tuition	Non-res. Tuition	Stipend	Offers:‡ 1	2	3	4
Connecticut											
University of Connecticut (Storrs)	18	Aug Jan	24, 15	Cert, BS	$6,816	$20,760					
Texas											
Univ of Texas Hlth Sci Ctr at San Antonio	14	Fall semester	11	Cert, BS	$7,500	$24,125				•	•
Univ of Texas M D Anderson Cancer Ctr (Houston)	17	Aug	12	Dipl, Cert, BS	$3,884	$16,672				•	

*Data are shown only for programs that completed the 2007 AMA Survey of Health Professions Education Programs.
‡Key to Offers: 1: Evening or weekend classes; 2: Non-English instruction; 3: Cultural competence instruction; 4: Distance education component.

Diagnostic Molecular Scientist

Programs*	Class Capacity	Begins	Length (months)	Award	Res. Tuition	Non-res. Tuition	Stipend	Offers:‡ 1	2	3	4
Kansas											
University of Kansas Medical Center (Kansas City)	12	Aug	24	BS	$6,522	$18,984					
Texas											
Univ of Texas M D Anderson Cancer Ctr (Houston)	20	Aug	12	Dipl, BS	$3,600	$15,916				•	

*Data are shown only for programs that completed the 2007 AMA Survey of Health Professions Education Programs.
‡Key to Offers: 1: Evening or weekend classes; 2: Non-English instruction; 3: Cultural competence instruction; 4: Distance education component.

Histotechnician

Arizona

Pima Community College
Histotechnician Prgm
2202 W Anklam
Tucson, AZ 85709-0215
www.pima.edu or http://wc.pima.edu/~jlindeberg
Prgm Dir: Jean Lindeberg, MS
Tel: 520 206-6031   *Fax:* 520 206-6902
E-mail: jean.lindeberg@pima.edu

Arkansas

Baptist Health Schools Little Rock
Histotechnician Prgm
11900 Colonel Glenn Rd
Little Rock, AR 72210-2820
www.baptist-health.org
Prgm Dir: S Shane Jones, BS HT(ASCP)
Tel: 501 202-6700   *Fax:* 501 202-7712
E-mail: shane.jones@baptist-health.org

California

TPMG Regional Laboratory
Histotechnician Prgm
1725 Eastshore Hwy
Berkeley, CA 94710
Prgm Dir: Carola Howe, MS MT(ASCP
Tel: 510 559-4923
E-mail: carola.howe@kp.org

Mt San Antonio College
Histotechnician Prgm
1100 N Grand Ave
Walnut, CA 91789-1399
Prgm Dir: Virginia Pascoe, MS
Tel: 909 594-5611, Ext 4218   *Fax:* 909 468-4170
E-mail: vpascoe@mtsac.edu

Connecticut

Goodwin College
Histotechnician Prgm
745 Burnside Ave
East Hartford, CT 06108
www.goodwincollege.org
Prgm Dir: Zoe Ann Durkin, MEd HT(ASCP)
Tel: 860 727-6917   *Fax:* 860 568-6209
E-mail: zdurkin@goodwin.edu

Delaware

Delaware Technical & Community College - Wilmington
Cosponsor: Christiana Care Health Services
Histotechnician Prgm
333 N Shipley St
WSE 308M
Wilmington, DE 19801
www.dtcc.edu/wilmington/ah/htt.html
Prgm Dir: Ray Lynch, MD
Tel: 302 571-5320   *Fax:* 302 577-6431
E-mail: wlynch@dtcc.edu

District of Columbia

Armed Forces Institute of Pathology
Histotechnician Prgm
6825 16th St NW, Bldg 54
Washington, DC 20306-6000
Prgm Dir: Julia Wilson, BS HT(ASCP)
Tel: 202 782-2194   *Fax:* 202 782-8150
E-mail: wilsonj@afip.osd.mil

Florida

Florida Community College - Jacksonville
Histotechnician Prgm
North Campus, 4501 Capper Rd
Jacksonville, FL 32218
Prgm Dir: Merry A Carter, MEd MT(ASCP) SC
Tel: 904 766-6511   *Fax:* 904 766-6654
E-mail: mcarter@fccj.edu

Miami Dade College
Histotechnician Prgm
950 NW 20th St
Miami, FL 33127-4693
www.mdc.edu
Prgm Dir: Caridad Ivis Gutierrez, MAEd HTL(ASCP)
Tel: 305 237-4231   *Fax:* 305 237-4278
E-mail: caridad.gutierrez@mdc.edu

Georgia

Darton College
Histotechnician Prgm
2400 Gillionville Rd
Albany, GA 31707
www.darton.edu
Prgm Dir: Nancy T Beamon, MS MT(ASCP)
Tel: 229 317-6846
E-mail: nancybeamon@darton.edu

Illinois

OSF St Francis Medical Center
Histotechnician Prgm
530 NE Glen Oak Ave
Peoria, IL 61637-0001
www.osfsaintfrancis.org
Prgm Dir: Carol E Becker, MS MT(ASCP) CLS(NCA)
Tel: 309 624-9021   *Fax:* 309 624-9150
E-mail: carol.e.becker@osfhealthcare.org

Indiana

Indiana University
Histotechnician Prgm
350 W 11th St
Rm 4083
Indianapolis, IN 46202
http://msa.iusm.iu.edu/hpp/admissions/histo/
Prgm Dir: Debra Wood, BS HT(ASCP)
Tel: 317 491-6410   *Fax:* 317 491-6411
E-mail: demwood@iupui.edu

Maryland

Harford Community College
Histotechnician Prgm
401 Thomas Run Rd
Bel Air, MD 21014
Prgm Dir: Floyd M Grimm III, MEd
Tel: 410 836-4372   *Fax:* 410 836-4485
E-mail: fgrimm@harford.edu

Michigan

Lansing Community College
Histotechnician Prgm
Ingham Intermediate School District
611 Hagadorn Rd
Mason, MI 48854-9592
Prgm Dir: Elizabeth Toy-Krummrey, MA HT(ASCP)
Tel: 517 244-1357   *Fax:* 517 676-3602
E-mail: bkrummre@inghamisd.org

William Beaumont Hospital
Histotechnician Prgm
3601 W 13 Mile Rd
Royal Oak, MI 48079-6769
www.beaumont.edu/alliedhealth
Prgm Dir: Peggy A Wenk, BA BS HTL(ASCP)SLS
Tel: 248 898-9079   *Fax:* 248 898-9054
E-mail: pwenk@beaumont.edu

Minnesota

Argosy University - Twin Cities
Histotechnician Prgm
Twin Cities Campus
1515 Central Parkway
Eagan, MN 55121
Prgm Dir: Joyce Sohrabian, BA HT(ASCP)
Tel: 952 844-0064   *Fax:* 952 844-0472
E-mail: jsohrabian@argosyu.edu

New York

SUNY at Cobleskill
Histotechnician Prgm
111 Schenectady Ave
Cobleskill, NY 12043
www.cobleskill.edu
Prgm Dir: Pamela Colony, PhD HT(ASCP)
Tel: 518 255-5417   *Fax:* 518 255-5113
E-mail: colonyp@cobleskill.edu

North Dakota

University of North Dakota
Histotechnician Prgm
School of Medicine & Health Sciences, Dept of Pathology
PO Box 9037
Grand Forks, ND 58202
Prgm Dir: Ruth Paur, MS MT(ASCP) CLS(NCA)
Tel: 701 777-2651
E-mail: ruthpaur@medicine.nodak.edu

Ohio

Columbus State Community College
Histotechnician Prgm
550 E Spring St
Columbus, OH 43215
www.cscc.edu/histology
Prgm Dir: Peggy Mayo, MEd MLT(ASCP)
Tel: 614 287-2608   *Fax:* 614 287-3854
E-mail: pmayo@cscc.edu

Youngstown State University
Histotechnician Prgm
Dept of Health Professions
One University Plaza
Youngstown, OH 44555
www.ysu.edu
Prgm Dir: Maria E Delost, PhD MT(ASCP) CLS(NCA)
Tel: 330 941-1761   *Fax:* 330 941-2921
E-mail: medelost@ysu.edu

Pennsylvania

Conemaugh Memorial Medical Center
Histotechnician Prgm
1086 Franklin St
Johnstown, PA 15905-4305
Prgm Dir: Gerard Campagna, PA (ASCP) BS HT (ASCP)
Tel: 814 534-9831   *Fax:* 814 534-9372
E-mail: gcampag@conemaugh.org

Texas

Tarleton State University
Histotechnician Prgm
1501 Enderly Place
Fort Worth, TX 76104
Prgm Dir: Glenda F Hood, BS HT(ASCP)
Tel: 817 926-1101, Ext 234   *Fax:* 817 922-8103
E-mail: hood@tarleton.edu

Houston Community College
Histotechnician Prgm
1900 Pressler
Houston, TX 77030
www.hccs.edu
Prgm Dir: Theresa Spain, MEd MT(ASCP) CLS(NCA)
Tel: 713 718-5518   *Fax:* 713 718-7653
E-mail: theresa.spain@hccs.edu

Univ of Texas M D Anderson Cancer Ctr
Histotechnician Prgm
1515 Holcombe Blvd, Box 206
Houston, TX 77030
www.mdanderson.org/healthsciences
Prgm Dir: Hazel V Dalton, MS HT(ASCP) QIHC
Tel: 713 563-3596   *Fax:* 713 745-0172
E-mail: hdalton@mdanderson.org

St Philip's College
Histotechnician Prgm
1801 Martin Luther King Dr
San Antonio, TX 78203
Prgm Dir: Jerri
Tel: 210 531-3449   *Fax:* 210 531-3459
E-mail: jreynolds@mail.accd.edu

Univ of Texas Hlth Sci Ctr at San Antonio
Histotechnician Prgm
7703 Floyd Curl Dr
San Antonio, TX 78284
Prgm Dir: Cynthia Morris, BS HTL/HT(ASCP)QIHC
Tel: 210 567-4059   *Fax:* 210 567-2478
E-mail: morrisc@uthscsa.edu

Wisconsin

St Joseph's Hospital
Cosponsor: Marshfield Clinic
Histotechnician Prgm
611 N St Joseph Ave
1000 N Oak
Marshfield, WI 54449-1898
www.marshfieldlaboratories.org/career.asp
Prgm Dir: Katherine Gorman, BS HT/HTL(ASCP)
Tel: 715 387-7790   *Fax:* 715 389-5353
E-mail: gorman.katherine@marshfieldclinic.org

Histotechnician

Programs*	Class Capacity	Begins	Length (months)	Award	Res. Tuition	Non-res. Tuition	Stipend	Offers:‡ 1	2	3	4
Arizona											
Pima Community College (Tucson)	28	Fall	20	Dipl, Cert, Assoc	$44	$75		•			
Arkansas											
Baptist Health Schools Little Rock	5	Jul	12	Cert	$4,800	$8,145					
Connecticut											
Goodwin College (East Hartford)	10	Sep Jan	12	Cert	$19,595	$19,595					
Delaware											
Delaware Technical & Community College - Wilmington	8	May	24	AAS	$2,070	$5,176					
Florida											
Miami Dade College	20	Aug	27	Dipl, AS	$60	$211		•			
Georgia											
Darton College (Albany)	12	Fall	8, 24	Cert, AS	$1,178	$4,655					
Illinois											
OSF St Francis Medical Center (Peoria)	2-3	Sep	7	Cert	$1,000	$2,000				•	
Indiana											
Indiana University (Indianapolis)	50	Aug	10	Cert	$5,000	$5,000					•
Maryland											
Harford Community College (Bel Air)	6	Sep	24, 10	Cert, AAS	$2,753	$8,258		•		•	
Michigan											
Lansing Community College (Mason)	12	Aug	20	Cert	$1,072	$2,880					
William Beaumont Hospital (Royal Oak)	2-3	Sep	7	Cert						•	
New York											
SUNY at Cobleskill	16	Aug Jan	24, 48	Dipl, AAS, BT	$4,350	$7,210				•	
Ohio											
Columbus State Community College	12	Every other yr	9	Cert	$79	$175				•	•
Youngstown State University	6	Aug	24	AAS	$6,468	$11,974		•			•
Pennsylvania											
Conemaugh Memorial Medical Center (Johnstown)		Jul Jan	12	Cert	$5,750	$5,750					
Texas											
Houston Community College	15	Fall	21	AAS	$2,000	$4,000				•	
Tarleton State University (Fort Worth)	16	Jan Jun Aug	12	Cert, AAS	$6,000	$15,000					•
Univ of Texas Hlth Sci Ctr at San Antonio	4	Aug	12	Cert							
Univ of Texas M D Anderson Cancer Ctr (Houston)	5	Aug	12	Cert	$3,576	$14,140				•	
Wisconsin											
St Joseph's Hospital (Marshfield)	2	Mar Sep	12	Cert							

*Data are shown only for programs that completed the 2007 AMA Survey of Health Professions Education Programs.
‡Key to Offers: 1: Evening or weekend classes; 2: Non-English instruction; 3: Cultural competence instruction; 4: Distance education component.

PROGRAMS

Histotechnologist

Florida

Barry University
Histotechnology Prgm
11300 NE Second Ave
Miami Shores, FL 33161-6695
Prgm Dir: Gerhild Packert, MT PhD
Tel: 305 899-3220   *Fax:* 305 899-3183
E-mail: gpackert@mail.barry.edu

Michigan

William Beaumont Hospital
Histotechnology Prgm
Anatomic Pathology Department
3601 W 13 Mile Rd
Royal Oak, MI 48073-6769
www.beaumont.edu/alliedhealth
Prgm Dir: Peggy Wenk, BA BS HTL(ASCP)SLS
Tel: 248 898-9079   *Fax:* 248 898-9054
E-mail: pwenk@beaumont.edu

South Carolina

Medical University of South Carolina
Histotechnology Prgm
165 Ashley Ave, Ste 309
PO Box 250908
Charleston, SC 29425
www.musc.edu/histoprogram
Prgm Dir: Nina Epps, MS/HPE MT(ASCP)
Tel: 843 792-1906   *Fax:* 843 792-7878
E-mail: eppsn@musc.edu

Pathologists' Assistant

Connecticut

Quinnipiac University
Pathologists' Assistant Prgm
275 Mt Carmel Ave
Hamden, CT 06518
www.quinnipiac.edu
Prgm Dir: Kenneth V Kaloustian, PhD
Tel: 203 582-8676   *Fax:* 203 582-8706
E-mail: kenneth.kaloustian@quinnipiac.edu

Illinois

Rosalind Franklin Univ of Medicine & Science
Pathologists' Assistant Prgm
3333 Green Bay Rd
North Chicago, IL 60064
http://finchcms.edu
Prgm Dir: John E Vitale, MHS PA(ASCP)
Tel: 847 578-8638
E-mail: john.vitale@rosalindfranklin.edu

Indiana

Indiana University
Pathologists' Assistant Prgm
350 W 11th St, Rm 4029A
Indianapolis, IN 46202
www.pathology.iupui.edu/htm/grad_programs.htm
Prgm Dir: Randy Stine, MS PA(ASCP)
Tel: 317 491-6356   *Fax:* 317 491-6419
E-mail: crstine@iupui.edu

Maryland

University of Maryland - Baltimore
Pathologists' Assistant Prgm
Dept of Pathology-UMMC
10 South Pine St
Baltimore, MD 21201
www.medschool.umaryland.edu/pathology
Prgm Dir: Raymond T Jones, PhD
Tel: 410 328-1221   *Fax:* 410 328-5508
E-mail: rjones@som.umaryland.edu

Michigan

Wayne State University
Cosponsor: Eugene Applebaum College of Pharmacy &
    Health Sci
Pathologists' Assistant Prgm
Department of Fundamental and Appl Sci, Mort Sci
5439 Woodward Ave
Detroit, MI 48202
www.wayne.edu
Prgm Dir: Peter D Frade, PhD
Tel: 313 577-7874   *Fax:* 313 577-4456
E-mail: ab8123@wayne.edu

North Carolina

Duke University Medical Center
Pathologists' Assistant Prgm
Box 3712
Durham, NC 27710
Prgm Dir: Kenneth R Broda, PhD
Tel: 919 681-4847   *Fax:* 919 668-2767
E-mail: broda001@mc.duke.edu

Ohio

Ohio State University
Pathologists' Assistant Prgm
410 W 10th Ave, N-308 Doan Hall
Columbus, OH 43210
www.pathology.medctr.ohio-state.edu/ext
Prgm Dir: Charles Hitchcock, MD PhD
Tel: 614 247-7469   *Fax:* 614 293-7273
E-mail: charles.hitchcock@osumc.edu

Pennsylvania

Drexel University
Pathologists' Assistant Prgm
College of Medicine, Division of Professional Grad
    Studies
245 N 15th St, MS 1009
Philadelphia, PA 19102
Prgm Dir: James Moore, MHS FAAPA PA(ASCP)
Tel: 610 988-8393
E-mail: James.Moore@DrexelMed.edu

Histotechnologist

Programs*	Class Capacity	Begins	Length (months)	Award	Res. Tuition	Non-res. Tuition	Stipend	Offers:‡ 1	2	3	4
Florida											
Barry University (Miami Shores)	14	Fall	30, 12	Dipl, Cert, BS	$20,000	$0	$5,000	•			
Michigan											
William Beaumont Hospital (Royal Oak)	4	Sep	12	Cert							•
South Carolina											
Medical University of South Carolina (Charleston)	4	Oct	12	Cert	$1,800	$1,800					

*Data are shown only for programs that completed the 2007 AMA Survey of Health Professions Education Programs.
‡Key to Offers: 1: Evening or weekend classes; 2: Non-English instruction; 3: Cultural competence instruction; 4: Distance education component.

Pathologists' Assistant

Programs*	Class Capacity	Begins	Length (months)	Award	Res. Tuition	Non-res. Tuition	Stipend	Offers:‡ 1	2	3	4
Connecticut											
Quinnipiac University (Hamden)	18	Jun	24	MHS	$25,000	$0		•			
Illinois											
Rosalind Franklin Univ of Medicine & Science (North Chicago)	23	Jun 1	22	MS	$17,210	$17,210					
Indiana											
Indiana University (Indianapolis)	8	Aug	12, 10	MS	$4,500	$13,100					
Maryland											
University of Maryland - Baltimore	10	Aug	22	Dipl, Cert, MS	$17,000	$27,000					
Michigan											
Wayne State University (Detroit)	10	Sep	24	BS	$461	$808					
North Carolina											
Duke University Medical Center (Durham)	8	Aug	24	Dipl, Cert, MHS	$22,000	$22,000					
Ohio											
Ohio State University (Columbus)	2-3	Jun 18	24	Dipl, MS	$12,584	$30,388					

*Data are shown only for programs that completed the 2007 AMA Survey of Health Professions Education Programs.
‡Key to Offers: 1: Evening or weekend classes; 2: Non-English instruction; 3: Cultural competence instruction; 4: Distance education component.

Phlebotomist

Arkansas

Phillips Community College/U of Arkansas
Phlebotomy Prgm
1000 Campus Dr, PO Box 785
Helena-West Helena, AR 72342
www.pccua.edu
Prgm Dir: Julie Byrd, MT(ASCP) MS
Tel: 870 338-6474, Ext 1109   *Fax:* 870 338-7542
E-mail: jbyrd@pccua.edu

California

Loma Linda University
Phlebotomy Prgm
School of Allied Health Professions
Dept of Clinical Lab Sci / NH A918
Loma Linda, CA 92350
Prgm Dir: Monique Gilbert, BS MT(ASCP)
Tel: 909 558-4966
E-mail: mgilbert@sahp.llu.edu

California State University - Long Beach
Phlebotomy Prgm
Dept of Biological Sciences
1250 Bellflower Blvd
Long Beach, CA 90840
Prgm Dir: Carol Ann Itatani, PhD MS MT(ASCP)
Tel: 562 985-4825   *Fax:* 562 985-8878
E-mail: citatani@csulb.edu

Florida

Florida Hospital
Phlebotomy Prgm
601 E Rollins St
Orlando, FL 32803
www.flhosp.org
Prgm Dir: Debra Pless, BS MT(ASCP)BB
Tel: 407 303-1855   *Fax:* 407 893-6943
E-mail: debra.pless@flhosp.org

Georgia

Dalton State College
Phlebotomy Prgm
650 College Dr
Dalton, GA 30720-3778
Prgm Dir: Doris M Shoemaker, EdS MLM MT(ASCP)
Tel: 706 272-4512   *Fax:* 706 272-2517
E-mail: dshoemaker@em.daltonstate.edu

Hawaii

Kapi'olani Community College
Phlebotomy Prgm
4303 Diamond Head Rd
Honolulu, HI 96816
Prgm Dir: Marcia A Armstrong, MS CLS(NCA) MT(ASCP)
Tel: 808 734-9231   *Fax:* 808 734-9126
E-mail: marciaa@hawaii.edu

Illinois

College of Lake County
Phlebotomy Prgm
19351 W Washington St
Grayslake, IL 60030-1198
www.clcillinois.edu
Prgm Dir: Remedios H Tesch, MSEd MT(ASCP)
Tel: 847 543-2878   *Fax:* 847 223-1357
E-mail: rtesch@clcillinois.edu

Moraine Valley Community College
Phlebotomy Prgm
9000 College Parkway
Palos Hills, IL 60465
www.morainevalley.edu/healthsciences
Prgm Dir: Susan E Phelan, MHS MT(ASCP)
Tel: 708 974-5743   *Fax:* 708 974-0185
E-mail: phelan@morainevalley.edu

South Suburban College
Phlebotomy Prgm
15800 S State St
South Holland, IL 60473
www.ssc.cc.il.us
Prgm Dir: Andrea Stone, MPA MT(ASCP)
Tel: 708 596-2000, Ext 2053
E-mail: astone@ingalls.org

Indiana

Indiana University Northwest
Phlebotomy Prgm
School of Health and Human Services
3400 Broadway
Gary, IN 46408
www.iun.edu
Prgm Dir: Susan A K Higgins, MS MT(ASCP)SC
Tel: 219 980-6923   *Fax:* 219 980-6649
E-mail: sahiggin@iun.edu

Ivy Tech Community College - South Bend
Phlebotomy Prgm
220 Dean Johnson Blvd
South Bend, IN 46619-3829
Prgm Dir: Pamela B Primrose, MLFSC MT(ASCP)
Tel: 574 289-7001, Ext 5401   *Fax:* 574 236-7166
E-mail: pprimros@ivytech.edu

Louisiana

Rapides Regional Medical Center
Phlebotomy Prgm
School of Phlebotomy
211 Fourth St
Alexandria, LA 71301-8421
Prgm Dir: E Ann Faircloth Dauzart, RN PBT(ASCP)
Tel: 318 473-3207   *Fax:* 318 473-3079
E-mail: Elizabeth.Faircloth@HCAHealthcare.com

Bossier Parish Community College
Phlebotomy Prgm
3220 East Texas St
Bossier City, LA 71111
Prgm Dir: Pam M Tully, MHS MT(ASCP) PBT(ASCP)
Tel: 318 678-6355   *Fax:* 318 678-6199
E-mail: ptully@bpcc.edu

L E Fletcher Technical Community College
Phlebotomy Prgm
310 St Charles St
PO Box 5033
Houma, LA 70360
Prgm Dir: Marcie Guidry, RN MSN
Tel: 985 876-8900
E-mail: mguidry@lefletcher.edu

Delgado Community College
Phlebotomy Prgm
615 City Park Ave
New Orleans, LA 70119
Prgm Dir: Erica Cassimere
Tel: 504 483-4328   *Fax:* 504 483-4198
E-mail: ecassi@dcc.edu

Maryland

Kaplan College
Phlebotomy Prgm
18618 Crestwood Dr
Hagerstown, MD 21742
Prgm Dir: Michele Buzard, MS MT (ASCP) BA
Tel: 301 739-2680, Ext 201   *Fax:* 301 791-7661
E-mail: mbuzard@hagerstownbusinesscol.edu

Michigan

Medright, Inc
Phlebotomy Prgm
427 Allen Rd
Ferndale, MI 48220
Prgm Dir: Gail Lucas, EMT-P BS
Tel: 248 547-0834   *Fax:* 248 543-8675
E-mail: medright1@aol.com

Mid Michigan Community College
Phlebotomy Prgm
Harrison, MI 48625
Prgm Dir: Cindy Fillmore, MBA

Baker College of Owosso
Phlebotomy Prgm
1020 S Washington St
Owosso, MI 48867
www.baker.edu
Prgm Dir: Diane Denard, BHSA MT(HHS) MLT(ASCP)
Tel: 989 729-3383   *Fax:* 989 729-3411
E-mail: diane.denard@baker.edu

Minnesota

College of St Catherine - Minneapolis
Phlebotomy Prgm
601 25th Ave S
Minneapolis, MN 55454
http://minerva.stkate.edu/offices/academic/
    phlebotomist.nsf
Prgm Dir: Julie Mumm, MT(ASCP) MBA
Tel: 651 690-7764
E-mail: jrmumm@stkate.edu

Missouri

Saint Luke's Hospital
Phlebotomy Prgm
4401 Wornall Rd
Kansas City, MO 64111
www.saintlukeshealthsystem.org
Prgm Dir: Brenna Ildza, MT(ASCP)SH PBT(ASCP)
Tel: 816 932-2074   *Fax:* 816 932-3822
E-mail: bildza@saint-lukes.org

New Jersey

Univ of Medicine & Dent of New Jersey
Phlebotomy Prgm
65 Bergen St
Bergen Bldg GB-159
Newark, NJ 07107
http://shrp.umdnj.edu/programs/cls/phlebotomy.htm
Prgm Dir: Nadine Fydryszewski, MS CLS(NCA)
    MT(ASCP)
Tel: 973 972-5089   *Fax:* 973 972-8527
E-mail: fydrysna@umdnj.edu

New York

Trocaire College
Phlebotomy Prgm
360 Choate Ave
Buffalo, NY 14220
www.trocaire.edu
Prgm Dir: Kathy L Smith, BS MT MS-ASCP NCA
Tel: 716 826-1200   *Fax:* 716 828-3595
E-mail: chernowskim@trocaire.edu

Nicholas H Noyes Memorial Hospital
Phlebotomy Prgm
111 Clara Barton St
Dansville, NY 14437
Prgm Dir: Dawn Kennedy
Tel: 585 335-4225   *Fax:* 585 335-4370
E-mail: dkennedy@noyes-hospital.org

Orange County Community College
Phlebotomy Prgm
115 South St
Middletown, NY 10940
www.sunyorange.edu
Prgm Dir: Rosamaria B Contarino, MS MT(ASCP)
    CLS(NCA)
Tel: 845 341-4136   *Fax:* 845 341-4122
E-mail: rcontari@sunyorange.edu

Rochester General Hospital
Phlebotomy Prgm
1425 Portland Ave
Rochester, NY 14621
Prgm Dir: Nancy C Mitchell, MS MT(ASCP)DLM
Tel: 585 922-4274   *Fax:* 585 922-2088
E-mail: nancy.mitchell@viahealth.org

North Carolina

Asheville-Buncombe Technical Comm College
Phlebotomy Prgm
340 Victoria Rd
Asheville, NC 28801
www.abtech.edu
Prgm Dir: Melissa Hyatt, BS MT(ASCP) MHS
Tel: 828 254-1921, Ext 266   *Fax:* 828 281-9734
E-mail: MHyatt@abtech.edu

Carolinas College of Health Sciences
Phlebotomy Prgm
PO Box 32861
Charlotte, NC 28232
www.carolinascollege.edu
Prgm Dir: Elizabeth T Anderson, MHDL MT(ASCP)
Tel: 704 355-4275   *Fax:* 704 355-5967
E-mail: banderson@carolinas.org

Fayetteville Technical Community College
Phlebotomy Prgm
2201 Hull Rd
PO Box 35236
Fayetteville, NC 28303
www.faytechcc.edu
Prgm Dir: Linda Starling, MT(ASCP) PBT (ASCP)
Tel: 910 678-8538   *Fax:* 910 678-8500
E-mail: starlinl@faytechcc.edu

Wake Technical Community College
Phlebotomy Prgm
9101 Fayetteville Rd
2901 Holston Lane
Raleigh, NC 27610
www.waketech.edu
Prgm Dir: Pamela B Horton, MEd MT(ASCP)
Tel: 919 212-3818   *Fax:* 919 250-4329
E-mail: pbhorton@waketech.edu

Nash Community College
Phlebotomy Prgm
522 N Old Carriage Rd, PO Box 7480
Rocky Mount, NC 27804
www.nashcc.edu
Prgm Dir: TaMeika Dickens, PBT (ASPT) BS Biology
Tel: 252 451-8336   *Fax:* 252 451-8201
E-mail: debg@nash.cc.nc.us

Brunswick Community College
Phlebotomy Prgm
PO Box 30
50 College Rd
Supply, NC 28462
Prgm Dir: Julianna Olsen, PBT(ASCP)
Tel: 910 755-7324   *Fax:* 910 754-9609
E-mail: olsenj@brunswickcc.edu

Southwestern Community College
Phlebotomy Prgm
447 College Dr
Sylva, NC 28779
Prgm Dir: Andrea L Kennedy, MBA MT(ASCP)
Tel: 828 586-4091, Ext 312   *Fax:* 828 586-3129
E-mail: andrea@southwesterncc.edu

Halifax Community College
Phlebotomy Prgm
PO Drawer 809
Hwy 158
Weldon, NC 27890
Prgm Dir: Lori M Howard, BSMT(ASCP)SM
Tel: 252 536-7284
E-mail: howardl@halifaxcc.edu

Rockingham Community College
Phlebotomy Prgm
PO Box 38
Wentworth, NC 27375-0038
www.rockinghamcc.edu
Prgm Dir: Darlene Vestal, MT(ASCP) PBT ASCP
Tel: 336 342-4261, Ext 2207   *Fax:* 336 634-1253
E-mail: dvastal@moorhead.org

Southeastern Community College
Phlebotomy Prgm
PO Box 151
Whiteville, NC 28472
www.sccnc.edu
Prgm Dir: Patricia Wright, MT(ASCP)
Tel: 910 642-7141, Ext 312   *Fax:* 910 642-3257
E-mail: pwright@sccnc.edu

Cape Fear Community College
Phlebotomy Prgm
411 N Front St
Wilmington, NC 28401-3993
Prgm Dir: Vickie Pridgen, MT(ASCP) AMT
Tel: 910 362-7162
E-mail: vpridgen@cfcc.edu

North Dakota

Bismarck State College
Phlebotomy Prgm
PO Box 5587
1500 Edwards Ave
Bismarck, ND 58506-5587
www.bismarckstate.edu
Prgm Dir: Angela Uhlich, MS MT(ASCP)SBB
Tel: 701 323-5482   *Fax:* 701 323-5831
E-mail: Angela.Uhlich@bsc.nodak.edu

Ohio

Collins Career Center
Phlebotomy Prgm
11627 State Route 243
Chesapeake, OH 45619
Prgm Dir: Shawn P Boggs, MT(ASCP)
Tel: 740 867-6641
E-mail: shawn.boggs@kdmc.net

Cuyahoga Community College
Phlebotomy Prgm
Metropolitan Campus
2900 Community College Ave
Cleveland, OH 44115-3196
Prgm Dir: Amy Gatautis, MBA MT(ASCP)SC
Tel: 216 987-4438   *Fax:* 216 987-4386
E-mail: amy.gatautis@tri-c.edu

Columbus State Community College
Phlebotomy Prgm
550 E Spring St
Columbus, OH 43215
www.cscc.edu/phlebotomy
Prgm Dir: Peggy Mayo, MEd MLT (ASCP)
Tel: 614 287-2608   *Fax:* 614 287-3854
E-mail: pmayo@cscc.edu

Lorain County Community College
Phlebotomy Prgm
1005 N Abbe Rd
Elyria, OH 44035
Prgm Dir: James E Daly, MEd MT(ASCP)
Tel: 800 995-5222, Ext 7194   *Fax:* 440 366-4116
E-mail: jdaly@lorainccc.edu

Edison Community College
Phlebotomy Prgm
1973 Edison Dr
Piqua, OH 45356
Prgm Dir: Cathy Chambers
Tel: 937 778-7994
E-mail: chambers@edisonohio.edu

Trumbull Memorial Hospital
Phlebotomy Prgm
1350 E Market St
Warren, OH 44482-1269
Prgm Dir: James Obermiyer, BA MT(ASCP)
Tel: 330 841-9128   *Fax:* 330 841-9110
E-mail: jobermiyer@forumhealth.org

Zane State College
Phlebotomy Prgm
1555 Newark Rd
Zanesville, OH 43701
Prgm Dir: Jane Poulson-Dunlap, MS MT(ASCP)
Tel: 740 588-1228
E-mail: jdunlap@zanestate.edu

Oklahoma

Tulsa Community College
Phlebotomy Prgm
909 S Boston Ave
10300 E 81st St, 74133
Tulsa, OK 74119
www.tulsacc.edu
Prgm Dir: Karen L Holmes, MT(ASCP)
Tel: 918 595-8666   *Fax:* 918 595-7091
E-mail: kholmes@tulsacc.edu

Pennsylvania

Montgomery County Community College
Phlebotomy Prgm
340 DeKalb Pike
PO Box 400
Blue Bell, PA 19422-0796
www.mc3.edu
Prgm Dir: Debra Eckman, MS MT(ASCP)
Tel: 215 641-6487   *Fax:* 215 619-7178
E-mail: deckman@mc3.edu

Community College of Beaver County
Phlebotomy Prgm
1 Campus Dr
Monaca, PA 15061
www.ccbc.edu
Prgm Dir: Estelle Del Principe, BA MEd MT(ASCP)
Tel: 724 775-8561, Ext 189   *Fax:* 724 775-3003
E-mail: estelle.delprincipe@ccbc.edu

Community College of Philadelphia
Phlebotomy Prgm
1700 Spring Garden St
Philadelphia, PA 19130
Prgm Dir: Robin Gaynor Krefetz, MEd MT(ASCP) CLS (NCA)
Tel: 215 751-8511   *Fax:* 215 751-8937
E-mail: rkrefetz@ccp.edu

Tennessee

Southwest Tennessee Community College
Phlebotomy Prgm
PO Box 780
761 Linden Ave
Memphis, TN 38101-0780
Prgm Dir: Darius Y Wilson, EdD MAT BS MT(ASCP)
Tel: 901 333-5407   *Fax:* 901 333-5391
E-mail: dwilson@southwest.tn.edu

Texas

Austin Community College
Phlebotomy Prgm
Eastview Campus
3401 Webberville Rd
Austin, TX 78702
www.austincc.edu/health/phb
Prgm Dir: Terry Kotrla, MS MT(ASCP)BB
Tel: 512 223-5932   *Fax:* 512 223-5898
E-mail: kotrla@austincc.edu

CHRISTUS Hospital - St Elizabeth
Phlebotomy Prgm
2830 Calder Ave
PO Box 5405
Beaumont, TX 77726-5405
www.christusste.org
Prgm Dir: Deborah R Zink, MBA MT(ASCP)
Tel: 409 899-7150, Ext 4002   *Fax:* 409 899-7991
E-mail: debbi.zink@christushealth.org

Wisconsin

Milwaukee Area Technical College
Phlebotomy Prgm
Health Occupations Division
700 W State St
Milwaukee, WI 53233
www.matc.edu
Prgm Dir: Dennis Schmidt, MS MT(ASCP)
Tel: 414 297-7142   *Fax:* 414 297-6851
E-mail: SchmidtD@matc.edu

Mid-State Technical College
Phlebotomy Prgm
933 Michigan Ave
Stevens Point, WI 54481-3141
www.mstc.edu
Prgm Dir: Lori Jasper, BSMT(ASCP) CMA
Tel: 715 342-3106   *Fax:* 715 342-3134
E-mail: lori.jasper@mstc.edu

Northcentral Technical College
Phlebotomy Prgm
1100 W Campus Dr
Wausau, WI 54401
Prgm Dir: Janice Miller, MS MT(ASCP)
Tel: 715 675-3331, Ext 1371
E-mail: millerja@ntc.edu

Phlebotomist

Programs*	Class Capacity	Begins	Length (months)	Award	Res. Tuition	Non-res. Tuition	Stipend	Offers:‡ 1	2	3	4
Arkansas											
Phillips Community College/U of Arkansas (Helena-West Helena)	8	Aug	9	Cert	$1,560	$2,970					
California											
California State University - Long Beach	16	Jun	2	Cert	$1,600	$0				•	
Loma Linda University	12	Jun 18	2	Cert	$2,000	$2,000		•		•	
Florida											
Florida Hospital (Orlando)	10	Jan May Sep	2	Cert	$300	$300				•	
Georgia											
Dalton State College	16	Aug Jan May	6	Cert	$1,656	$6,280				•	
Hawaii											
Kapi'olani Community College (Honolulu)	12	Jan Apr Jun Sep	2	Cert, CC	$950	$950		•			
Illinois											
College of Lake County (Grayslake)	20	Aug	3	Cert	$76	$201		•			
Moraine Valley Community College (Palos Hills)	60	Aug Jan May	8	Cert	$840	$0		•		•	
South Suburban College (South Holland)	16		4	Cert	$1,164	$3,840		•			
Indiana											
Indiana University Northwest (Gary)	18	Jan	5	Cert	$2,100	$5,100				•	
Ivy Tech Community College - South Bend	15	Fall Spring	4		$1,600	$3,200		•		•	•
Louisiana											
Rapides Regional Medical Center (Alexandria)	9	Apr Oct	6	Cert						•	

*Data are shown only for programs that completed the 2007 AMA Survey of Health Professions Education Programs.
‡Key to Offers: 1: Evening or weekend classes; 2: Non-English instruction; 3: Cultural competence instruction; 4: Distance education component.

Phlebotomist

Programs*	Class Capacity	Begins	Length (months)	Award	Res. Tuition	Non-res. Tuition	Stipend	Offers:‡ 1	2	3	4
Maryland											
Kaplan College (Hagerstown)	100	Quarterly	9	Cert	$13,853	$13,853		•			
Michigan											
Baker College of Owosso	16	Sep	8	Cert	$7,215	$7,215		•		•	•
Minnesota											
College of St Catherine - Minneapolis	12	Fall Winter	4	Cert	$2,214	$2,214				•	
Missouri											
Saint Luke's Hospital (Kansas City)	8	3-4x/yr	1	Cert	$700	$700				•	
New Jersey											
Univ of Medicine & Dent of New Jersey (Newark)	27	Sep	6	Cert	$950	$950		•		•	•
New York											
Orange County Community College (Middletown)	18	Fall Spring	4	Cert	$3,000	$6,000				•	
Rochester General Hospital	8	Jan Mar	3	Cert	$400	$0					
Trocaire College (Buffalo)	16	Mar Jun Oct	2	Cert	$0	$899		•			
North Carolina											
Asheville-Buncombe Technical Comm College	32	Aug	4	Cert	$608	$2,532					
Carolinas College of Health Sciences (Charlotte)	10	Jan May Sep	2	Cert	$505	$505					
Fayetteville Technical Community College	15	Aug Jan Mar	4	Cert	$543	$2,883					
Nash Community College (Rocky Mount)	15	Aug Jan	4	Cert	$498	$2,652				•	
Rockingham Community College (Wentworth)	18	Fall semester	5	Cert	$491	$2,526		•		•	
Southeastern Community College (Whiteville)	20	Jan 4	5	Cert	$632	$3,512					•
Southwestern Community College (Sylva)	12	Jan	4	Cert	$474	$2,634		•			•
Wake Technical Community College (Raleigh)	15	Jan Aug	4	Cert	$474	$2,634				•	
North Dakota											
Bismarck State College	10	Aug Jan	5	Cert	$3,240	$7,868		•		•	
Ohio											
Collins Career Center (Chesapeake)	30	Oct	11	Cert				•		•	
Columbus State Community College	15	Jun Jan	6	Cert	$79	$175				•	
Lorain County Community College (Elyria)	30	Aug	9	Cert	$1,753	$2,112					•
Trumbull Memorial Hospital (Warren)	14	2x/yr	2								
Oklahoma											
Tulsa Community College	30	Jun Aug Jan	4, 2	Cert	$600	$1,200					
Pennsylvania											
Community College of Beaver County (Monaca)	20	Sep Jan	4	Cert	$636	$1,236				•	
Montgomery County Community College (Blue Bell)	12	Sep Jan	4	Cert	$101	$197					
Tennessee											
Southwest Tennessee Community College (Memphis)	15	Sep 1 Jan 15	6	Cert	$1,324	$4,862					
Texas											
Austin Community College	14	Jan May Aug	3	Cert	$216	$532				•	
CHRISTUS Hospital - St Elizabeth (Beaumont)	10	Depends on need	2	Cert	$250	$250				•	
Wisconsin											
Mid-State Technical College (Stevens Point)	20	Jan Aug	7	Dipl	$92	$478		•	•	•	•
Milwaukee Area Technical College	35	Aug Jan	6	Dipl	$94	$543		•	•	•	•

*Data are shown only for programs that completed the 2007 AMA Survey of Health Professions Education Programs.
‡Key to Offers: 1: Evening or weekend classes; 2: Non-English instruction; 3: Cultural competence instruction; 4: Distance education component.

Includes:

- Career Counseling (CrC)
- College Counseling (ClC)
- Community Counseling (CC)
- Gerontological Counseling (GC)
- Marital, Couple and Family Counseling/Therapy (MFC/T)
- Mental Health Counselor (MHC)
- School Counseling (SC)
- Student Affairs (SA)
- Student Affairs-College Counseling (SACC)
- Student Affairs-Professional Practice (SAPP)
- Counselor Education and Supervision (CE)

Note: Career information and educational programs for rehabilitation counseling and genetic counseling are listed separately.

Career Description

The counseling profession differs from other human service professions in its developmental approach to problem solving. Counselors deal with human development concerns through support, therapeutic approaches, consultation, evaluation, teaching, and research. Simply stated, counseling is the art of helping people grow.

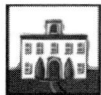

Employment Characteristics

Professional counselors can be found in a variety of settings, including:

- private practice
- elementary, middle, and secondary schools
- colleges/universities
- hospitals
- health maintenance organizations
- insurance firms
- drug and alcohol abuse rehabilitation agencies
- mental health agencies
- correctional institutions
- career development and vocational training facilities

Success in the counseling field requires motivation, a commitment to service, and skills in communication. Counselors will be faced with numerous challenges and opportunities in the future, including drug abuse, homelessness, disaster recovery, and the "graying of America" with an increasing percentage of Americans who are senior citizens. The foundations of the counseling profession have been intertwined with both social and educational reform movements in this century and will continue to be so in the future.

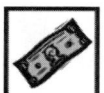

Salary

Median earnings for full-time educational and vocational counselors were about $42,110 a year in 2004. The bottom 10% earned less than $23,560 a year; the top 10% earned over $67,170 a year. As with most professions, pay scales differ based on education, prior experience, and geographical location. Refer to Section IV, Table 5 of this *Directory* for more information, or see www.ama-assn.org/go/hpsalary.

Educational Programs

Length. Career Counseling, College Counseling, Community Counseling, Gerontological Counseling, School Counseling, and Student Affairs programs are a minimum of 48 semester hours or 72 quarter hours. Mental Health Counseling and Marital, Couple and Family Counseling/Therapy programs are a minimum of 60 semester hours or 90 quarter hours.

Curriculum. Curricular experiences and demonstrated knowledge in each of the eight common core areas are required of all counseling students:

1. Professional Identity
2. Social and Cultural Diversity
3. Human Growth and Development
4. Career Development
5. Helping Relationships
6. Group Work
7. Assessment
8. Research and Program Evaluation

Clinical Requirements. Students must complete supervised practicum experiences that total a minimum of 100 clock hours. The practicum provides for the development of counseling skills under supervision. The student's practicum includes the following:

1. Forty hours of direct service with clients, including experience in individual counseling and group work.
2. Weekly interaction with an average of 1 hour per week of individual and/or triadic supervision, which occurs regularly over the course of one academic term by a programs faculty member or a supervisor working under the supervision of a program faculty member.
3. An average of 1 ½ hours per week of group supervision, provided on a regular schedule over the course of the student's practicum by a program faculty member or a supervisor under the supervision of a program faculty member.
4. Evaluation of the student's performance throughout the practicum, including a formal evaluation after the student completes the practicum.

The program requires students to complete a supervised internship of 600 clock hours after successful completion of the student's practicum. The internship provides an opportunity for the student to perform, under supervision, a variety of counseling activities that a professional counselor is expected to perform. The student's internship includes all of the following:

1. Two hundred and forty hours of direct service with clients appropriate to the programs of study.
2. Weekly interaction with an average of 1 hour per week of individual and/or triadic supervision, throughout the internship, usually performed by the on-site supervisor.
3. An average of 1 ½ hours per week of group supervision provided on a regular schedule throughout the internship, usually performed by a program faculty member.
4. The opportunity for the student to become familiar with a variety of professional activities in addition to direct service (eg, recordkeeping, supervision, information and referral, in-service and staff meetings).
5. The opportunity for the student to develop program-appropriate audio and/or videotapes of the student's interactions with clients for use in supervision.

6. The opportunity for the student to gain supervised experience in the use of a variety of professional resources, such as assessment instruments, technologies, print and nonprint media, professional literature, and research.
7. A formal evaluation of the student's performance during the internship by a program faculty member, in consultation with the site supervisor.

Certification

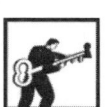 Some counselors elect to be nationally certified by the National Board for Certified Counselors, Inc. (NBCC), which grants the general practice credential "National Certified Counselor." To be certified, a counselor must hold a master's degree with a concentration in counseling from a regionally accredited college or university; must have at least 2 years of supervised field experience in a counseling setting (graduates from counselor education programs accredited by CACREP are exempted); must provide two professional endorsements, one of which must be from a recent supervisor; and must have a passing score on the NBCC's National Counselor Examination for Licensure and Certification (NCE). This national certification is voluntary and is distinct from state licensing. However, in some states, those who pass the national exam are exempted from taking a state certification exam. NBCC also offers specialty certifications in school, clinical mental health, and addiction counseling, which supplement the national certified counselor designation. These specialty certifications require passage of a supplemental exam. To maintain their certification, counselors retake and pass the NCE or complete 100 credit hours of acceptable continuing education every 5 years

 **Inquiries**

Careers
American Counseling Association
5999 Stevenson Avenue
Alexandria, VA 22304
703 823-9800
www.counseling.org

Certification
National Board for Certified Counselors
3 Terrace Way, Suite D
Greensboro, NC 27403
336 547-0607
www.nbcc.org

Program Accreditation
Council for Accreditation of Counseling and Related Educational Programs
5999 Stevenson Avenue
Alexandria, VA 22304
703 823-9800, x301
www.cacrep.org

Note: Adapted in part from the Bureau of Labor Statistics, U.S. Department of Labor, *Occupational Outlook Handbook*, 2006-07 Edition, Counselors, on the Internet at http://www.bls.gov/oco/ocos067.htm (visited November 6, 2007).

Counselor

Alabama

Auburn University
Counseling Prgm
2084 Haley Center
Auburn University, AL 36849-5222
Prgm Dir: Debra C Cobia
Tel: 334 844-5160   *Fax:* 334 844-2860
E-mail: cobiadc@auburn.edu

University of Montevallo
Counseling Prgm
CC, SC Programs
College of Education, Station 6380
Montevallo, AL 35115
Prgm Dir: Stephanie Puleo, PhD
Tel: 205 665-6371
E-mail: puleos@montevallo.edu

Troy University
Counseling Prgm
CC, MHC, SC Programs
One University Place
Phenix City, AL 36869
Prgm Dir: M Kathryn Ness
Tel: 334 448-5146   *Fax:* 334 448-5203
E-mail: kness@troy.edu

Troy University
Counseling Prgm
CC, SC Programs
10 McCartha Hall
Troy, AL 36082
Prgm Dir: Dianne Gossett, PhD
Tel: 334 670-3350
E-mail: dgossett@troy.edu

University of Alabama
Counseling Prgm
CC, SC, CE Programs
PO Box 870231
Tuscaloosa, AL 35487-0231
Prgm Dir: S Allen Wilcoxon
Tel: 205 348-7579   *Fax:* 205 348-7584
E-mail: awilcoxo@bamaed.ua.edu

Arizona

Northern Arizona University
Counseling Prgm
CC, SC Programs
Educational Psychology, PO Box 5774 - COE
Flagstaff, AZ 86011-5774
Prgm Dir: Eugene Moan, EdD
Tel: 928 523-9604   *Fax:* 928 523-9284
E-mail: Eugene.Moan@nau.edu

University of Phoenix
Counseling Prgm
CC Program
4605 E Elwood St (Mailstop Code AAC-704)
Phoenix, AZ 85040
Prgm Dir: Patricia L Kerstner, PhD
Tel: 480 537-2179   *Fax:* 480 929-7164
E-mail: patricia.kerstner@phoenix.edu

Arizona State University
Counseling Prgm
CC Program
PO Box 870611
Tempe, AZ 85287-0611
Prgm Dir: Sharon Kurpius
Tel: 480 965-6104   *Fax:* 480 965-8057
E-mail: sharon.kurpius@asu.edu

Arkansas

University of Arkansas
Counseling Prgm
CC, SC, CE Programs
136 Graduate Education Bldg
Fayetteville, AR 72701
Prgm Dir: Rebecca A Newgent
Tel: 479 575-3509   *Fax:* 479 575-2492
E-mail: newgent@uakron.alumlink.com

Arkansas State University
Counseling Prgm
SC Program
PO Box 1560
State University, AR 72467-1560
Prgm Dir: Nola Christenberry, PhD
Tel: 870 972-3064
E-mail: nchriste@astate.edu

British Columbia, Canada

Trinity Western University
Counseling Prgm
CC Program
7600 Glover Rd
Langley, BC V2Y 1Y1
Prgm Dir: Marvin McDonald, PhD RPsych
Tel: 604 513-2034, Ext 3223   *Fax:* 604 513-2150
E-mail: mcdonald@twu.ca

California

California State University - Fresno
Counseling Prgm
MFC/T Program
5005 N Maple Ave, M/S3
Fresno, CA 93740-8025
Prgm Dir: Sari H Dworkin
Tel: 559 278-0328   *Fax:* 559 278-0404
E-mail: sarid@csufresno.edu

California State University - Los Angeles
Counseling Prgm
MFC/T, SC Programs
5151 State University Dr
Los Angeles, CA 90032
Prgm Dir: Randy Campbell, PhD
Tel: 323 343-4250   *Fax:* 323 343-4252
E-mail: rcampbe@calstatela.edu

California State University - Northridge
Counseling Prgm
CrC, MFC/T, SACC, SC Programs
18111 Nordhoff St
Northridge, CA 91330-8265
Prgm Dir: Rie Rogers Mitchell, EdD
Tel: 818 677-2599   *Fax:* 818 677-2544
E-mail: rie.mitchell@csun.edu

Sonoma State University
Counseling Prgm
CC, SC Programs
1801 E Cotati Ave, Rm N220
Rohnert Park, CA 94928
Prgm Dir: Adam Hill, PhD
Tel: 707 664-2340
E-mail: adam.hill@sonoma.edu

San Francisco State University
Counseling Prgm
Dept of Counseling
1600 Holloway Ave
San Francisco, CA 94132
Prgm Dir: Robert C Chope, PhD
Tel: 415 338-2005   *Fax:* 415 338-0594
E-mail: rcchope@sfsu.edu

Colorado

Adams State College
Counseling Prgm
CC, SC Programs
Dept of Psychology
Alamosa, CO 81102
Prgm Dir: Susan C Varhely, PhD
Tel: 719 587-7224
E-mail: scvarhel@adams.edu

University of Colorado at Colorado Springs
Counseling Prgm
4120 Austin Bluffs Pkwy
PO Box 7150
Colorado Springs, CO 80933-7150
Prgm Dir: David Fenell, PhD
Tel: 719 262-4096
E-mail: dfenell@uccs.edu

U of Colorado (Denver) Health Sciences Center
Counseling Prgm
CC, MFC/T, SC Programs
Health Sciences Center, Campus Box 106,
    PO Box 173364
Denver, CO 80217-3364
Prgm Dir: Marsha Wiggins-Frame
Tel: 303 556-6032   *Fax:* 303 556-4479
E-mail: marsha.frame@cudenver.edu

Colorado State University
Counseling Prgm
CrC, CC, SC Programs
Education 215
Fort Collins, CO 80523-1588
Prgm Dir: John M Littrell, EdD
Tel: 970 491-5160
E-mail: John.Littrell@ColoState.edu

University of Northern Colorado
Counseling Prgm
CC, MFC/T, SC, CE Programs
Division of Professional Psychology
Greeley, CO 80639
Prgm Dir: Sandy Magnuson, EdD
Tel: 970 351-1627   *Fax:* 970 351-2625
E-mail: sandy.magnuson@unco.edu

Denver Seminary
Counseling Prgm
CC Program
Counseling Division
Littleton, CO 80120
Prgm Dir: Fred Gingrich, DMin
Tel: 303 783-3125   *Fax:* 303 762-6976
E-mail: fred.gingrich@denverseminary.edu

Connecticut

Western Connecticut State University
Counseling Prgm
CC, SC Programs
Education Dept
Danbury, CT 06810
Prgm Dir: Michael Gilles, PhD
Tel: 203 837-8513
E-mail: gillesm@wcsu.edu

Fairfield University
Counseling Prgm
CC, SC Programs
Graduate School of Ed & Allied Prof
Fairfield, CT 06430-7524
Prgm Dir: Virginia Kelly, PhD
Tel: 203 254-4000, Ext 3228   *Fax:* 203 254-4047
E-mail: Vkelly@mail.fairfield.edu

Southern Connecticut State University
Counseling Prgm
CC, SC Programs
Counseling & School Psychology Dept
New Haven, CT 06515
Prgm Dir: Patricia W De Barbieri
Tel: 203 392-5483   *Fax:* 203 392-5917
E-mail: debarbierip1@southernct.edu

Delaware

Wilmington College
Counseling Prgm
31 Read's Way
Wilson Graduate Center
New Castle, DE 19720
Prgm Dir: Richard C Williams, PhD
Tel: 302 295-1150
E-mail: r.craig.williams@wilmcoll.edu

District of Columbia

Gallaudet University
Counseling Prgm
MHC, SC Programs
800 Florida Ave NE
Washington, DC 20002
Prgm Dir: Roger Beach
Tel: 202 651-4511   *Fax:* 202 651-5657
E-mail: roger.beach@gallaudet.edu

George Washington University
Counseling Prgm
Graduate School of Edu and Human Dev
2134 G St NW
Washington, DC 20052
www.gwu.edu/~chaos
Prgm Dir: Pat Schwallie-Giddis, PhD
Tel: 202 994-6856   *Fax:* 202 994-3436
E-mail: drpat@gwu.edu

Florida

Florida Atlantic University
Counseling Prgm
MHC, SC Programs
777 Glades Rd
Boca Raton, FL 33431
Prgm Dir: Paul Peluso, PhD
Tel: 561 297-3625
E-mail: ppeluso@fau.edu

Stetson University
Counseling Prgm
MFC/T, MHC, SC Programs
421 N Woodland Blvd, Unit 8389
Deland, FL 32720
www.stetson.edu/artsci/counselor
Prgm Dir: Brigid Noonan, PhD LMHC
Tel: 386 822-7238   *Fax:* 386 740-3664
E-mail: bnoonan@stetson.edu

Florida Gulf Coast University
Counseling Prgm
MHC, SC Programs
10501 FGCU Blvd S
Fort Myers, FL 33965-6565
Prgm Dir: Madeyln Issacs, PhD
Tel: 239 590-7785
E-mail: misaacs@fgcu.edu

University of Florida
Counseling Prgm
Mental Health Counseling
Department of Counselor Education
Gainesville, FL 32611-7046
http://education.ufl.edu/counselor
Prgm Dir: Sondra Smith-Adcock, PhD
Tel: 352 392-0731, Ext 239   *Fax:* 352 846-2697
E-mail: ssmith@coe.ufl.edu

University of Florida
Counseling Prgm
Counselor Education Dept
1215 Norman Hall, PO Box 117046
Gainesville, FL 32611-7046
http://education.ufl.edu/counselor
Prgm Dir: Andrea Dixon Rayle, PhD
Tel: 352 392-0731, Ext 238   *Fax:* 352 846-2697
E-mail: rayle@ufl.edu

University of Florida
Counseling Prgm
Marriage and Family Counseling Program
Department of Counselor Education
Gainesville, FL 32611-7046
http://education.ufl.edu/counselor
Prgm Dir: Silvia Echevarria-Doan, PhD
Tel: 352 392-0731, Ext 237   *Fax:* 352 846-2697
E-mail: silvia@coe.ufl.edu

University of North Florida
Counseling Prgm
MHC, SC Programs
4567 St Johns Bluff Rd S
Jacksonville, FL 32224-2645
www.unf.edu
Prgm Dir: David Whittinghill
Tel: 904 620-1749   *Fax:* 904 620-2982
E-mail: dwhittin@unf.edu

Florida International University
Counseling Prgm
MHC, SC Programs
FIU University Park Campus
Miami, FL 33119
Prgm Dir: Adriana McEachern, PhD
Tel: 305 348-3202   *Fax:* 305 348-3205
E-mail: Adriana.Mceachern@fiu.edu

Barry University
Counseling Prgm
MHC, SC, MFC/T Programs
11300 NE 2nd Ave
Miami Shores, FL 33161-6695
Prgm Dir: Maureen Duffy, PhD
Tel: 305 899-3711
E-mail: mduffy@mail.barry.edu

University of Central Florida
Counseling Prgm
MHC, SC, CE programs
400 Central Blvd
Orlando, FL 32816
Prgm Dir: E H Robinson III, PhD
Tel: 407 823-2401   *Fax:* 407 823-3859
E-mail: erobinso@mail.ucf.edu

Florida State University
Counseling Prgm
CrC, MHC, SC Programs
215 Stone Bldg
Tallahassee, FL 32306
Prgm Dir: F Donald Kelly
Tel: 850 644-9439   *Fax:* 850 644-8776
E-mail: Railey@coe.fsu.edu

University of South Florida
Counseling Prgm
CrC, MHC, SC Programs
4202 E Fowler Ave EDU 162
Tampa, FL 33620-5650
Prgm Dir: Carlos Zalaquett, PhD
Tel: 813 974-8220   *Fax:* 813 974-5814
E-mail: zalaquet@tempest.coedu.usf.edu

Rollins College
Counseling Prgm
MHC, SC Programs
1000 Holt Ave, PO Box 2726
Winter Park, FL 32789-4499
Prgm Dir: Alicia Homrich
Tel: 407 646-2307
E-mail: jprovost@rollins.edu

Georgia

University of Georgia
Counseling Prgm
CC, SC Programs
402 Aderhold Hall
Athens, GA 30602-7142
Prgm Dir: Georgia Calhoun
Tel: 706 542-4130
E-mail: gcalhoun@uga.edu

Georgia State University
Counseling Prgm
CC, SC, CE programs
Professional Counseling Prgm
Atlanta, GA 30303-3083
www.gsu.edu
Prgm Dir: JoAnna White, PhD
Tel: 404 651-3427   *Fax:* 404 651-1160
E-mail: jwhite@gsu.edu

University of West Georgia
Counseling Prgm
CC, SC Programs
Dept of Counseling and Educational Psychology
Carrollton, GA 30118-5170
Prgm Dir: Brent M Snow
Tel: 770 836-6554
E-mail: bsnow@westga.edu

Columbus State University
Counseling Prgm
CC, SC Programs
4225 University Ave
Columbus, GA 31907-5645
Prgm Dir: Michael L Baltmore
Tel: 706 568-2222   *Fax:* 706 569-3434
E-mail: baltimore_michael@colstate.edu

Hawaii

University of Hawaii
Counseling Prgm
CC, SC Programs
Coll of Education
Honolulu, HI 96822
Prgm Dir: Brenda Cartwright, EdD
Tel: 808 956-7905   *Fax:* 808 956-3814
E-mail: bcartwri@hawaii.edu

Idaho

Boise State University
Counseling Prgm
Counseling Dept Ed Bldg, Rm 612
1910 University Dr
Boise, ID 83725-1710
Prgm Dir: Ken Coll
Tel: 208 426-1821   *Fax:* 208 426-2046
E-mail: kcoll@boisestate.edu

University of Idaho
Counseling Prgm
SC, CE programs
College of Education, Rm 206
Moscow, ID 83844-3083
Prgm Dir: Jerry Fischer
Tel: 208 885-6556   *Fax:* 208 885-6869
E-mail: jfischer@uidaho.edu

Northwest Nazarene University
Counseling Prgm
CC, SC, MFC Programs
623 Holly St
Nampa, ID 83686
www.nnu.edu/counseloreducation
Prgm Dir: Brenda Freeman, PhD LCPC NCC
Tel: 208 467-8428   *Fax:* 208 467-8339
E-mail: BJFreeman@nnu.edu

Idaho State University
Counseling Prgm
MHC, SC, SACC, CE, MFC/T Programs
PO Box 8120
Pocatello, ID 83209-8120
Prgm Dir: David M Kleist
Tel: 208 282-3156   *Fax:* 208 282-2583
E-mail: kleidavi@isu.edu

Illinois

Southern Illinois University Carbondale
Counseling Prgm
CC, MFC/T, SC, CE Programs
Wham Bldg, Rm 223
Carbondale, IL 62901-4618
Prgm Dir: Karen K Prichard
Tel: 618 536-7763   *Fax:* 618 453-7110
E-mail: prichard@siu.edu

Eastern Illinois University
Counseling Prgm
CC, SC programs
2102 Buzzard Hall
Charleston, IL 61920
Prgm Dir: Richard L Roberts, PhD
Tel: 217 581-2400   *Fax:* 217 581-7800
E-mail: rlroberts@eiu.edu

Chicago State University
Counseling Prgm
CC, SC Programs
9501 S King Dr
Chicago, IL 60629
Prgm Dir: Lindsay Bicknell-Hentges, PhD
Tel: 773 995-2359
E-mail: lbicknel@csu.edu

Northeastern Illinois University
Counseling Prgm
CC, SC, MFC/T Programs
5500 N St Louis Ave
Chicago, IL 60625-4699
Prgm Dir: Nan Giblin, PhD
Tel: 773 442-5552   *Fax:* 773 442-5559
E-mail: N-Giblin@neiu.edu

Roosevelt University
Counseling Prgm
CC, MHC Programs
Department of Counseling and Human Services
Chicago, IL 60605
Prgm Dir: Bruce F Dykeman, PhD
Tel: 847 619-8822   *Fax:* 847 619-8830
E-mail: bdykeman@roosevelt.edu

Northern Illinois University
Counseling Prgm
CC, SC, CE Programs
Graham Hall 223
DeKalb, IL 60115-2854
Prgm Dir: Francesca Giordano
Tel: 815 753-8462
E-mail: fgiordano@niu.edu

Western Illinois University
Counseling Prgm
CC, SC Programs
Quad Cities Counselor Education Department
Moline, IL 61265-5881
www.wiu.edu
Prgm Dir: Frank Main, EdD
Tel: 309 762-1876, Ext 273   *Fax:* 309 762-6989
E-mail: fo-main@wiu.edu

Bradley University
Counseling Prgm
1501 W Bradley Ave
Westlake Hall
Peoria, IL 61625
Prgm Dir: Jobie L Skaggs, PhD
Tel: 309 677-3193
E-mail: jskaggs@bradley.edu

Concordia University
Counseling Prgm
CC, SC Programs
Psychology Dept
River Forest, IL 60305-1499
Prgm Dir: Dale J Septeowski
Tel: 708 209-3059   *Fax:* 708 209-3176
E-mail: crfsepteodj@curf.edu

University of Illinois at Springfield
Counseling Prgm
CC, SC Programs
One University Plaza
Springfield, IL 62703
Prgm Dir: Bill Abler, PhD
Tel: 217 206-7567
E-mail: abler.william@uis.edu

Governors State University
Counseling Prgm
CC, MFC/T, SC Programs
College of Education
University Park, IL 60466
Prgm Dir: Cyrus Ellis
Tel: 708 534-4907   *Fax:* 708 255-2245
E-mail: c-ellis@govst.edu

Indiana

Indiana University - Bloomington
Counseling Prgm
School of Education 4003
201 N Rose Ave
Bloomington, IN 47405-1006
Prgm Dir: Jeff Daniels, PhD
Tel: 812 856-8304   *Fax:* 812 856-8333
E-mail: jedaniel@indiana.edu

Butler University/Clarian Health
Counseling Prgm
SC Program
4600 Sunset Dr
Indianapolis, IN 46208
Prgm Dir: John Bloom
Tel: 317 940-9490   *Fax:* 317 940-6481
E-mail: jbloom@butler.edu

Indiana Wesleyan University
Counseling Prgm
CC, MFC/T Programs
4201 S Washington St
Marion, IN 46953
Prgm Dir: Jerry E Davis
Tel: 765 677-2995   *Fax:* 765 677-2504
E-mail: jerry.davis@indwes.edu

Ball State University
Counseling Prgm
CC, SC Programs
Teachers College, Rm 622
Muncie, IN 47306-0585
Prgm Dir: Kristin Perrone-McGovern
Tel: 765 285-8040   *Fax:* 765 285-2067
E-mail: kperrone@bsu.edu

Indiana University South Bend
Counseling Prgm
CC, SC Programs
1700 Mishawaka Ave
South Bend, IN 46634
Prgm Dir: Jeremy Linton, PhD
Tel: 574 520-4244   *Fax:* 574 520-5550
E-mail: jmlinton@iusb.edu

Indiana State University
Counseling Prgm
MHC, SC Programs
School of Education, Rm 1517
Terre Haute, IN 47809
http://counseling.indstate.edu
Prgm Dir: James L Campbell, PhD
Tel: 812 237-4389   *Fax:* 812 237-2729
E-mail: jcampbell2@indstate.edu

Purdue University
Counseling Prgm
SC Program
Dept of Educational Studies
West Lafayette, IN 47907-2098
Prgm Dir: Jean Peterson, PhD LMHC NCC
Tel: 765 494-9742   *Fax:* 765 496-1228
E-mail: jeanp@purdue.edu

Iowa

University of Northern Iowa
Counseling Prgm
MHC, SC Programs
508 Schindler Education Center
Cedar Falls, IA 50614-0604
Prgm Dir: Jan Bartlett
Tel: 319 273-7979
E-mail: jan.bartlett@uni.edu

University of Iowa
Counseling Prgm
CC, CE, SC Programs
N338 Lindquist Center N
Iowa City, IA 52242-1529
Prgm Dir: Dennis R Maki
Tel: 319 335-5284   *Fax:* 319 335-5291
E-mail: dennis-maki@uiowa.edu

Kansas

Emporia State University
Counseling Prgm
MHC, SC, SA Programs
Campus Box 4036
Emporia, KS 66801-5087
Prgm Dir: Patricia J Neufeld
Tel: 620 341-5220   *Fax:* 316 341-6200
E-mail: pneufeld@emporia.edu

Pittsburg State University
Counseling Prgm
CC Program
Dept of Psychology & Counseling
Pittsburg, KS 66762-7551
Prgm Dir: Donald E Ward, PhD LCPC NCC ACS
Tel: 316 235-4530   *Fax:* 316 235-6102
E-mail: dward@pittstate.edu

Kentucky

Western Kentucky University
Counseling Prgm
MFC/T, MHC Programs
1906 College Heights Blvd
Bowling Green, KY 42101
Prgm Dir: Kelly M Burch-Ragan, PhD
Tel: 270 745-6317
E-mail: kelly.burch-ragan@wku.edu

Lindsey Wilson College
Counseling Prgm
MHC Program
210 Lindsey Wilson St
Columbia, KY 42728
Prgm Dir: John R Rigney, EdD NCC LPCC
Tel: 502 384-8520   *Fax:* 502 384-8152
E-mail: rigneyj@lindsey.edu

Eastern Kentucky University
Counseling Prgm
MHC, SC Programs
521 Lancaster Ave
Richmond, KY 40475
Prgm Dir: Kim A Naugle, PhD
Tel: 859 622-1863
E-mail: kim.naugle@eku.edu

Louisiana

Louisiana State University
Counseling Prgm
CC, SC Programs
122 Peabody Hall
Baton Rouge, LA 70803
Prgm Dir: Gary Gintner, PhD
Tel: 225 388-2199   *Fax:* 225 578-6918
E-mail: gintner@lsu.edu

Southeastern Louisiana University
Counseling Prgm
CC, SC, MFC/T Programs
SLU Box 10863
Hammond, LA 70402
Prgm Dir: Peter M Emerson
Tel: 985 549-2053
E-mail: pemerson@selu.edu

University of Louisiana at Monroe
Counseling Prgm
CC, MFC/T, SC Programs
700 University Ave
Monroe, LA 71209-0230
Prgm Dir: Pamela P Newman
Tel: 318 342-1256   *Fax:* 318 342-1213
E-mail: pnewman@ulm.edu

Northwestern State University
Counseling Prgm
CIC, SA Programs
College of Education
Natchitoches, LA 71497
Prgm Dir: Frances Pearson
Tel: 318 357-6915
E-mail: pearson@nsula.edu

Loyola University New Orleans
Counseling Prgm
CC Program
6363 St Charles Ave, Camp Box 66
New Orleans, LA 70118
Prgm Dir: Kevin A Fall, PhD
Tel: 504 864-7859   *Fax:* 504 864-7855
E-mail: kfall@loyno.edu

Our Lady of Holy Cross College
Counseling Prgm
MFC/T, CC Programs
4123 Woodland Dr
New Orleans, LA 70131
Prgm Dir: Carolyn C White, PhD
Tel: 504 398-2169   *Fax:* 504 391-2421
E-mail: cwhite@olhcc.edu

University of New Orleans
Counseling Prgm
CC, CE, SC Programs
348 Education Bldg
New Orleans, LA 70148-2515
www.uno.edu
Prgm Dir: Barbara Herlihy, PhD LPC NCC
Tel: 504 280-6662   *Fax:* 504 280-6453
E-mail: bherlihy@uno.edu

Maine

University of Southern Maine
Counseling Prgm
MHC, SC Programs
400D Bailey Hall
Gorham, ME 04038-1083
Prgm Dir: Reid D Stevens, PhD
Tel: 207 780-5079   *Fax:* 207 780-5043
E-mail: stevens@usm.maine.edu

Maryland

Loyola College of Maryland
Counseling Prgm
4501 N Charles St
Baltimore, MD 21210
Prgm Dir: Bradley T Erford, PhD NCC LCPC
Tel: 410 617-1509   *Fax:* 410 617-1708
E-mail: berford@loyola.edu

Univ of Maryland at College Park
Counseling Prgm
CE, SC Programs
College of Education
College Park, MD 20742
Prgm Dir: Courtland Lee, PhD
Tel: 301 405-8904   *Fax:* 301 405-9995
E-mail: clee5@umd.edu

Loyola College of Maryland
Counseling Prgm
Pastoral Counseling Department
8890 McGaw Rd, Ste 380
Columbia, MD 21045
www.loyola.edu/pastoralcounseling
Prgm Dir: David Newton
Tel: 410 617-7620   *Fax:* 410 617-7644
E-mail: dcnewton@Loyola.edu

Michigan

Andrews University
Counseling Prgm
Bell Hall 159
Berrien Springs, MI 49104-0104
www.educ.andrews.edu
Prgm Dir: Elvin Gabriel
Tel: 269 471-6223   *Fax:* 269 471-6374
E-mail: gabriel@andrews.edu

University of Detroit Mercy
Counseling Prgm
CC, SC Programs
444 Manning Hall
Detroit, MI 48219-0900
Prgm Dir: Nancy Calley
Tel: 313 578-0436
E-mail: calleyng@udmercy.edu

Wayne State University
Counseling Prgm
CC, SC, CE Programs
311 Education Bldg
Detroit, MI 48202
Prgm Dir: Daisy B Ellington
Tel: 313 577-2435   *Fax:* 313 577-5235
E-mail: ad4950@wayne.edu

Western Michigan University
Counseling Prgm
CC, CE, CIC, SC Programs
3102 Sangren Hall
Kalamazoo, MI 49008-5195
Prgm Dir: Carla Adkison-Bradley, PhD
Tel: 616 387-3504
E-mail: carla.bradley@wmich.edu

Oakland University
Counseling Prgm
CC, SC Programs
Dept of Counseling, 491B Pawley Hall
Rochester, MI 48309-4494
Prgm Dir: Luellen Ramey, PhD
Tel: 248 370-4169   *Fax:* 248 370-4141
E-mail: ramey@oakland.edu

Eastern Michigan University
Counseling Prgm
CC, SACC, SC Programs
304 Porter Bldg
Ypsilanti, MI 48197
Prgm Dir: Irene Mass Ametrano
Tel: 734 487-0255   *Fax:* 734 487-4608
E-mail: irene.ametrano@emich.edu

Minnesota

Minnesota State University - Mankato
Counseling Prgm
CC, SAPP, SC Programs
107 Armstrong Hall
Mankato, MN 56002-2423
Prgm Dir: Diane Coursol
Tel: 507 389-5656
E-mail: diane.coursol@mnsu.edu

Minnesota State University - Moorhead
Counseling Prgm
CC, SACC, SAPP Programs
Counseling & Student Affairs
Moorhead, MN 56563
Prgm Dir: Wes Erwin, PhD NCC
Tel: 218 477-2009   *Fax:* 218 477-2547
E-mail: erwin@mnstate.edu

Winona State University
Counseling Prgm
CC, SC Programs
University Center-Rochester
Rochester, MN 55904
Prgm Dir: Nicholas J Ruiz
Tel: 507 285-7136
E-mail: NRuiz@winona.edu

St Cloud State University
Counseling Prgm
SC Program
720 4th Ave S
St Cloud, MN 56301
Prgm Dir: Terrance Peterson
Tel: 320 308-2992
E-mail: tpeterson@stcloudstate.edu

Mississippi

Delta State University
Counseling Prgm
CC, SC Programs
Ewing 335
Cleveland, MS 38733
Prgm Dir: Matthew Buckley
Tel: 662 846-4357   *Fax:* 662 846-4402
E-mail: mbuckley@deltastate.edu

Mississippi College
Counseling Prgm
MFC/T, MHC, SC Programs
PO Box 4013
Clinton, MS 39058
Prgm Dir: Katherine Jones, PhD
Tel: 601 925-3803   *Fax:* 601 925-3951
E-mail: kjones@mc.edu

University of Southern Mississippi
Counseling Prgm
CC Program
Southern Station Box 05025
Hattiesburg, MS 39406-5025
Prgm Dir: Bonnie Nicholson
Tel: 601 266-4177   *Fax:* 601 266-5580
E-mail: Bonnie.Nicholson@usm.edu

Mississippi State University
Counseling Prgm
CC, SACC, SC, CE Programs
PO Box 9727
Mississippi State, MS 39762
Prgm Dir: E Joan Looby, PhD LPC NCC
Tel: 601 325-3426   *Fax:* 601 325-3263
E-mail: jlooby@colled.msstate.edu

University of Mississippi
Counseling Prgm
CC, SC, CE Programs
Ste 200, School of Education
University, MS 38677-1848
Prgm Dir: William B Kline
Tel: 662 915-2020
E-mail: wbk@olemiss.edu

Missouri

Southeast Missouri State University
Counseling Prgm
CC, SC Programs
Mail Stop 5550
Cape Girardeau, MO 63701-4799
Prgm Dir: A Zaidy MohdZain, EdD
Tel: 573 651-2399   *Fax:* 573 986-6812
E-mail: zmohdzain@semo.edu

University of Missouri - St Louis
Counseling Prgm
469 Marillac Hall
1 University Blvd
St Louis, MO 63121-4400
Prgm Dir: Mark Pope, EdD MAC LPC NCC
Tel: 314 516-7121   *Fax:* 314 516-5784
E-mail: PopeML@msx.umsl.edu

Montana

Montana State University
Counseling Prgm
MFC/T, MHC, SC Programs
218 Herrick Hall
Bozeman, MT 59717
Prgm Dir: Jill Thorngren, EdD
Tel: 406 994-3299   *Fax:* 406 994-2013
E-mail: jillt@montana.edu

University of Montana
Counseling Prgm
MHC, SC Programs
32 Campus Dr
Missoula, MT 59812-6356
Prgm Dir: Catherine Jenni, PhD
Tel: 406 243-2608
E-mail: cathy.jenni@umontana.edu

Nebraska

University of Nebraska - Kearney
Counseling Prgm
Dept of Counseling and School Psychology
College of Education Bldg
Kearney, NE 68849
Prgm Dir: Julie Ann Dinsmore
Tel: 308 865-8316   *Fax:* 308 865-8097
E-mail: dinsmoreja@unk.edu

University of Nebraska - Omaha
Counseling Prgm
CC, SC Programs
Kayser Hall 421
Omaha, NE 68182-0167
Prgm Dir: Jeannette Seaberry, PhD
Tel: 402 554-2728   *Fax:* 402 554-3684
E-mail: jseaberry@mail.unomaha.edu

Nevada

University of Nevada - Las Vegas
Counseling Prgm
CC, MFC/T, SC Programs
4505 S Maryland Pkwy
Las Vegas, NV 89154-3003
Prgm Dir: Pamela A Staples
Tel: 702 895-3253   *Fax:* 702 895-1658
E-mail: pamela.staples@unlv.edu

University of Nevada - Reno
Counseling Prgm
CC, SACC, SC, CE Programs
1664 N Virginia St
Reno, NV 89557-0213
Prgm Dir: Tom Harrison, PhD
Tel: 775 784-7318   *Fax:* 775 784-1990
E-mail: tch@unr.edu

New Jersey

College of New Jersey
Counseling Prgm
CC, SC Programs
Forcina Hall 322 / PO Box 7718
Ewing, NJ 08620-0718
Prgm Dir: Mark Woodford, PhD
Tel: 609 771-3018
E-mail: woodford@tcnj.edu

Rider University
Counseling Prgm
2083 Lawrenceville Rd
Lawrenceville, NJ 08648-3099
Prgm Dir: Jesse B Deesch
Tel: 609 895-5487   *Fax:* 609 896-5362
E-mail: deesch@rider.edu

Kean University
Counseling Prgm
CC, SC Programs
1000 Morris Ave
Union, NJ 07083
Prgm Dir: Juneau Gary, PhD
Tel: 908 737-3842
E-mail: jgary@kean.edu

William Paterson Univ of New Jersey
Counseling Prgm
Dept of Special Education and Counseling
300 Pompton Rd, Raubinger Hall
Wayne, NJ 07170
Prgm Dir: Paula R Danzinger, PhD LPC CCMHC
  NCGC ACS
Tel: 973 720-3085, Ext 3085
E-mail: danzingerp@wpunj.edu

New Mexico

University of New Mexico
Counseling Prgm
CC, SC, CE Programs
College of Education, Simpson Hall
Albuquerque, NM 87131-1246
Prgm Dir: Deborah Rifenbary
Tel: 505 277-8933
E-mail: divbse@unm.edu

New Mexico State University
Counseling Prgm
MHC Program
PO Box 30001
Las Cruces, NM 88003
Prgm Dir: Todd Savage
Tel: 505 646-4093
E-mail: tsavage@nmsu.edu

New York

SUNY Brockport
Counseling Prgm
350 New Campus Dr
Brockport, NY 14420-2953
http://brockport.edu
Prgm Dir: Susan R Seem, PhD LMHC NCC ACS
Tel: 585 395-2258   *Fax:* 585 395-2366
E-mail: sseem@brockport.edu

Long Island University - C W Post Campus
Counseling Prgm
MHC, SC Programs
Library Rm 320
Brookville, NY 11548-2814
Prgm Dir: Joseph Despres, EdD
Tel: 516 299-2814
E-mail: joseph.despres@liu.edu

St John's University
Counseling Prgm
SC Program
Jamaica & Staten Island Campus
Jamaica, NY 11439
Prgm Dir: Robert Eschenauer, PhD
Tel: 718 990-6455
E-mail: eschenar@stjohns.edu

SUNY College at Plattsburgh
Counseling Prgm
CC, SA, SC Programs
101 Broad St
Plattsburgh, NY 12901
Prgm Dir: Beverly A Burnell, PhD
Tel: 518 564-4177   *Fax:* 518 564-4161
E-mail: beverly.burnell@plattsburgh.edu

University of Rochester
Counseling Prgm
MHC, SC, CE Programs
Dewey Hall 1-314
Rochester, NY 14627
www.rochester.edu/Warner/
Prgm Dir: Deborah Erickson, PhD
Tel: 585 275-1007
E-mail: derickson@warner.rochester.edu

Syracuse University
Counseling Prgm
SACC, SC, CE, CC Programs
Counseling and Human Services
Syracuse, NY 13244-3240
http://soe.syr.edu/academics/grad/
  counseling_human_services/
Prgm Dir: Janine Bernard, PhD NCC ACS LMHC
Tel: 315 443-2266   *Fax:* 315 443-5732
E-mail: bernard@syr.edu

North Carolina

Appalachian State University
Counseling Prgm
CC, SC, CIC Programs
Boone, NC 28608
Prgm Dir: Lee Baruth
Tel: 704 262-3133
E-mail: baruthlg@appstate.edu

University of North Carolina - Chapel Hill
Counseling Prgm
SC Program
CB #3500 Peabody Hall
Chapel Hill, NC 27599-3500
Prgm Dir: John P Galassi, PhD
Tel: 919 962-9196
E-mail: jgalassi@email.unc.edu

Univ of North Carolina at Charlotte
Counseling Prgm
CC, CE, SC Programs
9201 University City Blvd
Charlotte, NC 28223-0001
Prgm Dir: Henry L Harry
Tel: 704 687-8971   *Fax:* 704 687-2916
E-mail: hharris2@uncc.edu

Western Carolina University
Counseling Prgm
CC, SC Programs
204 Killiam Bldg
Cullowhee, NC 28723
Prgm Dir: Mary Deck, PhD NCC LPC
Tel: 828 227-7207   *Fax:* 828 227-7388
E-mail: deck@email.wcu.edu

North Carolina A&T State University
Counseling Prgm
CC, SC Programs
Human Development & Services
Greensboro, NC 27411-1066
Prgm Dir: Patricia Bethea-Whitfield
Tel: 336 334-7916
E-mail: betheap@ncat.edu

University of North Carolina - Greensboro
Counseling Prgm
CC, CE, GC, MFC/T, SACC, SC Programs
PO Box 26171
Greensboro, NC 27402-6170
Prgm Dir: Diane L Borders, PhD
Tel: 336 334-3425   *Fax:* 336 334-3433
E-mail: borders@uncg.edu

North Carolina State University
Counseling Prgm
CC, SC, CIC, CE Programs
520 Poe Hall
Raleigh, NC 27695-7801
Prgm Dir: S Raymond Ting, PhD LPC NCC CDFI
Tel: 919 515-6362   *Fax:* 919 515-6891
E-mail: raymond_ting@ncsu.edu

Wake Forest University
Counseling Prgm
CC, SC Programs
PO Box 7406
Winston-Salem, NC 27109
http://wfu.edu/counseling
Prgm Dir: Sam Gladding, PhD LPC NCC CCMHC
Tel: 336 758-4882   *Fax:* 336 758-3129
E-mail: stg@wfu.edu

North Dakota

North Dakota State University
Counseling Prgm
CC, SC Programs
School of Education, 210 FLC
Fargo, ND 58105-5057
Prgm Dir: J Wade Hannon, EdD
Tel: 701 231-7204   *Fax:* 701 231-7416
E-mail: wade.hannon@ndsu.edu

Ohio

University of Akron
Counseling Prgm
Marriage and Family Therapy Programs
  (masters/doctoral)
127 Carroll Hall
Akron, OH 44325-5007
www.uakron.edu/colleges/educ/Counseling/
Prgm Dir: Patricia Parr, PhD
Tel: 330 972-8151   *Fax:* 330 972-5292
E-mail: pparr@uakron.edu

Ohio University
Counseling Prgm
CC, SC, CE Programs
201 McCracken Hall
Athens, OH 45701
www.coe.ohiou.edu
Prgm Dir: Dana Levitt, PhD
Tel: 740 593-4163   *Fax:* 740 593-0569
E-mail: Levitt@ohio.edu

University of Cincinnati
Counseling Prgm
PO Box 210002
Cincinnati, OH 45221
Prgm Dir: Geoffrey G Yager, PhD LPC
Tel: 513 556-3347   *Fax:* 513 556-3898
E-mail: Geof.Yager@uc.edu

Cleveland State University
Counseling Prgm
CC, SC Programs
1983 E 24th St
Cleveland, OH 44115
Prgm Dir: Kathryn C MacCluskie, EdD
Tel: 216 523-7147
E-mail: k.maccluskie@csuohio.edu

John Carroll University
Counseling Prgm
20700 North Park Blvd
University Heights
Cleveland, OH 44118-4581
www.jcu.edu/Graduate
Prgm Dir: Christopher Faiver, PhD
Tel: 216 397-3001   *Fax:* 216 397-3045
E-mail: faiver@jcu.edu

Wright State University
Counseling Prgm
CC, SC, MHC Programs
M052 Creative Arts Center
Dayton, OH 45435-0001
Prgm Dir: Stephen B Fortson
Tel: 937 775-2075
E-mail: stephen.fortson@wright.edu

Kent State University
Counseling Prgm
CC, SC, CE Programs
310 White Hall
Kent, OH 44242-0001
Prgm Dir: Jason McGlothlin, PhD
Tel: 330 672-2662   *Fax:* 330 672-3063
E-mail: jmcgloth@kent.edu

University of Toledo
Counseling Prgm
Counselor Education and School Psychology
Mail Stop 119
Toledo, OH 43606-3390
http://cesp.utoledo.edu
Prgm Dir: Martin Ritchie, EdD LPC NCC
Tel: 419 530-4775   *Fax:* 419 530-7879
E-mail: martin.ritchie@utoledo.edu

Youngstown State University
Counseling Prgm
CC, SC Programs
Department of Counseling, BCOE Rm 3305
Youngstown, OH 44555-0001
Prgm Dir: Victoria White Kress, PhD
Tel: 330 941-3257   *Fax:* 330 941-2369
E-mail: vewhite@ysu.edu

Oklahoma

Oklahoma State University
Counseling Prgm
CC, SC Programs
421 Willard Hall
Stillwater, OK 74078
Prgm Dir: Camille S DeBell, PhD
Tel: 405 744-9442
E-mail: dcamill@okstate.edu

Oregon

Oregon State University
Counseling Prgm
CC, SC, CE Programs
New School of Education
Corvallis, OR 97331
Prgm Dir: Cass Dykeman, PhD
Tel: 541 737-8204
E-mail: dykemanc@onid.orst.edu

Portland State University
Counseling Prgm
CC, SC Programs
PO Box 751
Portland, OR 97207-0751
Prgm Dir: Russell Miars, PhD
Tel: 503 725-4611   *Fax:* 503 725-5599
E-mail: miarsr@pdx.edu

Pennsylvania

Edinboro University of Pennsylvania
Counseling Prgm
SACC, SAPP, SC, CC Programs
128 Butterfield Hall
Edinboro, PA 16444
Prgm Dir: Salene Cowher
Tel: 814 732-1116   *Fax:* 814 732-2233
E-mail: scowher@edinboro.edu

Duquesne University
Counseling Prgm
CC, MFC/T, SC Programs
School of Education
Pittsburgh, PA 15282
www.education.duq.edu/counselored
Prgm Dir: Maura Krushinski, EdD
Tel: 412 396-5131   *Fax:* 412 396-1340
E-mail: Krushinski@duq.edu

Marywood University
Counseling Prgm
MHC, SC Programs
2300 Adams Ave
Scranton, PA 18509
Prgm Dir: John J Lemoncelli, EdD
Tel: 570 348-6211, Ext 2317
E-mail: lemoncelli@es.marywood.edu

University of Scranton
Counseling Prgm
CC, SC Programs
Dept of Counseling and Human Services
Scranton, PA 18510-4523
Prgm Dir: Kevin Wilkerson, PhD NCC ACS
Tel: 570 941-6649   *Fax:* 570 941-5882
E-mail: wilkersonk2@scranton.edu

Shippensburg University
Counseling Prgm
CC, MHC, SC, CIC, SA Programs
1871 Old Main Dr, Rm 115
Shippensburg, PA 17257
Prgm Dir: Todd Whitman, PhD
Tel: 717 477-1654   *Fax:* 717 530-4056
E-mail: tkwhit@ship.edu

Slippery Rock University of Pennsylvania
Counseling Prgm
CC Program
006 McKay Education Bldg
Slippery Rock, PA 16057
Prgm Dir: Donald Strano, PhD
Tel: 724 738-2274
E-mail: donald.strano@sru.edu

Penn State University
Counseling Prgm
Counselor Education
331 Cedar Bldg
University Park, PA 16828
www.ed.psu.edu/cned/ced.asp
Prgm Dir: Richard Hazler, PhD
Tel: 814 863-2415   *Fax:* 814 863-7750
E-mail: hazler@psu.edu

South Carolina

Clemson University
Counseling Prgm
CC, SACC, SAPP, SC Programs
Education and Human Development
Clemson, SC 29634-0710
Prgm Dir: Robert Urofsky, PhD
Tel: 864 656-0927
E-mail: rurofsk@clemson.edu

University of South Carolina
Counseling Prgm
MFC/T, SC, CE Programs
Family Counseling Program
Columbia, SC 29208
Prgm Dir: Joshua Gold, PhD NCC
Tel: 803 777-1936   *Fax:* 803 777-3045
E-mail: josgold@sc.edu

South Carolina State University
Counseling Prgm
SC Program
300 College St NE
Orangeburg, SC 29177
Prgm Dir: Philip M Scriven, PhD
Tel: 803 536-7147   *Fax:* 803 536-8841
E-mail: pscriven@scsu.edu

Winthrop University
Counseling Prgm
CC, SC Programs
143 Withers Bldg
Rock Hill, SC 29733
Prgm Dir: Johnny Sanders
Tel: 803 323-4757   *Fax:* 803 323-4755
E-mail: sandersj@winthrop.edu

South Dakota

South Dakota State University
Counseling Prgm
CC, SACC, SC Programs
PO Box 507
Brookings, SD 57007-0095
www.sdstate.edu
Prgm Dir: Jay Trenhaile, EdD
Tel: 605 688-4367   *Fax:* 605 688-5929
E-mail: jay_trenhaile@sdstate.edu

University of South Dakota
Counseling Prgm
Delzell School of Education
414 E Clark St
Vermillion, SD 57069
Prgm Dir: Frank Main
Tel: 605 677-5257   *Fax:* 605 677-5438
E-mail: Rita.Humphrey@usd.edu

Tennessee

University of Tennessee - Chattanooga
Counseling Prgm
CC, SC Programs
615 McCallie Ave
Chattanooga, TN 37403
Prgm Dir: Kristi Gibbs, PhD
Tel: 423 425-4106
E-mail: Kristi-Gibbs@utc.edu

East Tennessee State University
Counseling Prgm
CC, SC Programs
PO Box 70548
Johnson City, TN 37614-0548
Prgm Dir: Patricia Robertson, EdD
Tel: 423 439-7693   *Fax:* 423 439-7790
E-mail: robertpe@etsu.edu

University of Tennessee - Knoxville
Counseling Prgm
MHC, SC, CE Programs
College of Education
Knoxville, TN 37996-3400
Prgm Dir: Marianne Woodside, EdD
Tel: 865 974-0693   *Fax:* 865 974-0135
E-mail: mwoodsid@utk.edu

University of Memphis
Counseling Prgm
Ball Hall, Rm 100
Memphis, TN 38152-0001
Prgm Dir: Douglas C Strohmer, PhD
Tel: 901 678-5114   *Fax:* 901 678-5114
E-mail: dstrohmr@memphis.edu

Middle Tennessee State University
Counseling Prgm
SC Program
PO Box 87
Murfreesboro, TN 37132
Prgm Dir: Virginia Dansby
Tel: 615 898-2559
E-mail: vsdansby@mtsu.edu

Vanderbilt University
Counseling Prgm
CC, SC Programs
PO Box 322-GPC
Nashville, TN 37203
Prgm Dir: Camilla Benbow, EdD
Tel: 615 322-8407
E-mail: camilla.benbow@vanderbilt.edu

Texas

Texas A&M University - Commerce
Counseling Prgm
202 Education North
Commerce, TX 75429-3011
Prgm Dir: Richard E Lampe
Tel: 903 886-5631
E-mail: Richard_Lampe@tamu-commerce.edu

Texas A&M University - Corpus Christi
Counseling Prgm
CC, CE, MFC/T, SC Programs
6300 Ocean Dr
Corpus Christi, TX 78412
Prgm Dir: Robert Smith, PhD
Tel: 361 825-2307
E-mail: robert-l-smith@tamu.edu

Texas Woman's University
Counseling Prgm
CC, SC Programs
Dept of Family Sciences
Denton, TX 76204-5769
Prgm Dir: Susan Adams
Tel: 940 898-2692
E-mail: SAdams1@mail.twu.edu

University of North Texas
Counseling Prgm
CC, SC, CIC, CE Programs
PO Box 310829
Denton, TX 76203-0829
www.coe.unt.edu/che/coun
Prgm Dir: Dee Ray, PhD LPC-S NCC RPT-S
Tel: 940 369-7967   *Fax:* 940 565-2905
E-mail: dee.ray@unt.edu

Texas Tech University
Counseling Prgm
CC, SC, CE Programs
PO Box 41071
Lubbock, TX 79409-1071
Prgm Dir: Loretta J Bradley, PhD
Tel: 806 742-1997, Ext 263   *Fax:* 806 742-2179
E-mail: Loretta.Bradley@ttu.edu

Stephen F Austin State University
Counseling Prgm
CC, SC Programs
Department of Human Services
Nacogdoches, TX 75962-3019
www.sfasu.edu/hs/counseli.htm
Prgm Dir: David Lawson, PhD
Tel: 936 468-1079   *Fax:* 936 468-1342
E-mail: lawsondm@sfasu.edu

St Mary's University
Counseling Prgm
CC, CE, MHC Programs
One Camino Santa Maria
San Antonio, TX 78228-8527
Prgm Dir: Framcis Farrell, Jr
Tel: 210 436-3226   *Fax:* 210 431-6886
E-mail: ffarrell@stmarytx.edu

Texas State University - San Marcos
Counseling Prgm
CC, MFC/T, SACC, SC Programs
601 University Dr
San Marcos, TX 78666-4615
Prgm Dir: Linda Homeyer
Tel: 512 245-3757   *Fax:* 512 245-8872
E-mail: LH10@txstate.edu

Utah

University of Phoenix - Utah
Counseling Prgm
MHC Program
5373 S Green St
Salt Lake City, UT 84123
Prgm Dir: Donald E Beck, PhD
Tel: 801 263-1444, Ext 54222
E-mail: don.beck@phoenix.edu

Vermont

University of Vermont
Counseling Prgm
Mann Hall
208 Colchester Ave
Burlington, VT 05405-1757
www.uvm.edu/~cslgprog
Prgm Dir: Anne Geroski, EdD
Tel: 802 656-3888   *Fax:* 802 656-3173
E-mail: Anne.Geroski@uvm.edu

Virginia

Marymount University
Counseling Prgm
CC, SC Programs
2807 N Glebe Rd
Arlington, VA 22207
Prgm Dir: Lisa Jackson-Cherry
Tel: 703 284-1633
E-mail: lisa.jackson-cherry@marymount.edu

Virginia Polytechnic Inst & State Univ
Counseling Prgm
CC, SC, CE Programs
Counselor Education
Blacksburg, VA 24061-0302
Prgm Dir: Gerard Lawson, Asst Professor
Tel: 540 231-9703
E-mail: glawson@vt.edu

University of Virginia
Counseling Prgm
Counselor Ed-Ruffner Hall #160
405 Emmet St S, PO Box 400269
Charlottesville, VA 22904-2495
Prgm Dir: Harriet L Glosoff, PhD
Tel: 434 243-8717   *Fax:* 434 924-1433
E-mail: hlg2n@virginia.edu

James Madison University
Counseling Prgm
Department of Graduate Psychology
MSC 7401
Harrisonburg, VA 22807
Prgm Dir: Lennis Echterling, PhD
Tel: 540 568-6522   *Fax:* 540 568-3322
E-mail: echterlg@jmu.edu

Lynchburg College
Counseling Prgm
CC, SC Programs
1501 Lakeside Dr
Lynchburg, VA 24501-3199
www.lynchburg.edu
Prgm Dir: Jeanne Booth, PhD
Tel: 434 544-8551
E-mail: booth@lynchburg.edu

Old Dominion University
Counseling Prgm
CC, SC, SA Programs
College of Education
Norfolk, VA 23529
Prgm Dir: Nina Brown
Tel: 757 783-5308   *Fax:* 757 683-5756
E-mail: nbrown@odu.edu

Radford University
Counseling Prgm
PO Box 6994
Radford, VA 24142
Prgm Dir: Donald Anderson, EdD
Tel: 540 831-5214   *Fax:* 540 831-6755
E-mail: danderso@radford.edu

Regent University
Counseling Prgm
1000 Regent University Dr
Virginia Beach, VA 23464-9800
www.regent.edu/counseling
Prgm Dir: Rosemary Thompson, LPC NCC NCSC
Tel: 757 226-5000   *Fax:* 757 226-4263
E-mail: roseth1@regent.edu

College of William & Mary
Counseling Prgm
CC, SC, CE Programs
PO Box 8795
Williamsburg, VA 23187-8795
Prgm Dir: Victoria Foster, EdD LPC LMFT NCC
Tel: 757 221-2321   *Fax:* 757 221-2988
E-mail: vafost@wm.edu

Washington

Western Washington University
Counseling Prgm
Dept of Psychology
516 High St
Bellingham, WA 98225-9089
www.ac.wwu.edu/~psych/
Prgm Dir: Arleen C Lewis, PhD
Tel: 360 650-3523   *Fax:* 360 650-7305
E-mail: arleen.lewis@wwu.edu

Eastern Washington University
Counseling Prgm
MHC, SC Programs
705 W First Ave
Spokane, WA 99201
Prgm Dir: Mark Young, PhD
Tel: 509 623-4225   *Fax:* 509 359-4366
E-mail: Mark.Young@mail.ewu.edu

West Virginia

West Virginia University
Counseling Prgm
CC, SC Programs
3040 University Ave
Morgantown, WV 26506-6122
Prgm Dir: Ed Jacobs, PhD
Tel: 304 293-2177 *Fax:* 304 293-4082
E-mail: Ed.Jacobs@mail.wvu.edu

Wisconsin

University of Wisconsin - Oshkosh
Counseling Prgm
CC, SC Pgm, Department of Counselor Education
Nursing Education Building 001
Oshkosh, WI 54901
www.coehs.uwosh.edu/counselor_ed/
Prgm Dir: Alan Saginak, EdD Counselor Edu and
    Counseling
Tel: 920 424-1475 *Fax:* 920 424-0858
E-mail: saginak@uwosh.edu

University of Wisconsin - Superior
Counseling Prgm
CC, SC Programs
McCaskill Hall, Rm 111
Superior, WI 54880
Prgm Dir: James Holter
Tel: 715 394-8151 *Fax:* 715 394-8146
E-mail: jholter@uwsuper.edu

University of Wisconsin - Whitewater
Counseling Prgm
Counselor Educ Dept
800 W Main St
Whitewater, WI 53190
Prgm Dir: Brenda O'Beirne, PhD Licensed Psychologist
Tel: 262 472-1452 *Fax:* 262 472-2841
E-mail: obeirneb@uww.edu

Wyoming

University of Wyoming
Counseling Prgm
CC, SC, SA, CE Programs
PO Box 3374
Laramie, WY 82071
Prgm Dir: Serena Lambert, PhD
Tel: 307 766-5329 *Fax:* 307 766-2366
E-mail: slambert@uwyo.edu

Counselor

Programs*	Class Capacity	Begins	Length (months)	Award	Res. Tuition	Non-res. Tuition	Stipend	Offers:‡ 1	2	3	4
Arizona											
Northern Arizona University (Flagstaff)	60	Sep Jan	24, 18	MA	$5,214	$14,896	$9,151	•		•	
California											
San Francisco State University	100	Fall	24	MS	$3,000	$10,000		•		•	•
Colorado											
Colorado State University (Fort Collins)	25			MS				•		•	
Denver Seminary (Littleton)	85	Aug Jan	48	MA				•		•	
U of Colorado (Denver) Health Sciences Center	105	Every semester	36	Dipl, MA	$3,500	$0		•		•	
District of Columbia											
George Washington University	20	Sep Jan May	24	Dipl, Cert, MA, PhD	$1,012	$1,012		•		•	•
Florida											
Stetson University (Deland)	20	Fall Spring Summer	36	Dipl, MS	$500	$500		•			
University of Central Florida (Orlando)	30	Aug Jan	30	MA, PhD	$5,788	$21,927		•		•	
University of Florida (Gainesville)	Var	Fall Spring	36, 60	MEd EdS, PhD	$7,478	$22,603				•	
University of Florida (Gainesville)	Var	Fall Spring	36, 60	MEd EdS, PhD	$7,478	$22,603				•	
University of Florida (Gainesville)	Var	Fall Spring	48	MEd EdS, PhD	$7,478	$22,603				•	
University of North Florida (Jacksonville)	50	Aug May	24, 36	MEd, MA	$4,000	$0		•		•	
Georgia											
Georgia State University (Atlanta)	80	Aug	24	Dipl, MS	$4,000	$0		•		•	
Idaho											
Northwest Nazarene University (Nampa)				MS	$5,850	$5,850		•		•	
Illinois											
Eastern Illinois University (Charleston)	20	Aug	48	MS	$3,000	$0		•		•	
Western Illinois University (Moline)	50	Spring Fall	48	MSEd	$216	$433		•			
					Per credit hour						
Indiana											
Indiana State University (Terre Haute)	60	Jun Aug	24	MS, MEd	$5,086	$10,018	$5,200	•		•	
Purdue University (West Lafayette)	10	Fall	24	MSEd	$7,416	$22,224	$13,255	•		•	
Iowa											
University of Iowa (Iowa City)	30	Fall semester	24	MA	$6,759	$18,153		•		•	
Kansas											
Pittsburg State University	20	Each semester	24	MS	$4,831	$11,882	$4,410	•		•	
Louisiana											
University of New Orleans	140	Aug	24	MEd, PhD	$2,612	$0		•		•	•
Maryland											
Loyola College of Maryland (Columbia)	400	Sep Jan May	24, 48	Cert, MS, PhD	$10,560	$10,560					
Michigan											
Andrews University (Berrien Springs)	15	Aug	18, 24	MA	$16,800	$16,800	$4,000	•			
Oakland University (Rochester)	30	Sep Jan	24, 36	MA	$8,978	$15,476		•		•	•
Missouri											
University of Missouri - St Louis	20	Aug	30	MEd, PhD	$4,900	$8,900		•		•	
New Jersey											
William Paterson Univ of New Jersey (Wayne)		Ongoing	36	Dipl, MEd				•		•	

*Data are shown only for programs that completed the 2007 AMA Survey of Health Professions Education Programs.
‡Key to Offers: 1: Evening or weekend classes; 2: Non-English instruction; 3: Cultural competence instruction; 4: Distance education component.

Programs*	Class Capacity	Begins	Length (months)	Award	Res. Tuition	Non-res. Tuition	Stipend	Offers:‡ 1	2	3	4
New York											
SUNY Brockport		Fall Spring Summer		MSEd	$6,900	$10,920		•		•	
Syracuse University	25	Sep	24	MS				•		•	
University of Rochester	50	Rolling admission	24, 48	MS, PhD	$60,000	$60,000		•		•	
North Carolina											
North Carolina State University (Raleigh)	40	May Jul Aug	24, 48	MEd/BS, PhD	$5,636	$17,684	$9,000	•		•	•
Wake Forest University (Winston-Salem)	15	Aug	24	MA	$25,000	$25,000	$25,000			•	
Ohio											
John Carroll University (Cleveland)	30	Rolling admission	36	MA				•		•	
Ohio University (Athens)	90	Sep	24, 30	Dipl, MEd, PhD	$7,500	$7,500	$7,800	•		•	
University of Akron	15	Spring Fall	36, 48	Dipl, MA/MS, PhD	$8,000	$16,000	$11,000	•		•	
University of Toledo	20	Summer Fall Spring	24, 36	MA, PhD	$9,360	$18,172	$15,000	•		•	•
Pennsylvania											
Duquesne University (Pittsburgh)	65	Every semester	29	MSEd	$13,000	$13,000		•		•	
Penn State University (University Park)	30	Fall semester	22, 36	Dipl, Cert, MEd, PhD							
Shippensburg University					$1,734	$1,734		•			
South Dakota											
South Dakota State University (Brookings)	40	Sep Jan Jun	24, 36	MS	$125	$369		•			•
Texas											
Stephen F Austin State University (Nacogdoches)	20	Fall Spring Summer	36	MA	$5,000	$11,220	$8,000	•		•	•
University of North Texas (Denton)	23	Fall Spring Summer	24, 36	Cert, MEd MS, PhD				•		•	•
Vermont											
University of Vermont (Burlington)	20	Fall	36, 60	MS	$11,880	$27,764				•	
Virginia											
Lynchburg College	18	Fall Spring	30, 60	Dipl, MEd				•		•	
Regent University (Virginia Beach)	60	Fall	36, 30	Dipl, MA, PsyD	$575,695			•		•	
Washington											
Western Washington University (Bellingham)	6	Sep	24	Cert, MEd	$5,694	$16,221				•	
Wisconsin											
University of Wisconsin - Oshkosh	20	Fall	36	Dipl, MSEd				•		•	
University of Wisconsin - Whitewater	25	Sep		MS	$3,300	$8,600		•		•	

*Data are shown only for programs that completed the 2007 AMA Survey of Health Professions Education Programs.
‡Key to Offers: 1: Evening or weekend classes; 2: Non-English instruction; 3: Cultural competence instruction; 4: Distance education component.

Cytology is the study of the structure and the function of cells. Cytotechnologists are specially trained technologists who work with pathologists to evaluate cellular material from virtually all body sites primarily utilizing the microscope. Paramount to cytotechnologists is the microscopic recognition of normal and abnormal cytologic changes, including, but not limited to, malignant neoplasms, precancerous lesions, infectious agents, and inflammatory processes in gynecologic, non-gynecologic, and fine needle aspiration specimens. Cytotechnologists possess the technical skills for a wide variety of cytologic laboratory specimen preparations and a basic knowledge of contemporary procedures and technologies.

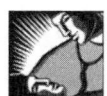

Career Description

Cell specimens may be obtained from various body sites, such as the female reproductive tract, the lung, or any body cavity shedding cells. Using special techniques, slides are first prepared from these specimens. Cytotechnologists then examine the slides microscopically, mark cellular changes that are most representative of a disease process, and submit to a pathologist for final evaluation. Using the findings of cytotechnologists, the pathologist is then able, in many instances, to diagnose cancer and other diseases long before they can be detected by other methods. In recent years, fine needles have been used to aspirate lesions, often deeply seated in the body, thus greatly enhancing the ability to diagnose tumors located in otherwise inaccessible sites.

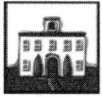

Employment Characteristics

Most cytotechnologists work in hospitals or in commercial laboratories. With experience, cytotechnologists may also work in private industry or in supervisory, research, and teaching capacities.

Salary

Employment opportunities and salaries vary depending on geographic location, experience, and ability. According to the ASCT, the average hourly pay for cytotechnologists was $30.35 in 2006. Refer to Section IV, Table 5 of this *Directory* for more information, or see www.ama-assn.org/go/hpsalary.

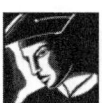

Educational Programs

Length. The length of the program depends significantly on its organizational structure. In general, after completion of the prerequisite course work, at least one calendar year of structured professional instruction in cytotechnology is necessary to achieve program objectives and to establish entry-level competencies.

Prerequisites. Applicants should be well grounded in the biological sciences and in basic chemistry. This entails that students have a minimum of 28 semester hours of biological sciences and chemistry upon completion of a cytotechnology program, and 3 semester hours of mathematics and/or statistics. In addition, applicants are also required to have a baccalaureate degree in order to qualify for the national certification exam.

Curriculum. The curriculum includes the principles of cytopreparation of cell samples, cytologic evaluation of cell samples from all body sites, introduction to principles of management, research, and education as they apply to the cytology laboratory, and cytology as applied in clinical medicine. Also, as molecular diagnostics becomes increasingly important in the field of pathology, programs are incorporating instruction in immunohistochemistry, cytogenetics, in situ hybridization, polymerase chain reaction, and flow cytometry. Upon completion of a cytotechnology program, graduates will possess the technical skills to evaluate a wide variety of cytologic preparations and have a basic knowledge of contemporary procedures and technologies used in cytopathology.

Inquiries

Careers/Curriculum
American Society of Cytopathology
400 West 9th Street, Suite 201
Wilmington, DE 19801
302 429-8802
302 429-8807 Fax
E-mail: asc@cytopathology.org

Certification/Registration
ASCP Board of Registry
PO Box 12270
Chicago, IL 60612
312 738-1336
E-mail: bor@ascp.org

Program Accreditation
Commission on Accreditation of Allied Health Education Programs (CAAHEP) in collaboration with:
Cytotechnology Programs Review Committee
American Society of Cytopathology
400 West 9th Street, Suite 201
Wilmington, DE 19801
302 429-8802
302 429-8807 Fax
E-mail: dmacintyre@cytopathology.org

eriate# Cytotechnologist

eriate## Cytotechnologist

Alabama

University of Alabama at Birmingham
Cytotechnology Prgm
Sch of Hlth Related Professions
UAB Station-RMSB 440
Birmingham, AL 35294-1212
www.uab.edu/ct
Prgm Dir: Vivian Pijuan-Thompson, PhD
Tel: 205 934-4863   *Fax:* 205 975-7302
E-mail: pijuan@uab.edu

Auburn University Montgomery
Cytotechnology Prgm
204B Moore Hall
PO Box 244023
Montgomery, AL 36124-4023
Prgm Dir: Sonya Griffin, MS SCT(ASCP) CT(IAC)
Tel: 334 244-3480   *Fax:* 334 244-3146
E-mail: sgriffi2@mail.aum.edu

Arkansas

University of Arkansas for Medical Sciences
Cytotechnology Prgm
College of Health Related Professions
4301 W Markham St, # 517
Little Rock, AR 72205-9985
www.uams.edu/chrp/cytotechnology/
Prgm Dir: Donald Simpson, PhD MPH CT(ASCP)CM
Tel: 501 686-8448   *Fax:* 501 686-8519
E-mail: simpsondonald@uams.edu

California

Loma Linda University
Cytotechnology Prgm
Dept of Clinical Laboratory Science
Anderson/Barton Rd
Loma Linda, CA 92350
www.llu.edu/llu/sahp
Prgm Dir: Marlene Ota, BS SCT(ASCP)
Tel: 909 558-4000, Ext 45386   *Fax:* 909 558-0458
E-mail: mota@sahp.llu.edu

Greater LA Cytotechnology Training Consortium
Cytotechnology Prgm
Department of Pathology
UCLA Medical Center, A3-231S
Los Angeles, CA 90095-1732
Prgm Dir: Mary Levin, SCT(ASCP)
Tel: 310 794-7135   *Fax:* 310 206-8108
E-mail: mlevin@mednet.ucla.edu

Connecticut

University of Connecticut Health Center
Cytotechnology Prgm
263 Farmington Ave
Department of Pathology MC-3985
Farmington, CT 06030
Prgm Dir: Nancy J Smith, MS SCT(ASCP)
Tel: 860 679-4215   *Fax:* 860 679-4334
E-mail: nsmith@nso1.uchc.edu
Notes: Affiliated with the University of Pittsburgh at Bradford, allowing graduate certified radiographers to transfer 50 credits toward a BS in Radiological Science

Indiana

Indiana University
Cytotechnology Prgm
Clarian Pathology Laboratory
350 West 11th St, Rm 6002J
Indianapolis, IN 46202
www.pathology.iupui.edu
Prgm Dir: William N Crabtree, PhD SCT(ASCP)
Tel: 317 491-6221   *Fax:* 317 491-6212
E-mail: wcrabtre@iupui.edu

Iowa

Mercy Medical Center
Cytotechnology Prgm
1111 6th Ave
Des Moines, IA 50314
www.mercydesmoines.org
Prgm Dir: Marty Boesenberg, BS SCT(ASCP)
Tel: 515 247-4466   *Fax:* 515 643-8810
E-mail: mboesenberg@mercydesmoines.org

Kansas

University of Kansas Medical Center
Cytotechnology Prgm
Mail Stop 4048
3901 Rainbow Blvd
Kansas City, KS 66160-7281
www.alliedhealth.kumc.edu/programs/cytotech.htm
Prgm Dir: Marilee Means, PhD SCT(ASCP)
Tel: 913 588-1179   *Fax:* 913 588-1160
E-mail: mmeans@kumc.edu

Louisiana

Nicholls State University
Cytotechnology Prgm
Dept of Allied Health Sciences
235 Civic Center Blvd
Houma, LA 70360
www.nicholls.edu
Prgm Dir: Celdrick Course, MS CT(ASCP)
Tel: 985 876-8850   *Fax:* 985 876-8856
E-mail: celdrick.course@nicholls.edu

Maryland

Johns Hopkins Hospital
Cytotechnology Prgm
600 N Wolfe St/406 Pathology Bldg
Baltimore, MD 21287-6940
www.pathology2.jhu.edu/cytopathology
Prgm Dir: Frances H Burroughs, SCT(ASCP)
Tel: 410 955-1180   *Fax:* 410 614-9556
E-mail: fburroug@jhmi.edu

Massachusetts

Berkshire Medical Center
Cytotechnology Prgm
725 North St
Pittsfield, MA 01201-4124
www.berkshirehealthsystems.org
Prgm Dir: Judith R Shaffer, SCT(ASCP) BS
Tel: 413 447-2590   *Fax:* 413 447-2097
E-mail: jshaffer@bhs1.org

Michigan

DMC University Laboratories
Cytotechnology Prgm
4707 St Antoine Blvd
Detroit, MI 48201
www.dmc.org/univlab
Prgm Dir: Mujtaba Husain, MD
Tel: 313 745-0831   *Fax:* 313 745-7158
E-mail: mhusain@dmc.org

Minnesota

Mayo School of Health Sciences
Cytotechnology Prgm
200 First St SW
Rochester, MN 55905
www.mayo.edu/education
Prgm Dir: Jill L Caudill, MEd SCT(ASCP)
Tel: 507 284-1142   *Fax:* 507 266-1578
E-mail: caudill.jill@mayo.edu

Mississippi

University of Mississippi Medical Center
Cytotechnology Prgm
Department of Diagnostic and Clinical Health Sciences
2500 N State St
Jackson, MS 39216
http://shrp.edu/programs/cyto.html
Prgm Dir: Zelma Cason, MS SCT(ASCP)
Tel: 601 984-6358   *Fax:* 601 815-1717
E-mail: zcason@shrp.umsmed.edu

Missouri

Barnes-Jewish Coll of Nursing/Allied Health
Cytotechnology Prgm
306 S Kingshighway Blvd
MS: 90-30-625
St Louis, MO 63110
www.barnesjewishcollege.edu
Prgm Dir: Linda Hoechst, MA SCT(ASCP)(IAC)
Tel: 314 454-8655   *Fax:* 314 454-5239
E-mail: lhoechst@bjc.org

Nebraska

University of Nebraska Medical Center
Cytotechnology Prgm
987549 Nebraska Medical Center
Omaha, NE 68198-7549
Prgm Dir: Amber Donnelly, SCT(ASCP)
Tel: 402 552-2043   *Fax:* 402 559-9044
E-mail: addonnelly@unmc.edu

Nevada

Quest Diagnostics - Las Vegas
Cytotechnology Prgm
4230 S Burnham Ave, Ste 250
Las Vegas, NV 89119
Prgm Dir: Robert Gay, CT(ASCP)
Tel: 702 733-7866, Ext 3200   *Fax:* 702 733-8941
E-mail: robert.w.gay@questdiagnostics.com

New Jersey

Univ of Medicine & Dent of New Jersey
Cytotechnology Prgm
School of Health Related Professions
1776 Raritan Rd
Scotch Plains, NJ 07076-2997
www.shrp.umdnj.edu/programs
Prgm Dir: Cecilia B Vallejo, MD
Tel: 908 889-2424   *Fax:* 908 889-2487
E-mail: vallejcb@umdnj.edu

New York

Albany College of Pharmacy
Cytotechnology Prgm
106 New Scotland Ave
Albany, NY 12208-3492
www.acp.edu
Prgm Dir: Indra Balachandran, PhD SCT(ASCP) CFIAC
Tel: 518 694-7390   *Fax:* 518 694-7063
E-mail: balachai@acp.edu

Memorial Sloan-Kettering Cancer Ctr
Cytotechnology Prgm
1275 York Ave C596
New York, NY 10065
www.mskcc.org/mskcc/html
Prgm Dir: Rose Marie Gatscha, SCT(ASCP)
Tel: 212 639-5902   *Fax:* 212 639-6318
E-mail: gatschar@mskcc.org

Stony Brook University
Cytotechnology Prgm
Sch of Health Tech and Management
HSC L-2, Rm 121A
Stony Brook, NY 11794-8207
www.hsc.stonybrook.edu/shtm/cyto/
Prgm Dir: Catherine M Murphy, MS SCT(ASCP) MT
Tel: 631 444-3180   *Fax:* 631 444-8821
E-mail: cvetter@notes.cc.sunysb.edu

SUNY Upstate Medical University
Cytotechnology Prgm
750 E Adams St, Silverman Hall
Syracuse, NY 13210
www.upstate.edu/chp/cyto
Prgm Dir: Susan B Stowell, MA SCT(ASCP)
Tel: 315 464-6900   *Fax:* 315 464-6914
E-mail: stowells@upstate.edu

St John's Riverside Hospital
Cytotechnology Prgm
967 N Broadway
Yonkers, NY 10701
Prgm Dir: Myron K Melamed, MD
Tel: 914 345-9395   *Fax:* 914 594-4163
E-mail: mikemelamed@verizon.net
Notes: Currently inactive

North Carolina

University of North Carolina - Chapel Hill
Cytotechnology Prgm
Department of Allied Health Sciences
CB 7135, Bondurant Hall
Chapel Hill, NC 27599-7135
www.med.unc.edu/ahs/cytotech/
Prgm Dir: Allen C Rinas, MS SCT(ASCP) CM(IAC)
Tel: 919 843-1065   *Fax:* 919 966-8384
E-mail: arinas@med.unc.edu

Central Piedmont Community College
Cytotechnology Prgm
PO Box 35009
Charlotte, NC 28235
http://www1.cpcc.edu/health_sciences/cytotechnology
Prgm Dir: M Arlene Parrish, MS SCT(ASCP) IAC
Tel: 704 330-6383   *Fax:* 704 330-6151
E-mail: arlene.parrish@cpcc.edu

North Dakota

University of North Dakota
Cytotechnology Prgm
School of Medicine and Health Sciences, Rm 3124
501 N Columbia Rd, Stop 9037
Grand Forks, ND 58202
Prgm Dir: Kathy Hoffman, MM SCT(ASCP)
Tel: 701 777-4466   *Fax:* 701 777-2404
E-mail: khoffman@medicine.nodak.edu

Ohio

Akron General Medical Center
Cytotechnology Prgm
400 Wabash Ave
Akron, OH 44307
Prgm Dir: Angela T Powell, MD
Tel: 330 344-6203   *Fax:* 330 344-6418
E-mail: jjohnson@agmc.org

Pennsylvania

Thomas Jefferson University
Cytotechnology Prgm
Jefferson Coll of Hlth Prof, Dept of Bioscience Tech
Edison Bldg, Ste 1924, 130 S Ninth St, Rm 1924
Philadelphia, PA 19107-5233
www.jefferson.edu/jchp/ls/
Prgm Dir: Shirley E Greening, MS JD CT(ASCP) CFIAC
Tel: 215 503-7844   *Fax:* 215 503-2189
E-mail: shirley.greening@jefferson.edu

Univ Health Center of Pittsburgh
Cytotechnology Prgm
Anisa I Kanbour Schol of Cytopathology
300 Halket St
Pittsburgh, PA 15213-3180
Prgm Dir: Anisa I Kanbour, MD
Tel: 412 641-4664   *Fax:* 412 641-6263
E-mail: akanbour@magee.edu

Puerto Rico

University of Puerto Rico
Cytotechnology Prgm
College of Allied Health Professions
PO Box 365067 Ofc 701
San Juan, PR 00936-5067
Prgm Dir: Alma J Camacho, CT (ASCP ASC) MBA
Tel: 787 758-2525, Ext 4604   *Fax:* 787 759-5095
E-mail: almacamacho@cprs.rcm.upr.edu

Rhode Island

University of Rhode Island
Cytotechnology Prgm
Office of Special Programs
80 Washington St
Providence, RI 02903
www.risschoolofcytotechnology.com
Prgm Dir: Barbara G Klitz, MSCT(ASCP)
Tel: 401 874-5210   *Fax:* 401 277-5060
E-mail: bgk@etal.uri.edu

South Carolina

Medical University of South Carolina
Cytotechnology Prgm
Health Prof, Department of Clinical Services
151B Rutledge Ave, Rm B102
Charleston, SC 29425
www.musc.edu/chp/cb
Prgm Dir: Karen B Geils, MS CT(ASCP) HT(ASCP)
Tel: 843 792-1913   *Fax:* 843 792-0506
E-mail: brinkerk@musc.edu

Tennessee

University of Tennessee Health Science Ctr
Cytotechnology Prgm
Coll of Allied Health Sciences
930 Madison Ave, Ste 674
Memphis, TN 38163
www.utmen.edu/allied/cytotechnology_home.html
Prgm Dir: Barbara Benstein, PhD SCT(ASCP)
Tel: 901 448-6304   *Fax:* 901 448-7545
E-mail: bbenstein@utmem.edu

Texas

Brooke Army Medical Center
Cytotechnology Prgm
Interservice Cytotechnology Program
Dept of Pathology and Area Laboratory Services
Fort Sam Houston, TX 78234-6200
Prgm Dir: HMC Jorge A Franco, MA Ed SCT(ASCP)IAC
Tel: 210 916-0499   *Fax:* 210 916-0877
E-mail: jorge.franco@cen.amedd.army.mil

Univ of Texas M D Anderson Cancer Ctr
Cytotechnology Prgm
School of Health Sciences
1515 Holcombe Blvd, Unit 206
Houston, TX 77030-4009
www.mdanderson.org/healthsciences
Prgm Dir: Christina M Alapat, MS SCT MP(ASCP) IAC
Tel: 713 794-5877   *Fax:* 713 745-0172
E-mail: calapat@mdanderson.org

Utah

University of Utah Health Science Center
Cytotechnology Prgm
ARUP Laboratory
500 Chipeta Way
Salt Lake City, UT 84108
www.path.utah.edu/MLS
Prgm Dir: Michael C Berry, SCT(ASCP)
Tel: 801 583-2787, Ext 2327   *Fax:* 801 584-5213
E-mail: berrymc@aruplab.com

Vermont

Fletcher Allen Health Care
Cytotechnology Prgm
111 Colchester Ave
Burlington, VT 05401
https://www.fahc.org/cytoschool
Prgm Dir: Sandra Giroux, MS SCT(ASCP) CFIAC
Tel: 802 847-5133   *Fax:* 802 847-3632
E-mail: Sandra.Giroux@vtmednet.org

Virginia

Old Dominion University
Cytotechnology Prgm
209 Spong Hall
Norfolk, VA 23529
Prgm Dir: Sophie K Thompson, MHS CT(ASCP)
Tel: 757 683-3016   *Fax:* 757 683-5028
E-mail: sxthomps@odu.edu

West Virginia

CAMC Health Education & Research Institute
Cytotechnology Prgm
3200 MacCorkle Ave SE
Charleston, WV 25304
www.cytologyschool.com
Prgm Dir: Carolyn H Stevens, CT(ASCP)
Tel: 304 388-5570   *Fax:* 304 388-9833
E-mail: carolyn.stevens@camc.org
Notes: Currently inactive

Cabell Huntington Hospital
Cytotechnology Prgm
1340 Hal Greer Blvd
Huntington, WV 25701
www.cabellhuntington.org
Prgm Dir: Margene Smith, SCT(ASCP)
Tel: 304 526-2155   *Fax:* 304 399-6877
E-mail: mjsmith@chhi.org

Wisconsin

State Laboratory of Hygiene
Cytotechnology Prgm
465 Henry Mall
Madison, WI 53706
www.slh.wisc.edu
Prgm Dir: John E Shalkham, MA SCT(ASCP)
Tel: 608 265-9191 *Fax:* 608 265-6294
E-mail: shalkham@wisc.edu

Marshfield Clinic
Cosponsor: St. Jospeph's Hospital
Cytotechnology Prgm
1000 N Oak Ave
Marshfield, WI 54449-5795
www.marshfieldlaboratories.org
Prgm Dir: Donald Schnitzler, BS CT(ASCP)
Tel: 715 387-7440 *Fax:* 715 389-5353
E-mail: schnitzler.donald@marshfieldclinic.org

University of Wisconsin - Milwaukee
Cytotechnology Prgm
College of Health Sciences
PO Box 413
Milwaukee, WI 53201
www.uwm.edu
Prgm Dir: Evelyn Dell, BS CT HT(ASCP)
Tel: 414 328-7914 *Fax:* 414 328-8505
E-mail: evelyn.dell@aurora.org

Cytotechnologist

Programs*	Class Capacity	Begins	Length (months)	Award	Res. Tuition	Non-res. Tuition	Stipend	Offers:‡ 1	2	3	4
Alabama											
University of Alabama at Birmingham	12	Aug	12	Cert, BS	$8,320	$20,800					
Arkansas											
University of Arkansas for Medical Sciences (Little Rock)	8	Aug	12	BS	$6,925	$15,165				•	
California											
Loma Linda University	12	Aug	12, 18	Cert, BS	$23,000	$23,000					
Indiana											
Indiana University (Indianapolis)	8	Aug	12	BS	$7,671	$22,538				•	
Iowa											
Mercy Medical Center (Des Moines)	4	Jul	12	Cert	$3,500	$3,500					
Kansas											
University of Kansas Medical Center (Kansas City)	4	Aug	12	BS	$7,166	$30,527					
Louisiana											
Nicholls State University (Houma)	6	May	12	BS	$4,253	$12,425					•
Maryland											
Johns Hopkins Hospital (Baltimore)	5	Aug	12	Cert	$8,650	$8,650				•	
Massachusetts											
Berkshire Medical Center (Pittsfield)	4	Sep	12	Cert, BS	$3,500	$3,500	$175				
Michigan											
DMC University Laboratories (Detroit)	5	Aug	12	Cert							
Minnesota											
Mayo School of Health Sciences (Rochester)	6	Jul	12	Cert	$3,500	$3,500				•	
Mississippi											
University of Mississippi Medical Center (Jackson)	12	Aug	18	BS	$2,301	$5,283					
Missouri											
Barnes-Jewish Coll of Nursing/Allied Health (St Louis)	12	Jun	12	Cert, BSCT	$15,200	$15,200				•	
New Jersey											
Univ of Medicine & Dent of New Jersey (Scotch Plains)	10	Late Aug	12	Cert, BSCLS, BSCLS	$9,590	$14,385					
New York											
Albany College of Pharmacy	14	Aug	12	Dipl, Cert, CT, BS	$12,550	$12,550					
Memorial Sloan-Kettering Cancer Ctr (New York)	6	Aug	12	Cert, CT	$8,000	$8,000					
Stony Brook University	6	Jul	24	BS	$4,358	$9,258					
SUNY Upstate Medical University (Syracuse)	11	Aug	12	BS	$6,526	$15,450					
North Carolina											
Central Piedmont Community College (Charlotte)	5	Aug	12	Cert	$1,896	$10,536					
University of North Carolina - Chapel Hill	5	May	12	Cert	$8,084	$17,748					•
Pennsylvania											
Thomas Jefferson University (Philadelphia)	24	Sep	12, 22	BS, MS	$29,750	$29,750		•		•	
Rhode Island											
University of Rhode Island (Providence)	8	Sep	11	Cert, CT, MS	$15,000	$15,000					
South Carolina											
Medical University of South Carolina (Charleston)	12	Aug	21	MS	$14,316	$29,445					
Tennessee											
University of Tennessee Health Science Ctr (Memphis)	6	Sep	21	MS	$7,960	$19,960					
Texas											
Univ of Texas M D Anderson Cancer Ctr (Houston)	6	Aug 27	12	Cert, BS	$3,240	$15,530				•	
Utah											
University of Utah Health Science Center (Salt Lake City)	4	Jun	12	Cert, BS	$6,900	$17,700					

*Data are shown only for programs that completed the 2007 AMA Survey of Health Professions Education Programs.
‡Key to Offers: 1: Evening or weekend classes; 2: Non-English instruction; 3: Cultural competence instruction; 4: Distance education component.

Cytotechnologist

Programs*	Class Capacity	Begins	Length (months)	Award	Res. Tuition	Non-res. Tuition	Stipend	Offers:‡ 1	2	3	4
Vermont											
Fletcher Allen Health Care (Burlington)	7	Sep	12	Cert, BS	$7,000	$7,000					
West Virginia											
Cabell Huntington Hospital	4	May	12	Cert, BS	$5,000	$5,000					
CAMC Health Education & Research Institute (Charleston)	6	Jun	12	Cert	$5,000	$5,000					
Wisconsin											
Marshfield Clinic	4	Jul	12	Cert	$850	$850					
State Laboratory of Hygiene (Madison)	12	Aug	12	Cert, BS	$5,500	$5,500					
University of Wisconsin - Milwaukee	6	Sep	12	BS	$8,700	$21,105					

*Data are shown only for programs that completed the 2007 AMA Survey of Health Professions Education Programs.
‡Key to Offers: 1: Evening or weekend classes; 2: Non-English instruction; 3: Cultural competence instruction; 4: Distance education component.

PROGRAMS

Emerging as a distinct profession in the 1940s, dance/movement therapy, a creative arts therapy, is rooted in the expressive nature of dance itself. Dance is the most fundamental of the arts, involving a direct expression and experience of oneself through the body. It is a basic form of authentic communication, and as such it is an especially effective medium for therapy. Based in the belief that the body, the mind, and the spirit are interconnected, dance/movement therapy is defined by the American Dance Therapy Association (ADTA) as "the psychotherapeutic use of movement as a process that furthers the emotional, cognitive, social, and physical integration of the individual."

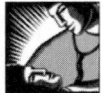

Career Description

Dance/movement therapists work with individuals of all ages, groups, and families in a wide variety of settings. They focus on helping their clients improve self-esteem and body image, develop effective communication skills and relationships, expand their movement vocabulary, and gain insight into patterns of behavior, as well as create new options for coping with problems. Dance/movement therapy can be a powerful tool for stress management and the prevention of physical and mental health problems. Movement is the primary medium that dance/movement therapists use for observation, assessment, research, therapeutic interaction, and interventions.

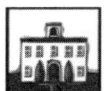

Employment Characteristics

Dance/movement therapists work in settings that include psychiatric and rehabilitation facilities, schools, nursing homes, drug treatment centers, counseling centers, medical facilities, crisis centers, and wellness and alternative health care centers. Dance/movement therapy is used with people of all ages, races, and ethnic backgrounds in individual, couples, family, and group therapy formats.

There are approximately 1,300 dance/movement therapists in 46 states and 41 foreign countries.

Educational Programs

Length. Professional training for US dance/movement therapists is on the graduate level. Graduates receive a master's degree in dance/movement therapy or related degree title. Graduates from an ADTA-approved dance/movement therapy program are eligible for the DTR (Dance Therapist Registered) credential upon completion of graduate studies. Approved programs have met the basic educational standards of the ADTA, which include that the program's parent institution is accredited by its regional accreditation association.

Prerequisites. Extensive dance experience and a liberal arts background with coursework in psychology are required. For specific prerequisites, contact each graduate program.

Registration

The ADTA distinguishes between dance/movement therapists prepared to work in professional settings within a team under supervision and those prepared for the responsibilities of working independently in private practice or providing supervision.

- *DTR: Dance Therapist Registered*—Therapists with this title have a master's degree and are fully qualified to work in a professional treatment system.
- *ADTR: Academy of Dance Therapists Registered*—Therapists with this title have met additional requirements and are fully qualified to teach, provide supervision, and engage in private practice.

Inquiries

American Dance Therapy Association
2000 Century Plaza, Suite 108
10632 Little Patuxent Parkway
Columbia, MD 21044-3263
412 624-6595
www.adta.org

Dance/Movement Therapist

Colorado

Naropa University
Dance/Movement Therapy Prgm
2130 Arapahoe Ave
Boulder, CO 80302
Prgm Dir: Z"e Avstreih, MA LPC ADTR
Tel: 303 245-4845   *Fax:* 303 245-4827
E-mail: zoe@naropa.edu

Illinois

Columbia College
Dance/Movement Therapy Prgm
600 S Michigan Ave
Chicago, IL 60605-9988
www.colum.graddance.edu
Prgm Dir: Susan Imus, MA ADTR LCPC GLCMA
Tel: 312 344-7097   *Fax:* 312 344-8054
E-mail: simus@colum.edu

Massachusetts

Lesley University
Dance/Movement Therapy Prgm
29 Everett St
Cambridge, MA 02138
Prgm Dir: Robyn Flaum Cruz, PhD ADTR NCC LPC
Tel: 617 349-8440   *Fax:* 617 349-8431
E-mail: rcruz@lesley.edu

New Hampshire

Antioch University New England
Dance/Movement Therapy Prgm
40 Avon St
Keene, NH 03431-3552
www.antiochne.edu/academics/appsy/dmt.html
Prgm Dir: Susan Loman, MA ADTR NCC
Tel: 603 283-2137, Ext 222   *Fax:* 603 357-0718
E-mail: sloman@antiochne.edu

New York

Pratt Institute
Dance/Movement Therapy Prgm
East 3, 200 Willoughby Ave
Brooklyn, NY 11205
Prgm Dir: Joan Wittig, MS LCAT ADTR
Tel: 718 636-3428
E-mail: jwittig@pratt.edu

Pennsylvania

Drexel University
Dance/Movement Therapy Prgm
Hahnemann Creative Arts in Therapy Program
1505 Race St
Philadelphia, PA 19102-1192
Prgm Dir: Ellen Schelly Hill, MMT ADTR NCC LPC
Tel: 215 762-7851   *Fax:* 215 762-6933
E-mail: es42@drexel.edu

Dance/Movement Therapist

	Class Capacity	Begins	Length (months)	Award	Res. Tuition	Non-res. Tuition	Stipend	Offers:‡ 1	2	3	4
Illinois											
Columbia College (Chicago)	28	Fall	30, 14	Dipl, Cert, MA, GLCMA	$16,000	$16,000				•	
New Hampshire											
Antioch University New England (Keene)	20	Fall semester	30	Cert, MA	$0	$18,750		•		•	
Pennsylvania											
Drexel University (Philadelphia)	40	Sep	21	Cert, MA	$17,960	$17,960				•	

*Data are shown only for programs that completed the 2007 AMA Survey of Health Professions Education Programs.
‡Key to Offers: 1: Evening or weekend classes; 2: Non-English instruction; 3: Cultural competence instruction; 4: Distance education component.

Career Description

Dentists diagnose, prevent, and treat problems with teeth or mouth tissue. They remove decay, fill cavities, examine x rays, place protective plastic sealants on children's teeth, straighten teeth, and repair fractured teeth. They also perform corrective surgery on gums and supporting bones to treat gum diseases. Dentists extract teeth and make models and measurements for dentures to replace missing teeth. They provide instruction on diet, brushing, flossing, the use of fluorides, and other aspects of dental care. They also administer anesthetics and write prescriptions for antibiotics and other medications.

Dentists use a variety of equipment, including x-ray machines; drills; and instruments such as mouth mirrors, probes, forceps, brushes, and scalpels. They wear masks, gloves, and safety glasses to protect themselves and their patients from infectious diseases.

Dentists in private practice oversee a variety of administrative tasks, including bookkeeping and buying equipment and supplies. They may employ and supervise dental hygienists, dental assistants, dental laboratory technicians, and receptionists.

More than 80% of dentists are general practitioners, handling a variety of dental needs. Other dentists practice in any of nine specialty areas.

- *Orthodontists*, the largest group of specialists, straighten teeth by applying pressure to the teeth with braces or retainers.
- *Oral and maxillofacial surgeons*, the next largest group, operate on the mouth and jaws.
- *Pediatric dentists* focus on dentistry for children
- *Periodontists* treat gums and bone supporting the teeth
- *Prosthodontists* replace missing teeth with permanent fixtures, such as crowns and bridges, or with removable fixtures such as dentures
- *Endodontists* perform root canal therapy
- *Public health dentists* promote good dental health and prevention of dental diseases within the community
- *Oral pathologists* study oral diseases
- *Oral and maxillofacial radiologists* diagnose diseases in the head and neck through the use of imaging technologies

Teaching, dental research and dental industry comprise additional rewarding career options for both general practitioners and dental specialists. Dentists also work in public health agencies, hospitals, the military and other settings.

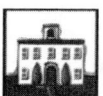

Employment Characteristics

Most dentists work 4 or 5 days a week. Some work evenings and weekends to meet their patients' needs.

Most full-time dentists work between 35 and 40 hours a week, but others work more. Initially, dentists may work more hours as they establish their practice. Experienced dentists often work fewer hours. Many continue in part-time practice well beyond the usual retirement age.

Most dentists are solo practitioners, meaning that they own their own businesses and work alone or with a small staff. Some dentists have partners, and a few work for other dentists as associate dentists.

Salary

In 2004, the average earnings for a general practitioner who owns his/her practice was over $185,940; the average earnings for a dental specialist was over $315,000. Dentists' average income places them in the highest 5% of US family income.

For more information, see www.ama-assn.org/go/hpsalary.

Employment Outlook

Employment of dentists is projected to grow about as fast as average for all occupations through 2014.

Although employment growth will provide some job opportunities, most jobs will result from the need to replace the large number of dentists expected to retire. Job prospects should be good as new dentists take over established practices or start their own.

Demand for dental care should grow substantially in the future. As members of the baby-boom generation advance into middle age, a large number will need complicated dental work, such as bridges. In addition, elderly people are more likely to retain their teeth than were their predecessors, so they will require much more care than in the past. The younger generation will continue to need preventive checkups despite treatments such as fluoridation of the water supply, which decreases the incidence of tooth decay. Employment of dentists, however, is not expected to grow as rapidly as the demand for dental services. As their practices expand, dentists are likely to hire more dental hygienists and dental assistants to handle routine services.

Dentists will increasingly provide care and instruction aimed at preventing the loss of teeth, rather than simply providing treatments such as fillings. Improvements in dental technology also will allow dentists to offer more effective and less painful treatment to their patients. For example, National Institute of Dental and Craniofacial Research (NIDCR) clinical and basic research that may revolutionize the practice of dentistry includes:

- Postnatal stem cell research aimed at tissue regeneration
- Salivary research, which is expected to yield new diagnostic tests
- Gene transfer therapy that may induce the salivary glands to produce hormones, antibodies, or other agents to prevent or treat oral and systemic disease
- Stem cells, possibly derived from the patient's own deciduous teeth, used to repair bone defects
- Small "labs-on-a-chip" placed intraorally to analyze hundreds of different components in oral fluids as early indicators of oral and systemic disease
- Restorative procedures and new dental materials to retain teeth

Need for Minority Dentists

There is a critical need in many underserved communities where minority and disadvantaged people are not getting the dental care they need. Only 12% of students entering dental school are minorities, while minorities make up 25% of the general population. Recent data shows that minority dentists treat a very high number of minority patients.

More underrepresented minority dentists (African American, Hispanic and American Indian) are necessary to eliminate the barriers to oral care. This need is expected to increase, in light of US

PROGRAMS

Census projections that minority populations will make up more than 50% of the US population by 2050.

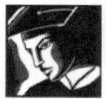

Educational Programs

Award, Length. Dental schools award the degree of Doctor of Dental Surgery (DDS) or Doctor of Dental Medicine (DMD); programs are 4 years.

Prerequisites. Those interested in a career in dentistry are encouraged to obtain broad exposure to science and math while in high school and to enroll in college preparatory classes in biology, algebra, and chemistry. In addition, it is recommended to continue taking natural science courses in college such as general biology, organic and inorganic chemistry, and physics. Majoring in science is not a must, but completion of pre-dental science requirements is necessary. A college undergraduate degree is recommended in preparation for dental school. Most dental students have completed four years of college.

Other good ways to learn more about the field and prepare for a career in dentistry:

- Ask to volunteer or job shadow at your family dentist's office, orthodontist's office and pediatric dentist's office
- Talk with admission officers about financial aid resources and dental school requirements
- Join the American Student Dental Association (ASDA)
- Take the Dental Admissions Test (DAT) a year before entering dental school

Curriculum. The four years of study leading to the DDS or DMD degree are divided into two components. Years 1 and 2 encompass:

- Classroom and laboratory instruction in basic health sciences (including anatomy, biochemistry, histology, microbiology, pharmacology, and physiology), with an emphasis on dental aspects
- Basic principles of oral diagnosis and treatment; students may practice on manikins and models, and may begin treating patients later in the second year

Years 3 and 4 cover the following:

- Treatment of patients under the supervision of licensed dental faculty. Procedures cover the broad scope of general dentistry

and include opportunities to work in a variety of settings, eg, community clinics, hospitals, and outpatient clinics
- Practice management courses, including instruction in effective communication skills, the use of allied dental personnel, and business management

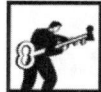

Licensure, Certification, Registration

All states require dentists to be licensed to practice. In most states, a candidate must graduate from a US dental school accredited by the ADA Commission on Dental Accreditation and pass written and practical examinations to qualify for licensure. In 2004, 17 states licensed or certified dentists who intended to practice in a specialty area. Requirements include 2 to 4 years of postgraduate education and, in some cases, the completion of a special state examination.

Inquiries

Education, Careers, Resources

American Dental Association
211 East Chicago Avenue
Chicago, IL 60611-2678
312 440-2500
www.ada.org

Program Accreditation

American Dental Association
Commission on Dental Accreditation (CODA)
211 East Chicago Avenue
Chicago, IL 60611-2678
312 440-2500
www.ada.org/prof/ed/accred/commission

Note: Adapted in part from the Bureau of Labor Statistics, U.S. Department of Labor, *Occupational Outlook Handbook*, 2006-07 Edition, Dentists, on the Internet at www.bls.gov/oco/ocos072.htm (visited August 24, 2007).

Dentist

Alabama

University of Alabama
Dentistry Prgm
School of Dentistry at UAB
1530 3rd Ave S
Birmingham, AL 35294
www.dental.uab.edu

Arizona

AT Still University of Health Sciences
Dentistry Prgm
Arizona School of Dentistry and Oral Health
5850 E Still Circle
Mesa, AZ 85206
www.atsu.edu/asdoh
Tel: 480 219-6000

California

Loma Linda University
Dentistry Prgm
School of Dentistry
Loma Linda, CA 92350

University of California - Los Angeles
Dentistry Prgm
School of Dentistry
Center for Health Science
Los Angeles, CA 90095
www.dent.ucla.edu

University of Southern California
Dentistry Prgm
School of Dentistry
925 W 34th St
Los Angeles, CA 90089
www.usc.edu/hsc/dental

University of California - San Francisco
Dentistry Prgm
School of Dentistry
513 Parnassus Ave
San Francisco, CA 94143
www.ucsf.edu

University of the Pacific
Dentistry Prgm
Arthur A Dugoni School of Dentistry
2155 Webster St
San Francisco, CA 94115
www.dental.pacific.edu
Tel: 415 929-6425

Colorado

U of Colorado (Denver) Health Sciences Center
Dentistry Prgm
School of Dentistry, Lazzara Center for Oral-Facial health
13065 E 17th Ave
Aurora, CO 80045
www.unmc.edu/dentistry
Tel: 303 724-7100

Connecticut

University of Connecticut
Dentistry Prgm
School of Dental Medicine
263 Farmington Ave
Farmington, CT 06030
http://sdm.uchc.edu

District of Columbia

Howard University
Dentistry Prgm
College of Dentistry
600 W Street, NW
Washington, DC 20059
www.howard.edu

Florida

Nova Southeastern University
Dentistry Prgm
College of Dental Medicine
3200 S University Dr
Fort Lauderdale, FL 33328
http://dental.nova.edu

University of Florida
Dentistry Prgm
College of Dentistry
1600 SW Archer Rd
Gainesville, FL 32610
http://dental.ufl.edu

Georgia

Medical College of Georgia
Dentistry Prgm
School of Dentistry
1120 15th St
Augusta, GA 30912
www.mcg.edu/SOD

Illinois

Southern Illinois University
Dentistry Prgm
School of Dental Medicine
2800 College Ave
Alton, IL 62002
www.siue.edu/sdm/

University of Illinois at Chicago
Dentistry Prgm
College of Dentistry
801 S Paulina St
Chicago, IL 60612
www.dentistry.uic.edu

Indiana

Indiana University
Dentistry Prgm
School of Dentistry
1121 W Michigan St
Indianapolis, IN 46202
www.iusd.iupui.edu

Iowa

University of Iowa
Dentistry Prgm
College of Dentistry
100 Dental Science Bldg
Iowa City, IA 52242
www.dentistry.uiowa.edu

Kentucky

University of Kentucky
Dentistry Prgm
College of Kentucky
800 Rose St
Lexington, KY 40536
www.mc.uky.edu/Dentistry

University of Louisville
Dentistry Prgm
School of Dentistry
501 S Preston St
Louisville, KY 40292
www.dental.louisville.edu/dental

Louisiana

Louisiana State University
Dentistry Prgm
School of Dentistry
LSU South Campus
Baton Rouge, LA 70820
www.lsusd.lsuhsc.edu

Maryland

University of Maryland
Dentistry Prgm
Baltimore College of Dental Surgery
650 W Baltimore St
Baltimore, MD 21201
www.dental.umaryland.edu

Massachusetts

Boston University
Dentistry Prgm
Goldman School of Dental Medicine
100 East Newton St
Boston, MA 02118
www.dentalshcool.bu.edu

Harvard Medical School
Dentistry Prgm
School of Dental Medicine
188 Longwood Ave
Boston, MA 02115
www.hsdm.med.harvard.edu

Tufts University
Dentistry Prgm
School of Dental Medicine
One Kneeland St
Boston, MA 02111
www.tufts.edu/dental

Michigan

University of Michigan
Dentistry Prgm
School of Dentistry
1011 N University Ave
Ann Arbor, MI 48109
www.dent.umich.edu

University of Detroit Mercy
Dentistry Prgm
School of Dentistry
8200 W Outer Dr
Detroit, MI 48219
www.udmercy.edu/dental

Minnesota

University of Minnesota - Minneapolis
Dentistry Prgm
School of Dentistry
Rm 15-209 Moos Tower
Minneapolis, MN 55455
www.dentistry.umn.edu

Mississippi

University of Mississippi Medical Center
Dentistry Prgm
School of Dentistry
2500 N State St
Jackson, MS 39216

Missouri

University of Missouri - Kansas City
Dentistry Prgm
School of Dentistry
650 E 25th St
Kansas City, MO 64108
www.umkc.edu/dentistry

Nebraska

University of Nebraska Medical Center
Dentistry Prgm
College of Dentistry
40th Holdrege St
Lincoln, NE 68583

Creighton University
Dentistry Prgm
School of Dentistry
2500 California Plaza
Omaha, NE 68178
http://cudental.creighton.edu

Nevada

University of Nevada - Las Vegas
Dentistry Prgm
School of Dental Medicine
Shadow Lane Campus, 1001 Shadow Lane
Las Vegas, NV 89106
http://dentalschool.unlv.edu/

New Jersey

Univ of Medicine & Dent of New Jersey
Dentistry Prgm
110 Bergen St
Rm B815
Newark, NJ 07103
www.umdnj.edu

New York

University at Buffalo - SUNY
Dentistry Prgm
School of Dental Medicine
325 Squire Hall
Buffalo, NY 14214
www.sdm.buffalo.edu

Columbia University
Dentistry Prgm
College of Dental Medicine
630 W 168th St
New York, NY 10032
http://cpmcnet.columbia.edu/dept/dental

New York University
Dentistry Prgm
College of Dentistry
345 East 24th St
New York, NY 10010
www.nyu.edu/dental

SUNY at Stony Brook
Dentistry Prgm
School of Dental Medicine
Health Sciences Center
Stony Brook, NY 11794
www.hsc.stonybrook.edu/dental

North Carolina

University of North Carolina Hospitals
Dentistry Prgm
School of Dentistry
UNC-CH CB#7450
Chapel Hill, NC 27599

Ohio

Case Western Reserve University
Dentistry Prgm
School of Dental Medicine
10900 Euclid Ave
Cleveland, OH 44106
http://dental.case.edu/

Ohio State University
Dentistry Prgm
College of Dentistry
305 W 12th Ave
Columbus, OH 43218
www.dent.ohio-state.edu

Oklahoma

University of Oklahoma Health Sciences Center
Dentistry Prgm
College of Dentistry
1201 N Stonewall Ave
Oklahoma City, OK 73117
http://dentistry.ouhsc.edu

Oregon

Oregon Health & Science University
Dentistry Prgm
School of Dentistry
611 SW Campus Dr
Portland, OR 97239
www.ohsu.edu/sod/admissions

Pennsylvania

Temple University
Dentistry Prgm
The Maurice H Kornberg School of Dentistry
3223 North Broad St
Philadelphia, PA 19140
www.temple.edu/dentistry

Univ of Penn School of Dental Medicine
Dentistry Prgm
240 S 40th St
Robert Shattner Center
Philadelphia, PA 19104
www.dental.upenn.edu

University of Pittsburgh
Dentistry Prgm
School of Dental Medicine
3501 Terrace St
Pittsburgh, PA 15261
www.dental.pitt.edu

Puerto Rico

University of Puerto Rico
Dentistry Prgm
School of Dentistry
Medical Sciences Campus
San Juan, PR 00936
www.dental.rcm.upr.edu/

South Carolina

Medical University of South Carolina
Dentistry Prgm
College of Dental Medicine
171 Ashley Ave
Charleston, SC 29425
www.gradstudies.musc.edu/dentistry/dental.html

Tennessee

University of Tennessee Health Science Ctr
Dentistry Prgm
College of Dentistry
875 Union Ave
Memphis, TN 38163
www.utmem.edu/dentistry

Meharry Medical College
Dentistry Prgm
School of Dentistry
1005 D B Todd Blvd
Nashville, TN 37208
www.dentistry.mmc.edu

Texas

Baylor College of Dentistry, Texas A&M HSC
Dentistry Prgm
3302 Gaston Ave
Dallas, TX 75246

Univ of Texas Hlth Sci Ctr at Houston
Dentistry Prgm
Dental Branch
6516 MD Anderson Blvd
Houston, TX 77225
www.db.uth.tmc.edu

Univ of Texas Hlth Sci Ctr at San Antonio
Dentistry Prgm
Dental School
7703 Floyd Curl Dr
San Antonio, TX 78284
www.dental.uthscsa.edu

Virginia

Virginia Commonwealth Univ/Health System
Dentistry Prgm
School of Dentistry
520 North 12th St
Richmond, VA 23298
www.dentistry.vcu.edu

Washington

University of Washington
Dentistry Prgm
Health Sciences School of Dentistry
D322 Health Sciences Bldg
Seattle, WA 98195
www.dental.washington.edu

West Virginia

West Virginia University
Dentistry Prgm
School of Dentistry
Robert C Byrd Health Science Center
Morgantown, WV 26506
www.hsc.wvu.edu/sod

Wisconsin

Marquette University
Dentistry Prgm
School of Dentistry
1801 W Wisconsin Ave
Milwaukee, WI 53233
www.dental.mu.edu

Includes:
- Dental assistant
- Dental hygienist
- Dental laboratory technician

Dental Assistant

The dental assistant increases the efficiency of the dental care team by aiding the dentist in the delivery of oral health care. The dental assistant performs a wide range of tasks requiring both interpersonal and technical skills. Duties range from aiding and educating patients to preparing and sterilizing dental instruments and performing administrative work.

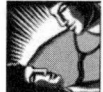

Job Description

Dental assistants are responsible for:
- Helping patients feel comfortable before, during, and after treatment
- Assisting the dentist during treatment
- Exposing and processing dental radiographs (x-rays)
- Recording the patient's medical history and taking blood pressure and pulse
- Preparing and sterilizing instruments and equipment for the dentist's use
- Providing patients with oral care instructions following such procedures as surgery or placement of a restoration (filling)
- Teaching patients proper brushing and flossing techniques
- Making impressions of patients' teeth for study casts
- Performing administrative and scheduling tasks, including using a personal computer, communicating by telephone, and maintaining an inventory supply system.

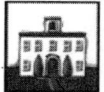

Employment Characteristics

Most of the more than 247,000 active dental assistants are employed by general dentists. In addition, dental specialists employ dental assistants. Most assistants work chairside, although they may also participate in the business aspects of the practice. Besides dental offices, other employment settings available to dental assistants include:
- Schools and clinics (public health dentistry)
- Hospitals (assisting dentists who are treating bedridden patients or in more elaborate dental procedures performed only in hospitals)
- Dental school clinics
- Insurance companies (processing dental insurance claims)
- Vocational schools, technical institutes, community colleges, and universities (teaching others to be dental assistants)

Among independent general practitioners, the average number of employees per dentist has remained relatively stable between 1997 and 1998, averaging 4.2 positions. In 1999, this number has increased to 4.3 positions.

Dental assisting also offers both flexibility and stability. Dental assistants have the flexibility to work full or part time. As of 2001, dental assistants had been working in their current practices for an average of 6.6 years.

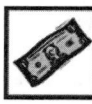

Salary

The salary of a dental assistant varies, depending on the responsibilities associated with the specific position, the individual's training, and the geographic location of employment. The average national wage of a full-time dental assistant employed by a general practitioner in 2004 was $15.48 per hour. Refer to Section IV, Table 5 of this *Directory* for more information, or see www.ama-assn.org/go/hpsalary.

In addition to salary, dental assistants may receive benefit packages from their employers, including health and disability insurance coverage, dues for membership in professional organizations, an allowance for uniforms, profit sharing plans, and paid vacations.

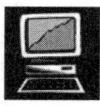

Employment Outlook

Most areas of the country are currently reporting shortages of dental assistants. Owing to the success of preventive dentistry in reducing the incidence of oral disease, senior citizens—a growing population—will retain their teeth longer and will be even more aware of the importance of regular dental care.

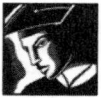

Educational Programs

Length. Nine to 11 months.

Prerequisites. High school diploma or equivalent.

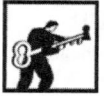

Certification

Dental assistants can become certified by passing the Certified Dental Assistant examination, administered by the Dental Assisting National Board (DANB). Passing this examination qualifies a dental assistant to use the designation Certified Dental Assistant (CDA). Dental assistants are eligible to take this examination if they have completed a dental assisting program accredited by the Commission on Dental Accreditation, or have 2 years full-time work experience, or are a graduate from a dental hygiene or dental program accredited by the Commission on Dental Accreditation. State regulations vary and some states offer registration or licensure in addition to this national certification program.

Miscellaneous Facts

- The 259 dental assisting education programs in the United States accredited by the American Dental Association's Commission on Dental Accreditation enrolled 7,240 students in 2004-2005.
- Women represented 96.4% of students enrolled in dental assisting programs in 2004-2005.
- Minority students represented 23% of enrollees in dental assisting programs in 2004-2005.
- Excellent career opportunities exist for nontraditional dental assisting students, seeking career change or job reentry after a period of unemployment, or from a culturally diverse background. Many dental assisting education programs offer more flexible program designs that meet the needs of nontraditional students by offering a variety of educational options, such as part-time or evening hours.

Dental Hygienist

Dental hygienists provide dental hygiene services as they work with dentists in the delivery of dental care to patients. Hygienists are licensed to use their knowledge and clinical skills to provide dental care to patients and their interpersonal skills to motivate and instruct patients on methods to prevent oral disease and maintain oral health.

Career Description

Although the range of services performed by dental hygienists varies from state to state, patient services rendered by dental hygienists frequently include:

- Performing patient screening procedures, such as assessing oral health conditions, reviewing health and dental history, and taking blood pressure, pulse, and temperature; oral cancer screening; head & neck inspection; and dental charting
- Exposing and developing dental radiographs (x-rays)
- Removing calculus and plaque (hard and soft deposits) from teeth
- Applying preventive materials to teeth (eg, sealants and fluorides)
- Teaching patients appropriate oral hygiene techniques
- Counseling patients regarding proper nutrition and its impact on oral health
- Making impressions of patients' teeth for study casts
- Administration of anesthesia (depending upon state practice act)

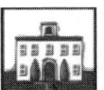

Employment Characteristics

Most of the approximately 158,000 licensed dental hygienists in the United States in 2004 are employed by general dentists. Additionally, dental specialists (such as periodontists or pediatric dentists) employ dental hygienists. Most hygienists work one to one with patients in providing dental hygiene services.

Dental hygienists also may be employed to provide dental hygiene care for patients in hospitals, nursing homes, public health clinics, and schools. Depending on the level of education and experience achieved, dental hygienists also can apply their skills and knowledge to other career activities, such as teaching. Research, public health, and business administration are other options. In addition, employment opportunities may be available with companies that market dental-related materials and equipment.

In some states, dental hygienists may also own their own dental hygiene business or practice on an independent contracting basis. These practitioners are not actually employed by dentists but provide dental hygiene services through contractual agreements.

Among independent general practitioners, the average number of employees per dentist has remained relatively stable between 1994 and 1998, averaging 4.2 positions. In 1999, the average number of employees increased to 4.3. Because 70.2% of solo general practitioners employ a dental hygienist, and 25.1% employ two or more hygienists, employment opportunities in this field are excellent.

As a career, dental hygiene also offers both stability and flexibility. As of 2001, for example, dental hygienists had been working in their current practices for an average of 7.3 years. Many hygienists also have considerable flexibility to undertake a full- or part-time schedule with evening or weekend hours.

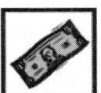

Salary

The salary of a dental hygienist varies, depending on the responsibilities associated with the specific position, the geographic location of employment, and the type of practice or other setting in which the hygienist works. Salary information from the American Dental Association indicates that the median salary for full-time dental hygienists in 2004 was $30.30 per hour. Refer to Section IV, Table 5 of this *Directory* for more information, or see www.ama-assn.org/go/hpsalary.

In addition, many full-time dental hygienists receive benefit packages from their dentist/employers, which may include health insurance coverage, dues for membership in professional organizations, paid vacations and sick leave, and tuition assistance for continuing education. Most state dental boards require mandatory continuing education for maintenance of the dental hygiene license.

Employment Outlook

According to the 2006-2007 edition of the *Occupational Outlook Handbook* and the *Monthly Labor Review,* published by the US Department of Labor's Bureau of Labor Statistics, dental hygiene is expected to increase 27% or more between 2004-2014. Some areas of the country are currently reporting shortages of dental hygienists.

Owing to the success of preventive dentistry in reducing the incidence of oral disease, senior citizens—a growing population—will retain their teeth longer and will require regular dental hygiene care.

Excellent career opportunities exist for nontraditional dental hygiene students, who might meet one or more of the following criteria: over 23 years of age, seeking career change or job reentry after a period of unemployment, or from a culturally diverse background. Some dental hygiene education programs offer more flexible program designs that meet the needs of nontraditional students by offering a variety of educational options, such as part-time or evening hours.

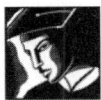

Educational Programs

Length. The majority of community college-based dental hygiene programs offer a 2-year associate degree. University-based dental hygiene programs may offer baccalaureate and master's degrees, which generally require at least 2 or more years of further education.

Prerequisites. Admission requirements vary, depending on the institution. High school-level courses such as health, biology, psychology, chemistry, mathematics, and speech will be beneficial in a dental hygiene career. Many programs prefer individuals who have completed at least 1 year of college, and some baccalaureate degree programs require applicants to have completed 2 years of college.

Curriculum. Dental hygiene education programs provide supervised patient care experiences. Programs also include courses in the liberal arts (English, speech, sociology, and psychology); basic sciences (anatomy, physiology, chemistry, biochemistry, immunology, nutrition, pharmacology, microbiology, and general pathology); and clinical sciences (dental hygiene; tooth morphology; head, neck, and oral anatomy; oral embryology and histology; oral pathology; radiography; periodontology; pain management; radiology; and dental materials). After completing a dental hygiene program, dental hygienists can pursue additional training in such areas as education, health administration, basic sciences, and public health.

Licensure

Dental hygienists are licensed by each state to provide dental hygiene care and patient education. Eligibility for state licensure usually includes graduation from a Commission-accredited dental hygiene education program. In addition to requiring a passing score on the state-authorized licensure examination, which tests candidates' clinical dental hygiene skills as well as their knowledge of dental hygiene and related subjects, almost all states require candidates for licensure to obtain a passing score on the Dental Hygiene National Board Examination (a comprehensive written examination).

Upon receipt of license, a dental hygienist may use RDH, signifying Registered Dental Hygienist, after his/her name.

Miscellaneous Facts

- The United States has approximately 290 dental hygiene education programs accredited by the American Dental Association's Commission on Dental Accreditation.
- Approximately 97.4% of the 13,895 students enrolled in dental hygiene programs in 2004-2005 were women.
- Minority students represented 17% of enrollees in dental hygiene programs in 2004-2005.

Dental Laboratory Technician

Dental laboratory technicians make dental prostheses—replacements for natural teeth, including dentures and crowns. The hallmarks of the qualified dental laboratory technician are skill in using small hand instruments, accuracy, artistic ability, and attention to detail to create practical and esthetically pleasing replacements.

Career Description

Dental laboratory technicians seldom interact directly with patients; rather, they work with dentists by following detailed written instructions to make dental prostheses, which are replacements for natural teeth that enable people who have lost some or all of their teeth to eat, chew, talk, and smile in a manner similar to the way they did before. The dental technician uses impressions (molds) of the patient's teeth or oral soft tissues to create full dentures, removable partial dentures or fixed bridges, crowns, and orthodontic appliances and splints.

Dental technicians use sophisticated instruments and equipment and work with a variety of materials for replacing damaged or missing tooth structure, including waxes, plastics, precious and nonprecious alloys, stainless steel, and porcelain.

Employment Characteristics

Most of the more than 43,000 active dental laboratory technicians in the United States today work in commercial dental laboratories, which on average employ between three to five technicians. In addition, some dentists employ dental technicians in their private dental offices. Other employment opportunities for dental technicians include dental schools, hospitals, the military, and companies that manufacture dental prosthetic materials. Dental laboratory technician education programs also offer teaching positions for qualified technicians.

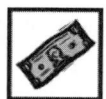

Salary

The starting salary of a dental technician varies depending on the responsibilities associated with the specific position and the geographic location of employment. Salary information from the American Dental Association indicates that the median salary for full-time dental technicians in 2003 was $15.40 per hour. Refer to Section IV, Table 5 of this *Directory* for more information, or see www.ama-assn.org/go/hpsalary. In addition to salary, many dental technicians receive benefit packages from their employers, which may include health and disability insurance coverage, reimbursement for continuing education programs, and paid vacations and holidays. Experienced technicians may become self-employed by opening their own dental laboratories, leading to greater financial rewards.

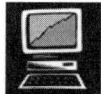

Employment Outlook

Since most dentists use laboratory services, employment opportunities in this field are excellent. Owing to the success of preventive dentistry in reducing the incidence of oral disease, senior citizens—a growing population—will retain their teeth longer and will require more sophisticated prostheses for longer periods, thus increasing the demand for dental laboratory services.

Excellent career opportunities exist for nontraditional dental technology students, who might be seeking career change or job reentry after a period of unemployment, or from a culturally diverse background.

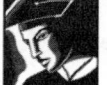

Educational Programs

Length. Most dental laboratory technicians receive their education and training through a 2-year program at a community college, vocational school, technical college, or dental school, for which they may receive a certificate or an associate degree.

Prerequisites. High school diploma or its equivalent, although the Commission strongly encourages formal college-level education.

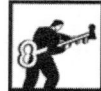

Certification

Dental laboratory technicians can become certified by passing an examination, administered by the National Board for Certification in Dental Laboratory Technology, that evaluates their technical skills and knowledge. Passing this examination qualifies a dental technician to use the designation Certified Dental Technician (CDT). A CDT specializes in one or more of five areas: complete dentures, partial dentures, crowns and bridges, ceramics, and orthodontics.

Dental technicians are eligible to take the examination if they have completed a dental laboratory technology program accredited by the Commission on Dental Accreditation and have 2 years of professional experience or have completed 5 years of work experience as dental technicians, or have graduated from a nonaccredited program and have 3 years of professional experience and passed a comprehensive examination.

Miscellaneous Facts

- In 2004-2005, 551 first-year dental laboratory technician students were enrolled in the approximately 23 dental technology education programs in the United States accredited by the American Dental Association's Commission on Dental Accreditation.
- Dental technology presents equal career opportunities for women and men. In 2004-2005, 47% of the students enrolled in dental technology programs were women, 53% were men.

- Minority students represented approximately 47.5% of enrollees in dental technology programs in the 2004-2005 graduating class.

 **Inquiries**

Careers/Curriculum
American Dental Association
211 E Chicago Avenue
Chicago, IL 60611-2678
312 440-2390
www.ada.org/prof/ed/careers

American Dental Education Association
1400 K Street NW, Suite 1100
Washington, DC 20005
202 289-7201
www.adea.org

American Dental Assistants Association
35 E Wacker Drive, Suite 1730
Chicago, IL 60601
312 541-1550
www.dentalassistant.org

American Dental Hygienists' Association
444 N Michigan Avenue, Suite 3400
Chicago IL 60611
312 440-8900
www.adha.org

Laboratory Conference Section Board of the American Dental Trade Association
4222 King Street W
Alexandria, VA 22302
703 379-7755

National Association of Dental Laboratories
325 John Knox Rd L103
Tallahassee, FL 32303
800 950-1150
www.nadl.org

Certification
Dental Assisting National Board, Inc
676 N St Clair, Suite 1880
Chicago, IL 60611
312 642-3368
800 FOR-DANB (367-3262)
312 642-1475 Fax
www.danb.org

National Board of Certification for Dental Laboratory Technicians
1530 Metropolitan Blvd
Tallahassee, FL 32308
850 224-0711
www.nadl.org

Program Accreditation
Commission on Dental Accreditation
American Dental Association
211 E Chicago Avenue
Chicago, IL 60611-2678
312 440-4653
312 440-2915 Fax
www.ada.org

Dental Assistant

Alabama

James H Faulkner State Community College
Dental Assisting Prgm
1900 Hwy 31 S
Bay Minette, AL 36507-2619
http://faulknerstate.edu
Prgm Dir: Michele Snider, CDA RDH AAS BA
Tel: 251 580-2110   *Fax:* 251 580-2228
E-mail: msnider@faulkner.edu

Calhoun Community College
Dental Assisting Prgm
PO Box 2216
Decatur, AL 35609-2216
Prgm Dir: Patricia Stueck, MA
Tel: 256 306-2812   *Fax:* 256 306-2525
E-mail: phs@calhoun.edu

Wallace State Community College
Dental Assisting Prgm
801 Main St NW
PO Box 2000
Hanceville, AL 35077-2000
Prgm Dir: Barbara Adams, RDH MA
Tel: 256 352-8380   *Fax:* 256 352-8382
E-mail: barbara.adams@wallacestate.edu

H Council Trenholm State Technical College
Dental Assisting Prgm
1225 Air Base Blvd
Montgomery, AL 36108
www.trenholmtech.cc.al.us
Prgm Dir: Cecile B Mathews, MS
Tel: 334 420-4427   *Fax:* 334 420-4269
E-mail: cmathews@trenholmtech.cc.al.us

Alaska

University of Alaska Anchorage
Dental Assisting Prgm
3211 Providence Dr, AHS 124
Anchorage, AK 99508-8371
Prgm Dir: Stephanie Olson, CDA BA
Tel: 907 786-6929   *Fax:* 907 786-6938
E-mail: afsmo1@uaa.alaska.edu

Arizona

Mesa Community College
Dental Assisting Prgm
1833 W Southern Ave
Mesa, AZ 85205
Prgm Dir: Monica Williamson Nenad, RDH MEd
Tel: 480 472-0806
E-mail: monica.nenad@mcmail.maricopa.edu

Phoenix College
Dental Assisting Prgm
1202 W Thomas Rd
Phoenix, AZ 85013
www.phoenixcollege.edu/dental
Prgm Dir: Rita Perry, CDA RDH MPA
Tel: 602 285-7326   *Fax:* 602 285-7330
E-mail: rita.perry@pcmail.maricopa.edu

Pima Community College
Dental Assisting Prgm
2202 W Anklam Rd
Tucson, AZ 85709
Prgm Dir: Pamela Horch
Tel: 520 206-3101   *Fax:* 520 206-3027
E-mail: pamela.horch@pima.edu

Arkansas

Arkansas Northeastern College
Dental Assisting Prgm
I-55 and Hwy 148
PO Box 36
Burdette, AR 72321
Prgm Dir: Kristi Austin, CDA RDA
Tel: 870 780-1210   *Fax:* 870 763-1496
E-mail: kmaustin@anc.edu

Pulaski Technical College
Dental Assisting Prgm
3000 W Scenic Dr
North Little Rock, AR 72118-3399
www.pulaskitech.edu
Prgm Dir: De Anna Davis, CDA RDA MEd
Tel: 501 812-2236   *Fax:* 501 812-2391
E-mail: ddavis@pulaskitech.edu

California

College of Alameda
Dental Assisting Prgm
555 Atlantic Ave
Alameda, CA 94501
Prgm Dir: Yvonne Carter, BA
Tel: 510 748-2262   *Fax:* 510 748-2156
E-mail: whycarter@aol.com

Heald College - Concord Campus
Dental Assisting Prgm
5130 Commercial Circle
Concord, CA 94520
www.heald.edu
Prgm Dir: Maria Pardorla, RDA CDA BA
Tel: 925 288-5800   *Fax:* 925 687-2428
E-mail: maria_pardorla@heald.edu

Orange Coast College
Dental Assisting Prgm
2701 Fairview Rd
Costa Mesa, CA 92628-0120
Prgm Dir: Judy Rose, MA CDA RDA
Tel: 714 432-5565   *Fax:* 714 432-5534
E-mail: jrose@mail.occ.cccd.edu

Cypress College
Dental Assisting Prgm
9200 Valley View St
Cypress, CA 90630
Prgm Dir: Mary Kay Davis, BS
Tel: 714 484-7293   *Fax:* 714 527-2175
E-mail: mdavis@cypress.cc.ca.us

College of the Redwoods
Dental Assisting Prgm
7351Tompkins Hill Rd
Eureka, CA 95501
www.redwoods.edu
Prgm Dir: Hillary Reed, RDA RDAEF CDA COA CDPMA
Tel: 707 476-4253   *Fax:* 707 476-4419
E-mail: hillary-reed@redwoods.edu

Citrus College
Dental Assisting Prgm
1000 W Foothill
Glendora, CA 91741
www.citruscollege.edu
Prgm Dir: Claudia Pohl, CDA RDA BVEd
Tel: 626 914-8728   *Fax:* 626 914-8724
E-mail: cpohl@citruscollege.edu

Heald College - Hayward Campus
Dental Assisting Prgm
25500 Industrial Blvd
Hayward, CA 94545
Prgm Dir: Evangeline Tenchavez
Tel: 510 783-2100
E-mail: evangeline_tenchavez@heald.edu

College of Marin
Dental Assisting Prgm
835 College Ave
Kentfield, CA 94904
Prgm Dir: Grace Hom, CDA RDAEF MA
Tel: 415 485-9327   *Fax:* 415 485-9328
E-mail: grace.hom@marin.edu

Hacienda LaPuente Adult Education
Dental Assisting Prgm
14101 E Nelson Ave
La Puente, CA 91746
Prgm Dir: Gretchen Richardson
Tel: 626 934-2890   *Fax:* 626 934-5723
E-mail: grichardson@hlpusd.k12.ca.us

Foothill Community College
Dental Assisting Prgm
12345 El Monte Rd
Los Altos Hills, CA 94022
Prgm Dir: Cara Miyasaki-Ching, RDHEF MS
Tel: 650 949-7351   *Fax:* 650 949-9788
E-mail: miyasakicara@fhda.edu

Modesto Junior College
Dental Assisting Prgm
435 College Ave
Modesto, CA 95350
Prgm Dir: Robert Keach, CDA RDA
Tel: 209 575-6914   *Fax:* 209 575-6593
E-mail: keachr@mjc.edu

Monterey Peninsula College
Dental Assisting Prgm
980 Fremont St
Monterey, CA 93940
Prgm Dir: Patricia A Lewis, BS
Tel: 831 646-4137   *Fax:* 831 645-1353
E-mail: plewis@mpc.edu

Cerritos College
Dental Assisting Prgm
11110 E Alondra Blvd
Norwalk, CA 90650
Prgm Dir: Donna Wedell
Tel: 562 860-2451, Ext 2575   *Fax:* 562 467-5077
E-mail: dwedell@cerritos.edu

Pasadena City College
Dental Assisting Prgm
1570 E Colorado Blvd
Pasadena, CA 91106
www.pasadena.edu
Prgm Dir: Lori Gagliardi, EdD
Tel: 626 585-7542   *Fax:* 626 585-7966
E-mail: ligagliardi@pasadena.edu

Diablo Valley College
Dental Assisting Prgm
321 Golf Club Rd
Pleasant Hill, CA 94523
Prgm Dir: Marylou Pineda, MA CDA RDA
Tel: 925 685-1230, Ext 2351   *Fax:* 925 689-6529
E-mail: MPineda@dvc.edu

Chaffey College
Dental Assisting Prgm
5885 Haven Ave
Rancho Cucamonga, CA 91737-3002
http://http:www.chaffey.edu
Prgm Dir: Beverly Cox, MAEd BS
Tel: 909 652-6678   *Fax:* 909 652-6688
E-mail: Beverly.Cox@chaffey.edu

Sacramento City College
Dental Assisting Prgm
3835 Freeport Blvd
Sacramento, CA 95822
www.scc.losrios.edu
Prgm Dir: Sandra Lo, DDS
Tel: 916 558-2650   *Fax:* 916 538-2067
E-mail: los@scc.losrios.edu

San Diego Mesa College
Dental Assisting Prgm
7250 Mesa College Dr
San Diego, CA 92111-4999
www.sdmesa.edu
Prgm Dir: Margaret Fickess, RDA CDA MEd
Tel: 619 388-2697   *Fax:* 619 388-2677
E-mail: mfickess@sdccd.edu

City College of San Francisco
Dental Assisting Prgm
50 Phelan Ave
San Francisco, CA 94112
www.ccsf.edu
Prgm Dir: Anna Nelson, CDA RDA MA
Tel: 415 239-3479   *Fax:* 415 239-3719
E-mail: anelson@ccsf.edu

San Jose City College
Dental Assisting Prgm
2100 Moorpark Ave
San Jose, CA 95128-2799
Prgm Dir: Laura sanchez, AA
Tel: 408 288-3712, Ext 3254   *Fax:* 408 275-9386
E-mail: laura.sanchez@sjcc.edu

Palomar Community College
Dental Assisting Prgm
1140 W Mission Rd
San Marcos, CA 92069
Prgm Dir: Denise Rudy
Tel: 760 744-1150, Ext 2573   *Fax:* 760 744-1150
E-mail: drudy@palomar.edu

College of San Mateo
Dental Assisting Prgm
1700 W Hillsdale Blvd
San Mateo, CA 94402-3795
Prgm Dir: Audrey Behrens, CDA RDA BA
Tel: 650 574-6212   *Fax:* 650 574-6485
E-mail: audb2@pacbell.net

Contra Costa College
Dental Assisting Prgm
2600 Mission Bell Dr
San Pablo, CA 94806
Prgm Dir: Sandra Everhart, BA
Tel: 510 235-7800, Ext 4385   *Fax:* 510 236-6768
E-mail: severhart@contracosta.cc.ca.us

Santa Rosa Junior College
Dental Assisting Prgm
1501 Mendocino Ave
Santa Rosa, CA 95401-4395
www.santarosa.edu
Prgm Dir: Doni Bird, MA
Tel: 707 522-2828   *Fax:* 707 527-4426
E-mail: dbird@santarosa.edu

Heald College - Stockton Campus
Dental Assisting Prgm
1605 E March Lane
Stockton, CA 95210
Prgm Dir: Levy Pineda, CDT DMD
Tel: 209 473-5200, Ext 5244   *Fax:* 209 477-2739
E-mail: levy_pineda@heald.edu

Colorado

T H Pickens Technical Center
Dental Assisting Prgm
500 Airport Blvd
Aurora, CO 80011
Prgm Dir: Karen Einsle, BA CDA EDDA
Tel: 303 344-4910, Ext 27787   *Fax:* 303 326-1277
E-mail: karene@pickens.aps.k12.co.us

IntelliTec Medical Institute
Dental Assisting Prgm
2345 N Academy Blvd
Colorado Springs, CO 80909
Prgm Dir: Ed Rito
Tel: 719 596-7400

Pikes Peak Community College
Dental Assisting Prgm
11195 Highway 83
Campus Box R13
Colorado Springs, CO 80921-3602
www.ppcc.edu
Prgm Dir: Frank Delgesso, CO Career & Tech Edu
Credential
Tel: 719 502-3347 *Fax:* 719 502-3330
E-mail: frank.delgesso@ppcc.edu

Emily Griffith Opportunity School
Dental Assisting Prgm
1250 W Welton St
Denver, CO 80204
Prgm Dir: Brenda D Stevens
Tel: 720 423-4736 *Fax:* 303 575-4762
E-mail: Brenda_Stevens@dpsk12.org

Front Range Comm College
Dental Assisting Prgm
Larimer Campus/4616 S Shields
Fort Collins, CO 80526-8312
www.frontrange.edu
Prgm Dir: Dana Quiller, DDS
Tel: 970 204-8220 *Fax:* 970 204-8118
E-mail: dana.quiller@frontrange.edu

Pueblo Community College
Dental Assisting Prgm
900 W Orman Ave, MT Rm 122B
Pueblo, CO 81004
www.pueblocc.edu
Prgm Dir: Janet Trujillo, CDA EFDA BS
Tel: 719 549-3263 *Fax:* 719 549-3381
E-mail: janet.trujillo@pueblocc.edu

Connecticut

Porter and Chester Institute - Enfield
Dental Assisting Prgm
132 Weymouth Rd
Enfield, CT 06082
Prgm Dir: Susan M Corriveau, BA CDA
Tel: 860 253-6100 *Fax:* 860 741-0234
E-mail: pcidentassist@aol.com

Tunxis Community College
Dental Assisting Prgm
271 Scott Swamp Rd
Farmington, CT 06032-3187
Prgm Dir: Erin Annecharico, CDA RDH BS MS
Tel: 860 255-3673 *Fax:* 860 255-3675
E-mail: eannecharico@txcc.commnet.edu

Eli Whitney Vocational Technical School
Dental Assisting Prgm
71 Jones Rd
Hamden, CT 06514
Prgm Dir: Angela Macolino, CDA
Tel: 203 397-4031, Ext 344 *Fax:* 203 397-4129
E-mail: Angela.Macolino@ct.gov

A I Prince Technical High School
Dental Assisting Prgm
500 Bookfield St
Hartford, CT 06106
Prgm Dir: Janice Ferrara, CDA
Tel: 860 951-7112, Ext 323 *Fax:* 860 951-1529
E-mail: Janice.Ferrara@po.state.ct.us

Briarwood College
Dental Assisting Prgm
2279 Mt Vernon Rd
Southington, CT 06489
Prgm Dir: Rosemary Ryan
Tel: 800 952-2444, Ext 69 *Fax:* 860 628-6444
E-mail: ryanr@briarwood.edu

Windham Regional Vocational Tech School
Dental Assisting Prgm
210 Birch St
Willimantic, CT 06226
Prgm Dir: Susan Dolliver, BA
Tel: 860 456-3879, Ext 322 *Fax:* 860 450-0630
E-mail: susan.dolliver@po.state.ct.us

Florida

South Florida Community College
Dental Assisting Prgm
600 W College Dr
Avon Park, FL 33825
www.southflorida.edu
Prgm Dir: Rebecca Sroda, RDH MS
Tel: 863 784-7021 *Fax:* 863 453-9442
E-mail: srodar@southflorida.edu

Manatee Technical Institute
Dental Assisting Prgm
5520 Lakewood Ranch Blvd
Bradenton, FL 34211
www.manateetechnicalinstitute.org
Prgm Dir: Kimberly Bland, CDA BS
Tel: 941 752-8100, Ext 210 *Fax:* 941 727-6254
E-mail: blandk@manateeschools.net

Brevard Community College
Dental Assisting Prgm
1519 Clearlake Rd
Cocoa, FL 32922
Prgm Dir: Holly Kahler, CDA RDH EdD
Tel: 321 433-7571 *Fax:* 321 433-7599
E-mail: kahlerh@brevardcc.edu

Daytona Beach Community College
Dental Assisting Prgm
1200 W International Speedway Blvd
Daytona Beach, FL 32120
Prgm Dir: Pamela Ridilla, CDA RDH MS
Tel: 386 785-2093 *Fax:* 386 785-2090
E-mail: ridillp@dbcc.edu

Americare School of Nursing
Dental Assisting Prgm
7275 Estapona Circle
Fern Park, FL 32730
Prgm Dir: Dana Wickman
Tel: 407 262-8101

Broward Community College
Dental Assisting Prgm
3501 SW Davie Rd, Bldg 8
Fort Lauderdale, FL 33314
www.broward.edu
Prgm Dir: Joyce Abraham, CDA RDH BA
Tel: 954 201-6904 *Fax:* 954 201-6397
E-mail: jabraham@broward.edu

Edison College
Dental Assisting Prgm
PO Box 60210
Fort Myers, FL 33906-6210
www.edison.edu
Prgm Dir: Karen Molumby, CDA RDH MBA
Tel: 239 985-8322 *Fax:* 239 985-8352
E-mail: kmolumby@edison.edu

Indian River Community College
Dental Assisting Prgm
3209 Virginia Ave
Fort Pierce, FL 34981-5599
Prgm Dir: Karen Allen, MEd
Tel: 772 462-7530 *Fax:* 772 462-4900
E-mail: kallen@ircc.edu

Santa Fe Community College
Dental Assisting Prgm
3000 NW 83rd St, Bldg W
Gainesville, FL 32606
Prgm Dir: Karen Autrey, BHS MEd
Tel: 352 395-5705 *Fax:* 352 395-5662
E-mail: karen.autrey@sfcc.edu

Palm Beach Community College
Dental Assisting Prgm
4200 Congress Ave
Lake Worth, FL 33461
http://pbcc.edu
Prgm Dir: Colleen Bradshaw, CDA MHS
Tel: 561 868-3196 *Fax:* 561 868-3753
E-mail: bradshac@pbcc.edu

Traviss Career Center
Dental Assisting Prgm
3225 Winter Lake Rd
Lakeland, FL 33803
www.travisstech.org
Prgm Dir: Susan Rexroat, CDA CDPMA BA
Tel: 863 499-2715, Ext 286 *Fax:* 863 413-2067
E-mail: susan.rexroat@polk-fl.net

Lindsey Hopkins Tech Education Center
Dental Assisting Prgm
750 NW 20th St
Miami, FL 33127
Prgm Dir: Debra Morales
Tel: 305 324-6070 *Fax:* 305 324-6249
E-mail: dmorales@dadeschools.net

Robert Morgan Educational Center
Dental Assisting Prgm
18180 SW 122nd Ave
Miami, FL 33177
http://rmec.dadeschools.net
Prgm Dir: Aurea Hurtado, CDA BS
Tel: 305 253-9920, Ext 2212 *Fax:* 305 259-3270
E-mail: ahurtado@dadeschools.net

Lorenzo Walker Institute of Technology
Dental Assisting Prgm
3702 Estey Ave
Naples, FL 34104
www.lwit.edu
Prgm Dir: Linda Rae Flood, CDA RDH BS
Tel: 239 377-0932 *Fax:* 239 377-1004
E-mail: floodli@collier.k12.fl.us

Okaloosa-Walton College
Dental Assisting Prgm
100 College Blvd
Niceville, FL 32578
Prgm Dir: Mary E Thomas
Tel: 850 729-6444
E-mail: thomasm@owc.edu

Central Florida Community College
Dental Assisting Prgm
3001 SW College Rd
PO Box 1388
Ocala, FL 34479
Prgm Dir: Deanna Stentiford
Tel: 352 854-2322, Ext 1529
E-mail: stentifd@cf.edu

Orlando Tech
Dental Assisting Prgm
301 W Amelia St
Orlando, FL 32801
www.orlandotech.ocps.net
Prgm Dir: Cynthia K Bradley, CDA CDPMA EFDA
Tel: 407 246-7060, Ext 4923 *Fax:* 407 317-3372
E-mail: bradlec@ocps.k12.fl.us

Gulf Coast Community College
Dental Assisting Prgm
5230 W US Hwy 98
Panama City, FL 32401-1041
Prgm Dir: Kim Herremans, RDH MS
Tel: 850 769-1551, Ext 5832 *Fax:* 850 747-3246
E-mail: kherremans@gulfcoast.edu

Pensacola Junior College
Dental Assisting Prgm
5555 Hwy 98 W
Pensacola, FL 32507
Prgm Dir: Teresa Lucas
Tel: 850 484-2348 *Fax:* 850 484-2390
E-mail: tlucas@pjc.edu

Charlotte Technical Center
Dental Assisting Prgm
18300 Toledo Blade Blvd
Port Charlotte, FL 33948-3399
Prgm Dir: Lance Petersen, DDS
Tel: 941 255-7500, Ext 140 *Fax:* 941 255-7509
E-mail: Lance_Petersen@ccps.k12.fl.us

Pinellas Tech Educ Ctr - St Petersburg
Dental Assisting Prgm
901 34th St S
St Petersburg, FL 33711
Prgm Dir: Barbara Thomas, BS CDA MA
Tel: 727 893-2500, Ext 1073 *Fax:* 727 552-1613
E-mail: bthomas@ptec.pinellas.k12.fl.us

Tallahassee Community College
Dental Assisting Prgm
444 Appleyard Dr
Tallahassee, FL 32304
Prgm Dir: Cynthia R Biron, RDH MA
Tel: 850 201-8577 *Fax:* 850 201-8575
E-mail: bironc@tcc.fl.edu

Erwin Technical Center
Dental Assisting Prgm
2010 E Hillsborough Ave
Tampa, FL 33610
Prgm Dir: Darcy Abel Hunter, MEd
Tel: 813 231-1800, Ext 1323 *Fax:* 813 231-1812
E-mail: hunter_d@firn.edu

Hillsborough Community College
Dental Assisting Prgm
Dale Mabry Campus
PO Box 30030
Tampa, FL 33614
Prgm Dir: Connie Gore, CDA BS
Tel: 813 253-7279 *Fax:* 813 253-7377
E-mail: cgore@hccfl.edu

Georgia

Albany Technical College
Dental Assisting Prgm
1704 S Slappey Blvd
Albany, GA 31701-3514
Prgm Dir: Linda Cauley
Tel: 229 430-3544 *Fax:* 229 430-5115
E-mail: lcauley@albanytech.edu

Athens Technical College
Dental Assisting Prgm
Allied Health and Nursing
800 US Hwy 29 N
Athens, GA 30601
Prgm Dir: Tina A Grile, MHS RDH CDA
Tel: 706 355-5142
E-mail: tgrile@athenstech.edu

Atlanta Technical College
Dental Assisting Prgm
1560 Metropolitan Pkwy SW, Rm 2157
Atlanta, GA 30310-4446
www.atlantatech.edu
Prgm Dir: Dorothy Smith, CDA EFDA BA
Tel: 404 756-3723, Ext 3723 *Fax:* 404 758-8522
E-mail: dsmith@atlantatech.edu

Augusta Technical College
Dental Assisting Prgm
3200 Augusta Tech Dr
Augusta, GA 30906
Prgm Dir: Beverly Dalber, BS CDA
Tel: 706 771-4178 *Fax:* 706 771-4181
E-mail: bdalber@augustatech.edu

Columbus Technical College
Dental Assisting Prgm
928 Manchester Expwy
Columbus, GA 31904
www.columbustech.edu
Prgm Dir: Jan J Jones, CDA RDH MPA
Tel: 706 649-1977 *Fax:* 706 649-1599
E-mail: jjones@columbustech.edu

Gwinnett Technical College
Dental Assisting Prgm
5150 Sugarloaf Pkwy
Lawrenceville, GA 30043
Prgm Dir: Lea Anna Harding, BS Ed
Tel: 770 962-7580 *Fax:* 770 962-1338
E-mail: lharding@gwinnetttech.edu

Lanier Technical College
Dental Assisting Prgm
2990 Landrum Education Dr
Oakwood, GA 30566
Prgm Dir: Liza Charlton, BA
Tel: 770 531-6370 *Fax:* 770 531-6306
E-mail: lcharlto@laniertech.edu

Coosa Valley Technical College
Dental Assisting Prgm
466 Brock Rd
Rockmart, GA 30153
www.coosavalleytech.edu
Prgm Dir: Donna Sutton, RDH MS CDA
Tel: 770 684-3128 *Fax:* 770 684-8710
E-mail: dsutton@coosavalleytech.edu

Savannah Technical College
Dental Assisting Prgm
5717 White Bluff Rd
Savannah, GA 31405-5521
www.savannahtech.edu
Prgm Dir: Debi Yawn, CDA EFDA
Tel: 912 443-5812
E-mail: dyawn@savannahtech.edu

Medix School
Dental Assisting Prgm
2108 Cobb Pkwy
Smyrna, GA 30080
www.medixschool.com
Prgm Dir: Terroll Farries, AS CDA
Tel: 770 980-0002 *Fax:* 770 980-0811
E-mail: terrellfarries@yahoo.com

Ogeechee Technical College
Dental Assisting Prgm
1 Joe Kennedy Blvd
Statesboro, GA 30458-8049
Prgm Dir: Denise Campopiano, BS RDA CDA
Tel: 912 486-7614 *Fax:* 912 486-7604
E-mail: dcampopiano@ogeecheetech.edu

Valdosta Technical College
Dental Assisting Prgm
PO Box 928-4089 Val Tech Rd
Valdosta, GA 31603-0928
Prgm Dir: Sandi Woodward, RDH CDA BSED
Tel: 229 259-5533 *Fax:* 229 259-5567
E-mail: swoodward@valdostatech.edu

Middle Georgia Technical College
Dental Assisting Prgm
80 Cohen Walker Dr
Warner Robins, GA 31088-2729
Prgm Dir: Debbie Wrenn, CDA EFDA
Tel: 478 988-6800, Ext 4026 *Fax:* 478 988-6875
E-mail: dwrenn@middlegatech.edu

Hawaii

Maui Community College
Dental Assisting Prgm
310 Kaahumana Ave
Kahului, HI 96732
Prgm Dir: June M Wolken-Vierra
E-mail: jwvierra@hawaii.edu

Idaho

Apollo College - Boise
Dental Assisting Prgm
1200 N Liberty St
Boise, ID 83704
Prgm Dir: Erlinda Hiles, BA CDA
Tel: 208 377-8080, Ext 17 *Fax:* 208 322-7658
E-mail: ehiles@apolloboise.com

Boise State University
Dental Assisting Prgm
College of Technology
1910 University Dr
Boise, ID 83725
Prgm Dir: Bonnie Tollinger, CDA
Tel: 208 426-2169 *Fax:* 208 426-5659
E-mail: btollinger@boisestate.edu

Illinois

John A Logan College
Dental Assisting Prgm
700 Logan College Rd
Carterville, IL 62918
Prgm Dir: Kathy Gibson, MS
Tel: 618 985-3741, Ext 8389 *Fax:* 618 985-9181
E-mail: kathy.gibson@jal.cc.il.us

Kaskaskia College
Dental Assisting Prgm
27210 College Rd
Centralia, IL 62801
www.kaskaskia.edu
Prgm Dir: Lori Schmidt, RDA RDH AAS BS
Tel: 618 545-3320 *Fax:* 618 545-3389
E-mail: lschmidt@kc.cc.il.us

Elgin Community College
Dental Assisting Prgm
1700 Spartan Dr
Elgin, IL 60123
Prgm Dir: Kim Plate, CDA
Tel: 847 214-7351 *Fax:* 847 622-3063
E-mail: kplate@elgin.edu

Lewis & Clark Community College
Dental Assisting Prgm
5800 Godfrey Rd, RiverBend Arena RM 235
Godfrey, IL 62035
www.lc.edu
Prgm Dir: Constance Pero-Fox, CDA BS
Tel: 618 468-4411 *Fax:* 618 468-2394
E-mail: cperofox@lc.edu

Illinois Valley Community College
Dental Assisting Prgm
815 N Orlando Smith Ave
Oglesby, IL 61348-9691
Prgm Dir: Patricia Pearson, CDA
Tel: 815 224-2720, Ext 359 *Fax:* 815 224-3033
E-mail: Pat_Pearson@ivcc.edu

Indiana

Ivy Tech Community College - Anderson
Dental Assisting Prgm
104 W 53rd St
Anderson, IN 46013
www.ivytech.edu/anderson
Prgm Dir: Teresa Macauley, CDA EFDA MS
Tel: 765 643-7133, Ext 2369
E-mail: tmacaule@ivytech.edu

Columbus Area Career Connection/Ivy Tech St
Dental Assisting Prgm
230 S Marr Rd
Columbus, IN 47201
Prgm Dir: Christy Ross, CDA
Tel: 812 376-4202   *Fax:* 812 376-4358
E-mail: rossc@bcsc.k12.in.us

University of Southern Indiana
Dental Assisting Prgm
8600 University Blvd
Evansville, IN 47712
Prgm Dir: Kimberly Hite, CDA EFDA RDH BS
Tel: 812 465-1155   *Fax:* 812 465-1071
E-mail: kghite@usi.edu

Indiana Univ - Purdue Univ Ft Wayne
Dental Assisting Prgm
2101 Coliseum Blvd E
Fort Wayne, IN 46805
Prgm Dir: Connie Kracher, MSD CDA BSEd
Tel: 260 481-6567   *Fax:* 260 481-4162
E-mail: kracher@ipfw.edu

Indiana University Northwest
Dental Assisting Prgm
3400 Broadway St
Gary, IN 46408
www.iun.edu
Prgm Dir: Juanita Robinson, CDA EFDA LDH MSEd
Tel: 219 980-6734   *Fax:* 219 981-4249
E-mail: jurobin@iun.edu

Indiana University
Dental Assisting Prgm
1121 W Michigan St
Indianapolis, IN 46202-5186
www.iusd.iupui.edu
Prgm Dir: Pamela Ford, CDA EFDA RDH MSW
Tel: 317 278-2814   *Fax:* 317 274-1363
E-mail: ptavenne@iupui.edu

Kaplan College
Dental Assisting Prgm
7302 Woodland Dr
Indianapolis, IN 46278
Prgm Dir: Shannon Irvin, BS
Tel: 317 299-6001   *Fax:* 317 298-6342
E-mail: sirvin@kaplan.edu

Ivy Tech Community College - Kokomo
Dental Assisting Prgm
700 E Firmin St
Kokomo, IN 46902
Prgm Dir: Darci Post
Tel: 765 457-0858, Ext 123

Ivy Tech Community College - Lafayette
Dental Assisting Prgm
3101 S Creasy Ln
PO Box 6299
Lafayette, IN 47903-6299
Prgm Dir: Judith Buckles
Tel: 765 269-5205   *Fax:* 765 269-5248
E-mail: jbuckles@ivytech.edu

Indiana University South Bend
Dental Assisting Prgm
1700 Mishawaka Ave
South Bend, IN 46634
Prgm Dir: Nanci Genich-Yokom, CDA RDH MBA
Tel: 574 237-4154   *Fax:* 574 237-4854
E-mail: nyokom@iusb.edu

Iowa

Des Moines Area Community College
Dental Assisting Prgm
2006 Ankeny Blvd
Ankeny, IA 50023-3993
Prgm Dir: Deborah P Bell, AA
Tel: 515 964-6308   *Fax:* 515 964-6640
E-mail: dpbell@dmacc.edu

Scott Community College
Dental Assisting Prgm
500 Belmont Rd
Bettendorf, IA 52722-5649
www.eicc.edu
Prgm Dir: Tina Ford-Ball, CDA RDA EFDA
Tel: 563 441-4260   *Fax:* 563 441-4204
E-mail: tball@eicc.edu

Kirkwood Community College
Dental Assisting Prgm
6301 Kirkwood Blvd SW, PO Box 2068
Cedar Rapids, IA 52406-9973
Prgm Dir: Pam Hanson
Tel: 319 398-5560   *Fax:* 319 398-1293
E-mail: phanson@kirkwood.edu

Iowa Western Community College
Dental Assisting Prgm
2700 College Rd/PO Box 4C
Council Bluffs, IA 51503
www.iwcc.edu
Prgm Dir: Sue Norman, BA CDA RDA
Tel: 712 325-3469   *Fax:* 712 325-3736
E-mail: snorman@iwcc.edu

Vatterott College - Des Moines Campus
Dental Assisting Prgm
6100 Thornton Ave, Ste 290
Des Moines, IA 50321
www.vatterott-college.edu
Prgm Dir: Sarah Bouma, RDA CDA
Tel: 515 309-9000   *Fax:* 515 309-0366
E-mail: sarah.bouma@vatterott-college.edu

Marshalltown Community College
Dental Assisting Prgm
3700 S Center St
Marshalltown, IA 50158
Prgm Dir: Elaine B Peterson, BA CDA RDA EFDA
Tel: 641 752-7106, Ext 294   *Fax:* 641 752-8149
E-mail: elaine.peterson@iavalley.edu

Northeast Iowa Community College
Dental Assisting Prgm
10250 Sundown Rd
Peosta, IA 52068
www.nicc.edu
Prgm Dir: Gloria Kluesner, CDA BLS RDA EFDA
Tel: 800 728-7367, Ext 227   *Fax:* 319 556-5058
E-mail: kluesneg@nicc.edu

Western Iowa Tech Community College
Dental Assisting Prgm
4647 Stone Ave, PO Box 5199
Sioux City, IA 51102-5199
www.witcc.edu
Prgm Dir: Jackie Krueger, CDA RDA
Tel: 712 274-8733, Ext 1267   *Fax:* 712 274-6448
E-mail: kruegej@witcc.edu

Hawkeye Community College
Dental Assisting Prgm
1501 E Orange Rd
PO Box 8015
Waterloo, IA 50704
www.hawkeyecollege.edu
Prgm Dir: Suzanne Van Syoc, CDA RDA BA
Tel: 319 296-2320, Ext 1355   *Fax:* 319 296-2874
E-mail: svansyoc@hawkeyecollege.edu

Kansas

Flint Hills Technical College
Dental Assisting Prgm
3301 W 18th Ave
Emporia, KS 66801
Prgm Dir: Monica Jones, CDA MBE
Tel: 620 341-2300, Ext 1314   *Fax:* 620 343-4611
E-mail: mjones@fhtc.edu

Salina Area Technical School
Dental Assisting Prgm
2562 Centennial Rd
Salina, KS 67401
Prgm Dir: Janet Fisher, CDA MS
Tel: 785 309-3126   *Fax:* 785 309-3101
E-mail: janet.fisher@usd305.com

Wichita Area Technical College
Dental Assisting Prgm
324 N Emporia St
Wichita, KS 67202
Prgm Dir: Melanie Mitchell, CDA
Tel: 316 677-1355, Ext 71368   *Fax:* 316 677-1332
E-mail: mmitchell@watc.edu

Kentucky

Bluegrass Community and Technical College
Dental Assisting Prgm
164 Opportunity Way
Lexington, KY 40511-1020
www.bluegrass.kctcs.edu
Prgm Dir: Olivia "Libby" Ritchie, CDA EDDA AA
Tel: 859 246-6622   *Fax:* 859 246-6618
E-mail: olivia.ritchie@kctcs.edu

West Kentucky Community & Technical College
Dental Assisting Prgm
4810 Alben Barkley Dr
Paducah, KY 42001
www.westkentucky.kctcs.edu
Prgm Dir: Darlene Daniel, BS
Tel: 270 534-3358, Ext 43358   *Fax:* 270 554-6260
E-mail: Darlene.Daniel@kctcs.edu

Maine

University College of Bangor
Dental Assisting Prgm
Lincoln Hall, 29 Texas Ave
Bangor, ME 04401-4324
Prgm Dir: Diana L Olsen, CDA CDPMA RDH MS
Tel: 207 262-7878   *Fax:* 207 262-7751
E-mail: dolsen@maine.edu

Maryland

Medix School
Dental Assisting Prgm
700 York Rd
Towson, MD 21204
Prgm Dir: Linda Einolf
Tel: 410 337-5155   *Fax:* 410 337-5104
E-mail: info@medixschool.com

Massachusetts

Massasoit Community College
Dental Assisting Prgm
900 Randolph St
Canton, MA 02021
Prgm Dir: Mary A Frohn, BS
Tel: 781 821-2222, Ext 2754   *Fax:* 781 575-9428
E-mail: mfrohn@massasoit.mass.edu

Northern Essex Community College
Dental Assisting Prgm
45 Franklin St
Lawrence, MA 01841
www.necc.mass.edu/healthprofessions
Prgm Dir: Kerin Hamidiani, MEd
Tel: 978 738-7427   *Fax:* 978 738-7450
E-mail: khamidiani@necc.mass.edu

Middlesex Community College - Lowell
Dental Assisting Prgm
33 Kearney Square
Lowell, MA 01852
Prgm Dir: Margaret Bloy, MS
Tel: 978 656-3053, Ext 3053   *Fax:* 978 656-3078
E-mail: bloyp@middlesex.mass.edu

Charles H McCann Technical School
Dental Assisting Prgm
70 Hodges Cross Rd
North Adams, MA 01247
Prgm Dir: Denice Kozak, CDA AS
Tel: 413 663-5383, Ext 183   *Fax:* 413 664-9424
E-mail: dkozak@mccanntech.org

Southeastern Technical Institute
Dental Assisting Prgm
250 Foundry St
South Easton, MA 02375
Prgm Dir: Audrey Beaudoin, MEd
Tel: 508 238-1860   *Fax:* 508 230-1558
E-mail: abeaudoin@sersd.org

Springfield Technical Community College
Dental Assisting Prgm
One Armory Sq
PO Box 9000
Springfield, MA 01102
http://stcc.edu
Prgm Dir: Carol A Giaquinto, CDA RDH MEd
Tel: 413 755-4861   *Fax:* 413 755-6312
E-mail: giaquinto@stcc.edu

Quinsigamond Community College
Dental Assisting Prgm
670 W Boylston St
Worcester, MA 01606
Prgm Dir: Adrienne Nichols, MEd
Tel: 508 854-2742   *Fax:* 508 854-2704
E-mail: anichols@qcc.mass.edu

Michigan

Washtenaw Community College
Dental Assisting Prgm
4800 E Huron River Dr
Ann Arbor, MI 48106
www.wccnet.edu/health/dental.php
Prgm Dir: Kathleen Weber, CDA RDA BAS
Tel: 734 973-3338   *Fax:* 734 677-5334
E-mail: weber@wccnet.edu

Lake Michigan College
Dental Assisting Prgm
2755 E Napier Ave
Benton Harbor, MI 49022
Prgm Dir: Deborah Burch, CDA RDA MS
Tel: 616 927-8100, Ext 5100   *Fax:* 616 927-8186
E-mail: burch@lakemichigancollege.edu

Wayne County Community College District
Dental Assisting Prgm
8551 Greenfield, Rm 308A
Detroit, MI 48228
www.wcccd.edu
Prgm Dir: Pamela Zarb, CDA RDA RDH MA LPC
Tel: 313 943-4045   *Fax:* 313 943-4025
E-mail: pzarb1@wcccd.edu

Mott Community College
Dental Assisting Prgm
1401 E Court St
Flint, MI 48503
Prgm Dir: Darlene Boersema, MA
Tel: 810 762-0496   *Fax:* 810 232-8874
E-mail: csmith@mcc.edu

Grand Rapids Community College
Dental Assisting Prgm
143 Bostwick St NE
Grand Rapids, MI 49503
Prgm Dir: Eve Sidney
Tel: 616 234-4240   *Fax:* 616 234-4317
E-mail: bvliem@grcc.edu

Northwestern Michigan College
Dental Assisting Prgm
1701 E Front St
Traverse City, MI 49686
Prgm Dir: Sallie Donovan, MS
Tel: 231 995-1240   *Fax:* 231 995-1950
E-mail: sdonovan@nmc.edu

Delta College
Dental Assisting Prgm
1961 Delta Rd
University Center, MI 48710
Prgm Dir: Pamela Smith, CDA RDA MAT
Tel: 989 686-9565, Ext 9565   *Fax:* 989 686-8736
E-mail: pamelasmith@delta.edu

Minnesota

Northwest Technical College - Bemidji
Dental Assisting Prgm
905 Grant Ave SE
Bemidji, MN 56601
www.ntcmn.edu
Prgm Dir: Julie Dokken, RDA CDA
Tel: 218 333-6657   *Fax:* 218 333-6694
E-mail: julie.dokken@ntcmn.edu

Central Lakes College
Dental Assisting Prgm
501 W College Dr
Brainerd, MN 56401
Prgm Dir: LeAnn Schoenle
Tel: 218 855-8106, Ext 8106   *Fax:* 218 855-8220
E-mail: lschoenl@clcmn.edu

Minnesota West Comm & Tech College
Dental Assisting Prgm
1011 First St W
Canby, MN 56220
Prgm Dir: Daniel Prust, DDS MS
Tel: 507 223-7252, Ext 139   *Fax:* 507 223-5291
E-mail: danp@cb.mnwest.mnscu.edu

Herzing College - Lakeland Academy Division
Dental Assisting Prgm
5700 W Broadway Ave
Crystal, MN 55428
http://herzing.edu
Prgm Dir: Linda R Boyum, CDA RDA
Tel: 763 231-3177   *Fax:* 763 535-9205
E-mail: lboyum@mpls.herzing.edu

Hennepin Technical College
Dental Assisting Prgm
13100 College View Dr
Eden Prairie, MN 55347
Prgm Dir: Susan Thaemert, BS
Tel: 763 995-1593
E-mail: susan.thaemert@hennepintech.edu

Hibbing Community College
Dental Assisting Prgm
1515 E 25th St
Hibbing, MN 55747
www.hcc.mnscu.edu
Prgm Dir: Anne Badanjak, MEd
Tel: 218 262-7242   *Fax:* 218 262-7257
E-mail: annebadanjak@hibbing.edu

Minneapolis Community & Technical Coll
Dental Assisting Prgm
1501 Hennepin Ave S
Minneapolis, MN 55403
Prgm Dir: Kathleen Lapham
Tel: 612 659-6071   *Fax:* 612 659-6825
E-mail: kathleen.lapham@minneapolis.edu

Minnesota State Comm & Tech Coll - Moorhead
Dental Assisting Prgm
1900 28th Ave S
Moorhead, MN 56560-4899
www.minnesota.edu
Prgm Dir: Thomas Boe, DDS MBA
Tel: 218 299-6819, Ext 6819   *Fax:* 218 299-6532
E-mail: thomas.boe@minnesota.edu

South Central College
Dental Assisting Prgm
1920 Lee Blvd
North Mankato, MN 56003
Prgm Dir: Karon Metz, CDA RDA RF BS
Tel: 507 389-5846   *Fax:* 507 389-5850
E-mail: karon.metz@southcentral.edu

Rochester Community & Technical College
Dental Assisting Prgm
851 30th Ave SE
Rochester, MN 55904
Prgm Dir: Bonnie Crawford, CDA RDA
Tel: 507 280-3149   *Fax:* 507 280-3180
E-mail: Bonnie.Crawford@roch.edu

Dakota County Technical College
Dental Assisting Prgm
1300 145th St E
Rosemount, MN 55068
www.dctc.edu
Prgm Dir: Diana Sullivan, MS
Tel: 651 423-8483   *Fax:* 651 423-8775
E-mail: diana.sullivan@dctc.edu

St Cloud Technical College
Dental Assisting Prgm
1540 Northway Dr
St Cloud, MN 56303-1240
www.sctc.edu
Prgm Dir: Rita Peterson, BS CDA RDA
Tel: 320 308-5031   *Fax:* 320 308-5055
E-mail: rpeterson@sctc.edu

Century College
Dental Assisting Prgm
3300 Century Ave N
White Bear Lake, MN 55110
Prgm Dir: Arlene Retzer, CDA RDA
Tel: 651 779-5778   *Fax:* 651 799-5779
E-mail: a.retzer@century.mnscu.edu

Mississippi

Pearl River Community College
Dental Assisting Prgm
5448 US Hwy 49 S
Hattiesburg, MS 39401
http://www/prcc/edu
Prgm Dir: Emily Addison, CDA BS
Tel: 601 544-5483   *Fax:* 601 545-5548
E-mail: eaddison@prcc.edu

Hinds Community College
Dental Assisting Prgm
1750 Chadwick Dr
Jackson, MS 39204
Prgm Dir: Richard Gavant, DMD
Tel: 601 371-3526   *Fax:* 601 371-3703
E-mail: rgavant@hindscc.edu

Missouri

Nichols Career Center
Dental Assisting Prgm
605 Union St
Jefferson City, MO 65101
www.jcps.k12.mo.us
Prgm Dir: Kathy Jeffries, CDA EFDA BA MBA
Tel: 573 659-3112   *Fax:* 573 659-3154
E-mail: kathy.jeffries@jcps.k12.mo.us

Concorde Career College - Kansas City
Dental Assisting Prgm
3239 Broadway Blvd
Kansas City, MO 64111
http://ww.concorde.edu
Prgm Dir: Robert Pruitt, CDA
Tel: 816 531-5223   *Fax:* 816 756-3231
E-mail: rpruitt@concorde.edu

Metropolitan Community College - Penn Valley
Dental Assisting Prgm
3201 SW Trafficway
Kansas City, MO 64111-2764
www.mcckc.edu
Prgm Dir: Rose Gupta, BDS
Tel: 816 759-4237   *Fax:* 816 759-4553
E-mail: Rose.Gupta@mcckc.edu

Ozarks Technical Community College
Dental Assisting Prgm
1001 E Chestnut Expressway
Springfield, MO 65802
Prgm Dir: Kelly Tillery, MEd RDH CDA
Tel: 417 895-7124, Ext 7124   *Fax:* 417 895-7057
E-mail: tilleryk@otc.edu

Missouri College
Dental Assisting Prgm
10121 Manchester Rd
St Louis, MO 63122-1583
Prgm Dir: Patricia Frank
Tel: 314 909-5568

St Louis Community College - Forest Park
Dental Assisting Prgm
5600 Oakland Ave
St Louis, MO 63110-1393
Prgm Dir: Mary Ann Taylor, CDA MSN
Tel: 314 644-9332   *Fax:* 314 951-9490
E-mail: mtaylor@stlcc.edu

Montana

Montana State Univ - Great Falls Coll of Tech
Dental Assisting Prgm
2100 16th Ave S
Great Falls, MT 59405
www.msugf.edu
Prgm Dir: Carmen Perry, BS MEd CDA
Tel: 406 771-4354   *Fax:* 406 771-4317
E-mail: cperry@msugf.edu

Salish Kootenai College
Dental Assisting Prgm
Box 70
52000 Hwy 93
Pablo, MT 59855
www.skc.edu
Prgm Dir: Donna Kotyk, RDH CDA MA
Tel: 406 275-4912   *Fax:* 406 275-4816
E-mail: donna_kotyk@skc.edu

Nebraska

Central Community College
Dental Assisting Prgm
PO Box 1024
Hastings, NE 68902-1024
www.cccneb.edu
Prgm Dir: Marie Cecil, CDA MAT
Tel: 402 461-2467   *Fax:* 402 460-2138
E-mail: mcecil@cccneb.edu

Southeast Community College
Dental Assisting Prgm
8800 O St
Lincoln, NE 68520-1299
Prgm Dir: Susan Asher, CDA BS
Tel: 402 437-2740   *Fax:* 402 437-2404
E-mail: sasher@southeast.edu

Mid-Plains Community College
Dental Assisting Prgm
1101 Halligan Dr
North Platte, NE 69101
Prgm Dir: Rose White, AAS
Tel: 308 535-3650   *Fax:* 308 534-5767
E-mail: whiter@mpcc.edu

Metropolitan Community College
Dental Assisting Prgm
PO Box 3777
Omaha, NE 68103-0777
Prgm Dir: Karen Finley, CDA BGS
Tel: 402 738-4676   *Fax:* 402 738-4554
E-mail: kfinley@mccneb.edu

Vatterott College - Omaha Campus
Dental Assisting Prgm
11818 I St
Omaha, NE 68137
Prgm Dir: Wendy Simon
Tel: 402 891-9411, Ext 142
E-mail: wsimon@vatterott-college.edu

Nevada

College of Southern Nevada
Dental Assisting Prgm
6375 W Charleston Blvd
Las Vegas, NV 89146
www.ccsn.nevada.edu
Prgm Dir: Carole Brew, BS
Tel: 702 651-5851   *Fax:* 702 651-7453
E-mail: carole.brew@csn.edu

Truckee Meadows Community College
Dental Assisting Prgm
7000 Dandini Blvd
Reno, NV 89512-3999
Prgm Dir: Julie Muhle, CDA AA AAS
Tel: 775 673-7125   *Fax:* 775 673-7034
E-mail: jmuhle@tmcc.edu

New Hampshire

New Hampshire Technical Institute
Dental Assisting Prgm
31 College Dr
Concord, NH 03301-7412
www.nhti.edu
Prgm Dir: Lynnea Adams, CDA BA
Tel: 603 271-7149   *Fax:* 603 271-7182
E-mail: ladams@nhctc.edu

New Jersey

Camden County College
Dental Assisting Prgm
PO Box 200
Blackwood, NJ 08012
www.camdencc.edu
Prgm Dir: Sandra Rodier, CDA RDA BSHS
Tel: 856 227-7200, Ext 4471   *Fax:* 856 374-5048
E-mail: srodier@camdencc.edu

Cumberland County Technical Education Center
Dental Assisting Prgm
601 Bridgeton Ave
Bridgeton, NJ 08302
Prgm Dir: Judy Zirkle, CDA RDA MEd
Tel: 856 451-9000, Ext 346   *Fax:* 856 451-1118
E-mail: JZirkle@cumberland.tec.nj.us

Cape May County Technical Institute
Dental Assisting Prgm
188 Crest Haven Rd
Cape May Courthouse, NJ 08210
Prgm Dir: Candida J Ditzler, CDA RDA
Tel: 609 465-2161, Ext 432   *Fax:* 609 465-4962
E-mail: cditzler@capemaytech.com

The Institute for Health Education
Dental Assisting Prgm
7 Spielman Rd
Fairfield, NJ 07004
Prgm Dir: Theresa Lennon, CDA RDA
Tel: 973 808-1110   *Fax:* 973 808-1130
E-mail: Healthcareer@gmail.com

Atlantic County Institute of Technology
Dental Assisting Prgm
5080 Atlantic Ave
Mays Landing, NJ 08330
www.acitech.org
Prgm Dir: Stefanie J White, CDA RDA LRT(D) RDH BS
Tel: 609 625-2249, Ext 1316   *Fax:* 609 625-8622
E-mail: swhite@acitech.org
Notes: Currently inactive

Univ of Medicine & Dent of New Jersey
Dental Assisting Prgm
1776 Raritan Rd
Scotch Plains, NJ 07076
www.shrp.umdnj.edu
Prgm Dir: Carolyn Breen, EdD CDA RDA RDH
Tel: 908 889-2419   *Fax:* 908 889-2477
E-mail: breen@umdnj.edu

Technical Institute of Camden County
Cosponsor: Camden County Technical Schools
Dental Assisting Prgm
343 Berlin-Cross Keys Rd
Sicklerville, NJ 08081-9709
www.ccts.tec.nj.us/
Prgm Dir: Susan Michaleski, BA CDA CDPMA
Tel: 609 767-7000, Ext 5553   *Fax:* 609 767-6625
E-mail: smichaleski@ccts.tec.nj.us

Berdan Institute
Dental Assisting Prgm
201 Willowbrook Blvd 2nd Fl
Wayne, NJ 07470
www.berdaninstitute.com
Prgm Dir: Helene Pizzuta, CDA RDA
Tel: 973 837-1818, Ext 212   *Fax:* 973 837-1840
E-mail: hpizzuta@edaff.com

New Mexico

Central New Mexico Community College
Dental Assisting Prgm
525 Buena Vista SE
Albuquerque, NM 87106
www.tvi.edu
Prgm Dir: Melanie Upshaw, BSDH CDA
Tel: 505 224-4111, Ext 5247   *Fax:* 505 224-5201
E-mail: mupshaw@cnm.edu

University of New Mexico - Gallup
Dental Assisting Prgm
200 College Rd
Gallup, NM 87301
www.gallup.unm.edu
Prgm Dir: Jean Martinez-Welles, MS CDA
Tel: 505 863-7515   *Fax:* 505 863-7513
E-mail: jmwelles@unm.edu

Dona Ana Community College
Dental Assisting Prgm
3400 S Espina St
Las Cruces, NM 88007
http://dabcc.nmsu.edu
Prgm Dir: Martha McCaslin
Tel: 505 527-7653
E-mail: mmccasli@nmsu.edu

Santa Fe Community College
Dental Assisting Prgm
6401 Richards Ave, Rm 421B
Santa Fe, NM 87509
www.sfccnm.edu/dental
Prgm Dir: Aamna Nayyar, BSc BDS
Tel: 505 428-1258, Ext 258   *Fax:* 505 428-1327
E-mail: anayyar@sfccnm.edu

New York

SUNY Educational Opportunity Center
Dental Assisting Prgm
465 Washington St
Buffalo, NY 14203
Prgm Dir: Susan Camizzi
Tel: 716 849-6727, Ext 181   *Fax:* 716 849-6755

Columbia University
Dental Assisting Prgm
College of Dental Medicine
630 W 168th St
New York, NY 10032
http://dental.columbia.edu/odma/
Prgm Dir: Dennis A Mitchell, DDS MPH
Tel: 212 342-3716   *Fax:* 212 305-1034
E-mail: DML48@columbia.edu

Monroe Community College
Dental Assisting Prgm
1000 E Henrietta Rd
Rochester, NY 14623-5780
Prgm Dir: David B Lawrence, DDS
Tel: 585 292-2761   *Fax:* 585 424-5703
E-mail: dlawrence@monroecc.edu

North Carolina

Asheville-Buncombe Technical Comm College
Dental Assisting Prgm
340 Victoria Rd
Asheville, NC 28801
www.abtech.edu
Prgm Dir: Shaun Tate, RDH MAEd
Tel: 828 254-1921, Ext 271   *Fax:* 828 281-9792
E-mail: state@abtech.edu

University of North Carolina - Chapel Hill
Dental Assisting Prgm
CB 7450
Chapel Hill, NC 27599-7450
Prgm Dir: Ethel Campbell, RDH MS
Tel: 919 966-2777   *Fax:* 919 966-6761
E-mail: ethel_campbell@dentistry.unc.edu

Central Piedmont Community College
Dental Assisting Prgm
3210 CPCC West Campus Dr
Charlotte, NC 28208
Prgm Dir: Jane Lavin, BSDH RDH
Tel: 704 330-4614   *Fax:* 704 330-4641
E-mail: jane_lavin@cpcc.cc.nc.us

Fayetteville Technical Community College
Dental Assisting Prgm
2201 Hull Rd
PO Box 35236
Fayetteville, NC 28303
www.faytechcc.edu
Prgm Dir: Angela Simmons, CDA BS
Tel: 910 678-9858   *Fax:* 910 678-8500
E-mail: simmonsa@faytechcc.edu

Wayne Community College
Dental Assisting Prgm
3000 Wayne Memorial Dr
Goldsboro, NC 27533
www.waynecc.edu
Prgm Dir: Christie Smith, CDA BS
Tel: 919 735-5152, Ext 287   *Fax:* 919 581-1013
E-mail: christie@waynecc.edu

Alamance Community College
Dental Assisting Prgm
PO Box 8000
Graham, NC 27253-8000
www.alamance.cc.nc.us
Prgm Dir: Janelle Christopher, BS CDA
Tel: 336 506-4162   *Fax:* 336 578-7047
E-mail: christopherj@alamance.cc.nc.us

Coastal Carolina Community College
Dental Assisting Prgm
444 Western Blvd
Jacksonville, NC 28546
Prgm Dir: Elise Beall, BS
Tel: 910 938-6276   *Fax:* 910 455-4989
E-mail: bealle@coastal.cc.nc.us

Guilford Technical Community College
Dental Assisting Prgm
PO Box 309
601 High Point Rd
Jamestown, NC 27282
www.gtcc.edu
Prgm Dir: Lynda Snider, CDA BS
Tel: 336 334-4822, Ext 2212   *Fax:* 336 819-2041
E-mail: lfsnider@gtcc.edu

Western Piedmont Community College
Dental Assisting Prgm
1001 Burkemont Ave
Morganton, NC 28655
www.wp.cc.nc.us
Prgm Dir: Tammy Glover, CDA RDH
Tel: 828 438-6129   *Fax:* 828 430-7183
E-mail: tglover@wp.cc.nc.us

Wake Technical Community College
Dental Assisting Prgm
9101 Fayetteville Rd
Raleigh, NC 27603-5696
Prgm Dir: Trudy Clark, BS
Tel: 919 212-3811   *Fax:* 919 250-4329
E-mail: tsclark@waketech.edu

Rowan-Cabarrus Community College
Dental Assisting Prgm
PO Box 1595
1333 Jake Alexander Blvd
Salisbury, NC 28145-1595
Prgm Dir: Linda Kamp, CDA BS
Tel: 704 637-0760, Ext 308   *Fax:* 704 642-0750
E-mail: kampl@rowancabarrus.edu

Wilkes Community College
Dental Assisting Prgm
PO Box 120
Wilkesboro, NC 28697-0120
www.wilkescc.edu
Prgm Dir: Martha Townes, CDA RDH MEd
Tel: 336 838-6253   *Fax:* 336 838-6255
E-mail: martha.townes@wilkescc.edu

Martin Commuity College
Dental Assisting Prgm
1161 Kehukee Park Rd
Williamston, NC 27892-9988
www.martincc.edu
Prgm Dir: Susan Cutler
Tel: 252 792-1521, Ext 299   *Fax:* 252 792-4425
E-mail: scutler@martincc.edu

Cape Fear Community College
Dental Assisting Prgm
411 N Front St
Wilmington, NC 28401-3993
http://cfcc.edu
Prgm Dir: Nancy Fetter, CDA RDH BS BEd
Tel: 910 362-7416   *Fax:* 910 362-7418
E-mail: nfetter@cfcc.edu

Forsyth Technical Community College
Dental Assisting Prgm
2100 Silas Creek Pkwy
Winston-Salem, NC 27103
Prgm Dir: Jannette Whisenhunt, PhD
Tel: 336 734-7414   *Fax:* 336 734-7444
E-mail: jwhisenhunt@forsythtech.edu

North Dakota

North Dakota State College of Science
Dental Assisting Prgm
800 N 6th St
Wahpeton, ND 58076
Prgm Dir: Susan Swanson, DDS
Tel: 701 671-2333   *Fax:* 701 671-2570
E-mail: Susan.Swanson@ndscs.edu

Ohio

Polaris Career Center
Dental Assisting Prgm
7285 Old Oak Blvd
Middleburg Heights, OH 44130-3375
www.polaris.edu
Prgm Dir: Kathy Becker, CDA EFDA
Tel: 440 891-7600   *Fax:* 440 243-3952
E-mail: kbecker@polaris.edu

Jefferson Community College
Dental Assisting Prgm
4000 Sunset Blvd
Steubenville, OH 43952
www.jcc.edu
Prgm Dir: Donna Robinson, BA CDA EFDA
Tel: 740 264-5591, Ext 164   *Fax:* 740 264-9504
E-mail: drobinson@jcc.edu

Choffin Career & Technical Center
Dental Assisting Prgm
200 E Wood St
Youngstown, OH 44501
Prgm Dir: Paula J Oliver, CDA CDPMA CODA
Tel: 330 744-8749   *Fax:* 330 744-8749
E-mail: natasha1059@aol.com

Oklahoma

Rose State College
Dental Assisting Prgm
6420 SE 15th St
Midwest City, OK 73110
www.rose.edu
Prgm Dir: Janet Turley, RDH CDA MEd
Tel: 405 733-7337   *Fax:* 405 736-0389
E-mail: jturley@rose.edu

Moore Norman Technology Center
Dental Assisting Prgm
4701 12th Ave NW
Norman, OK 73069
www.mntechnology.com
Prgm Dir: Pat Trent, RDH BS CDA
Tel: 405 364-5763, Ext 6523   *Fax:* 405 447-6289
E-mail: ptrent@mntechnology.com

Metro Technology Centers
Dental Assisting Prgm
1720 Springlake Dr
Oklahoma City, OK 73111
Prgm Dir: Erica Hannah
Tel: 405 605-4613   *Fax:* 405 424-9403
E-mail: ehannah@metrotech.org

Oregon

Linn-Benton Community College
Dental Assisting Prgm
6500 SW Pacific Blvd
Albany, OR 97321
http://linnbenton.edu
Prgm Dir: Sheri Billetter, CDA EFDA MADAA
Tel: 541 917-4496   *Fax:* 541 917-4508
E-mail: billets@linnbenton.edu

Central Oregon Community College
Dental Assisting Prgm
2600 NW College Way
Bend, OR 97701
Prgm Dir: Deb Davies, RDH AAS
Tel: 541 330-4368   *Fax:* 541 317-3064
E-mail: ddavies@cocc.edu

Lane Community College
Dental Assisting Prgm
4000 E 30th Ave
Eugene, OR 97405
Prgm Dir: Sandra Stice, COA
Tel: 541 463-5638   *Fax:* 541 463-5616
E-mail: stices@lanecc.edu

Blue Mountain Community College
Dental Assisting Prgm
2411 NW Carden
PO Box 100
Pendleton, OR 97801
www.bluecc.edu
Prgm Dir: Crystal D Patton-Doherty, CDA EFDA BS
Tel: 541 278-5876   *Fax:* 541 278-5874
E-mail: cpatton@bluecc.edu

Concorde Career Institute - Portland
Dental Assisting Prgm
1425 NE Irving St, Bldg 300
Portland, OR 97232
Prgm Dir: Tracy Cook, BS CDA EFDA EFODA
Tel: 503 281-4181, Ext 130   *Fax:* 503 281-6739
E-mail: tcook@concorde.edu

Portland Community College
Dental Assisting Prgm
PO Box 19000
Portland, OR 97280-0990
www.pcc.edu
Prgm Dir: Josette Beach, RDH MS
Tel: 503 977-4235   *Fax:* 503 977-8300
E-mail: jbeach@pcc.edu

Chemeketa Community College
Dental Assisting Prgm
4000 Lancaster Dr NE
PO Box 14007
Salem, OR 97309-7070
Prgm Dir: Joyce Vaughan
Tel: 503 399-5265   *Fax:* 503 399-5496
E-mail: joycev@chemeketa.edu

Pennsylvania

Harcum College
Dental Assisting Prgm
750 Montgomery Ave
Bryn Mawr, PA 19010
Prgm Dir: Dorothea Cavallucci, MS
Tel: 610 526-6029   *Fax:* 610 526-6182
E-mail: dcavallucci@harcum.edu

Harrisburg Area Community College
Dental Assisting Prgm
One HACC Dr
Harrisburg, PA 17110-2999
Prgm Dir: Debra Nickey, CDA RDH MAEd
Tel: 717 221-1731   *Fax:* 717 780-1110
E-mail: danickey@hacc.edu

Manor College
Dental Assisting Prgm
Expanded Functions Dental Assististing Program
700 Fox Chase Rd
Jenkintown, PA 19046-3399
www.manor.edu/.com
Prgm Dir: Diane Meehan, CDA EFDA
Tel: 215 885-2360, Ext 288   *Fax:* 215 885-6084
E-mail: dmeehan@manor.edu

**Commonwealth Tech Inst at
Hiram G Andrews Ctr**
Dental Assisting Prgm
727 Goucher St
Johnstown, PA 15905
Prgm Dir: James Howanek, DDS
Tel: 814 255-8281   *Fax:* 814 255-3406
E-mail: jhowanek@state.pa.us

Luzerne County Community College
Dental Assisting Prgm
1333 S Prospect St
Nanticoke, PA 18634-3899
www.luzerne.edu
Prgm Dir: Cathryn M Brown, CDA RDH MEd
Tel: 570 740-0447   *Fax:* 570 740-0265
E-mail: CBrown@luzerne.edu

Bradford School - Pittsburgh
Dental Assisting Prgm
125 W Station Square Dr, Ste 129
Pittsburgh, PA 15219
Prgm Dir: Linda DeFalle, MEd
Tel: 412 319-6361   *Fax:* 412 471-6714
E-mail: ldefalle@bradfordpittsburgh.edu

Westmoreland County Community College
Dental Assisting Prgm
145 Pavilion Ln
Youngwood, PA 15697-1895
Prgm Dir: Angela Rinchuse, RDH MEd
Tel: 724 925-4163   *Fax:* 724 925-5808
E-mail: rinchusea@wccc-pa.edu

Puerto Rico

University of Puerto Rico
Dental Assisting Prgm
Medical Sciences Campus
PO Box 365067
San Juan, PR 00936-5067
Prgm Dir: Angel Rafael Aja, DDS
Tel: 787 758-2525, Ext 1157   *Fax:* 787 751-3061
E-mail: angela@cprs.rcm.upr.edu

Rhode Island

Community College of Rhode Island
Dental Assisting Prgm
1762 Louisquisset Pike
Lincoln, RI 02865
www.ccri.edu
Prgm Dir: Donna Medas Patton, CDA RDH MEd
Tel: 401 333-7220   *Fax:* 401 333-7146
E-mail: dmedaspatton@ccri.edu

South Carolina

Aiken Technical College
Dental Assisting Prgm
PO Drawer 696
Aiken, SC 29802
Prgm Dir: Amelia Capers, BS
Tel: 803 593-9231   *Fax:* 803 593-6526
E-mail: capersa@atc.edu

Trident Technical College
Dental Assisting Prgm
PO Box 118067
Charleston, SC 29423-8067
www.tridenttech.edu
Prgm Dir: Barbara Jarrett, MS
Tel: 843 574-6294   *Fax:* 843 574-6585
E-mail: Barbara.Jarrett@tridenttech.edu

Midlands Technical College
Dental Assisting Prgm
Expanded Duty Dental Assisting
PO Box 2408
Columbia, SC 29202
Prgm Dir: Maria Marchant, BHS
Tel: 803 822-3453   *Fax:* 803 822-3079
E-mail: marchantm@midlandstech.edu

Horry - Georgetown Technical College
Dental Assisting Prgm
2050 Hwy 501 E, Box 261966
Conway, SC 29528-6066
www.hgtc.edu
Prgm Dir: Pamela Moyers, CDA AS
Tel: 843 349-5331   *Fax:* 843 349-7576
E-mail: pamela.moyers@hgtc.edu

Florence-Darlington Technical College
Dental Assisting Prgm
PO Box 100548
Florence, SC 29501-0548
www.fdtc.edu
Prgm Dir: J Richard Moore, DMD
Tel: 843 661-8223   *Fax:* 843 292-0851
E-mail: richard.moore@fdtc.edu

Greenville Technical College
Dental Assisting Prgm
South Pleasanburg Ave
PO Box 5616 - Station B
Greenville, SC 29606-5616
Prgm Dir: Cynthia Baker, DDS
Tel: 864 250-8000, Ext 8074   *Fax:* 864 250-8588
E-mail: cynthia.baker@gvltec.edu

Tri-County Technical College
Dental Assisting Prgm
PO Box 587
Pendleton, SC 29670
www.tctc.edu
Prgm Dir: Donna Shannon, CDA RDH BS
Tel: 864 646-1347, Ext 1347 *Fax:* 864 646-1892
E-mail: dshanno1@tctc.edu

York Technical College
Dental Assisting Prgm
Expanded Duty DA Program
452 S Anderson Rd
Rock Hill, SC 29730
Prgm Dir: Kathleen Peter, RDH MHA
Tel: 803 981-7068 *Fax:* 803 327-8059
E-mail: kpeter@yorktech.com

Spartanburg Community College
Dental Assisting Prgm
PO Drawer 4386, Highway I-85
Spartanburg, SC 29305-4386
Prgm Dir: Kim Golightly
Tel: 864 592-4872 *Fax:* 864 591-3881
E-mail: golightlyk@sccsc.edu

South Dakota

Lake Area Technical Institute
Dental Assisting Prgm
230 11th St NE
Watertown, SD 57201
http://sweb.lakeareatech.edu/dental/
Prgm Dir: Rhonda Bradberry, CDA
Tel: 605 882-5284, Ext 214 *Fax:* 605 882-6299
E-mail: bradberr@lati.tec.sd.us

Tennessee

Chattanooga State Technical Comm College
Dental Assisting Prgm
4501 Amnicola Hwy
Chattanooga, TN 37406-1097
Prgm Dir: Karen Castleberry, CDA RDA BS
Tel: 423 697-4474 *Fax:* 423 697-2629
E-mail: karen.castleberry@chattanoogastate.edu

Tennessee Technology Center - Dickson
Dental Assisting Prgm
740 Hwy 46 South
Dickson, TN 37055
www.ttcdickson.edu
Prgm Dir: Vanessa Pilkinton, CDA RDA
Tel: 615 441-6220, Ext 121 *Fax:* 615 441-6223
E-mail: vanessa.pilkinton@ttcdickson.edu

Northeast State Technical Comm College
Dental Assisting Prgm
1000 W Jason Witten Way
Elizabethton, TN 37643
www.northeaststate.edu
Prgm Dir: Paulette Kehm-Yelton, MPA CDA EFDA
Tel: 423 547-4910 *Fax:* 423 543-2266
E-mail: pkyelton@NortheastState.edu

Volunteer State Community College
Dental Assisting Prgm
Nashville Pike
Gallatin, TN 37066
Prgm Dir: Desiree Sutphen, CDA RDA BA
Tel: 615 452-8600, Ext 3439 *Fax:* 615 230-3344
E-mail: Desiree.Sutphen@volstate.edu

Tennessee Technology Center - Knoxville
Dental Assisting Prgm
1100 Liberty St
Knoxville, TN 37919
Prgm Dir: Mary Vaughn, BS CDA RDA
Tel: 865 546-5567, Ext 131 *Fax:* 865 971-4474
E-mail: mvaughn@knoxville.tec.tn.us

Concorde Career College - Memphis
Dental Assisting Prgm
5100 Poplar Ave, Ste 132
Memphis, TN 38137
Prgm Dir: Shay Ashford
Tel: 901 761-9494 *Fax:* 901 761-3293
E-mail: sashford@concorde.edu

Tennessee Technology Center - Memphis
Dental Assisting Prgm
550 Alabama Ave
Memphis, TN 38105-3604
www.ttcmemphis.edu
Prgm Dir: Bettie J Brooks
Tel: 901 543-6143 *Fax:* 901 543-6126
E-mail: bettie.brooks@ttcmemphis.edu

Tennessee Technology Center - Murfreesboro
Dental Assisting Prgm
1303 Old Fort Pkwy
Murfreesboro, TN 37129
www.ttcmurfreesboro.edu
Prgm Dir: Suzanne Dowdle, CDA RDA
Tel: 615 898-8010, Ext 133 *Fax:* 615 893-4194
E-mail: sdowdle@ttcmurfreesboro.edu

Texas

Del Mar College
Dental Assisting Prgm
101 Baldwin Blvd
Corpus Christi, TX 78404-3897
www.delmar.edu/da
Prgm Dir: David G Arreguin, DDS
Tel: 361 698-2859 *Fax:* 361 698-2811
E-mail: darreguin@delmar.edu

Grayson County College
Dental Assisting Prgm
6101 Grayson Dr
Box 48
Denison, TX 75020-8299
Prgm Dir: Gwen Kirk, CDA AS BBM RDA
Tel: 903 463-8780
E-mail: kirkgw@grayson.edu

El Paso Community College
Dental Assisting Prgm
PO Box 20500
El Paso, TX 79998
Prgm Dir: Sharon Dickinson, CDA CDPMA RDA
Tel: 915 831-4065 *Fax:* 915 831-4445
E-mail: sdickins@epcc.edu

Texas State Technical College - Harlingen
Dental Assisting Prgm
1902 N Loop 499
Harlingen, TX 78550-3697
Prgm Dir: Robert Bennett, DMD
Tel: 956 364-4690 *Fax:* 956 364-5148
E-mail: bob.bennett@harlingen.tstc.edu

Houston Community College
Dental Assisting Prgm
1900 Pressler Dr
Houston, TX 77030
www.hccs.edu
Prgm Dir: Rosalva Perez, BS CDA RDA
Tel: 713 718-7350 *Fax:* 713 718-7608
E-mail: rosie.perez@hccs.edu

Lamar State College - Orange
Dental Assisting Prgm
410 Front St
Orange, TX 77630
www.lsco.edu
Prgm Dir: Carolyn Flippen, CDA RDA
Tel: 409 882-3022 *Fax:* 409 882-5000
E-mail: Carolyn.Flippen@lsco.edu

San Antonio College
Dental Assisting Prgm
1300 San Pedro Ave, NTC 125
San Antonio, TX 78212-4299
Prgm Dir: Stella Lovato, MA Ed MS
Tel: 210 785-6184 *Fax:* 210 733-2926
E-mail: slovato@accd.edu

882d Training Group
Dental Assisting Prgm
917 Missile Rd
Sheppard AFB, TX 76311
Prgm Dir: Thomas Grimm, DDS
Tel: 940 676-6932 *Fax:* 940 676-8104
E-mail: thomas.grimm@sheppard.af.mil

Texas State Technical College - Waco
Dental Assisting Prgm
3801 Campus Dr
Waco, TX 76705
http://waco.tstc.edu
Prgm Dir: Donna Estes, AAS
Tel: 254 867-4864 *Fax:* 254 867-2239
E-mail: donna.estes@tstc.edu

Utah

Davis Applied Technology College
Dental Assisting Prgm
550 East 300 South
Kaysville, UT 84037
Prgm Dir: Cathleen Turnbow, CDA
Tel: 801 593-2349 *Fax:* 801 593-7849
E-mail: turnboc@datc.net

Bridgerland Applied Technology College
Dental Assisting Prgm
1301 West 600 North
Logan, UT 84321
Prgm Dir: Wendi Wilde, ASC
Tel: 435 750-3121 *Fax:* 435 750-2016
E-mail: wwilde@bridgerlandatc.org

Ogden-Weber Applied Technology College
Dental Assisting Prgm
200 N Washington Blvd
Ogden, UT 84404-6704
Prgm Dir: Brenda Fell, CDA CDPMA AS
Tel: 801 627-8444 *Fax:* 801 395-3703
E-mail: fellb@owatc.edu

Careers Unlimited
Dental Assisting Prgm
575 E University Pkwy, Ste 163
Orem, UT 84097
Prgm Dir: Krista McClure
Tel: 801 787-3223

AmeriTech College
Dental Assisting Prgm
1675 N Freedom Blvd Ste 3B
Provo, UT 84604
www.ameritech.edu
Prgm Dir: Lynn Tyler, BS CDA
Tel: 801 377-2900, Ext 109 *Fax:* 801 375-3077
E-mail: ltyler@ameritech.edu

Provo College
Dental Assisting Prgm
1450 W 820 N
Provo, UT 84604
www.provocollege.com
Prgm Dir: Judy Simpson, AAS
Tel: 801 818-8915 *Fax:* 801 375-9728
E-mail: judys@provocollege.edu

Vermont

Center for Technology - Essex
Dental Assisting Prgm
3 Educational Dr
Essex Junction, VT 05452
www.go-cte.org
Prgm Dir: Beth Ladd, CDA EFDA
Tel: 802 879-8153   *Fax:* 802 879-5593
E-mail: bladd@ccsuvt.org

Virginia

Tidewater Tech
Dental Assisting Prgm
7020 N Military Hwy
Norfolk, VA 23518-4202
Prgm Dir: Linda Hamilton
Tel: 757 853-2121   *Fax:* 757 852-9017

J Sargeant Reynolds Community College
Dental Assisting Prgm
PO Box 85622
Richmond, VA 23285-5622
www.jsr.vccs.edu
Prgm Dir: Nancy L Daniel, BS
Tel: 804 523-5380   *Fax:* 804 786-5298
E-mail: ndaniel@jsr.vccs.edu

Washington

Bellingham Technical College
Dental Assisting Prgm
3028 Lindbergh Ave
Bellingham, WA 98225
www.btc.ctc.edu
Prgm Dir: Jenny Shuler, CDA BS
Tel: 360 752-8408   *Fax:* 360 752-7208
E-mail: jshuler@btc.ctc.edu

Lake Washington Technical College
Dental Assisting Prgm
11605 132nd Ave NE
Kirkland, WA 98034
www.lwtc.ctc.edu/dental
Prgm Dir: Scarlet Kendrick, CDA MAOM
Tel: 425 739-8369   *Fax:* 425 739-8292
E-mail: scarlet.kendrick@lwtc.edu

Clover Park Technical College
Dental Assisting Prgm
4500 Steilacoom Blvd SW
Lakewood, WA 98498-4098
Prgm Dir: Roberta Wirth
Tel: 253 589-6023   *Fax:* 253 589-5866
E-mail: roberta.wirth@cptc.edu

South Puget Sound Community College
Dental Assisting Prgm
2011 Mottman Rd SW
Olympia, WA 98512-6292
www.spscc.ctc.edu
Prgm Dir: Joan Martin, CDA BA MAED
Tel: 360 596-5295   *Fax:* 360 596-5707
E-mail: jmartin@spscc.ctc.edu

Renton Technical College
Dental Assisting Prgm
3000 NE Fourth St
Renton, WA 98056
Prgm Dir: Kathy Leviton, BS CDA
Tel: 425 235-2352, Ext 5560   *Fax:* 425 235-2436
E-mail: kleviton@rtc.edu

Seattle Vocational Institute
Dental Assisting Prgm
2120 S Jackson St
Seattle, WA 98144
Prgm Dir: Jeanne Nichols, BA
Tel: 206 587-4930   *Fax:* 206 587-4949
E-mail: jnichols@sccd.ctc.edu

Spokane Community College
Dental Assisting Prgm
N 1810 Greene St, MS 2090
Spokane, WA 99207
Prgm Dir: Donna Phinney, MEd
Tel: 509 533-7300   *Fax:* 509 533-8621
E-mail: dphinney@scc.spokane.edu

Bates Technical College
Dental Assisting Prgm
1101 S Yakima Ave
Tacoma, WA 98405
www.bates.ctc.edu
Prgm Dir: Dave Dailey, Dean
Tel: 253 680-7212   *Fax:* 253 680-7211
E-mail: ddailey@bates.ctc.edu

West Virginia

Mercer County Technical Education Center
Dental Assisting Prgm
1397 Stafford Dr
Princeton, WV 24740
Prgm Dir: Bertha Robertson, CDA RDA
Tel: 304 425-9551, Ext 127   *Fax:* 304 425-0833

Wisconsin

Fox Valley Technical College
Dental Assisting Prgm
1825 N Bluemound Dr
Appleton, WI 54913
www.fvtc.edu
Prgm Dir: Harold Peaslee, CDA BA MS
Tel: 920 735-5666   *Fax:* 920 735-2582
E-mail: peaslee@fvtc.edu

Northeast Wisconsin Technical College
Dental Assisting Prgm
2740 W Mason St, PO Box 19042
Green Bay, WI 54307-9042
Prgm Dir: Carol Johnson, CDA BS
Tel: 920 498-5472, Ext 5472   *Fax:* 920 498-5673
E-mail: carol.johnson@nwtc.edu

Blackhawk Technical College
Dental Assisting Prgm
6004 Prairie Rd
PO Box 5009
Janesville, WI 53547-5009
Prgm Dir: Lois D Swanson, CDA RDH MS
Tel: 608 757-7732   *Fax:* 608 743-4407
E-mail: ldswanson@blackhawk.edu

Gateway Technical College
Dental Assisting Prgm
3520 30th Ave
Kenosha, WI 53144-1690
www.gtc.edu
Prgm Dir: Heidi Gottfried, BA CDA
Tel: 262 564-2544   *Fax:* 262 564-2299
E-mail: gottfriedh@gtc.edu

Western Technical College
Dental Assisting Prgm
304 N Sixth St, PO Box C-908
La Crosse, WI 54601
www.westerntc.edu
Prgm Dir: Sue Harpstreith
Tel: 608 785-9137   *Fax:* 608 785-9087
E-mail: harpstreiths@wwtc.edu

Dental Assistant

	Class Capacity	Begins	Length (months)	Award	Res. Tuition	Non-res. Tuition	Stipend	Offers:‡ 1	2	3	4
Alabama											
H Council Trenholm State Technical College (Montgomery)	30	Aug	12, 18	Cert, AAT	$4,320	$7,644					
James H Faulkner State Community College (Bay Minette)	30	Aug	12, 24	Cert, AAS	$5,859	$10,322				•	
Wallace State Community College (Hanceville)	30	Aug	12	Cert	$2,052	$4,104				•	
Arizona											
Phoenix College	24	Aug Jan	9, 24	Cert, AAS	$2,145	$0				•	
Arkansas											
Pulaski Technical College (North Little Rock)	26	Aug	9	Cert	$2,886	$4,641					
California											
Chaffey College (Rancho Cucamonga)	55	Every 8 wks	9, 18	Cert, AS	$954	$5,600	$4,000	•		•	
Citrus College (Glendora)	30	Sep Feb	9	Cert	$725	$4,500					
City College of San Francisco	36	Aug	10, 20	Cert, AS	$670	$4,790					
College of the Redwoods (Eureka)	24	Aug	9, 24	Cert, AS	$884	$6,222		•		•	
Cypress College	32	Aug	8	Cert	$1,279	$4,149					
Heald College - Concord Campus	24	Jan Apr Jul Oct	18	AAS	$10,800	$10,800		•		•	
Heald College - Stockton Campus	24	Jul	18	AAS	$24,000	$0		•			

*Data are shown only for programs that completed the 2007 AMA Survey of Health Professions Education Programs.
‡Key to Offers: 1: Evening or weekend classes; 2: Non-English instruction; 3: Cultural competence instruction; 4: Distance education component.

Dental Assistant

Dental Assistant

	Class Capacity	Begins	Length (months)	Award	Res. Tuition	Non-res. Tuition	Stipend	1	2	3	4
Pasadena City College	30	Aug	10	Cert	$650	$2,610				•	
Sacramento City College	30	Aug	11	Cert, AS	$540	$5,200					
San Diego Mesa College	24	Jun	10	Cert, AS	$900	$4,098					
Santa Rosa Junior College	30	Aug	11	Cert	$975	$5,317					
Colorado											
Front Range Comm College (Fort Collins)	24	Aug Jan	11	Cert	$3,315	$9,945		•			
Pikes Peak Community College (Colorado Springs)	30	Aug	11, 19	Cert, AAS	$3,816	$16,534		•			
Pueblo Community College	18	Aug	11, 24	Cert, AAS	$8,335	$17,380	$3,935			•	
Connecticut											
Eli Whitney Vocational Technical School (Hamden)	18	Aug	9	Cert	$2,750	$2,750					
Tunxis Community College (Farmington)	24	Aug	11	Cert	$3,000	$8,100		•		•	
Florida											
Broward Community College (Fort Lauderdale)	36	Aug	10	Cert	$3,500	$9,500					
Edison College (Fort Myers)	12	Aug	10	Cert	$2,545	$9,554					
Erwin Technical Center (Tampa)	14	Every 18 wks	12	Dipl	$2,238	$7,854					
Lorenzo Walker Institute of Technology (Naples)	16	Jun	14	Cert	$2,362	$8,900		•			
Manatee Technical Institute (Bradenton)	20	Aug	11, 15	Cert	$2,325	$4,700		•		•	
Orlando Tech	25	Aug Jan	10	Cert	$2,450	$0		•		•	
Palm Beach Community College (Lake Worth)	25	Aug	9	Cert	$2,500	$7,500				•	
Pinellas Tech Educ Ctr - St Petersburg	15	Quarterly	13	Cert	$2,349	$9,422					
Robert Morgan Educational Center (Miami)	20	Sep Jan Apr	12	Cert	$2,188	$7,660				•	
Santa Fe Community College (Gainesville)	30	Aug	10	Cert	$2,001	$8,007				•	
South Florida Community College (Avon Park)	12	Aug	11	Dipl	$4,500	$9,000				•	•
Traviss Career Center (Lakeland)	16	Aug	10	Cert	$2,313	$9,274					
Georgia											
Atlanta Technical College	25	Spring Fall quarters	15	Dipl, Cert	$3,265	$6,000					
Columbus Technical College	14	Jan Jul	15	Dipl	$2,821	$0					
Coosa Valley Technical College (Rockmart)	15	Jan	12	Dipl	$2,100	$4,200					
Medix School (Smyrna)	90	Every 5 wks	10	Dipl	$11,702	$11,702		•		•	
Middle Georgia Technical College (Warner Robins)	16	Winter quarter	12	Dipl	$1,636	$1,636					•
Savannah Technical College	25	Apr	12	Dipl	$1,116	$2,124					
Valdosta Technical College	14	Oct	12	Dipl	$1,856	$3,712				•	
Illinois											
Kaskaskia College (Centralia)	24	Aug	9	Cert	$4,189	$6,597	$1,000			•	
Lewis & Clark Community College (Godfrey)	30	Aug Jan	9	Cert	$3,315	$8,906				•	
Indiana											
Columbus Area Career Connection/Ivy Tech St	20	Aug	9	Cert	$3,276	$3,276					
Indiana University (Indianapolis)	35	Aug	10	Cert	$6,850	$18,904				•	•
Indiana University Northwest (Gary)	20	Aug	12	Cert	$5,077	$13,423				•	
Ivy Tech Community College - Anderson	20	Jan	12	Cert	$6,000	$9,000					
Kaplan College (Indianapolis)	30	Nov	11	Cert, DA	$12,000	$12,000		•			
University of Southern Indiana (Evansville)	24	Aug	9, 18	Cert, AS	$5,085	$12,442					
Iowa											
Hawkeye Community College (Waterloo)	24	Aug	11	Dipl	$5,236	$10,472					
Iowa Western Community College (Council Bluffs)	12	Aug	10	Dipl	$5,280	$7,464					
Marshalltown Community College	20	Aug	11	Dipl	$5,088	$7,200				•	•
Northeast Iowa Community College (Peosta)	25	Aug	11	Dipl	$5,824	$5,824				•	
Scott Community College (Bettendorf)	20	Aug	9	Dipl	$3,783	$5,655					
Vatterott College - Des Moines Campus		Every 10 wks	17	AOS	$24,974	$0				•	
Western Iowa Tech Community College (Sioux City)	40	Aug	9	Dipl	$3,995	$5,049		•		•	•
Kansas											
Flint Hills Technical College (Emporia)	30	Aug	9	Cert	$4,586	$4,586					
Salina Area Technical School	18	Aug	9	Cert	$3,332	$3,332					
Wichita Area Technical College	18	Aug	9	Cert, AAS	$3,316	$14,922				•	
Kentucky											
Bluegrass Community and Technical College (Lexington)	50	Aug	11	Dipl	$4,508	$13,708					
West Kentucky Community & Technical College (Paducah)	20	Aug	11	Dipl	$5,290	$15,870					•
Massachusetts											
Middlesex Community College - Lowell	20	Sep	10	Cert, AS	$4,572	$5,004					
Northern Essex Community College (Lawrence)	30	Sep	9	Cert	$5,000	$6,000					
Quinsigamond Community College (Worcester)	12	Sep	9	Cert	$7,060	$15,103				•	
Springfield Technical Community College	25	Jun	12	Cert	$4,404	$13,084					
Michigan											
Grand Rapids Community College	24	Aug Sep	10, 24	Cert, AAAS	$4,170	$7,500				•	
Washtenaw Community College (Ann Arbor)	24	Sep	12	Cert	$5,402	$6,845					•
Wayne County Community College District (Detroit)	24	Aug	11	Dipl, Cert	$2,004	$3,367				•	•

*Data are shown only for programs that completed the 2007 AMA Survey of Health Professions Education Programs.
‡Key to Offers: 1: Evening or weekend classes; 2: Non-English instruction; 3: Cultural competence instruction; 4: Distance education component.

Dental Assistant

	Class Capacity	Begins	Length (months)	Award	Res. Tuition	Non-res. Tuition	Stipend	Offers:‡ 1	2	3	4
Minnesota											
Century College (White Bear Lake)	30	Aug Jan Jun	15, 24	Dipl, AAS	$9,477	$17,986					
Dakota County Technical College (Rosemount)	45	Aug	12	Dipl, AAS	$4,173	$8,346				•	
Herzing College - Lakeland Academy Division (Crystal)	180	Jan Jun Sep	12, 21	Dipl, AAS	$17,500	$18,300				•	
Hibbing Community College	32	Sep	9	Dipl	$5,800	$7,200					
Minnesota State Comm & Tech Coll - Moorhead	24	Aug	11	Dipl	$5,192	$10,384					
Northwest Technical College - Bemidji	30	Aug	11	Dipl	$6,745	$6,745					
South Central College (North Mankato)	24	Jun - Aug	12, 24	Dipl, AAS	$6,500	$6,500					
St Cloud Technical College	30	Aug	20	Dipl, AAS	$5,087	$5,087					
Mississippi											
Pearl River Community College (Hattiesburg)	15	Aug	12	Dipl, Cert	$2,200	$2,200					
Missouri											
Concorde Career College - Kansas City	15	Jan-Nov	8	Dipl	$10,950	$10,950		•			
Metropolitan Community College - Penn Valley (Kansas City)	20	Jun	12, 24	Cert, AS	$5,800	$11,000					
Nichols Career Center (Jefferson City)	18	Aug	9	Cert	$5,650	$5,650					
Montana											
Montana State Univ - Great Falls Coll of Tech	18	Sep	11	Cert	$2,496	$8,162		•		•	•
Salish Kootenai College (Pablo)	30	Varies	12, 24	Cert, AAS	$5,361	$9,933				•	
Nebraska											
Central Community College (Hastings)	22	Aug	10, 18	Dipl, AAS	$3,066	$4,452		•			
Nevada											
College of Southern Nevada (Las Vegas)	24	Sep Jan	9	Cert	$1,808	$4,962		•			
New Hampshire											
New Hampshire Technical Institute (Concord)	30	Sep	11	Cert	$5,160	$11,868					
New Jersey											
Atlantic County Institute of Technology (Mays Landing)			10								
Berdan Institute (Wayne)	15	Every 6-9 wks	9, 12	Cert	$14,000	$0		•			
Camden County College (Blackwood)	22	Sep	9, 24	Cert, AAS	$5,600	$6,200					
Cape May County Technical Institute (Cape May Courthouse)	18	Sep	10	Cert	$1,865	$3,865					
Cumberland County Technical Education Center (Bridgeton)	20	Sep	10	Cert	$2,535	$4,000					
Technical Institute of Camden County (Sicklerville)	24	Sep	10, 15	Cert	$3,484	$3,660					
Univ of Medicine & Dent of New Jersey (Scotch Plains)	24	Jan	10	Cert	$5,842	$0				•	
New Mexico											
Central New Mexico Community College (Albuquerque)	24	Aug	12	Cert	$497	$7,960				•	
Dona Ana Community College (Las Cruces)	20	Jan	12	Cert	$2,200	$0		•		•	
Santa Fe Community College	14	Aug	10, 24	Cert, AAS	$1,560	$3,114		•		•	
University of New Mexico - Gallup	10	Aug	12	Cert	$1,464	$3,724		•	•	•	
New York											
Columbia University (New York)	25	Sep Mar	12	Cert							
Monroe Community College (Rochester)	14	Sep	10	Cert	$2,700	$5,400					
North Carolina											
Alamance Community College (Graham)	30	Aug	15	Dipl	$1,496	$8,156		•			
Asheville-Buncombe Technical Comm College	30	Aug	12	Dipl	$2,016	$11,194					•
Cape Fear Community College (Wilmington)	18	Aug	12	Dipl	$1,859	$9,893				•	
Coastal Carolina Community College (Jacksonville)	28	Aug	12	Dipl	$1,764	$9,802					
Fayetteville Technical Community College	42	Aug	12	Dipl	$1,770	$9,748				•	
Forsyth Technical Community College (Winston-Salem)	20	Fall	11	Dipl	$1,920	$3,520					
Guilford Technical Community College (Jamestown)	36	Aug	11	Dipl	$1,580	$8,780					
Martin Commuity College (Williamston)	15	Aug	12	Dipl	$1,900	$1,900			•	•	•
Wayne Community College (Goldsboro)	24	Aug	12	Dipl	$1,580	$8,560					
Western Piedmont Community College (Morganton)	16	Aug	12	Dipl	$1,866	$7,120					
Wilkes Community College (Wilkesboro)	15	Aug	12	Dipl	$1,680	$9,332					
North Dakota											
North Dakota State College of Science (Wahpeton)	18	Aug	10	Cert	$4,500	$8,860					
Ohio											
Choffin Career & Technical Center (Youngstown)	24	Aug	9	Cert	$4,550	$4,550	$3,300			•	
Jefferson Community College (Steubenville)	24	Aug	10	Cert	$2,419	$2,624					
Polaris Career Center (Middleburg Heights)	20	Aug	9	Cert	$5,505	$0		•			
Oklahoma											
Moore Norman Technology Center	12	Aug	9	Cert	$1,060	$1,565					
Rose State College (Midwest City)	12	Aug	10	Cert, AAS	$2,772	$6,511					
Oregon											
Blue Mountain Community College (Pendleton)	17	Sep	9	Cert	$3,464	$6,982					
Concorde Career Institute - Portland	15	Nov Jan Feb Mar Apri	8	Dipl	$12,100	$0		•			
Linn-Benton Community College (Albany)	24	Sep	11, 24	Cert, AS	$3,705	$10,488				•	

*Data are shown only for programs that completed the 2007 AMA Survey of Health Professions Education Programs.
‡Key to Offers: 1: Evening or weekend classes; 2: Non-English instruction; 3: Cultural competence instruction; 4: Distance education component.

	Class Capacity	Begins	Length (months)	Award	Res. Tuition	Non-res. Tuition	Stipend	Offers:‡ 1	2	3	4
Portland Community College	45	Sep	9	Cert	$2,943	$8,695				•	•
Pennsylvania											
Bradford School - Pittsburgh	45	Sep	16	AST	$13,640	$13,640					
Commonwealth Tech Inst at Hiram G Andrews Ctr (Johnstown)	10	Jan May Sep	12	Dipl	$11,900	$0					
Harcum College (Bryn Mawr)	30	Sep	10, 24	Cert, AS	$15,450	$15,450					
Harrisburg Area Community College	26	Aug	10	Cert	$3,900	$7,320					
Luzerne County Community College (Nanticoke)	24	Jul	10	Cert	$2,800	$5,600					
Manor College (Jenkintown)	18	Sep	19, 10	Cert, AS	$11,398	$11,398		•			
Rhode Island											
Community College of Rhode Island (Lincoln)	24	Sep	9	Cert	$2,550	$7,470				•	
South Carolina											
Florence-Darlington Technical College	18	Aug	12	Dipl	$3,100	$5,200					
Greenville Technical College	40	Aug	12, 9	Dipl, Cert	$4,530	$9,480		•		•	
Horry - Georgetown Technical College (Conway)	18	Aug	12	Dipl	$4,200	$6,396					
Tri-County Technical College (Pendleton)	20	Aug	12	Dipl	$4,104	$9,342				•	
Trident Technical College (Charleston)	24	Aug	12	Dipl	$4,671	$8,847					
York Technical College (Rock Hill)	20	Aug	12	Dipl	$4,350	$4,896					
South Dakota											
Lake Area Technical Institute (Watertown)	42	Aug	11, 24	Dipl, AAS	$3,071	$3,071					
Tennessee											
Chattanooga State Technical Comm College	36	Aug	10	Cert	$4,052	$14,700				•	•
Northeast State Technical Comm College (Elizabethton)	16	Aug	12	Cert, AAS	$3,592	$9,396					
Tennessee Technology Center - Dickson	15	May	12	Dipl	$2,058	$2,058				•	
Tennessee Technology Center - Memphis	30	May	12	Dipl	$2,058	$0		•			
Tennessee Technology Center - Murfreesboro	24	Sep	12	Dipl	$4,300	$4,300					
Volunteer State Community College (Gallatin)	24	Aug	12	Cert	$3,550	$13,195					
Texas											
882d Training Group (Sheppard AFB)	24	Varies	20	Cert							
Del Mar College (Corpus Christi)	24	Sep	12	Cert, AAS	$965	$2,165					
El Paso Community College	10	Aug	12, 24	Cert, AAS	$2,103	$2,781		•			
Houston Community College	30	Aug	12	Cert	$2,065	$5,007				•	
Lamar State College - Orange	30	Aug	11	Cert	$4,120	$15,120				•	
Texas State Technical College - Waco	220	Open entry	12	Cert	$4,184	$8,747		•			
Utah											
AmeriTech College (Provo)	40	Every 5 wks	9	Dipl	$9,213	$9,213					
Provo College	30	Every 5 wks	18, 24	Dipl, Cert, AAS	$6,000	$0					
Vermont											
Center for Technology - Essex (Essex Junction)	32	Aug	9	Cert	$7,300	$7,300					
Virginia											
J Sargeant Reynolds Community College (Richmond)	20	Aug Jan	12	Cert	$3,588	$10,850				•	
Washington											
Bates Technical College (Tacoma)	15	Sep Jan Apr	11	Cert, AS	$4,448	$12,798				•	
Bellingham Technical College	22	Jan Mar	11	Cert	$3,917	$10,283				•	
Lake Washington Technical College (Kirkland)	30	Mar Sep	11, 17	Cert, AAS	$3,774	$3,774				•	
Renton Technical College	44	Sep Jan	10	Cert, AAS, AAST	$3,291	$3,291				•	
Seattle Vocational Institute	15	Open entry	12	Cert	$3,981	$0					
South Puget Sound Community College (Olympia)	32	Sep	11	Cert, ATA	$3,949	$3,991				•	
Spokane Community College	42	Sep	9, 18	Cert, AAS	$3,416	$8,617				•	
Wisconsin											
Fox Valley Technical College (Appleton)	25	Jan Aug	9	Dipl	$3,503	$14,200					
Gateway Technical College (Kenosha)	18	Aug	10	Dipl	$3,022	$13,668					•
Western Technical College (La Crosse)	24	Aug	10	Dipl	$2,030	$12,151				•	

*Data are shown only for programs that completed the 2007 AMA Survey of Health Professions Education Programs.
‡Key to Offers: 1: Evening or weekend classes; 2: Non-English instruction; 3: Cultural competence instruction; 4: Distance education component.

Dental Hygienist

Alabama

Wallace State Community College
Dental Hygiene Prgm
PO Box 2000
Hanceville, AL 35077-2000
Prgm Dir: Barbara Adams, AAS MA
Tel: 256 352-8380   *Fax:* 256 352-8382
E-mail: Barbara.adams@wallacestate.edu

Alaska

University of Alaska Anchorage
Dental Hygiene Prgm
3211 Providence Dr, AHS 124
Anchorage, AK 99508-8371
Prgm Dir: Sandra Pence, BS RDH
Tel: 907 786-6925   *Fax:* 907 786-6938
E-mail: pence@uaa.alaska.edu

Arizona

Mohave Community College
Dental Hygiene Prgm
3400 Highway 95
Bullhead City, AZ 86442
www.mohave.edu
Prgm Dir: Tracy Gift, RDH MS
Tel: 928 704-7793   *Fax:* 928 704-7790
E-mail: tgift@mohave.edu

Northern Arizona University
Dental Hygiene Prgm
Box 15065
Flagstaff, AZ 86011-5065
www.nau.edu/hp/dept/dh/
Prgm Dir: Denise Helm, MA
Tel: 928 523-7425   *Fax:* 928 523-6195
E-mail: denise.helm@nau.edu

Mesa Community College
Dental Hygiene Prgm
7110 E McKellips Rd
Mesa, AZ 85207
www.maricopa.edu
Prgm Dir: Phebe Blitz, RDH CDA MS
Tel: 480 654-7772   *Fax:* 480 654-7372
E-mail: phebeblitz@mail.mc.maricopa.edu

Phoenix College
Dental Hygiene Prgm
1202 W Thomas Rd
Phoenix, AZ 85013
Prgm Dir: Maria Fidazzo, CDA RDH MEd
Tel: 602 285-7329   *Fax:* 602 285-7330
E-mail: maria.fidazzo@pcmail.maricopa.edu

Rio Salado College
Dental Hygiene Prgm
2323 W 14th St
Temple, AZ 85281-6950
Prgm Dir: Mary (Liz) Elizabeth Kaz, RDH MS
Tel: 480 517-8020   *Fax:* 480 517-8029
E-mail: liz.kaz@riomail.maricopa.edu

Pima Community College
Dental Hygiene Prgm
2202 W Anklam Rd
Tucson, AZ 85709
Prgm Dir: Joyce Flieger
Tel: 520 206-3102   *Fax:* 520 206-3027
E-mail: joyce.flieger@pima.edu

Arkansas

University of Arkansas - Fort Smith
Dental Hygiene Prgm
5210 Grand Ave, PO Box 3649
Fort Smith, AR 72913-3649
Prgm Dir: Carol Amerine, RDH BS
Tel: 479 788-7272   *Fax:* 479 788-7273
E-mail: camerine@uafortsmith.edu

University of Arkansas for Medical Sciences
Dental Hygiene Prgm
4301 W Markham St Slot 609
Little Rock, AR 72205
Prgm Dir: Susan Long, RDH EdD
Tel: 501 686-5735   *Fax:* 501 686-8519
E-mail: longsusanl@uams.edu

California

Cabrillo College
Dental Hygiene Prgm
6500 Soquel Dr
Aptos, CA 95003
www.cabrillo.edu
Prgm Dir: Bridgete H Clark, RhD DDS
Tel: 831 479-6471   *Fax:* 831 477-5687
E-mail: brclark@cabrillo.edu

Southwestern College
Dental Hygiene Prgm
900 Otay Lakes Rd
Chula Vista, CA 91910
Prgm Dir: Teresa Poulos, MEd
Tel: 619 216-6665, Ext 4860   *Fax:* 619 216-6678
E-mail: tpoulos@swccd.edu

West Los Angeles College
Dental Hygiene Prgm
9000 Overland Ave
Culver City, CA 90230
Prgm Dir: Ulla E Lemborn, MS
Tel: 310 287-4242   *Fax:* 310 287-4461
E-mail: lemboru@wlac.edu

Cypress College
Dental Hygiene Prgm
9200 Valley View St
Cypress, CA 90630
http://CypressCollege.edu
Prgm Dir: Carol Green, RDH MA
Tel: 714 484-7292
E-mail: cgreen@cypresscollege.edu

Fresno City College
Dental Hygiene Prgm
1101 E University Ave
Fresno, CA 93741
Prgm Dir: Monta Denver RDH MS; Jean Kulbeth, RDH MS
Tel: 559 244-2601   *Fax:* 559 244-2614
E-mail: jean.kulbeth@fresnocitycollege.edu

Chabot College
Dental Hygiene Prgm
25555 Hesperian Blvd
Hayward, CA 94545
http://chabotweb.clpccd.cc.ca.us/
Prgm Dir: JoAnn Galliano, MEd RDH
Tel: 510 723-6866   *Fax:* 510 723-7089
E-mail: jgalliano@chabotcollege.edu

Loma Linda University
Dental Hygiene Prgm
School of Dentistry
11092 Anderson St
Loma Linda, CA 92350
Prgm Dir: Joni Stephens, EdS RDH
Tel: 909 558-4631, Ext 48234   *Fax:* 909 558-0313
E-mail: jstephens@llu.edu

Foothill Community College
Dental Hygiene Prgm
12345 El Monte Rd
Los Altos Hills, CA 94022
Prgm Dir: Phyllis Spragge, MA
Tel: 650 949-7467   *Fax:* 650 947-9788
E-mail: spraggephyllis@fhda.edu

University of Southern California
Dental Hygiene Prgm
University Park MC0641
Los Angeles, CA 90089-6041
Prgm Dir: Diane Melrose
Tel: 213 740-1086   *Fax:* 213 740-1094
E-mail: mmelrose@usc.edu

Riverside Comm Coll - Moreno Valley Campus
Dental Hygiene Prgm
16130 Lasselle St
Moreno Valley, CA 92551
www.rcc.edu
Prgm Dir: Donna Lesser
Tel: 951 571-6425
E-mail: donna.lesser@rcc.edu

Cerritos College
Dental Hygiene Prgm
11110 E Alondra Blvd
Norwalk, CA 90650
Prgm Dir: Patricia J Stewart, RDH PhD
Tel: 562 860-2451, Ext 2557   *Fax:* 562 467-5077
E-mail: pstewart@cerritos.edu

Oxnard College
Dental Hygiene Prgm
4000 S Rose Ave
Oxnard, CA 93033-6699
Prgm Dir: Betsy Lindbergh, RDH DDS
Tel: 805 986-5823   *Fax:* 805 986-5867
E-mail: blindbergh@vcccd.net

Pasadena City College
Dental Hygiene Prgm
1570 E Colorado Blvd
Pasadena, CA 91106
Prgm Dir: Jeanne Porush, RDH
Tel: 626 585-7537   *Fax:* 626 585-7966
E-mail: jkporush@pasadena.edu

Diablo Valley College
Dental Hygiene Prgm
321 Golf Club Rd
Pleasant Hill, CA 94523
Prgm Dir: Gay Teel, RDH MA
Tel: 925 685-1230, Ext 2345   *Fax:* 925 689-6529
E-mail: gteel@dvc.edu

Shasta College
Dental Hygiene Prgm
11555 Old Oregon Trail
PO Box 496006
Redding, CA 96049-6006
www.shastacollege.edu
Prgm Dir: Charles Cort, RDH MA
Tel: 530 245-7334, Ext 205   *Fax:* 530 245-7333
E-mail: ccort@shastacollege.edu

Sacramento City College
Dental Hygiene Prgm
3835 Freeport Blvd
Sacramento, CA 95822
www.scc.losrios.edu
Prgm Dir: Sandra Lo, DDS
Tel: 916 558-2650   *Fax:* 916 558-2067
E-mail: los@scc.losrios.edu

Western Career College - Sacramento
Dental Hygiene Prgm
8909 Folsom Blvd
Sacramento, CA 95826
Prgm Dir: Dorothy J Rowe, PhD
Tel: 916 361-5163   *Fax:* 916 361-6666
E-mail: djrowe@westerncollege.com

PROGRAMS

Santa Rosa Junior College
Dental Hygiene Prgm
1501 Mendocino Ave
Santa Rosa, CA 95401-4395
Prgm Dir: Doni Bird, MA
Tel: 707 522-2828   *Fax:* 707 527-4426
E-mail: dbird@santarosa.edu

Taft College
Dental Hygiene Prgm
29 Emmons Park Dr, Box 1437
Taft, CA 93268
Prgm Dir: Stacy Eastman, RDH DDS
Tel: 661 763-7706   *Fax:* 661 763-7808
E-mail: seastman@taft.org

San Joaquin Valley College - Visalia
Dental Hygiene Prgm
8400 W Mineral King
Visalia, CA 93291
Prgm Dir: Cindy Callaghan, RDH
Tel: 559 622-1947   *Fax:* 559 651-3645
E-mail: cindyc@sjvc.edu

Colorado

University of Colorado at Denver
Dental Hygiene Prgm
School of Dental Medicine
13065 E 17th Ave, Rm 104P
Aurora, CO 80045
www.uchsc.edu/sod
Prgm Dir: Terri Tilliss, PhD Donna Stach, RDH, RDH
MEd
Tel: 303 724-7040   *Fax:* 303 724-7049
E-mail: Terri.Tilliss@UCHSC.edu,
Donna.Stach@UCHSC.edu

Community College of Denver
Dental Hygiene Prgm
Bldg 753 1062 Akron Way
Denver, CO 80230
www.ccd.edu/dental
Prgm Dir: Stephanie Harrison, RDH MA
Tel: 303 365-8334   *Fax:* 303 365-8330
E-mail: stephanie.harrison@ccd.edu

Pueblo Community College
Dental Hygiene Prgm
900 W Orman Ave
Pueblo, CO 81004
www.pueblocc.edu
Prgm Dir: Sue Kochevar, RDH MA
Tel: 719 549-3286   *Fax:* 719 549-3136
E-mail: Sue.Kochevar@pueblocc.edu

Colorado Northwestern Community College
Dental Hygiene Prgm
500 Kennedy Dr
Rangley, CO 81648
Prgm Dir: Mark Patterson, RDH BS
Tel: 800 562-1105, Ext 247   *Fax:* 970 675-3330
E-mail: mark.patterson@cncc.edu

Connecticut

U of Bridgeport/Fones Sch of Dental Hygiene
Dental Hygiene Prgm
30 Hazel St
Bridgeport, CT 06601
Prgm Dir: Meg Zayan
Tel: 203 576-4138   *Fax:* 203 576-4220
E-mail: mzayan@bridgeport.edu

Tunxis Community College
Dental Hygiene Prgm
271 Scott Swamp Rd
Farmington, CT 06032-3187
Prgm Dir: Mary A Bencivengo, RDH MS
Tel: 860 255-3626   *Fax:* 860 255-3649
E-mail: mbencivengo@txcc.commnet.edu

University of New Haven
Dental Hygiene Prgm
300 Orange Ave
West Haven, CT 06516
Prgm Dir: Sandra D'Amato-Palambo, MPS
Tel: 203 931-6023   *Fax:* 203 931-6083
E-mail: spalumbo@newhaven.edu

Delaware

Delaware Technical & Community College - Wilmington
Dental Hygiene Prgm
333 Shipley St
Wilmington, DE 19801
Prgm Dir: Judith A Hall, RDH BS
Tel: 302 657-5177   *Fax:* 302 577-6431
E-mail: jhall@dtcc.edu

District of Columbia

Howard University
Dental Hygiene Prgm
600 W Street NW, Rm 401
Washington, DC 20059
www.howard.edu
Prgm Dir: Marie Varley Gillis, RDH MS
Tel: 202 806-0079   *Fax:* 202 806-0354
E-mail: mgillis@howard.edu

Florida

South Florida Community College
Dental Hygiene Prgm
600 W College Dr
Avon Park, FL 33825
www.southflorida.edu
Prgm Dir: Rebecca Sroda, MS
Tel: 863 784-7021   *Fax:* 863 453-9442
E-mail: srodar@southflorida.edu

Manatee Community College
Dental Hygiene Prgm
5840 26th St W
Bradenton, FL 34207
www.mccfl.edu
Prgm Dir: Anita J Weaver, MS
Tel: 941 752-5350   *Fax:* 941 747-6643
E-mail: weavera@mccfl.edu

Brevard Community College
Dental Hygiene Prgm
1519 Clearlake Rd
Cocoa, FL 32922
www.brevardcc.edu
Prgm Dir: Janice Elkins, MEd RDH
Tel: 321 632-1111, Ext 7568   *Fax:* 321 433-7599
E-mail: elkinsj@brevardcc.edu

Daytona Beach Community College
Dental Hygiene Prgm
1155 County Rd 4139
DeLand, FL 32724
Prgm Dir: Pamela S Ridilla
Tel: 386 785-2093   *Fax:* 386 785-2090
E-mail: ridillp@dbcc.edu

Broward Community College
Dental Hygiene Prgm
3501 SW Davie Rd
Fort Lauderdale, FL 33314
www.broward.edu
Prgm Dir: Joyce Abraham, CDA RDH BA
Tel: 954 201-6904   *Fax:* 954 201-6397
E-mail: jabraham@broward.edu

Edison College
Dental Hygiene Prgm
8099 College Pkwy SW
Fort Myers, FL 33906-6210
www.edison.edu
Prgm Dir: Karen Molumby, CDA RDH MBA
Tel: 239 985-8322   *Fax:* 239 985-8352
E-mail: kmolumby@edison.edu

Indian River Community College
Dental Hygiene Prgm
3209 Virginia Ave
Fort Pierce, FL 34981-5599
Prgm Dir: Marta Ferguson, EdD
Tel: 772 462-7523   *Fax:* 772 462-4900
E-mail: mferguso@ircc.edu

Santa Fe Community College
Dental Hygiene Prgm
3000 NW 83rd St, Bldg W81
Gainesville, FL 32606
Prgm Dir: Karen Autrey, BHS MEd
Tel: 352 395-5705   *Fax:* 352 395-5758
E-mail: karen.autrey@sfcc.edu

Florida Community College - Jacksonville
Dental Hygiene Prgm
4501 Capper Rd
Jacksonville, FL 32218
Prgm Dir: Jeffrey Smith, DMD
Tel: 904 766-6655   *Fax:* 904 713-4856
E-mail: jesmith@fccj.edu

Palm Beach Community College
Dental Hygiene Prgm
4200 Congress Ave
Lake Worth, FL 33461
www.pbcc.edu
Prgm Dir: Beth Kuzmirek, RDH BS Ed
Tel: 561 868-3752   *Fax:* 561 868-3753
E-mail: kuzmireb@pbcc.edu

Miami Dade College
Dental Hygiene Prgm
Medical Ctr Campus
950 NW 20th St
Miami, FL 33127
Prgm Dir: Susan Kass, EdD
Tel: 305 237-4029   *Fax:* 305 237-4278
E-mail: skass@mdc.edu

Pasco-Hernando Community College
Dental Hygiene Prgm
10230 Ridge Rd, M-144
New Port Richey, FL 34654-5199
Prgm Dir: James Hall, DDS
Tel: 727 816-3281   *Fax:* 727 816-3478
E-mail: hallj@phcc.edu

Valencia Community College
Dental Hygiene Prgm
1800 S Kirkman Rd
Orlando, FL 32811
Prgm Dir: Pamela Sandy, RDH MA
Tel: 407 582-1544   *Fax:* 407 582-1295
E-mail: PSandy@valenciacc.edu

Gulf Coast Community College
Dental Hygiene Prgm
5230 W US Hwy 98
Panama City, FL 32401-1041
Prgm Dir: Mary Benjamin, RDH DDS
Tel: 850 769-1551, Ext 5832   *Fax:* 850 747-3246
E-mail: mbenjamin@gulfcoast.edu

Pensacola Junior College
Dental Hygiene Prgm
5555 Hwy 98 W
Pensacola, FL 32507
Prgm Dir: Linda Lambert, RDH MS
Tel: 850 484-2244   *Fax:* 850 484-2390
E-mail: llambert@pjc.edu

St Petersburg College
Dental Hygiene Prgm
PO Box 13489
St Petersburg, FL 33781
Prgm Dir: Tami Grzesikowski, RDH
Tel: 727 341-3671   *Fax:* 727 341-3744
E-mail: grzesikowskit@spjc.edu

Tallahassee Community College
Dental Hygiene Prgm
444 Appleyard Dr
Tallahassee, FL 32304-2895
Prgm Dir: Cynthia R Biron, MA
Tel: 850 201-8577   *Fax:* 850 201-8575
E-mail: bironc@tcc.fl.edu

Hillsborough Community College
Dental Hygiene Prgm
4001 Tampa Bay Blvd
Tampa, FL 33614-2754
Prgm Dir: Donna Solovan-Gleason, RDH PhD
Tel: 813 253-7426
E-mail: dsolovangleason@hccfl.edu

Georgia

Darton College
Dental Hygiene Prgm
2400 Gillionville Rd
Albany, GA 31707
www.darton.edu/Programs/AlliedHealth/denthyg.htm
Prgm Dir: Stacey Marshall, RDH MSEd DMD
Tel: 229 317-6840   *Fax:* 229 317-6620
E-mail: stacey.marshall@darton.edu

Athens Technical College
Dental Hygiene Prgm
800 US Hwy 29 N
Athens, GA 30601-1500
Prgm Dir: Tina Grile, MHS RDH CDA
Tel: 706 355-5142   *Fax:* 706 425-3104
E-mail: tgrile@athenstech.edu

Medical College of Georgia
Dental Hygiene Prgm
1120 15th St, AD3103
Augusta, GA 30912-0200
www.mcg.edu
Prgm Dir: Marie Collins, RDH EdD
Tel: 706 721-2938   *Fax:* 706 721-8857
E-mail: mcollins@mcg.edu

Columbus Technical College
Dental Hygiene Prgm
928 Manchester Expwy
Columbus, GA 31904-6572
Prgm Dir: Jan Jones, CDA RDH MPA
Tel: 706 649-1977   *Fax:* 706 649-1599
E-mail: jjones@columbustech.edu

West Central Technical College
Dental Hygiene Prgm
4600 Timber Ridge Dr
Douglasville, GA 30135
www.westcentral.org
Prgm Dir: Carol C Johnson, RDH MSHA
Tel: 770 947-7225   *Fax:* 770 947-7377
E-mail: cjohnson@westcentraltech.edu

Georgia Perimeter College
Dental Hygiene Prgm
2101 Womack Rd
Dunwoody, GA 30338-4497
Prgm Dir: Linda D Boyd, RDH RD EdD
Tel: 770 551-3096   *Fax:* 770 604-3797
E-mail: lboy2@gpc.edu

Central Georgia Technical College
Dental Hygiene Prgm
300 Macon Tech Dr
Macon, GA 31206
http://centralgatech.edu
Prgm Dir: Marsha R McCrimmon, RDH BST MPH
Tel: 478 757-3487   *Fax:* 478 757-3489
E-mail: mccrimmon@centralgatech.edu

Clayton State University
Dental Hygiene Prgm
2000 Clayton State Blvd W
Ste T-105
Morrow, GA 30260
www.clayton.edu
Prgm Dir: Susan Duley, RDH EdD LPC CEDS
Tel: 678 466-4911   *Fax:* 678 466-4669
E-mail: susanduley@clayton.edu

Lanier Technical College
Dental Hygiene Prgm
2990 Landrum Education Dr
Oakwood, GA 30566
Prgm Dir: David Byers, DMD
Tel: 770 535-6905   *Fax:* 770 531-6306
E-mail: dbyers@laniertech.edu

Georgia Highlands College
Dental Hygiene Prgm
415 E Third Ave
Rome, GA 30161
www.highlands.edu/dental
Prgm Dir: Donna Miller, RDH MS
Tel: 706 295-6760   *Fax:* 706 802-5140
E-mail: dmiller@highlands.edu

Armstrong Atlantic State University
Dental Hygiene Prgm
11935 Abercorn St
Savannah, GA 31419-1997
Prgm Dir: Suzanne Edenfield, EdD RDH
Tel: 912 921-7440   *Fax:* 912 921-7466
E-mail: suzanne.edenfield@armstrong.edu

Valdosta State University
Cosponsor: Valdosta Technical College
Dental Hygiene Prgm
4089 Val Tech Rd, PO Box 928
Valdosta, GA 31603
Prgm Dir: Renee' Graham, BSEd RDH
Tel: 912 245-3716   *Fax:* 912 259-5567
E-mail: rgraham@valdostatech.org

Valdosta Technical College
Dental Hygiene Prgm
4089 Val Tech Rd
Valdosta, GA 31603-0928
Prgm Dir: Rene Graham, BS
Tel: 229 259-5534   *Fax:* 229 259-5567
E-mail: rgraham@valdostatech.edu

Middle Georgia Technical College
Dental Hygiene Prgm
80 Cohen Walker Dr
Warner Robins, GA 31088-2729
www.middlegatech.edu
Prgm Dir: Barbara Jansen, DDS
Tel: 478 988-6800, Ext 4024   *Fax:* 478 988-6875
E-mail: bjansen@middlegatech.edu

Hawaii

University of Hawaii
Dental Hygiene Prgm
2445 Campus Rd, Rm 200-B
Honolulu, HI 96822
Prgm Dir: Carolyn Kuba, MEd
Tel: 808 956-8821   *Fax:* 808 956-5707
E-mail: ckuba@hawaii.edu

Idaho

Apollo College - Boise
Dental Hygiene Prgm
1200 N Liberty St
Boise, ID 83704
www.apollocollege.edu
Prgm Dir: David Reff, DDS
Tel: 208 672-0742   *Fax:* 208 947-6822
E-mail: Dreff@apollocollege.edu

Idaho State University
Dental Hygiene Prgm
Box 8048
Pocatello, ID 83209-8380
Prgm Dir: Kathleen Hodges, RDH MS
Tel: 208 282-2744   *Fax:* 208 282-4071
E-mail: hodgkat1@isu.edu

Illinois

Southern Illinois University Carbondale
Dental Hygiene Prgm
School of Allied Health
Mail Code 6615
Carbondale, IL 62901
www.siu.edu/~sah/dh/home.htm
Prgm Dir: Dwayne Summers, DMD
Tel: 618 453-7213   *Fax:* 618 453-7020
E-mail: dsummers@siu.edu

John A Logan College
Dental Hygiene Prgm
700 Logan College Rd
Carterville, IL 62918
Prgm Dir: Pamela Karns, RDH BSDH
Tel: 618 985-2828, Ext 8639   *Fax:* 618 985-4654
E-mail: pamkarns@jalc.edu

Parkland College
Dental Hygiene Prgm
2400 W Bradley Ave
Champaign, IL 61821
Prgm Dir: Mary L Emmons, MEd
Tel: 217 373-3717   *Fax:* 217 373-3830
E-mail: MEmmons@parkland.edu

Kennedy-King College
Dental Hygiene Prgm
UIC College of Dentistry, Rm 201 S, Mail Code 621
801 S Paulina St
Chicago, IL 60612
Prgm Dir: Shirley M Beaver, RDH PhD
Tel: 312 996-8071   *Fax:* 312 996-1023
E-mail: sbeaver@uic.edu

Prairie State College
Dental Hygiene Prgm
202 S Halsted St
Chicago Heights, IL 60411
Prgm Dir: Barbara Gorbitz, RDH BS
Tel: 708 709-3714, Ext 3714   *Fax:* 708 709-3777
E-mail: bgorbitz@prairiestate.edu

Carl Sandburg College
Dental Hygiene Prgm
2400 Tom L Wilson Blvd
209 E Main St
Galesburg, IL 61401
Prgm Dir: Kim Norris, RDH MS
Tel: 309 344-2595   *Fax:* 309 344-2611
E-mail: kimnorris@sandburg.edu

College of DuPage
Dental Hygiene Prgm
425 Fawell Blvd
Glen Ellyn, IL 60137
Prgm Dir: Patricia S Wellner
Tel: 630 942-4237   *Fax:* 630 858-5409
E-mail: wellner@cdnet.cod.edu

Lewis & Clark Community College
Dental Hygiene Prgm
5800 Godfrey Rd
Godfrey, IL 62035
www.lc.edu
Prgm Dir: Michelle Singley, RDH EdM
Tel: 618 468-4413   *Fax:* 618 468-2394
E-mail: msingley@lc.edu

College of Lake County
Dental Hygiene Prgm
19351 W Washington St
Grayslake, IL 60030-1198
Prgm Dir: Sue Nierstheimer, RDH
Tel: 847 543-2638   *Fax:* 847 223-1357
E-mail: snierstheimer@clcillinois.edu

Lake Land College
Dental Hygiene Prgm
5001 Lake Land Blvd
Mattoon, IL 61938-9366
http://lakeland.cc.il.us
Prgm Dir: Jane Slaughter, RDH BS
Tel: 217 234-5202   *Fax:* 217 234-5248
E-mail: jslaught@lakeland.cc.il.us

Harper College
Dental Hygiene Prgm
1200 W Algonquin Rd
Palatine, IL 60067
Prgm Dir: Kathleen Hock, M Ad
Tel: 847 925-6543   *Fax:* 847 925-6077
E-mail: khock@harper.cc.il.us

Illinois Central College
Dental Hygiene Prgm
201 SW Adams St
Peoria, IL 61635-0001
Prgm Dir: Debra Spears, BS
Tel: 309 999-4662   *Fax:* 309 673-9626
E-mail: dspears@icc.edu

Rock Valley College
Dental Hygiene Prgm
3301 N Mulford Rd
Rockford, IL 61114-5699
www.rockvalleycollege.edu
Prgm Dir: Marie Navickis, BSDH RDH
Tel: 815 921-3206   *Fax:* 815 921-3249
E-mail: m.navickis@rockvalleycollege.edu

Indiana

University of Southern Indiana
Dental Hygiene Prgm
8600 University Blvd
Evansville, IN 47712
Prgm Dir: D Carl, RDH MEd
Tel: 812 464-1702   *Fax:* 812 465-7092
E-mail: dcarl@usi.edu

Indiana Univ - Purdue Univ Ft Wayne
Dental Hygiene Prgm
2101 Coliseum Blvd E
Fort Wayne, IN 46805
Prgm Dir: Elaine S Foley, RDH MSEd
Tel: 219 481-6837   *Fax:* 219 481-4162
E-mail: foley@ipfw.edu

Indiana University Northwest
Dental Hygiene Prgm
3400 Broadway St
Gary, IN 46408
www.iun.edu
Prgm Dir: Juanita Robinson, CDA EFDA LDH MSEd
Tel: 219 980-6734   *Fax:* 219 981-4249
E-mail: jurobin@iun.edu

Indiana University
Dental Hygiene Prgm
School of Dentistry
1121 W Michigan St
Indianapolis, IN 46202-5186
Prgm Dir: Nancy Young, MEd
Tel: 317 274-7801   *Fax:* 317 274-1363
E-mail: nayoung@iupui.edu

Indiana University South Bend
Dental Hygiene Prgm
1700 Mishawaka Ave
South Bend, IN 46634
Prgm Dir: Nanci Genich-Yokom, CDA RDH MBA
Tel: 219 237-4154   *Fax:* 219 237-4854
E-mail: nyokom@iusb.edu

Iowa

Des Moines Area Community College
Dental Hygiene Prgm
2006 Ankeny Blvd
Ankeny, IA 50023-3993
www.dmacc.edu/programs/dentalhygiene/
Prgm Dir: Deborah A Penney, DH MS
Tel: 515 964-6582   *Fax:* 515 964-6582
E-mail: dapenney@dmacc.edu

Kirkwood Community College
Dental Hygiene Prgm
6301 Kirkwood Blvd SW, PO Box 2068
Cedar Rapids, IA 52406
www.kirkwoodcollege.com
Prgm Dir: Shaunda Clark, CDA RDH BS MED
Tel: 319 398-5514   *Fax:* 319 398-1293
E-mail: shaunda.clark@kirkwood.edu

Iowa Western Community College
Dental Hygiene Prgm
2700 College Rd/PO Box 4C
Council Bluffs, IA 51502-3004
www.iwcc.edu
Prgm Dir: Janet Hillis, RDH MA
Tel: 712 325-3738, Ext 3738   *Fax:* 712 325-3736
E-mail: jhillis@iwcc.edu

Hawkeye Community College
Dental Hygiene Prgm
1501 E Orange Rd
PO Box 8015
Waterloo, IA 50704
www.hawkeyecollege.edu
Prgm Dir: Tonya Knautz, RDH MEd
Tel: 319 296-2320, Ext 1121   *Fax:* 319 296-4450
E-mail: tknautz@hawkeyecollege.edu

Kansas

Johnson County Community College
Dental Hygiene Prgm
12345 College Blvd
Overland Park, KS 66210-1299
www.jccc.edu
Prgm Dir: Margaret LoGiudice, RDH MS
Tel: 913 469-2582   *Fax:* 913 469-2378
E-mail: mlog@jccc.edu

Wichita State University
Dental Hygiene Prgm
1845 N Fairmount
Wichita, KS 67260-0144
Prgm Dir: Denise Maseman, RDH MS
Tel: 316 978-3614   *Fax:* 316 978-5459
E-mail: denise.maseman@wichita.edu

Kentucky

Western Kentucky University
Dental Hygiene Prgm
Academic Complex, Rm 201
Bowling Green, KY 42101
Prgm Dir: Lynn Austin, RDH MPH
Tel: 270 745-2427   *Fax:* 270 745-6869
E-mail: lynn.austin@wku.edu

Henderson Community College
Dental Hygiene Prgm
2660 S Green St
Henderson, KY 42420
Prgm Dir: Kim Conley, RDH MS
Tel: 270 831-9707   *Fax:* 270 831-9745
E-mail: kim.conley@kctcs.net

Bluegrass Community and Technical College
Dental Hygiene Prgm
Rm 250 Oswald Bldg
Cooper Dr
Lexington, KY 40506
www.bluegrass.kctcs.edu/LCC/DHY
Prgm Dir: Laura Justice, RDH MSED
Tel: 859 246-6233   *Fax:* 859 246-4667
E-mail: laura.justice@kctcs.edu

University of Louisville
Dental Hygiene Prgm
School of Dentistry
501 S Preston St
Louisville, KY 40292
Prgm Dir: Susan Crim, PhD
Tel: 502 852-1229   *Fax:* 502 852-1317
E-mail: sjbail02@louisville.edu

Big Sandy Community & Technical College
Dental Hygiene Prgm
1 Bert T Combs Dr
Prestonsburg, KY 41653
www.bigsandy.kctcs.edu
Prgm Dir: Eric Dixon, DMD
Tel: 606 886-3863, Ext 67352   *Fax:* 606 889-0742
E-mail: edixon0001@kctcs.edu

Louisiana

Louisiana State University
Dental Hygiene Prgm
8000 GSRI Ave, Building 3110
Baton Rouge, LA 70820
www.lsuhsc.edu
Prgm Dir: Caroline Mason, RDH BS MEd
Tel: 225 334-1792   *Fax:* 225 334-1794
E-mail: cmason@lsuhsc.edu

University of Louisiana at Monroe
Dental Hygiene Prgm
700 University Ave
Monroe, LA 71209
Prgm Dir: Beverly B Jarrell, RDH MED
Tel: 318 342-1619   *Fax:* 318 342-1687
E-mail: jarrell@ulm.edu

Southern Univ at Shreveport
Dental Hygiene Prgm
3050 Martin Luther King Jr Dr
Shreveport, LA 71107
www.susla.edu
Prgm Dir: Kheysia Washington, BS
Tel: 318 678-4690   *Fax:* 318 678-4627
E-mail: kwashington@susla.edu

Maine

University College of Bangor
Dental Hygiene Prgm
29 Texas Ave
Bangor, ME 04401-4324
www.uma.maine.edu
Prgm Dir: Ann Curtis, RDH RD MS CAS
Tel: 207 262-7870   *Fax:* 207 262-7871
E-mail: curtisa@maine.edu

University of New England
Dental Hygiene Prgm
Westbrook College Campus
716 Stevens Ave
Portland, ME 04103-2670
www.une.edu
Prgm Dir: Bernice Mills, RDH MS
Tel: 207 221-4314   *Fax:* 207 221-4889
E-mail: bamills@une.edu

Maryland

Baltimore City Community College
Dental Hygiene Prgm
2901 Liberty Heights Ave
Baltimore, MD 21215
Prgm Dir: Annette Russell, RDH BS MS
Tel: 410 462-7718   *Fax:* 410 462-7682
E-mail: arussell@bccc.edu

University of Maryland
Dental Hygiene Prgm
Division of Dental Hygiene
650 W Baltimore St, Rm 1202
Baltimore, MD 21201
www.umaryland.edu
Prgm Dir: Jacquelyn Fried, RDH MS
Tel: 410 706-7773   *Fax:* 410 706-0349
E-mail: jfried@umaryland.edu

Allegany College of Maryland
Dental Hygiene Prgm
12401 Willowbrook Rd SE
Cumberland, MD 21502-2596
Prgm Dir: J Steven Skupas, DDA
Tel: 301 784-5580   *Fax:* 301 784-5015
E-mail: sskupas@ac.cc.md.us

Massachusetts

Mass College of Pharmacy & Health Sciences
Dental Hygiene Prgm
179 Longwood Ave
Boston, MA 02115-5896
Prgm Dir: Gail Barnes
Tel: 617 892-8229
E-mail: gail.barnes@mcphs.edu

Bristol Community College
Dental Hygiene Prgm
777 Elsbree St
Fall River, MA 02720
www.bristol.mass.edu
Prgm Dir: Kristine Bishop Chapman, RDH MA
Tel: 508 678-2811, Ext 2143   *Fax:* 508 730-3281
E-mail: kchapman@bristol.mass.edu

Middlesex Community College - Lowell
Dental Hygiene Prgm
33 Kearney Square
Lowell, MA 01852
Prgm Dir: Kathleen Sweeney, RDH BS MS
Tel: 978 656-3096   *Fax:* 978 656-3078
E-mail: sweeneyk@middlesex.mass.edu

Mt Ida College
Dental Hygiene Prgm
777 Dedham St
Newton Centre, MA 02459
Prgm Dir: Jacyn Stultz, RDH MS
Tel: 617 928-7343   *Fax:* 617 928-7370
E-mail: JStultz@mountida.edu

Springfield Technical Community College
Dental Hygiene Prgm
One Armory Sq, Ste 1
PO Box 9000
Springfield, MA 01102-9000
www.stcc.edu
Prgm Dir: Carol B Szlachetka, CDA RDH MNS
Tel: 413 755-4858   *Fax:* 413 755-4926
E-mail: szlachetka@stcc.edu

Cape Cod Community College
Dental Hygiene Prgm
2240 Lyanough Rd
West Barnstable, MA 02668-1599
www.capecod.edu
Prgm Dir: Elaine Madden, RDH BS MEd
Tel: 508 362-2131, Ext 4628   *Fax:* 508 375-4008
E-mail: emadden@capecod.edu

Quinsigamond Community College
Dental Hygiene Prgm
670 W Boylston St
Worcester, MA 01606
Prgm Dir: Jane Gauthier, RDH MEd
Tel: 508 854-4231   *Fax:* 508 852-2704
E-mail: jgauthier@qcc.mass.edu

Michigan

University of Michigan
Dental Hygiene Prgm
1011 N University
Ann Arbor, MI 48109-1078
Prgm Dir: Wendy Kerschbaum, RDH MA MPH
Tel: 734 763-3392   *Fax:* 734 763-5503
E-mail: wendyek@umich.edu

Kellogg Community College
Dental Hygiene Prgm
450 North Ave
Battle Creek, MI 49017
www.kellogg.edu
Prgm Dir: Paula Sullivan, RDH MHP
Tel: 269 965-3931, Ext 2303   *Fax:* 269 565-2055
E-mail: sullivanp@kellogg.edu

Ferris State University
Dental Hygiene Prgm
200 Ferris Dr
Big Rapids, MI 49307-2740
www.ferris.edu
Prgm Dir: Kimberly Beistle, BA RDH MSA CDA
Tel: 231 591-2224   *Fax:* 231 591-2325
E-mail: beistlk@ferris.edu

University of Detroit Mercy
Dental Hygiene Prgm
8200 W Outer Dr
PO Box 19900
Detroit, MI 48219-0900
Prgm Dir: Kathi R Shepherd, RDH MS
Tel: 313 494-6693   *Fax:* 313 494-6697
E-mail: shephekr@udmercy.edu

Wayne County Community College District
Dental Hygiene Prgm
8551 Greenfield, Rm 310
Detroit, MI 48228
Prgm Dir: Jo Ann Allen Nyquist, BSDH MA EDS
Tel: 919 943-4055   *Fax:* 919 943-4025
E-mail: jnyquis1@wcccd.edu

Mott Community College
Dental Hygiene Prgm
1401 E Court St
Flint, MI 48503
Prgm Dir: Catherine Smith, RDH MA
Tel: 810 762-0328   *Fax:* 810 232-8874
E-mail: csmith@email.mcc.edu

Grand Rapids Community College
Dental Hygiene Prgm
143 Bostwick St NE
Grand Rapids, MI 49503
www.grcc.edu/dental
Prgm Dir: Eve Sidney
Tel: 616 234-4240   *Fax:* 616 234-4317
E-mail: esidney@grcc.edu

Kalamazoo Valley Community College
Dental Hygiene Prgm
6767 West O Ave, Box 4070
Kalamazoo, MI 49003-4070
Prgm Dir: Wanda Scott, MA
Tel: 269 488-4267   *Fax:* 269 488-4720
E-mail: wscott@kvcc.edu

Lansing Community College
Dental Hygiene Prgm
MC 3100D Health and Human Service Careers
PO Box 40010
Lansing, MI 48901-7210
www.lcc.edu/humanhealth/dental/
Prgm Dir: Sherry Kohlmann, MA RDH RDA
Tel: 517 483-1457   *Fax:* 517 483-9925
E-mail: skohlman@lcc.edu

Baker College of Port Huron
Dental Hygiene Prgm
3403 Lapeer Rd
Port Huron, MI 48060
www.baker.edu
Prgm Dir: Sharon Walby, RDH MS
Tel: 810 985-7000, Ext 104   *Fax:* 810 985-7066
E-mail: sharon.walby@baker.edu

Delta College
Dental Hygiene Prgm
1961 Delta Rd
University Center, MI 48710
www.delta.edu
Prgm Dir: Mary Jo Miller, RDH MA
Tel: 989 686-9383   *Fax:* 989 667-2210
E-mail: maryjomiller@delta.edu

Oakland Community College
Dental Hygiene Prgm
7350 Cooley Lake Rd
Waterford, MI 48327
www.oaklandcc.edu
Prgm Dir: Stephanie Markwardt
Tel: 248 942-3267   *Fax:* 248 942-3113
E-mail: sjmarkwa@oaklandcc.edu

Minnesota

Normandale Community College
Dental Hygiene Prgm
9700 France Ave S
Bloomington, MN 55431
www.normandale.edu
Prgm Dir: Carol R Larsen, RDH MEd
Tel: 952 487-8368   *Fax:* 952 487-7022
E-mail: carol.larsen@normandale.edu

Lake Superior College
Dental Hygiene Prgm
2101 Trinity Rd
Duluth, MN 55811
www.lsc.edu
Prgm Dir: Kathy Griffin, RDH BS MEd RF
Tel: 218 733-5938   *Fax:* 218 723-4921
E-mail: k.griffin@lsc.edu

Argosy University - Twin Cities
Dental Hygiene Prgm
1515 Cental Parkway
Eagan, MN 55121
www.argosyu.edu
Prgm Dir: Dinah Bunn, RDH EdD
Tel: 651 846-3416   *Fax:* 651 994-0885
E-mail: dbunn@argosyu.edu

Minnesota State University - Mankato
Dental Hygiene Prgm
3 Morris Hall
Mankato, MN 56001
Prgm Dir: Lynnette M Engeswick, RDH MS
Tel: 507 389-5848   *Fax:* 507 389-5850
E-mail: lynnette.engeswick@mnsu.edu

Herzing College - Lakeland Academy Division
Dental Hygiene Prgm
Lakeland Academy Division
5700 W Broadway Ave
Minneapolis, MN 55428
www.herzing.edu
Prgm Dir: Sandra Johnston, RDH BS
Tel: 763 535-3000   *Fax:* 763 535-9205
E-mail: sjohnston@mpls.herzing.edu

University of Minnesota - Minneapolis
Dental Hygiene Prgm
9-372 Moos Tower
515 Delaware St SE
Minneapolis, MN 55455
www.dentistry.umn.edu
Prgm Dir: Christine Blue, MS
Tel: 612 625-5954   *Fax:* 612 625-1605
E-mail: bluex005@umn.edu

Minnesota State Comm & Tech Coll - Moorhead
Dental Hygiene Prgm
Allied Dental Careers Dept
1900 28th Ave S
Moorhead, MN 56560-4899
www.minnesota.edu
Prgm Dir: Thomas Boe, DDS MBA
Tel: 218 299-6819   *Fax:* 218 299-6532
E-mail: thomas.boe@minnesota.edu

Rochester Community & Technical College
Dental Hygiene Prgm
851 30th Ave SE
Rochester, MN 55904
Prgm Dir: Anne M High, RDH MS
Tel: 507 280-3114   *Fax:* 507 280-3180
E-mail: anne.high@roch.edu

St Cloud Technical College
Dental Hygiene Prgm
1540 Northway Dr
St Cloud, MN 56303-1240
www.sctc.edu
Prgm Dir: Barbara L Henkemeyer, RDH MS
Tel: 320 308-5933   *Fax:* 320 308-5960
E-mail: bhenkemeyer@sctc.edu

Century College
Dental Hygiene Prgm
3300 Century Ave N
White Bear Lake, MN 55110
www.century.cc.mn.us
Prgm Dir: Linda Jorgenson, RDH BS
Tel: 651 779-3983   *Fax:* 651 779-3401
E-mail: linda.jorgenson@century.edu

Mississippi

Northeast Mississippi Community College
Dental Hygiene Prgm
Cunningham Blvd
Booneville, MS 38829
Prgm Dir: Nick Alexander
Tel: 662 720-7283   *Fax:* 662 278-1165
E-mail: nalexan@necc.cc.ms.us

Pearl River Community College
Dental Hygiene Prgm
5448 US Hwy 49 S
Hattiesburg, MS 39401
www.prcc.edu
Prgm Dir: Stanley L Hill, DMD
Tel: 601 554-5509   *Fax:* 601 554-5548
E-mail: slhill@prcc.edu

University of Mississippi Medical Center
Dental Hygiene Prgm
2500 N State St
SHRP
Jackson, MS 39216-4505
http://shrp.umc.edu
Prgm Dir: Beckie Barry, MEd
Tel: 601 984-6310   *Fax:* 601 815-1717
E-mail: bbarry@shrp.umsmed.edu

Meridian Community College
Dental Hygiene Prgm
910 Hwy 19 N
Meridian, MS 39307
www.meridiancc.edu
Prgm Dir: William Lindsay, DDS
Tel: 601 484-8751, Ext 751   *Fax:* 601 484-8704
E-mail: blindsay@mcc.cc.ms.us

Mississippi Delta Community College
Dental Hygiene Prgm
PO Box 668
Highway 3 at Cherry St
Moorhead, MS 38761
Prgm Dir: Melissa-Marble Warrington, RDH BS
Tel: 662 246-6511   *Fax:* 662 246-6299
E-mail: mwarrington@msdelta.edu

Missouri

Missouri Southern State University
Dental Hygiene Prgm
3950 E Newman and Duquesne Rds
Joplin, MO 64801-1595
www.mssu.edu
Prgm Dir: Sandra Scorse, DDS
Tel: 417 625-9709   *Fax:* 417 625-3078
E-mail: scorse-s@mssu.edu

University of Missouri - Kansas City
Dental Hygiene Prgm
650 E 25th St
Kansas City, MO 64108
www.umkc.edu/dentistry
Prgm Dir: Kimberly Bray, RDH MS
Tel: 816 235-2050   *Fax:* 816 235-2157
E-mail: brayk@umkc.edu

State Fair Community College
Dental Hygiene Prgm
3201 W 16th St
Sedalia, MO 65301
www.sfccmo.edu
Prgm Dir: Renee Fiquet-Freeman, RDH BS
Tel: 660 596-7234, Ext 7234
E-mail: rfiquet@sfccmo.edu

Ozarks Technical Community College
Dental Hygiene Prgm
1001 E Chestnut Expressway
Springfield, MO 65802
Prgm Dir: Kelly Tillery, MEd RDH CDA
Tel: 417 447-8829   *Fax:* 417 447-8806
E-mail: tilleryk@otc.edu

St Louis Community College - Forest Park
Dental Hygiene Prgm
5600 Oakland Ave
4th Fl, Tower A
St Louis, MO 63110-1393
http://stlcc.edu
Prgm Dir: Mario Conte, DMD
Tel: 314 644-9334   *Fax:* 314 951-9490
E-mail: mconte@stlcc.edu

Montana

Montana State Univ - Great Falls Coll of Tech
Dental Hygiene Prgm
2100 16th Ave S
Great Falls, MT 59405
www.msugf.edu
Prgm Dir: Kim L Woloszyn, RDH BA
Tel: 406 771-4365   *Fax:* 406 771-4317
E-mail: kwoloszyn@msugf.edu

Nebraska

Central Community College
Dental Hygiene Prgm
PO Box 1024
Hastings, NE 68902-1024
www.cccneb.edu
Prgm Dir: Wanda Cloet, RDH MS
Tel: 402 461-2470   *Fax:* 402 460-2128
E-mail: wcloet@cccneb.edu

University of Nebraska - Lincoln
Dental Hygiene Prgm
40th and Holdrege Sts
Lincoln, NE 68583-0740
Prgm Dir: Gwen Hlava, RDH
Tel: 402 472-1433   *Fax:* 402 472-6681
E-mail: ghlava@unmc.edu

Nevada

College of Southern Nevada
Dental Hygiene Prgm
6375 W Charleston Blvd
W1A
Las Vegas, NV 89146
Prgm Dir: Doreen Craig, RDH MA
Tel: 702 651-5593   *Fax:* 702 651-7401
E-mail: doreen.craig@csn.edu

Truckee Meadows Community College
Dental Hygiene Prgm
7000 Dandini Blvd, RMDT 417-H
Reno, NV 89512-3999
www.tmcc.edu
Prgm Dir: Vickie Kimbrough, RDH MBA
Tel: 775 674-7554   *Fax:* 775 673-8242
E-mail: vkimbrough@tmcc.edu

New Hampshire

New Hampshire Technical Institute
Dental Hygiene Prgm
31 College Dr
Concord, NH 03301-7412
www.nhti.edu
Prgm Dir: Donna Clougherty, RDH MEd
Tel: 603 271-7164   *Fax:* 603 271-7182
E-mail: dclougherty@ccsnh.edu

New Jersey

Camden County College
Dental Hygiene Prgm
PO Box 200
Blackwood, NJ 08012
Prgm Dir: Catherine Boos, DMD
Tel: 856 227-7200, Ext 4472   *Fax:* 856 374-5048
E-mail: cboos@camdencc.edu

Middlesex County College
Dental Hygiene Prgm
2600 Woodbridge Ave, PO Box 3050
Edison, NJ 08818-3050
Prgm Dir: Hope-Claire Holbeck, RDH MS
Tel: 732 906-2580   *Fax:* 732 906-2633
E-mail: HHolbeck@middlesexcc.edu

Bergen Community College
Dental Hygiene Prgm
400 Paramus Rd, S-337
Paramus, NJ 07652
Prgm Dir: Susan Callahan Barnard, DHSc RDH
Tel: 201 447-7937   *Fax:* 201 612-3876
E-mail: sbarnard@bergen.edu

Burlington County College
Dental Hygiene Prgm
601 Pemberton-Browns Mills Rd
Pemberton, NJ 08068
Prgm Dir: Linda Hecker, CDA RDH BS MA
Tel: 609 894-9311, Ext 1419
E-mail: lhecker@bcc.edu

Univ of Medicine & Dent of New Jersey
Dental Hygiene Prgm
1776 Raritan Rd
Scotch Plains, NJ 07076
Prgm Dir: Carolyn K Breen, EdD CDA RDA RDH
Tel: 908 889-2419   *Fax:* 908 889-2477
E-mail: breen@umdnj.edu

New Mexico

University of New Mexico
Dental Hygiene Prgm
Health Science Center
Division of Dental Hygiene
Albuquerque, NM 87131-1391
Prgm Dir: Demetra Logothethis, MS
Tel: 505 272-4513   *Fax:* 505 272-5584
E-mail: dlogothetis@salud.unm.edu

San Juan College
Dental Hygiene Prgm
4601 College Blvd
Farmington, NM 87402-4699
www.sanjuancollege.edu
Prgm Dir: Julius Manz, DDS
Tel: 505 566-3018   *Fax:* 505 566-3790
E-mail: manzj@sanjuancollege.edu

New York

Broome Community College
Dental Hygiene Prgm
PO Box 1017
Binghamton, NY 13902
Prgm Dir: Maureen Hankin, RDH MPH
Tel: 607 778-5393   *Fax:* 607 778-5467
E-mail: hankin_m@sunybroome.edu

Eugenio Maria De Hostos Community College
Dental Hygiene Prgm
475 Grand Concourse
Bronx, NY 10451
Prgm Dir: Mary Errico, DDS
Tel: 718 518-4234   *Fax:* 718 518-4194
E-mail: merrico@hostos.cuny.edu

New York City College of Technology
Dental Hygiene Prgm
Dental Hygiene Department P201
300 Jay St
Brooklyn, NY 11201-2983
Prgm Dir: Leonard Fiedman, DMD
Tel: 718 260-5074   *Fax:* 718 260-5069
E-mail: lfriedman@citytech.cuny.edu

SUNY at Canton
Dental Hygiene Prgm
34 Cornell Dr
Canton, NY 13617-1096
www.canton.edu/can/can_start.taf?oage=study_school_
    healthmed
Prgm Dir: Pamela P Quinn, RDH BSE MSEd
Tel: 607 222-2910
E-mail: quinnp@canton.edu

Farmingdale State College, SUNY
Dental Hygiene Prgm
2350 Broadhollow Rd
Farmingdale, NY 11735
www.farmingdale.edu
Prgm Dir: Laura Joseph, RDH MS EdD
Tel: 631 420-2060   *Fax:* 631 420-2582
E-mail: laura.joseph@farmingdale.edu

Orange County Community College
Dental Hygiene Prgm
115 South St
Middletown, NY 10940
www.sunyorange.edu
Prgm Dir: Roberta Smith, MPS
Tel: 845 341-4306   *Fax:* 845 341-4799
E-mail: rsmith@sunyorange.edu

New York University
Dental Hygiene Prgm
345 E 24th St
New York, NY 10010
www.nyu.edu/dental
Prgm Dir: Cheryl Westphal, RDH
Tel: 212 998-9390   *Fax:* 212 995-4593
E-mail: cmw1@nyu.edu

Monroe Community College
Dental Hygiene Prgm
1000 E Henrietta Rd
Rochester, NY 14623-5780
Prgm Dir: David B Lawrence, DDS
Tel: 585 292-2761   *Fax:* 585 424-5703
E-mail: dlawrence@monroecc.edu

Hudson Valley Community College
Dental Hygiene Prgm
80 Vandenburgh Ave
Troy, NY 12180
Prgm Dir: J Romano, RDH BS MA
Tel: 518 629-7442   *Fax:* 518 629-8191
E-mail: romanjud@hvcc.edu

Erie Community College - North Campus
Dental Hygiene Prgm
6205 Main St
Williamsville, NY 14221-7095
www.ecc.edu
Prgm Dir: Joseph Sowinski, DDS
Tel: 716 851-1390   *Fax:* 716 851-1392
E-mail: sowinski@ecc.edu

North Carolina

Asheville-Buncombe Technical Comm College
Dental Hygiene Prgm
340 Victoria Rd
Asheville, NC 28801
www.abtech.edu
Prgm Dir: Shaun Tate, RDH MAEd
Tel: 828 254-1921, Ext 271   *Fax:* 828 281-9792
E-mail: state@abtech.edu

University of North Carolina - Chapel Hill
Dental Hygiene Prgm
Dental Hygiene Prgms
3220 Old Dental Bldg, CB 7450
Chapel Hill, NC 27599-7450
www.dent.unc.edu
Prgm Dir: Sally Mauriello, RDH EdD
Tel: 919 966-2800   *Fax:* 919 966-6761
E-mail: sally_mauriello@dentistry.unc.edu

Central Piedmont Community College
Dental Hygiene Prgm
1201 Elizabeth Ave, Kings Dr
Charlotte, NC 28204
Prgm Dir: Judith Qualtieri, RDH MS
Tel: 704 330-6365   *Fax:* 704 330-6533
E-mail: judy.qualtieri@cpcc.edu

Fayetteville Technical Community College
Dental Hygiene Prgm
2201 Hull Rd
PO Box 35236
Fayetteville, NC 28303
www.faytechcc.edu
Prgm Dir: Susan Ellis, RDH MEd
Tel: 910 678-8575   *Fax:* 910 678-8500
E-mail: elliss@faytechcc.edu

Wayne Community College
Dental Hygiene Prgm
3000 Wayne Memorial Dr
Goldsboro, NC 27533
www.waynecc.edu
Prgm Dir: Sue Fowler, BS
Tel: 919 735-5152, Ext 206   *Fax:* 919 581-1013
E-mail: suef@waynecc.edu

Catawba Valley Community College
Dental Hygiene Prgm
2550 Hwy 70 SE
Hickory, NC 28602
www.cvcc.edu
Prgm Dir: Luis E Arzola, DMD
Tel: 828 327-7000, Ext 4339   *Fax:* 828 624-5205
E-mail: larzola@cvcc.edu

Coastal Carolina Community College
Dental Hygiene Prgm
444 Western Blvd
Jacksonville, NC 28546
Prgm Dir: Joseph Hewitt, DDS
Tel: 910 938-6271   *Fax:* 910 455-4989
E-mail: hewittj@coastal.cc.nc.us

Guilford Technical Community College
Dental Hygiene Prgm
PO Box 309
Jamestown, NC 27282
Prgm Dir: Lois Smith, RDH CDA MS
Tel: 336 334-4822, Ext 2452   *Fax:* 336 819-2015
E-mail: lhsmith@gtcc.edu

Wake Technical Community College
Dental Hygiene Prgm
2901 Holston Lane
Raleigh, NC 27610
www.waketech.edu
Prgm Dir: Brenda Maddox, RDH MS
Tel: 919 212-3263   *Fax:* 919 212-3261
E-mail: bpmaddox@waketech.edu

Halifax Community College
Dental Hygiene Prgm
PO Drawer 809
Weldon, NC 27890-0809
www.hcc.cc.nc.us
Prgm Dir: Doris Markham, RDH MSEd
Tel: 252 538-4305
E-mail: markhamdj@halifaxcc.edu

Cape Fear Community College
Dental Hygiene Prgm
411 N Front St
Wilimington, NC 28401-3993
Prgm Dir: Mary Ellen Naylor
Tel: 910 362-7193   *Fax:* 910 362-7418
E-mail: mnaylor@cfcc.edu

Forsyth Technical Community College
Dental Hygiene Prgm
2100 Silas Creek Pkwy
Winston-Salem, NC 27103-5197
Prgm Dir: Janette Whisenhunt, PhD (RDH CDA BS MEd)
Tel: 336 734-7414   *Fax:* 336 734-7444
E-mail: jwhisenhunt@forsythtech.edu

North Dakota

North Dakota State College of Science
Dental Hygiene Prgm
800 N 6th St
Wahpeton, ND 58076
Prgm Dir: Susan Swanson, DDS
Tel: 701 671-2334   *Fax:* 701 671-2570
E-mail: Susan.Swanson@ndscs.edu

Ohio

University of Cincinnati
Cosponsor: Raymond Walters College
Dental Hygiene Prgm
9555 Plainfield Rd
Cincinnati, OH 45236
Prgm Dir: Janelle Schierling, EdD
Tel: 513 745-5631   *Fax:* 513 792-8623
E-mail: schierjm@ucrwcu.rwc.uc.edu

Cuyahoga Community College
Dental Hygiene Prgm
2900 Community College Ave
Cleveland, OH 44115
Prgm Dir: Mary Lou Gerosky
Tel: 216 987-4494   *Fax:* 216 987-4386
E-mail: mary-lou.gerosky@tri-c.cc.oh.us

Columbus State Community College
Dental Hygiene Prgm
550 E Spring St, PO Box 1609
Union Hall 410
Columbus, OH 43216
Prgm Dir: Connie Grossman, MEd RDH
Tel: 614 287-5645   *Fax:* 614 287-5198
E-mail: cgrossma@cscc.edu

Ohio State University
Dental Hygiene Prgm
305 W 12th Ave
PO Box 182357
Columbus, OH 43218-2357
www.dent.osu.edu/dhy
Prgm Dir: Michele Carr, RDH MA
Tel: 614 292-2228   *Fax:* 614 292-8013
E-mail: carr.3@osu.edu

Sinclair Community College
Dental Hygiene Prgm
444 W Third St
Dayton, OH 45402
Prgm Dir: Rena Shuchat, MS
Tel: 937 512-2779   *Fax:* 937 512-4175
E-mail: rena.shuchat@sinclair.edu

Lorain County Community College
Dental Hygiene Prgm
1005 N Abbe Rd
Elyria, OH 44035-1691
Prgm Dir: Denise Price
Tel: 440 365-5222, Ext 7196   *Fax:* 440 366-4116
E-mail: dprice@lorainccc.edu

Lakeland Community College
Dental Hygiene Prgm
7700 Clocktower Dr
Kirtland, OH 44094-5198
Prgm Dir: Cathy Patterson
Tel: 440 525-7190   *Fax:* 440 525-7433
E-mail: cpatterson@lakelandcc.edu

Rhodes State College
Dental Hygiene Prgm
4240 Campus Dr
Lima, OH 45804
Prgm Dir: Denise Bowers, MSEd
Tel: 419 995-8385   *Fax:* 419 995-8162
E-mail: bowers.d@rhodesstate.edu

Stark State College of Technology
Dental Hygiene Prgm
6200 Frank Ave NW
North Canton, OH 44720-7299
www.starkstate.edu
Prgm Dir: Nichole Oocumma, RDH MA CHES
Tel: 330 966-5458, Ext 4707   *Fax:* 330 966-6586
E-mail: noocumma@starkstate.edu

Shawnee State University
Dental Hygiene Prgm
940 Second St
Portsmouth, OH 45662
www.shawnee.edu
Prgm Dir: Nancy Bentley, RDH MS
Tel: 740 351-3236, Ext 3273   *Fax:* 740 351-3354
E-mail: nbentley@shawnee.edu

Owens Community College
Dental Hygiene Prgm
PO Box 10,000
Toledo, OH 43699
Prgm Dir: Elizabeth Tronolone, MS
Tel: 419 661-7290   *Fax:* 419 661-7304
E-mail: elizabeth_tronolone@owens.edu

Youngstown State University
Dental Hygiene Prgm
Dept of Health Professions
One University Plaza
Youngstown, OH 44555
Prgm Dir: Madeleine Haggerty, RDH
Tel: 330 941-1766   *Fax:* 330 941-1767
E-mail: mbhaggerty@ysu.edu

Oklahoma

Rose State College
Dental Hygiene Prgm
6420 SE 15th St
Midwest City, OK 73110
www.rose.edu
Prgm Dir: Janet Turley, RDH CDA MEd
Tel: 405 733-7337   *Fax:* 405 736-0389
E-mail: jturley@rose.edu

Univ of Oklahoma Health Sciences Center
Dental Hygiene Prgm
PO Box 26901
Oklahoma City, OK 73117
Prgm Dir: Jane A Bowers
Tel: 405 271-4436   *Fax:* 405 271-4785
E-mail: jane-bowers@ouhsc.edu

Tulsa Community College
Dental Hygiene Prgm
909 S Boston Ave, Rm MP 458
Tulsa, OK 74119-2094
www.tulsacc.edu
Prgm Dir: Denise Lysikowski, RDH MPH
Tel: 918 595-7019   *Fax:* 918 595-8300
E-mail: dlysikow@tulsacc.edu

Oregon

Lane Community College
Dental Hygiene Prgm
4000 E 30th Ave
Eugene, OR 97405
Prgm Dir: Sharon Hagan, RDH MS
Tel: 541 463-5616   *Fax:* 541 463-5616
E-mail: hagans@lanecc.edu

Mt Hood Community College
Dental Hygiene Prgm
26000 SE Stark St
Gresham, OR 97030
Prgm Dir: T Tong, RDH MS
Tel: 503 491-7691   *Fax:* 503 491-6005
E-mail: tongt@mhcc.edu

Oregon Institute of Technology
Dental Hygiene Prgm
3201 Campus Dr
Semon Hall #222
Klamath Falls, OR 97601
Prgm Dir: Terri Armstrong, MS
Tel: 541 885-1886   *Fax:* 541 885-1849
E-mail: armstrot@oit.edu

Portland Community College
Dental Hygiene Prgm
PO Box 19000
Portland, OR 97219-0990
www.pcc.edu
Prgm Dir: Josette Beach, RDH MS
Tel: 503 977-4235   *Fax:* 503 977-8300
E-mail: jbeach@pcc.edu

Pennsylvania

Northampton Community College
Dental Hygiene Prgm
3835 Green Pond Rd
Bethlehem, PA 18020
Prgm Dir: Terry Sigal Greene, RDH MEd
Tel: 610 861-5440   *Fax:* 610 861-4139
E-mail: tsigalgreene@northampton.edu

Montgomery County Community College
Dental Hygiene Prgm
340 DeKalb Pike
Blue Bell, PA 19422-0758
Prgm Dir: Jenny Sheaffer, RDH MS
Tel: 215 641-6623   *Fax:* 215 619-7171
E-mail: jsheaffe@mc3.edu

Harcum College
Dental Hygiene Prgm
750 Montgomery Ave
Bryn Mawr, PA 19010
https://www.harcum.edu
Prgm Dir: Jean Byrnes-Ziegler, MA
Tel: 610 526-6110, Ext 6046   *Fax:* 610 526-6182
E-mail: jbyrnes-ziegler@harcum.edu

Tri-State Business Institute
Dental Hygiene Prgm
5757 W Ridge Rd
Erie, PA 16506
Prgm Dir: Susan Gorman, RDH BS Ed
Tel: 814 838-7673, Ext 266   *Fax:* 814 838-4276
E-mail: sgorman@tsbi.edu

Harrisburg Area Community College
Dental Hygiene Prgm
One HACC Dr, SM-102
Harrisburg, PA 17110-2999
www.hacc.edu
Prgm Dir: Sandra Zagar, RDH MSA
Tel: 717 221-1733   *Fax:* 717 780-1170
E-mail: szzagar@hacc.edu

Manor College
Dental Hygiene Prgm
700 Fox Chase Rd
Jenkintown, PA 19046-3399
Prgm Dir: Virginia Saunders, RDH BS MEd
Tel: 215 885-2360, Ext 284   *Fax:* 215 576-6564
E-mail: vsaunders@manor.edu

Luzerne County Community College
Dental Hygiene Prgm
1333 S Prospect St
Nanticoke, PA 18634-3899
www.luzerne.edu
Prgm Dir: Cathryn Brown, CDA RDH MEd
Tel: 570 740-0447   *Fax:* 570 740-0265
E-mail: cbrown@luzerne.edu

Community College of Philadelphia
Dental Hygiene Prgm
1700 Spring Garden St
Philadelphia, PA 19130
www.ccp.edu
Prgm Dir: Theresa M Grady
Tel: 215 751-8927   *Fax:* 215 751-8937
E-mail: tgrady@ccp.edu

University of Pittsburgh
Dental Hygiene Prgm
3501 Terrace St
B-82 Salk Hall
Pittsburgh, PA 15261
www.dental.pitt.edu/students/dental_hygiene.php
Prgm Dir: Angelina Riccelli, RDH MS
Tel: 412 648-8432   *Fax:* 412 383-8737
E-mail: riccelli@pitt.edu

Pennsylvania College of Technology
Dental Hygiene Prgm
One College Ave
Williamsport, PA 17701
Prgm Dir: Shawn Kiser, RDH BS MEd
Tel: 570 320-8007   *Fax:* 570 320-2401
E-mail: skiser@pct.edu

Westmoreland County Community College
Dental Hygiene Prgm
145 Pavilion Ln
Youngwood, PA 15697-1895
Prgm Dir: Angela S Rinchuse, RDH MEd
Tel: 724 925-4163   *Fax:* 724 925-5808
E-mail: rinchusea@wccc-pa.edu

Rhode Island

Community College of Rhode Island
Dental Hygiene Prgm
1762 Louisquisset Pike
Lincoln, RI 02865-4585
www.ccri.edu
Prgm Dir: Kathleen Gazzola, RDH EMT CDA BS MA
Tel: 401 333-7227   *Fax:* 401 333-7146
E-mail: kgazzola@ccri.edu

South Carolina

Trident Technical College
Dental Hygiene Prgm
PO Box 118067
Charleston, SC 29423-8067
Prgm Dir: Barbara Ankersen, RDH MS
Tel: 843 574-6439   *Fax:* 843 574-6585
E-mail: barbara.ankersen@tridenttech.edu

Midlands Technical College
Dental Hygiene Prgm
PO Box 2408
Columbia, SC 29202
Prgm Dir: Martha H Hanks, DDS
Tel: 803 822-3451   *Fax:* 803 822-3079
E-mail: hanksm@midlandstech.edu

Horry - Georgetown Technical College
Dental Hygiene Prgm
PO Box 261966
2050 Highway 501 East
Conway, SC 29528-6066
www.hgtc.edu
Prgm Dir: Alice Derouen, RDH MEd
Tel: 843 349-5371   *Fax:* 843 349-7576
E-mail: alice.derouen@hgtc.edu

Florence-Darlington Technical College
Dental Hygiene Prgm
PO Box 100548
Florence, SC 29501-0548
Prgm Dir: Richard Moore, DMD
Tel: 843 661-8223   *Fax:* 843 292-0851
E-mail: richard.moore@fdtc.edu

Greenville Technical College
Dental Hygiene Prgm
PO Box 5616
Greenville, SC 29606-5616
Prgm Dir: Debra Grubbs, RDH BSHSE
Tel: 864 250-8588   *Fax:* 864 250-8261
E-mail: debra.grubbs@gvltec.edu

York Technical College
Dental Hygiene Prgm
452 S Anderson Rd
Rock Hill, SC 29730
Prgm Dir: Kathleen Peter, RDH MHA
Tel: 803 327-8039   *Fax:* 803 327-8059
E-mail: kpeter@york.tech.com

South Dakota

University of South Dakota
Dental Hygiene Prgm
East Hall 414, E Clark St
Vermillion, SD 57069
Prgm Dir: Ann Brunick, RDH MS
Tel: 605 677-5379   *Fax:* 605 677-5638
E-mail: abrunick@usd.edu

Tennessee

Chattanooga State Technical Comm College
Dental Hygiene Prgm
4501 Amnicola Hwy
Chattanooga, TN 37406-1097
Prgm Dir: William Johnson
Tel: 423 697-4768   *Fax:* 423 634-3071
E-mail: william.johnson@chattanoogastate.edu

East Tennessee State University
Dental Hygiene Prgm
PO Box 70690
Johnson City, TN 37614-0690
www.etsu.edu/cpah/dental
Prgm Dir: Charles Faust, RDH EdD
Tel: 423 439-4497   *Fax:* 423 439-4030
E-mail: faust@etsu.edu

University of Tennessee Health Science Ctr
Dental Hygiene Prgm
930 Madison Ave, Ste 600
Memphis, TN 38163
www.utmem.edu/allied/dental_hygiene_home.html
Prgm Dir: Cassandra Holder-Ballard, RDH MPA EdD
Tel: 901 448-4252   *Fax:* 901 448-7545
E-mail: cballard@utmem.edu

Tennessee State University
Dental Hygiene Prgm
3500 John A Merritt Blvd
Nashville, TN 37209-1561
Prgm Dir: Marian W Patton, RDH EdD
Tel: 615 963-5801   *Fax:* 615 963-5836
E-mail: mpatton@tnstate.edu

Roane State Community College
Dental Hygiene Prgm
701 Briarcliff Ave
Oak Ridge, TN 37830-8795
Prgm Dir: Michael D Curran, DDS
Tel: 865 483-0816, Ext 2127   *Fax:* 865 481-2019
E-mail: Curranm@roanestate.edu

Texas

Amarillo College
Dental Hygiene Prgm
PO Box 447
Amarillo, TX 79178
Prgm Dir: Donna Cleere, RDH BSOE MEd
Tel: 806 354-6064   *Fax:* 806 354-6076
E-mail: cleere-dk@actx.edu

Austin Community College
Dental Hygiene Prgm
Highland Business Center
5930 Middle Fiskville Rd
Austin, TX 78702
Prgm Dir: Renee Cornett
Tel: 512 223-5711   *Fax:* 512 223-5906
E-mail: rcornett@austincc.edu

Lamar Institute of Technology
Dental Hygiene Prgm
PO Box 10061
Beaumont, TX 77710
Prgm Dir: Betty Reynard, RDH EdD
Tel: 409 880-8846   *Fax:* 409 880-8955
E-mail: betty.reynard@lit.edu

Coastal Bend College
Dental Hygiene Prgm
3800 Charco Rd
Beeville, TX 78102
http://coastalbend.edu
Prgm Dir: Andrea Westmoreland, RDH MEd
Tel: 361 354-2556   *Fax:* 361 354-2540
E-mail: andygump@coastalbend.edu

Howard College
Dental Hygiene Prgm
1001 Birdwell Ln
Big Spring, TX 79720
Prgm Dir: Jeri Farmer, RDH MEd
Tel: 915 264-5075   *Fax:* 915 264-5630
E-mail: jfarmer@howardcollege.edu

Blinn College
Dental Hygiene Prgm
PO Box 6030
Bryan, TX 77805-6030
Prgm Dir: Lisa Wiese, RDH MS
Tel: 979 209-7272   *Fax:* 979 209-7289
E-mail: Lwiese@blinn.edu

Del Mar College
Dental Hygiene Prgm
101 Baldwin Blvd
Corpus Christi, TX 78404
www.delmar.edu/dh
Prgm Dir: David G Arreguin, DDS
Tel: 361 698-2859   *Fax:* 361 698-2811
E-mail: darreguin@delmar.edu

Baylor College of Dentistry, Texas A&M HSC
Dental Hygiene Prgm
The Texas A & M University System Health Science
   Center
PO Box 660677
Dallas, TX 75266-0677
Prgm Dir: Janice Dewald, BSDH DDS MS
Tel: 214 828-8340   *Fax:* 214 828-8196
E-mail: jdewald@bcd.tamhsc.edu

Texas Woman's University
Dental Hygiene Prgm
Box 425648 TWU Station
Denton, TX 76204
Prgm Dir: Nahid Nikpour, PhD
Tel: 940 898-2874   *Fax:* 940 898-2869
E-mail: nnikpour@mail.twu.edu

El Paso Community College
Dental Hygiene Prgm
PO Box 20500
El Paso, TX 79998
www.epcc.edu
Prgm Dir: William Ekvall, DDS
Tel: 915 831-4060   *Fax:* 915 831-4445
E-mail: williame@epcc.edu

Texas State Technical College - Harlingen
Dental Hygiene Prgm
1902 N Loop 499
Harlingen, TX 78550-3697
Prgm Dir: Barbara L Bennett, CDA
Tel: 956 364-4697   *Fax:* 956 364-5162
E-mail: bbennett@harlingen.tstc.edu

Univ of Texas Hlth Sci Ctr at Houston
Dental Hygiene Prgm
PO Box 20068
Houston, TX 77225-0068
www.db.uth.tmc.edu
Prgm Dir: Jayne McWherter, RDH MEd
Tel: 713 500-4399   *Fax:* 713 500-0410
E-mail: Jayne.A.McWherter@uth.tmc.edu

Tarrant County College - Northeast Campus
Dental Hygiene Prgm
828 Harwood Rd
Hurst, TX 76054
Prgm Dir: Cindy A O'Neal, RDH BS
Tel: 817 515-6640   *Fax:* 817 515-6700
E-mail: cindy.oneal@tccd.edu

Kingwood College - NHMCCD
Dental Hygiene Prgm
20000 Kingwood Dr
Health & Science Building 118A
Kingwood, TX 77339
www.nhmccd.edu
Prgm Dir: Maribeth Stitt, RDH MEd
Tel: 281 312-1517   *Fax:* 281 312-1722
E-mail: Maribeth.Stitt@nhmccd.edu

Collin County Community College
Dental Hygiene Prgm
2200 W University Dr
McKinney, TX 75069-8001
Prgm Dir: Joanne Fletcher, RDH MS
Tel: 972 548-6738   *Fax:* 972 548-6536
E-mail: jfletcher@ccccd.edu

Univ of Texas Hlth Sci Ctr at San Antonio
Dental Hygiene Prgm
7703 Floyd Curl Dr MSC 6244
San Antonio, TX 78229-3900
www.uthscsa.edu
Prgm Dir: Taline Infante, MS RDH
Tel: 210 567-8820   *Fax:* 210 567-8843
E-mail: dadian@uthscsa.edu

Temple College
Dental Hygiene Prgm
2600 S First St
Temple, TX 76504-7435
Prgm Dir: Norma Maedgen, RDH PhD
Tel: 254 298-8677   *Fax:* 254 298-8676
E-mail: norma.maedgen@templejc.edu

Tyler Junior College
Dental Hygiene Prgm
PO Box 9020
Tyler, TX 75711
Prgm Dir: Carrie Hobbs, RDH BS MEd
Tel: 903 510-2341   *Fax:* 903 510-2879
E-mail: chob@tjc.edu

Wharton County Junior College
Dental Hygiene Prgm
911 Boling Hwy
Wharton, TX 77488
Prgm Dir: Leigh Ann Collins, MAI
Tel: 979 532-6398   *Fax:* 979 532-6489
E-mail: lacollins@wcjc.edu

Midwestern State University
Dental Hygiene Prgm
3410 Taft Blvd
Wichita Falls, TX 76308-2099
www.mwsu.edu
Prgm Dir: Barbara DeBois, RDH MS
Tel: 940 397-4764   *Fax:* 940 397-4973
E-mail: dental.hygiene@mwsu.edu

Utah

Weber State University
Dental Hygiene Prgm
3920 University Circle
Ogden, UT 84408-3920
Prgm Dir: Stephanie Bossenberger, MS RDH
Tel: 801 626-6130   *Fax:* 801 626-7304
E-mail: bossenberger@weber.edu

Utah Valley State College
Dental Hygiene Prgm
800 W University Pkwy
Orem, UT 84058
Prgm Dir: George Veit, DDS
Tel: 801 764-7592   *Fax:* 800 764-7595
E-mail: veitge@uvsc.edu

Dixie State College of Utah
Dental Hygiene Prgm
225 South 700 East
St George, UT 84770
Prgm Dir: Gordon Jennings, DDS
Tel: 435 652-7869   *Fax:* 435 656-4031
E-mail: jennings@dixie.edu

Salt Lake Community College
Dental Hygiene Prgm
3491 Wights Fort Rd
Jordan HTC 115R
West Jordan, UT 84088
www.slcc.edu/dentalhygiene/
Prgm Dir: Marie Frankos, RDH BS
Tel: 801 957-2621   *Fax:* 801 957-2819
E-mail: marie.frankos@slcc.edu

Vermont

Vermont Technical College
Dental Hygiene Prgm
301 Lawrence Pl
Williston Campus
Williston, VT 05495
Prgm Dir: Ellen Grimes, EdD
Tel: 802 879-5632   *Fax:* 802 879-2317
E-mail: ellen.grimes@vtc.edu

Virginia

Old Dominion University
Dental Hygiene Prgm
Gene W Hirschfeld School of Dental Hygiene
2011 Health Science Building, 4608 Hampton Blvd
Norfolk, VA 23529-0499
www.odu.edu/dental
Prgm Dir: Deborah Bauman, BSDH MS
Tel: 757 683-3338   *Fax:* 757 683-5239
E-mail: dbauman@odu.edu

Virginia Commonwealth University
Dental Hygiene Prgm
School of Dentistry
PO Box 980566
Richmond, VA 23298-0566
www.dentistry.vcu.edu
Prgm Dir: Kim Isringhausen, BSDH RDH MPH
Tel: 804 828-9096   *Fax:* 804 827-0969
E-mail: ktisring@vcu.edu

Virginia Western Community College
Dental Hygiene Prgm
3097 Colonial Ave
Roanoke, VA 24015
www.vw.vccs.edu/health/denthome.htm
Prgm Dir: Martha Roberson, RDH MSHA
Tel: 540 857-6282   *Fax:* 540 857-6224
E-mail: mroberson@vw.vccs.edu

Northern Virginia Community College
Dental Hygiene Prgm
6699 Springfield Center Dr
Springfield, VA 22150
www.nvcc.edu
Prgm Dir: Cynthia Hebert, CDA RDH BSDH
Tel: 703 822-6686   *Fax:* 703 822-6610
E-mail: chebert@nvcc.edu

Wytheville Community College
Dental Hygiene Prgm
1000 E Main St
Wytheville, VA 24382
Prgm Dir: Elaine Smith, RDH BS
Tel: 276 223-4840   *Fax:* 276 227-0411
E-mail: wcsmite@wcc.vccs.edu

Washington

Lake Washington Technical College
Dental Hygiene Prgm
11605 132nd Ave NE
Kirkland, WA 98034
www.lwtc.ctc.edu/dental
Prgm Dir: Mary Young, RDH BS MHA
Tel: 425 739-8403   *Fax:* 425 739-8292
E-mail: mary.young@lwtc.edu

Pierce College
Dental Hygiene Prgm
9401 Farwest Dr SW
Lakewood, WA 98498-1999
http://pierce.ctc.edu
Prgm Dir: Sharon S Golightly, RDH BS MS EdD
Tel: 253 964-6661   *Fax:* 253 964-6313
E-mail: sgolight@pierce.ctc.edu

Columbia Basin College
Dental Hygiene Prgm
2600 N 20th Ave
Pasco, WA 99301
www.columbiabasin.edu
Prgm Dir: Lynn Stedman, RDH BSDH MEd MA
Tel: 509 547-0511, Ext 2991   *Fax:* 509 544-2025
E-mail: lynn.stedman@columbiabasin.edu

Seattle Central Community College
Dental Hygiene Prgm
1701 Broadway, BE3210
Seattle, WA 98122
http://seattlecentral.edu/programs/dental.php
Prgm Dir: Ona Canfield, RDH MEd
Tel: 206 587-6922   *Fax:* 206 587-6337
E-mail: scccdh@sccd.ctc.edu

Shoreline Community College
Dental Hygiene Prgm
16101 Greenwood Ave N
Shoreline, WA 98133
http://success.shore.ctc.edu/dental/
Prgm Dir: Marianne Baker, RDH MEd
Tel: 206 546-4709   *Fax:* 206 546-5830
E-mail: mbaker@shoreline.edu

Eastern Washington University
Dental Hygiene Prgm
310 N Riverpoint Blvd Box E
Spokane, WA 99202
Prgm Dir: Rebecca Stolberg, RDH MS
Tel: 509 368-6528   *Fax:* 509 368-6514
E-mail: rstolberg@mail.ewu.edu

Clark College
Dental Hygiene Prgm
1933 Fort Vancouver Way
Vancouver, WA 98663
Prgm Dir: D Wittmayer, RDH MS
Tel: 360 992-2474   *Fax:* 360 992-2880
E-mail: dwittmayer@clark.edu

Yakima Valley Community College
Dental Hygiene Prgm
PO Box 22520
Yakima, WA 98907-2520
www.yvcc.edu
Prgm Dir: Patricia Hakala, RDH BA
Tel: 509 574-4918   *Fax:* 509 574-6875
E-mail: phakala@yvcc.edu

West Virginia

Community & Technical College at WVU Tech
Dental Hygiene Prgm
604 Davis Hall
Montgomery, WV 25136
Prgm Dir: Melissa France, RDH MA
Tel: 304 442-3345   *Fax:* 304 442-3093
E-mail: melissa.france@mail.wvu.edu

West Virginia University
Dental Hygiene Prgm
Health Science Ctr N, PO Box 9425
Morgantown, WV 26506-9425
www.hsc.wvu.edu/sod/departments/Hygiene/
Prgm Dir: Amy Funk, MSDH
Tel: 304 293-3417   *Fax:* 304 293-4882
E-mail: afunk@hsc.wvu.edu

Southern West Virginia Comm & Tech College
Dental Hygiene Prgm
Dempsey Branch Rd
Mount Gay, WV 25637
Prgm Dir: Lisa Haddox-Heston
Tel: 304 792-7098, Ext 259
E-mail: lisah@southern.wvnet.edu

West Liberty State College
Dental Hygiene Prgm
PO Box 295
CSC 121
West Liberty, WV 26074-0295
Prgm Dir: Margaret Six, RDH MSDH
Tel: 304 336-8030   *Fax:* 304 336-8905
E-mail: sixmj@wlsc.edu

Wisconsin

Fox Valley Technical College
Dental Hygiene Prgm
1825 Bluemound Dr
Appleton, WI 54914
www.fvtc.edu
Prgm Dir: Joan Rohrer, RDH BS
Tel: 920 735-2452   *Fax:* 920 831-4314
E-mail: rohrer@fvtc.edu

Northeast Wisconsin Technical College
Dental Hygiene Prgm
2740 W Mason St, PO Box 19042
Green Bay, WI 54307-9042
Prgm Dir: Sheila Gross, RDH MS
Tel: 920 498-6839   *Fax:* 920 498-6890
E-mail: sheila.gross@nwtc.edu

Madison Area Technical College
Dental Hygiene Prgm
211 N Carroll St
Madison, WI 53703
www.matcmadison.edu
Prgm Dir: E Lynn Goetsch, RDH MS
Tel: 608 258-2470   *Fax:* 608 258-2482
E-mail: egoetsch@matcmadison.edu

Milwaukee Area Technical College
Dental Hygiene Prgm
700 W State St
Milwaukee, WI 53233
Prgm Dir: Laurie Klos, MS
Tel: 414 297-7126   *Fax:* 414 297-7205
E-mail: klosl@matc.edu

Waukesha County Technical College
Dental Hygiene Prgm
800 Main St
Pewaukee, WI 53072
Prgm Dir: Pamela Brilowski, RDH MS
Tel: 262 691-5561, Ext 5561   *Fax:* 262 691-5077
E-mail: pbrilowski@wctc.edu

Northcentral Technical College
Dental Hygiene Prgm
1000 Campus Dr
Wausau, WI 54401
www.ntc.edu
Prgm Dir: Michelle Hilts, RDH MAE
Tel: 715 675-3331, Ext 1329   *Fax:* 715 675-3772
E-mail: hilts@ntc.edu

Wyoming

Laramie County Community College
Dental Hygiene Prgm
1400 E College Dr
Cheyenne, WY 82007-3299
Prgm Dir: Connie Henry
Tel: 307 778-1386   *Fax:* 307 772-7304
E-mail: chenry@lccc.wy.edu

Sheridan College
Dental Hygiene Prgm
3059 Coffeen Ave
Sheridan, WY 82801
www.sheridan.edu
Prgm Dir: Jan Dill, RDH BSDH MS
Tel: 307 674-6446, Ext 3405   *Fax:* 307 674-3352
E-mail: jldill@sheridan.edu

Dental Hygienist

	Class Capacity	Begins	Length (months)	Award	Res. Tuition	Non-res. Tuition	Stipend	Offers:‡ 1	2	3	4
Alabama											
Wallace State Community College (Hanceville)	30	Aug	21	AAS	$2,430	$4,860				•	
Alaska											
University of Alaska Anchorage	12	Aug	18	AAS	$3,300	$11,570					
Arizona											
Mesa Community College	18	Aug	18	AAS	$60	$85		•		•	
Mohave Community College (Bullhead City)	18	Aug	20	AAS	$1,682	$4,872				•	
Northern Arizona University (Flagstaff)	30	Aug	30	BS	$9,188	$28,856		•		•	•
Phoenix College	22	Aug	18	AAS	$1,950	$8,400				•	
Arkansas											
University of Arkansas for Medical Sciences (Little Rock)	34	Aug	19	AS, BS	$6,800	$0				•	
California											
Cabrillo College (Aptos)	22	Jun	24	AS	$1,615	$12,026					
Chabot College (Hayward)	20	Aug	24	AA	$780	$7,320				•	
Cypress College	18	Aug	18	Cert, AS	$377	$2,166				•	
Fresno City College	30	Aug	18	AS	$264	$3,036				•	
Loma Linda University	42	Sep	21	BS	$25,515	$25,515				•	
Riverside Comm Coll - Moreno Valley Campus	22	Fall	24	Dipl, AS	$20	$0		•		•	
Sacramento City College	24	Aug	20	AS	$480	$3,667				•	
Santa Rosa Junior College	24	Aug	24	AS	$26	$171				•	
Shasta College (Redding)	14	Sep	24	AA							
Colorado											
Community College of Denver	24	Aug	22, 34	Cert, AAS	$4,282	$10,853				•	
Pueblo Community College	15	Aug	18	AAS	$4,500	$10,500				•	

*Data are shown only for programs that completed the 2007 AMA Survey of Health Professions Education Programs.
‡Key to Offers: 1: Evening or weekend classes; 2: Non-English instruction; 3: Cultural competence instruction; 4: Distance education component.

Dental Hygienist

	Class Capacity	Begins	Length (months)	Award	Res. Tuition	Non-res. Tuition	Stipend	Offers:‡ 1	2	3	4
University of Colorado at Denver (Aurora)	18	Jul	24	BS	$11,063	$25,197				•	
District of Columbia											
Howard University (Washington)	20	Aug	20	Cert	$15,925	$15,925				•	
Florida											
Brevard Community College (Cocoa)	12	Aug	24	Cert, AS	$2,980	$10,868		•		•	•
Broward Community College (Fort Lauderdale)	16	Aug	12	AS	$4,000	$10,000				•	
Edison College (Fort Myers)	18	Aug	24	AS	$3,500	$12,000					
Manatee Community College (Bradenton)	14	Aug	24	AS	$1,260	$4,708				•	
Miami Dade College	50	Aug	19	AS	$2,347	$8,201				•	
Palm Beach Community College (Lake Worth)	24	Aug	21	AS	$11,000	$33,000				•	
Pensacola Junior College	36	May	24	AAS	$3,000	$14,825					•
Santa Fe Community College (Gainesville)	24	Aug	24, 16	AS	$5,575	$20,658				•	
South Florida Community College (Avon Park)	12	Aug	21	AAS	$4,100	$20,000				•	•
Valencia Community College (Orlando)	24	May	24	AS	$2,550	$0				•	•
Georgia											
Armstrong Atlantic State University (Savannah)	26	Aug	21	Dipl, AS	$4,611	$16,134				•	•
Central Georgia Technical College (Macon)	18	Aug	21	AS	$1,457	$2,945					
Clayton State University (Morrow)	28	Aug	60	BSDH	$3,582	$12,186		•		•	•
Columbus Technical College	14	Oct	20	ADH	$3,751	$3,751				•	
Darton College (Albany)	24	Aug	24	AS	$2,110	$7,350					
Georgia Highlands College (Rome)	14	Aug	20	AS						•	
Medical College of Georgia (Augusta)	28	Aug	21	BS	$6,485	$20,127				•	
Middle Georgia Technical College (Warner Robins)	14	Oct	21	AAS	$1,860	$3,720					
West Central Technical College (Douglasville)	14	Jul	24	AAS	$1,828	$1,828				•	
Idaho											
Apollo College - Boise	30		20	AAS	$50,000	$50,000				•	
Illinois											
Carl Sandburg College (Galesburg)	30	Aug	24	AAS	$3,760	$3,760				•	
College of Lake County (Grayslake)	24	Fall semester	24	AAS	$3,600	$5,000					
Lake Land College (Mattoon)	30	Aug	21	AAS	$2,600	$5,600				•	
Lewis & Clark Community College (Godfrey)	24	Aug	18	AAS	$5,480	$16,408					
Prairie State College (Chicago Heights)	36	May	24	AAS	$6,700	$9,500					
Rock Valley College (Rockford)	22	Aug	24	AAS	$2,494	$15,319				•	
Southern Illinois University Carbondale	36	Aug	32	BS	$4,254	$7,356					
Indiana											
Indiana University (Indianapolis)	50	Aug	21	AS, BS	$6,668	$18,675				•	•
Indiana University Northwest (Gary)	24	Aug	24	AS	$8,610	$22,722				•	
University of Southern Indiana (Evansville)	24	Aug	16	BS	$4,905	$11,694				•	
Iowa											
Des Moines Area Community College (Ankeny)	24	Aug	19	AAS	$3,927	$7,854				•	
Hawkeye Community College (Waterloo)	22	Aug	21	AAS	$3,488	$6,976				•	•
Iowa Western Community College (Council Bluffs)	18	Aug	21	AAS	$1,800	$0				•	
Kirkwood Community College (Cedar Rapids)	24	Fall	18	AAS	$3,708	$3,708				•	
Kansas											
Johnson County Community College (Overland Park)	26	Aug	24	AAS	$1,985	$4,536				•	
Wichita State University	36	Aug	19	AS, BSDH	$4,500	$12,000				•	
Kentucky											
Big Sandy Community & Technical College (Prestonsburg)	16	Aug	24	AAS	$3,724	$11,324					•
Bluegrass Community and Technical College (Lexington)	24	Jun	24	AAS	$4,370	$13,110				•	
University of Louisville	30	Aug	20	BS	$4,000	$6,000				•	
Western Kentucky University (Bowling Green)	26	Aug	17, 33	Dipl, AS, BS	$3,500	$8,350					
Louisiana											
Louisiana State University (Baton Rouge)	42	Aug	18	BS	$3,008	$0				•	•
Southern Univ at Shreveport	12	Aug	21	AAS	$3,452	$4,800				•	
University of Louisiana at Monroe	26	Aug	24, 48	BS	$5,039	$13,967				•	
Maine											
University College of Bangor	24	Sep	27	AS, BS	$4,985	$11,124				•	
University of New England (Portland)	50	Sep	27, 36	AS, BS	$24,440	$24,440		•		•	
Maryland											
University of Maryland (Baltimore)	36	Aug	24	Dipl, BS, MS	$4,900	$14,800		•		•	•
Massachusetts											
Bristol Community College (Fall River)	22	Sep	16	AS	$4,550	$12,173				•	
Cape Cod Community College (West Barnstable)	22	Sep	18	AS	$3,660	$9,840				•	•
Middlesex Community College - Lowell	42	Sep	24	AS	$4,320	$11,736				•	•
Mt Ida College (Newton Centre)	24	Aug	20	Dipl, AA	$19,800	$19,800				•	
Quinsigamond Community College (Worcester)	30	Sep	18	AS	$8,495	$16,399				•	

*Data are shown only for programs that completed the 2007 AMA Survey of Health Professions Education Programs.
‡Key to Offers: 1: Evening or weekend classes; 2: Non-English instruction; 3: Cultural competence instruction; 4: Distance education component.

Dental Hygienist

	Class Capacity	Begins	Length (months)	Award	Res. Tuition	Non-res. Tuition	Stipend	Offers:‡ 1	2	3	4
Springfield Technical Community College	20	Sep	18	AS	$5,715	$13,419					
Michigan											
Baker College of Port Huron	24	Sep	27	AAS	$10,800	$10,800				•	
Delta College (University Center)	18	Aug Sep	18	AAS	$2,734	$5,407				•	
Ferris State University (Big Rapids)	60	Fall semester	21	AS	$6,400	$12,500					•
Grand Rapids Community College	32	Aug Sep	22	AAAS	$4,031	$7,250				•	
Kellogg Community College (Battle Creek)	20	Sep	24	AAS	$4,322	$6,142				•	
Lansing Community College	24	Aug	21	AAS	$6,201	$8,793				•	
Oakland Community College (Waterford)	30	Sep	18	AAS	$2,865	$5,511					•
Minnesota											
Argosy University - Twin Cities (Eagan)	48	Sep	19	AS							
Century College (White Bear Lake)	24	Aug	20	AAS	$2,632	$7,498		•		•	
Herzing College - Lakeland Academy Division (Minneapolis)	36	Every other semester	24	AAS	$23,250	$0					
Lake Superior College (Duluth)	18	Aug	18	AAS	$7,375	$13,275				•	
Minnesota State Comm & Tech Coll - Moorhead	18	Sep	20	AAS	$10,210	$15,470					
Normandale Community College (Bloomington)	30	Aug	18	AS	$4,806	$4,806		•		•	•
Rochester Community & Technical College	18	Jun	24	AAS	$5,700	$11,400		•		•	
St Cloud Technical College	14	Aug	18	AAS	$9,600	$9,600					
University of Minnesota - Minneapolis	24	Sep	27	BS	$8,000	$20,000				•	•
Mississippi											
Meridian Community College	14	Aug	21	AAS	$1,450	$2,740					
Pearl River Community College (Hattiesburg)	16	Aug	20	AAS	$1,900	$2,900					
University of Mississippi Medical Center (Jackson)	22	Late May, Early Jun	22	BS	$4,611	$10,574				•	
Missouri											
Missouri Southern State University (Joplin)	30	Aug	22	AS	$3,510	$7,020					
St Louis Community College - Forest Park	32	Aug	21	AAS	$1,470	$2,345				•	
State Fair Community College (Sedalia)	10	Fall	24	AAS	$70	$150				•	
University of Missouri - Kansas City	30	Aug	20	BS, MSDH	$12,947	$17,122				•	
Montana											
Montana State Univ - Great Falls Coll of Tech	14	Aug	22	AAS	$2,496	$8,162					
Nebraska											
Central Community College (Hastings)	15	Aug	24	AAS	$2,664	$3,774				•	
Nevada											
College of Southern Nevada (Las Vegas)	30	Aug Sep	21	AS, BSDH	$1,600	$5,000				•	
Truckee Meadows Community College (Reno)	12	Fall	24	AS	$1,567	$3,803					•
New Hampshire											
New Hampshire Technical Institute (Concord)	48	Aug	21, 29	AS	$7,010	$14,038					
New Jersey											
Bergen Community College (Paramus)	44	Sep	18	AAS	$3,060	$5,934			•		•
Camden County College (Blackwood)	22	Sep	24	AAS	$4,000	$4,800					
Middlesex County College (Edison)	30	Sep	15	AAS	$2,965	$5,993					
Univ of Medicine & Dent of New Jersey (Scotch Plains)	44	Jan	32	AAS	$6,480	$9,720		•		•	
New Mexico											
San Juan College (Farmington)	12	Fall	18	AAS	$30	$40				•	
New York											
Erie Community College - North Campus (Williamsville)	60	Sep Jan	24	AAS	$2,987	$5,974				•	
Farmingdale State College, SUNY	52	Sep	16	AS	$4,350	$10,300				•	
Hudson Valley Community College (Troy)	45	Aug	20	Dipl, AAS	$2,700	$8,100		•		•	
Monroe Community College (Rochester)	48	Sep	24	AAS	$2,700	$5,400					
New York University	100	Sep	20, 40	Dipl, AAS, BS	$39,000	$39,000		•			
Orange County Community College (Middletown)	20	Sep	9	AAS	$3,000	$6,000				•	
SUNY at Canton	30	Aug	24	AAS	$4,350	$7,210				•	•
North Carolina											
Asheville-Buncombe Technical Comm College	20	Aug	21	AAS	$2,016	$11,194				•	•
Cape Fear Community College (Wilimington)	12	Aug	22	AAS	$1,344	$7,465				•	
Catawba Valley Community College (Hickory)	20	Aug	24	AS	$1,896	$10,536				•	
Central Piedmont Community College (Charlotte)	30	May	24	AAS	$1,850	$9,450				•	
Coastal Carolina Community College (Jacksonville)	24	Aug	23	AAS	$1,497	$8,156					
Fayetteville Technical Community College	34	Aug	22	AAS	$1,932	$10,731				•	
Forsyth Technical Community College (Winston-Salem)	12	Aug	21	AAS	$1,920	$10,560					
Guilford Technical Community College (Jamestown)	36	Aug	22	AAS	$2,174	$9,734				•	
Halifax Community College (Weldon)	18	Aug	21	AAS	$1,775	$8,874				•	
University of North Carolina - Chapel Hill	36	Aug	18	Cert, BS, MS	$5,448	$21,096				•	
Wake Technical Community College (Raleigh)	24	Aug	22	AAS	$1,580	$8,780				•	
Wayne Community College (Goldsboro)	30	Aug	20	AAS	$1,556	$8,577			•	•	

*Data are shown only for programs that completed the 2007 AMA Survey of Health Professions Education Programs.
‡Key to Offers: 1: Evening or weekend classes; 2: Non-English instruction; 3: Cultural competence instruction; 4: Distance education component.

Dental Hygienist

	Class Capacity	Begins	Length (months)	Award	Res. Tuition	Non-res. Tuition	Stipend	Offers: 1	2	3	4
North Dakota											
North Dakota State College of Science (Wahpeton)	28	Aug	20	AAS	$4,600	$8,860					
Ohio											
Ohio State University (Columbus)	32	Sep	33	BSDH	$8,676	$21,285				•	
Rhodes State College (Lima)	24	Sep	21	AAS	$6,200	$12,400				•	
Shawnee State University (Portsmouth)	24	Aug	22	Dipl, AAS	$5,628	$9,972				•	
Sinclair Community College (Dayton)	35	Sep	21	AAS	$2,886	$4,715					
Stark State College of Technology (North Canton)	20	Aug	22	AAS	$3,556	$4,676				•	
Oklahoma											
Rose State College (Midwest City)	12	Aug	24	AAS	$2,340	$6,780					
Tulsa Community College	14	Aug	16	AAS	$1,673	$4,488				•	
Oregon											
Lane Community College (Eugene)	26	Sep	18	AAS	$5,400	$0		•		•	•
Portland Community College	20	Sep	18	AAS	$4,860	$14,800				•	
Pennsylvania											
Community College of Philadelphia	32	Jul	24	AAS	$8,600	$22,000					
Harcum College (Bryn Mawr)	32	Sep	20	AS	$16,000	$16,000					
Harrisburg Area Community College	34	Aug	20	AA	$7,298	$10,701				•	
Luzerne County Community College (Nanticoke)	30	Jul	24	AAS	$3,440	$6,880					
Northampton Community College (Bethlehem)	40	Aug	17	AAS	$3,600	$11,484				•	
University of Pittsburgh	36	Aug	22, 21	Cert, BSDH	$18,159	$32,424				•	
Rhode Island											
Community College of Rhode Island (Lincoln)	36	Sep	24	AAS	$2,800	$7,296		•		•	
South Carolina											
Florence-Darlington Technical College	18	Aug	22	AAS	$3,500	$6,700					
Horry - Georgetown Technical College (Conway)	16	Aug	21	AS	$7,000	$10,660					
Trident Technical College (Charleston)	24	Jan	21	AS	$4,830	$9,150		•			•
York Technical College (Rock Hill)	20	Aug	21	AHS	$4,350	$4,896					
Tennessee											
East Tennessee State University (Johnson City)	24	Aug	19	BSDH	$3,678	$9,633					•
Tennessee State University (Nashville)	36	Aug	18, 24	AAS	$2,207	$6,863				•	
University of Tennessee Health Science Ctr (Memphis)	34	Sep	21	Dipl, BS	$6,295	$16,393				•	
Texas											
Baylor College of Dentistry, Texas A&M HSC (Dallas)	30	Aug	21	BS, MS	$3,700	$13,000				•	
Coastal Bend College (Beeville)	30	Aug	19	Dipl, AAS	$5,784	$6,576				•	
Del Mar College (Corpus Christi)	24	Sep	16	AAS	$1,655	$1,855					
El Paso Community College	16	Aug	21	AAS	$1,496	$2,615					
Kingwood College - NHMCCD	12	Fall semester	21	AAS	$2,016	$7,920				•	
Midwestern State University (Wichita Falls)	18	Aug Sep	18	BS	$5,200	$14,300				•	
Tarrant County College - Northeast Campus (Hurst)	30	Aug	24	AAS	$1,900	$5,956				•	
Temple College	12	May	24	AAS	$4,280	$6,290				•	
Texas Woman's University (Denton)	28	Aug	36	BS	$3,690	$10,170					
Univ of Texas Hlth Sci Ctr at Houston	40	Aug	20	Cert, BS	$4,488	$13,563				•	•
Univ of Texas Hlth Sci Ctr at San Antonio	30	Aug	22, 48	BS, MS	$3,926	$11,792				•	•
Utah											
Salt Lake Community College (West Jordan)	26	Aug	16	Dipl, AAS, AS	$2,312	$7,232				•	
Virginia											
Northern Virginia Community College (Springfield)	74	Aug	22	AAS	$2,970	$9,262		•		•	•
Old Dominion University (Norfolk)	48	Aug	37	BS, MS	$6,516	$18,252		•		•	•
Virginia Commonwealth University (Richmond)	18+	Jul	20	BSDH	$6,899	$19,443				•	
Virginia Western Community College (Roanoke)	18	Aug	24	AAS	$2,943	$9,252				•	•
Wytheville Community College	20	Aug	21	AAS	$2,500	$7,332					
Washington											
Clark College (Vancouver)	26	Sep	19	AAS	$2,900	$12,680					
Columbia Basin College (Pasco)	18	Fall quarter	22	AAS	$3,072	$9,808				•	
Eastern Washington University (Spokane)	36	Sep	38	BS	$4,905	$13,749				•	
Lake Washington Technical College (Kirkland)	30	Sep	21	AAS	$5,715	$5,715		•	•		
Pierce College (Lakewood)	26	Sep	21	AAS	$2,672	$3,129				•	•
Seattle Central Community College	18	Fall quarter	21	AAS-T	$3,460	$10,882				•	
Shoreline Community College	24	Sep	20	AAAS	$6,786	$12,369				•	•
Yakima Valley Community College	36	Sep	18	AAS	$2,970	$8,178				•	
West Virginia											
Community & Technical College at WVU Tech (Montgomery)	24	Aug	24	AS	$5,042	$11,135					
West Virginia University (Morgantown)	24	Aug	43	BSDH, MSDH	$6,140	$18,745				•	
Wisconsin											
Fox Valley Technical College (Appleton)	18	Aug	36	AS	$2,500	$12,000		•		•	•

*Data are shown only for programs that completed the 2007 AMA Survey of Health Professions Education Programs.
‡Key to Offers: 1: Evening or weekend classes; 2: Non-English instruction; 3: Cultural competence instruction; 4: Distance education component.

	Class Capacity	Begins	Length (months)	Award	Res. Tuition	Non-res. Tuition	Stipend	Offers:‡ 1	2	3	4
Madison Area Technical College	36	Aug	18	AAS	$1,802	$10,200					
Milwaukee Area Technical College	48	Aug Jan	18	AAS	$2,933	$17,789		•	•	•	
Northcentral Technical College (Wausau)	24	Aug	24, 27	AS	$5,962	$20,104					•
Wyoming											
Sheridan College	24	Aug	18	AAS	$1,368	$4,104					

*Data are shown only for programs that completed the 2007 AMA Survey of Health Professions Education Programs.
‡Key to Offers: 1: Evening or weekend classes; 2: Non-English instruction; 3: Cultural competence instruction; 4: Distance education component.

Dental Laboratory Technician

Alabama

H Council Trenholm State Technical College
Dental Lab Technician Prgm
1225 Air Base Blvd
Montgomery, AL 36108
Prgm Dir: Roosevelt Daniel, DDS
Tel: 334 420-4428
E-mail: rdaniel@trenholmtech.cc.al.us

Arizona

Pima Community College
Dental Lab Technician Prgm
2202 W Anklam Rd, HRP 220
Tucson, AZ 85709-0080
Prgm Dir: Max Atwell, BS
Tel: 520 206-3100   *Fax:* 520 206-3027
E-mail: Max.Atwell@pima.edu

California

Los Angeles City College
Dental Lab Technician Prgm
855 N Vermont Ave
Los Angeles, CA 90029
Prgm Dir: Arax S Cohen, BSB
Tel: 323 953-4000, Ext 2501   *Fax:* 323 953-4013
E-mail: cohenas@lacitycollege.edu

Pasadena City College
Dental Lab Technician Prgm
1570 E Colorado Blvd, R505
Pasadena, CA 91106
Prgm Dir: Anita M Bobich, BA AA CDT
Tel: 626 585-7884   *Fax:* 626 585-3168
E-mail: ambobich@pasadena.edu

Florida

McFatter Technical Center
Dental Lab Technician Prgm
6500 Nova Dr
Davie, FL 33317
http://mcfattertech.com
Prgm Dir: Fred Isaac
Tel: 754 321-3023, Ext 3022   *Fax:* 754 321-5820
E-mail: fred.isaac@browardschools.com

Indian River Community College
Dental Lab Technician Prgm
3209 Virginia Ave
Fort Pierce, FL 34981-5599
Prgm Dir: Don Symington, EdS
Tel: 772 462-7527   *Fax:* 772 462-4900
E-mail: dsymingt@ircc.edu

Georgia

Atlanta Technical College
Dental Lab Technician Prgm
1560 Metropolitan Pkwy SW
Atlanta, GA 30310-4446
Prgm Dir: Becky Tolson, CDT
Tel: 404 225-4561   *Fax:* 404 758-8522
E-mail: btolson@atlantatech.edu

Idaho

Idaho State University
Dental Lab Technician Prgm
Dental Lab Tech Box 8380
Pocatello, ID 83209-8380
Prgm Dir: Diane Edmunds
Tel: 208 282-3141   *Fax:* 208 282-3975
E-mail: edmudian@isu.edu

Indiana

Indiana Univ - Purdue Univ Ft Wayne
Dental Lab Technician Prgm
2101 Coliseum Blvd E
Fort Wayne, IN 46805
Prgm Dir: Brends Valliere
Tel: 260 481-6837   *Fax:* 260 481-5767
E-mail: valliereb@ipfw.edu

Iowa

Kirkwood Community College
Dental Lab Technician Prgm
6301 Kirkwood Blvd SW, PO Box 2068
Cedar Rapids, IA 52406-9973
www.kirkwood.edu
Prgm Dir: Betty Mitchell, BS CDT
Tel: 319 398-5400   *Fax:* 319 398-1293
E-mail: betty.mitchell@kirkwood.edu

Kentucky

Bluegrass Community and Technical College
Dental Lab Technician Prgm
470 Cooper Dr, 330 Oswald Bldg
Lexington, KY 40506-0235
www.bluegrass.kctcs.edu/ahDLT/
Prgm Dir: Robin Gornto, MSEd CDT
Tel: 859 246-6244   *Fax:* 859 246-4671
E-mail: robin.gornto@kctcs.edu

Louisiana

Louisiana State University
Dental Lab Technician Prgm
School of Dentistry
1100 Florida Ave
New Orleans, LA 70119
www.lsusd.lsumc.edu/academic/lab_tech.htm
Prgm Dir: Leonard Aucoin, Jr, CDT MEd
Tel: 225 334-5853   *Fax:* 225 334-5145
E-mail: laucoi@lsuhsc.edu

Massachusetts

Middlesex Community College - Lowell
Dental Lab Technician Prgm
33 Kearney Square
Lowell, MA 01852
Prgm Dir: Jerry Kessler, BS
Tel: 978 656-3056, Ext 3056   *Fax:* 978 656-3078
E-mail: kesslerj@middlesex.cc.ma.us

New York

New York City College of Technology
Dental Lab Technician Prgm
300 Jay St
Brooklyn, NY 11201-2983
Prgm Dir: Nicholas Manos
Tel: 718 260-5137   *Fax:* 718 260-5995
E-mail: NManos@citytech.cuny.edu

Erie Community College - South Campus
Dental Lab Technician Prgm
4041 Southwestern Blvd
Orchard Park, NY 14127-2199
https://www.ecc.edu
Prgm Dir: Marvin Herman, MD
Tel: 716 851-1759   *Fax:* 716 851-1704
E-mail: herman@ecc.edu

North Carolina

Durham Technical Community College
Dental Lab Technician Prgm
1637 Lawson St
Durham, NC 27703
www.durhamtech.edu
Prgm Dir: Michael Patrick, AA AAS CDT
Tel: 919 686-3399   *Fax:* 919 686-3737
E-mail: patrickm@durhamtech.edu

Oregon

Portland Community College
Dental Lab Technician Prgm
PO Box 19000
Portland, OR 97280-0990
Prgm Dir: Josette Beach, RDH MS
Tel: 503 977-4235   *Fax:* 503 977-8300
E-mail: jbeach@pcc.edu

Texas

Univ of Texas Hlth Sci Ctr at San Antonio
Dental Lab Technician Prgm
Dental Laboratory Sciences
7703 Floyd Curl Dr
San Antonio, TX 78284-7914
www.uthscsa.edu/sah/dlt.html
Prgm Dir: Roosevelt Davis, MS
Tel: 210 567-3056   *Fax:* 210 567-3061
E-mail: davisrd@uthscsa.edu

School of Health Care Sciences - Air Force
Dental Lab Technician Prgm
381 TRS/XWAE
917 Missile Rd
Sheppard AFB, TX 76311-2246
Prgm Dir: Lt Col Thomas S Bingham III
Tel: 940 676-6967   *Fax:* 940 676-6928

Virginia

J Sargeant Reynolds Community College
Dental Lab Technician Prgm
PO Box 85622
Richmond, VA 23285-5622
Prgm Dir: Ernie Wolfe, CDT AAS BS MEd
Tel: 804 523-5931   *Fax:* 804 786-5298
E-mail: ewolfe@jsr.vccs.edu

Washington

Bates Technical College
Dental Lab Technician Prgm
1101 S Yakima Ave
Tacoma, WA 98405
Prgm Dir: Jean Watley
Tel: 253 680-7215   *Fax:* 253 680-7293
E-mail: jwatley@bates.ctc.edu

Dental Laboratory Technician

	Class Capacity	Begins	Length (months)	Award	Res. Tuition	Non-res. Tuition	Stipend	1	2	3	4
Florida											
McFatter Technical Center (Davie)	24	Aug	18	Cert	$5,041	$10,000					
Iowa											
Kirkwood Community College (Cedar Rapids)	15	Aug	22	AAS	$4,183	$8,366				•	
Kentucky											
Bluegrass Community and Technical College (Lexington)	15	Aug	16	Cert, AAS	$2,760	$8,280					
Louisiana											
Louisiana State University (New Orleans)	12	Aug	24, 36	AS, BS	$2,304	$3,604					
New York											
Erie Community College - South Campus (Orchard Park)	30	Sep	24	AAS	$2,500	$5,000		•		•	
North Carolina											
Durham Technical Community College	24	Aug	12, 21	Cert, AAS	$2,106	$11,198					
Texas											
Univ of Texas Hlth Sci Ctr at San Antonio	12	Aug	18, 21	BS	$3,700	$12,226					

*Data are shown only for programs that completed the 2007 AMA Survey of Health Professions Education Programs.
‡Key to Offers: 1: Evening or weekend classes; 2: Non-English instruction; 3: Cultural competence instruction; 4: Distance education component.

Diagnostic Medical Sonographer

The diagnostic medical sonographer provides patient services using medical ultrasound (high-frequency sound waves that produce images of internal structures). Working under the supervision of a physician responsible for the use and interpretation of ultrasound procedures, the sonographer helps gather sonographic data to diagnose a variety of conditions and diseases, as well as monitor fetal development.

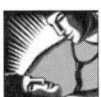

Job Description

The sonographer provides patient services in a variety of medical settings in which the physician is responsible for the use and interpretation of ultrasound procedures. In assisting physicians in gathering sonographic data, the diagnostic medical sonographer is able to

- Obtain, review, and integrate pertinent patient history and supporting clinical data to facilitate optimum diagnostic results
- Perform appropriate procedures and record anatomical, pathological, and/or physiological data for interpretation by a physician
- Record and process sonographic data and other pertinent observations made during the procedure for presentation to the interpreting physician
- Exercise discretion and judgment in the performance of sonographic services
- Provide patient education related to medical ultrasound
- Promote principles of good health

Employment Characteristics

Diagnostic medical sonographers may be employed in hospitals, clinics, private offices, and industry. Most full-time sonographers work about 40 hours a week; they may have evening weekend hours and times when they are on call and must be ready to report to work on short notice.

The demand for sonographers, including suitably qualified educators, researchers, and administrators, continues to exceed the supply, with faster than average job growth anticipated. The supply and demand ratio affects salaries, depending on experience and responsibilities.

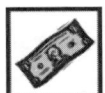

Salary

According to the Society of Diagnostic Medical Sonographers, the hourly salary for diagnostic medical sonographers is $29.00; median income in 2005 was $61,984. Refer to Section IV, Table 5 of this *Directory* for more information, or see www.ama-assn.org/go/hpsalary.

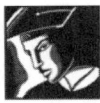

Educational Programs

Length. Accredited programs are between 1 and 4 years (certificate, associate, and baccalaureate level), depending on program design, objectives, and the degree or certificate awarded.

Prerequisites. Applicants to a 1-year program must possess qualifications in a clinically related allied health profession. Applicants to 2-year programs must be high school graduates (or equivalent) with an educational background in basic science, general physics, and algebra. All applicants must demonstrate satisfactory completion of the following courses at college level: general physics, biological science, algebra, and communication skills.

Skills potential and practicing sonographers should exhibit include social perceptiveness, learning strategies, critical thinking skills, instructional skills, active listening, active learning, reading comprehension, and written/oral expression.

Curriculum. Curricula of accredited programs include physical sciences, applied biological sciences, patient care, clinical medicine, applications of ultrasound, instrumentation, related diagnostic procedures, and image evaluation. A plan for well-structured, competency-based clinical education is an essential part of the curriculum of all sonography programs.

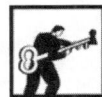

Registration

Although no state requires licensure in diagnostic medical sonography, organizations such as the American Registry for Diagnostic Medical Sonography (ARDMS) certify the competency of sonographers through registration. Because registration provides an independent, objective measure of an individual's professional standing, many employers prefer to hire registered sonographers. Registration with ARDMS requires passing a general physical principles and instrumentation examination, in addition to passing an exam in a specialty such as obstetric and gynecologic sonography, abdominal sonography, or neurosonography. To keep their registration current, sonographers must complete continuing education to stay abreast of technological advances related to the occupation.

Inquiries

Careers/Curriculum
Society of Diagnostic Medical Sonography
2745 Dallas Parkway, Suite 350
Plano, TX 75093-4706
214 473-8057
214 473-8563 Fax
E-mail: info@sdms.org
www.sdms.org

Society for Vascular Ultrasound
4601 Presidents Drive, Suite 260
Lanham, MD 20706-4365
301 459-7550 or 800 SVT- VEIN
301 459-5651 Fax
www.svtnet.org

American Society of Echocardiography
1500 Sunday Drive, Suite 102
Raleigh, NC 27607
919 861-5574
919 787-4916 Fax
www.asecho.org

Registration
American Registry for Diagnostic Medical Sonography
51 Monroe Street, Plaza East Ore
Rockville, MD 20852
301 738-8401
www.ardms.org

American Registry of Radiologic Technologists
1255 Northland Drive
St Paul, MN 55120-1155
651 687-0048
www.arrt.org

Program Accreditation
Commission on Accreditation of Allied Health Education Programs
(CAAHEP) in collaboration with:
Joint Review Committee on Education in Diagnostic Medical
Sonography

2025 Woodlane Drive
St Paul, MN 55125
651 731-1582
E-mail: jrc-dms@jcahpo.org

Note: Adapted in part from the Bureau of Labor Statistics, US
Department of Labor, *Occupational Outlook Handbook*, 2006-07
Edition, Diagnostic Medical Sonographers, on the Internet at
www.bls.gov/oco/ocos273.htm (visited November 06, 2007).

Diagnostic Medical Sonographer

Alabama

Wallace State Community College
Diagnostic Med Sonography Prgm
General concentration
PO Box 2000
Hanceville, AL 35077-2000
www.wallacestate.edu
Prgm Dir: Janet E Money, RDMS CNMT
Tel: 256 352-8318   *Fax:* 256 352-8320
E-mail: janet.money@wallacestate.edu

Institute of Ultrasound Diagnostics
Diagnostic Med Sonography Prgm
General concentration
1230 Montlimar Dr, Ste A
Mobile, AL 36609
www.iudmed.com
Prgm Dir: Kathryn A Gill, MS RT RDMS
Tel: 251 460-2485   *Fax:* 251 460-0672
E-mail: kgill@iudmed.com

Baptist Medical Center South
Diagnostic Med Sonography Prgm
General concentration
School of Diagnostic Ultrasound
Montgomery, AL 36111
www.baptistfirst.org
Prgm Dir: Brandi S Merrill, BS RT(R) RDMS (AB
   OB/GYN) RVT
Tel: 334 281-3470, Ext 2   *Fax:* 334 281-3671
E-mail: bmerrill@baptistfirst.org

Arizona

GateWay Community College
Diagnostic Med Sonography Prgm
General concentration
108 N 40th St
Phoenix, AZ 85034
Prgm Dir: Kathleen Murphy
Tel: 602 286-8490   *Fax:* 602 288-8003
E-mail: Murphy@gatewaycc.edu

Arkansas

University of Arkansas for Medical Sciences
Diagnostic Med Sonography Prgm
General, Cardiac, Vascular
4301 W Markham St Mail Slot 563-B
Little Rock, AR 72205
www.uams.edu/chrp/sonography/
Prgm Dir: Terry DuBose, MS RDMS FAIUM FSDMS
Tel: 501 686-5948   *Fax:* 501 686-6513
E-mail: duboseterryj@uams.edu

Arkansas State University
Diagnostic Med Sonography Prgm
General concentration
PO Box 910
State University, AR 72467
Prgm Dir: Jennifer DeClerk, BSRS RDMS RT(R)
Tel: 870 972-2914   *Fax:* 870 972-2004
E-mail: jdeclerk@astate.edu

California

Orange Coast College
Diagnostic Med Sonography Prgm
General concentration
2701 Fairview Rd
Costa Mesa, CA 92628-5005
Prgm Dir: Joan M Clasby, BVE RDMS
Tel: 714 432-5893   *Fax:* 714 432-5534
E-mail: jclasby@mail.occ.cccd.edu

Cypress College
Diagnostic Med Sonography Prgm
General concentration
9200 Valley View
Cypress, CA 90630
Prgm Dir: Lynn Mitts, MA RT ARDMS
Tel: 714 484-7283, Ext 48901   *Fax:* 714 527-2175
E-mail: lmitts@cypresscollege.edu

Loma Linda University
Diagnostic Med Sonography Prgm
General concentration
Sch of Allied Hlth Profs
Loma Linda, CA 92354
Prgm Dir: Marie T DeLange, BS RT RDMS RDCS
Tel: 909 558-4000, Ext 43027   *Fax:* 909 558-4166
E-mail: mdelange@ahs.llumc.edu

Foothill Community College
Diagnostic Med Sonography Prgm
General concentration
12345 El Monte Rd
Los Altos Hills, CA 94022-4599
www.foothill.edu
Prgm Dir: Kathleen Austin, BS RDMS RT
Tel: 650 949-7304   *Fax:* 650 949-7686
E-mail: austinkathleen@fhda.edu

Merced College
Diagnostic Med Sonography Prgm
General and Cardiac concentrations
3600 M Street
Merced, CA 95348-2806
Prgm Dir: Joy Guthrie, DHSc RDMS RDCS RVT
Tel: 209 384-6057
E-mail: guthriej@hotmail.com

Kaiser Permanente Sch of Allied Hlth Sciences
Diagnostic Med Sonography Prgm
General concentration
938 Marina Way South
Richmond, CA 94804
Prgm Dir: Carmelo Fernandez, MD RDMS
Tel: 510 231-5055   *Fax:* 510 231-5103
E-mail: Carmelo.F.Fernandez@kp.org

Univ of California San Diego Med Ctr
Diagnostic Med Sonography Prgm
General concentration
200 W Arbor Dr
San Diego, CA 92103-8759
http://radtech.ucsd.edu
Prgm Dir: Nannette Forsythe, BA RDMS RVT
Tel: 619 543-6617   *Fax:* 619 543-7464
E-mail: nforsythe@ucsd.edu

Colorado

U of Colorado (Denver) Health Sciences Center
Diagnostic Med Sonography Prgm
General concentration
Univ of Colorado Hosp, Anhschutz Center of Advanced
   Med
Aurora, CO 80045
www.uchsc.edu/radiology/
Prgm Dir: James Cacari, BS RT RVT RDMS
Tel: 720 848-1872   *Fax:* 720 848-1882
E-mail: James.Cacari@uch.edu

Connecticut

St Francis Hospital & Medical Center
Cosponsor: The Hofman Heart Institute of Connecticut
Diagnostic Med Sonography Prgm
Cardiac concentration
114 Woodland St
Hartford, CT 06105
Prgm Dir: Richard Palma, BS RDCS APS FASE
Tel: 860 714-4569
E-mail: rpalma@stfranciscare.org

Delaware

Delaware Technical & Community College - Wilmington
Diagnostic Med Sonography Prgm
General, Cardiac, and Vascular concentrations
333 Shipley St
Wilmington, DE 19801
www.dtcc.edu/wilmington/ah
Prgm Dir: Lily O Lee, BS RDMS RVT
Tel: 302 765-4588   *Fax:* 302 765-4599
E-mail: lillee@christianacare.org

District of Columbia

George Washington University
Diagnostic Med Sonography Prgm
General, Cardiac, and Vascular concentrations
900 23rd St NW, #6180
Washington, DC 20037
Prgm Dir: Catheeja Ismail, MA RDMS
Tel: 202 994-8697   *Fax:* 202 994-1073
E-mail: cismail@gwu.edu

Florida

Broward Community College
Diagnostic Med Sonography Prgm
General and Cardiac concentrations
North Campus Bldg 41
Coconut Creek, FL 33066
Prgm Dir: Sharon Calton, MS RDMS RDCS FSDMS
Tel: 954 201-2089   *Fax:* 954 201-2348
E-mail: scalton@broward.edu

Keiser University - Daytona Beach
Diagnostic Med Sonography Prgm
General concentration
1800 Business Park Blvd
Daytona Beach, FL 32114
www.keiseruniversity.edu
Prgm Dir: Marianne Peiffer, RDMS
Tel: 386 274-5060, Ext 123   *Fax:* 386 274-2725
E-mail: mariannep@keiseruniversity.edu

Keiser University
Diagnostic Med Sonography Prgm
General concentration
1500 NW 49th St
Fort Lauderdale, FL 33309
Prgm Dir: Rosy Silverman, RDMS
Tel: 954 776-4456, Ext 524   *Fax:* 954 776-5157
E-mail: rsilverman@keiseruniversity.edu

Nova Southeastern University
Diagnostic Med Sonography Prgm
Vascular concentration
3200 S University Dr
Fort Lauderdale, FL 33328
Prgm Dir: Terrence D Case, MEd RVT
Tel: 954 262-1220
E-mail: tcase@nova.edu

St Vincent's Medical Center
Diagnostic Med Sonography Prgm
General, Vascular
1800 Barrs St
Jacksonville, FL 32204
www.jaxhealth.com
Prgm Dir: Chemene Wilson, RT(R) RDMS RVT
Tel: 904 308-8272   *Fax:* 904 308-5109
E-mail: cwils002@stvincentshealth.com

Miami Dade College
Diagnostic Med Sonography Prgm
General and Cardiac concentrations
Medical Center Campus
Miami, FL 33127-4693
Prgm Dir: Dalia Sanchez-Suarez, BS RDMS RDCS
Tel: 305 237-4245   *Fax:* 305 237-4278
E-mail: dsanche1@mdc.edu

Valencia Community College
Diagnostic Med Sonography Prgm
General concentration
PO Box 3028
Orlando, FL 32811
www.valenciacc.edu/Sonography
Prgm Dir: Barbara Ball, BA RT(R) RDMS
Tel: 407 582-1191   *Fax:* 407 582-1278
E-mail: bball@valenciacc.edu

Palm Beach Community College
Diagnostic Med Sonography Prgm
General concentration
3160 PGA Blvd
Palm Beach Gardens, FL 33410
Prgm Dir: Patty Moraino-Braga, BS RDMS RVT RDCS RT(R)
Tel: 561 207-5053   *Fax:* 561 207-5011
E-mail: bragap@pbcc.edu

Hillsborough Community College
Diagnostic Med Sonography Prgm
General concentration
PO Box 30030
Tampa, FL 33630-3030
Prgm Dir: Louis J Gomez, RDMS RVT
Tel: 813 253-7412   *Fax:* 813 253-7473
E-mail: lgomez@hccfl.edu

Georgia

Grady Health System
Diagnostic Med Sonography Prgm
General concentration
80 Jesse Hill Jr Dr SE, PO Box 26095
Atlanta, GA 30303-3050
www.gradyhealthsystem.org
Prgm Dir: Judy K Billings, BS RT(R) RDMS
Tel: 404 616-5032   *Fax:* 404 616-3512
E-mail: jbillings@gmh.edu

Sanford-Brown Institute
Diagnostic Med Sonography Prgm
General concentration
1140 Hammond Dr, Ste A 1150
Atlanta, GA 30328
Prgm Dir: B Dwight Gunter
Tel: 770 576-6451
E-mail: dgunter@sb-atlanta.com

Medical College of Georgia
Diagnostic Med Sonography Prgm
General concentration
1120 15th St, AE1003
Augusta, GA 30912
Prgm Dir: Eric L Meaders
Tel: 706 721-2759   *Fax:* 706 721-8293
E-mail: emeaders@mcg.edu

Coosa Valley Technical College
Diagnostic Med Sonography Prgm
General, Vascular, and Echocardiography concentrations
1 Maurice Culberson Dr
Rome, GA 30161
http://test.cvtcollege.org/Ac_Programs/dms_vascular/
Prgm Dir: Leif Penrose, BA RDMS RDCS RVT
Tel: 706 295-6970   *Fax:* 706 295-6894
E-mail: lpenrose@coosavalleytech.edu

Ogeechee Technical College
Diagnostic Med Sonography Prgm
General concentration
1 Joe Kennedy Blvd
Statesboro, GA 30458
Prgm Dir: Tina W Welch, AS RDMS RVT RT(R)
Tel: 912 688-6019   *Fax:* 912 486-7604
E-mail: twelch@ogeecheetech.edu

Idaho

Boise State University
Diagnostic Med Sonography Prgm
General concentration
Radiologic Sciences Department
Boise, ID 83725-1845
http://radsci.boisestate.edu
Prgm Dir: Joie Burns, MS RT(R)(S) RDMS RVT
Tel: 208 426-1996   *Fax:* 208 426-4459
E-mail: jburns@boisestate.edu

Illinois

Southern Illinois University Carbondale
Diagnostic Med Sonography Prgm
General concentration
1365 Douglas Dr, Mailcode 6615
Carbondale, IL 62901
www.siuc.edu/~sah/RADS/rads.html
Prgm Dir: Karen Having, MS Ed RT(R) RDMS
Tel: 618 453-4980   *Fax:* 618 453-7020
E-mail: khaving@siu.edu

John A Logan College
Diagnostic Med Sonography Prgm
Cardiac concentration
700 Logan College Rd
Carterville, IL 62918
www.jalc.edu
Prgm Dir: Valerie Newberry, RVT RDCS
Tel: 618 985-2828, Ext 8622   *Fax:* 618 985-4654
E-mail: valerienewberry@jalc.edu

Northwestern Memorial Hospital
Diagnostic Med Sonography Prgm
General concentration
676 N St Clair St, Ste 550
Chicago, IL 60611
Prgm Dir: Casey Clarke, BSRT RT(R) RDMS RDCS
Tel: 312 926-1196   *Fax:* 312 926-1741
E-mail: cclarke@nmh.org

Rush University
Diagnostic Med Sonography Prgm
Vascular concentration
600 S Paulina St, Ste 440
Chicago, IL 60612
Prgm Dir: Eileen French-Sherry, MA RVT
Tel: 312 942-7286
E-mail: eileen_french-sherry@rush.edu

College of DuPage
Diagnostic Med Sonography Prgm
General and Vascular concentrations
425 Fawell Blvd
Glen Ellyn, IL 60137
www.cod.edu
Prgm Dir: Terrie Ciez, MS RDMS RDCS RT CNMT
Tel: 630 942-2436   *Fax:* 630 858-5409
E-mail: ciezte@cod.edu

Triton College
Diagnostic Med Sonography Prgm
General concentration
2000 N Fifth Ave
River Grove, IL 60171
Prgm Dir: Debra L Krukowski, BS RDMS RT(R)
Tel: 708 456-0300, Ext 3979   *Fax:* 708 583-3336
E-mail: dkrukows@triton.edu

South Suburban College
Diagnostic Med Sonography Prgm
General concentration
15800 S State St
South Holland, IL 60473
Prgm Dir: Casey Clark, RDMS RDCS RT(R)
Tel: 708 596-2000, Ext 2318
E-mail: dms@southsuburbancollege.edu
Notes: Currently inactive

Iowa

Mercy College of Health Sciences
Diagnostic Med Sonography Prgm
General and Cardiovascular concentrations
928 Sixth Ave
Des Moines, IA 50309-1239
Prgm Dir: Kathleen Lane, MSE S RDCS RVT
Tel: 515 643-6610   *Fax:* 515 643-6698
E-mail: klane@mercydesmoines.org

University of Iowa Hospitals & Clinics
Diagnostic Med Sonography Prgm
General, Cardiac, and Vascular concentrations
C-723 Radiology
Iowa City, IA 52242-1077
http://radiology.uiowa.edu/RadTech/
    SonographyBrochure.htm
Prgm Dir: Stephanie Ellingson, MS RDMS RDCS RVT
    RTR
Tel: 319 356-4871   *Fax:* 319 384-9574
E-mail: stephanie-ellingson@uiowa.edu

Kansas

University of Kansas Medical Center
Diagnostic Med Sonography Prgm
Cardiac concentration
Mid-American Cardiology
Kansas City, KS 66160
Prgm Dir: Mary Chivington, BS RDCS RVT
Tel: 913 588-9635   *Fax:* 913 588-1605
E-mail: mchivington@mac.md

University of Kansas Medical Center
Diagnostic Med Sonography Prgm
General and Vascular concentrations
2105 Bell Memorial Hospital
Kansas City, KS 66160
Prgm Dir: Candace S Spalding, BA RDMS RVT RT(R)
Tel: 913 588-6802
E-mail: cpaldin@kumc.edu

Washburn University
Diagnostic Med Sonography Prgm
General, Cardiac, and Vascular concentrations
1700 SW College Ave
Topeka, KS 66621
Prgm Dir: Doug James
Tel: 785 231-1010, Ext 2170
E-mail: doug.james@washburn.edu

Kentucky

St Catharine College
Diagnostic Med Sonography Prgm
General, Cardiac, and Vascular concentrations
310 Xavier Dr
Bardstown, KY 40004
Prgm Dir: Dennis Walter, AAS RRT RVT
Tel: 502 348-0475   *Fax:* 502 348-0466
E-mail: dwalters@bardstowncable.net

Bowling Green Technical College
Diagnostic Med Sonography Prgm
General concentration
1845 Loop Dr
Bowling Green, KY 42101-3601
www.bowlinggreen.kctcs.edu
Prgm Dir: Becky Stevens, BS RT(R)(M) RDMS
Tel: 270 901-1082   *Fax:* 270 901-1139
E-mail: becky.stevens@kctcs.edu

Morehead State University
Diagnostic Med Sonography Prgm
General concentration
150 University Blvd
Morehead, KY 40351
Prgm Dir: Wretha G Goodpaster, MSRS
    RT(M)(QM)(CT) RDMS RVT
Tel: 606 783-2647   *Fax:* 606 783-5051
E-mail: w.goodpaster@moreheadstate.edu

**West Kentucky Community & Technical
    College**
Diagnostic Med Sonography Prgm
General concentration
4810 Alben Barkley Dr, PO Box 7380
Paducah, KY 42002-7308
Prgm Dir: Alice Robertson, BS RT(R) RDMS
Tel: 270 534-3487, Ext 43487   *Fax:* 270 534-3498
E-mail: alice.vaughn@kctcs.edu

Louisiana

Louisiana State University - Eunice
Diagnostic Med Sonography Prgm
General concentration
PO Box 1129
Eunice, LA 70535
Prgm Dir: Drew Thibodeaux
Tel: 337 550-1431
E-mail: dthibode@lsue.edu

Delgado Community College
Diagnostic Med Sonography Prgm
General concentration
615 City Park Ave
New Orleans, LA 70119
www.dcc.edu
Prgm Dir: John Geshner, BA RDMS RDCS
Tel: 504 568-6473   *Fax:* 504 568-5494
E-mail: jgeshn@dcc.edu

Maryland

Johns Hopkins Hospital
Diagnostic Med Sonography Prgm
General concentration
Radiology Admin B-179
Baltimore, MD 21287
http://radiologycareers.rad.jhmi.edu
Prgm Dir: Carol Iversen, MS RDMS
Tel: 410 528-8263   *Fax:* 410 528-8308
E-mail: cblank1@jhmi.edu

University of Maryland Baltimore County
Diagnostic Med Sonography Prgm
Cardiac, General, and Vascular concentrations
South Campus, Technology Center
Baltimore, MD 21227
www.umbctrainingcenters.com
Prgm Dir: Lyna El-Khoury Rumbarger, BS RDCS
Tel: 443 543-5423   *Fax:* 443 543-5410
E-mail: lrumbarger@umbctrainingcenters.com

Montgomery College
Diagnostic Med Sonography Prgm
General, Cardiac, and Vascular concentrations
7977 Georgia Ave
Silver Spring, MD 20910
http://montgomerycollege.edu/dms
Prgm Dir: Linda Zanin, EdD RDMS
Tel: 301 567-5569   *Fax:* 301 562-5569
E-mail: linda.zanin@montgomerycollege.edu

Massachusetts

Middlesex Community College - Bedford
Diagnostic Med Sonography Prgm
General concentration
Springs Rd, Bldg 6
Bedford, MA 01730
www.middlesex.mass.edu
Prgm Dir: Thomas Walsh, MA RDMS RVS
Tel: 781 280-3983   *Fax:* 781 280-3845
E-mail: walsht@middlesex.mass.edu

Bunker Hill Community College
Diagnostic Med Sonography Prgm
General and Cardiac concentrations
250 New Rutherford Ave
Boston, MA 02129-2991
Prgm Dir: Michelle Gagnon, BS RDCS RVT
Tel: 617 228-2407   *Fax:* 617 228-2052
E-mail: mgagnon@bhcc.mass.edu

Springfield Technical Community College
Diagnostic Med Sonography Prgm
General concentration
One Armory Square
Springfield, MA 01102-9000
www.stcc.edu
Prgm Dir: David J Sloan, BA RDMS RVT
Tel: 413 755-4915   *Fax:* 413 755-4764
E-mail: djsloan@stcc.edu

Michigan

Henry Ford Hospital
Diagnostic Med Sonography Prgm
General concentration
2799 W Grand Blvd
Detroit, MI 48202
www.henryfordhealth.org
Prgm Dir: Michael Moffatt, MA RDMS
Tel: 313 916-3519   *Fax:* 313 916-9480
E-mail: mike@rad.hfh.edu

Jackson Community College
Diagnostic Med Sonography Prgm
General, Cardiac, and Vascular concentrations
2111 Emmons Rd
Jackson, MI 49201
Prgm Dir: Lynne Schreiber, MS RDMS RT(R)
Tel: 517 796-8494   *Fax:* 517 768-7004
E-mail: lynne_schreiber@jccmi.edu

Lansing Community College
Diagnostic Med Sonography Prgm
General concentration
PO Box 40010
Lansing, MI 48901-7210
Prgm Dir: Julie A Atkinson, BBA RDMS
Tel: 517 483-1410   *Fax:* 517 483-1508
E-mail: atkinsoj@lcc.edu

Oakland Community College - Southfield
Diagnostic Med Sonography Prgm
General concentration
22322 Rutland Dr
Southfield, MI 48075
Prgm Dir: Carolyn E Nacy, RDMS
Tel: 248 233-2918   *Fax:* 248 233-2891
E-mail: ceoneill@oaklandcc.edu

Providence Hospital
Diagnostic Med Sonography Prgm
General, Vascular
16001 W Nine Mile Rd
Southfield, MI 48075
www.stjohn.org/AlliedHealth/Sonography/
Prgm Dir: Janette Jablonski, BAS RDMS RVT RDCS
Tel: 248 849-5385   *Fax:* 248 849-5395
E-mail: janette.jablonski@providence-stjohnhealth.org

Delta College
Diagnostic Med Sonography Prgm
General concentration
1961 Delta Rd
University Center, MI 48710
Prgm Dir: Kim Boldt, BS RMS RVT RDCS RT
Tel: 989 686-9361   *Fax:* 989 667-2230
E-mail: kboldt@alpha.delta.edu

Minnesota

Argosy University - Twin Cities
Diagnostic Med Sonography Prgm
General and Echocardiography concentrations
1515 Central Parkway
Eagan, MN 55121
Prgm Dir: Susan D Hummel, BS RT(R) RDMS
Tel: 651 846-3405   *Fax:* 651 994-0144
E-mail: shummel@argosyu.edu

College of St Catherine - Minneapolis
Diagnostic Med Sonography Prgm
General concentration
601 25th Ave S
Minneapolis, MN 55454
Prgm Dir: Dick Mabbs, BA RVT RDMS
Tel: 612 690-7889   *Fax:* 612 690-7765
E-mail: dvmabbs@stkate.edu

Mayo School of Health Sciences
Diagnostic Med Sonography Prgm
General, Cardiac, and Vascular concentrations
200 First St SW
Rochester, MN 55905
www.mayo.edu/mshs
Prgm Dir: Kathryn Kuntz, BS RT RDMS RVT
Tel: 507 284-6520   *Fax:* 507 284-0656
E-mail: dms.admissions@mayo.edu

St Cloud Technical College
Diagnostic Med Sonography Prgm
General concentration
1540 Northway Dr
St Cloud, MN 56303
www.sctc.edu
Prgm Dir: Jeff Gunderson, BS RT(R) RDMS RVT
Tel: 320 308-0971   *Fax:* 320 308-6172
E-mail: jgunderson@sctc.edu

Mississippi

Hinds Community College
Diagnostic Med Sonography Prgm
General concentration
1750 Chadwick Dr
Jackson, MS 39204
Prgm Dir: Melissa K Mabry, RT(R) RDMS RVT
Tel: 601 371-3536   *Fax:* 601 371-3508
E-mail: mmabry@hindscc.edu

Itawamba Community College
Diagnostic Med Sonography Prgm
General concentration
2176 S Eason Blvd
Tupelo, MS 38804
Prgm Dir: Nita Megginson, RT(R) RDMS
Tel: 662 620-5145
E-mail: nmmegginson@iccms.edu

Missouri

University of Missouri - Columbia
Diagnostic Med Sonography Prgm
General and Vascular concentrations
605 Lewis Hall
Columbia, MO 65211
www.missouri.edu
Prgm Dir: Moses Hdeib
Tel: 573 884-2994   *Fax:* 573 884-8000
E-mail: hdeibm@health.missouri.edu

CoxHealth
Diagnostic Med Sonography Prgm
General, Cardiac, and Vascular concentrations
3801 S National Ave
Springfield, MO 65807
Prgm Dir: Tammy J Stearns, BSRT(R) RDMS RVT
Tel: 417 269-8669   *Fax:* 417 269-8900
E-mail: Tammy.Stearns@CoxHealth.com

St Louis Community College - Forest Park
Diagnostic Med Sonography Prgm
General, Cardiac, and Vascular concentrations
5600 Oakland Ave
St Louis, MO 63110
Prgm Dir: Beth Anderhub, MEd RDMS RT
Tel: 314 644-9399   *Fax:* 314 644-9752
E-mail: banderhub@stlcc.edu

Nebraska

NE Methodist Coll Nursing & Allied Hlth
Diagnostic Med Sonography Prgm
General, Cardiac, and Vascular concentrations
8501 W Dodge Rd
Omaha, NE 68114
Prgm Dir: Patricia Sullivan, MA RDMS RT
Tel: 402 354-4851   *Fax:* 402 354-8875
E-mail: psulliv@methodistcollege.edu

University of Nebraska Medical Center
Diagnostic Med Sonography Prgm
General concentration
Division of Radiation Sciences Technology Educ
Omaha, NE 68198-4545
www.unmc.edu/alliedhealth/rste
Prgm Dir: Kim Michael, MA RT(R) RDMS RVT
Tel: 402 559-1189   *Fax:* 402 559-4667
E-mail: kkmichael@unmc.edu

Nevada

College of Southern Nevada
Diagnostic Med Sonography Prgm
General, Cardiac, and Vascular concentrations
6375 W Charleston Blvd, W3K
Las Vegas, NV 89146
Prgm Dir: Tracy Lopez, MEd RDMS RDCS RVT
Tel: 702 651-5925   *Fax:* 702 651-7459
E-mail: tracy.lopez@csn.edu

New Hampshire

New Hampshire Technical Institute
Diagnostic Med Sonography Prgm
General concentration
31 College Dr
Concord, NH 03301-7412
www.nhti.edu
Prgm Dir: Kevin P Barry, MEd RT(R) RDMS RDCS
Tel: 603 271-7154   *Fax:* 603 271-7182
E-mail: kbarry@nhctc.edu

New Jersey

Sanford-Brown Institute
Diagnostic Med Sonography Prgm
General concentration
675 US 1 Plaza Gill Ln, 2nd Fl
Iselin, NJ 08830
www.sbinj.com
Prgm Dir: Anthony Rodriguez, RVT RDMS
Tel: 732 623-5740   *Fax:* 866 759-5357
E-mail: arodriguez@sb-nj.com

Bergen Community College
Diagnostic Med Sonography Prgm
General and Cardiac concentrations
400 Paramus Rd
Paramus, NJ 07652-1595
Prgm Dir: Katherine Benz-Campbell, MA BS RDMS
Tel: 201 447-7944, Ext 7939   *Fax:* 201 612-3876
E-mail: kbcampbell@bergen.edu

Muhlenberg Regional Medical Center
Diagnostic Med Sonography Prgm
General concentration
Harold B and Dorothy A Snyder Schools
Plainfield, NJ 07061
Prgm Dir: Harry H Holdorf, MPA RT(ARRT) RDMS
Tel: 908 668-2884   *Fax:* 908 226-4568
E-mail: hholdorf@solarishs.org

Univ of Medicine & Dent of New Jersey
Diagnostic Med Sonography Prgm
General concentration
School of Health Related Professions
Scotch Plains, NJ 07076
http://shrp.umdnj.edu
Prgm Dir: Cynthia Silkowski, MA RDMS RVT
Tel: 908 889-2521   *Fax:* 908 889-2527
E-mail: silkowcy@umdnj.edu

Gloucester County College
Diagnostic Med Sonography Prgm
General concentration
1400 Tanyard Rd
Sewell, NJ 08080
Prgm Dir: Michael Keith, BSRT RDMS
Tel: 856 415-2195   *Fax:* 856 464-8463
E-mail: mkeith@gccnj.edu

New Mexico

Central New Mexico Community College
Diagnostic Med Sonography Prgm
General concentration
525 Buena Vista SE
Albuquerque, NM 87106
Prgm Dir: Darlene Blagg
Tel: 505 224-4127   *Fax:* 505 224-4120
E-mail: DBlagg@cnm.edu

Dona Ana Community College
Diagnostic Med Sonography Prgm
General concentration
MSC3DA PO Box 30001
Las Cruces, NM 88003-8001
http://dabcc.nmsu.edu/sonography
Prgm Dir: Darla Matthew, RT RDMS
Tel: 505 582-7047   *Fax:* 505 527-7765
E-mail: dmatthew@nmsu.edu

New York

Long Island University
Diagnostic Med Sonography Prgm
Vascular concentration
1 University Plaza (M-101)
Brooklyn, NY 11201-5372
www.brooklyn.liu.edu
Prgm Dir: Lydia Thomas
Tel: 718 488-3639
E-mail: lydia.thomas@liu.edu

SUNY Downstate Medical Center
Diagnostic Med Sonography Prgm
General and Cardiac concentrations
College of Health-Related Professions
Brooklyn, NY 11203
Prgm Dir: Joyce Miller, EdD RDMS
Tel: 718 270-7765   *Fax:* 718 270-7746
E-mail: joyce.miller@downstate.edu

New York University
Diagnostic Med Sonography Prgm
General and Cardiac concentrations
726 Broadway, Rm 652
New York, NY 10003-6688
www.scps.nyu.edu/degcert/
  degree_info.jsp?stDegType=AS
Prgm Dir: Kerry Weinberg, MPA RT RDMS RDCS
Tel: 212 992-8723   *Fax:* 212 995-4890
E-mail: kerry.weinberg@nyu.edu

Western Suffolk BOCES
Diagnostic Med Sonography Prgm
General, Cardiac, and Vascular concentrations
152 Laurel Hill Rd
Northport, NY 11768
Prgm Dir: John Thomas, MS BED RDMS RVT RDCS RT
Tel: 631 261-3730   *Fax:* 631 623-4908
E-mail: jthomas@wsboces.org

Rochester Institute of Technology
Diagnostic Med Sonography Prgm
General and Echocardiography concentrations
153 Lomb Memorial Dr
Rochester, NY 14623
Prgm Dir: Hamad Ghazle, MS BS RDMS
Tel: 585 475-2241   *Fax:* 585 475-5809
E-mail: hhgscl@rit.edu

Hudson Valley Community College
Diagnostic Med Sonography Prgm
General and Cardiac concentrations
80 Vandenburgh Ave
Troy, NY 12180
Prgm Dir: Sheila Hughes, BPS LRT RDMS RVT
Tel: 518 629-7345   *Fax:* 518 629-4871
E-mail: hugheshe@hvcc.edu

North Carolina

Asheville-Buncombe Technical Comm College
Diagnostic Med Sonography Prgm
General and Vascular concentrations
340 Victoria Rd
Asheville, NC 28801
Prgm Dir: Chastity Coates Case, RT(R) RDMS RVT
Tel: 828 254-1921, Ext 470   *Fax:* 828 251-6355
E-mail: ccase@asheville.cc.nc.us

Pitt Community College
Diagnostic Med Sonography Prgm
General and Cardiac concentrations
PO Drawer 7007
Greenville, NC 27835-7007
Prgm Dir: Ruggie MacKenzie, RDMS RDCS
Tel: 252 321-4453   *Fax:* 252 321-4451
E-mail: rmackenz@email.pittcc.edu

Caldwell Comm College & Tech Institute
Diagnostic Med Sonography Prgm
General and Cardiac concentrations
2855 Hickory Blvd
Hudson, NC 28638
www.cccti.edu
Prgm Dir: Kimberlee B Watts, MS RDMS
Tel: 828 726-2322   *Fax:* 828 726-2489
E-mail: kwatts@cccti.edu

Johnston Community College
Diagnostic Med Sonography Prgm
General, Cardiac, and Vascular concentrations
PO Box 2350
Smithfield, NC 27577
www.johnstoncc.edu
Prgm Dir: Cathy Godwin, BS RTR RDMS RDCS RVT
Tel: 919 209-2158   *Fax:* 919 209-2153
E-mail: godwinc@johnstoncc.edu

Cape Fear Community College
Diagnostic Med Sonography Prgm
General concentration
411 N Front St
Wilmington, NC 28401
Prgm Dir: Kellee Stacks
Tel: 910 362-7482   *Fax:* 910 602-3151
E-mail: kstacks@cfcc.edu

Forsyth Technical Community College
Diagnostic Med Sonography Prgm
General concentration
2100 Silas Creek Pkwy
Winston-Salem, NC 27103
Prgm Dir: Wendy Barnhardt, BS RDMS RDCS
Tel: 336 734-7157   *Fax:* 336 734-7444
E-mail: wbarnhardt@forsythtech.edu

Ohio

Mercy Medical Center
Diagnostic Med Sonography Prgm
General concentration
1320 Mercy Dr NW
Canton, OH 44708
Prgm Dir: Susan Black, RDMS
Tel: 330 489-1000, Ext 6609   *Fax:* 330 580-4726
E-mail: susan.black@csauh.com

Cincinnati State Tech & Comm College
Diagnostic Med Sonography Prgm
General, Cardiac, and Vascular concentrations
3250 Central Pkwy
Cincinnati, OH 45223
www.cincinnatistate.edu
Prgm Dir: Susan Gomien, RDMS
Tel: 513 569-1665   *Fax:* 513 569-1659
E-mail: susan.gomien@cincinnatistate.edu

Lorain County Community College
Diagnostic Med Sonography Prgm
General concentration
1005 N Abbe Rd
Elyria, OH 44035
www.lorainccc.edu
Prgm Dir: Craig Peneff, BSAS RDMS RVT
Tel: 800 995-5222, Ext 7189   *Fax:* 440 366-4116
E-mail: cpeneff@lorainccc.edu

Kettering College of Medical Arts
Diagnostic Med Sonography Prgm
General, Cardiac, and Vascular concentrations
3737 Southern Blvd
Kettering, OH 45429
Prgm Dir: Joyce Grube, MS RDMS
Tel: 937 298-3399, Ext 55656   *Fax:* 937 395-8635
E-mail: joyce.grube@kcma.edu

Sanford-Brown Institute
Diagnostic Med Sonography Prgm
General concentration
17535 Rosbough Dr
Middleburg Heights, OH 44130
Prgm Dir: Renato M Agustin, MD RDMS RVT
Tel: 440 202-3236   *Fax:* 440 239-9648
E-mail: ragustin@sbc-cleveland.com

Central Ohio Technical College
Diagnostic Med Sonography Prgm
General, Cardiac, and Vascular concentrations
1179 University Dr
Newark, OH 43055-1767
Prgm Dir: Cathie Scholl, RDMS RVT
Tel: 740 366-9274   *Fax:* 740 366-5047
E-mail: cscholl@cotc.edu

Cuyahoga Community College
Diagnostic Med Sonography Prgm
General, Cardiac, and Vascular concentrations
11000 Pleasant Valley Rd
Parma, OH 44130
Prgm Dir: Denise M Kinches, BS RT RDMS
Tel: 216 987-5564   *Fax:* 216 987-5066
E-mail: denise.kinches@tri-c.edu

University of Rio Grande
Cosponsor: Rio Grande Community College
Diagnostic Med Sonography Prgm
General concentration
PO Box 500
Rio Grande, OH 45674-0500
www.rio.edu
Prgm Dir: Stephanie Sanunders, BS RDCS RVT
Tel: 740 245-7139   *Fax:* 740 245-5266
E-mail: ssaunders@rio.edu

Owens Community College
Diagnostic Med Sonography Prgm
General concentration
PO Box 10,000, Oregon Rd
Toledo, OH 43699-1947
Prgm Dir: Susan Perry, RDMS BSRT
Tel: 419 661-7560   *Fax:* 419 661-7251
E-mail: sperry@owens.edu

Oklahoma

Moore Norman Technology Center
Diagnostic Med Sonography Prgm
General concentration
4701 12th Ave NW
Norman, OK 73069
www.mntechnology.com
Prgm Dir: Meleah Meadows, BSRT RDMS RVT
Tel: 405 364-5763, Ext 7200
E-mail: mmeadows@mntechnology.com

Univ of Oklahoma Health Sciences Center
Diagnostic Med Sonography Prgm
General and Cardiac concentrations
PO Box 26901
Oklahoma City, OK 73190
Prgm Dir: Kari Boyce, PhD RDMC RDCS
Tel: 405 271-6477   *Fax:* 405 271-1424
E-mail: kari-boyce@ouhsc.edu

Pennsylvania

Northampton Community College
Diagnostic Med Sonography Prgm
General concentration
3835 Green Pond Rd
Bethlehem, PA 18020
www.northampton.edu
Prgm Dir: Catherine Rienzo, MS RT(R) RDMS
Tel: 610 332-6177   *Fax:* 610 861-4581
E-mail: crienzo@northampton.edu

Misericordia Unversity
Diagnostic Med Sonography Prgm
General concentration
301 Lake St
Dallas, PA 18612
Prgm Dir: Sheryl E Goss, MS RT RDMS RDCS RVT
Tel: 570 674-6790   *Fax:* 570 674-3052
E-mail: sgoss@misericordia.edu

Great Lakes Institute of Technology
Diagnostic Med Sonography Prgm
General concentration
5100 Peach St
Erie, PA 16509
Prgm Dir: Doug McCraney, RDMS RVT
Tel: 814 864-6666, Ext 264   *Fax:* 814 868-1717
E-mail: dougm@glit.edu

Harrisburg Area Community College
Diagnostic Med Sonography Prgm
General concentration
1 HACC Dr
Harrisburg, PA 17110-2999
Prgm Dir: Julia R Imboden
Tel: 717 221-1322   *Fax:* 717 909-4010
E-mail: jrimbode@hacc.edu

Lancaster Gen Coll of Nursing & Hlth Sciences
Diagnostic Med Sonography Prgm
General concentration
410 N Lime St
Lancaster, PA 17602
www.LancasterGeneral.org
Prgm Dir: Robert M Hess, BS RDMS
Tel: 717 544-5637   *Fax:* 717 544-5970
E-mail: rmhess@LancasterGeneral.org

Comm College of Allegheny County
Diagnostic Med Sonography Prgm
General and Cardiac concentrations
595 Beatty Rd
Monroeville, PA 15146
http://ccac.edu
Prgm Dir: Lynn Gigandet, MSEd RDMS
Tel: 724 325-6731   *Fax:* 724 325-6701
E-mail: lgigandet@ccac.edu

Thomas Jefferson University
Diagnostic Med Sonography Prgm
General, Cardiac, and Vascular concentrations
130 S Ninth St, Ste 1011
Philadelphia, PA 19107
Prgm Dir: Michael J Hartman, MS RDMS RVT RT(R)
Tel: 215 503-8724   *Fax:* 215 503-1031
E-mail: michael.hartman@jefferson.edu

Western School of Health & Business -
  Pittsburgh
Diagnostic Med Sonography Prgm
General concentration
421 Seventh Ave
Pittsburgh, PA 15219
Prgm Dir: Sandra M Gosnell, RDMS
Tel: 412 209-0472   *Fax:* 412 281-0319
E-mail: sgosnell@western-school.com

Lackawanna College
Diagnostic Med Sonography Prgm
General and Vascular concentrations
501 Vine St
Scranton, PA 18509
Prgm Dir: Janine Oliveri, MSEd BSRT RDMS RVT
Tel: 570 504-7920   *Fax:* 570 961-7832
E-mail: oliverij@lackawanna.edu

Crozer-Keystone Medical Center
Diagnostic Med Sonography Prgm
General concentration
North Campus Rm 214A
Upland, PA 19013
www.crozer.org
Prgm Dir: Barbara Annunziato, BS RT RDMS RVT
Tel: 610 447-2502, Ext 2   *Fax:* 610 447-2296
E-mail: barbara.annunziato@crozer.org

Wilkes-Barre General Hospital
Cosponsor: Wyoming Valley Health Care System
Diagnostic Med Sonography Prgm
General concentration
575 N River St
Wilkes-Barre, PA 18764
Prgm Dir: Lisa Capizzi, BS RT(R)(M) RDMS RVT
Tel: 570 552-4654   *Fax:* 570 552-4653
E-mail: lcapizzi@wvhcs.org

Rhode Island

Rhode Island Hospital
Diagnostic Med Sonography Prgm
General concentration
4 Davol Square, Building "A" , Box 162
Providence, RI 02903
www.lifespan.org/diagimag
Prgm Dir: Paul Maria, RDMS RVT
Tel: 401 528-8531, Ext 228   *Fax:* 401 457-0219
E-mail: pmaria@lifespan.org

South Carolina

Greenville Technical College
Diagnostic Med Sonography Prgm
General concentration
PO Box 5616
Greenville, SC 29606
Prgm Dir: Ronda Keller, RT(R) RDMS RVT
Tel: 864 250-8110   *Fax:* 864 250-8462
E-mail: ronda.keller@gvltec.edu

South Dakota

Southeast Technical Institute
Diagnostic Med Sonography Prgm
General concentration
2320 N Career Ave
Sioux Falls, SD 57107
Prgm Dir: Jo Ellen Hagemeyer, RT(R) RDMS
Tel: 605 367-7624
E-mail: jo.ellen.hagemeyer@southeasttech.com

Tennessee

Chattanooga State Technical Comm College
Diagnostic Med Sonography Prgm
General concentration
HPF 177
Chattanooga, TN 37406
www.chattanoogastate.edu
Prgm Dir: Jody Hancock, MAEd RDMS RVT RT(R)
Tel: 423 697-3341   *Fax:* 423 697-3324
E-mail: jody.hancock@chattanoogastate.edu

Volunteer State Community College
Diagnostic Med Sonography Prgm
General concentration
1480 Nashville Pike
Gallatin, TN 37066-3188
Prgm Dir: Gene Spain, BBA RDMS
Tel: 615 452-8600, Ext 3339   *Fax:* 615 230-3574
E-mail: gene.spain@volstate.edu

Baptist College of Health Sciences
Diagnostic Med Sonography Prgm
General and Vascular Sonography concentrations
1003 Monroe Ave
Memphis, TN 38104
www.bchs.edu
Prgm Dir: Mitzi Roberts, MS RT RDMS
Tel: 901 572-2653   *Fax:* 901 572-2750
E-mail: mitzi.roberts@bchs.edu

Methodist Le Bonheur Healthcare
Diagnostic Med Sonography Prgm
General concentration
Dept of Radiology
Memphis, TN 38104
Prgm Dir: Dawn L Driver, RDMS RDCS RVT
Tel: 901 516-8099   *Fax:* 901 516-2870
E-mail: driverd@methodisthealth.org

Vanderbilt University Medical Center
Diagnostic Med Sonography Prgm
General concentration
1161 21st Ave S
Nashville, TN 37232-2675
Prgm Dir: Jill D Herzog, BS RT(R) RDMS RVT
Tel: 615 343-0905   *Fax:* 615 322-3764
E-mail: jill.herzog@vanderbilt.edu

Texas

Alvin Community College
Diagnostic Med Sonography Prgm
Echocardiography and Vascular concentrations
3110 Mustang Rd
Alvin, TX 77511-4898
Prgm Dir: Jessica L Murphy, BS RRT-NPS RDCS RVT
Tel: 281 756-5650   *Fax:* 281 756-5606
E-mail: jmurphy@alvincollege.edu

Austin Community College
Diagnostic Med Sonography Prgm
General and Cardiac concentrations
3401 Webberville Rd
Austin, TX 78702
Prgm Dir: Regina Swearengin, AAS BS RDMS
Tel: 512 223-5944   *Fax:* 512 223-5895
E-mail: ginas@austincc.edu

Lamar Institute of Technology
Diagnostic Med Sonography Prgm
General concentration
PO Box 10061
Beaumont, TX 77710
www.lit.edu
Prgm Dir: Sheila Trahan, RDMS RT
Tel: 409 839-2924   *Fax:* 409 880-8955
E-mail: sheila.trahan@lit.edu

Univ Tx at Brownsville/Tx Southmost Coll
Diagnostic Med Sonography Prgm
General concentration
80 Fort Brown
Brownsville, TX 78620
Prgm Dir: Marti Flores, MS RDMS RDCS RT(R)
Tel: 956 882-5011   *Fax:* 956 882-5012
E-mail: marti.flores@utb.edu

Del Mar College
Diagnostic Med Sonography Prgm
General concentration
101 Baldwin and Ayers Sts
Corpus Christi, TX 78404
Prgm Dir: Rita S Orchard, MS RT(R) RDMS
Tel: 361 698-2833   *Fax:* 361 698-2811
E-mail: rorchard@delmar.edu

Cy-Fair College
Diagnostic Med Sonography Prgm
General concentration
9191 Barker-Cypress Rd
Cypress, TX 77433
Prgm Dir: Christina Hagerty, MEd RT(R) RDMS
Tel: 281 290-3971
E-mail: christina.hagerty@nhmccd.edu

El Centro College
Diagnostic Med Sonography Prgm
General concentration
Main and Lamar Sts
Dallas, TX 75202
Prgm Dir: Jan Bryant, MS RDMS
Tel: 214 860-2300   *Fax:* 214 860-2268
E-mail: jdb5529@dcccd.edu

Sanford-Brown Institute - Dallas
Diagnostic Med Sonography Prgm
General concentration
1250 W Mockingbird Ln
Dallas, TX 75247
Prgm Dir: Amjad Majeed, MB BS DMRD RDMS
Tel: 214 459-8490, Ext 8517   *Fax:* 214 638-6006
E-mail: amajeed@sbdallas.com

El Paso Community College
Diagnostic Med Sonography Prgm
General concentration
PO Box 20500
El Paso, TX 79998
Prgm Dir: Nora M Balderas, BS RT(R) RDMS
Tel: 915 831-4108, Ext 4141   *Fax:* 915 831-4114
E-mail: norab@epcc.edu

Houston Community College
Diagnostic Med Sonography Prgm
General concentration
1900 Pressler Dr
Houston, TX 77030
Prgm Dir: William Richardson, MPA RT(R) RDMS
Tel: 713 718-7343
E-mail: william.richardson@hccs.edu

Sanford-Brown Institute - Houston
Diagnostic Med Sonography Prgm
General concentration
10500 Forum Place Dr #200
Houston, TX 77036
Prgm Dir: Wendy Fuller
Tel: 713 779-1110   *Fax:* 713 779-2408
E-mail: wfuller@sbhouston.com

Midland College
Diagnostic Med Sonography Prgm
General concentration
3600 N Garfield
Midland, TX 79705
Prgm Dir: Elizabeth Brown
Tel: 432 685-4600   *Fax:* 432 685-4762
E-mail: lbrown@midland.edu

Tyler Junior College
Diagnostic Med Sonography Prgm
General concentration
PO Box 9020
Tyler, TX 75711
Prgm Dir: Pam Brower, RVT RVS
Tel: 903 510-2668   *Fax:* 903 510-2889
E-mail: pbro@tjc.edu

Virginia

Southwest Virginia Community College
Diagnostic Med Sonography Prgm
General concentration
PO Box SVCC (A-139)
Richlands, VA 24641-1510
Prgm Dir: Linda Brewster, BS RDMS RT(R)
Tel: 540 964-7642   *Fax:* 540 964-7715
E-mail: linda_brewster@sw.cc.va.us

Tidewater Community College
Diagnostic Med Sonography Prgm
General concentration
1700 College Crescent
Virginia Beach, VA 23453
www.tcc.edu/healthprofessions/
Prgm Dir: Felicia Toreno, PhD RDMS RVT
Tel: 757 822-7271   *Fax:* 757 822-7556
E-mail: ftoreno@tcc.edu

Washington

Bellevue Community College
Diagnostic Med Sonography Prgm
General and Cardiac concentrations
3000 Landerholm Circle SE, Rm B243
Bellevue, WA 98007-6484
Prgm Dir: Ann Polin, MSRS RDMS
Tel: 425 564-4181   *Fax:* 425 564-3128
E-mail: apolin@bcc.ctc.edu

Seattle University
Diagnostic Med Sonography Prgm
General, Cardiac, and Vascular concentrations
901 12th Ave, PO Box 222000
Seattle, WA 98122-4360
Prgm Dir: Carolyn Coffin, MPH RDMS RDCS RVT
Tel: 206 296-5960   *Fax:* 206 296-6429
E-mail: coffinc@seattleu.edu

West Virginia

Mountain State University
Diagnostic Med Sonography Prgm
General concentration
PO Box 9003
Beckley, WV 25802-9003
Prgm Dir: Robert Lilly, MS RDCS RDMS
Tel: 304 929-1389, Ext 1389   *Fax:* 304 253-3485
E-mail: boblilly@mountainstate.edu

West Virginia University Hospitals
Diagnostic Med Sonography Prgm
General concentration
PO Box 8062
Morgantown, WV 26506
Prgm Dir: Debra L Williams, RDMS
Tel: 304 598-4187   *Fax:* 304 598-4072
E-mail: williamsd@rcbhsc.wvu.edu

Wisconsin

Chippewa Valley Technical College
Diagnostic Med Sonography Prgm
General concentration
620 W Clairemont Ave
Eau Claire, WI 54701
Prgm Dir: Tina Salava, RT(R) RDMS RVT
Tel: 715 833-6430   *Fax:* 715 833-6430
E-mail: tsalava@cvtc.edu

Northeast Wisconsin Technical College
Diagnostic Med Sonography Prgm
General concentration
2740 W Mason St
Green Bay, WI 54307-9042
www.nwtc.edu
Prgm Dir: Lori Suddick
Tel: 920 498-5513   *Fax:* 920 491-2660
E-mail: lori.suddick@nwtc.edu

University of Wisconsin Hospital and Clinics
Diagnostic Med Sonography Prgm
General and Cardiac concentrations
Dept of Radiology
Madison, WI 53792
www.uwhealth.org/ultrasoundschool
Prgm Dir: Carol Mitchell, PhD RDMS RDCS RVT RT(R)
Tel: 608 263-9033   *Fax:* 608 263-9208
E-mail: cc.mitchell@hosp.wisc.edu

Aurora St Luke's Medical Center
Diagnostic Med Sonography Prgm
General and Vascular concentrations
180 W Grange Ave
Milwaukee, WI 53207
www.aurora.org/sonography
Prgm Dir: Laura Sorenson, RT(R)(M) RDMS RVT
Tel: 414 747-4352   *Fax:* 414 747-4366
E-mail: laura.woodruff@aurora.org

Columbia St Mary's Hospitals
Diagnostic Med Sonography Prgm
General and Vascular concentrations
2121 E Newport Ave
Milwaukee, WI 53211
http://ccon.edu
Prgm Dir: Rosemarie Fridrick, RDMS RT(R)
Tel: 414 961-3945   *Fax:* 414 961-4205
E-mail: rfridric@columbia-stmarys.org

Wheaton Franciscan Healthcare - St Francis
Diagnostic Med Sonography Prgm
General concentration
3237 S 16th St
Milwaukee, WI 53215
www.wfhealthcare.org/stellent/groups/public/documents
 /www/cmke_118270.hcsp
Prgm Dir: Marc Wojciechowski, RDMS RDCS RVT MS
Tel: 414 647-5711   *Fax:* 414 647-5732
E-mail: marc.wojciechowski@WFHC.org

Diagnostic Medical Sonographer

	Class Capacity	Begins	Length (months)	Award	Res. Tuition	Non-res. Tuition	Stipend	Offers:‡ 1	2	3	4
Alabama											
Baptist Medical Center South (Montgomery)	10	Oct	12	Cert	$5,450	$5,450					
Insitute of Ultrasound Diagnostics (Mobile)	30	Jan Jul	12	Cert	$9,500	$9,500					•
Wallace State Community College (Hanceville)	25	Aug	18	Dipl AAS	$3,600	$7,200				•	
Arkansas											
University of Arkansas for Medical Sciences (Little Rock)	21	Aug	22, 18	Cert, BS DMS, AC DMS	$6,630	$14,820				•	•
California											
Foothill Community College (Los Altos Hills)	30	Jun	15	Cert, AS	$2,500	$9,744				•	•
Kaiser Permanente Sch of Allied Hlth Sciences (Richmond)	15	Oct	18	Cert	$9,000	$9,000				•	
Univ of California San Diego Med Ctr	6	Jan	12	Cert	$12,000	$12,000					
Colorado											
U of Colorado (Denver) Health Sciences Center (Aurora)	14	Sep	12	Cert	$3,000	$3,000					
Delaware											
Delaware Technical & Community College - Wilmington	14	May	24	AAS	$3,105	$7,764				•	
Florida											
Keiser University (Fort Lauderdale)	14	Jan May Sep	24	AS	$12,000	$0					
Keiser University - Daytona Beach	14	Jan May Sep	24	Dipl, AS	$18,660	$18,660					
Palm Beach Community College (Palm Beach Gardens)	15	May	24, 14	Cert, AS, CCC	$1,995	$0					
St Vincent's Medical Center (Jacksonville)	6	Jul	18	Cert	$3,500	$3,500					

*Data are shown only for programs that completed the 2007 AMA Survey of Health Professions Education Programs.
‡Key to Offers: 1: Evening or weekend classes; 2: Non-English instruction; 3: Cultural competence instruction; 4: Distance education component.

	Class Capacity	Begins	Length (months)	Award	Res. Tuition	Non-res. Tuition	Stipend	Offers:‡ 1	2	3	4
Valencia Community College (Orlando)	12	Aug	22	AS	$2,379	$8,929				•	
Georgia											
Coosa Valley Technical College (Rome)	46	Fall	18	Dipl, AAT	$1,088	$2,176					
Grady Health System (Atlanta)	10	Sep	12	Cert	$8,000	$8,000				•	
Idaho											
Boise State University	6	Aug	12	Cert, BS	$6,400	$14,000					
Illinois											
College of DuPage (Glen Ellyn)	38	Fall	15, 6	Cert	$5,500	$12,000		•			
John A Logan College (Carterville)	7	Aug	18, 30	Dipl, Cert, AS	$64	$255	$1,160				•
Northwestern Memorial Hospital (Chicago)	6	Jul	18	Cert	$7,500	$7,500				•	
Southern Illinois University Carbondale	20	Aug	12	Cert, BS	$4,500	$9,000				•	•
Iowa											
University of Iowa Hospitals & Clinics (Iowa City)	12	Sep	18	Cert, BS	$4,500	$6,750				•	
Kentucky											
Bowling Green Technical College	8	Aug	13	Dipl, Cert, AAS	$4,830	$4,830				•	
Morehead State University	12	Jul	13	BS	$4,320	$11,480					
West Kentucky Community & Technical College (Paducah)	12	Aug	12	Dipl, AAS	$3,724	$11,172		•			
Louisiana											
Delgado Community College (New Orleans)	12	Aug	16	Cert	$3,200	$8,600					
Maryland											
Johns Hopkins Hospital (Baltimore)	10	Jun	14	Cert	$9,000	$9,000					
Montgomery College (Silver Spring)	30	Jul	24	Dipl, Cert, AAS	$2,625	$4,550		•		•	•
University of Maryland Baltimore County	40	Jul	13	Cert, BS/BA	$17,995	$17,995				•	
Massachusetts											
Bunker Hill Community College (Boston)	13	Sep	24	AS	$4,500	$8,000		•		•	•
Middlesex Community College - Bedford	24	Sep	12, 24	Cert, AS	$3,060	$3,366		•			
Springfield Technical Community College	10	Sep	22	AS	$3,888	$11,266					
Michigan											
Henry Ford Hospital (Detroit)	16	Sep	17	Cert	$1,000	$1,000				•	
Providence Hospital (Southfield)	5	Sep	16	Cert	$2,500	$2,500					
Minnesota											
Mayo School of Health Sciences (Rochester)	24	Sep	18	Cert	$11,025	$11,025				•	
St Cloud Technical College	12	Aug	27	AAS	$2,497	$4,994					
Missouri											
University of Missouri - Columbia	15	Jun	24	BHS/MH	$6,960	$9,126				•	
Nebraska											
University of Nebraska Medical Center (Omaha)	8	Aug	12	BS	$6,910	$21,168				•	
New Hampshire											
New Hampshire Technical Institute (Concord)	8	Sep	16	Cert	$7,090	$14,051					
New Jersey											
Muhlenberg Regional Medical Center (Plainfield)		Sep	28	Dipl, Cert, AS	$15,651	$15,651				•	•
Sanford-Brown Institute (Iselin)	22	Aug Feb	18	Cert							
Univ of Medicine & Dent of New Jersey (Scotch Plains)	19	Sep	15	Cert, BSAHT	$11,176	$16,764				•	
New Mexico											
Dona Ana Community College (Las Cruces)	14	Jan	17, 19	Cert, AAS	$1,368	$3,552					
New York											
Long Island University (Brooklyn)	20	Sep Jan	12	Cert	$20,000	$20,000					
New York University	20	Sep	30	AAS	$23,205	$23,205				•	
North Carolina											
Caldwell Comm College & Tech Institute (Hudson)	30	Aug	21	AAS	$1,896	$10,536				•	
Forsyth Technical Community College (Winston-Salem)	10	Aug	21	AAS	$1,562	$8,668				•	
Johnston Community College (Smithfield)	20	Aug	16, 21	Dipl, AAS	$49	$233					
Ohio											
Cincinnati State Tech & Comm College	24	Sep	24	Cert, AAS	$4,210	$8,421		•			•
Kettering College of Medical Arts	20	Aug	36, 48	Dipl, AS, BS	$18,000	$18,000				•	
Lorain County Community College (Elyria)	11	Jan	17	AAS	$4,061	$9,878				•	
Sanford-Brown Institute (Middleburg Heights)	24	Jul Dec	18	Dipl	$16,700	$16,700		•			
University of Rio Grande	14	Jun	15	AS	$11,851	$11,851					
Oklahoma											
Moore Norman Technology Center	10	Varies	15	Dipl	$2,025	$3,036				•	
Pennsylvania											
Comm College of Allegheny County (Monroeville)	32	Aug	20	Cert, AS	$2,108	$6,324				•	•
Crozer-Keystone Medical Center (Upland)	8	Sep	18	Cert	$8,000	$8,000				•	
Harrisburg Area Community College	12	Jan	12, 24	Cert, AAS	$7,029	$10,278					
Lancaster Gen Coll of Nursing & Hlth Sciences	16	Aug	24	Dipl, AS	$13,550	$13,550				•	

*Data are shown only for programs that completed the 2007 AMA Survey of Health Professions Education Programs.
‡Key to Offers: 1: Evening or weekend classes; 2: Non-English instruction; 3: Cultural competence instruction; 4: Distance education component.

	Class Capacity	Begins	Length (months)	Award	Res. Tuition	Non-res. Tuition	Stipend	Offers:‡ 1	2	3	4
Northampton Community College (Bethlehem)	11	Fall semester	24, 18	Dipl, AAS	$3,145	$9,879					
Wilkes-Barre General Hospital	4	Sep 7	18	Cert	$0	$10,000					
Rhode Island											
Rhode Island Hospital (Providence)	6	Jul	14	Cert	$6,500	$6,500					
Tennessee											
Baptist College of Health Sciences (Memphis)	12	Sep	48	BS	$7,472	$7,472					
Chattanooga State Technical Comm College	25	Aug	12	Cert	$3,345	$12,261					•
Texas											
Alvin Community College	30	Jan May	18, 24	Cert, ATC, AAS	$1,500	$3,500			•	•	
Austin Community College	30	Summer	22, 28	AAS	$54	$274			•	•	
Del Mar College (Corpus Christi)	13	Aug Sep	18	AAS	$1,500	$4,000					
El Paso Community College	10	Jul	18, 24	Dipl, Cert, AAS	$4,996	$7,215		•		•	
Houston Community College	15	Aug	16	Cert	$2,028	$4,914					
Lamar Institute of Technology (Beaumont)	20	Jun	18	Cert, AAS	$1,280	$5,460					
Tyler Junior College	12	Aug	16	AAS	$3,533	$5,759	$1,500				
Virginia											
Tidewater Community College (Virginia Beach)	15	Aug	21	AAS	$6,516	$19,127				•	
West Virginia											
Mountain State University (Beckley)	29	May	18, 30	Cert, AAS, BS	$21,070	$21,070					•
Wisconsin											
Aurora St Luke's Medical Center (Milwaukee)	14	Sep	18	Cert	$3,400	$3,400					
Columbia St Mary's Hospitals (Milwaukee)	5	Sep	18	Cert	$3,000	$3,000					
Northeast Wisconsin Technical College (Green Bay)	8	Aug	24	AAS	$3,458	$19,727					•
University of Wisconsin Hospital and Clinics (Madison)	16	Sep	24	Dipl, Cert, BS	$6,860	$16,428					
Wheaton Franciscan Healthcare - St Francis (Milwaukee)	5	Aug	18	Cert	$3,000	$3,000					

*Data are shown only for programs that completed the 2007 AMA Survey of Health Professions Education Programs.
‡Key to Offers: 1: Evening or weekend classes; 2: Non-English instruction; 3: Cultural competence instruction; 4: Distance education component.

PROGRAMS

Includes:
- Registered dietitian/nutritionist
- Dietetic technician, registered

Registered Dietitian/Nutritionist

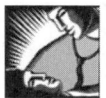

Career Description

Dietetics is the science of applying food and nutrition to health. Registered Dietitians are nutritionists who integrate and apply the principles derived from the sciences of food, nutrition, biochemistry, physiology, food management, and behavior to achieve and maintain the health status of the public they serve.

Employment Characteristics

Clinical registered dietitians are a vital part of the medical team in hospitals, nursing homes, health maintenance organizations, and other health care facilities. As a key member of the health care team, the clinical RD provides medical nutrition therapy and the use of specific nutrition services to treat chronic conditions, illnesses, or injuries. Opportunities for advancement are available by choosing a particular area of nutrition practice, such as diabetes, heart disease, or pediatrics, or by expanding into hospital administration.

Community registered dietitians work in public and home health agencies, day care centers, health and recreation clubs, and in government-funded programs that feed and counsel families, the elderly, pregnant women, children, and individuals with special needs. Wherever proper nutrition can help improve quality of life, community RDs reach out to the public to teach, monitor, and advise.

Educator registered dietitians work in colleges, universities, and medical centers, teaching future physicians, nurses, dietitians, and dietetic technicians the science of foods and nutrition.

Research registered dietitians work in government agencies, food and pharmaceutical companies, and major universities and medical centers. They conduct or direct experiments to answer critical nutrition questions, find alternative foods, and form dietary recommendations for the public.

Consultant registered dietitians work under contract with health care or food companies or in their own business. In private practice, they perform nutrition screening and assessment of their own clients and those referred to them by physicians. They counsel on weight loss, cholesterol reduction, and a variety of other diet-related concerns. Those under contract with health care facilities consult with food service or restaurant managers, food vendors or distributors, athletes, nursing home residents, or company employees.

Management registered dietitians work in health care institutions, schools, cafeterias, and restaurants, playing a key role where food is served. They are responsible for personnel management, menu planning, budgeting, and purchasing.

Business registered dietitians work in food- and nutrition-related industries, in such areas as communications, consumer affairs, product development, sales, marketing, advertising, and public relations.

Salary

According to the American Dietetic Association (ADA) 2007 Dietetics Compensation and Benefits Survey, among registered dietitians employed full time in dietetics in their primary position for less than 5 years, half earn between $42,000 and $55,000 per year. Salary levels may vary with location, scope of responsibility, and supply of job applicants. Salary also increases as experience increases; many RDs, particularly those in management and business earn incomes between $60,000 and $91,000 per year. Refer to Section IV, Table 5 of this *Directory* for more information, or see www.ama-assn.org/go/hpsalary.

Employment Outlook

According to the US Bureau of Labor Statistics, employment of dietitians is expected to grow faster than the average profession through the year 2015, especially in the community, consulting, and business areas.

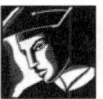

Educational Programs

Length. The professional component is a minimum of 2 years at the baccalaureate or graduate degree level. Postbaccalaureate dietetic internship programs vary from 6 months to 2 years, depending on study design and integration in a graduate program. Following completion of academic and supervised practice requirements, individuals are eligible to take a national certification examination for registered dietitians. Most states also regulate dietitians and nutritionists. National certification as a RD will meet state requirements.

Prerequisites. Variable for programs at the baccalaureate and graduate degree levels, depending on the degree offered and institutional requirements. Applicants to postbaccalaureate dietetic internship programs must have completed a baccalaureate degree from a US regionally accredited college or university or equivalent foreign degree and Commission on Accreditation for Dietetics Education (CADE)-approved didactic coursework.

Curriculum. Didactic curriculum requirements focus on food and nutrition sciences and management, supported by the physical and biological as well as behavioral and social sciences, in addition to business, economics, and communication. The supervised practice curriculum provides experiences to develop the skills and competence to practice dietetics.

Program Types
Coordinated Program in Dietetics (CP)
- An academic program in a regionally accredited college or university granting a baccalaureate or graduate degree
- Includes didactic instruction and a minimum of 900 hours of supervised practice experiences, which may be planned concurrently with or following the didactic component
- Graduates are eligible to write the registration examination for dietitians

Didactic Program in Dietetics (DPD)
- An academic program in a regionally accredited college or university granting a baccalaureate or graduate degree
- Graduates can apply for a dietetic internship program leading to eligibility to write the registration examination for dietitians

Dietetic Internship (DI)

- A supervised practice program sponsored by a health care facility, college or university, federal or state agency, business, or corporation
- Minimum of 900 hours of supervised practice experiences
- Entry requires completion of CADE-approved Didactic Program in Dietetics and at least a baccalaureate degree from a US regionally accredited college or university or foreign equivalent
- May be full-time or part-time and vary from 6 months to 2 years
- Graduates are eligible to write the registration examination for dietitians

Dietetic Technician, Registered

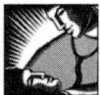

Career Description
Dietetic technicians assist in shaping the public's food choices and provide nutrition assessment and counseling to persons with illnesses or injuries. Technicians work under the supervision of the registered dietitian. They often screen patients to identify nutrition problems, provide patient education and counseling to individuals and groups, develop menus and recipes, supervise food service personnel, purchase food, and monitor inventory and food quality.

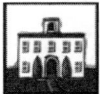

Employment Characteristics
As an integral part of the nutrition care team, dietetic technicians work with registered dietitians in a number of different settings, such as hospitals, public health nutrition programs, and long-term care facilities. Technicians also work in child nutrition and school lunch programs, community wellness centers, health clubs, nutrition programs for the elderly, food companies, restaurants, and food service management.

Salary
According to the ADA's 2007 Dietetics compensation and benefit survey, half of all registered dietetic technicians employed full-time in their primary position for 5 years or less earn annual incomes of between $30,000 and $40,000. Salary levels may vary based on location, scope of responsibility, and supply of DTRs. Refer to Section IV, Table 5 of this *Directory* for more information, or see www.ama-assn.org/go/hpsalary.

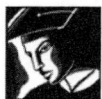

Educational Programs
Length. Two years (associate degree), combining classroom and supervised practical experience, at a US regionally accredited college or university. After completing this program, individuals are eligible to take the registration examination for dietetic technicians. Those who pass the exam become Dietetic Technicians, Registered, and can use the initials "DTR" after their names.

Prerequisites. Applicants must have a high school diploma or equivalency and must meet institutional entrance requirements.

Curriculum. Didactic instruction and a minimum of 450 hours of supervised practice experiences make up the curriculum. Food, nutrition, and management courses are emphasized, supported by the sciences, especially biology, anatomy, and chemistry. Mathematics, english, sociology, psychology, communications, and business courses are also important.

Inquiries

Careers
Inquiries regarding careers in dietetics and nutrition should be addressed to:
Accreditation and Education Programs
American Dietetic Association
120 S Riverside Plaza, Suite 2000
Chicago, IL 60606-6995
312 899-0040, Ext 5400
E-mail: education@eatright.org

Certification/Registration
Inquiries regarding dietitian and dietetic technician registration should be addressed to:
Commission on Dietetic Registration
120 S Riverside Plaza, Suite 2000
Chicago, IL 60606-6995
312 899-0040, Ext 5500
E-mail: cdr@eatright.org

Program Accreditation and Approval
Accreditation and Education Programs
American Dietetic Association
120 S Riverside Plaza, Suite 2000
Chicago, IL 60606-6995
312 899-0040, Ext 5400
E-mail: education@eatright.org

Accredited and Approved Programs
A list of accredited and approved programs with selected information is available on the ADA Web site at:
www.eatright.org/cade

Dietitian/Nutritionist

Alabama

Auburn University
Dietetics-Didactic Prgm
Nutrition and Food Science
328 Spidle Hall
Auburn, AL 36849-5605
www.humsci.auburn.edu

Samford University
Dietetics-Didactic Prgm
Family and Consumer Educ
800 Lakeshore Dr
Birmingham, AL 35229-2239
www.samford.edu

University of Alabama at Birmingham
Dietetic Internship Prgm
Dept of Nutrition Sciences
Webb Bldg Rm 212
Birmingham, AL 35294
www.uab.edu/nutrition

Oakwood College
Dietetic Internship Prgm
Family and Consumer Science
7000 Adventist Blvd
Huntsville, AL 35896
www.oakwood.edu

Oakwood College
Dietetics-Didactic Prgm
Family and Consumer Science
7000 Adventist Blvd
Huntsville, AL 35896
www.oakwood.edu/fcs

Jacksonville State University
Dietetics-Didactic Prgm
Family and Consumer Sciences
125 E Mason Hall
Jacksonville, AL 36265
www.jsu.edu

University of Montevallo
Dietetics-Didactic Prgm
Family and Consumer Sciences
Station 6385 Bloch Hall
Montevallo, AL 35115-6000
www.montevallo.edu

Alabama A&M University
Dietetics-Didactic Prgm
Nutrition and Hospitality Mgmt
Div of Family & Consumer Serv PO Box 639
Normal, AL 35762-0639
www.aamu.edu/

University of Alabama
Dietetics-Coordinated Prgm
Human Nutrition and Hosp Mgmt
PO Box 870158, 206 Doster Hall
Tuscaloosa, AL 35487-0158
www.ches.ua.edu

University of Alabama
Dietetics-Didactic Prgm
Human Nutrition and Hosp Mgmt
PO Box 870158
Tuscaloosa, AL 35487-0158
www.ches.ua.edu

Tuskegee University
Dietetics-Didactic Prgm
Food and Nutrition Sciences
204 Campbell Hall
Tuskegee, AL 36088
www.tuskegee.edu

Alaska

University of Alaska Anchorage
Dietetic Internship Prgm
3211 Providence Dr
108 Cuddy Center
Anchorage, AK 99508
www.uaa.alaska.edu/

Arizona

Arizona State University at the Polytechnic Campus
Dietetic Internship Prgm
Department of Nutrition
7001 E Williams Field Rd, Bldg 20
Mesa, AZ 85212
www.east.asu.edu/ecollege/nutrition

Arizona State University at the Polytechnic Campus
Dietetics-Didactic Prgm
Department of Nutrition
7001 E Williams Field Rd
Mesa, AZ 85212
www.east.asu.edu/ecollege/nutrition

Arizona Department of Health Services
Dietetic Internship Prgm
150 N 18th Ave, Ste 310
Phoenix, AZ 85007

Maricopa County Dept of Public Health
Dietetic Internship Prgm
Office of Nutrition Services
4041 North Central, Ste 700 C
Phoenix, AZ 85012

Paradise Valley Unified School District
Dietetic Internship Prgm
20621 N 32nd St
Phoenix, AZ 85050
www.pvusd.k12.az.us

Southwestern DI Consortium (PhD)
Dietetic Internship Prgm
Phoenix Indian Medical Center
Phoenix, AZ 85016

Yavapai County Health Department
Dietetic Internship Prgm
930 Division St
Prescott, AZ 86301

Carondelet St Mary's Hospital
Dietetic Internship Prgm
Morrisons Custom Mgmt Co
1601 W St Mary's Rd
Tucson, AZ 85745
www.azdpac.org/programinfo.cfm?PID=100020

University Medical Center
Dietetics-Didactic Prgm
Dept of Nutritional Sciences
PO Box 210038, Shantz 309
Tucson, AZ 85721-0038
www.ag.arizona.edu/NSC/nschome.htm

University of Arizona
Dietetic Internship Prgm
University Medical Center Support Services
1501 N Campbell Ave
Tucson, AZ 85724-5088
www.arizona.edu/

Arkansas

Henderson State University
Dietetics-Didactic Prgm
Dept of Family and Consumer Sciences
PO Box 7504
Arkadelphia, AR 71999-0001
www.hsu.edu

Ouachita Baptist University
Dietetics-Didactic Prgm
Dept of Biology
PO Box 3769
Arkadelphia, AR 71998-0001
www.obu.edu/biology/program_in_dietetics.htm

University of Central Arkansas
Dietetic Internship Prgm
Family and Consumer Sciences
McAlister Hall 100
Conway, AR 72035
www.uca.edu/divisions/academic/chas/diet.html

University of Central Arkansas
Dietetics-Didactic Prgm
Family and Consumer Sciences
McAlister Hall 100
Conway, AR 72035
www.uca.edu/divisions/academic/chas/diet.html

University of Arkansas
Dietetics-Didactic Prgm
Human Environmental Sciences
118 HOEC
Fayetteville, AR 72701
www.uark.edu/depts/hesweb

University of Arkansas for Medical Sciences
Dietetic Internship Prgm
Veterans Affairs Med Ctr
4301 W Markham St, Slot 627
Little Rock, AR 72205-7199
www.uams.edu/chrp/dietnutrition/

University of Arkansas at Pine Bluff
Dietetics-Didactic Prgm
Dept of Home Economics
1200 N University Dr, PO Box 4971
Pine Bluff, AR 71601

Harding University
Dietetics-Didactic Prgm
Family and Consumer Sciences
900 E Center Ave, Box 12233
Searcy, AR 72149-0001

California

Clinica Sierra Vista
Dietetic Internship Prgm
1430 Truxtun Ave, Ste 120
Bakersfield, CA 93301-3834

University of California - Berkeley
Dietetics-Didactic Prgm
Dept of Nutritional Sciences and Toxicology
119 Morgan Hall
Berkeley, CA 94720-3104
http://nutrition.berkeley.edu

California State University - Chico
Dietetics-Didactic Prgm
Dept of Biological Sciences
Tehama Hall 124
Chico, CA 95929-0002

California State University - Chico
Dietetic Internship Prgm
Nutrition and Food Sciences
Dept of Biological Sciences
Chico, CA 95929-0002
www.csuchico.edu/biol/nfsc

University of California - Davis
Dietetics-Didactic Prgm
Dept of Nutrition
One Shields Ave
Davis, CA 95616-8669
www.ucdavis.edu

California State University - Fresno
Dietetics-Didactic Prgm
Dept of Ecology Food Science and Nutrition
5300 N Campus Dr MS FF17
Fresno, CA 93740-8019
http://cast.csufresno.edu/fsn

California State University - Fresno
Dietetic Internship Prgm
Dept of Ecology Food Science and Nutrition
5300 N Campus Dr MS FF17
Fresno, CA 93740-8019
http://cast.csufresno.edu/fsn

Glendale Memorial Hospital and Health Center
Dietetic Internship Prgm
Food and Nutrition Services
1420 S Central Ave
Glendale, CA 91204-2594
www.glendalememorial.com/dietary

Public Health Foundation Enterprises
Dietetic Internship Prgm
WIC Program
12781 Schabarum Ave
Irwindale, CA 91706-6802
www.phfewic.org

Loma Linda University
Dietetics-Coordinated Prgm
School of Public Health, Nutrition Dept
Nichol Hall, Rm 1102
Loma Linda, CA 92350
www.llu.edu/llu/nutrition

Loma Linda University
Dietetics-Coordinated Prgm
School of Allied Health Professions
Dept of Nutrition & Dietetics
Loma Linda, CA 92354
www.llu.edu/llu/nutrition

California State University - Long Beach
Dietetic Internship Prgm
Family and Consumer Sciences
1250 N Bellflower Blvd
Long Beach, CA 90840-0501
www.csulb.edu/~gcfrank

California State University - Long Beach
Dietetics-Didactic Prgm
Family and Consumer Sciences
1250 Bellflower Blvd
Long Beach, CA 90840-0501
www.csulb.edu

California State University - Los Angeles
Dietetics-Coordinated Prgm
Kinesiology and Nutritional Science
5151 State University Dr
Los Angeles, CA 90032-8172
www.calstatela.edu/dept/hnut_sci/dept_pro.htm

California State University - Los Angeles
Dietetics-Didactic Prgm
Health and Nutritional Sciences
5151 State University Dr
Los Angeles, CA 90032-8162
www.calstatelal.edu/dept/hnut_sci/dept_pro.htm

Center for Child Development/Disabilities/UAP
Cosponsor: Children's Hosp of Los Angeles
Dietetic Internship Prgm
Child Development and Developmental Disorders
Mailstop 53, PO Box 54700
Los Angeles, CA 90054-0700

Los Angeles County+USC Healthcare Network
Dietetic Internship Prgm
Morrison Management Specialists
1200 N State St, Rm 1506
Los Angeles, CA 90033-4525

VA Greater Los Angeles Healthcare System
Dietetic Internship Prgm
Nutrition and Food Dept 120
11301 Wilshire Blvd
Los Angeles, CA 90073

Pepperdine University
Dietetics-Didactic Prgm
RAC108C, Nutritional Sciences
24255 Pacific Coast Hwy
Malibu, CA 90263-4325
www.pepperdine.edu

Napa State Hospital
Dietetic Internship Prgm
2100 Napa Vallejo Hwy
Napa, CA 94558-6293

California State University - Northridge
Dietetics-Didactic Prgm
Family Environmental Sciences
18111 Nordhoff St
Northridge, CA 91330-8308
www.csun.edu

California State University - Northridge
Dietetic Internship Prgm
Family Environmental Sciences
18111 Nordhoff St
Northridge, CA 91330-8308
www.csundi.com

Patton State Hospital
Dietetic Internship Prgm
3102 E Highland Ave
Patton, CA 92369

California State Polytechnic University
Dietetics-Didactic Prgm
Foods and Nutrition Dept
3801 W Temple Ave
Pomona, CA 91768-2557
www.csupomona.edu

California State Polytechnic University
Dietetic Internship Prgm
Foods and Nutri/Home Economics
3801 W Temple Ave
Pomona, CA 91768-2557
www.csupomona.edu/~kcaldwellfreeman

Porterville Development Center
Dietetic Internship Prgm
PO Box 2000
Porterville, CA 93258-2000

Central Valley WIC Dietetic Internship
Dietetic Internship Prgm
1560 E Manning Ave
Reedley, CA 93654

California State University - Sacramento
Dietetic Internship Prgm
6000 J Street
Sacramento, CA 95819-6053
www.cce.csus.edu/programs/di/

California State University - Sacramento
Dietetics-Didactic Prgm
Human Environmental Sciences
6000 J St
Sacramento, CA 95819-6053
www.csus.edu

UC Davis Medical Center
Dietetic Internship Prgm
2315 Stockton Blvd
Sacramento, CA 95817

California State University - San Bernardino
Dietetics-Didactic Prgm
Health Science and Human Ecology
5500 University Pkwy
San Bernardino, CA 92407-2318
http://health.csusb.edu/dchen

Point Loma Nazarene University (PhD)
Dietetics-Didactic Prgm
3900 Lomaland Dr
San Diego, CA 92106

San Diego State University
Dietetic Internship Prgm
WIC Dietetic Internship
5500 Campanile Dr
San Diego, CA 92111
www.rohan.sdsu.edu

San Diego State University
Dietetics-Didactic Prgm
Exercise and Nutritional Sciences
5500 Campanile Dr
San Diego, CA 92182-7251
www.sdsu.edu

VA San Diego Healthcare System
Dietetic Internship Prgm
Dietetics and Clinical Nutrition Serv 120
3350 La Jolla Village Dr
San Diego, CA 92161-0002

Northeast Valley Health Corporation
Dietetic Internship Prgm
1172 N Maclay Ave
San Fernando, CA 91340

San Francisco State University
Dietetics-Didactic Prgm
Cons and Fam Studies
1600 Holloway Ave
San Francisco, CA 94132-1722
www.sfsu.edu

San Francisco State University
Dietetic Internship Prgm
Cons and Fam Studies
1600 Holloway Ave
San Francisco, CA 94132
www.sfsu.edu

University of California - San Francisco
Dietetic Internship Prgm
Medical Center, Box 0212 Rm M-294
Dept of Nutrition & Dietetics
San Francisco, CA 94143-0212
www.ucsf.edu/

San Jose State University
Dietetic Internship Prgm
Nutrition Food and Science
One Washington Square
San Jose, CA 95192-0058

San Jose State University
Dietetics-Didactic Prgm
Nutrition and Food Science
San Jose, CA 95192-0058

California Polytechnic State University
Dietetic Internship Prgm
San Luis Obispo, CA 93407

California Polytechnic State University
Dietetics-Didactic Prgm
Food Science and Nutrition
San Luis Obispo, CA 93407
www.calpoly.edu

Olive View/UCLA Medical Center
Dietetic Internship Prgm
Dept of Food and Nutrition
14445 Olive View Dr, Rm 1C112
Sylmar, CA 91342-1438

Colorado

Centura Health/Penrose-St Francis Hlth Serv
Dietetic Internship Prgm
Nutrition Services
PO Box 7021
Colorado Springs, CO 80933-7021

University of Colorado at Colorado Springs
Dietetics-Didactic Prgm
1420 Austin Bluffs Parkway
Colorado Springs, CO 80933

Johnson & Wales University
Dietetics-Didactic Prgm
7150 Montview Blvd
Denver, CO 80220

Colorado State University
Dietetic Internship Prgm
Food Sci and Human Nutrition
Fort Collins, CO 80523-1571
www.colostate.edu

Colorado State University
Dietetics-Coordinated Prgm
Food Sci and Human Nutrition
Gifford Bldg 205
Fort Collins, CO 80523-1571
www.fshn.cahs.colostate.edu

University of Northern Colorado
Dietetics-Didactic Prgm
Community Health and Nutrition
CHN, Box 93-501 20th St
Greeley, CO 80639
www.univnorthco.edu

University of Northern Colorado
Dietetic Internship Prgm
Community Health and Nutrition
CHN Box 93-501 20th St
Greeley, CO 80639
www.unco.edu/dietetic

Tri-County Health Department
Dietetic Internship Prgm
Nutrition Services
4857 S Broadway
Greenwood Village, CO 80111

Connecticut

Danbury Hospital
Dietetic Internship Prgm
24 Hospital Ave
Danbury, CT 06810-6077
www.danburyhospital.org

Yale-New Haven Hospital
Dietetic Internship Prgm
Food and Nutrition
20 York St GBB
New Haven, CT 06504
www.ynhh.org/general/training.html#diet

University of Connecticut
Dietetics-Coordinated Prgm
School of Allied Health
358 Mansfield Rd, Unit 2101
Storrs, CT 06269-2101
www.alliedhealth.uconn.edu

University of Connecticut
Dietetic Internship Prgm
School of Allied Health
358 Mansfield Rd, Unit 2101
Storrs, CT 06269-2101
www.alliedhealth.uconn.edu

University of Connecticut
Dietetics-Didactic Prgm
Nutritional Sciences U-4017
3624 Horsebarn Rd Extension
Storrs, CT 06269
www.canr.uconn.edu/nusci

Saint Joseph College
Dietetics-Didactic Prgm
Nutrition and Family Studies
1678 Asylum Ave
West Hartford, CT 06117-2700
www.sjc.edu

Saint Joseph College
Dietetic Internship Prgm
Nutrition and Family Studies
1678 Asylum Ave
West Hartford, CT 06117-2700

Saint Joseph College
Dietetics-Coordinated Prgm
Nutrition and Family Studies
1678 Asylum Ave
West Hartford, CT 06117-2700
www.sjc.edu

University of New Haven
Dietetics-Didactic Prgm
College of Arts and Sciences
300 Orange Ave
West Haven, CT 06516-1916
www.newhaven.edu

Delaware

Delaware State University
Dietetics-Didactic Prgm
Dept of Family and Consumer Sciences
1200 N Dupont Hwy
Dover, DE 19901-2277
www.desu.edu/

University of Delaware
Dietetic Internship Prgm
Nutrition and Dietetics
315 Alison Hall
Newark, DE 19716
www.udel.edu

University of Delaware
Dietetics-Didactic Prgm
Dept of Nutrition and Dietetics
234A Alison Hall
Newark, DE 19716-3301
www.udel.edu

District of Columbia

Howard University
Dietetics-Coordinated Prgm
Nutritional Sciences
6th and Bryant Sts NW, Annex I
Washington, DC 20059
www.howard.edu

University of the District of Columbia
Dietetics-Didactic Prgm
Biological and Environmental Sciences
Bldg 44 Rm 200-2, 4200 Connecticut Ave NW
Washington, DC 20008-1173

Florida

Bay Pines VA Medical Center
Dietetic Internship Prgm
Bay Pines, FL 33744

University of Florida
Dietetics-Didactic Prgm
Food Sci and Human Nutrition
PO Box 110370
Gainesville, FL 32611-0370
www.ufl.edu

University of Florida
Dietetic Internship Prgm
Food Sci and Human Nutrition
359 FSB, PO Box 110370
Gainesville, FL 32611
http://fshn.ifas.ufl.edu

St Luke's Hosp/Mayo Clinic Jacksonville
Dietetic Internship Prgm
4500 San Pablo Rd
Jacksonville, FL 32224

University of North Florida
Dietetic Internship Prgm
Dept of Health Science
4567 St Johns Bluff Rd S
Jacksonville, FL 32224-2646
www.unf.edu/coh

University of North Florida
Dietetics-Didactic Prgm
College of Health
4567 St Johns Bluff Rd S
Jacksonville, FL 32224-2645
www.unf.edu

Florida International University
Dietetics-Didactic Prgm
Dietetics and Nutrition
11200 SW 8th St
Miami, FL 33199
http://w3.fiu.edu/

Florida International University
Dietetics-Coordinated Prgm
Dept of Dietetics and Nutrition
11200 SW 8th St
Miami, FL 33199
www.fiu.edu/

Pasco County Health Department
Dietetic Internship Prgm
Nutrition Div
10841 Little Rd
New Port Richey, FL 34654-2533
www.doh.state.fl.us/chdpasco/default.html

Sarasota District Schools
Dietetic Internship Prgm
Food and Nutrition Services
101 Old Venice Rd
Osprey, FL 34229-9023
www.sarasota.k12.fl.us/~fns

Sarasota Memorial Hospital
Dietetic Internship Prgm
Food and Nutrition Services
1700 S Tamiami Trail
Sarasota, FL 34239-3555
www.smh.com

Florida Department of Education
Dietetic Internship Prgm
325 W Gaines St, Rm 1032
Tallahassee, FL 32399-0400

Florida State University
Dietetic Internship Prgm
Nutrition Food and Exercise Sciences
400 Sandels Bldg
Tallahassee, FL 32306-1493
www.fsu.edu

Florida State University
Dietetics-Didactic Prgm
Nutrition Food and Exercise Sciences
436 Sandels Bldg
Tallahassee, FL 32306-1493
www.fsu.edu

James A Haley Veteran's Hospital
Dietetic Internship Prgm
13000 N Bruce B Downs Blvd
Tampa, FL 33612-4745

Georgia

University of Georgia
Dietetics-Didactic Prgm
Dept of Foods and Nutrition
Dawson Hall
Athens, GA 30602

University of Georgia
Dietetic Internship Prgm
Dept of Foods and Nutrition
Dawson Hall
Athens, GA 30602
www.fcs.uga.edu

Div of Pub Hlth/Georgia Dept of Hum Res
Dietetic Internship Prgm
Office of Nutrition
Two Peachtree St NW, Ste 11-254
Atlanta, GA 30303-3142
http://health.state.ga.us/

Emory University Hospital
Dietetic Internship Prgm
Food and Nutrition Services
1364 Clifton Rd NE, Rm FG06
Atlanta, GA 30322
http://medshare.emory.org/EHC/FNSWeb.nsf

Georgia State University
Dietetics-Didactic Prgm
Dept of Nutrition and Dietetics
MSC2A0880, 33 Gilmer St SE, Unit 2
Atlanta, GA 30303-3083
www.gsu.edu

Georgia State University
Dietetics-Coordinated Prgm
PO Box 3999
Atlanta, GA 30302

Georgia State University
Dietetic Internship Prgm
Dept of Nutrition and Dietetics
University Plaza
Atlanta, GA 30303-3083
www.gsu.edu

Augusta Area Dietetic Internship
Cosponsor: Morrison Health Care Foodservice
Dietetic Internship Prgm
University Hospital
1350 Walton Way
Augusta, GA 30901-2629
https://www.universityhealth.org

Fort Valley State University
Dietetics-Didactic Prgm
Family and Consumer Sciences
1005 State University Dr, PO Box 4622 FVSU
Fort Valley, GA 31030

Life University
Dietetic Internship Prgm
1269 Barclay Circle SE
110 Annex B
Marietta, GA 30060-2903

Life University
Dietetics-Didactic Prgm
Dept of Nutrition
1269 Barclay Circle
Marietta, GA 30060-2903

Southern Regional Medical Center
Dietetic Internship Prgm
11 Upper Riverdale Rd SW
Riverdale, GA 30274-2600
www.southernregional.org

Georgia Southern University
Dietetics-Didactic Prgm
Family and Consumer Sciences
Box 8034
Statesboro, GA 30460
www.georgiasouthern.edu

Hawaii

University of Hawaii
Dietetics-Didactic Prgm
Food Sci and Human Nutrition
Ag Sciences III, 1955 East West Rd, Rm 3141
Honolulu, HI 96822-2218
www.hawaii.edu/dietetics

Idaho

University of Idaho
Dietetics-Coordinated Prgm
Family and Consumer Science
College of Agriculture
Moscow, ID 83844-3183
www.uidaho.edu/fcs

Idaho State University
Dietetics-Didactic Prgm
Health and Nutrition Science
Campus Box 8109, 1291 East Terry, MLK Way
Pocatello, ID 83209-8109
www.isu.edu

Idaho State University
Dietetic Internship Prgm
Health and Nutrition Sciences
Campus Box 8109
Pocatello, ID 83209-8109
www.isu.edu

Illinois

Olivet Nazarene University
Dietetics-Didactic Prgm
Family and Consumer Sciences
One University Dr
Bourbonnais, IL 60914
http://web.olivet.edu/facs

Southern Illinois University Carbondale
Dietetics-Didactic Prgm
Animal Sci Food and Nutrition
Mailcode 4317
Carbondale, IL 62901-4317

Southern Illinois University Carbondale
Dietetic Internship Prgm
Food and Nutrition
Mail Code 4317
Carbondale, IL 62901-4317
www.siu.edu/cwis

Eastern Illinois University
Dietetic Internship Prgm
Family and Consumer Sciences
600 Lincoln Ave, Klehm Hall 1433
Charleston, IL 61920-3099
www.eiu.edu/~dietetic

Eastern Illinois University
Dietetics-Didactic Prgm
Family and Consumer Sci, Klehm Hall 109-B
600 Lincoln Ave, Klehm Hall 1433
Charleston, IL 61920-3099
www.eiu.edu/~famsci

Rush University Medical Center
Dietetic Internship Prgm
1653 W Congress Pkwy
425 Triangle Office Bldg
Chicago, IL 60612-3864
www.rushu.rush.edu/health/dept.html

University of Illinois at Chicago
Dietetics-Coordinated Prgm
Human Nutrition and Dietetics
1919 W Taylor St, M/C 517
Chicago, IL 60612-7256

University of Illinois at Chicago
Dietetics-Didactic Prgm
Chicago, IL 60612

Northern Illinois University
Dietetic Internship Prgm
Family Consumer and Nutri Sciences
DeKalb, IL 60115-2854
www.fcns.niu.edu

Northern Illinois University
Dietetics-Didactic Prgm
Family Consumer and Nutri Sciences
DeKalb, IL 60115-2854
www.niu.edu

Ingalls Memorial Hospital
Dietetic Internship Prgm
One Ingalls Dr
Harvey, IL 60426
www.ingalls.org

Edward Hines Jr VA Hospital
Dietetic Internship Prgm
Nutrition and Food Service (120D)
PO Box 5000
Hines, IL 60141
www.hines.med.va.gov/

Benedictine University
Dietetics-Didactic Prgm
Dept of Nutrition
5700 College Rd
Lisle, IL 60532-0900
www.ben.edu/nutrition

Benedictine University
Dietetic Internship Prgm
Dept of Nutrition
5700 College Rd Birck-329
Lisle, IL 60532-0900
www.ben.edu

Western Illinois University
Dietetics-Didactic Prgm
Family and Consumer Sciences
Macomb, IL 61455
www.wiu.edu/users/mifcs

Loyola University of Chicago
Dietetic Internship Prgm
2160 S First Ave
2873 Maguire Center
Maywood, IL 60153
www.luc.edu

Illinois State University
Dietetics-Didactic Prgm
Family and Consumer Sciences
Campus Box 5060
Normal, IL 61790-5060
www.cast.ilstu.edu/fcs

Illinois State University
Dietetic Internship Prgm
Dept of Family and Consumer Sciences
Campus Box 5060
Normal, IL 61790-5060
www.cast.ilstu.edu/isudi

Bradley University
Dietetics-Didactic Prgm
Family and Consumer Sciences
1501 W Bradley Ave
Peoria, IL 61625-0015
www.bradley.edu

OSF St Francis Medical Center
Dietetic Internship Prgm
530 NE Glen Oak Ave
Peoria, IL 61637-0001
www.osfsaintfrancis.org

Dominican University
Dietetics-Coordinated Prgm
7900 W Division
River Forest, IL 60305

Dominican University
Dietetics-Didactic Prgm
Dept of Nutrition Sciences
7900 W Division St
River Forest, IL 60305-1066
www.dom.edu

Univ of Illinois at Urbana-Champaign
Dietetics-Didactic Prgm
Food Sci and Human Nutri, 345 Bevier Hall
905 S Goodwin Ave
Urbana, IL 61801-3852
www.fshn.uiuc.edu/Dietetics

Univ of Illinois at Urbana-Champaign
Dietetic Internship Prgm
Dept of Food Science and Human Nutrition
443 Bevier Hall, 905 S Goodwin Ave
Urbana, IL 61801
www.aces.uiuc.edu/~dietetic

Indiana

Indiana University - Bloomington
Dietetics-Didactic Prgm
Applied Health Science
HPER 116
Bloomington, IN 47405-7109

Indiana University
Dietetic Internship Prgm
Nutrition/Diet Prgm, Sch of Allied Hlth
Ball Residence, Rm 114
Indianapolis, IN 46202-5180

Ball State University
Dietetic Internship Prgm
Family and Consumer Sciences
150 Applied Technology Bldg
Muncie, IN 47306
www.bsu.edu

Ball State University
Dietetics-Didactic Prgm
Family and Consumer Sciences
Muncie, IN 47306-0250
www.bsu.edu

Indiana State University
Dietetics-Coordinated Prgm
Family and Consumer Sciences
Terre Haute, IN 47809

Purdue University
Dietetics-Didactic Prgm
Dept of Foods and Nutrition
1264 Stone Hall
West Lafayette, IN 47907-1264
www.purdue.edu/

Purdue University
Dietetics-Coordinated Prgm
Dept of Foods and Nutrition
700 W State St
West Lafayette, IN 47907-2059
www.cfs.purdue.edu

Iowa

Iowa State University
Dietetic Internship Prgm
Food Sci and Human Nutrition
220 MacKay Hall
Ames, IA 50011
www.dietetics.iastate.edu

Iowa State University
Dietetics-Didactic Prgm
Food Sci and Human Nutrition
220 MacKay Hall
Ames, IA 50011-1120
www.dietetics.iastate.edu

University of Iowa Hospitals & Clinics
Dietetic Internship Prgm
200 Hawkins Dr, W146GH
Iowa City, IA 52242-1051
www.uihealthcare.com/

Kansas

University of Kansas Medical Center
Dietetic Internship Prgm
Dept of Dietetics and Nutrition
3901 Rainbow Blvd
Kansas City, KS 66160-7250
http://www2.kumc.edu/sah/dn/

Kansas State University
Dietetics-Coordinated Prgm
Hotel Rest Inst Mgmt and Diet
Justin Hall 104
Manhattan, KS 66506-1404
www.ksu.edu/humec/hrimd

Kansas State University
Dietetics-Didactic Prgm
Hotel Rest Inst Mgmt and Diet
Justin Hall 104
Manhattan, KS 66506-1404
www.ksu.edu/humec/hrimd

Kentucky

Western Kentucky University
Dietetics-Didactic Prgm
Consumer and Family Sci, Acad Complex 302F
One Big Red Way
Bowling Green, KY 42101-3576
www.wku.edu/dietetics

Univ of Kentucky Hospital
Dietetic Internship Prgm
Nutrition Services
H507 UKCMC, 800 Rose St
Lexington, KY 40536-0293
www.hes.eku.edu

University of Kentucky
Dietetic Internship Prgm
Human Environmental Sciences
204 Funkhouser Bldg
Lexington, KY 40506-0054
www.uky.edu

University of Kentucky
Dietetics-Coordinated Prgm
Nutrition and Food Science
210C Erikson Hall
Lexington, KY 40506-0050
www.uky.edu

University of Kentucky
Dietetics-Didactic Prgm
Nutrition and Food Science
204 Funkhouser Bldg
Lexington, KY 40506-0050
www.uky.edu

Morehead State University
Dietetics-Didactic Prgm
Science and Technology
Reed Hall 246, UPO 721
Morehead, KY 40351-1689

Murray State University
Dietetics-Didactic Prgm
Food Serv Systems Management
200 N Oakley, Applied Sciences Bldg
Murray, KY 42071-3345
www.murraystate.edu

Murray State University
Dietetic Internship Prgm
Nutrition Dietetics and Food Management
200 N Oakley, Applied Sciences Bldg
Murray, KY 42071-3345
www.murraystate.edu

Eastern Kentucky University
Dietetics-Didactic Prgm
Human Environmental Sciences
102 Burrier
Richmond, KY 40475
www.fcs.eku.edu

Eastern Kentucky University
Dietetic Internship Prgm
Human Environmental Sciences
102 Burrier Bldg, 521 Lancaster Ave
Richmond, KY 40475-3107
www.fcs.eku.edu

Louisiana

Louisiana State University
Dietetics-Didactic Prgm
School of Human Ecology
Baton Rouge, LA 70803-4300
http://sun.huec.lsu.edu

Southern Univ and A&M College
Dietetics-Didactic Prgm
Agriculture and Home Econ
PO Box 11342
Baton Rouge, LA 70813-1342
www.subr.edu

Southern Univ and A&M College
Dietetic Internship Prgm
PO Box 11342
Baton Rouge, LA 70813-1342
www.subr.edu

North Oaks Medical Center
Dietetic Internship Prgm
Nutritional Services
PO Box 2668
Hammond, LA 70404-2668
www.northoaks.org

University of Louisiana at Lafayette
Dietetics-Didactic Prgm
Coll of Applied Life Sciences
Sch of Human Res, Box 40399, McKinley St
Lafayette, LA 70504-0399
www.sustainablelouisiana/humr.org

University of Louisiana at Lafayette
Dietetic Internship Prgm
School of Human Resources
PO Box 40399, McKinley St
Lafayette, LA 70504-0399
www.louisiana.edu

McNeese State University
Dietetics-Didactic Prgm
PO Box 92820
Lake Charles, LA 70609

McNeese State University
Dietetic Internship Prgm
PO Box 92820 MSU
Lake Charles, LA 70609-2820

Touro Infirmary
Dietetic Internship Prgm
1401 Foucher St
New Orleans, LA 70115-3515

Tulane University
Dietetic Internship Prgm
Pub Hlth and Comm Hlth Sciences
1440 Canal St, Ste 2317
New Orleans, LA 70112-2699

Louisiana Tech University
Dietetics-Didactic Prgm
College of Human Ecology
PO Box 3167
Ruston, LA 71272
www.latech.edu/ans/human-ecology/index.shtml

Louisiana Tech University
Dietetic Internship Prgm
College of Human Ecology
PO Box 3167
Ruston, LA 71272
www.latech.edu/ans/human-ecology/index.shtml

Nicholls State University
Dietetics-Didactic Prgm
Family and Consumer Sciences
Box 2014
Thibodaux, LA 70310

Nicholls State University
Dietetic Internship Prgm
PO Box 2001
Thibodaux, LA 70310

Maine

University of Maine - Orono
Dietetics-Didactic Prgm
Food Sci and Human Nutrition
5735 Hitchner Hall
Orono, ME 04469-5735
www.fsn.umaine.edu

University of Maine - Orono
Dietetic Internship Prgm
Food Sci and Human Nutrition
5735 Hitchner Hall, Rm 113
Orono, ME 04469-5749
www.umaine.edu/

Maryland

Johns Hopkins Bayview Medical Center
Dietetics-Coordinated Prgm
4940 Eastern Ave
Baltimore, MD 21224

Johns Hopkins Bayview Medical Center
Dietetic Internship Prgm
Clinical Nutrition Dept
4940 Eastern Ave
Baltimore, MD 21224-2735
www.jhbmc.jhu.edu/nutri

Morgan State University
Dietetics-Didactic Prgm
Dept of Family and Consumer Sci, Jenkins Bldg,
    Rm 403-A
1700 E Cold Spring Ln
Baltimore, MD 21251
www.morgan.edu

University of Maryland Medical System
Dietetic Internship Prgm
Food and Nutrition Services
22 S Greene St
Baltimore, MD 21201-1595

National Institutes of Health
Dietetic Internship Prgm
Nutrition Dept, Clinical Ctr, Bldg 10 Rm B1S-234
10 Center Dr MSC 1078
Bethesda, MD 20892-1078
www.cc.nih.gov/nutr

Univ of Maryland at College Park
Dietetics-Didactic Prgm
Dept of Nutrition and Food Science
College Park, MD 20742-7521
www.nfsc.umd.edu/

Univ of Maryland at College Park
Dietetic Internship Prgm
Dept of Nutrition and Food Science
0112 Skinner Bldg
College Park, MD 20742
www.nfsc.umd.edu/

Sodexho Health Care Services, Mid Atlantic
Dietetic Internship Prgm
10500 Little Patuxent Pkwy, Ste 620
Columbia, MD 21044
www.dieteticintern.com/

University of Maryland Eastern Shore
Dietetics-Didactic Prgm
Dept of Human Ecology
Princess Anne, MD 21853-1299
www.umes.edu/ecology/ap4.htm

University of Maryland Eastern Shore
Dietetic Internship Prgm
Dept of Human Ecology
Princess Anne, MD 21853-1299
www.umes.edu/ecology/ap4.htm

Massachusetts

University of Massachusetts - Amherst
Dietetics-Didactic Prgm
Dept of Nutrition Box 31420
213 Chenoweth Laboratory, 100 Holdsworth Way
Amherst, MA 01003-9282
www.umass.edu

Beth Israel Deaconess Medical Center
Dietetic Internship Prgm
330 Brookline Ave
Boston, MA 02215-5491
www.bidmc.harvard.edu/dietetic

Boston University/Sargent College
Dietetics-Coordinated Prgm
One Sherborn St
Boston, MA 02215

Boston University/Sargent College
Dietetics-Didactic Prgm
635 Commonwealth Ave
Boston, MA 02215-1605
www.bu.edu/sargent

Boston University/Sargent College
Dietetic Internship Prgm
Graduate Nutrition Div
635 Commonwealth Ave
Boston, MA 02215-1605
www.bu.edu/sargent

Brigham & Women's Hospital
Dietetic Internship Prgm
75 Francis St
Boston, MA 02115-6195
www.brighamandwomens.org/

Frances Stern Nutrition Center
Dietetic Internship Prgm
New England Medical Center, Tufts University
750 Washington St, Box 783
Boston, MA 02111-1533
www.tufts.edu/nutrition/program/dietetic_internship

Massachusetts General Hospital
Dietetic Internship Prgm
Dept of Dietetics
Boston, MA 02114
www.massgeneral.org

Simmons College
Dietetics-Didactic Prgm
Dept of Nutrition
300 The Fenway
Boston, MA 02115-5898
www.simmons.edu

Simmons College
Dietetic Internship Prgm
Dept of Nutrition
300 The Fenway
Boston, MA 02115
www.simmons.edu

Mount Auburn Hospital
Dietetic Internship Prgm
330 Mount Auburn St
Cambridge, MA 02138
www.mountauburnhospital.org/

Framingham State College
Dietetics-Coordinated Prgm
Family and Consumer Sciences
100 State St
Framingham, MA 01701-9101
www.framingham.edu

Framingham State College
Dietetics-Didactic Prgm
Family and Consumer Sciences
100 State St
Framingham, MA 01701-9101
www.framingham.edu

University of Massachusetts - Amherst
Dietetic Internship Prgm
Academic Programs
100 Venture Way, Ste 201
Hadley, MA 01035
www.umass.edu/contined

Sodexho Health Care Services
Dietetic Internship Prgm
Southcoast Hospitals Group
101 Page St
New Bedford, MA 02740-3464
www.southcoast.org/jobs/interns-dietary.html

Sodexho Health Care Services
Dietetic Internship Prgm
101 Page St
Waltham, MA 02451
www.dieteticintern.com

Michigan

University of Michigan
Dietetics-Didactic Prgm
School of Public Health
Human Nutrition Prgm
Ann Arbor, MI 48109-2029

University of Michigan
Dietetic Internship Prgm
School of Public Health
1420 Washington Heights M6150
Ann Arbor, MI 48109-2029

University of Michigan Hospitals & Health Ctr
Dietetic Internship Prgm
UH2C227/0056
1500 E Medical Ctr Dr
Ann Arbor, MI 48109-0056
www.med.umich.edu/pfans/internship

Andrews University
Dietetic Internship Prgm
Dept of Nutrition
Berrien Springs, MI 49104-0210
www.andrews.edu

Andrews University
Dietetics-Didactic Prgm
Dept of Nutrition
Berrien Springs, MI 49104-0210
www.andrews.edu.

Detroit Dept of Hlth & Wellness Promotions
Dietetic Internship Prgm
Nutrition Div
1151 Taylor St
Detroit, MI 48202-1732

Harper University Hospital
Dietetic Internship Prgm
Dept of Nutrition and Food Svcs
3901 Beaubien Ave
Detroit, MI 48201-2018
www.harperhospital.org/harper/diet/intro

Henry Ford Hospital
Dietetic Internship Prgm
Dept of Food and Nutrition Services
2799 W Grand Blvd
Detroit, MI 48202-2689

Wayne State University
Dietetics-Coordinated Prgm
Nutrition and Food Science
3009 Science Hall
Detroit, MI 48202
www.wayne.edu/

Michigan State University
Dietetics-Didactic Prgm
Food Science and Human Nutrition
210 Trout FSHN Bldg
East Lansing, MI 48824-1224
www.msu.edu/unit/fshn

Michigan State University
Dietetic Internship Prgm
Dept of Food Science and Human Nutrition
2100 Anthony Hall
East Lansing, MI 48824-1225
www.msu.edu/unit/fshn/grad/intern.html

Hurley Medical Center
Dietetic Internship Prgm
Nutrition Service Dept
One Hurley Plaza
Flint, MI 48503-5993

Western Michigan University
Dietetic Internship Prgm
Family and Consumer Sciences
3025 Kohrman Hall
Kalamazoo, MI 49008-5067
www.wmich.edu

Western Michigan University
Dietetics-Didactic Prgm
Family and Consumer Sciences
3024 Kohrman Hall
Kalamazoo, MI 49008
www.wmich.edu

Madonna University
Dietetics-Didactic Prgm
Dept of Biological and Health Sciences
36600 Schoolcraft Rd
Livonia, MI 48150-1173
www.madonna.edu

Central Michigan University
Dietetic Internship Prgm
Human Environmental Studies
205 Wightman Hall
Mount Pleasant, MI 48859-3652
http://nutrition.cmich.edu

Central Michigan University
Dietetics-Didactic Prgm
Human Environmental Studies
205 Wightman Hall
Mount Pleasant, MI 48859
http://nutrition.cmich.edu/

Eastern Michigan University
Dietetics-Coordinated Prgm
206 Roosevelt Hall
Ypsilanti, MI 48197
www.emich.edu

Minnesota

Minnesota State University - Mankato
Dietetics-Didactic Prgm
Family Consumer Sciences Department
102 Wiecking Center
Mankato, MN 56001
www.mnsu.edu

University of Minnesota Med Ctr - Fairview
Dietetic Internship Prgm
2450 Riverside Ave
Minneapolis, MN 55454
www.fairview-university.fairview.org/

Veterans Affairs Medical Center
Dietetic Internship Prgm
Nutrition and Food Service
One Veterans Dr
Minneapolis, MN 55417
www.va.gov/nfs

Concordia College - Moorhead
Dietetic Internship Prgm
Dept of Family and Nutrition Sciences
901 S 8th St
Moorhead, MN 56562
www.cord.edu

Concordia College - Moorhead
Dietetics-Didactic Prgm
Family and Nutrition Sciences
Moorhead, MN 56562
www.cord.edu

St Mary's Hospital
Cosponsor: Mayo Medical Center
Dietetic Internship Prgm
1216 2nd St SW
Rochester, MN 55902-1906
www.mayo.edu

College of St Benedict/St John's University
Dietetics-Didactic Prgm
Nutrition Dept
37 S College Ave
St Joseph, MN 56374-2099
www.csbsju.edu/nutrition

College of St Catherine - St Paul
Dietetics-Didactic Prgm
Family Consumer and Nutri Sci, MC 4182
2004 Randolph Ave
St Paul, MN 55105-1750
www.stkate.edu

University of Minnesota - St Paul
Dietetics-Didactic Prgm
225 Food Science and Nutrition
1334 Eckles Ave
St Paul, MN 55108-6099
http://www1.umn.edu/twincities/index.php

University of Minnesota - St Paul
Dietetic Internship Prgm
225 Food Science and Nutrition
1334 Eckles Ave
St Paul, MN 55108-6099
http://fscn.che.umn.edu/index.html

Mississippi

Alcorn State University
Dietetics-Didactic Prgm
Family and Consumer Sciences
1000 ASU Dr #839
Alcorn State, MS 39096-7500
www.alcorn.edu/HumanSciences

Delta State University
Dietetics-Coordinated Prgm
Div of Family and Consumer Sciences
PO Box 3273
Cleveland, MS 38733
www.deltastate.edu/pages/1.asp

University of Southern Mississippi
Dietetics-Didactic Prgm
Family and Consumer Science
118 College Dr #5172
Hattiesburg, MS 39406
www.usm.edu/nfs

University of Southern Mississippi
Dietetic Internship Prgm
Family and Consumer Sciences
PO Box 5172
Hattiesburg, MS 39406-5035
www.usm.edu/nfs/

St Dominic-Jackson Memorial Hospital
Dietetic Internship Prgm
969 Lakeland Dr
Jackson, MS 39216-4699
www.stdom.com

Mississippi State University
Dietetic Internship Prgm
School of Human Sciences Box 9745
128 Lloyd Ricks
Mississippi State, MS 39762-9745
www.msstate.edu

Mississippi State University
Dietetics-Didactic Prgm
School of Human Sciences
PO Box 9805, 107 Herzer, Stone Blvd
Mississippi State, MS 39762-9745
www.msstate.edu

University of Mississippi
Dietetics-Didactic Prgm
Family and Consumer Sciences
110 Meek Hall, PO Box 1848
University, MS 38677-1848

Missouri

Southeast Missouri State University
Dietetic Internship Prgm
Dept of Human Enviromental Studies
One University Plaza
Cape Girardeau, MO 63701-4799
www5.semo.edu/dietetic_internship

Southeast Missouri State University
Dietetics-Didactic Prgm
Dept of Human Environmental Studies
One University Plaza MS 5750
Cape Girardeau, MO 63701-4799
www.semo.edu

University of Missouri - Columbia
Dietetics-Coordinated Prgm
106 McKee
Columbia, MO 65211-0001
www.missouri.edu/~nutsci

Missouri Dept of Health & Senior Service
Dietetic Internship Prgm
PO Box 570
Jefferson City, MO 65102-0570

ARAMARK Healthcare Kansas City
Dietetic Internship Prgm
St Joseph Health System
1000 Carondelet Dr
Kansas City, MO 64114-4802
www.aramark.com

Northwest Missouri State University
Dietetics-Didactic Prgm
Coll of Educ and Human Services
Family and Consumer Sciences, Rm 309 Admin Bldg
Maryville, MO 64468-6001
www.nwmissouri.edu

College of the Ozarks
Dietetics-Didactic Prgm
Dietetics and Nutrition Educ
PO Box 17
Point Lookout, MO 65726-0017
www.cofo.edu/

Cox College of Nursing and Health Services
Dietetic Internship Prgm
Springfield, MO 65802

Missouri State University
Dietetics-Didactic Prgm
Dept of Biomedical Sciences
901 S National Ave
Springfield, MO 65804
www.missouristate.edu

DVA Medical Center
Dietetic Internship Prgm
Jefferson Barracks Div-Nutri and Food Serv 120/JB
One Jefferson Barracks Dr
St Louis, MO 63125
www.va.gov/nfs/StLouisVA

Fontbonne University
Dietetics-Didactic Prgm
Human Environmental Sciences
6800 Wydown Blvd
St Louis, MO 63105-3098

Saint Louis University Doisy College of Health Sciences
Dietetics-Didactic Prgm
Dept of Nutri and Diet, Rm 3076
3437 Caroline St
St Louis, MO 63104-1111
www.slu.edu/x2270.xml

Saint Louis University Doisy College of Health Sciences
Dietetic Internship Prgm
Dept of Nutri and Diet, Rm 3076
3437 Caroline St
St Louis, MO 63104-1111
www.slu.edu/colleges/AH

University of Central Missouri
Dietetics-Didactic Prgm
Dept of Health and Human Performance
Morrow 100
Warrensburg, MO 64093
www.cmsu.edu/dietetics

Montana

Montana State University
Dietetics-Didactic Prgm
Health and Human Development
101 MH H&PE Complex
Bozeman, MT 59717
www.montana.edu/wwwhhd

Nebraska

University of Nebraska - Lincoln
Dietetics-Didactic Prgm
Nutrition Science and Dietetics
104H Ruth Leverton Hall
Lincoln, NE 68583-0806
www.unl.edu

University of Nebraska - Lincoln
Dietetic Internship Prgm
Nutrition Science and Dietetics
120 Ruth Leverton Hall
Lincoln, NE 68583-0806
http://cehs.unl.edu/nhs/internships/dieteticintern.shtml

University of Nebraska Medical Center
Dietetic Internship Prgm
981200 Nebraska Medical Center
Omaha, NE 68198-1200
www.unmc.edu/alliedhealth/mne

Nevada

University of Nevada - Las Vegas
Dietetic Internship Prgm
4505 Maryland Pkwy
Las Vegas, NV 89154

University of Nevada - Las Vegas
Dietetics-Didactic Prgm
Box 453026
4505 S Maryland Pkwy
Las Vegas, NV 89154-3026

University of Nevada - Reno
Dietetics-Didactic Prgm
Dept of Nutrition
SFB Mail Stop 142
Reno, NV 89557
www.unr.edu

University of Nevada - Reno
Dietetic Internship Prgm
Dept of Nutrition
Mail Stop 142
Reno, NV 89557-0132
www.cabnr.unr.edu/nutrition

New Hampshire

University of New Hampshire
Dietetics-Didactic Prgm
Animal and Nutri Sci Human Nutrition Ctr
Kendall Hall
Durham, NH 03824
www.anscandnutr.unh.edu

University of New Hampshire
Dietetic Internship Prgm
Nutrition Assessment and Counseling Services
Kendall Hall
Durham, NH 03824
www.dieteticinternship.unh.edu

Keene State College
Dietetic Internship Prgm
229 Main St, M2903
Keene, NH 03431
www.keene.edu/academics/dietetics

Keene State College
Dietetics-Didactic Prgm
Health Sciences/Nutrition
Joslin House MS 2903
Keene, NH 03435-2903
www.keene.edu/programs/hlsc

New Jersey

College of St Elizabeth
Dietetic Internship Prgm
Dept of Foods and Nutrition
Henderson Hall, 2 Convent Rd
Morristown, NJ 07960-6989
www.cse.edu

College of St Elizabeth
Dietetics-Didactic Prgm
Dept of Foods and Nutrition
2 Convent Rd
Morristown, NJ 07960-6989
www.cse.edu

Rutgers University
Dietetics-Didactic Prgm
Nutrition Sci, 229B Davison Hall
26 Nichol Ave
New Brunswick, NJ 08901-2882
www.rutgers.edu

Univ of Medicine & Dent of New Jersey
Dietetic Internship Prgm
School of Health Related Professions
1776 Raritan Rd
Scotch Plains, NJ 07076
http://shrp.umdnj.edu/programs/dietetic

Univ of Medicine & Dent of New Jersey
Dietetics-Coordinated Prgm
School of Health Related Profs Primary Care Dept
1776 Raritan Rd
Scotch Plains, NJ 07076
http://shrp.umdnj.edu/programs/dietetic

Montclair State University
Dietetics-Didactic Prgm
Dept of Human Ecology
111 Finley
Upper Montclair, NJ 07043
www.montclair.edu

Montclair State University
Dietetic Internship Prgm
Dept of Home Ecology
University Hall
Upper Montclair, NJ 07043

South Jersey Healthcare Regional Med Center
Dietetic Internship Prgm
1505 West Sherman Ave
Vineland, NJ 08360

New Mexico

University of New Mexico
Dietetic Internship Prgm
Individual Family and Community Education
Nutrition MSC05 3040
Albuquerque, NM 87131-1231
www.unm.edu/

University of New Mexico
Dietetics-Didactic Prgm
Individual Family and Community Education
Nutrition MSC05 3040
Albuquerque, NM 87131-1231
www.unm.edu/

New Mexico State University
Dietetics-Didactic Prgm
Dept of Family and Consumer Sciences
Box 30003, MSC 3470
Las Cruces, NM 88003-8003
www.nmsu.edu/~famcon

New York

CUNY Herbert H Lehman College
Dietetics-Didactic Prgm
Dept of Health Serv Dietetics Food and Nutri
Bedford Park Blvd W
Bronx, NY 10468-1589
www.lehman.cuny.edu

CUNY Herbert H Lehman College
Dietetic Internship Prgm
Dept of Health Services
250 Bedford Park Blvd W
Bronx, NY 10468-1589
www.lehman.cuny.edu/deannss/healthsci/di/info.html

James J Peters VA Medical Center
Dietetic Internship Prgm
Nutrition and Food Program (120)
130 W Kingsbridge Rd
Bronx, NY 10468-3904
www.va.gov/visns/visn03/diethome.asp

CUNY Brooklyn College
Dietetics-Didactic Prgm
Dept of Health and Nutrition Sciences
2900 Bedford Ave
Brooklyn, NY 11210-2889
http://academic.brooklyn.cuny.edu/hns

CUNY Brooklyn College
Dietetic Internship Prgm
Dept of Health and Nutrition Sciences
2900 Bedford Ave
Brooklyn, NY 11210-2889
http://academic.brooklyn.cuny.edu/hns

Long Island University - C W Post Campus
Dietetic Internship Prgm
Dept of Nutrition
720 Northern Blvd
Brookville, NY 11548
www.cwpost.liu.edu/nutrit

Long Island University - C W Post Campus
Dietetics-Didactic Prgm
Dept of Nutrition, Life Science Bldg
720 Northern Blvd
Brookville, NY 11548
www.liu.edu/nutrit

Buffalo State, SUNY
Dietetics-Didactic Prgm
Dietetics and Nutrition Dept
1300 Elmwood Ave
Buffalo, NY 14222-1095
www.buffalostate.edu

Buffalo State, SUNY
Dietetics-Coordinated Prgm
Dietetics and Nutrition Dept, Caudell Hall 207
1300 Elmwood Ave
Buffalo, NY 14222-1095
www.buffalostate.edu

D'Youville College
Dietetics-Coordinated Prgm
320 Porter Ave
Buffalo, NY 14201-1084
www.dyc.edu

University at Buffalo - SUNY
Dietetic Internship Prgm
15 Farber Hall
3435 Main St
Buffalo, NY 14214
www.phhp.buffalo.edu/ens/nutrition/ntr-internship.html

Sodexho Health Care Services
Cosponsor: NY Metropolitan Dietetic Internship
Dietetic Internship Prgm
90 Merrick Ave, Ste 210
East Meadow, NY 11554
http://dieteticintern.com/NYmetro/

CUNY Queens College
Dietetic Internship Prgm
Family Nutri and Exercise Sciences
65-30 Kissena Blvd
Flushing, NY 11367-1597
www.qc.edu/FNES/dietintern.html

CUNY Queens College
Dietetics-Didactic Prgm
Dept of Family, Nutri and Exercise Sciences
65-30 Kissena Blvd
Flushing, NY 11367-1597
www.qc.edu

Cornell University
Dietetic Internship Prgm
Division of Nutritional Sciences
225 Savage Hall
Ithaca, NY 14853-4401
www.nutrition.cornell.edu/dns7_dieteticintern.html

Cornell University
Dietetics-Didactic Prgm
Div of Nutritional Sciences
373 MVR Hall
Ithaca, NY 14853-4401
www.nutrition.cornell.edu/dns7_dietetic.html

ARAMARK Healthcare
Cosponsor: Metropolitan New York DI Program
Dietetic Internship Prgm
90-15 158th Ave
Jamaica, NY 11414
www.aramark.com/careers.asp

North Shore-Long Island Jewish Hlth System
Dietetic Internship Prgm
300 Community Dr
Manhasset, NY 11030

Columbia University Teachers College
Dietetic Internship Prgm
Dept of Health and Behavior Studies
525 W 120th St, Box 137
New York, NY 10027-6625
www.tc.columbia.edu/hbs/nutrition

CUNY Hunter College
Dietetics-Didactic Prgm
Brookdale Hlth Science Ctr
425 E 25th St
New York, NY 10010-2590

CUNY Hunter College
Dietetic Internship Prgm
School of Health Sciences
425 E 25th St, Box 896
New York, NY 10010-2590
www.hunter.cuny.edu/schoolhp/phn/dietetic_internship

New York University
Dietetic Internship Prgm
Nutrition and Food Studies
35 W 4th St, 10th Fl
New York, NY 10011-1172
www.nyu.edu/education/nutrition

New York University
Dietetics-Didactic Prgm
Nutrition and Food Studies
35 W 4th St, 10th Fl, Rm 1077
New York, NY 10012-1172
www.nyu.edu/education/nutrition

New York-Presbyterian Hospital
Dietetic Internship Prgm
525 E 68th St AN-833
Box 92
New York, NY 10021-4873
www.nyp.org/nutrition

New York Institute of Technology
Dietetics-Didactic Prgm
Clinical Nutrition Dept
NYCOM II, Rm 334
Old Westbury, NY 11568-8000
www.nyit.edu

SUNY College at Oneonta
Dietetics-Didactic Prgm
Dept of Human Ecology
104C Human Ecology
Oneonta, NY 13820-4015
www.oneonta.edu/academics/huec/dietetics4.asp

SUNY College at Oneonta
Dietetic Internship Prgm
Dept of Human Ecology
39 Denison Hall
Oneonta, NY 13820
www.oneonta.edu/academics/dieteticinternship

SUNY College at Plattsburgh
Dietetics-Didactic Prgm
Nutrition and Food Studies
101 Broad St
Plattsburgh, NY 12901-2681
www.plattsburgh.edu/

Rochester Institute of Technology
Dietetics-Didactic Prgm
Hospitality and Service Management
14 Lomb Memorial Dr
Rochester, NY 14623-5604
www.rit.edu

Stony Brook University
Dietetic Internship Prgm
Department of Family Medicine
Health Sciences Center Level 4, Rm 050
Stony Brook, NY 11794-8461
www.hsc.stonybrook.edu/SOM/fammed/intern_program

Syracuse University
Dietetics-Didactic Prgm
Nutrition and Foodservice Mgmt
034 Slocum Hall
Syracuse, NY 13244-1250

Syracuse University
Dietetics-Coordinated Prgm
Nutrition and Foodservice Mgmt
034 Slocum Hall
Syracuse, NY 13244-1250
www.hshp.syr.edu/schools/nhm

Syracuse University
Dietetic Internship Prgm
Nutrition and Foodservice Mgmt
034 Slocum Hall
Syracuse, NY 13244-1250
www.hshp.syr.edu/schools/nhm/academics/grad/mams/
 dietetic

Marymount College of Fordham University
Dietetics-Didactic Prgm
Dept of Human Ecology
100 Marymount Ave
Tarrytown, NY 10591
www.fordham.edu

The Sage Colleges
Dietetic Internship Prgm
45 Ferry St
Troy, NY 12180-4115
www.sage.edu

The Sage Colleges
Dietetics-Didactic Prgm
Div of Health and Rehab Sciences, Ackerman Hall
45 Ferry St
Troy, NY 12180-4115
www.sage.edu

North Carolina

Appalachian State University
Dietetic Internship Prgm
Family and Consumer Sciences
PO Box 32056
Boone, NC 28608-2056
www.appstate.edu

Appalachian State University
Dietetics-Didactic Prgm
Family and Consumer Sciences
Boone, NC 28608-2630
www.appstate.edu

University of North Carolina - Chapel Hill
Dietetics-Coordinated Prgm
McGavran-Greenberg Hall
Dept of Nutrition CB 7461
Chapel Hill, NC 27599-7461
www.sph.unc.edu/nutr

University of North Carolina - Chapel Hill
Dietetics-Didactic Prgm
McGavran-Greenburg Hall
Dept of Nutrition CB 7461
Chapel Hill, NC 27599-7461
www.sph.unc.edu/nutr

Western Carolina University
Dietetics-Didactic Prgm
Dept of Health Sciences
Cullowhee, NC 28723
www.wcu.edu/

Western Carolina University
Dietetic Internship Prgm
Nutrition/Sciences
Dept of Health Sciences
Cullowhee, NC 28723
www.wcu.edu/

North Carolina Central University
Dietetics-Didactic Prgm
Dept of Human Sciences
PO Box 19615
Durham, NC 27707-0099
www.nccu.edu

North Carolina Central University
Dietetic Internship Prgm
Dept of Human Sciences
PO Box 19615
Durham, NC 27707-0099
www.nccu.edu

North Carolina A&T State University
Dietetics-Didactic Prgm
Dept of Human Environment and Families
102 Benbow Hall, 1601 E Market St
Greensboro, NC 27411-1064
www.ag.ncat.edu/academics/fcs/dietetics/index.htm

University of North Carolina - Greensboro
Dietetics-Didactic Prgm
Nutrition and Foodservice Systems
PO Box 26170
Greensboro, NC 27402-6170
www.uncg.edu/nutrition

University of North Carolina - Greensboro
Dietetic Internship Prgm
Dept of Nutrition and Food Service Systems
1000 Spring Garden St
Greensboro, NC 27402-6170
www.uncg.edu/nutrition

East Carolina University
Dietetic Internship Prgm
School of Human Environmental Sciences
Nutrition & Hospitality Mgmt
Greenville, NC 27858-4353
www.ecu.edu

East Carolina University
Dietetics-Didactic Prgm
School of Human Environmental Sciences
Nutrition & Hospitality Mgmt
Greenville, NC 27858-4353
www.ecu.edu

Meredith College
Dietetics-Didactic Prgm
Human Environmental Sciences
3800 Hillsborough St
Raleigh, NC 27607-5298

Meredith College
Dietetic Internship Prgm
Human Environmental Sciences
3800 Hillsborough St
Raleigh, NC 27607-5298
www.meredith.edu/

North Dakota

North Dakota State University
Dietetics-Coordinated Prgm
Dept of Health, Nutrition, and Exercise Science
PO Box 5057
Fargo, ND 58105-5057
www.ndsu.nodak.edu

North Dakota State University
Dietetics-Didactic Prgm
Dept of Health, Nutrition, and Exercise Science
PO Box 5057
Fargo, ND 58105
www.ndsu.nodak.edu

University of North Dakota
Dietetics-Coordinated Prgm
Nutrition and Dietetics
PO Box 8237
Grand Forks, ND 58202-8237
www.und.edu

Ohio

University of Akron
Dietetics-Coordinated Prgm
Home Econ and Family Ecology
215 Schrank Hall S
Akron, OH 44325-6103
www.uakron.edu/fcs

University of Akron
Dietetics-Didactic Prgm
School of Family and Consumer Sciences
215 Schrank Hall S
Akron, OH 44325-6103
www3.uakron.edu/fcs

Ohio University
Dietetics-Didactic Prgm
Human and Consumer Sciences
Grover Center W324
Athens, OH 45701-2979
www.ohiou.edu

Bluffton College
Dietetics-Didactic Prgm
Family and Consumer Sciences
1 University Dr, Box 1346
Bluffton, OH 45817-1196
www.bluffton.edu/fcs

Bowling Green State University
Dietetic Internship Prgm
Family and Consumer Sciences
Bowling Green, OH 43403-0254
www.bgsu.edu

Bowling Green State University
Dietetics-Didactic Prgm
Family and Consumer Sciences
206 Johnston Hall
Bowling Green, OH 43403-0254
www.bgsu.edu/colleges/edhd/FCS

Christ Hospital
Dietetic Internship Prgm
Food and Nutrition Services
2139 Auburn Ave
Cincinnati, OH 45219-2906
www.health-alliance.com

Good Samaritan Hospital
Dietetic Internship Prgm
Nutrition Dept
375 Dixmyth Ave
Cincinnati, OH 45220-2489

University of Cincinnati
Dietetics-Didactic Prgm
Dept of Health Sciences
363C Hastings & William French Bldg, Box 670394
Cincinnati, OH 45267-0394
www.cahs.uc.edu

University of Cincinnati
Dietetics-Coordinated Prgm
PO Box 210063
Cincinnati, OH 45267

Case Western Reserve University
Dietetic Internship Prgm
Dept of Nutrition, School of Medicine
10900 Euclid Ave
Cleveland, OH 44106-1712

Case Western Reserve University
Dietetics-Didactic Prgm
Dept of Nutrition
10900 Euclid Ave
Cleveland, OH 44106-4906
www.case.edu/

Cleveland Clinic Foundation
Dietetic Internship Prgm
Nutrition Therapy M17
9500 Euclid Ave
Cleveland, OH 44195
www.clevelandclinic.org/education/diet

Louis Stokes Cleveland VA Med Ctr
Dietetic Internship Prgm
10701 East Blvd
Cleveland, OH 44106-1702
www.cwru.edu/med/nutrition/clevamc.html

MetroHealth Medical Center
Dietetic Internship Prgm
2500 MetroHealth Dr
Cleveland, OH 44109-1998
www.metrohealth.org/

University Hospitals Case Medical Center
Dietetic Internship Prgm
11100 Euclid Ave
Lakeside 5021
Cleveland, OH 44106-5000
www.cwru.edu/med/nutrition/uhocle.html

Mt Carmel College of Nursing
Dietetic Internship Prgm
127 S Davis Ave
Columbus, OH 43222-1504
www.mccn.edu/

Ohio State University
Dietetics-Didactic Prgm
Dept of Human Nutrition and Food Management
1787 Neil Ave
Columbus, OH 43210-1220
http://hec.osu.edu/hn

Ohio State University
Dietetic Internship Prgm
Dept of Human Nutrition and Food Managemnt
325 Campbell Hall, 1787 Neil Ave
Columbus, OH 43210-1220
http://hec.osu.edu/hn

Ohio State University
Dietetic Internship Prgm
School of Allied Medical Profs
Med Dietetics, 1583 Perry St
Columbus, OH 43210-1234
www.osu.edu/

Ohio State University
Dietetics-Coordinated Prgm
Sch of Allied Medical Profs
1583 Perry St
Columbus, OH 43210-1234
www.osu.edu/

Miami Valley Hospital
Dietetic Internship Prgm
One Wyoming St
Dayton, OH 45409-2793
www.miamivalleyhospital.com

University of Dayton
Dietetics-Didactic Prgm
Health and Sports Science
300 College Park Ave
Dayton, OH 45469-1210
www.udayton.edu/

Kent State University
Dietetic Internship Prgm
100 Nixson Hall
Kent, OH 44242
www.kent.edu

Kent State University
Dietetics-Didactic Prgm
Family and Consumer Studies
Nixson Hall, Nutrition & Dietetics
Kent, OH 44242
www.dept.kent.edu/f&cs

Miami University
Dietetics-Didactic Prgm
Phys Ed Hlth and Sports Studies
100A Phillips Hall
Oxford, OH 45056
www.miami.muohio.edu/

Youngstown State University
Dietetics-Coordinated Prgm
One University Plaza
Youngstown, OH 44555-0001
www.ysu.edu

Youngstown State University
Dietetics-Didactic Prgm
Human Ecology Dept
One University Plaza
Youngstown, OH 44555-0001
www.ysu.edu

Oklahoma

University of Central Oklahoma
Dietetic Internship Prgm
Human Environmental Sciences
100 N University Dr
Edmond, OK 73034
www.educ.ucok.edu

University of Central Oklahoma
Dietetics-Didactic Prgm
College of Education
Human Environmental Sciences
Edmond, OK 73034
www.ucok.edu/

Langston University
Dietetics-Didactic Prgm
Dept of Home Ecology
302 Jones Hall
Langston, OK 73050
www.lunet.edu

Univ of Oklahoma Health Sciences Center
Dietetics-Didactic Prgm
College of Allied Health
Nutritional Sci, PO Box 26901
Oklahoma City, OK 73190
www.ah.ouhsc.edu/main

Univ of Oklahoma Health Sciences Center
Dietetic Internship Prgm
College of Allied Hlth, Dept of Nutri Sci
PO Box 26901 CHB
Oklahoma City, OK 73190
www.ah.ouhsc.edu/main

Univ of Oklahoma Health Sciences Center
Dietetics-Coordinated Prgm
Dept of Nutritional Sciences
801 NE 13th, PO Box 26901
Oklahoma City, OK 73190
www.ouhsc.edu

Oklahoma State University
Dietetics-Didactic Prgm
Nutritional Sciences Dept
301 HES
Stillwater, OK 74078-6141
http://ches.okstate.edu/nsci/

Oklahoma State University
Dietetic Internship Prgm
Dept of Nutritional Sciences
HES 301
Stillwater, OK 74078-6337
http://ches.okstate.edu/nsci/

Northeastern State University
Dietetics-Didactic Prgm
Coll of Business and Technology
600 N Grand, 210A PA Bldg
Tahlequah, OK 74464-2399
http://arapaho.nsuok.edu/~fcs

Oregon

Oregon State University
Dietetics-Didactic Prgm
Nutrition and Food Mgmt
212 Milam Hall
Corvallis, OR 97331-5103
www.oregonstate.edu

Oregon Health & Science University
Dietetic Internship Prgm
EJH-10-FM 10
3181 SW Sam Jackson Park Rd
Portland, OR 97201-3098
www.ohsu.edu/dietetic

Mid Willamette Valley Dietetic Internship
Dietetic Internship Prgm
1955 Dallas Hwy NW, Ste 1200
Salem, OR 97304
www.capitalmanor.com/internship.htm

Pennsylvania

Cedar Crest College
Dietetics-Didactic Prgm
100 College Dr
Allentown, PA 18104-6196
www.cedarcrest.edu/Redesign/homepage5/index.htm

Sodexho Health Care Services
Dietetics-Preprofessional Practice Prgm
6081 Hamilton Blvd
PO Box 3501
Allentown, PA 18106-0501
www.woodco.com

Geisinger Medical Center
Dietetic Internship Prgm
100 N Academy Ave
Danville, PA 17822-0115
www.geisinger.org

Edinboro University of Pennsylvania
Cosponsor: Pennsylvania Consortium
Dietetics-Coordinated Prgm
Biology and Health Services
Edinboro, PA 16444

Gannon University
Cosponsor: Pennsylvania Consortium
Dietetics-Coordinated Prgm
Sciences Engineering and Health Science
109 University Square
Erie, PA 16541-0001
www.gannon.edu

Mercyhurst College
Cosponsor: Pennsylvania Consortium
Dietetics-Coordinated Prgm
Dept of Human Ecology
501 E 38th St
Erie, PA 16546
www.mercyhurst.edu

Messiah College
Dietetics-Didactic Prgm
Dept of Natural Sciences
One College Ave
Grantham, PA 17027
www.messiah.edu

Seton Hill University
Dietetics-Coordinated Prgm
Family and Consumer Sciences
Seton Hill Dr
Greensburg, PA 15601-1599
www.setonhill.edu

Immaculata University
Dietetic Internship Prgm
Nutrition Educ
Box 500, Graduate Div
Immaculata, PA 19345-0901
www.immaculata.edu

Immaculata University
Dietetics-Didactic Prgm
Fashion Foods and Nutrition
Box 722
Immaculata, PA 19345-0722
www.immaculata.edu

Indiana University of Pennsylvania
Dietetics-Didactic Prgm
Dept of Food and Nutrition
911 South Dr
Indiana, PA 15705-1087
www.hhs.iup.edu/fn

Indiana University of Pennsylvania
Dietetic Internship Prgm
Dept of Food and Nutrition
Ackerman Hall 14
Indiana, PA 15705-1087
www.hhs.iup.edu/fn

Mansfield University
Dietetics-Didactic Prgm
203C Elliott Hall
Dept of Health Sciences
Mansfield, PA 16933
www.mnsfld.edu/~health/index.htm

ARAMARK Healthcare
Dietetic Internship Prgm
1717 Arch St, 42nd Fl
Philadelphia, PA 19103
www.aramark.com/Careers.asp

Drexel University
Dietetics-Didactic Prgm
Nutrition and Food Sciences
3141 Chestnut St
Philadelphia, PA 19104-2875
www.drexel.edu/

La Salle University
Dietetics-Coordinated Prgm
1900 W Olney Ave
Philadelphia, PA 19141-1199
www.lasalle.edu

La Salle University
Dietetics-Didactic Prgm
1900 W Olney Ave
Philadelphia, PA 19141-1199
www.lasalle.edu

Adajio Health
Dietetic Internship Prgm
960 Penn Ave, Ste 600
Pittsburgh, PA 15222-1417
www.adagiohealth.org

University of Pittsburgh
Dietetics-Didactic Prgm
Health and Rehab Science
4048 Forbes Tower
Pittsburgh, PA 15260-1802
www.pitt.edu/

University of Pittsburgh
Dietetics-Coordinated Prgm
Health and Rehab Sciences
4048 Forbes Tower
Pittsburgh, PA 15260-1802
www.shrs.pitt.edu/cdn

UPMC Presbyterian Shadyside
Dietetic Internship Prgm
5230 Centre Ave
Pittsburgh, PA 15232-1304
www.upmc.edu/shadyside/Dieteticinternship

Marywood University
Dietetics-Didactic Prgm
Dept of Nutrition and Dietetics
2300 Adams Ave
Scranton, PA 18509-1514
www.marywood.edu/departments/nutr_diet/home.html

Marywood University
Dietetic Internship Prgm
Dept of Nutrition and Dietetics
2300 Adams Ave
Scranton, PA 18509-1514
www.marywood.edu/departments/nutr_diet/home.html

Marywood University
Dietetics-Coordinated Prgm
Dept of Nutrition and Dietetics
2300 Adams Ave
Scranton, PA 18509-1598
www.marywood.edu/departments/nutr_diet/home.html

Penn State University
Dietetic Internship Prgm
Nutrition Dept Coll of Hlth and Human Dev
5126 Henderson Bldg
University Park, PA 16802
http://nutrition.hhdev.psu.edu/internship/index.html

Penn State University
Dietetics-Didactic Prgm
Nutrition Dept
Coll of Hlth & Human Development
University Park, PA 16802-6500
http://nutrition.hhdev.psu.edu/internship/index.html

Sodexho Health Care Services
Dietetic Internship Prgm
Fuld Campus
Rte 532 & General Sullivan Rd
Washington Cross, PA 18977
www.dieteticintern.com/NJ-Phila

West Chester University
Dietetics-Didactic Prgm
H302 Department of Health
Sturzebecker Health Sciences Center
West Chester, PA 19383
www.wcupa.edu

Puerto Rico

Universidad Del Turabo
Dietetics-Coordinated Prgm
Gurabo, PR 00778

Puerto Rico Department of Health
Dietetic Internship Prgm
PO Box 70184
San Juan, PR 00936

University of Puerto Rico
Dietetics-Didactic Prgm
Box 23347 UPR Station
Rio Piedras Campus
San Juan, PR 00931-3347

University of Puerto Rico
Dietetic Internship Prgm
College of Health Related Professions
Med Sci Campus, PO Box 365067
San Juan, PR 00936-5067
http://cprsweb.rcm.upr.edu

VA Caribbean Healthcare System
Dietetic Internship Prgm
10 Calle Casia
San Juan, PR 00921

Rhode Island

University of Rhode Island
Dietetics-Didactic Prgm
Food Science and Nutrition
110 Ranger Hall
Kingston, RI 02881-0804
www.uri.edu/cels/fsn

University of Rhode Island
Dietetic Internship Prgm
Food Science and Nutrition
106 Ranger Hall
Kingston, RI 02881
www.uri.edu/cels/fsn

Johnson & Wales University
Dietetics-Didactic Prgm
College of Culinary Arts
One Washington Square
Providence, RI 02905
www.jwu.edu

South Carolina

Medical University of South Carolina
Dietetic Internship Prgm
96 Jonathan Lucas St, Ste 219K
PO Box 250327
Charleston, SC 29425
www.musc.edu/dieteticinternship

Clemson University
Dietetics-Didactic Prgm
Dept of Food Science
223 Poole, Agricultural Center
Clemson, SC 29634-0371
www.clemson.edu/foodscience

SC Dept of Health & Environmental Control
Dietetic Internship Prgm
Mills Complex
PO Box 101106
Columbia, SC 29211-0106
www.scdhec.gov

South Carolina State University
Dietetics-Didactic Prgm
Staley Hall PO Box 7657
300 College Ave
Orangeburg, SC 29117-0001

Winthrop University
Dietetics-Didactic Prgm
Dept of Human Nutrition
302 Life Sciences Bldg
Rock Hill, SC 29733
www.winthrop.edu/nutrition

Winthrop University
Dietetic Internship Prgm
Dept of Human Nutrition
302 Life Sciences Bldg
Rock Hill, SC 29733
www.winthrop.edu/nutrition/dietetic.htm

South Dakota

South Dakota State University
Dietetics-Didactic Prgm
Family and Consumer Sciences
PO Box 2275A
Brookings, SD 57007-0497
www3.sdstate.edu

University of South Dakota
Dietetic Internship Prgm
School of Medicine
1400 W 22nd St
Sioux Falls, SD 57105
www.usd.edu/cd/dieteticinternship

Tennessee

University of Tennessee - Chattanooga
Dietetics-Didactic Prgm
Dept of Human Ecology, #4204
615 McCallie Ave
Chattanooga, TN 37403
www.utc.edu/

Tennessee Technological University
Dietetics-Didactic Prgm
School of Home Economics
Box 5035
Cookeville, TN 38505
www.tntech.edu/

Carson-Newman College
Dietetics-Didactic Prgm
PO Box 71881
2130 Branner Ave
Jefferson City, TN 37760-7001
www.cn.edu/

East Tennessee State University
Dietetics-Didactic Prgm
Applied Human Sciences
PO Box 70671
Johnson City, TN 37614-0671
www.etsu.edu

East Tennessee State University
Dietetic Internship Prgm
Applied Human Sciences-STAT
PO Box 70671
Johnson City, TN 37614-0671
www.etsu.edu/scitech/ahsc/ahsc.htm

University of Tennessee - Knoxville
Dietetics-Didactic Prgm
Dept of Nutrition
1215 W Cumberland Ave
Knoxville, TN 37996-1920

University of Tennessee - Knoxville
Dietetic Internship Prgm
Human Ecology, Dept of Nutrition
1215 Cumberland Ave, Rm 229
Knoxville, TN 37996-1920
http://nutrition.utk.edu

University of Tennessee - Martin
Dietetic Internship Prgm
Human Environmental Sciences
340 Gooch Hall
Martin, TN 38238-5045
www.utm.edu/

University of Tennessee - Martin
Dietetics-Didactic Prgm
Dept of Family and Consumer Sci
340 Gooch Hall
Martin, TN 38238-5045
www.utm.edu/

University of Memphis
Dietetics-Didactic Prgm
Consumer Science and Education
Fieldhouse 1611
Memphis, TN 38152
http://hss.memphis.edu

University of Memphis
Dietetic Internship Prgm
Dept of Health and Sport Science
161A Fieldhouse
Memphis, TN 38152
www.memphis.edu/

Middle Tennessee State University
Dietetics-Didactic Prgm
Dept of Human Sciences
PO Box 86
Murfreesboro, TN 37132
www.mtsu.edu

National HealthCare LP
Dietetic Internship Prgm
PO Box 1398
Murfreesboro, TN 37133-1398
www.nhccare.com/di.htm

Lipscomb University
Dietetic Internship Prgm
3901 Granny White Pike
Nashville, TN 37204-3951
www.lipscomb.edu

Lipscomb University
Dietetics-Didactic Prgm
Family and Consumer Sciences
3901 Granny White Pike
Nashville, TN 37204-3951
www.lipscomb.edu

Tennessee State University
Dietetics-Didactic Prgm
Family Consumer Sciences PO Box 9538
3500 John A Merritt Blvd
Nashville, TN 37209-1561
www.tnstate.edu/sacs

Vanderbilt University Medical Center
Dietetic Internship Prgm
B-802TVC
1301 22nd Ave S
Nashville, TN 37232-5510
www.mc.vanderbilt.edu/alliedhealth

Texas

Abilene Christian University
Dietetics-Didactic Prgm
Family and Consumer Sciences
ACU Box 28155
Abilene, TX 79699
www.acu.edu/

Texas WIC
Dietetic Internship Prgm
Bureau of Nutrition Services
1100 W 49th St
Austin, TX 78756
www.dshs.state.tx.us/

University of Texas at Austin
Dietetics-Coordinated Prgm
Dept of Human Ecology
1 University Station, A2700
Austin, TX 78712-1097
www.he.utexas.edu/

University of Texas at Austin
Dietetics-Didactic Prgm
Dept of Human Ecology
1 University Station, A2700
Austin, TX 78712
www.utexas.edu/depts/he

Lamar University
Dietetic Internship Prgm
Family and Consumer Sciences
PO Box 10035
Beaumont, TX 77710-0035
www.lamar.edu

Lamar University
Dietetics-Didactic Prgm
Family and Consumer Sciences
PO Box 10035
Beaumont, TX 77710-0035
www.lamar.edu

Texas A&M University
Dietetic Internship Prgm
Dept of Animal Science
2253 TAMU
College Station, TX 77843-2253
http://nfs.tamu.edu/

Texas A&M University
Dietetics-Didactic Prgm
Human Nutrition Section
2253 TAMU
College Station, TX 77843-2471
http://nfs.tamu.edu

Baylor University Med Center
Dietetic Internship Prgm
3500 Gaston Ave
Dallas, TX 75246-2045
www.baylorhealth.com/locations/bumc/

Presbyterian Hospital of Dallas
Dietetic Internship Prgm
8200 Walnut Hill Ln
Dallas, TX 75231-4402
www.phscare.org/phd/dietetics

Univ of Texas Southwestern Med Ctr
Dietetics-Coordinated Prgm
Dept of Clinical Nutrition
5323 Harry Hines Blvd
Dallas, TX 75390-8877
www.utsouthwestern.edu/clinnut

Texas Woman's University
Dietetics-Didactic Prgm
Nutrition and Food Sciences
304 Administration Dr, Clock Tower
Denton, TX 76201
www.twu.edu/hs/nfs

Texas Woman's University
Dietetic Internship Prgm
Nutrition and Food Sciences
PO Box 425888
Denton, TX 76204-5888
www.twu.edu/hs/nfs/intern.htm

Univ of Texas - Pan American
Dietetics-Coordinated Prgm
Health and Human Services
1201 W University Dr
Edinburg, TX 78539-2909
www.panam.edu

US Military Dietetic Internship Consortium
Dietetic Internship Prgm
Nutrition Care Div
3851 Roger Brooke Dr
Fort Sam Houston, TX 78234-6200
www.amsc.amedd.army.mil/training.asp

Texas Christian University
Dietetics-Coordinated Prgm
Dept of Nutrition and Dietetics
TCU Box 298600
Fort Worth, TX 76129
www.tcu.edu/

Texas Christian University
Dietetics-Didactic Prgm
Dept of Nutrition and Dietetics
TCU Box 298600
Fort Worth, TX 76129
www.tcu.edu/

Michael E DeBakey VA Medical Center
Dietetic Internship Prgm
2002 Holcombe Blvd
Houston, TX 77030-4298
www.va.gov/nfs/HoustonVAMC

Texas Southern University
Dietetics-Didactic Prgm
Human Svcs and Consumer Sci
3100 Cleburne Ave
Houston, TX 77004-4575
www.tsu.edu

Texas Woman's University
Dietetic Internship Prgm
1130 John Freeman Blvd
Houston, TX 77030-2897
www.twu.edu/hs/nfs/hintern.htm

Univ of Texas Hlth Sci Ctr at Houston
Dietetic Internship Prgm
Sch of Public Hlth, E619 RAS Bldg
1200 Herman Pressler St
Houston, TX 77030
www.sph.uth.tmc.edu

University of Houston
Dietetics-Didactic Prgm
Human Development and Consumer Sci
4800 Calhoun Rd
Houston, TX 77204-6861
http://hhp.uh.edu/nutrition

University of Houston
Dietetic Internship Prgm
Human Development and Consumer Sci
4800 Calhoun Rd
Houston, TX 77204-6020
www.hhp.uh.edu/internship

Sam Houston State University
Dietetic Internship Prgm
PO Box 2177
1700 Sam Houston Ave
Huntsville, TX 77341-2177
www.shsu.edu/~hec_www

Sam Houston State University
Dietetics-Didactic Prgm
Food Science and Nutrition
SHSU Box 2177
Huntsville, TX 77341-2177
www.shsu.edu/~hec_www

Texas A&M University - Kingsville
Dietetics-Didactic Prgm
Dept of Human Sciences
MSC 168, 700 University Blvd
Kingsville, TX 78363
www.tamu.edu

Texas A&M University - Kingsville
Dietetic Internship Prgm
Dept of Human Sciences
MSC 168, 700 University Blvd
Kingsville, TX 78363-8202
www.tamu.edu

Texas Tech University
Dietetics-Didactic Prgm
Educ Nutri and Rest Hotel Mgmt
PO Box 41162, 15th and Akron St
Lubbock, TX 79409-1162
www.hs.ttu.edu

Texas Tech University
Dietetic Internship Prgm
Dept of Educ, Nutr, Rest, and Hotel Mgmt
PO Box 41162, 15th and Akron St
Lubbock, TX 79409-1162
www.hs.ttu.edu/intern

Stephen F Austin State University
Dietetics-Didactic Prgm
Dept of Human Sciences
SFA Station 13014
Nacogdoches, TX 75962-3014
www.sfasu.edu

Stephen F Austin State University
Dietetic Internship Prgm
Dept of Human Sciences
SFA Station PO Box 13014
Nacogdoches, TX 75962-3014
www.sfasu.edu/di

Prairie View A&M University
Dietetics-Didactic Prgm
Dept of Human Sciences
PO Box 4329
Prairie View, TX 77446-4329
www.pvamu.edu

Prairie View A&M University
Dietetic Internship Prgm
Box 4329
Prairie View, TX 77446
www.pvamu.edu

University of the Incarnate Word
Dietetics-Didactic Prgm
4301 Broadway St
San Antonio, TX 78209-6318
www.uiw.edu

University of the Incarnate Word
Dietetic Internship Prgm
4301 Broadway Box 311
San Antonio, TX 78209
www.uiw.edu

US Military Consortium
Dietetic Internship Prgm
Wilford Hall Medical Center/USAF
San Antonio, TX 78236

Texas State University - San Marcos
Dietetic Internship Prgm
Family and Consumer Sciences
601 University Dr
San Marcos, TX 78666-4616
www.txstate.edu/

Texas State University - San Marcos
Dietetics-Didactic Prgm
Family and Consumer Sciences
601 University Dr
San Marcos, TX 78666-4616
www.txstate.edu/

Baylor University
Dietetics-Didactic Prgm
Family and Consumer Sciences
BU Box 97346
Waco, TX 76798-7346

Utah

Utah State University
Dietetics-Coordinated Prgm
Nutrition and Food Science
Logan, UT 84322-8700
www.usu.edu/~dietetic

Utah State University
Dietetics-Didactic Prgm
8700 Old Main Hill
Logan, UT 84322-8700
www.usu.edu/~dietetic

Brigham Young University
Dietetics-Didactic Prgm
Food Science and Nutrition
S219 ESC, PO Box 24620
Provo, UT 84602-4620
http://ndfs.byu.edu

Brigham Young University
Dietetic Internship Prgm
Food Science and Nutrition
S219 ESC, PO Box 24620
Provo, UT 84602-4620
http://ndfs.byu.edu

University of Utah
Dietetics-Coordinated Prgm
Div of Foods and Nutrition
250 South 1850 East #214
Salt Lake City, UT 84112
www.health.utah.edu/nutr/

Utah State University - Salt Lake
Dietetic Internship Prgm
5250 S Commerce Dr Ste 300
Salt Lake City, UT 84107
http://extension.usu.edu/intern

Vermont

University of Vermont
Dietetics-Coordinated Prgm
349 Waterman Bldg
Burlington, VT 05405

University of Vermont
Dietetics-Didactic Prgm
Dept of Nutritional Sciences
Terrill Hall
Burlington, VT 05405
http://nutrition.uvm.edu

Virginia

Virginia Polytechnic Inst & State Univ
Dietetics-Didactic Prgm
Human Nutrition Foods and Exercise
College of Agriculture and Life Sciences
Blacksburg, VA 24061-0430
www.hnfe.vt.edu

Virginia Polytechnic Inst & State Univ
Dietetic Internship Prgm
338 Wallace Hall
Blacksburg, VA 24061-0430
www.hnfe.vt.edu

University of Virginia Health System
Dietetic Internship Prgm
Box 800673
Charlottesville, VA 22908
http://hsc.virginia.edu/internet/dietetics

James Madison University
Dietetics-Didactic Prgm
Dept of Health Sciences MSC 4301
HHS 3140
Harrisonburg, VA 22807
www.jmu.edu

James Madison University
Dietetic Internship Prgm
MSC 4301
800 S Main St
Harrisonburg, VA 22807
www.healthsci.jmu.edu/dietetics/graduate.htm

Norfolk State University
Dietetics-Didactic Prgm
700 Park Ave
Norfolk, VA 23504

Virginia State University
Dietetics-Didactic Prgm
Dept of Human Ecology, Box 9211
Petersburg, VA 23806-0001
www.vsu.edu

Virginia State University
Dietetic Internship Prgm
PO Box 9211
Petersburg, VA 23806
www.vsu.edu

Radford University
Dietetics-Didactic Prgm
Dept of Health Services
PO Box 6962
Radford, VA 24142-5826
www.radford.edu/~fdsn-web

Virginia Commonwealth Univ/Health System
Dietetic Internship Prgm
PO Box 980294
Richmond, VA 23298-0294
http://views.vcu.edu/dietetic

Virginia Department of Health
Dietetic Internship Prgm
Div of WIC and Community Nutrition Services
109 Governor St, 9th Fl
Richmond, VA 23219

Washington

Central Washington University
Dietetics-Didactic Prgm
Family and Consumer Sciences
400 E University Way
Ellensburg, WA 98926-7565
www.cwu.edu

Central Washington University
Dietetic Internship Prgm
Family and Consumer Sciences
400 E University Way
Ellensburg, WA 98929-7565
www.cwu.edu/~fandcs/internship.html

Bastyr University
Dietetic Internship Prgm
Nutrition Program
14500 Juanita Dr NE
Kenmore, WA 98028-4966

Bastyr University
Dietetics-Didactic Prgm
14500 Juanita Dr NE
Kenmore, WA 98028-4966
www.bastyr.edu

Washington State University
Dietetics-Coordinated Prgm
106 FSHN Bldg
PO Box 646376
Pullman, WA 99164-6376
http://fshn.wsu.edu

Washington State University
Dietetics-Didactic Prgm
Food Sci and Human Nutrition
FSHN 120, PO Box 646376
Pullman, WA 99164-6376
http://fshn.wsu.edu

Sea Mar Community Health Center
Dietetic Internship Prgm
8915 14th Ave S
Seattle, WA 98108-4807
www.seamar.org

Seattle Pacific University
Dietetics-Didactic Prgm
Family and Consumer Sciences
3307 3rd Ave W
Seattle, WA 98119-1997
www.spu.edu/depts/fcs

University of Washington
Dietetic Internship Prgm
Box 353410
305 Raitt Hall
Seattle, WA 98195
http://depts.washington.edu/nutr

University of Washington
Dietetics-Didactic Prgm
305 Raitt Hall, Box 353410
Seattle, WA 98195-3410
http://depts.washington.edu/nutr

Washington State University - Spokane
Dietetics-Coordinated Prgm
310 N Riverpoint Blvd Box M
Spokane, WA 99210
www.wsu.edu/

West Virginia

Marshall University
Dietetic Internship Prgm
Corbly Hall 203 Family and Consumer Sci
One John Marshall Dr
Huntington, WV 25755-9521
www.marshall.edu

Marshall University
Dietetics-Didactic Prgm
One John Marshall Dr
Huntington, WV 25755-9521
www.marshall.edu

West Virginia University
Dietetics-Didactic Prgm
Coll of Agriculture and Forestry
PO Box 6108
Morgantown, WV 26506-6124
www.caf.wvu.edu

West Virginia University
Dietetic Internship Prgm
Coll of Agriculture and Forestry
PO Box 6108
Morgantown, WV 26506-6124
www.caf.wvu.edu

West Virginia University Hospitals
Dietetic Internship Prgm
Dept of Nutrition and Environmental Serv
Medical Center Dr, PO Box 8016
Morgantown, WV 26506-8016
www.hsc.wvu.edu/di

Wisconsin

University of Wisconsin - Green Bay
Dietetics-Didactic Prgm
Human Biology Dept LS 423
2420 Nicolet Dr
Green Bay, WI 54311-7001
www.uwgb.edu/humbio/program/Majors.htm

University of Wisconsin - Green Bay
Dietetic Internship Prgm
2420 Nicolet Dr
Human Biology Dept ES 301
Green Bay, WI 54311-7001
www.uwgb.edu/humbio/dietetics/Index.htm

Viterbo College
Dietetic Internship Prgm
Nutrition and Dietetics Dept
900 Viterbo Dr
La Crosse, WI 54601-4797
www.viterbo.edu/

Viterbo College
Dietetics-Coordinated Prgm
Nutrition and Dietetics Dept
900 Viterbo Dr
La Crosse, WI 54601-4797
www.viterbo.edu/

University of Wisconsin - Madison
Dietetics-Coordinated Prgm
Dept of Nutritional Sciences
1415 Linden Dr
Madison, WI 53706-1571
www.nutrisci.wisc.edu/

University of Wisconsin - Madison
Dietetics-Didactic Prgm
Dept of Nutritional Sciences
1415 Linden Dr
Madison, WI 53706-1571
http://nutrisci.wisc.edu

University of Wisconsin Hospital and Clinics
Dietetic Internship Prgm
Food and Nutrition Services F4/120
600 Highland Ave
Madison, WI 53792-1510
www.uwhealth.org

University of Wisconsin - Stout
Dietetic Internship Prgm
Dept of Food and Nutrition
222 Home Economics Bldg
Menomonie, WI 54751
www.uwstout.edu/programs/msfns/intern

University of Wisconsin - Stout
Dietetics-Didactic Prgm
College of Human Development
415 E 10th Ave
Menomonie, WI 54751-0790
www.uwstout.edu/programs/bsd

Mount Mary College
Dietetics-Coordinated Prgm
Dept of Dietetics
2900 N Menomonee River Pkwy
Milwaukee, WI 53222-4597
www.mtmary.edu

Mount Mary College
Dietetic Internship Prgm
Graduate Program in Dietetics
2900 N Menomonee River Pkwy
Milwaukee, WI 53222-4597
www.mtmary.edu/dietetics.htm

University of Wisconsin - Stevens Point
Dietetics-Didactic Prgm
Health Promotion and Human Development
202 CPS
Stevens Point, WI 54481
www.uwsp.edu

Wyoming

University of Wyoming
Dietetics-Didactic Prgm
Dept of Family and Consumer Sciences
1000 E University Ave
Laramie, WY 82071-3354
www.uwyo.edu/family

Dietetic Technician

Arizona

Chandler-Gilbert Community College
Dietetic Technician-AD Prgm
2626 East Pecos Rd
Chandler, AZ 85225
cgcmail.maricopa.edu

Central Arizona College
Dietetic Technician-AD Prgm
8470 N Overfield Rd
Coolidge, AZ 85228-9030
www.centralaz.edu

Paradise Valley Community College
Dietetic Technician-AD Prgm
18401 N 32nd St
Phoenix, AZ 85032
www.pvc.maricopa.edu

Arkansas

Black River Technical College
Dietetic Technician-AD Prgm
PO Box 468
Pocahontas, AR 72455
www.blackrivertech.org

California

Orange Coast College
Dietetic Technician-AD Prgm
2701 Fairview Rd
Costa Mesa, CA 92628-0120

Loma Linda University
Dietetic Technician-AD Prgm
Nutrition and Dietetics
School of Allied Hlth Profs
Loma Linda, CA 92350
www.llu.edu/llu/nutrition

Long Beach City College
Dietetic Technician-AD Prgm
Fam and Consumer Studies Div
Liberal Arts Campus
Long Beach, CA 90808-1706

Los Angeles City College
Dietetic Technician-AD Prgm
Family and Consumer Studies
855 N Vermont Ave
Los Angeles, CA 90029-3590
www.lacc.cc.ca.us

Merritt College
Dietetic Technician-AD Prgm
12500 Campus Dr
Oakland, CA 94619-3107

Chaffey College
Dietetic Technician-AD Prgm
Food Service Management
5885 Haven Ave
Rancho Cucamonga, CA 91737-3002
www.chaffey.edu

Cosumnes River Community College
Dietetic Technician-AD Prgm
8401 Center Pkwy
Sacramento, CA 95823-5799
http://crc.losrios.edu/~diettech

Colorado

Front Range Comm College
Dietetic Technician-AD Prgm
3645 W 112th Ave, #23
Westminster, CO 80031-2199
www.frontrange.edu

Connecticut

Gateway Community College
Dietetic Technician-AD Prgm
88 Bassett Rd
New Haven, CT 06473
www.gwctc.commnet.edu

Briarwood College
Dietetic Technician-AD Prgm
2279 Mt Vernon Rd
Southington, CT 06489-1007
www.briarwoodcollege.com/

Florida

Florida Community College - Jacksonville
Dietetic Technician-AD Prgm
North Campus, 4501 Capper Rd
Jacksonville, FL 32218-4436
www.fccj.org

Pensacola Junior College
Dietetic Technician-AD Prgm
1000 College Blvd
Pensacola, FL 32504-8998
www.pjc.edu

Illinois

Harper College
Dietetic Technician-AD Prgm
1200 W Algonquin Rd
Palatine, IL 60067-7398
www.harpercollege.edu

Louisiana

Delgado Community College
Dietetic Technician-AD Prgm
615 City Park Ave
New Orleans, LA 70119
www.dcc.edu

Maine

Southern Maine Community College
Dietetic Technician-AD Prgm
2 Fort Rd
South Portland, ME 04106
www.smccme.edu

Maryland

Baltimore City Community College
Dietetic Technician-AD Prgm
Dept of Allied Health
2901 Liberty Heights Ave
Baltimore, MD 21215-7893
www.bccc.state.md.us

Massachusetts

Caritas Labour, College
Dietetic Technician-AD Prgm
2120 Dorchester Ave
Boston, MA 02124-5698
www.laboure.edu

Michigan

Wayne County Community College District
Dietetic Technician-AD Prgm
Northwest Campus
8551 Greenfield Rd
Detroit, MI 48226
wcccd.edu

Minnesota

Normandale Community College
Dietetic Technician-AD Prgm
9700 France Ave S
Bloomington, MN 55431-4309
www.normandale.mnscu.edu

University of Minnesota - Crookston
Dietetic Technician-AD Prgm
Center for Health and Human Serv
2900 University Ave
Crookston, MN 56716-5001
www.crk.umn.edu

Missouri

St Louis Community College - Florissant Valley
Dietetic Technician-AD Prgm
3400 Pershall Rd
St Louis, MO 63135-1499
www.stlcc.edu

Nebraska

Southeast Community College
Dietetic Technician-AD Prgm
8800 O St
Lincoln, NE 68520-1227
www.southeast.edu

Nevada

Truckee Meadows Community College
Dietetic Technician-AD Prgm
7000 Dandini Blvd, RDMT 334J
Reno, NV 89512-3999
www.tmcc.edu

New Hampshire

University of New Hampshire
Dietetic Technician-AD Prgm
Thompson School of Applied Sci
6A Putnam Hall
Durham, NH 03824
www.unh.edu

New Jersey

Camden County College
Dietetic Technician-AD Prgm
PO Box 200
College Dr
Blackwood, NJ 08012-0200
www.camdencc.edu

Middlesex County College
Dietetic Technician-AD Prgm
2600 Woodbridge Ave, PO Box 3050
Edison, NJ 08818-3050
www.middlesex.cc.nj.us

New York

LaGuardia Community College
Dietetic Technician-AD Prgm
City University of New York
31-10 Thomson Ave, Rm E300
Long Island City, NY 11101-3071
www.lagcc.cuny.edu

SUNY at Morrisville
Dietetic Technician-AD Prgm
Bailey Annex
Morrisville, NY 13408

Suffolk County Community College - Eastern Campus
Dietetic Technician-AD Prgm
Eastern Campus
121 Speonk-Riverhead Rd
Riverhead, NY 11901-3499
www.sunysuffolk.edu

Westchester Community College
Dietetic Technician-AD Prgm
75 Grasslands Rd
Student Center Building, Rm 215
Valhalla, NY 10595-1698
www.sunywcc.edu

Erie Community College - North Campus
Dietetic Technician-AD Prgm
6205 Main St
Williamsville, NY 14221-7095
www.ecc.edu

North Carolina

Gaston College - Lincolnton
Dietetic Technician-AD Prgm
PO Box 600
Lincolnton, NC 28093
www.gaston.edu

Ohio

Cincinnati State Tech & Comm College
Dietetic Technician-AD Prgm
Health Technologies Div
3520 Central Pkwy
Cincinnati, OH 45223-2690
www.cincinnatistate.edu

Cuyahoga Community College
Dietetic Technician-AD Prgm
2900 Community College Ave
Cleveland, OH 44115-3196
www.tri-c.edu

Columbus State Community College
Dietetic Technician-AD Prgm
550 E Spring St, PO Box 1609
Columbus, OH 43216-1609
www.cscc.edu

Sinclair Community College
Dietetic Technician-AD Prgm
444 W Third St
Dayton, OH 45402-1460
www.sinclair.edu

Hocking College
Dietetic Technician-AD Prgm
3301 Hocking Pkwy
Nelsonville, OH 45764-9704
www.hocking.edu

Owens Community College
Dietetic Technician-AD Prgm
PO Box 10000
Oregon Rd
Toledo, OH 43699-1947
www.owens.edu

Youngstown State University
Dietetic Technician-AD Prgm
Dept of Human Ecology
One University Plaza
Youngstown, OH 44555-3344
www.ysu.edu

Pennsylvania

Comm College of Allegheny County
Dietetic Technician-AD Prgm
808 Ridge Ave
Pittsburgh, PA 15212-6097
www.ccac.edu

Penn State University
Dietetic Technician-AD Prgm
Coll of Health and Human Development
Hotel Rest & Recreation Mgmt
University Park, PA 16802-1307
www.worldcampus.psu.edu

Westmoreland County Community College
Dietetic Technician-AD Prgm
400 Armbrust Rd
Youngwood, PA 15697
www.wccc.edu

Tennessee

Southwest Tennessee Community College
Dietetic Technician-AD Prgm
PO Box 780
Union A-106
Memphis, TN 38101-0780
www.southwest.tn.edu

Texas

Tarrant County Jr College - South
Dietetic Technician-AD Prgm
2100 Southeast Pkwy
Arlington, TX 76018
www.tccd.edu/campus/default.asp?menu=3

San Jacinto College Central
Dietetic Technician-AD Prgm
8060 Spencer Hwy
PO Box 2007
Pasadena, TX 77505-2007
www.sjcd.edu

Washington

Shoreline Community College
Dietetic Technician-AD Prgm
16101 Greenwood Ave N, Rm 5334
Seattle, WA 98133-5696
www.shoreline.ctc.edu

Wisconsin

Madison Area Technical College
Dietetic Technician-AD Prgm
3550 Anderson St
Madison, WI 53704-2599
www.matcmadison.edu

Milwaukee Area Technical College
Dietetic Technician-AD Prgm
1200 S 71st St
West Allis, WI 53214-3110
www.matc.edu

Electroneurodiagnostic Technologist

Electroneurodiagnostics is the allied health care profession centered around recording, monitoring, and analyzing nervous system function to promote the effective treatment of pathologic conditions.

Electroneurodiagnostic or END professionals
- Are credentialed
- Have met a minimum education level and related educational and performance standards
- Meet continuing education requirements
- Perform within a code of ethics and defined scope of practice
- Are recognized by physicians, employers, the public, governmental agencies, payors and other health care professionals
- Form a national society whose activities include lobbying for the profession
- Contribute to the advancement of knowledge in neuroscience

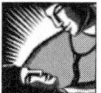

Career Description

Technologists record electrical activity arising from the brain, spinal cord, peripheral nerves, and somatosensory or motor nerve systems using a variety of techniques and instruments. Technologists prepare data and documentation for interpretation by a physician. Considerable individual initiative, reasoning skill, and sound judgment are all expected of the electroneurodiagnostic professional. The most common electroneurodiagnostic procedures include:
- Electroencephalogram (EEG)
- Intraoperative Neuromonitoring (IONM)
- Long Term Monitoring (LTM)
- Polysomnogram (PSG)
- Evoked Potential (EP)
- Nerve Conduction Studies (NCS)

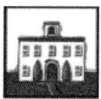

Employment Characteristics

END personnel work primarily in neurology-related departments of hospitals, but many also work in clinics and the private offices of neurologists and neurosurgeons. Growth in employment within the profession is expected to be greater than average, owing to the increased use of EEG and EP techniques in surgery; in diagnosing and monitoring patients with epilepsy; and in diagnosing sleep disorders. Technologists generally work a 40-hour week, but may work 12-hour days for sleep studies and be on-call for emergencies and intraoperative monitoring.

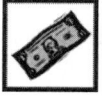

Salary

According to the American Society of Electroneurodiagnostic Technologists, Inc (ASET), 2006 entry-level salaries average $35,610. Refer to Section IV, Table 5 of this *Directory* for more information, or see www.ama-assn.org/go/hpsalary.

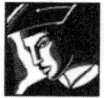

Educational Programs

Length. Programs may be 12 to 24 months and are typically integrated into a community college-sponsored program leading to an associate degree.

Prerequisites. High school diploma or equivalent.

Curriculum. The curriculum includes anatomy, physiology, and neuroanatomy (with major emphasis on the brain), as well as instrumentation, personal and patient safety, recording techniques, clinical electroneurodiagnostics, and correlations. Clinical rotations are conducted in medical centers.

Inquiries

Careers
American Society of Electroneurodiagnostic Technologists, Inc
6501 East Commerce Avenue
Suite 120
Kansas City, MO 64120
816 931-1120
816 931-1145 Fax
E-mail: info@aset.org
www.aset.org

Certification/Registration (Credentials R EEG T®, R EP T®, CNIM®)
American Board of Registration of Electroencephalographic and
    Evoked Potential Technologists (ABRET)
1904 Croydon Drive
Springfield, IL 62703
217 553-3758
217 585-6663 Fax
E-mail: abreteo@aol.com
www.abret.org

Certification/Registration (Credentials R NCS T)
American Association of Electrodiagnostic Technologists (AAET)
28 Sabins Lane
North Chatham, MA 02650
508 945-2781 Phone/Fax
E-mail: rta1@aol.com
www.aaet.info

Certification/Registration (Credentials RPSGT™)
The Board of Registered Polysomnographic Technologists (BRPT)
8201 Greensboro Drive, Suite 300
McLean, VA 22102
703 610-9020
703 610-9005 Fax
E-mail: info@brpt.org
www.brpt.org

Program Accreditation
Commission on Accreditation of Allied Health Education Programs
    (CAAHEP) in collaboration with:
Committee on Accreditation for Education in
    Electroneurodiagnostic Technology
6654 S Sycamore Street
Littleton, CO 80120
303 738-0770
303 738-3223 Fax
E-mail: office@coa-end.org
www.coa-end.org

Electroneurodiagnostic Technologist

California

Orange Coast College
Electroneurodiagnostic Tech Prgm
2701 Fairview Rd
PO Box 5005
Costa Mesa, CA 92626
www.orangecoastcollege.com
Prgm Dir: Walt Banoczi, R EEG/EP T CNIM RPSGT
Tel: 714 432-5591   *Fax:* 714 432-5534
E-mail: wbanoczi@cccd.edu

Florida

Erwin Technical Center
Electroneurodiagnostic Tech Prgm
2010 E Hillsborough Ave
Tampa, FL 33610
Prgm Dir: Henry Coet III, R EEG T
Tel: 813 231-1800, Ext 1341   *Fax:* 813 231-1820
E-mail: coet_h@firn.edu

Illinois

St John's Hospital
Cosponsor: Lincoln Land Community College
Electroneurodiagnostic Tech Prgm
School of ENDT
800 E Carpenter St
Springfield, IL 62769
Prgm Dir: Diane Liesen, R EEG T
Tel: 217 544-6464, Ext 44707   *Fax:* 217 535-3695
E-mail: diane.liesen@st-johns.org

Indiana

Clarian Health Partners Inc
Electroneurodiagnostic Tech Prgm
Clarian Health Partners, Wile Hall Rm 604
I-65 at 21st St
Indianapolis, IN 46206-1367
Prgm Dir: Debby Ferguson, MSEd REEG/EPT RPSGT
   RNCST
Tel: 317 962-1291   *Fax:* 317 963-5518
E-mail: dferguson@clarian.org

Iowa

Scott Community College
Electroneurodiagnostic Tech Prgm
500 Belmont Rd
Bettendorf, IA 52722
www.eicc.edu
Prgm Dir: Sherry Kelly, R EEG/EP T RPSGT
Tel: 563 441-4268   *Fax:* 563 441-4204
E-mail: skelly@eicc.edu

Kirkwood Community College
Cosponsor: Univ of Iowa Hosp and Clinics
Electroneurodiagnostic Tech Prgm
Dept of Neurology
6301 Kirkwood Blvd SW, PO Box 2068
Cedar Rapids, IA 52406-9973
Prgm Dir: Elizabeth Meng, R EEG/EPT
Tel: 319 356-8768   *Fax:* 319 351-1209
E-mail: elizabeth-meng@uiowa.edu

Massachusetts

Caritas Labour, College
Electroneurodiagnostic Tech Prgm
2120 Dorchester Ave
Boston, MA 02124
Prgm Dir: Jean Wilkins Farley, MA R EEG T
Tel: 617 296-8300, Ext 4043   *Fax:* 617 296-7947
E-mail: Jean.Farley@caritaschristi.org

Michigan

Carnegie Institute
Electroneurodiagnostic Tech Prgm
550 Stephenson Hwy, Stes 100-110
Troy, MI 48083
www.carnegie-institute.edu
Prgm Dir: Lisa Lovely, BA R EEG/EPT CNIMI
Tel: 248 589-1078   *Fax:* 248 589-1631
E-mail: lisalovely@umich.edu

Minnesota

Mayo School of Health Sciences
Electroneurodiagnostic Tech Prgm
Clinical Neurophysiology Technology Program
200 First St SW
Rochester, MN 55905
www.mayo.edu/mshs
Prgm Dir: Jan M Buss, R NCS T
Tel: 507 284-1255   *Fax:* 507 284-0656
E-mail: buss.jan@mayo.edu

North Carolina

Pamlico Community College
Electroneurodiagnostic Tech Prgm
PO Box 185
Grantsboro, NC 28529-0185
Prgm Dir: Mary Ellen Washington, MS REEG T REDT
Tel: 252 249-1851, Ext 3049   *Fax:* 252 249-2377
E-mail: Mwetherington@pamlicocc.edu

Pennsylvania

Crozer-Keystone Medical Center
Electroneurodiagnostic Tech Prgm
One Medical Ctr Blvd
Upland, PA 19013
Prgm Dir: Michele Carley, R EEG/EPT
Tel: 610 447-2691   *Fax:* 610 447-2696
E-mail: michele.carley@crozer.org

Texas

McLennan Community College
Electroneurodiagnostic Tech Prgm
1400 College Dr
Waco, TX 76708
www.mclennan.edu
Prgm Dir: Mary Feltman, BS REEGT
Tel: 254 299-8525   *Fax:* 254 299-8747
E-mail: mfeltman@mclennan.edu

Virginia

Naval School of Health Sciences
Electroneurodiagnostic Tech Prgm
1001 Holcomb Rd
Portsmouth, VA 23708-5200
Prgm Dir: Michael McNamara, R EEGT/ R EPT
Tel: 757 953-2144
E-mail: End@hsp.med.navy.mil

Wisconsin

Western Technical College
Electroneurodiagnostic Tech Prgm
304 N Sixth St, PO Box C-908
La Crosse, WI 54602-0908
www.westerntc.edu
Prgm Dir: Stacey Austin, R EEG/EP T RPSGT
Tel: 608 789-6141, Ext 96141   *Fax:* 608 785-9879
E-mail: austins@westerntc.edu

PROGRAMS

Electroneurodiagnostic Technologist

	Class Capacity	Begins	Length (months)	Award	Res. Tuition	Non-res. Tuition	Stipend	Offers:‡ 1	2	3	4
California											
Orange Coast College (Costa Mesa)	24	Aug (even years)	22	AS	$1,520	$15,500					
Indiana											
Clarian Health Partners Inc (Indianapolis)	6	Varies	18	Cert	$4,000	$4,000				•	
Iowa											
Scott Community College (Bettendorf)	15	Aug	22	AAS	$97	$145		•			
Michigan											
Carnegie Institute (Troy)	12	Sep	12	Dipl	$9,935	$9,935		•		•	
Minnesota											
Mayo School of Health Sciences (Rochester)	8	Aug	24	Cert, AAS	$5,880	$5,880					
North Carolina											
Pamlico Community College (Grantsboro)	30	Aug	24	Cert, AAS	$720	$5,868				•	•
Pennsylvania											
Crozer-Keystone Medical Center (Upland)	12	Sep	21	Cert	$4,500	$4,500				•	
Texas											
McLennan Community College (Waco)	20	Sep	12, 24	Cert, AA	$1,960	$2,380				•	
Wisconsin											
Western Technical College (La Crosse)	28	Jun	24	AAS	$2,311	$15,411					•

*Data are shown only for programs that completed the 2007 AMA Survey of Health Professions Education Programs.
‡Key to Offers: 1: Evening or weekend classes; 2: Non-English instruction; 3: Cultural competence instruction; 4: Distance education component.

Emergency Medical Technician-Paramedic

Emergency Medical Technicians (EMTs) and EMT-Paramedics are trained to provide emergency care to people who have suffered from an illness or an injury outside of the hospital setting. EMTs and Paramedics work under protocols approved by a physician medical director to recognize, assess, and manage medical emergencies and transport patients to definitive medical care. EMTs provide basic life support, and EMT-Paramedics provide advanced life support.

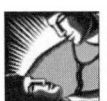
Career Description
EMTs and EMT-Paramedics may be employed by a private ambulance company, fire department, police department, public EMS agency, private ambulance company, hospital, or combination of the above. EMS responders may be paid or volunteers in the community.

EMTs must be proficient in First Aid, and training is centered on recognizing and treating life-threatening conditions outside the hospital environment. EMTs learn the basics of how to handle cardiac and respiratory arrest, heart attacks, seizures, diabetic emergencies, respiratory problems, and other medical emergencies. They also learn how to manage traumatic injuries such as falls, fractures, lacerations, and burns. EMTs also are introduced into patient assessment, history taking, and vital signs.

EMTs perform CPR, artificial ventilations, oxygen administration, basic airway management, defibrillation using an AED, spinal immobilization, vital signs, bandaging/splinting, and may administer Nitroglycerin, Glucose, Epinephrine, and Albuterol in special circumstances.

EMT-Paramedics perform all of the skills performed by an EMT-Basic. In addition, they perform advance airway management, such as endotracheal intubation, under medical supervision and from a base station, usually in a hospital emergency room. They obtain electrocardiographs (ECGs), introduce intravenous lines, and administer numerous emergency medications. EMT-Paramedics assess ECG tracings and defibrillate. They have extensive training in patient assessment and are exposed to a variety of clinical experiences during training.

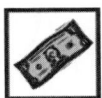
Salary
Earnings of EMTs and paramedics depend on the employment setting and geographic location as well as the individual's training and experience. Median annual earnings of EMTs and paramedics were $25,310 in May 2004. The middle 50 percent earned between $19,970 and $33,210. The lowest 10 percent earned less than $16,090, and the highest 10 percent earned more than $43,240. Median annual earnings in the industries employing the largest numbers of EMTs and paramedics in May 2004 were:

Local government	$27,710
General medical and surgical hospitals	$26,590
Other ambulatory health care services	$23,130

Those in emergency medical services who are part of fire or police departments receive the same benefits as firefighters or police officers. For example, many are covered by pension plans that provide retirement at half pay after 20 or 25 years of service or if the worker is disabled in the line of duty.

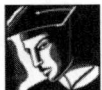
Educational Programs
In most locations in the United States, the minimum level of education that most EMS professionals have before entering the workforce is that of a Basic-Level EMT. Individuals who work as firefighters or police officers may perform some emergency medical work when trained as first responders. Some Paramedic programs provide an all-inclusive program that includes both EMT and Paramedic training in one program. All levels of EMS training are set by the federal government through the National Highway Traffic Safety Administration (NHTSA).

EMT training is offered at community colleges, technical schools, hospitals, and universities as well as EMS, fire, and police academies. Those interested in EMT training should contact their state's EMS Office. Those interested in Paramedic training should contact the Committee on Accreditation for EMS Professionals (CoAEMSP). Both of these agencies can help potential students find local training.

Length. EMT training varies from 2 to 6 months, depending on the training site and hours of class scheduled per week. There are training programs that have class every day for several months for those interested in quick completion. Longer programs are available to accommodate students who have family, a full-time job, or other responsibilities that limit their available time for education. Approximate training requirements are:

- First Responder   40 hours of training
- EMT-Basic   110 hours of training
- EMT-Intermediate   200-400 hours of training
- Paramedic   1,000 or more hours of training

Prerequisites. An EMT student is expected to be a high school graduate or the equivalent and to meet the physical and mental demands of the occupation. EMT-Paramedic students must have completed their EMT training prior to enrollment in most EMT-Paramedic courses unless they are enrolled in a joint EMT and Paramedic program. Some Paramedic programs are part of Associate of Applied Science (AAS) or Bachelor of Science (BS) degree programs offered at colleges and universities. Generally, a Certificate of Completion is offered for those who do not receive a college degree.

Curriculum. EMT and Paramedic training are composed of in-classroom, didactic instruction; in-hospital clinical practice; and a supervised field internship on an ambulance. Courses typically are competency-based and supported by performance assessments. Instruction provides students with knowledge of acute and critical changes in physiology and psychological and clinical symptoms that they might encounter in an emergency medical situation.

Inquiries
Careers
National Association of Emergency Medical Technicians (NAEMT)
PO Box 1400
Clinton, MS 39060-1400
800 34-NAEMT
www.naemt.org

Certification/Licensure
National Registry of Emergency Medical Technicians (NREMT)
Rocco V. Morando Bldg
Box 29233
6610 Busch Blvd
Columbus, OH 43229-0233
614 888-4484
www.nremt.org

Program Accreditation
Commission on Accreditation of Allied Health Education Programs
    (CAAHEP) in collaboration with:
Committee on Accreditation of Educational Programs for the EMS
    Professions (CoAEMSP)
1248 Harwood Road
Bedford, TX 76021-4244
817 283-9403
E-mail: george@coaemsp.org

Note: Adapted in part from the Bureau of Labor Statistics, US Department of Labor, *Occupational Outlook Handbook*, 2006-07 Edition, Emergency Medical Technicians and Paramedics, on the Internet at www.bls.gov/oco/ocos101.htm (visited November 6, 2007).

Emergency Medical Technician-Paramedic

Alabama

Lurleen B Wallace Junior College
Emergency Med Tech-Paramedic Prgm
PO Box 1418
Andalusia, AL 36420
Prgm Dir: Wayne Godwin
Tel: 334 881-2210   *Fax:* 334 881-2300
E-mail: wgodwin@lbwcc.edu

University of Alabama at Birmingham
Emergency Med Tech-Paramedic Prgm
Department of Emergency Medicine
912 18th St S
Birmingham, AL 35205
Prgm Dir: Randal E Gray, MA NREMT-P CCEMT-P
Tel: 205 934-3611   *Fax:* 205 975-7573
E-mail: rgray@uab.edu

Calhoun Community College
Emergency Med Tech-Paramedic Prgm
PO Box 2216 Hwy 31 N
Decatur, AL 35609
Prgm Dir: Jarrod Taylor, BS RN NREMT-P
Tel: 256 306-2781   *Fax:* 256 306-2909
E-mail: jwt@calhoun.edu

George C Wallace Community College
Emergency Med Tech-Paramedic Prgm
1141 Wallace Dr
Dothan, AL 36303
Prgm Dir: Rebecca Burke, BS Ed NREMT-P
Tel: 334 556-2442   *Fax:* 334 556-2405
E-mail: rburke@wallace.edu

Gadsden State Community College
Emergency Med Tech-Paramedic Prgm
PO Box 227
Gadsden, AL 35902-0227
Prgm Dir: Patrick T Brown, BS NREMT-P
Tel: 256 549-8654   *Fax:* 256 549-8276
E-mail: pbrown@gadsdenstate.edu

Wallace State Community College
Emergency Med Tech-Paramedic Prgm
301 Main St NW, PO Box 2000
Hanceville, AL 35077
Prgm Dir: Cindy Durham
Tel: 205 352-8335   *Fax:* 205 352-8337
E-mail: ems@wallacestate.edu

University of South Alabama
Emergency Med Tech-Paramedic Prgm
2002 Old Bay Front Dr
Mobile, AL 36615
www.usouthal.edu
Prgm Dir: David W Burns, MPH ScD(c) EMT-P
Tel: 251 431-6418   *Fax:* 251 431-6525
E-mail: dburns@usouthal.edu

H Council Trenholm State Technical College
Emergency Med Tech-Paramedic Prgm
1225 Air Base Blvd
Montgomery, AL 36108
Prgm Dir: Becky A Morris, BS NREMT-P
Tel: 334 420-4432   *Fax:* 334 420-4437
E-mail: bmorris@trenholmtech.cc.al.us

Northwest-Shoals Community College
Emergency Med Tech-Paramedic Prgm
PO Box 2545
Muscle Shoals, AL 35662
Prgm Dir: J Bret McGill, MS NREMT-P
Tel: 256 331-5435   *Fax:* 256 331-5371
E-mail: mcgillb@nwscc.edu

Southern Union State Community College
Emergency Med Tech-Paramedic Prgm
1701 Lafayette Pkwy
Opelika, AL 36801
www.suscc.edu
Prgm Dir: Steven Simpson, BSBA NREMT-P
Tel: 334 745-6437, Ext 5533   *Fax:* 334 741-9795
E-mail: ssimpson@suscc.edu

Northeast Alabama Community College
Emergency Med Tech-Paramedic Prgm
PO Box 159
Rainsville, AL 35986-0159
www.nacc.edu
Prgm Dir: Roger Wootten, BS NREMT-P
Tel: 256 228-6001, Ext 355   *Fax:* 256 228-3309
E-mail: woottenr@nacc.edu

Bevill State Community College
Emergency Med Tech-Paramedic Prgm
101 S State St
Sumiton, AL 35148
Prgm Dir: Scott Karr, MEd NREMT-P
Tel: 205 648-3271, Ext 5570   *Fax:* 205 384-4581
E-mail: skarr@mail.bscc.edu

Shelton State Community College
Cosponsor: Alabama Fire College
Emergency Med Tech-Paramedic Prgm
2501 Phoenix Dr
Tuscaloosa, AL 35405
Prgm Dir: Julie L Coffman, BS AD
Tel: 205 391-3743   *Fax:* 205 391-3771
E-mail: jcoffman@alabamafirecollege.org

Arkansas

Univ of Arkansas Comm Coll - Batesville
Emergency Med Tech-Paramedic Prgm
2005 White Dr, PO Box 3350
Batesville, AR 72501
Prgm Dir: Wesley Gay, NREMT-P
Tel: 870 612-2070
E-mail: wgay@uaccb.edu

NorthWest Arkansas Community College
Emergency Med Tech-Paramedic Prgm
1 College Dr
Bentonville, AR 72712
http://nwacc.edu
Prgm Dir: Jamin Snarr, NREMT-P bEd
Tel: 479 619-4251   *Fax:* 479 619-4254
E-mail: jsnarr@nwacc.edu

Arkansas Northeastern College
Emergency Med Tech-Paramedic Prgm
I-55 and Hwy 148
Burdette, AR 72321
Prgm Dir: Kathy Arnold, NREMT-P
Tel: 870 780-1221   *Fax:* 870 763-1496
E-mail: karnold@anc.edu

U of Arkansas-Monticello Coll of Tech-McGehee
Emergency Med Tech-Paramedic Prgm
700 W Gaines
PO Box 620
Dermott, AR 71638
Prgm Dir: Gursam Singh, BS NREMT-P
Tel: 870 538-0248, Ext 5504   *Fax:* 870 538-5666
E-mail: singh@seark.net

East Arkansas Community College
Emergency Med Tech-Paramedic Prgm
1700 Newcastle Rd
Forrest City, AR 72335
www.eacc.edu
Prgm Dir: Tami Jo Jones, BSEd NREMT-P
Tel: 870 633-4480, Ext 269   *Fax:* 870 633-7222
E-mail: tjjones@eacc.edu

North Arkansas College
Emergency Med Tech-Paramedic Prgm
1515 Pioneer Dr
Harrison, AR 72601
Prgm Dir: K C Jones, BSE NREMT-P
Tel: 870 391-3125   *Fax:* 870 391-3250
E-mail: kcjones@northark.edu

National Park Community College
Emergency Med Tech-Paramedic Prgm
101 College Dr
Hot Springs, AR 71913
www.npcc.edu
Prgm Dir: John Dodd, MS NREMT-P/I
Tel: 501 760-4158   *Fax:* 501 760-4141
E-mail: jdodd@npcc.edu

University of Arkansas for Medical Sciences
Emergency Med Tech-Paramedic Prgm
4301 W Markham St Slot 635
Little Rock, AR 72205
www.uams.edu
Prgm Dir: Danny Bercher, MEd
Tel: 501 686-5773   *Fax:* 501 686-6513
E-mail: dlbercher@uams.edu

Arkansas Tech University - Ozark Campus
Emergency Med Tech-Paramedic Prgm
PO Box 506
Ozark, AR 72956
Prgm Dir: Lisa Robles, NREMT-P
Tel: 479 667-2117, Ext 326   *Fax:* 479 667-2106
E-mail: lisa.robles@mail.atu.edu

Southeast Arkansas College
Emergency Med Tech-Paramedic Prgm
1900 Hazel St
Pine Bluff, AR 71603
Prgm Dir: Floyd Nutter, EMT-P AAS
Tel: 870 543-5917   *Fax:* 870 543-5912
E-mail: fnutter@seark.edu

Black River Technical College
Emergency Med Tech-Paramedic Prgm
PO Box 468
Pocahontas, AR 72455
www.blackrivertech.org
Prgm Dir: Kimeron J Hubbard, NREMT-P BS
Tel: 870 888-5750   *Fax:* 870 886-7481
E-mail: captdiver@earthlink.net

California

Bakersfield College
Emergency Med Tech-Paramedic Prgm
1801 Panorama Dr
Bakersfield, CA 93305
Prgm Dir: Myron Smith
Tel: 661 395-4284
E-mail: smithm@hallamb.com

Southwestern College
Emergency Med Tech-Paramedic Prgm
School of Technology and Human Services, Rm 570B
900 Otay Lakes Rd
Chula Vista, CA 91910
Prgm Dir: Joanne Stonecipher, RN MSN
Tel: 619 421-6700, Ext 5599   *Fax:* 619 216-6616
E-mail: jstonecipher@swc.cc.ca.us

Los Angeles County Paramedic Training Inst
Emergency Med Tech-Paramedic Prgm
5555 Ferguson Dr, Ste 220
Commerce, CA 90022
http://ladhs.org/ems/
Prgm Dir: Terry Crammer, RN BSN
Tel: 323 890-7506   *Fax:* 323 890-8528
E-mail: tcrammer@ladhs.org

Palomar Community College
Emergency Med Tech-Paramedic Prgm
1951 E Valley Pkwy
Escondido, CA 92056
Prgm Dir: Mary Reed
Tel: 760 744-1150, Ext 8150   *Fax:* 760 432-0353
E-mail: mreed@palomar.edu

North Coast Emergency Medical Services
Emergency Med Tech-Paramedic Prgm
3340 Glenwood St
Eureka, CA 95501
Prgm Dir: Douglas Boileau, MBA EMT-P
Tel: 707 445-2081
E-mail: amra@norcalsafety.com

California EMS Academy Inc
Emergency Med Tech-Paramedic Prgm
1098 Foster City Blvd, Ste 106 PMB 708
Foster City, CA 94404
Prgm Dir: Nancy L Black, RN MS
Tel: 866 577-9197   *Fax:* 650 701-1968
E-mail: Nancy@caems-academy.com

Fresno City College
Emergency Med Tech-Paramedic Prgm
1901 E Shields, Ste 250
Fresno, CA 93726
Prgm Dir: Mark Allen, EMT-P BA
Tel: 559 256-0188   *Fax:* 559 256-0199
E-mail: mark.allen@fresnocitycollege.edu

Fresno County Paramedic Program
Emergency Med Tech-Paramedic Prgm
1221 Fulton Mall
Fresno, CA 93721
Prgm Dir: Debra Becker, RN
Tel: 559 445-3387   *Fax:* 559 445-3205
E-mail: dbecker@co.fresno.ca.us

Imperial Valley Community College
Emergency Med Tech-Paramedic Prgm
380 E Aten Rd
Imperial, CA 92251
Prgm Dir: Jackilyn E Cypher, RN CEN MICN NREMT-P
Tel: 760 355-6275   *Fax:* 760 355-6346
E-mail: jcypher@imperial.cc.ca.us

UCLA Center for Prehospital Care
Emergency Med Tech-Paramedic Prgm
Daniel Freeman Memorial Hospital
333 N Prairie Ave
Inglewood, CA 90301
Prgm Dir: William Dunne, MS NREMT-P
Tel: 310 674-7050, Ext 3580   *Fax:* 310 680-8640
E-mail: wdunne@mednet.ucla.edu

California Paramedic Institute
Emergency Med Tech-Paramedic Prgm
23141 Lake Center Dr
Lake Forest, CA 92630
Prgm Dir: Robert Nieblas
E-mail: rnieblas@cpimedic.com

Antelope Valley College
Emergency Med Tech-Paramedic Prgm
44201 10th St W
Lancaster, CA 93534
Prgm Dir: Marco Johnson, BA EMT-P
Tel: 661 726-1911
E-mail: lhodge@avc.edu

Northern California Training Institute - Bay Area Counties
Emergency Med Tech-Paramedic Prgm
7503 Southfront Rd #A
Livermore, CA 94550
Prgm Dir: Kenneth Reed, BS EMT-P
Tel: 925 454-6184   *Fax:* 925 454-6297
E-mail: kenneth_reed@amr-ems.com

Saddleback College
Emergency Med Tech-Paramedic Prgm
28000 Marguerite Pkwy
Mission Viejo, CA 92692
Prgm Dir: Barbara Penland, RN MA
Tel: 949 582-4385
E-mail: bpenland@saddleback.edu

Butte College
Emergency Med Tech-Paramedic Prgm
3536 Butte Campus Dr
Oroville, CA 95965
Prgm Dir: Michael Boyd
Tel: 530 879-4310   *Fax:* 530 895-2472
E-mail: boydmi@butte.edu

Foothill Community College
Emergency Med Tech-Paramedic Prgm
4000 Middlefield Rd, Ste 1
Palo Alto, CA 94303
Prgm Dir: Mary Jane Arlene Green, NREMT-P AA
Tel: 650 949-6972   *Fax:* 650 949-6979
E-mail: greenmary@foothill.edu

Riverside Comm Coll - Moreno Valley Campus
Emergency Med Tech-Paramedic Prgm
Ben Clark Training Center
3423 Davis Ave
Riverside, CA 92518
www.rcc.edu/academicPrograms/ems/
Prgm Dir: Chris Nollette, EdD NREMTP LP
Tel: 951 571-6100, Ext 4609   *Fax:* 951 656-7520
E-mail: chris.nollette@rcc.edu

Northern California Training Institute - Placer County
Emergency Med Tech-Paramedic Prgm
333 Sunrise Ave, Ste 500
Roseville, CA 95661
Prgm Dir: Vickie Wolf, RN
Tel: 916 960-6284   *Fax:* 916 960-6296
E-mail: vwolf@amr-ems.com

American River College
Emergency Med Tech-Paramedic Prgm
4700 College Oak Dr
Sacramento, CA 95841-4217
www.arc.losrios.edu
Prgm Dir: Grant Goold, EdD
Tel: 916 484-8843
E-mail: GooldG@arc.losrios.edu

City College of San Francisco
Emergency Med Tech-Paramedic Prgm
John Adams Campus
1860 Hayes St
San Francisco, CA 94117
Prgm Dir: Megan Corry, MA EMTP
Tel: 415 561-1938   *Fax:* 415 561-1999
E-mail: mcorry@ccsf.edu

WestMed College
Emergency Med Tech-Paramedic Prgm
5300 Stevens Creek Blvd, Ste 200
San Jose, CA 95129
Prgm Dir: Jolyn Camacho
Tel: 408 977-0723   *Fax:* 408 977-1396
E-mail: vershep@aol.com

Hospital Consortium Education Network
Emergency Med Tech-Paramedic Prgm
222 W 39th Ave 3A09
San Mateo Medical Center
San Mateo, CA 94403
Prgm Dir: Art Hsieh
Tel: 650 573-3930
E-mail: ahsieh@hospitalconsort.org

Emergency Training Services Inc
Emergency Med Tech-Paramedic Prgm
3050 Paul Sweet Rd
Santa Cruz, CA 95065
Prgm Dir: Mary Foraker, BSN
Tel: 831 476-8813   *Fax:* 831 477-4914
E-mail: info@emergencytraining.com

Northern California Training Institute - Santa Barbara County
Emergency Med Tech-Paramedic Prgm
800 S College Ave
Santa Maria, CA 93454
Prgm Dir: Vicki Wolf, EMT-P
Tel: 805 688-6550
E-mail: vwolf@amr-ems.com

Emergency Medical Sciences Training Institute
Cosponsor: San Joaquin County EMS Agency
Emergency Med Tech-Paramedic Prgm
343 E Main St #906
Stockton, CA 95202
Prgm Dir: Craig Stroup, BS NREMT-P
Tel: 209 461-5550   *Fax:* 209 461-5553
E-mail: Emstiservices@aol.com

Mendocino Community College
Emergency Med Tech-Paramedic Prgm
1000 Hensley Creek Rd
Ukiah, CA 95482
Prgm Dir: Bill Webster, BS
Tel: 707 468-3005
E-mail: bwebster@mendocino.cc.ca.us

Ventura College
Emergency Med Tech-Paramedic Prgm
4667 Telegraph Rd
Ventura, CA 93003
Prgm Dir: Meredith H Mundell, BSN RN
Tel: 805 654-6364   *Fax:* 805 654-6328
E-mail: MMundell@vcccd.net

Victor Valley Community College District
Emergency Med Tech-Paramedic Prgm
18422 Bear Valley Rd
Victorville, CA 92395
www.vvc.edu
Prgm Dir: Scott C Jones, MBA EMT-P
Tel: 760 245-4271, Ext 2338   *Fax:* 760 951-5861
E-mail: joness@vvc.edu

Mt San Antonio College
Emergency Med Tech-Paramedic Prgm
1100 N Grand Ave
Walnut, CA 91789
Prgm Dir: Stephen A Williams, RN MEd NREMT
Tel: 909 594-5611, Ext 4750   *Fax:* 909 468-3938
E-mail: swilliam@mtsac.edu

Santa Rosa Junior College
Emergency Med Tech-Paramedic Prgm
5743 Skylane Blvd
Windsor, CA 95492
www.santarosa.edu/ps
Prgm Dir: Linda V Anderson, RN
Tel: 707 836-2919   *Fax:* 707 836-2948
E-mail: landerson@santarosa.edu

Crafton Hills College
Emergency Med Tech-Paramedic Prgm
11711 Sand Canyon Rd
Yucaipa, CA 92399
Prgm Dir: Kathy Crow, BVE NREMT-P
Tel: 909 389-3220   *Fax:* 909 389-3253
E-mail: kcrow@craftonhills.edu

Colorado

Pikes Peak Community College
Emergency Med Tech-Paramedic Prgm
5675 S Academy Blvd, CC-13
Colorado Springs, CO 80906
Prgm Dir: Jeff Force, EMT-P
Tel: 719 540-7697   *Fax:* 719 540-7699
E-mail: jeff.force@ppcc.edu

Centura Health-St Anthony Hospitals
Emergency Med Tech-Paramedic Prgm
4231 W 16th Ave, Ste 413
Denver, CO 80204
Prgm Dir: Scott Phillips, BS NREMT-P
Tel: 303 629-4478   *Fax:* 303 629-3622
E-mail: scottphillips@centura.org

Community College of Aurora
Emergency Med Tech-Paramedic Prgm
9235 E 10th Dr, Rm 154
Denver, CO 80230
www.ccaurora.edu/ems
Prgm Dir: Bob Matoba
Tel: 303 340-7212   *Fax:* 303 340-7209
E-mail: bob.matoba@ccaurora.edu

Denver Health Medical Center
Emergency Med Tech-Paramedic Prgm
190 W 6th Ave
Mail Code 3652
Denver, CO 80204
Prgm Dir: James Manson, NREMT-P
Tel: 303 436-5347   *Fax:* 303 436-8844
E-mail: jmanson@dhha.org

Colorado Mountain College
Emergency Med Tech-Paramedic Prgm
150 Miller Ranch Rd
Edwards, CO 81632
Prgm Dir: Michael Trujillo
Tel: 970 569-2922
E-mail: mtrujillo@coloradomtn.edu

HealthONE EMS
Cosponsor: Arapahoe Community College
Emergency Med Tech-Paramedic Prgm
333 W Hampden Ave #200
Englewood, CO 80110
www.healthoneems.com
Prgm Dir: Patricia Tritt, RN MA
Tel: 303 788-6236   *Fax:* 303 788-7656
E-mail: patricia.tritt@healthonecares.com

Pueblo Community College
Emergency Med Tech-Paramedic Prgm
900 W Orman Ave
Pueblo, CO 81004
Prgm Dir: Dawnelle Mathis, BS NREMT-P
Tel: 719 549-3489   *Fax:* 719 549-3147
E-mail: dawnelle.mathis@pueblocc.edu

Connecticut

Capital Community College
Emergency Med Tech-Paramedic Prgm
950 Main St
Hartford, CT 06103
Prgm Dir: Terry DeVito, RN MEd CEN EMT-P
Tel: 860 906-5153, Ext 1009   *Fax:* 860 906-5148
E-mail: tdevito@ccc.commnet.edu

Delaware

Delaware Technical & Community College - Dover
Emergency Med Tech-Paramedic Prgm
100 Campus Dr
ETB 706
Dover, DE 19904
Prgm Dir: Aaron Z Royston, MS NREMT-P
Tel: 302 857-1325   *Fax:* 302 857-1398
E-mail: aroyston@college.dtcc.edu

District of Columbia

George Washington University
Emergency Med Tech-Paramedic Prgm
900 23rd St NW
Washington, DC 20037
Prgm Dir: Keith Monosky, MPM EMT-P
Tel: 703 726-3739   *Fax:* 202 741-2946
E-mail: monosky@gwu.edu

Florida

Manatee Technical Institute
Emergency Med Tech-Paramedic Prgm
5603 34th St W
Bradenton, FL 34210
Prgm Dir: Jim Cena
Tel: 941 752-8100, Ext 228   *Fax:* 941 727-6254
E-mail: cenaj@fc.manatee.k12.fl.us

Brevard Community College
Emergency Med Tech-Paramedic Prgm
1519 Clearlake Rd
Cocoa, FL 32922
www.brevard.cc.fl.us
Prgm Dir: John C Smoot, BAAS NREMT-P
Tel: 321 632-1111, Ext 7710   *Fax:* 321 634-3731
E-mail: smootj@brevardcc.edu

Broward Community College
Emergency Med Tech-Paramedic Prgm
3501 SW Davie Rd
Davie, FL 33314
Prgm Dir: Elizabeth Jordan, MN NREMT-P
Tel: 954 201-6776   *Fax:* 954 201-6397
E-mail: ejordan@broward.edu

Daytona Beach Community College
Emergency Med Tech-Paramedic Prgm
PO Box 2811
Daytona Beach, FL 32120-2811
Prgm Dir: Martha Driscoll, AS NREMT-P
Tel: 386 255-3000, Ext 3249   *Fax:* 386 506-3222
E-mail: Driscom@dbcc.edu

Lake Technical Center
Emergency Med Tech-Paramedic Prgm
2001 Kurt St
Eustis, FL 32726
Prgm Dir: L Johnson
Tel: 352 589-2250, Ext 220   *Fax:* 352 357-4776
E-mail: johnsonl@lake.k12.fl.us

Edison College
Emergency Med Tech-Paramedic Prgm
8099 College Pkwy SW, PO Box 06210
Fort Myers, FL 33906-6210
Prgm Dir: Joe Crutcher
Tel: 239 985-8308   *Fax:* 239 489-9331
E-mail: jcrutcher@edison.edu

Indian River Community College
Emergency Med Tech-Paramedic Prgm
3209 Virginia Ave
Fort Pierce, FL 34981-5599
www.ircc.edu
Prgm Dir: Marjorie Bowers, EdD RN EMT-P
Tel: 772 462-7533   *Fax:* 772 462-7816
E-mail: mbowers@ircc.edu

Santa Fe Community College
Emergency Med Tech-Paramedic Prgm
3737 NE 39th Ave
Institute of Public Safety
Gainesville, FL 32609
Prgm Dir: Louis Mallory, MBA REMT-P
Tel: 352 334-0300   *Fax:* 352 334-0329
E-mail: louis.mallory@sfcc.edu

Florida Community College - Jacksonville
Emergency Med Tech-Paramedic Prgm
North Campus, 4501 Capper Rd
Jacksonville, FL 32218
Prgm Dir: Marjorie Fisher, MA EMT-P
Tel: 904 766-6513   *Fax:* 904 766-5573
E-mail: mfisher@fccj.edu

Lake City Community College
Emergency Med Tech-Paramedic Prgm
149 SE College Place
Lake City, FL 32025
Prgm Dir: Alan Espinosa, AS EMT-P
Tel: 386 754-4292   *Fax:* 386 754-4792
E-mail: espinosaa@lakecitycc.edu

Palm Beach Community College
Emergency Med Tech-Paramedic Prgm
4200 S Congress Ave, MS60
Lake Worth, FL 33461
Prgm Dir: Shari Turner, NREMT-P MEd
Tel: 561 868-3873   *Fax:* 561 868-3814
E-mail: turners@pbcc.edu

Miami Dade College
Emergency Med Tech-Paramedic Prgm
Medical Center Campus
950 NW 20th St
Miami, FL 33127
Prgm Dir: Michael A Yoder, RN EMT-P
Tel: 305 237-4337   *Fax:* 305 237-4278
E-mail: myoder@mdcc.edu

Pasco-Hernando Community College
Emergency Med Tech-Paramedic Prgm
10230 Ridge Rd
New Port Richey, FL 34654-5199
www.phcc.edu
Prgm Dir: Toni Vineyard, EMT-P
Tel: 727 816-3733   *Fax:* 727 816-3417
E-mail: vineyat@phcc.edu

Central Florida Community College
Emergency Med Tech-Paramedic Prgm
PO Box 1388
Ocala, FL 34478
Prgm Dir: Wayne Ramsey, REMT-P
Tel: 352 237-2111, Ext 1252
E-mail: ramseyw@cf.edu

Valencia Community College
Emergency Med Tech-Paramedic Prgm
PO Box 3028
Orlando, FL 32802-3028
Prgm Dir: Andrea Brody, BS RN NREMT-P
Tel: 407 299-5000, Ext 1595   *Fax:* 407 582-1278
E-mail: abrody@valenciacc.edu

Gulf Coast Community College
Emergency Med Tech-Paramedic Prgm
5230 W US Hwy 98
Panama City, FL 32401
Prgm Dir: Daniel Finley, PhD NREMT-P
Tel: 850 913-3315   *Fax:* 850 747-3246
E-mail: dfinley@gulfcoast.edu

Pensacola Junior College
Emergency Med Tech-Paramedic Prgm
Warrington Campus
5555 W Hwy 98
Pensacola, FL 32507-1097
Prgm Dir: Donald Lee, CP BS Management
Tel: 850 484-2225   *Fax:* 850 484-2364
E-mail: dlee@pjc.edu

Seminole Community College
Emergency Med Tech-Paramedic Prgm
100 Weldon Blvd
Sanford, FL 32773-6199
Prgm Dir: Robert D Holborn, MEd EMT-P
Tel: 407 328-2200   *Fax:* 407 328-2098
E-mail: holbornr@scc-fl.edu

Sarasota County Technical Institute
Emergency Med Tech-Paramedic Prgm
4748 Beneva Rd
Sarasota, FL 34233
Prgm Dir: Linda W Swisher, EdD RN
Tel: 941 924-1365, Ext 381   *Fax:* 941 361-6886
E-mail: linda_swisher@sarasota.k12.fl.us

St Petersburg College
Emergency Med Tech-Paramedic Prgm
Health Education Ctr
PO Box 13489
St Petersburg, FL 33733
Prgm Dir: Nerina Stepanovsky, MSN RN EMT-P
Tel: 727 341-3680   *Fax:* 727 341-3784
E-mail: stepanovskyn@spcollege.edu

Tallahassee Community College
Emergency Med Tech-Paramedic Prgm
444 Appleyard Dr
Tallahassee, FL 32304
www.tcc.fl.edu
Prgm Dir: Brian P Dunmyer, BA RP
Tel: 850 201-8328   *Fax:* 850 201-8329
E-mail: dunmyerb@tcc.fl.edu

Hillsborough Community College
Emergency Med Tech-Paramedic Prgm
PO Box 30030
Tampa, FL 33630
Prgm Dir: William D Corso, RN EMT-P MA
Tel: 813 253-7454   *Fax:* 813 253-7464
E-mail: bcorso@hccfl.edu

Polk Community College
Emergency Med Tech-Paramedic Prgm
999 Avenue H NE
Winter Haven, FL 33881-4299
Prgm Dir: Don Guillette, AS-EMS AS-Fire Science
    EMT-P RN
Tel: 863 669-2902   *Fax:* 863 297-1036
E-mail: dguillette@polk.edu

Georgia

Gwinnett Technical College
Emergency Med Tech-Paramedic Prgm
5150 Sugarloaf Pkwy
Lawrenceville, GA 30043-5702
Prgm Dir: Steven Moyers, NREMT-P MA
Tel: 678 226-6732   *Fax:* 770 685-1280
E-mail: smoyers@GwinnettTech.edu

Idaho

Idaho State University
Emergency Med Tech-Paramedic Prgm
College of Technology
Box 8380
Pocatello, ID 83209-8380
www.isu.edu
Prgm Dir: Jeff Bates, EMT-P
Tel: 208 373-1787   *Fax:* 208 373-1795
E-mail: batejef2@isu.edu

College of Southern Idaho
Emergency Med Tech-Paramedic Prgm
315 Falls Ave
Twin Falls, ID 83301
www.csi.edu/paramedic
Prgm Dir: Gordon Kokx, MS NREMT-P
Tel: 208 732-6710   *Fax:* 208 736-4743
E-mail: gkokx@csi.edu

Illinois

Loyola University Medical Center
Emergency Med Tech-Paramedic Prgm
2160 S First Ave
Bldg 110LL
Maywood, IL 60153
Prgm Dir: Lauri Beechler, RN BS
Tel: 708 327-2547   *Fax:* 708 327-2548
E-mail: lbeechler@lumc.edu

Trinity College of Nursing & Health Sciences
Emergency Med Tech-Paramedic Prgm
2122 25th Ave
Rock Island, IL 61201
www.trinitycollegeqc.edu
Prgm Dir: Karen Wilson, MSN RN
Tel: 309 779-7728   *Fax:* 309 779-7796
E-mail: wilsonk@trinityqc.com

Indiana

St Francis Hospital & Health Centers
Emergency Med Tech-Paramedic Prgm
1600 Albany St
Beech Grove, IN 46107
Prgm Dir: Brad Sparks, NREMT-P
Tel: 317 782-6480   *Fax:* 317 783-6481
E-mail: brad.sparks@ssfhs.org

Ivy Tech Community College - Columbus
Emergency Med Tech-Paramedic Prgm
4475 Central Ave
Columbus, IN 47203
Prgm Dir: Charles B Sims Jr
Tel: 812 372-9925, Ext 5221
E-mail: csims@ivytech.edu

Elkhart General Hospital
Emergency Med Tech-Paramedic Prgm
600 East Blvd
Elkhart, IN 46514
Prgm Dir: Anthony Hartman
Tel: 574 523-3127   *Fax:* 574 523-3458
E-mail: thartman@egh.org

Ivy Tech Community College - Evansville
Cosponsor: St Mary's Medical Center and Deaconess
    Hospital
Emergency Med Tech-Paramedic Prgm
3501 First Ave
Evansville, IN 47710
Prgm Dir: Timothy J Vollmer, BS BA MS-Ed
Tel: 812 429-9870   *Fax:* 812 429-1495
E-mail: tvollmer@ivytech.edu

Methodist Hospitals Inc
Emergency Med Tech-Paramedic Prgm
Midlake Campus
2269 W 2269th Ave
Gary, IN 46404
www.methodisthospitals.org
Prgm Dir: Joseph Paunicka, BS EMT-P
Tel: 219 944-4160   *Fax:* 219 944-4174
E-mail: jpaunicka@methodisthospitals.org

Clarian Health Partners Inc
Cosponsor: Methodist Hospital
Emergency Med Tech-Paramedic Prgm
Wile Hall Rm 631
1701 N Senate Blvd
Indianapolis, IN 46206
Prgm Dir: Lindi Holt, MS NREMT-P
Tel: 317 962-3327   *Fax:* 317 962-2102
E-mail: lholt@clarian.org

Ivy Tech Community College - Kokomo
Emergency Med Tech-Paramedic Prgm
700 E Firmin St
PO Box 1373
Kokomo, IN 46903-1373
Prgm Dir: Donnie Woodyard, BA NREM-P PL
Tel: 765 457-0858, Ext 121
E-mail: dwoodyard@ivytech.edu

Iowa

Kirkwood Community College
Emergency Med Tech-Paramedic Prgm
6301 Kirkwood Blvd SW
Cedar Rapids, IA 52406
Prgm Dir: Cathy Ross-Garron, BSN NREMT-P
Tel: 319 398-5672
E-mail: cgarron@kirwood.edu

Mercy Medical Center
Emergency Med Tech-Paramedic Prgm
207 Crocker, Ste 100
Des Moines, IA 50309
Prgm Dir: Fritz Nordengern
Tel: 515 643-7499   *Fax:* 515 643-7492
E-mail: ems@mercydesmoines.org

University of Iowa Hospitals & Clinics
Emergency Med Tech-Paramedic Prgm
200 Hawkins Dr, S608-1 GH
Iowa City, IA 52242
Prgm Dir: Douglas K York, REMT-P
Tel: 319 356-2597   *Fax:* 319 353-7508
E-mail: douglas-york@uiowa.edu

Kansas

Coffeyville Community College
Emergency Med Tech-Paramedic Prgm
400 W 11th St
Coffeyville, KS 67337
Prgm Dir: Kacia Adams, MICT I/C AS
Tel: 620 251-7700, Ext 2174   *Fax:* 620 252-7059
E-mail: kacia@coffeyville.edu

Flint Hills Technical College
Emergency Med Tech-Paramedic Prgm
3301 W 18th St
Emporia, KS 66801
Prgm Dir: Carman Allen, MICT I/C BA
Tel: 620 343-4600, Ext 265   *Fax:* 620 343-4610
E-mail: callen@fhtc.net

Garden City Community College
Emergency Med Tech-Paramedic Prgm
801 Campus Dr
Penka Bldg
Garden City, KS 67846
Prgm Dir: Lenora Cook
Tel: 316 276-9560   *Fax:* 316 276-9569
E-mail: lenora.cook@gcccks.edu

Barton County Community College
Emergency Med Tech-Paramedic Prgm
245 NE 30th Rd
Great Bend, KS 67530
Prgm Dir: Chy Miller
Tel: 620 792-9347
E-mail: millerc@bartonccc.edu

Kansas City Kansas Community College
Emergency Med Tech-Paramedic Prgm
7250 State Ave
Kansas City, KS 66112
Prgm Dir: Donna Olafson
Tel: 913 288-7179   *Fax:* 913 288-7677
E-mail: dolafson@toto.net

Johnson County Community College
Emergency Med Tech-Paramedic Prgm
12345 College Blvd
Overland Park, KS 66210-1299
Prgm Dir: Ray Wright, MICT
Tel: 913 469-8500, Ext 3175   *Fax:* 913 469-2315
E-mail: rwright@jccc.net

Cowley County Community College
Emergency Med Tech-Paramedic Prgm
1406 E 8th St
Winfield, KS 67156
www.cowley.edu/departments/allied/ems/
Prgm Dir: Slade Griffiths, MEd MICT IC
Tel: 620 441-6584   *Fax:* 620 441-6589
E-mail: griffiths@cowley.edu

Kentucky

Eastern Kentucky University
Emergency Med Tech-Paramedic Prgm
Dizney 225
Richmond, KY 40475-3135
www.emc.eku.edu
Prgm Dir: Nancye Davis, RN MSN
Tel: 859 622-1028   *Fax:* 859 622-6333
E-mail: nancye.davis@eku.edu

Louisiana

Bossier Parish Community College
Emergency Med Tech-Paramedic Prgm
6220 E Texas St
Bossier City, LA 71111
Prgm Dir: Austin Beard, BS EMT-P
Tel: 318 678-6135   *Fax:* 318 678-6199
E-mail: abeard@bpcc.edu

Delgado Community College
Emergency Med Tech-Paramedic Prgm
615 City Park Ave
New Orleans, LA 70119
Prgm Dir: Eric Randall, RN BS EMT
Tel: 504 483-4646   *Fax:* 504 485-2361
E-mail: eranda@dcc.edu

Maryland

Anne Arundel Community College
Emergency Med Tech-Paramedic Prgm
101 College Pkwy
101 College Pkwy
Arnold, MD 21012-1895
http://myaacc.edu
Prgm Dir: Sally Gresty, MS RN NREMT-P
Tel: 410 777-7084   *Fax:* 410 777-7099
E-mail: sjgresty@aacc.edu

Community College of Baltimore County - Essex Campus
Emergency Med Tech-Paramedic Prgm
7201 Rossville Blvd
Baltimore, MD 21237
Prgm Dir: Robert M Henderson, Jr, BS NREMT-P
Tel: 410 780-6477   *Fax:* 410 780-6405
E-mail: rhenderson@ccbcmd.edu

University of Maryland Baltimore County
Emergency Med Tech-Paramedic Prgm
Dept of Emergency Health Services
1000 Hilltop Circle
Baltimore, MD 21250
www.umbc.edu/ehs
Prgm Dir: Dwight A Polk, MSW NREMT-P
Tel: 410 455-3782   *Fax:* 410 455-3045
E-mail: polk@umbc.edu

Howard Community College
Emergency Med Tech-Paramedic Prgm
10901 Little Patuxent Parkway
Columbia, MD 21044
Prgm Dir: Angel Clark Burba, MS EMT-P
Tel: 410 772-4948   *Fax:* 410 772-4494
E-mail: aburba@howardcc.edu

Associates in Emergency Care
Emergency Med Tech-Paramedic Prgm
PO Box 490
Damascus, MD 20872
Prgm Dir: Sal E Marini, NREMT-P MA
Tel: 301 865-8880   *Fax:* 301 865-8881
E-mail: aecare911@aol.com

Michigan

Huron Valley Ambulance
Emergency Med Tech-Paramedic Prgm
1200 State Circle
Ann Arbor, MI 48108
Prgm Dir: Shaun Pochik, BS EMT-P
Tel: 734 477-6731   *Fax:* 734 477-6927
E-mail: spochik@hva.org

Lansing Community College
Emergency Med Tech-Paramedic Prgm
3100-HHPS Division
500 N Washington, PO Box 40010
Lansing, MI 48901-7210
Prgm Dir: Tim Cooper, EMT-P I/C AAS
Tel: 517 483-1410   *Fax:* 517 483-1508
E-mail: tcooper@lcc.edu

Minnesota

Northland Community & Technical College
Emergency Med Tech-Paramedic Prgm
2022 Central Ave NE
East Grand Forks, MN 56721
Prgm Dir: Dan Sponsler, BS NREMT-P
Tel: 218 773-4634   *Fax:* 218 773-4502
E-mail: dan.sponsler@northlandcollege.edu

Greater Minnesota Paramedic Consortium
Emergency Med Tech-Paramedic Prgm
PO Box 1014
214 E Junius Ave
Fergus Falls, MN 56537
www.ringdahlems.com
Prgm Dir: Dennis A Ehrichs, NREMT-P
Tel: 218 998-2739   *Fax:* 218 998-3299
E-mail: eta@eot.com

Inver Hills Community College
Emergency Med Tech-Paramedic Prgm
2500 E 80th St
Inver Grove Heights, MN 55076-3224
Prgm Dir: Marti Breiter
Tel: 651 450-8675   *Fax:* 651 450-8579
E-mail: mbreite@inverhills.edu

South Central College
Emergency Med Tech-Paramedic Prgm
1920 Lee Blvd
North Mankato, MN 56003
http://southcentral.edu
Prgm Dir: Laurie Oelslager, EdD NREMT-P
Tel: 507 389-7306   *Fax:* 507 388-9951
E-mail: laurie.oelslager@southcentral.edu

Rochester Community & Technical College
Emergency Med Tech-Paramedic Prgm
851 30th Ave SE
Rochester, MN 55904
Prgm Dir: Richard Peterson
Tel: 800 247-1296
E-mail: richard.peterson@roch.edu

St Cloud Technical College
Emergency Med Tech-Paramedic Prgm
1540 Northway Dr
St Cloud, MN 56303
Prgm Dir: Larry R Starks
Tel: 320 308-5405   *Fax:* 320 255-2595
E-mail: lstarks@sctc.edu

Century College
Emergency Med Tech-Paramedic Prgm
3300 Century Ave N
White Bear Lake, MN 55110
Prgm Dir: Denise Howard
Tel: 651 779-5794   *Fax:* 651 779-5797
E-mail: l.goerisch@century.mnscu.edu

Mississippi

East Central Community College
Emergency Med Tech-Paramedic Prgm
PO Box 129
Decatur, MS 39327
Prgm Dir: S Bush
Tel: 601 635-2111, Ext 214   *Fax:* 601 635-4031
E-mail: sbush@eccc.edu

Jones County Junior College
Emergency Med Tech-Paramedic Prgm
900 S Court St
Ellisville, MS 39437
www.jcjc.edu
Prgm Dir: Gregory M Cole, BS NREMT-P CCEMT-P FP-C
Tel: 601 477-4074   *Fax:* 601 477-4152
E-mail: mike.cole@jcjc.edu

Itawamba Community College
Emergency Med Tech-Paramedic Prgm
602 W Hill St
Fulton, MS 38843
Prgm Dir: Deborah Roebuck, RN REMT-P
Tel: 601 620-5270   *Fax:* 601 862-8150
E-mail: dmroebuck@iccms.edu

Mississippi Gulf Coast Community College
Emergency Med Tech-Paramedic Prgm
2226 Switzer Rd
Gulfport, MS 39507
Prgm Dir: Gary Shirley, REMT-P BS ThM
Tel: 228 896-2554   *Fax:* 228 897-3918
E-mail: gary.shirley@mgccc.edu

University of Mississippi Medical Center
Emergency Med Tech-Paramedic Prgm
2500 N State St
Jackson, MS 39216
www.shrp.umc.edu
Prgm Dir: Clyde Deschamp, PhD NREMT-P
Tel: 601 984-5585   *Fax:* 601 815-1715
E-mail: cdeschamp@shrp.umsmed.edu

Holmes Community College
Emergency Med Tech-Paramedic Prgm
412 W Ridgeland Ave
Ridgeland, MS 39157
Prgm Dir: Blaine Riggleman, BA BS MPA
Tel: 601 856-5400   *Fax:* 601 605-3410
E-mail: briggleman@holmescc.edu

Northwest Mississippi Community College
Emergency Med Tech-Paramedic Prgm
4975 Hwy 51 N
Drawer 7020
Senatobia, MS 38668
www.northwestms.edu
Prgm Dir: Brenda Hood, RN BSN NREMT
Tel: 662 562-3986   *Fax:* 662 560-1107
E-mail: bjhood@northwestms.edu

Missouri

IHM Health Studies Center
Emergency Med Tech-Paramedic Prgm
2500 Abbott Pl
St Louis, MO 63143
Prgm Dir: John F Elder, NREMT-P
Tel: 314 768-1234, Ext 1128   *Fax:* 314 768-1595
E-mail: ihm@abbottems.org

Montana

Montana State University - Billings
Emergency Med Tech-Paramedic Prgm
3803 Central Ave
Billings, MT 59102
Prgm Dir: David J Gurchiek, MS NREMT-P
Tel: 406 247-3076   *Fax:* 406 652-1729
E-mail: dgurchiek@msubillings.edu

Nebraska

Creighton University
Emergency Med Tech-Paramedic Prgm
2514 Cuming St
Omaha, NE 68131
http://ems.creighton.edu
Prgm Dir: William Raynovich, NREMT-P EdD
Tel: 402 280-1280   *Fax:* 402 280-1288
E-mail: billr@creighton.edu

Nevada

College of Southern Nevada
Emergency Med Tech-Paramedic Prgm
6375 W Charleston Blvd
Las Vegas, NV 89146
Prgm Dir: Rod Hackwith, BS NREMT-P
Tel: 702 651-7385   *Fax:* 702 651-5077
E-mail: rod.hackwith@csn.edu

New Hampshire

New Hampshire Technical Institute
Emergency Med Tech-Paramedic Prgm
31 College Dr
Concord, NH 03001-7412
www.nhti.edu
Prgm Dir: Nancy L Brubaker, MEd EMT-P RN
Tel: 603 271-7157   *Fax:* 603 271-7148
E-mail: nbrubaker@ccsnh.edu

New England EMS Institute
Emergency Med Tech-Paramedic Prgm
One Elliot Way
Manchester, NH 03103
Prgm Dir: William Thorpe, Jr, BS NREMT-P I/C
Tel: 603 663-2641   *Fax:* 603 663-2110
E-mail: thorpe@elliot-hs.org

New Mexico

University of New Mexico
Emergency Med Tech-Paramedic Prgm
School of Medicine
2700 Yale Blvd SE
Albuquerque, NM 87106
Prgm Dir: Larry A Cobb, RN CEN EMT-P
Tel: 505 272-5757   *Fax:* 505 244-1505
E-mail: larryc@unm.edu

Dona Ana Community College
Emergency Med Tech-Paramedic Prgm
Box 30001, Dept 3DA
Las Cruces, NM 88003
Prgm Dir: Joyce S Bradley, NREMT-P AAS BHCS
Tel: 505 527-7645   *Fax:* 505 527-7765
E-mail: jobradle@nmsu.edu

Eastern New Mexico University - Roswell
Emergency Med Tech-Paramedic Prgm
PO Box 6000
52 University Blvd
Roswell, NM 88202-6000
Prgm Dir: Mike Buldra, MEd NREMT-P
Tel: 505 624-7239   *Fax:* 505 624-7100
E-mail: mike.buldra@roswell.enmu.edu

New York

New York Methodist Hospital
Emergency Med Tech-Paramedic Prgm
2009 85th St
Brooklyn, NY 11214
Prgm Dir: Jerry Rozenberg, PA-C EMT-P
Tel: 718 333-2273   *Fax:* 718 654-2092
E-mail: ecpmedic@aol.com

Bassett Healthcare Center for Rural EMS Educ
Cosponsor: State University of New York
Emergency Med Tech-Paramedic Prgm
College of Agriculture and Technology
State Rte 7
Cobleskill, NY 12043
www.CREMSE.org
Prgm Dir: Richard Beebe, MEd RN EMTP
Tel: 518 255-5367
E-mail: BeebeRW@Cobleskill.edu

CUNY Borough of Manhattan Community Coll
Emergency Med Tech-Paramedic Prgm
199 Chambers St
Dept of Allied Hlth Sciences
New York, NY 10007
Prgm Dir: Everett W Flannery, MPS RRT
Tel: 212 346-8731   *Fax:* 212 346-8738
E-mail: eflannery@bmcc.cuny.edu

Monroe Community College
Emergency Med Tech-Paramedic Prgm
1190 Scottsville Rd, Ste 216
Rochester, NY 14624
www.mccparamedic.com
Prgm Dir: Peter Bonadonna, EMT-P NYS
Tel: 585 753-3713   *Fax:* 585 753-3850
E-mail: pbonadonna@monroecc.edu

SUNY Ulster
Emergency Med Tech-Paramedic Prgm
Cottekill Rd
Stone Ridge, NY 12484
Prgm Dir: Douglas Sandbrook
Tel: 845 687-5276   *Fax:* 845 687-5133
E-mail: sandbrod@sunyulster.edu

SUNY Upstate Medical University
Emergency Med Tech-Paramedic Prgm
750 E Adams St
Syracuse, NY 13210
Prgm Dir: Gail J Weinstein
Tel: 315 464-4858   *Fax:* 315 464-4854
E-mail: weinsteg@upstate.edu

Hudson Valley Community College
Emergency Med Tech-Paramedic Prgm
80 Vandenburgh Ave
Troy, NY 12180
Prgm Dir: Gregory Chapman, RRT REMT-P
Tel: 518 629-4899   *Fax:* 518 629-4881
E-mail: chapmgre@hvcc.edu

Dutchess Community College
Emergency Med Tech-Paramedic Prgm
31 Marshall Rd
Wappingers Falls, NY 12590
Prgm Dir: Michele Lieberman
Tel: 845 298-0717
E-mail: lieberman@sunydutchess.edu

North Carolina

Western Carolina University
Emergency Med Tech-Paramedic Prgm
122 Moore
Cullowhee, NC 28723
Prgm Dir: Michael W Hubble, PhD
Tel: 828 227-7113, Ext 3516   *Fax:* 828 227-7446
E-mail: mhubble@email.wcu.edu

Joint Special Operations Medical Training Ctr
Emergency Med Tech-Paramedic Prgm
Uniformed Services University of the Health Sciences
Fort Bragg, NC 28310
Prgm Dir: Gerald Depold, PA
Tel: 910 396-0089, Ext 236   *Fax:* 910 396-5395
E-mail: depoldg@soc.mil

Catawba Valley Community College
Emergency Med Tech-Paramedic Prgm
2550 Hwy 70 SE
Hickory, NC 28602-9699
www.cvcc.edu
Prgm Dir: Martha McCrea, RN PA BSN EMT-P
Tel: 828 327-7000, Ext 4347   *Fax:* 828 327-7276
E-mail: mmccrea@cvcc.edu

North Dakota

University of Mary/St Alexius Medical Ctr
Emergency Med Tech-Paramedic Prgm
PO Box 5510
Bismarck, ND 58506-5510
Prgm Dir: Mark Haugen, NREMT-P EMS
Tel: 701 530-7700   *Fax:* 701 530-7701
E-mail: mhaugen@primecare.org

Ohio

Akron General Medical Center
Emergency Med Tech-Paramedic Prgm
400 Wabash Ave
Akron, OH 44307
Prgm Dir: Scott W Martin, MEd NREMT-P
Tel: 330 344-6655   *Fax:* 330 253-8293
E-mail: smartin@agmc.org

Summa Health System
Emergency Med Tech-Paramedic Prgm
444 N Main St
Akron, OH 44310
Prgm Dir: Brian Tritchler, RN BSN EMT-P
Tel: 330 379-5966   *Fax:* 330 379-9543
E-mail: tritchlb@summa-health.org

University of Cincinnati
Emergency Med Tech-Paramedic Prgm
9555 Plainfield Rd
Cincinnati, OH 45236-0086
Prgm Dir: Alan F Mistler, MEd RN REMT-P
Tel: 513 936-7131   *Fax:* 513 745-0363
E-mail: alan.mistler@uc.edu

Columbus State Community College
Emergency Med Tech-Paramedic Prgm
550 E Spring St
Columbus, OH 43215
Prgm Dir: Carolyn Steffl, EMT-P AS
Tel: 614 227-2510   *Fax:* 614 287-5490
E-mail: csteffl@cscc.edu

Parma Community General Hospital
Emergency Med Tech-Paramedic Prgm
7300 State Rd
Parma, OH 44134
www.parmahospital.org
Prgm Dir: Joseph W Toth, REMT-P
Tel: 440 743-4970   *Fax:* 440 743-4966
E-mail: jtoth@parmahospital.org

Youngstown State University
Emergency Med Tech-Paramedic Prgm
Department of Health Professions
One University Plaza
Youngstown, OH 44555-3327
Prgm Dir: Randall W Benner, MEd NREMT-P
Tel: 330 941-3327   *Fax:* 330 941-2921
E-mail: rwbenner@cc.ysu.edu

Oklahoma

Oklahoma City Community College
Emergency Med Tech-Paramedic Prgm
7777 S May Ave
Oklahoma City, OK 73159
Prgm Dir: Romeo L Opichka, BBA REMT-P
Tel: 405 682-1611, Ext 7343   *Fax:* 405 682-7826
E-mail: ropichka@okccc.edu

Oregon

College of Emergency Services (CESWA)
Emergency Med Tech-Paramedic Prgm
9735 SW Sunshine Ct, Ste 1000
Beaverton, OR 97005
Prgm Dir: Carl T Miller, MS EMT-P
Tel: 503 644-9999   *Fax:* 503 644-1672
E-mail: ces@ces-ems.org

Chemeketa Community College
Emergency Med Tech-Paramedic Prgm
4000 Lancaster Dr NE
PO Box 14007
Salem, OR 97309-7070
www.chemeketa.edu/programs/ems
Prgm Dir: Gregg W Lander, BS NREMT-P
Tel: 503 399-2664   *Fax:* 503 588-6438
E-mail: greggl@chemeketa.edu

Oregon Health & Science University
Cosponsor: Oregon Institute of Technology
Emergency Med Tech-Paramedic Prgm
Paramedic Education Program
12400 SW Tonquin Rd
Sherwood, OR 97140
www.oit.edu/paramedic
Prgm Dir: Suzann Schmele, BA NREMT-P
Tel: 503 625-4721   *Fax:* 503 625-2497
E-mail: schmelse@tvfr.com

Pennsylvania

Lehigh Valley Hospital
Emergency Med Tech-Paramedic Prgm
2166 S 12th, Ground Floor
Allentown, PA 18103
www.emi-lvh.com or www.lccc.edu
Prgm Dir: Marianne Kostenbader
Tel: 610 969-0258
E-mail: marianne.kostenbader@lvh.com

Harrisburg Area Community College
Emergency Med Tech-Paramedic Prgm
One HACC Dr
Harrisburg, PA 17110-2999
Prgm Dir: Craig Davis, MEd EMT-P
Tel: 717 780-2564   *Fax:* 717 780-2551
E-mail: cadavis@hacc.edu

Ctr for Emer Med of Western Pennsylvania
Emergency Med Tech-Paramedic Prgm
230 McKee Pl
Ste 500
Pittsburgh, PA 15213
Prgm Dir: Thomas E Platt, MEd NREMT-P
Tel: 412 647-4665   *Fax:* 412 647-4670
E-mail: plattt@pitt.edu

Pennsylvania College of Technology
Emergency Med Tech-Paramedic Prgm
One College Ave
Williamsport, PA 17701
www.pct.edu/schools/hs/paramedic
Prgm Dir: Mark A Trueman, BS NREMT-P
Tel: 570 329-4931   *Fax:* 570 320-4432
E-mail: mtrueman@pct.edu

South Carolina

Trident Technical College
Emergency Med Tech-Paramedic Prgm
7000 Rivers Ave
PO Box 118067
Charleston, SC 29423-8067
Prgm Dir: Edward Lee, BA AAS NREMT-P CCEMT-P
Tel: 843 722-5533
E-mail: edward.lee@tridentech.edu

Greenville Technical College
Emergency Med Tech-Paramedic Prgm
506 S Pleasantburg Dr, 106D #702
Greenville, SC 29607
www.gvltec.edu/academics/health_nursing/emergency_
medical_technolo_degr.html
Prgm Dir: Michael Fisher, NREMT-P CCEMT-P AHS
Tel: 864 250-8490   *Fax:* 864 250-8218
E-mail: Mike.Fisher@gvltec.edu

South Dakota

Avera McKennan Hospital
Emergency Med Tech-Paramedic Prgm
800 E 21st St
Sioux Falls, SD 57117
www.sdparamedics.org
Prgm Dir: Don Jones, BS NREMT-P
Tel: 605 322-2086   *Fax:* 605 322-2090
E-mail: don.jones@mckennan.org

Tennessee

Northeast State Technical Comm College
Emergency Med Tech-Paramedic Prgm
PO Box 246
Blountville, TN 37617-0246
Prgm Dir: Darren K Ellenburg, BS EMT-P
Tel: 423 323-0238   *Fax:* 423 323-0213
E-mail: dkellenburg@NorteastState.edu

Chattanooga State Technical Comm College
Emergency Med Tech-Paramedic Prgm
4501 Amnicola Hwy
Chattanooga, TN 37406
Prgm Dir: Curtis Aukerman, MAEd NREMT-P
Tel: 423 697-3332   *Fax:* 423 697-3324
E-mail: curtis.aukerman@chattanoogastate.edu

Columbia State Community College
Emergency Med Tech-Paramedic Prgm
PO Box 1315
Columbia, TN 38402
Prgm Dir: Richard Beck, BS EMT-P
Tel: 931 540-2792
E-mail: rbeck4@columbiastate.edu

Volunteer State Community College
Emergency Med Tech-Paramedic Prgm
1480 Nashville Pike
Gallatin, TN 37066
Prgm Dir: Richard A Collier, BSN CEN EMT-P
Tel: 615 230-3346   *Fax:* 615 230-3344
E-mail: ric.collier@volstate.edu

Jackson State Community College
Emergency Med Tech-Paramedic Prgm
2046 N Parkway St
Jackson, TN 38301-3797
Prgm Dir: Thomas H Coley, BEd EMT-P
Tel: 901 424-3520, Ext 296   *Fax:* 901 425-9551
E-mail: tcoley@jscc.edu

Roane State Community College
Emergency Med Tech-Paramedic Prgm
132 Hayfield Rd
Knoxville, TN 37922-2301
Prgm Dir: Danny Sheckles, MS NREMT-P
Tel: 423 539-6905   *Fax:* 423 539-6907
E-mail: shecklesdm@roanestate.edu

Southwest Tennessee Community College
Emergency Med Tech-Paramedic Prgm
PO Box 780
Memphis, TN 38101
Prgm Dir: Glenn Faught, MS EMT-P
Tel: 901 333-5414, Ext 5414   *Fax:* 901 333-5431
E-mail: gfaught@southwest.tn.edu

Walters State Community College
Emergency Med Tech-Paramedic Prgm
500 S Davy Crockett Pkwy
Morristown, TN 37813-6899
Prgm Dir: Tim Strange, BS EMT-P I/C
Tel: 423 585-2672   *Fax:* 423 318-2738
E-mail: tim.strange@ws.edu

Texas

Austin Community College
Emergency Med Tech-Paramedic Prgm
3401 Webberville Rd
Austin, TX 78702
Prgm Dir: Kyle Pierce, LP BA
Tel: 512 223-5918   *Fax:* 512 223-5898
E-mail: kpierce@austincc.edu

Univ of Texas Southwestern Med Ctr
Cosponsor: El Centro College
Emergency Med Tech-Paramedic Prgm
5323 Harry Hines Blvd
Dallas, TX 75390-9134
Prgm Dir: Debra Cason, RN MS EMT-P
Tel: 214 648-5246   *Fax:* 214 648-5245
E-mail: debra.cason@UTSouthwestern.edu

Galveston College
Emergency Med Tech-Paramedic Prgm
4015 Ave Q
Galveston, TX 77550
Prgm Dir: Rory Prue, BS NREMT-P LP
Tel: 409 944-4242, Ext 494   *Fax:* 409 944-1511
E-mail: rprue@gc.edu

Houston Community College
Emergency Med Tech-Paramedic Prgm
1900 Galen Dr, MC 1637/H232
Houston, TX 77030
Prgm Dir: George W Hatch, Jr, EdD EMT-P
Tel: 713 718-7692, Ext 102   *Fax:* 713 718-7697
E-mail: george.hatch@hccs.edu

North Harris College
Emergency Med Tech-Paramedic Prgm
2700 W W Thorne Dr, Ste WN174
Houston, TX 77073
www.northharriscollege.com
Prgm Dir: Steven L Kolar, MBA RN LP EMSC
Tel: 281 618-5783   *Fax:* 281 618-1155
E-mail: steven.kolar@nhmccd.edu

San Jacinto College North
Emergency Med Tech-Paramedic Prgm
5800 Uvalde Rd
Houston, TX 77049-4599
Prgm Dir: Joseph J Hamilton, MS LP EMS-C
Tel: 281 459-7151   *Fax:* 281 459-7603
E-mail: joe.hamilton@sjcd.edu

Tarrant County College - Northeast Campus
Emergency Med Tech-Paramedic Prgm
828 Harwood Rd
Hurst, TX 76054-3299
Prgm Dir: Jeff McDonald, AA LP
Tel: 817 515-6448   *Fax:* 817 515-6700
E-mail: jeff.mcdonald@tccd.edu

Brazosport College
Emergency Med Tech-Paramedic Prgm
500 College Dr
Lake Jackson, TX 77568
Prgm Dir: John Creech, AAS LP
Tel: 979 230-3426   *Fax:* 979 230-3390
E-mail: jcreech@brazosport.edu

South Plains College
Emergency Med Tech-Paramedic Prgm
1401 S College Ave
Levelland, TX 79336
www.southplainscollege.edu
Prgm Dir: Mike DeLoach, BS NREMT-P
Tel: 806 885-3048, Ext 4627   *Fax:* 806 897-5295
E-mail: mdeloach@southplainscollege.edu

San Jacinto College Central
Emergency Med Tech-Paramedic Prgm
8060 Spencer Hwy
PO Box 2007
Pasadena, TX 77501-2007
Prgm Dir: Joseph J Hamilton, MS LP
Tel: 281 476-1501, Ext 1862   *Fax:* 281 478-2754
E-mail: Joe.Hamilton@sjcd.edu

Univ of Texas Hlth Sci Ctr at San Antonio
Emergency Med Tech-Paramedic Prgm
7703 Floyd Curl Dr
San Antonio, TX 78229
www.uthscsa.edu/emt
Prgm Dir: Lance Villers, PhD
Tel: 210 567-8760   *Fax:* 210 567-8749
E-mail: villers@uthscsa.edu

College of the Mainland
Emergency Med Tech-Paramedic Prgm
1200 Amburn Rd
Texas City, TX 77591
www.com.edu
Prgm Dir: Cissy Matthews, MBA LP EMSC
Tel: 409 938-1211, Ext 461   *Fax:* 409 938-3146
E-mail: cmatthews@com.edu

Wharton County Junior College
Emergency Med Tech-Paramedic Prgm
911 Boling Hwy
Wharton, TX 77488
Prgm Dir: Maggie Mejorado, LP EMT-P AAA AAS
Tel: 979 532-6540   *Fax:* 979 532-6541
E-mail: maggiem@wcjc.edu

Utah

Weber State University
Emergency Med Tech-Paramedic Prgm
3902 University Circle
Ogden, UT 84408-3902
Prgm Dir: Vapory Quick, MSN MREMT-P
Tel: 801 626-6521   *Fax:* 801 626-6610
E-mail: vquick@weber.edu

Utah Valley State College
Emergency Med Tech-Paramedic Prgm
3131 Mike Jense Parkway
Provo, UT 84601
Prgm Dir: Barry Stone, PA-C MPAS RN EMT-P
Tel: 801 863-7700, Ext 7747   *Fax:* 801 863-7738
E-mail: stoneba@uvsc.edu

Unified Fire Authority/Utah Valley State Coll
Emergency Med Tech-Paramedic Prgm
3380 South 900 West
Salt Lake City, UT 84119
Prgm Dir: Karla Holmes, RN
Tel: 801 743-7200
E-mail: kholmes@ufa-slco.org

Dixie State College of Utah
Emergency Med Tech-Paramedic Prgm
225 South 700 East
St George, UT 84770
Prgm Dir: Betty Wallis, RN MN
Tel: 435 752-7876   *Fax:* 435 656-4025
E-mail: wallis@dixie.edu

Virginia

Piedmont Virginia Community College
Cosponsor: University of Virginia Dept of Emergency
Medicine
Emergency Med Tech-Paramedic Prgm
501 College Dr
Charlottesville, VA 22902
Prgm Dir: Rita Krenz, BA BS NREMT-P
Tel: 434 961-5227   *Fax:* 434 961-5428
E-mail: rkrenz@pvcc.edu

Loudoun County Dept of Fire-Rescue
Emergency Med Tech-Paramedic Prgm
16600 Courage Court
Leesburg, VA 20175
Prgm Dir: Jose V Salazar
Tel: 703 777-0333   *Fax:* 703 777-0451
E-mail: jsalazar@loudoun.gov

Southwest Virginia Community College
Emergency Med Tech-Paramedic Prgm
PO Box SVCC
US Hwy 19
Richlands, VA 24641
www.sw.edu
Prgm Dir: Bill Akers Jr, MS NREMT-P
Tel: 276 964-7729   *Fax:* 276 964-7531
E-mail: Bill.Akers@sw.edu

J Sargeant Reynolds Community College
Emergency Med Tech-Paramedic Prgm
PO Box 85622
Richmond, VA 23285
Prgm Dir: Gregory S Neiman, BA NREMT-P
Tel: 804 523-5768   *Fax:* 804 786-5298
E-mail: gneiman@jsr.vccs.edu

Virginia Commonwealth Univ/Health System
Emergency Med Tech-Paramedic Prgm
PO Box 980044
Richmond, VA 23298-0044
Prgm Dir: Daniel P Barry, MHA NREMT-P
Tel: 804 828-3687
E-mail: dbarry@hsc.vcu.edu

Jefferson College of Health Sciences
Emergency Med Tech-Paramedic Prgm
PO Box 13186
Roanoke, VA 24031-3186
www.jchs.edu
Prgm Dir: Glen Mayhew, NREMT-P DHS
Tel: 540 985-8398   *Fax:* 540 985-9722
E-mail: cigrm1@jchs.edu

Northern Virginia Community College
Emergency Med Tech-Paramedic Prgm
6699 Springfield Center Dr, Office 239
Springfield, VA 22150
Prgm Dir: Holly C Frost, MS NREMT-P
Tel: 703 822-6557   *Fax:* 703 822-6614
E-mail: hfrost@nvcc.edu

Tidewater Community College
Emergency Med Tech-Paramedic Prgm
1700 College Crescent
Virginia Beach, VA 23453
Prgm Dir: Lorna Ramsey, RN MSN NREMT-P
Tel: 757 822-7335   *Fax:* 757 822-7460
E-mail: lramsey@tcc.edu

Washington

Bellingham Technical College
Emergency Med Tech-Paramedic Prgm
3028 Lindbergh Ave
Bellingham, WA 98225
Prgm Dir: Roger Christensen
Tel: 360 676-6830   *Fax:* 360 738-7312
E-mail: Rchristensen@btc.ctc.edu

Central Washington University
Emergency Med Tech-Paramedic Prgm
Dept of Health, Human Performance and Nutrition
400 E University Way
Ellensburg, WA 98926
Prgm Dir: Carolyn E Booth, RN MPH
Tel: 509 963-1451   *Fax:* 509 963-1848
E-mail: boothc@cwu.edu

Columbia Basin College
Emergency Med Tech-Paramedic Prgm
2600 N 20th Ave
Mailstop R-2
Pasco, WA 99301
www.cbc2.org
Prgm Dir: Troy Stratford, BS EMT-P
Tel: 509 547-0511, Ext 4020   *Fax:* 509 542-5675
E-mail: tstratford@columbiabasin.edu

Harborview Med Ctr - Univ of Washington
Emergency Med Tech-Paramedic Prgm
325 Ninth Ave, Mailbox 359727
Seattle, WA 98104
Prgm Dir: Roy D Waugh, EMT-P
Tel: 206 521-1215   *Fax:* 206 521-1914
E-mail: rwaugh@u.washington.edu

Spokane Community College
Emergency Med Tech-Paramedic Prgm
N 1810 Greene St, MS 2090
Spokane, WA 99217
Prgm Dir: R Mark Zandhuisen, EMT-P
Tel: 509 533-8129   *Fax:* 509 533-8621
E-mail: RMZandhuisen@scc.spokane.edu

Tacoma Community College
Emergency Med Tech-Paramedic Prgm
6501 S 19th St
Tacoma, WA 98466
Prgm Dir: Michael Smith, BS MICP
Tel: 253 566-5220   *Fax:* 253 566-5273
E-mail: msmith@tcc.ctc.edu

Tacoma Fire Department
Cosponsor: Pierce College
Emergency Med Tech-Paramedic Prgm
2124 E Marshall Ave
Tacoma, WA 98421
www.tacomafiredepartment.org
Prgm Dir: Lisa Breitinger, RN
Tel: 253 591-5149   *Fax:* 253 591-5417
E-mail: lbreitinger@ci.tacoma.wa.us

Northwest Regional Training Center
Emergency Med Tech-Paramedic Prgm
11606 NE 66th St, Ste 103
Vancouver, WA 98662
www.nwrtc.org
Prgm Dir: David Anderson, BS EMT-P
Tel: 360 759-4404   *Fax:* 360 892-4350
E-mail: davea@nwrtc.org

Emergency Medical Technician-Paramedic

	Class Capacity	Begins	Length (months)	Award	Res. Tuition	Non-res. Tuition	Stipend	Offers:‡ 1	2	3	4
Alabama											
Northeast Alabama Community College (Rainsville)	20	Jan	17	Cert, AAS	$3,468	$6,060				•	
Southern Union State Community College (Opelika)	15	Sep	18	Cert, AS	$3,240	$6,480		•			
University of South Alabama (Mobile)	20	Jan May Sep	18	Cert, BS EMS	$4,020	$7,920		•			
Arkansas											
Black River Technical College (Pocahontas)	25	Aug	24	Cert, AAS	$2,518	$6,497					
East Arkansas Community College (Forrest City)	Open	Aug	16	Cert, AAS	$1,372	$1,680					
National Park Community College (Hot Springs)	20	Aug	24	AAS	$1,350	$1,560					
NorthWest Arkansas Community College (Bentonville)	16	May	12, 24	Cert, AAS	$2,146	$4,663					
University of Arkansas for Medical Sciences (Little Rock)	20	Aug	17, 6	Cert, AS	$4,270	$24,381				•	•
California											
American River College (Sacramento)	200	Jan Aug	24, 12	Dipl, Cert, AS	$1,800	$5,580		•		•	•
Los Angeles County Paramedic Training Inst (Commerce)	40	Jan Apr Jul Oct	6	Cert	$660	$4,960					
Riverside Comm Coll - Moreno Valley Campus	40	Aug	12	Dipl, Cert, AAS	$990	$0					
Santa Rosa Junior College (Windsor)	28	Aug	12	Cert, AS	$2,500	$7,000				•	
Victor Valley Community College District (Victorville)	45	Jan Jun	12	Cert	$925	$4,615					
Colorado											
Community College of Aurora (Denver)	30	Jan Aug	18	Cert	$6,100	$16,875	$86	•			
HealthONE EMS (Englewood)	25	Jan Jun	6, 12	Cert, Assoc	$5,500	$5,500					
Florida											
Brevard Community College (Cocoa)	40	Aug Jan	11	Cert, AS	$2,915	$5,850		•			
Hillsborough Community College (Tampa)	40	Aug Jan May	10	Cert, AS, AAS	$3,400	$10,200		•			
Indian River Community College (Fort Pierce)	32	Aug Jan	10	Cert, AS	$4,013	$16,052					
Miami Dade College	54	Aug Jan May	12	Cert, AS	$3,002	$10,242		•			
Pasco-Hernando Community College (New Port Richey)	30	Aug	11	Cert, ATD	$2,754	$10,315		•			
Pensacola Junior College	20	Jul	12, 24	Cert, AAS	$3,200	$9,000		•		•	
Polk Community College (Winter Haven)	24	Aug	12, 24	Cert, AS, AAS	$2,900	$9,900					
Tallahassee Community College	15	Aug	11, 23	Cert, AS	$1,550	$4,650					
Georgia											
Gwinnett Technical College (Lawrenceville)	30	Sep	24	Dipl, AAS	$1,500	$2,748					
Idaho											
College of Southern Idaho (Twin Falls)	12	Jan	18	Cert, AAS, TC	$2,100	$5,900				•	
Idaho State University (Pocatello)	30	Aug	24	AS/ATC	$4,688	$9,376					
Illinois											
Trinity College of Nursing & Health Sciences (Rock Island)	20	Aug	10, 24	Cert, AAS	$9,150	$9,150				•	
Indiana											
Ivy Tech Community College - Columbus	24	Aug	24	AS	$3,993	$3,993					
Ivy Tech Community College - Evansville	24	Aug	20	Cert, AAS	$3,510	$6,092		•			•
Methodist Hospitals Inc (Gary)	20	Aug	17	Cert, AS	$3,500	$3,500					

*Data are shown only for programs that completed the 2007 AMA Survey of Health Professions Education Programs.
‡Key to Offers: 1: Evening or weekend classes; 2: Non-English instruction; 3: Cultural competence instruction; 4: Distance education component.

Emergency Medical Technician-Paramedic

	Class Capacity	Begins	Length (months)	Award	Res. Tuition	Non-res. Tuition	Stipend	Offers:‡ 1	2	3	4
Iowa											
Kirkwood Community College (Cedar Rapids)	30	Jan	19	AAS	$99	$0		•			
Kansas											
Cowley County Community College (Winfield)	40	Jan	12, 18	AAS	$3,470	$6,117		•		•	
Kentucky											
Eastern Kentucky University (Richmond)	20	Aug	12, 24	Cert, AS, BS	$2,236	$6,136		•			
Maryland											
Anne Arundel Community College (Arnold)	25	Aug	18, 24	Cert, AAS	$5,500	$5,500		•		•	•
University of Maryland Baltimore County	15	Sep	48	BS, MS	$8,622	$17,354				•	
Michigan											
Huron Valley Ambulance (Ann Arbor)	30	Sep Jan	12	Cert	$4,513	$4,513		•			
Minnesota											
Greater Minnesota Paramedic Consortium (Fergus Falls)	20	Jun Sep	12	Cert	$8,000	$9,000		•			
South Central College (North Mankato)	25	Aug	16	Dipl, AAS	$2,216	$4,432		•		•	
Mississippi											
Jones County Junior College (Ellisville)	15	Aug Jan	18	AAS	$1,800	$2,952		•			
Mississippi Gulf Coast Community College (Gulfport)	30	Aug	12	Cert, AAS	$2,235	$5,004					
Northwest Mississippi Community College (Senatobia)	25	Aug	16	AS	$1,700	$2,000					
University of Mississippi Medical Center (Jackson)	25	Aug	12	Cert	$2,250	$2,913				•	
Nebraska											
Creighton University (Omaha)	50	Aug	12	Dipl, Cert, BS EMS, AS	$25,000	$25,000		•	•	•	•
New Hampshire											
New Hampshire Technical Institute (Concord)	14	Aug 29	18	AS	$4,200	$0					
New York											
Bassett Healthcare Center for Rural EMS Educ (Cobleskill)	30	Sep	12, 24	Cert, AAS, AS	$4,000	$5,500		•			
Monroe Community College (Rochester)	30	Jan	18	Dipl, Cert AAS	$3,000	$6,000		•			
North Carolina											
Catawba Valley Community College (Hickory)	25	Aug	24	AAS	$1,829	$9,864				•	
Joint Special Operations Medical Training Ctr (Fort Bragg)	72	Every 6 wks	6	Cert							
Ohio											
Parma Community General Hospital	50	Jan Sep	12	Cert	$3,000	$3,000					
Summa Health System (Akron)	35	Jan	10	Cert	$3,500	$3,500		•		•	
Youngstown State University	25	Aug	11, 21	Cert, AAS	$6,400	$9,750					
Oregon											
Chemeketa Community College (Salem)	24	Sep Apr	18	AAS	$2,852	$9,338				•	
Oregon Health & Science University (Sherwood)	24	Sep	12	Dipl, AAS	$14,800	$18,009					
Pennsylvania											
Lehigh Valley Hospital (Allentown)	30	Jan Mar	12, 10	Cert, AS	$2,650	$2,650					
Pennsylvania College of Technology (Williamsport)	32	Aug	24, 15	Cert, AAS	$10,360	$13,061					
South Carolina											
Greenville Technical College	36	Aug (day) Jan (eve)	21	Cert, AS	$4,125	$8,625		•		•	
Trident Technical College (Charleston)	24	Aug	21	AS	$2,950	$3,276					•
South Dakota											
Avera McKennan Hospital (Sioux Falls)	25	Feb Sep	10, 12	Dipl, Cert, AA, BS	$5,750	$5,750		•		•	•
Tennessee											
Northeast State Technical Comm College (Blountville)	25	Jun	15	Cert	$3,000	$12,000					
Roane State Community College (Knoxville)	20	Aug	12	Cert, AAS	$3,200	$11,000		•			
Southwest Tennessee Community College (Memphis)	75	Sep	12	Cert	$1,536	$6,144		•			
Texas											
College of the Mainland (Texas City)	20	Jun	12	Cert, AAS	$950	$1,795		•			
North Harris College (Houston)	50	Aug	21	Cert, AAS	$852	$1,692		•		•	•
San Jacinto College Central (Pasadena)	60	Jan Sep	17	Cert, AAS	$750	$1,125		•	•	•	•
San Jacinto College North (Houston)	25	Jan Sep	17, 24	Cert, AAS	$750	$1,125		•	•	•	
South Plains College (Levelland)	40	Jan Aug	24	Cert, AAS				•			•
Univ of Texas Hlth Sci Ctr at San Antonio	30	Varies	9, 18	Cert	$3,400	$12,243					
Univ of Texas Southwestern Med Ctr (Dallas)	38	Aug Feb	6, 13	Cert	$2,203	$4,168					
Virginia											
Jefferson College of Health Sciences (Roanoke)	30	Aug	21	AAS	$15,500	$0		•			
Southwest Virginia Community College (Richlands)	75	Aug	22	AAS	$2,500	$7,500		•		•	
Washington											
Columbia Basin College (Pasco)	24	Jan	18	Dipl, Cert, AAS	$2,800	$4,000		•		•	
Harborview Med Ctr - Univ of Washington (Seattle)	20	Oct	10	Cert	$8,000	$0					
Northwest Regional Training Center (Vancouver)	24	Aug	12	Cert	$8,675	$8,675				•	
Tacoma Fire Department	25	Sep	9	Cert	$5,400	$0					

*Data are shown only for programs that completed the 2007 AMA Survey of Health Professions Education Programs.
‡Key to Offers: 1: Evening or weekend classes; 2: Non-English instruction; 3: Cultural competence instruction; 4: Distance education component.

Includes:
- Exercise physiology (clinical and applied)
- Exercise science
- Personal fitness training

Exercise Physiology

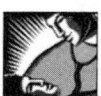

Career Description

Exercise physiology is a discipline that includes clinical exercise physiology and applied exercise physiology. Applied exercise physiologists manage programs to assess, design, and implement individual and group exercise and fitness programs for apparently healthy individuals and individuals with controlled disease. Clinical exercise physiologists work under the direction of a physician to apply physical activity and behavioral interventions in clinical situations where they have been scientifically proven to provide therapeutic or functional benefit.

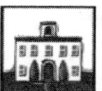

Employment Characteristics

As a clinical part of the health and wellness team, exercise physiologists can work with personal fitness trainers, exercise science professionals, and physicians in cardiac rehabilitation, typically in a hospital or clinical setting. Exercise physiologists work with clients who have been diagnosed with a chronic metabolic, pulmonary, or cardiac disease.

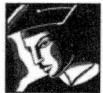

Educational Programs

Length: Exercise physiologist programs can be completed in a 2-year master's degree level program.
Prerequisites: Applicants should have a high school diploma or equivalent, meet the specific institutional entrance requirements, and have a bachelor's degree in exercise science.
   Curriculum: Exercise physiologist programs will include a comprehensive academic curriculum and at least one culminating internship experience.

Exercise Science

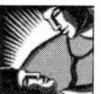

Career Description

Exercise science encompasses a wide variety of disciplines including, but not limited to, biomechanics, sports nutrition, sport psychology, motor control/development, and exercise physiology. The study of these disciplines is integrated into the academic preparation of exercise science professionals. Exercise science professionals work in the health and fitness industry and are skilled in evaluating health behaviors and risk factors, conducting fitness assessments, writing appropriate exercise prescriptions, and motivating individuals to modify negative health habits and maintain positive lifestyle behaviors for health promotion.

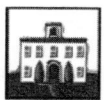

Employment Characteristics

As an integral part of the health and wellness team, exercise science professionals can work with personal fitness trainers and exercise physiologists in a number of different settings, such as corporate, clinical, community, and commercial fitness and wellness centers. Exercise science professionals work with the apparently healthy population and clients with controlled disease, leading and demonstrating these clients in safe and effective methods of exercise. The exercise science professional can also assess risk factors and identify the health status of clients.

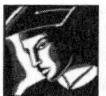

Educational Programs

Length: Exercise science programs can be completed in a 4-year bachelor's degree level program.
Prerequisites: Applicants should have a high school diploma or equivalent and meet the specific institutional entrance requirements.
   Curriculum: Exercise science programs include a comprehensive academic curriculum and at least one culminating internship experience.

Personal Fitness Training

Career Description

Personal fitness trainers are skilled practitioners who work with a wide variety of client demographics in one-to-one and small group environments. They are familiar with multiple forms of exercise used to improve and maintain health-related components of physical fitness and performance. They are knowledgeable in basic assessment and development of exercise recommendations. In addition, they are proficient in leading and demonstrating safe and effective methods of exercise and motivating individuals to begin and to continue with healthy behaviors. They consult with and refer to other appropriate allied health professionals when client conditions exceed the personal trainer's education, training, and experience.

Employment Characteristics

As an integral part of the health and wellness team, personal fitness trainers can work with exercise science professionals and exercise physiologists in a number of different settings, such as corporate, clinical, community, and commercial fitness and wellness centers. Personal fitness training involves working with the apparently healthy population, leading and demonstrating these clients in safe and effective methods of exercise.

Educational Programs

Length: Personal fitness training programs can be completed in a 1-year certificate program or in a 2-year associate's degree level program.
   Prerequisites: Applicants should have a high school diploma or equivalent and meet the specific institutional entrance requirements.
   Curriculum: Personal fitness training programs will include a comprehensive academic curriculum and at least one culminating internship experience.

 **Inquiries**

Careers

American Alliance for Health, Physical Education, Recreation, and Dance (AAHPERD)
1900 Association Drive
Reston, VA 20191-1598
800 213-7193
www.aahperd.org

American Association of Cardiovascular and Pulmonary Rehabilitation (AACVPR)
401 North Michigan Avenue, Suite 2200
Chicago, IL 60611
312 321-5146
www.aacvpr.org

Medical Fitness Association (MFA)
PO Box 73103
Richmond, VA 23235-8026
804 327-0330
www.medicalfitness.org

American Kinesiotherapy Association (AKTA)
CCB-KT
PO Box 1390
Hines, IL 60141-1390
800 296-2582
www.akta.org

Certification

American College of Sports Medicine (ACSM)
401 West Michigan Street
Indianapolis, IN 46202
317 637-9200
www.acsm.org

National Strength and Conditioning Association (NSCA)
1885 Bob Johnson Drive
Colorado Springs, CO 80906
800 815-6826
www.nsca.com

National Academy of Sports Medicine (NASM)
26632 Agoura Road
Calabasas, CA 91302
800 460-6276
www.nasm.org

The Cooper Institute
12330 Preston Road
Dallas, TX 75230
972 341-3200
www.cooperinst.org

Program Accreditation

Commission on Accreditation of Allied Health Education Programs (CAAHEP) in collaboration with:
Committee on Accreditation of the Exercise Sciences (CoAES)
401 West Michigan Street
Indianapolis, IN 46202
317 352-3826
www.coaes.org

Exercise Physiologist

Louisiana

University of Louisiana at Monroe
Exercise Physiology Prgm
Department of Kinesiology
700 University Ave
Monroe, LA 71209
www.ulm.edu
Prgm Dir: Lisa Colvin, PhD
Tel: 318 342-1306   *Fax:* 318 342-1308
E-mail: lcolvin@ulm.edu

Pennsylvania

East Stroudsburg University
Exercise Physiology Prgm
Exercise Physiology
Koehler Fieldhouse
East Stroudsburg, PA 18301
Prgm Dir: Donald Cummings
Tel: 570 422-3302
E-mail: dcummings@po-box.esu.edu

Exercise Science Professional

Alabama

Samford University
Exercise Science Prgm
800 Lakeshore Dr
Birmingham, AL 35229
Prgm Dir: Alan P Jung, PhD HFI CSCS
Tel: 205 726-4026
E-mail: apjung@samford.edu

Louisiana

University of Louisiana at Monroe
Exercise Science Prgm
Department of Kinesiology
700 University Ave
Monroe, LA 71209
www.ulm.edu
Prgm Dir: Luke Thomas, PhD
Tel: 318 342-1309   *Fax:* 318 342-1308
E-mail: lthomas@ulm.edu

Maryland

Salisbury University
Exercise Science Prgm
Maggs Physical Acitivity Center
Salisbury, MD 21801
Prgm Dir: Susan Muller, MD
Tel: 410 548-5555
E-mail: smmuller@salisbury.edu

Massachusetts

Westfield State College
Exercise Science Prgm
Department of Movement Sciences
577 Western Ave
Westfield, MA 01086
Prgm Dir: Theresa Fitts, DPE
Tel: 413 572-5368
E-mail: tfitts@wsc.ma.edu

North Dakota

North Dakota State University
Exercise Science Prgm
Bentson Bunker Fieldhouse
Fargo, ND 58105
Prgm Dir: Donna Terbizan
Tel: 701 231-7792   *Fax:* 701 231-8872
E-mail: d.terbizan@ndsu.edu

Pennsylvania

East Stroudsburg University
Exercise Science Prgm
Koehler Fieldhouse
East Stroudsburg, PA 18301
Prgm Dir: Donald Cummings, PhD
Tel: 570 422-3302
E-mail: dcummings@po-box.esu.edu

Slippery Rock University of Pennsylvania
Exercise Science Prgm
128 E Gym, Stoner Complex
Slippery Rock, PA 16057
Prgm Dir: Patricia Pierce, FACSM
Tel: 724 738-2830
E-mail: patricia.pierce@sru.edu

Virginia

Old Dominion University
Exercise Science Prgm
140 HPE Bldg
Norfolk, VA 23529
Prgm Dir: J David Branch, PhD
Tel: 757 683-4995   *Fax:* 757 683-4270
E-mail: dbranch@odu.edu

Exercise Physiologist

	Class Capacity	Begins	Length (months)	Award	Res. Tuition	Non-res. Tuition	Stipend	Offers:‡ 1	2	3	4
Louisiana											
University of Louisiana at Monroe	20	Each semester	12	MS				•			

*Data are shown only for programs that completed the 2007 AMA Survey of Health Professions Education Programs.
‡Key to Offers: 1: Evening or weekend classes; 2: Non-English instruction; 3: Cultural competence instruction; 4: Distance education component.

Exercise Science Professional

	Class Capacity	Begins	Length (months)	Award	Res. Tuition	Non-res. Tuition	Stipend	Offers:‡ 1	2	3	4
Louisiana											
University of Louisiana at Monroe	25	Each semester		BS				•			
North Dakota											
North Dakota State University (Fargo)	50	Fall semester	48	BS							

*Data are shown only for programs that completed the 2007 AMA Survey of Health Professions Education Programs.
‡Key to Offers: 1: Evening or weekend classes; 2: Non-English instruction; 3: Cultural competence instruction; 4: Distance education component.

Genetic Counselor

Genetic counselors are specialized health care professionals who work at the crossroads of medicine, technology, and bioethics. They facilitate the translation of genetic discoveries to everyday medical care by working with individuals and families seeking information about medical conditions that have a genetic contribution.

Career Description

As health care professionals, genetic counselors interpret and provide clear and comprehensive information about the risk of any medical condition that may have a genetic contribution. This involves collecting and interpreting family, medical, and psychosocial history information. Analysis of this history information together with an understanding of genetic principles and the knowledge of current technologies provide individuals and their families with information about risk, prognosis, medical management, and diagnostic and prevention options. Genetic counselors facilitate an informed decision-making process that elicits and respects the spectrum of personal beliefs and values that exist in society.

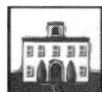

Employment Characteristics

Genetic counselors practice as part of a health care team. The settings in which genetic counselors work include hospitals and medical centers, public health agencies, colleges and universities, diagnostic laboratories, biotechnology companies, research institutions, private practice, and governmental agencies.

According to the 2006 Professional Status Survey (PSS), conducted by the National Society of Genetic Counselors (NSGC), 69% of all genetic counselors work in university medical centers, private hospitals, and medical facilities.

Prenatal, cancer, pediatric, and adult are the most common specialty areas in which genetic counselors work, according to the 2006 PSS. Examples of other specialty areas include neurogenetics, psychiatry, cardiology, infertility, laboratory testing/screening, and disease-specific clinics.

In addition to health care, advances made by the Human Genome Project have relevance in many other areas. As a result, genetic counselors have expanded and adapted their skills into areas such as research, industry, education, policy, pubic health, administration, and advocacy work.

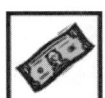

Salary

According to the 2006 PSS, the yearly gross salaries reported by survey respondents range from $20,000 to $150,000, with an average of $59,000. Salaries vary by location and are highest in California, New York, and New Jersey and lowest in the southeastern United States. Refer to Section IV, Table 5 of this *Directory* for more information, or see www.ama-assn.org/go/hpsalary.

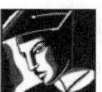

Educational Programs

Length. Genetic counselors have a master's degree from a graduate program specifically designed to prepare individuals for a career as a genetic counselor. The training is specialized and includes coursework and hands-on supervised clinical experiences.

Curriculum. The coursework includes instruction in the following general content areas:

- Human, medical, and clinical genetics
- Psychosocial theory and techniques
- Social, ethical, and legal issues
- Health care delivery systems and public health principles
- Teaching techniques
- Research methods

The supervised clinical experiences provide students with diversified clinical training and give them experience working with individuals and families affected with a broad range of genetic disorders and counseling situations. This clinical training is important in exposing students to the natural history and management of and psychosocial issues associated with common genetic conditions and birth defects. Students also obtain experience in teaching, laboratory methods, and research.

The American Board of Genetic Counseling accredits graduate programs in genetic counseling.

Inquiries

Careers
Kristen Smith, CAE, Executive Director
National Society of Genetic Counselors
401 North Michigan Avenue
Chicago, IL 60611
312 321-6834
312 673-6972 Fax
E-mail: nsgc@nsgc.org
www.nsgc.org

Credentialing/ Program Accreditation
Sheila O'Neil, Executive Director
American Board of Genetic Counseling
18000 West 105th Street
Olathe, KS 66061
913 895-4617
913 895-4652
E-mail: info@abgc.net
www.abgc.net

Genetic Counselor

Arkansas

University of Arkansas for Medical Sciences
Genetic Counseling Prgm
College of Health Related Professions
Department of Genetic Counseling
Little Rock, AR 72205
www.uams.edu/chrp/genetics/
Prgm Dir: Bruce Haas, MS CGC
Tel: 501 526-7700   *Fax:* 501 526-7711
E-mail: GeneticCounseling@uams.edu

British Columbia, Canada

University of British Columbia
Genetic Counseling Prgm
Department of Medical Genetics
Children's and Women's Hlth Centre of BC
Vancouver, BC V6H 3NI
www.medgen.ubc.ca/academics/mast_gen.htm
Prgm Dir: Anita Dircks, MSc CGC CCGC
Tel: 604 875-2832   *Fax:* 604 875-3490
E-mail: adircks@cw.bc.ca

California

California State University - Northridge
Genetic Counseling Prgm
18111 Nordhoff St
Northridge, CA 91330
Prgm Dir: Aida Metzenberg, PhD
Tel: 818 677-3355   *Fax:* 818 677-6692
E-mail: aida.metzenberg@csun.edu

University of CA - Irvine School of Medicine
Genetic Counseling Prgm
Div of Human Genetics
Dept of Pediatrics, UCIMC-ZOT 4482
Orange, CA 92868
Prgm Dir: Ann P Walker, MA CGC
Tel: 714 456-5789   *Fax:* 714 456-5330
E-mail: awalker@uci.edu

Colorado

U of Colorado (Denver) Health Sciences Center
Genetic Counseling Prgm
Education 2 South, L28, 4107
13121 E 17th Ave
Aurora, CO 80045
www.uchsc.edu/gs/gs
Prgm Dir: Carol Walton, MS CGC
Tel: 303 724-2356   *Fax:* 720 777-7322
E-mail: Walton.Carol@tchden.org

District of Columbia

Howard University
Genetic Counseling Prgm
520 W St NW, Box 75
Washington, DC 20059
Prgm Dir: Verle Headings, MD PhD
Tel: 202 806-9814   *Fax:* 202 806-7058
E-mail: vheadings@howard.edu

Illinois

Northwestern University
Genetic Counseling Prgm
Feinberg School of Medicine
676 N St Clair St, #1280
Chicago, IL 60611
Prgm Dir: Kelly Ormond, MS
Tel: 312 926-7726   *Fax:* 312 926-3553
E-mail: geneticcounseling@northwestern.edu

Indiana

Indiana University
Genetic Counseling Prgm
School of Medicine
Dept of Medical and Molecular Genetics
Indianapolis, IN 46202-5251
www.iupui.edu/~medgen/
Prgm Dir: Paula Delk, MS
Tel: 317 278-8837   *Fax:* 317 274-2387
E-mail: pwinter@iupui.edu

Maryland

University of Maryland
Genetic Counseling Prgm
660 W Redwood St, Ste 570
Baltimore, MD 21201
Prgm Dir: Shannon DeLany Dixon, MS CGC
Tel: 410 706-4713   *Fax:* 410 706-1644
E-mail: sdelany@som.umaryland.edu

Johns Hopkins University
Cosponsor: National Human Genome Research Institute
Genetic Counseling Prgm
Social and Behavioral Research Branch NHGRI/NIH
2 Center Dr MSC0249, Bldg 2, Rm 4W17
Bethesda, MD 20892
Prgm Dir: Barbara Biesecker, MS
Tel: 301 496-3979   *Fax:* 301 480-3108
E-mail: barbarab@nhgri.nih.gov

Massachusetts

Boston University
Genetic Counseling Prgm
Center for Human Genetics
715 Albany St, W408
Boston, MA 02118
Prgm Dir: MaryAnn Whalen, MS
Tel: 617 638-7170
E-mail: maryann@bu.edu

Brandeis University
Genetic Counseling Prgm
Biology Dept MS008
Waltham, MA 02454
www.bio.brandeis.edu/gc01/
Prgm Dir: Judith Tsipis, PhD
Tel: 781 736-3165   *Fax:* 781 736-3107
E-mail: tsipis@brandeis.edu

Michigan

University of Michigan
Genetic Counseling Prgm
Dept of Human Genetics
4909 Buhl
Ann Arbor, MI 48109-0618
www.hg.med.umich.edu
Prgm Dir: Beverly M Yashar, PhD
Tel: 734 763-2933   *Fax:* 734 763-3784
E-mail: yashar@umich.edu

Wayne State University
Genetic Counseling Prgm
540 E Canfield, 3216 Scott Hall
Detroit, MI 48201
Prgm Dir: Anne Greb, MS
Tel: 313 577-6298   *Fax:* 313 577-9137
E-mail: agreb@genetics.wayne.edu

Minnesota

University of Minnesota - Minneapolis
Genetic Counseling Prgm
University of Minnesota Institute of Human Genetics
Department of Genetics, Cell Biology & Development
Minneapolis, MN 55455
www.cbs.umn.edu/gc/
Prgm Dir: Bonnie S LeRoy, MS CGC
Tel: 612 624-7193   *Fax:* 612 625-4490
E-mail: leroy001@umn.edu

New York

Sarah Lawrence College
Genetic Counseling Prgm
One Mead Way
Bronxville, NY 10708-5999
Prgm Dir: Caroline Lieber, MS
Tel: 914 395-2371   *Fax:* 914 395-2664
E-mail: clieber@sarahlawrence.edu

Mt Sinai School of Medicine
Genetic Counseling Prgm
Dept of Genetics and Genomic Sciences, Box 1497
One Gustave Levy Pl
New York, NY 10029
www.mssm.edu
Prgm Dir: Randi Zinberg, MS CGC
Tel: 212 241-6947, Ext 212-24   *Fax:* 212 860-3316
E-mail: randi.zinberg@mssm.edu

North Carolina

University of North Carolina - Greensboro
Genetic Counseling Prgm
119 McIver St
Greensboro, NC 27402
www.uncg.edu/gen
Prgm Dir: Nancy Callanan, MS CGC
Tel: 336 256-0175   *Fax:* 336 256-0174
E-mail: nancy_callanan@uncg.edu

Ohio

Cincinnati Children's Hospital Medical Center
Genetic Counseling Prgm
Division of Human Genetics
3333 Burnet Ave, ML 4006
Cincinnati, OH 45229
Prgm Dir: Nancy Steinberg Warren, MS CGC
Tel: 513 636-4475   *Fax:* 513 636-0543
E-mail: Nancy.Warren@UC.Edu

Case Western Reserve University
Genetic Counseling Prgm
10900 Euclid Ave
Cleveland, OH 44106-4955
Prgm Dir: Anne Matthews, RN PhD
Tel: 216 368-1821   *Fax:* 216 368-3432
E-mail: anne.mathews@case.edu

Oklahoma

Univ of Oklahoma Health Sciences Center
Genetic Counseling Prgm
940 NE 13th St, Rm 2B2418
Oklahoma City, OK 73104
Prgm Dir: Susan J Hassed, MS
Tel: 405 271-8001, Ext 42182   *Fax:* 405 271-8697
E-mail: susan-hassed@ouhsc.edu

Ontario, Canada

University of Toronto
Genetic Counseling Prgm
1 King's College Circle
Toronto, ON M5S 1A8
Prgm Dir: Cheryl Shuman, MS CGC
Tel: 416 813-6374   *Fax:* 416 813-5345
E-mail: cshuman@sickkids.on.ca

Pennsylvania

Arcadia University
Genetic Counseling Prgm
450 S Easton Rd
Glenside, PA 19038
Prgm Dir: Kathleen Valverde, MS CGC
Tel: 215 572-4058   *Fax:* 215 881-8758
E-mail: valverde@arcadia.edu

University of Pittsburgh
Genetic Counseling Prgm
Dept of Human Genetics
A300 Crabtree Hall, 130 DeSoto St
Pittsburgh, PA 15261
Prgm Dir: Jeanette Norbut
Tel: 412 624-3018   *Fax:* 412 624-3020
E-mail: jeanette.norbut@hgen.pitt.edu

Quebec, Canada

McGill University
Genetic Counseling Prgm
1205 Dr Penfield Ave, Rm N5/13
Montreal, QC H3A 1B1
www.mcgill.ca/humgenet
Prgm Dir: Jennifer Fitzpatrick, MS
Tel: 514 398-3600   *Fax:* 514 398-2430
E-mail: jennifer.fitzpatrick@mcgill.ca

South Carolina

University of South Carolina
Genetic Counseling Prgm
Dept of OB/GYN
Two Medical Park
Columbia, SC 29203
http://geneticcounseling.med.sc.edu/
Prgm Dir: Janice G Edwards, MS
Tel: 803 779-4928, Ext 227   *Fax:* 803 434-4596
E-mail: jedwards@gw.mp.sc.edu

Texas

Univ of Texas Medical School at Houston
Genetic Counseling Prgm
Graduate School of Biomedical Sciences, Dept of
    Pediatrics
PO Box 20708
Houston, TX 77225
http://gsbs.uth.tmc.edu
Prgm Dir: Claire Singletary, MS CGC
Tel: 713 500-5760   *Fax:* 713 500-5689
E-mail: Claire.N.Singletary@uth.tmc.edu

Utah

University of Utah Health Science Center
Genetic Counseling Prgm
15 North 2030 East #2100
Salt Lake City, UT 84112
Prgm Dir: Bonnie J Baty, MS CGC LGC
Tel: 801 581-6914   *Fax:* 801 585-7252
E-mail: bonnie.baty@hsc.utah.edu

Virginia

Virginia Commonwealth Univ/Health System
Genetic Counseling Prgm
Dept of Human Genetics
PO Box 980033
Richmond, VA 23298-0033
Prgm Dir: Rachel Gannaway, MS
Tel: 804 828-9632, Ext 132   *Fax:* 804 828-7094
E-mail: rgannaway@vcu.edu

Wisconsin

University of Wisconsin - Madison
Genetic Counseling Prgm
445 Henry Mall, Rm 118
Madison, WI 53706
Prgm Dir: Catherine A Reiser, MS CGC
Tel: 608 262-9722   *Fax:* 608 263-3496
E-mail: reiser@waisman.wisc.edu

Genetic Counselor

	Class Capacity	Begins	Length (months)	Award	Res. Tuition	Non-res. Tuition	Stipend	Offers:‡ 1	2	3	4
Arkansas											
University of Arkansas for Medical Sciences (Little Rock)	<12	Fall semester	22	MS						•	•
British Columbia, Canada											
University of British Columbia (Vancouver)	6	Sep of each year	20	MSc	$15,300	$15,300				•	
Colorado											
U of Colorado (Denver) Health Sciences Center (Aurora)	6-8	Aug	21	Dipl, MS	$8,500	$13,500				•	
Illinois											
Northwestern University (Chicago)	10	Sep	18	Dipl, MS	$44,000	$44,000	$6,600			•	
Indiana											
Indiana University (Indianapolis)	6	Aug	22	Dipl, MS	$4,300	$12,400				•	
Massachusetts											
Boston University	6	Sep	21	MS	$30,000	$30,000	$3,500			•	
Brandeis University (Waltham)	10	Aug	20	MS						•	
Michigan											
University of Michigan (Ann Arbor)	6	Sep	20	MS	$12,149	$24,415	$900			•	
Minnesota											
University of Minnesota - Minneapolis	8	Sep	21	MS	$9,302	$16,400				•	
New York											
Mt Sinai School of Medicine (New York)	5-7	Aug	20	MS	$12,000	$12,000				•	
North Carolina											
University of North Carolina - Greensboro	8	Aug	21	MS	$5,700	$18,000				•	
Ohio											
Cincinnati Children's Hospital Medical Center	20	Sep	21	MS	$11,661	$21,495	$4,000	•		•	•
Oklahoma											
Univ of Oklahoma Health Sciences Center (Oklahoma City)	4	Fall	21	MS						•	
Ontario, Canada											
University of Toronto	4	Sep	18	MSc	$6,147	$10,560				•	
Quebec, Canada											
McGill University (Montreal)	4	Sep 1	20	MSc	$3,500	$10,000			•	•	
South Carolina											
University of South Carolina (Columbia)	8	Aug	21	MS						•	
Texas											
Univ of Texas Medical School at Houston	6-8	Aug	21	MS	$1,500	$9,000					
Virginia											
Virginia Commonwealth Univ/Health System (Richmond)	5	Aug	21	MS	$8,320	$17,562				•	

*Data are shown only for programs that completed the 2007 AMA Survey of Health Professions Education Programs.
‡Key to Offers: 1: Evening or weekend classes; 2: Non-English instruction; 3: Cultural competence instruction; 4: Distance education component.

Health Information Management

Includes:
- Health information administrator
- Health information technician

Definition of the Profession

The health information management profession includes managers, technicians, and specialists expert in systems and processes for health information management, including:

- Planning: Formulating strategic, functional, and user requirements for health information
- Engineering: Designing information flow, data models, and definitions
- Administration: Managing data collection and storage, information retrieval, and release
- Application: Analyzing, interpreting, classifying, and coding data and facilitating information use by others
- Policy: Establishing and implementing security, confidentiality, retention, integrity, and access standards

Health Information Administrator

Graduates of baccalaureate degree educational programs in health information management are known as health information administrators and apply their training and expertise in both science and management to develop, implement, and/or provide oversight to health care data collection and reporting systems to assure the integrity and availability of the information resources needed to support authorized users and decision-makers. Health information managers have expertise in developing and managing effective processes and systems to assure the integrity of health care data and to preserve the complete, accurate, and legal source of patient data (patient medical records), as well as expertise in developing and managing effective processes and systems to preserve patient privacy, confidentiality, and the security of health information maintained in paper or computerized systems. Common job titles held by health information administrators in today's job market are related to line, staff, and/or technical positions such as director, assistant director, manager, privacy officer, compliance officer, claims analyst, clinical information specialist, HIM educator, etc. It is anticipated that job titles will change (eg, health information engineer, clinical information coordinator, data administrator, information security officer) as health care enterprises expand their reliance on information systems and technology. Health information administrators have, and will continue to assume, roles that directly contribute to the development of computer-based patient record systems and a national health information infrastructure.

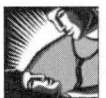

Career Description

The tasks or functions performed by health information administrators are numerous and are continually changing within the work environment. Although the job title and work setting will dictate the actual tasks performed by the health information administrator, in general this individual performs tasks related to the management of health information and the systems used to collect, store, process, retrieve, analyze, disseminate, and communicate that information, regardless of the physical medium in which information is maintained. In addition, health information administrators assess the uses of information and identify what information is available and where there are inconsistencies, gaps, and duplications in health data sources. They are capable of planning and designing systems and serving as pivotal team members in the development of computer-based patient record systems and other enterprise-wide information systems. Their responsibilities also include serving as brokers of information services. Among the information services provided are a design and requirements definition for clinical and administrative systems development, data administration, data quality management, data security management, decision support design and data analyses, and management of information-intensive areas such as clinical quality/performance assessment and utilization and case management.

Employment Characteristics

Presently, opportunities for practice are found in numerous settings such as acute care general hospitals, managed care organizations, consulting firms, claims and reimbursement organizations, accounting firms, home health care agencies, long-term care facilities, corrections facilities, drug companies, behavioral health care organizations, insurance companies, state and federal health care agencies, and public health care computing industries. Practice opportunities are unlimited.

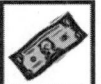

Salary

According to the American Health Information Management Association (AHIMA), entry-level salaries average between $40,000 and $75,000. Refer to Section IV, Table 5 of this *Directory* for more information, or see www.ama-assn.org/go/hpsalary.

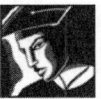

Educational Programs

Length. Baccalaureate degree programs are 4 years. Postbaccalaureate and other certificate programs are generally 1 year.

Prerequisites. Applicants for the 4-year baccalaureate degree program should have a high school diploma or equivalent. Applicants for the 1-year post-baccalaureate certificate program should have a baccalaureate degree that includes coursework in science and statistics, as specified.

Curriculum. The preprofessional curriculum should include appropriate general education credit predicated on the requirements of the academic institution. The professional curriculum requires:

- Biomedical sciences (anatomy, physiology, language of medicine, pharmacology, and disease processes)
- Information technology (microcomputer applications, programming, system architectures and operating systems, introduction to database concepts, and data communications)
- Health care delivery systems
- Legal aspects of health care and ethical issues
- Organization and management (managerial principles, human resources management and development, financial management for health care, organizational behavior, and interpersonal skills)

- Quantitative methods and research methodologies (introductory and advanced health care statistics/epidemiology, research methods in health care)
- Health care information requirements and standards
- Health care information systems (computer applications in health care, systems analysis and design)
- Health data content and structures, classification, nomenclature and reimbursement systems, clinical quality assessment, and performance improvement
- Biomedical and health services research support
- Health information services management
- A capstone experience/practicum/project

Health Information Technician

Graduates of associate degree programs are known as health information technicians and conduct health data collection, monitoring, maintenance, and reporting activities in accordance with established data quality principles, legal and regulatory standards, and professional best practice guidelines. These functions encompass, among other areas, monitoring electronic and paper-based documentation and processing and using health data for billing and reporting purposes through use of various electronic systems. Common job titles held by health information technicians in today's job market include reimbursement specialist, information access and disclosure specialist, coder, medical record technician, data quality coordinator, supervisor, etc. It is anticipated that job titles will change as health care enterprises expand their reliance on information systems and technology. Health information technicians have, and will continue to assume, roles that support efforts toward the development of computer-based patient record systems and a national health information infrastructure.

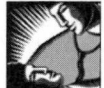

Career Description

The tasks or functions performed by health information technicians are numerous and continually changing within the work environment. The job title and work setting will dictate the actual tasks performed by the health information technician. However, in general, these individuals perform tasks related to the use, analysis, validation, presentation, data abstracting, analysis, coding, release of information, data privacy and security, retrieval, quality measurement, and control of health care data regardless of the physical medium in which information is maintained. Their task responsibilities may also include supervising personnel.

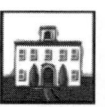

Employment Characteristics

Presently, opportunities for practice are found in numerous settings such as acute care general hospitals, managed care organizations, physician office practices, home health care agencies, long-term care facilities, correctional facilities, behavioral health care organizations, insurance companies, ambulatory settings, and state and federal health care agencies, and public health departments. Practice opportunities are unlimited.

Salary

According to AHIMA, entry-level salaries average between $25,000 and $50,000. Refer to Section IV, Table 5 of this *Directory* for more information, or see www.ama-assn.org/go/hpsalary.

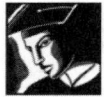

Educational Programs

Length. Programs are generally 2 years, offering an associate degree.

Prerequisites. High school diploma or equivalent.

Curriculum. In addition to general education courses, the professional component of the technician program requires:

- Biomedical sciences (anatomy, physiology, language of medicine, disease processes, and pharmacology)
- Information technology (microcomputer applications and computers in health care)
- Health data content and structure
- Health care delivery systems, organization and supervision, health care statistics, and data literacy
- Clinical quality assessment and performance improvement
- Clinical classification systems
- Reimbursement methodologies
- Legal and ethical issues
- Supervised professional practice experiences in health information departments of health care facilities and agencies

Inquiries

Careers and Credentialing
American Health Information Management Association
233 N Michigan Avenue, Suite 2150
Chicago, IL 60601-5800
312 233-1100
www.ahima.org

Program Accreditation
Commission on Accreditation for Health Informatics and Information Management Education (CAHIIM)
233 N Michigan Avenue, Suite 2150
Chicago, IL 60601-5800
312 233-1129
312 233-1429 Fax
E-mail: george.payan@cahiim.org
www.cahiim.org

Health Information Administrator

Alabama

University of Alabama at Birmingham
Health Information Admin Prgm
1675 University Blvd
Webb 550
Birmingham, AL 35294-3361
www.uab.edu/him
Prgm Dir: Kay R Clements, MA RHIA CCS
Tel: 205 975-0809   *Fax:* 205 934-5980
E-mail: kclement@uab.edu

Alabama State University
Health Information Admin Prgm
PO Box 271
Montgomery, AL 36101-0271
Prgm Dir: Nina Vick-Abro, MEd RHIA
Tel: 334 229-5058   *Fax:* 334 229-5880
E-mail: nabro@alasu.edu

Arkansas

Arkansas Tech University
Health Information Admin Prgm
1311 N El Paso Ave, T5
Russellville, AR 72801
www.atu.edu
Prgm Dir: Melinda Wilkins, MEd RHIA
Tel: 479 968-0441   *Fax:* 479 964-0504
E-mail: mwilkins@atu.edu

California

Loma Linda University
Health Information Admin Prgm
1905 Nichol Hall
Loma Linda, CA 92350
www.llu.edu/llu/sahp/health/#program
Prgm Dir: Marilyn R Davidian, MA RHIA
Tel: 909 558-4976   *Fax:* 909 558-0404
E-mail: mdavidian@llu.edu

Colorado

Regis University
Health Information Admin Prgm
3333 Regis Blvd
Denver, CO 80221-1099
Prgm Dir: Sheila A Carlon, PhD RHIA
Tel: 303 458-4108   *Fax:* 303 964-5533
E-mail: scarlon@regis.edu

Florida

Florida International University
Health Information Admin Prgm
11200 SW 8th St, HLS 146
Miami, FL 33199
Prgm Dir: Sandra McDonald, MHSA RHIA
Tel: 305 348-0406   *Fax:* 305 348-0437
E-mail: mcdons@fiu.edu

University of Central Florida
Health Information Admin Prgm
PO Box 162200
Orlando, FL 32816-2205
www.cohpa.ucf.edu/health.pro/him/
Prgm Dir: Alice Noblin, MBA RHIA
Tel: 407 823-2353   *Fax:* 407 823-6138
E-mail: anoblin@mail.ucf.edu

Florida A&M University
Health Information Admin Prgm
324 Lewis-Beck Allied Health Building
Tallahassee, FL 32307
www.famu.edu
Prgm Dir: Marjorie H McNeill, PhD RHIA CCS
Tel: 850 561-2021   *Fax:* 850 561-2457
E-mail: marjorie.mcneill@famu.edu

Georgia

Medical College of Georgia
Health Information Admin Prgm
Bldg AL-130
1120 15th St
Augusta, GA 30912-0400
Prgm Dir: Carol A Campbell, DBA RHIA
Tel: 706 721-3436   *Fax:* 706 721-6067
E-mail: cacampbe@mail.mcg.edu

Macon State College
Health Information Admin Prgm
100 College Station Dr
Macon, GA 31206-5144
Prgm Dir: Nanette Sayles, EdD RHIA CCS CHP
Tel: 478 471-2788   *Fax:* 478 417-2787
E-mail: nsayles@mail.maconstate.edu

Illinois

Chicago State University
Health Information Admin Prgm
9501 S King Dr, BHS 610
Chicago, IL 60628-1598
Prgm Dir: Leona M Thomas, MHS RHIA
Tel: 773 995-2593   *Fax:* 773 995-4484
E-mail: lmthomas@msn.com

University of Illinois at Chicago
Health Information Admin Prgm
College of Applied Health Sciences
1919 W Taylor St, M/C 250
Chicago, IL 60612
Prgm Dir: Karen Patena, MBA RHIA
Tel: 312 996-1444   *Fax:* 312 996-8342
E-mail: patena@uic.edu

Illinois State University
Health Information Admin Prgm
5220 Health Sciences
Normal, IL 61790-5220
www.healthsciences.ilstu.edu/health_info_management/
Prgm Dir: Francis L Waterstraat, Jr, PhD RHIA
Tel: 309 438-8809   *Fax:* 309 438-2450
E-mail: fwaterst@ilstu.edu

Indiana

Indiana University
Health Information Admin Prgm
School of Informatics
ICTC 475, 535 W Michigan St
Indianapolis, IN 46202
Prgm Dir: Danita Forgey, MIS RHIA CCS-P CCS
Tel: 317 278-4113   *Fax:* 317 278-7859
E-mail: dforgey@iupui.edu

Kansas

University of Kansas Medical Center
Health Information Admin Prgm
Taylor 1012, Mail Stop 2008
3901 Rainbow Blvd
Kansas City, KS 66160
www.him.kumc.edu
Prgm Dir: Karl Koob, MMIS RHIA CPEHR
Tel: 913 588-2423   *Fax:* 913 588-2428
E-mail: kkoob@kumc.edu

Kentucky

Eastern Kentucky University
Health Information Admin Prgm
521 Lancaster Ave
Richmond, KY 40475-3102
Prgm Dir: Dawn W Jackson, MAEd RHIA
Tel: 859 622-1915   *Fax:* 859 622-2013
E-mail: dawn.jackson@eku.edu

Louisiana

University of Louisiana at Lafayette
Health Information Admin Prgm
College of Sciences
PO Box 41007
Lafayette, LA 70504
http://him.louisiana.edu
Prgm Dir: Carol Venable, MPH RHIA FAHIMA
Tel: 337 482-6629   *Fax:* 337 482-5902
E-mail: venable@louisiana.edu

Louisiana Tech University
Health Information Admin Prgm
Health Information Management Program
PO Box 3171
Ruston, LA 71272
Prgm Dir: Angela Kennedy, MBA RHIA CPHQ
Tel: 318 257-2854   *Fax:* 318 257-4896
E-mail: kennedy@him.latech.edu

Michigan

Ferris State University
Health Information Admin Prgm
Coll of Allied Health Sciences
200 Ferris Dr, VFS 402
Big Rapids, MI 49307-2740
www.ferris.edu/htmls/colleges/alliedhe/MR/
Prgm Dir: Ellen J Haneline, PhD RHIA
Tel: 231 591-2269   *Fax:* 231 591-2325
E-mail: haneline@ferris.edu

Minnesota

College of St Scholastica
Health Information Admin Prgm
1200 Kenwood Ave
Duluth, MN 55811
Prgm Dir: Kathleen M LaTour, MA RHIA FAHIMA
Tel: 218 723-6011   *Fax:* 218 733-2239
E-mail: klatour@css.edu

Mississippi

University of Mississippi Medical Center
Health Information Admin Prgm
Health Information Management Program
2500 N State St
Jackson, MS 39216
Prgm Dir: Rebecca J Yates, MEd RHIA
Tel: 601 984-6305   *Fax:* 601 815-1717
E-mail: byates@shrp.umsmed.edu

Missouri

Stephens College
Health Information Admin Prgm
Campus Box 2083
1200 East Broadway
Columbia, MO 65215
Prgm Dir: Darla D Branda, MA RHIA
Tel: 573 876-7125   *Fax:* 573 876-2320
E-mail: dbranda@stephens.edu

Saint Louis University Doisy College of Health Sciences
Health Information Admin Prgm
Department of Health Informatics and Information Management
3437 Caroline St
St Louis, MO 63104
Prgm Dir: Jody Smith, PhD RHIA FAHIMA
Tel: 314 977-8516   *Fax:* 314 977-8503
E-mail: smithjk@slu.edu

Nebraska

College of Saint Mary
Health Information Admin Prgm
7000 Mercy Rd
Omaha, NE 68106
Prgm Dir: Ellen B Jacobs, MEd RHIA
Tel: 402 399-2611   *Fax:* 402 399-2657
E-mail: ejacobs@csm.edu

New Jersey

Kean University
Cosponsor: University of Medicine and Dentistry of New Jersey
Health Information Admin Prgm
Health Information Management Program
65 Bergen St, SB 350
Newark, NJ 07107
www.umdnj.edu
Prgm Dir: Barbara Manger, MPA RHIA CCS FAHIMA
Tel: 973 972-6499
E-mail: mangerbj@umdnj.edu

New York

Long Island University - C W Post Campus
Health Information Admin Prgm
720 Northern Blvd
School of Health Professions
Brookville, NY 11548
Prgm Dir: Kerry Kimmins-Lawrence, MHA RHIA
Tel: 516 299-2485   *Fax:* 516 299-2527
E-mail: kkimmins@nshs.edu

SUNY Institute of Tech - Utica/Rome
Health Information Admin Prgm
PO Box 3050
Utica, NY 13504-3050
Prgm Dir: Donna L Silsbee, PhD RHIA
Tel: 315 792-7391   *Fax:* 315 792-7555
E-mail: Donna.Silsbee@sunyit.edu

North Carolina

Western Carolina University
Health Information Admin Prgm
126 Moore Hall
Cullowhee, NC 28723
http://hs.wcu.edu/HS_UG-hia.htm
Prgm Dir: Irene Mueller, EdD RHIA
Tel: 828 227-3510   *Fax:* 828 227-7446
E-mail: imueller@email.wcu.edu

East Carolina University
Health Information Admin Prgm
School of Allied Hlth Sciences
Health Sciences Building 4340-D
Greenville, NC 27858
www.ecu.edu/cs-dhs/hsim/him.cfm
Prgm Dir: Elizabeth J Layman, PhD RHIA FAHIMA
Tel: 252 744-6177   *Fax:* 252 744-6179
E-mail: laymane@ecu.edu

Ohio

University of Cincinnati
Health Information Admin Prgm
College of Allied Health Sciences, French East Bldg
3202 Eden Ave
Cincinnati, OH 45267
Prgm Dir: Gail Smith, MA RHIA CCS-P
Tel: 513 558-8512
E-mail: gail.smith@uc.edu

Ohio State University
Health Information Admin Prgm
453 W 10th Ave, Rm 543
Columbus, OH 43210-1234
Prgm Dir: Melanie Brodnik, PhD RHIA
Tel: 614 292-0567   *Fax:* 614 292-0210
E-mail: melanie.brodnik@osumc.edu

University of Toledo
Health Information Admin Prgm
2801 W Bancroft St
Mail Stop 119
Toledo, OH 43606-3390
Prgm Dir: Maria A Janes, MEd RHIA
Tel: 419 530-4523
E-mail: marie.janes@utoledo.edu

Oklahoma

East Central University
Health Information Admin Prgm
Department of Health Information Management
1100 E 14th St
Ada, OK 74820
Prgm Dir: Sandra A Dixon, MEd MCE RHIA
Tel: 580 310-5555   *Fax:* 580 310-5606
E-mail: sdixon@mailclerk.ecok.edu

Southwestern Oklahoma State University
Health Information Admin Prgm
100 Campus Dr
Weatherford, OK 73096
https://www.swosu.edu
Prgm Dir: Marion Prichard, MEd RHIA
Tel: 580 774-3287, Ext 3287   *Fax:* 580 774-7159
E-mail: marion.prichard@swosu.edu

Pennsylvania

Gwynedd-Mercy College
Health Information Admin Prgm
1325 Sumneytown Pike
Gwynedd Valley, PA 19437
Prgm Dir: Christine Staropoli, MS RHIA CCS
Tel: 215 542-4660   *Fax:* 215 641-5559
E-mail: staropoli.c@gmc.edu

Temple University
Health Information Admin Prgm
College of Health Professions
3307 N Broad St
Philadelphia, PA 19140
Prgm Dir: Laurinda B Harman, PhD RHIA
Tel: 215 707-4823   *Fax:* 215 707-5852
E-mail: Laurinda.Harman@temple.edu

Duquesne University
Health Information Admin Prgm
Dept of Health Mgmt Systems
431 Fisher Hall
Pittsburgh, PA 15282-0001
Prgm Dir: Kathleen Begler, MPM RHIA
Tel: 412 396-4772   *Fax:* 412 396-5554
E-mail: begler@duq.edu

University of Pittsburgh
Health Information Admin Prgm
6051 Forbes Tower
Pittsburgh, PA 15260
www.him.pitt.edu
Prgm Dir: Mervat Abdelhak, PhD RHIA
Tel: 412 383-6650   *Fax:* 412 383-6655
E-mail: abdelhak@pitt.edu

Puerto Rico

University of Puerto Rico
Health Information Admin Prgm
GPO Box 365067
San Juan, PR 00936-5067
http://cprsweb.rcm.upr.edu/adminfsalud.asp
Prgm Dir: Anna Orabona-Ocasio, EdD RHIA CCS
Tel: 787 758-2525, Ext 4507   *Fax:* 787 764-3609
E-mail: anaorabona@cprs.rcm.upr.edu

South Dakota

Dakota State University
Health Information Admin Prgm
East Hall
Madison, SD 57042-1799
www.dsu.edu
Prgm Dir: Dorine Bennett, MBA RHIA
Tel: 605 256-5137   *Fax:* 605 256-5060
E-mail: dorine.bennett@dsu.edu

Tennessee

University of Tennessee Health Science Ctr
Health Information Admin Prgm
Dept of Health Information Management
920 Madison Ave, Ste 518
Memphis, TN 38163
Prgm Dir: Elizabeth Bowman, MPA RHIA
Tel: 901 448-6486   *Fax:* 901 448-1629
E-mail: ebowman@utmem.edu

Tennessee State University
Health Information Admin Prgm
3500 John A Merritt Blvd
Nashville, TN 37209-1561
Prgm Dir: Elizabeth I Kunnu, MEd RHIA
Tel: 615 963-7441   *Fax:* 615 963-7498
E-mail: ekunnu@tnstate.edu

Texas

Texas Southern University
Health Information Admin Prgm
3100 Cleburne Ave
Houston, TX 77004
Prgm Dir: Fanny Hawkins, EdD RRA RHIA CPHQ
Tel: 713 313-7341   *Fax:* 713 313-1094
E-mail: Hawkins_FC@tsu.edu

Texas State University - San Marcos
Health Information Admin Prgm
601 University Dr
San Marcos, TX 78666
www.health.txstate.edu/him
Prgm Dir: Sue E Biedermann, MSHP RHIA
Tel: 512 245-8242   *Fax:* 512 245-8258
E-mail: sb02@txstate.edu

Utah

Weber State University
Health Information Admin Prgm
3911 University Circle
Ogden, UT 84408-3911
Prgm Dir: Patricia L Shaw, MEd RHIA
Tel: 801 626-7989   *Fax:* 801 626-6475
E-mail: pshaw@weber.edu

Washington

University of Washington
Health Information Admin Prgm
Health Informatics and Health Information Management
1100 NE 45th, Ste 405, Box F
Seattle, WA 98105
http://depts.washington.edu/hihim/
Prgm Dir: Gretchen Murphy, MEd RHIA FAHIMA
Tel: 206 543-8810   *Fax:* 206 616-5249
E-mail: gcmurphy@u.washington.edu

Health Information Administrator

	Class Capacity	Begins	Length (months)	Award	Res. Tuition	Non-res. Tuition	Stipend	Offers:‡ 1	2	3	4
Alabama											
University of Alabama at Birmingham	30	Fall	21, 45	Cert, BS	$6,327	$12,654		•			•
Arkansas											
Arkansas Tech University (Russellville)	30	Aug	37	BS	$3,432	$6,864		•			
California											
Loma Linda University	60	Sep	26, 9	Cert, BS	$21,000	$21,000				•	
Florida											
Florida A&M University (Tallahassee)	30	Aug	48	BS	$101	$498		•		•	
University of Central Florida (Orlando)	32	Aug	24	BS	$2,211	$12,870					•
Illinois											
Illinois State University (Normal)	30	Aug	24	BS	$6,500	$13,500					
Kansas											
University of Kansas Medical Center (Kansas City)	24	Aug	24	BS	$6,818	$17,909					•
Louisiana											
University of Louisiana at Lafayette	45	Aug	48	BS	$3,424	$9,604					
Michigan											
Ferris State University (Big Rapids)	20	Aug	48	BS	$7,200	$14,640		•		•	
Minnesota											
College of St Scholastica (Duluth)	40	Sep	24	BA, MA	$23,434	$0					•
Missouri											
Saint Louis University Doisy College of Health Sciences (St Louis)	25	Aug Jan	48	BS	$26,250	$26,250					
New Jersey											
Kean University (Newark)	25	Sep	48, 60	BS, BS/MS	$3,753	$5,069		•			•
North Carolina											
East Carolina University (Greenville)	30	Aug	18	BS	$4,003	$14,517				•	•
Western Carolina University (Cullowhee)	18	Aug	20	BS	$4,871	$14,454					
Ohio											
Ohio State University (Columbus)	25	Sep	18	Cert, BS	$4,383	$12,732					
University of Cincinnati			27	Dipl, BS	$262	$272					•
Oklahoma											
Southwestern Oklahoma State University (Weatherford)	16	Aug	24	BS	$3,680	$8,480			•		
Pennsylvania											
Duquesne University (Pittsburgh)	30	Aug Jan May	48, 60	BS, MHMS	$17,000	$17,000		•			
University of Pittsburgh	35	Sep Jan Apr	18, 24	BS, MS/PhD	$14,308	$26,290					
Puerto Rico											
University of Puerto Rico (San Juan)	10	Aug	21	MS	$6,029	$6,029		•		•	•
South Dakota											
Dakota State University (Madison)	30	Sep	48	BS	$2,643	$3,963					•
Texas											
Texas State University - San Marcos	50	Aug	22	BS	$7,000	$16,000				•	•
Utah											
Weber State University (Ogden)	20	Open	24	Dipl, BS	$2,988	$10,495		•		•	
Washington											
University of Washington (Seattle)	40	Jun	12	Cert, BS	$15,200	$15,200		•			

*Data are shown only for programs that completed the 2007 AMA Survey of Health Professions Education Programs.
‡Key to Offers: 1: Evening or weekend classes; 2: Non-English instruction; 3: Cultural competence instruction; 4: Distance education component.

Health Information Technician

Alabama

Wallace State Community College
Health Information Tech Prgm
Bevill Health Education Bldg
PO Box 2000
Hanceville, AL 35077-9080
Prgm Dir: Donna S Stanley, EdS RHIA
Tel: 256 352-8327   *Fax:* 256 352-8320
E-mail: donna.stanley@wallacestate.edu

Bishop State Community College
Health Information Tech Prgm
1365 Martin Luther King Ave
Mobile, AL 36603
Prgm Dir: Annalesia Sharp, RHIA
Tel: 334 405-4451   *Fax:* 334 405-4505
E-mail: asharp@bishop.edu

Alaska

University of Alaska Southeast
Health Information Tech Prgm
UAS Sitka Campus
1332 Seward Ave
Sitka, AK 99835-9498
www.uas.alaska.edu
Prgm Dir: Leslie Gordon, RHIA
Tel: 907 747-9474   *Fax:* 907 747-7731
E-mail: leslie.gordon@uas.alaska.edu

Arizona

Phoenix College
Health Information Tech Prgm
1202 W Thomas Rd
Phoenix, AZ 85013
Prgm Dir: Bonnie Petterson, PhD RHIA
Tel: 602 285-7149   *Fax:* 602 285-7528
E-mail: b.petterson@pcmail.maricopa.edu

Arkansas

National Park Community College
Health Information Tech Prgm
101 College Dr
Hot Springs, AR 71913-9174
Prgm Dir: Valerie Bond, MA RHIA
Tel: 501 760-4294   *Fax:* 501 760-4141
E-mail: vbond@npcc.edu

University of Arkansas for Medical Sciences
Health Information Tech Prgm
4301 W Markham St, Slot 733
Little Rock, AR 72205
Prgm Dir: Kathy C Trawick, EdD RHIA
Tel: 501 686-8613   *Fax:* 501 686-8519
E-mail: trawickkathyc@uams.edu

California

Cypress College
Health Information Tech Prgm
9200 Valley View St
Cypress, CA 90630
www.cypresscollege.edu
Prgm Dir: Rosalie Majid, RHIA
Tel: 714 484-7289   *Fax:* 714 484-7300
E-mail: rmajid@cypresscollege.edu

Fresno City College
Health Information Tech Prgm
1101 E University Ave
Fresno, CA 93741
Prgm Dir: Sarah Edwards, RHIA
Tel: 559 244-2640   *Fax:* 559 244-2626
E-mail: sarah.edwards@fresnocitycollege.edu

Chabot College
Health Information Tech Prgm
25555 Hesperian Blvd
Hayward, CA 94545-5001
Prgm Dir: Wanda Ziemba, MFA RHIT BA
Tel: 510 723-7496   *Fax:* 510 656-7492
E-mail: wziemba@chabotcollege.edu

Charles R Drew Univ of Med & Science
Health Information Tech Prgm
1731 E 120th St
Los Angeles, CA 90059
Prgm Dir: Dorothy Hendrix, MEd RHIT
Tel: 323 563-5888   *Fax:* 323 563-5898
E-mail: dohendri@cdrewu.edu

East Los Angeles College
Health Information Tech Prgm
1301 Avenida Cesar Chavez
Monterey Park, CA 91754-6099
Prgm Dir: Elizabeth Garcia
Tel: 323 265-8883   *Fax:* 323 265-8876
E-mail: garciaea@elac.edu

DeVry University - Pomona Campus
Health Information Tech Prgm
901 Corporate Center Dr
Pomona, CA 91768
Prgm Dir: Shirley Lewis, MHA RHIA CPHQ
Tel: 909 868-4023
E-mail: slewis@devry.edu

Cosumnes River Community College
Health Information Tech Prgm
8401 Center Pkwy
Sacramento, CA 95823-5799
Prgm Dir: George Hines, RHIA RHIT
Tel: 916 691-7452   *Fax:* 916 691-7146
E-mail: hinesg@crc.losrios.edu

San Diego Mesa College
Health Information Tech Prgm
7250 Mesa College Dr
San Diego, CA 92111
www.sdmesa.sdccd.cc.ca.us
Prgm Dir: Teddy L Scribner, MS RHIA
Tel: 619 388-2606   *Fax:* 619 279-5668
E-mail: tscribne@sdccd.edu

City College of San Francisco
Health Information Tech Prgm
John Adams Campus
1860 Hayes St
San Francisco, CA 94117
Prgm Dir: Marie T Conde, MPA RHIT CCS
Tel: 415 561-1818   *Fax:* 415 561-1861
E-mail: mconde@ccsf.edu

Santa Barbara City College
Health Information Tech Prgm
721 Cliff Dr
Santa Barbara, CA 93109-2394
www.sbcc.edu
Prgm Dir: Kathleen Peterson, MS RHIA CCS
Tel: 805 965-0581, Ext 2851   *Fax:* 805 963-7222
E-mail: petersok@sbcc.edu

Colorado

Arapahoe Community College
Health Information Tech Prgm
5900 S Santa Fe Dr, POB 9002
Littleton, CO 80160-9002
Prgm Dir: Annette Bigalk, RHIA
Tel: 303 795-5795   *Fax:* 303 797-5842
E-mail: annette.bigalk@arapahoe.edu

Connecticut

Briarwood College
Health Information Tech Prgm
2279 Mt Vernon Rd
Southington, CT 06489
Prgm Dir: Phyllis Hilt, MBA RHIA
Tel: 860 628-4751, Ext 186   *Fax:* 860 276-8838
E-mail: hiltp@briarwood.edu

Florida

Broward Community College
Health Information Tech Prgm
Ctr for Hlth Science Educ
1000 Coconut Creek Blvd
Coconut Creek, FL 33066
Prgm Dir: Charline Bumgardner, BA RHIT
Tel: 954 201-2086   *Fax:* 954 201-2348
E-mail: cbumgard@broward.edu

Daytona Beach Community College
Health Information Tech Prgm
PO Box 2811
Daytona Beach, FL 32120-2811
www.dbcc.edu
Prgm Dir: Nancy Thomas, EdD RHIA
Tel: 386 506-3748   *Fax:* 386 506-3300
E-mail: thomasn@dbcc.edu

International College
Health Information Tech Prgm
4501 Colonial Blvd
Fort Myers, FL 33912
Prgm Dir: Deborah Howard, MA RHIA CCS
Tel: 239 482-0019
E-mail: dhoward@internationalcollege.edu

Indian River Community College
Health Information Tech Prgm
3209 Virginia Ave
Fort Pierce, FL 34981-5599
Prgm Dir: Claudia Keating, MEd RHIA
Tel: 772 462-4911   *Fax:* 772 462-4900
E-mail: ckeating@ircc.edu

Santa Fe Community College
Health Information Tech Prgm
Health Information Management Program
3000 NW 83rd St, A07K
Gainesville, FL 32606
www.santafe.edu
Prgm Dir: Karen Bakuzonis, MSHA RHIA
Tel: 352 381-3835   *Fax:* 352 395-5286
E-mail: karen.bakuzonis@sfcc.edu

Florida Community College - Jacksonville
Health Information Tech Prgm
4501 Capper Rd
Jacksonville, FL 32218
Prgm Dir: Eudelia S Thomas, MS RHIA
Tel: 904 766-6663   *Fax:* 904 766-5565
E-mail: ethomas@fccj.edu

Lake-Sumter Community College
Health Information Tech Prgm
9501 US Hwy 441
Leesburg, FL 34788-8751
www.lscc.edu
Prgm Dir: Brandy G Ziesemer, MA RHIA CCS
Tel: 352 435-6414
E-mail: ziesemerb@lscc.edu

Miami Dade College
Health Information Tech Prgm
Medical Center Campus
950 NW 20th St
Miami, FL 33127
www.mdc.edu/medical/
Prgm Dir: Mary Worsley, RHIA
Tel: 305 237-4156   *Fax:* 305 237-4278
E-mail: mworsley@mdc.edu

Central Florida Community College
Health Information Tech Prgm
3001 SW College Rd
Ocala, FL 34474
Prgm Dir: Suzanne B Garrett, MSA RHIA
Tel: 352 854-2322, Ext 1466   *Fax:* 352 873-5870
E-mail: garretts@cf.edu

St Johns River Community College
Health Information Tech Prgm
Orange Park Campus
283 College Dr
Orange Park, FL 32065
Prgm Dir: Sheila Newberry, MEd RHIT
Tel: 904 276-6758   *Fax:* 904 276-6888
E-mail: SheilaNewberry@sjrcc.edu

Pensacola Junior College
Health Information Tech Prgm
Dept of Allied Health
1000 College Blvd
Pensacola, FL 32504
Prgm Dir: Donna M Shumway, MEd RHIA
Tel: 904 484-2213   *Fax:* 904 484-2375
E-mail: dshumway@pjc.edu

St Petersburg College
Health Information Tech Prgm
PO Box 13489
St Petersburg, FL 33733
Prgm Dir: Angela Picard, MEd RHIA
Tel: 727 341-3623   *Fax:* 727 341-3455
E-mail: picard.angela@spcollege.edu

Polk Community College
Health Information Tech Prgm
999 Avenue H NE
Winter Haven, FL 33881
www.polk.edu
Prgm Dir: Hertencia Bowe, MSA RHIA
Tel: 863 297-1010, Ext 5370   *Fax:* 863 297-1034
E-mail: hbowe@polk.edu

Georgia

Darton College
Health Information Tech Prgm
2400 Gillionville Rd
Albany, GA 31707
Prgm Dir: Linda Parks, MA RHIT CCS
Tel: 229 317-6894   *Fax:* 229 317-6682
E-mail: linda.parks@darton.edu

DeVry University - Atlanta
Health Information Tech Prgm
250 N Arcadia Ave
Decatur, GA 30030-2198
Prgm Dir: Kristyn Murphy-Rodvill, MHA RHIA
Tel: 404 292-7900, Ext 2123
E-mail: kmurphy-rodvill@faculty.atl.devry.edu

Macon State College
Health Information Tech Prgm
100 College Station Dr
Macon, GA 31206-5145
Prgm Dir: Nanette Sayles, EdD RHIA CCS CHP
Tel: 478 471-2788   *Fax:* 478 471-2787
E-mail: nsayles@mail.maconstate.edu

Ogeechee Technical College
Health Information Tech Prgm
1 Joe Kennedy Blvd
Statesboro, GA 30458
Prgm Dir: Lisa Parker Kagay, MBA RHIA
Tel: 912 486-7792   *Fax:* 912 486-7604
E-mail: lkagay@ogeecheetech.edu

Idaho

Boise State University
Health Information Tech Prgm
College of Health Science
1910 University Dr
Boise, ID 83725
Prgm Dir: Patricia Elison-Bowers, PhD RHIA
Tel: 208 426-1130   *Fax:* 208 426-2199
E-mail: pelison@boisestate.edu

Idaho State University
Health Information Tech Prgm
Campus Box 8380
Pocatello, ID 83209-8380
Prgm Dir: Glenna Young, RHIA CCS
Tel: 208 282-4524   *Fax:* 208 282-3975
E-mail: younglen@isu.edu

Illinois

Southwestern Illinois College
Health Information Tech Prgm
2500 Carlyle Ave
Belleville, IL 62221
www.swic.edu
Prgm Dir: Wendy Holder, RHIA
Tel: 618 235-2700, Ext 5385   *Fax:* 618 235-2052
E-mail: wendy.holder@swic.edu

DeVry University - Chicago
Health Information Tech Prgm
3300 N Campbell Ave
Chicago, IL 60618
Prgm Dir: Patricia Hertel, MA RHIT
Tel: 773 697-2147
E-mail: phertel@chi.devry.edu

Northwestern Business College
Health Information Tech Prgm
4811 N Milwaukee Ave
Chicago, IL 60630
Prgm Dir: Joni Rudd, RHIA
Tel: 773 777-4200, Ext 2319   *Fax:* 708 237-5005
E-mail: jrudd@nwbc.edu

Danville Area Community College
Health Information Tech Prgm
2000 E Main St
Danville, IL 61832
www.dacc.cc.il.us/
Prgm Dir: Janet M Westberg, MS RHIA
Tel: 217 443-8574   *Fax:* 217 443-8595
E-mail: janwest@dacc.edu

Oakton Community College
Health Information Tech Prgm
1600 E Golf Rd
Des Plaines, IL 60016
www.oakton.edu/acad/dept/hit/
Prgm Dir: Anita Taylor, MEd RHIA CCS
Tel: 847 635-1957   *Fax:* 847 635-1764
E-mail: anitat@oakton.edu

College of DuPage
Health Information Tech Prgm
425 Fawell Blvd
Glen Ellyn, IL 60137-6599
Prgm Dir: Kim D Pack, MS RHIA
Tel: 630 942-2532   *Fax:* 630 858-9399
E-mail: packki@cod.edu

College of Lake County
Health Information Tech Prgm
19351 W Washington St
Grayslake, IL 60030-1198
Prgm Dir: Margaret Kyriakos, MBA RHIA
Tel: 847 543-2879   *Fax:* 847 223-1357
E-mail: mkyriakos@clcillinois.edu

Southern Illinois Collegiate Common Market
Health Information Tech Prgm
3213 S Park Ave
Herrin, IL 62948
www.siccm.com
Prgm Dir: Mary J Sullivan, PhD RHIA
Tel: 618 942-6902   *Fax:* 618 942-6658
E-mail: sullivan@siccm.com
Notes: Currently inactive

DeVry University - Naperville
Health Information Tech Prgm
1200 E Diehl Rd
Naperville, IL 60563
Prgm Dir: Natasha Freeman Cauley, MPH RHIA
Tel: 404 494-9417
E-mail: ncauley@devry.edu

Moraine Valley Community College
Health Information Tech Prgm
10900 S 88th Ave
Palos Hills, IL 60465
Prgm Dir: Donna Schnepp, RHIA
Tel: 708 974-5315   *Fax:* 708 974-0185
E-mail: schnepp@morainevalley.edu

Indiana

Indiana University Northwest
Health Information Tech Prgm
3400 Broadway St
Gary, IN 46408
Prgm Dir: Margaret A Skurka, MS RHIA CCS
Tel: 219 980-6654   *Fax:* 219 980-6649
E-mail: mskurk@iun.edu

Vincennes University
Health Information Tech Prgm
1002 N First St
Vincennes, IN 47591-9986
www.vinu.edu
Prgm Dir: Sharon O'Neill, MS RHIA
Tel: 812 888-4411   *Fax:* 812 888-4550
E-mail: soneill@vinu.edu

Iowa

Scott Community College
Health Information Tech Prgm
500 Belmont Rd
Bettendorf, IA 52722
www.eicc.edu/highschool/programs/career/
Prgm Dir: Barbara A Foster, BA RHIA CTR
Tel: 563 441-4157   *Fax:* 563 441-4204
E-mail: bfoster@eicc.edu

Northeast Iowa Community College
Health Information Tech Prgm
1625 Hwy 150 South
PO Box 400
Calmar, IA 52132
Prgm Dir: Shawna Sweeney, RHIA
Tel: 563 562-3263, Ext 345   *Fax:* 563 562-4357
E-mail: sweeneys@nicc.edu

Kirkwood Community College
Health Information Tech Prgm
6301 Kirkwood Blvd SW, PO Box 2068
Cedar Rapids, IA 52406-9973
Prgm Dir: Betty Haar, BS RHIA
Tel: 319 398-4923 *Fax:* 319 398-1293
E-mail: betty.haar@kirkwood.edu

Indian Hills Community College
Health Information Tech Prgm
Health Occupations Division Arts and Science Center
525 Grandview Ave, Bldg 6
Ottumwa, IA 52501
Prgm Dir: Heidi Jones, BS RHIA
Tel: 641 683-5163 *Fax:* 641 683-5254
E-mail: hjones@indianhills.edu

Northwest Iowa Community College
Health Information Tech Prgm
603 W Park St
Sheldon, IA 51201
Prgm Dir: Mari Beth Lane, RHIA
Tel: 712 324-5061, Ext 223 *Fax:* 712 324-4136
E-mail: MLane@nwicc.edu

Kansas

Hutchinson Community College
Health Information Tech Prgm
Area Voc School
1300 N Plum
Hutchinson, KS 67501
www.hutchcc.edu
Prgm Dir: Loretta A Horton, MEd RHIA
Tel: 316 694-2455 *Fax:* 316 665-4988
E-mail: hortonl@hutchcc.edu

Washburn University
Health Information Tech Prgm
1700 College Ave SW
Topeka, KS 66621
Prgm Dir: Michelle Shipley, MS RHIA CCS
Tel: 785 670-2174
E-mail: michelle.shipley@washburn.edu

Kentucky

Western Kentucky University
Health Information Tech Prgm
South Campus
Bowling Green, KY 42101
Prgm Dir: Karen C Sansom, MS RHIA
Tel: 270 780-2567 *Fax:* 270 780-2591
E-mail: karen.sansom@wku.edu

Jefferson Community and Technical College
Health Information Tech Prgm
109 E Broadway St
Louisville, KY 40202
Prgm Dir: Elizabeth Neichter, EdD RHIA
Tel: 502 213-2199 *Fax:* 502 213-2343
E-mail: elizabeth.neichter@kctcs.edu

National College - Louisville
Health Information Tech Prgm
4205 Dixie Hwy
Louisville, KY 40216
http://national-college.edu
Prgm Dir: Kristie Couch, RHIA
Tel: 502 447-7634 *Fax:* 502 447-7665
E-mail: kcouch@national-college.edu

Louisiana

Delgado Community College
Health Information Tech Prgm
615 City Park Ave
New Orleans, LA 70119-4399
Prgm Dir: Melissa LaCour, RHIA
Tel: 504 671-6219 *Fax:* 504 483-4609
E-mail: mlacou@dcc.edu

Louisiana Tech University
Health Information Tech Prgm
PO Box 3171
Ruston, LA 71272
Prgm Dir: Helen Baxter, MA RHIA
Tel: 318 257-2854 *Fax:* 318 257-4896
E-mail: baxter@him.latech.edu

Southern Univ at Shreveport
Health Information Tech Prgm
610 Texas St, Ste 328A
Shreveport, LA 71101
Prgm Dir: Kimberly Madden, RHIA
Tel: 318 674-3487 *Fax:* 318 676-3454
E-mail: kmadden@susla.edu

Maine

Kennebec Valley Community College
Health Information Tech Prgm
92 Western Ave
Fairfield, ME 04937
Prgm Dir: Sharon S Veilleux, MPA RHIT
Tel: 207 453-5156 *Fax:* 207 453-5197
E-mail: sveilleux@kvcc.me.edu

Maryland

Baltimore City Community College
Health Information Tech Prgm
2901 Liberty Heights Ave
Baltimore, MD 21215-7893
Prgm Dir: Betty Neely Mitchell, RHIA
Tel: 410 462-7735 *Fax:* 410 462-7734
E-mail: bmitchell@bccc.edu

Kaplan College
Health Information Tech Prgm
18618 Crestwood Dr
Hagerstown, MD 21742
Prgm Dir: Beth Shanholtzer, RHIA
Tel: 301 739-2680, Ext 152 *Fax:* 301 791-7661
E-mail: bshanholtzer@hagerstownbusinesscol.edu

Prince George's Community College
Health Information Tech Prgm
Health Information Management Program
301 Largo Rd
Largo, MD 20774-2199
http://academic.pgcc.edu/alliedhealth
Prgm Dir: Muriel Adams, RHIA CCS
Tel: 301 322-0735 *Fax:* 301 386-7528
E-mail: madams@pgcc.edu

Montgomery College
Health Information Tech Prgm
Health Information Management Program
7600 Takoma Ave
Takoma Park, MD 20912
Prgm Dir: Shirley Suzanne Meiskey, MSA RHIA
Tel: 240 567-5519 *Fax:* 240 567-5585
E-mail: sue.meiskey@montgomerycollege.edu

Massachusetts

Caritas Labour, College
Health Information Tech Prgm
2120 Dorchester Ave
Boston, MA 02124
www.laboure.edu
Prgm Dir: Nancy Entwistle, MPA RHIT CCS
Tel: 617 296-8300, Ext 4063
E-mail: Nancy_Entwistle@laboure.edu

Bristol Community College
Health Information Tech Prgm
777 Elsbree St
Fall River, MA 02777
Prgm Dir: Edward J Dobbs, BBA RHIA
Tel: 508 678-2811, Ext 2329 *Fax:* 508 675-2318
E-mail: edobbs@bristol.mass.edu

Fisher College
Health Information Tech Prgm
451 Elm St
North Attleboro, MA 02760
Prgm Dir: Patricia Parkes, RHIA
Tel: 508 699-6200
E-mail: pparkes@fisher.edu

Michigan

Baker College of Allen Park
Health Information Tech Prgm
4500 Enterprise Dr
Allen Park, MI 48101
Prgm Dir: Charmaine Irvin, MEd RHIA RHIT CCS
Tel: 313 425-3732
E-mail: charmaine.irvin@baker.edu

Ferris State University
Health Information Tech Prgm
Coll of Allied Health Sciences
200 Ferris Dr, VFS 402
Big Rapids, MI 49307-2740
Prgm Dir: Ellen J Haneline, PhD RHIA
Tel: 231 591-2269 *Fax:* 231 591-2325
E-mail: haneline@ferris.edu

Baker College of Flint
Health Information Tech Prgm
1050 W Bristol Rd
Flint, MI 48507
Prgm Dir: Amy Savage, MAT RHIA CCS
Tel: 810 766-4147 *Fax:* 810 766-2055
E-mail: amy.savage@baker.edu

Schoolcraft College
Health Information Tech Prgm
1751 Radcliff St
Garden City, MI 48135-1197
Prgm Dir: Patricia A Rubio, MSA RHIA
Tel: 734 462-4770, Ext 6025 *Fax:* 734 462-4775
E-mail: prubio@schoolcraft.edu

**Davenport University - Grand Rapids
(Fulton St)**
Health Information Tech Prgm
415 Fulton St E
Grand Rapids, MI 49503
www.davenport.edu
Prgm Dir: Susan Slajus, BS RHIA
Tel: 616 451-3511
E-mail: susan.slajus@davenport.edu

Minnesota

Anoka Technical College
Health Information Tech Prgm
1355 W Hwy 10
Anoka, MN 55303
Prgm Dir: Mary Ann Jackels, BA RHIA
Tel: 763 576-4970
E-mail: mjackels@ank.tec.mn.us

Rasmussen Colleges - Brooklyn Park
Health Information Tech Prgm
8301 93rd Ave N
Brooklyn Park, MN 55445
Prgm Dir: Cindy Glewwe, RHIA
Tel: 651 687-9000
E-mail: cindyg@rasmussen.edu

Rasmussen Colleges - Eagan
Health Information Tech Prgm
3500 Federal Dr
Eagan, MN 55122
Prgm Dir: Cindy Glewwe, RHIA
Tel: 651 687-9000 *Fax:* 651 687-0507
E-mail: cindyg@rasmussen.edu

College of St Catherine
Health Information Tech Prgm
601 25th Ave S
Minneapolis, MN 55454
Prgm Dir: Marsha Holey, RHIA
Tel: 651 690-7795   *Fax:* 651 690-7849
E-mail: mkholey@stkate.edu

Minnesota State Comm & Tech Coll - Moorhead
Health Information Tech Prgm
1900 28th Ave S
Moorhead, MN 56560
Prgm Dir: Susan Hanna, RHIT
Tel: 218 299-6558   *Fax:* 218 236-0342
E-mail: susan.hanna@minnesota.edu

Rochester Community & Technical College
Health Information Tech Prgm
851 30th Ave SE
Rochester, MN 55904
Prgm Dir: Judy Gust, MEd BA RHIT
Tel: 507 285-7456
E-mail: judy.gust@roch.edu

Ridgewater College - Willmar Campus
Health Information Tech Prgm
2101 15th Ave NW
Willmar, MN 56201-2098
Prgm Dir: Mary Juenemann, RHIA CCS
Tel: 320 231-2949   *Fax:* 320 231-7690
E-mail: mary.juenemann@ridgewater.edu

Mississippi

Hinds Community College
Health Information Tech Prgm
1750 Chadwick Dr
Jackson, MS 39204
www.hindscc.edu
Prgm Dir: Michelle McGuffee, RHIA
Tel: 601 376-4823   *Fax:* 601 376-4962
E-mail: mlmcguffee@hindscc.edu

Meridian Community College
Health Information Tech Prgm
910 Hwy 19 N
Meridian, MS 39307
www.mcc.cc.ms.us/healthinfo
Prgm Dir: Robin Allen Jones, RHIA
Tel: 601 484-8759   *Fax:* 601 484-8824
E-mail: rjones@meridiancc.edu

Itawamba Community College
Health Information Tech Prgm
2176 S Eason Blvd
Tupelo, MS 38801
Prgm Dir: Nena Scott, MSEd RHIA CCS CCSP
Tel: 662 620-5123   *Fax:* 662 620-5077
E-mail: npscott@iccms.edu

Missouri

Metropolitan Community College - Penn Valley
Health Information Tech Prgm
3201 SW Trafficway
Kansas City, MO 64111
http://mcckc.edu
Prgm Dir: Jennifer Scott, MLA RHIA
Tel: 816 759-4245   *Fax:* 816 759-4553
E-mail: Jennifer.Scott@mcckc.edu

Ozarks Technical Community College
Health Information Tech Prgm
1001 E Chestnut Expressway
Springfield, MO 65802-3625
www.otc.edu
Prgm Dir: Sue Kirk, BGS RHIT
Tel: 417 447-8821   *Fax:* 417 447-8806
E-mail: kirks@otc.edu

Missouri Western State University
Health Information Tech Prgm
4525 Downs Dr
St Joseph, MO 64507
Prgm Dir: Marsha Dolan, MBA RHIA
Tel: 816 271-5949   *Fax:* 816 271-5849
E-mail: dolan@missouriwestern.edu

St Charles Community College
Health Information Tech Prgm
4601 Mid Rivers Mall Dr
St Peters, MO 63376
www.stchas.edu/divisions/msh/hitindex.shtml
Prgm Dir: Candace E Neu, MDE RHIA CCS
Tel: 636 922-8292   *Fax:* 636 922-8478
E-mail: cneu@stchas.edu

Montana

Montana State Univ - Great Falls Coll of Tech
Health Information Tech Prgm
2100 16th Ave S
Great Falls, MT 59405
Prgm Dir: Lynn Ward, RHIA
Tel: 406 771-4358   *Fax:* 406 771-4317
E-mail: lynn.ward@msugf.edu

Nebraska

Central Community College
Health Information Tech Prgm
PO Box 1024
Hastings, NE 68902-1024
www.cccneb.edu
Prgm Dir: Shawna Stump, RHIA
Tel: 402 461-2514   *Fax:* 402 461-2506
E-mail: sstump@cccneb.edu

Clarkson College
Health Information Tech Prgm
101 S 42nd St
Omaha, NE 68131-2739
Prgm Dir: Mary Miller, RHIA
Tel: 402 552-6216   *Fax:* 402 552-6019
E-mail: millerm@clarksoncollege.edu

College of Saint Mary
Health Information Tech Prgm
7000 Mercy Rd
Omaha, NE 68106
Prgm Dir: Ellen B Jacobs, MEd RHIA
Tel: 402 399-2611   *Fax:* 402 399-2657
E-mail: ejacobs@csm.edu

Western Nebraska Community College
Health Information Tech Prgm
1601 E 27th St
Scottsbluff, NE 69361-1899
Prgm Dir: Peg Wolff, MBA RHIA
Tel: 308 635-6064   *Fax:* 308 635-6100
E-mail: pwolff@wncc.net

Nevada

College of Southern Nevada
Health Information Tech Prgm
6375 W Charleston Blvd
Las Vegas, NV 89146
www.csn.edu/health
Prgm Dir: Cassie Gentry, MEd RHIA CHP
Tel: 702 651-5896   *Fax:* 702 651-5077
E-mail: cassie.gentry@csn.edu

New Jersey

Camden County College
Health Information Tech Prgm
200 N Broadway
Attn: Health Information Technology College Hill
Camden, NJ 08012
Prgm Dir: Lynette M Williamson, MBA RHIA CCS CPC
Tel: 856 968-1331
E-mail: lwilliamson@camdencc.edu

Hudson County Community College
Health Information Tech Prgm
870 Bergen Ave
Cudari Bldg, Rm 209
Jersey City, NJ 07306
Prgm Dir: Judith Hall, RHIA
Tel: 201 360-4225
E-mail: jhall@hccc.edu

Passaic County Community College
Health Information Tech Prgm
One College Blvd
Paterson, NJ 07505-1179
Prgm Dir: Lisa DeLiberto, BS RRA
Tel: 973 684-6297   *Fax:* 973 684-6627
E-mail: LDeLiberto@pccc.edu

Burlington County College
Health Information Tech Prgm
601 Pemberton Browns Mills Rd
Pemberton, NJ 08068-1599
Prgm Dir: Susan Scully, RHIA CCS CCS-P
Tel: 609 894-9311, Ext 1257   *Fax:* 609 894-4712
E-mail: sscully@bcc.edu

New Mexico

Central New Mexico Community College
Health Information Tech Prgm
525 Buena Vista SE
BIT
Albuquerque, NM 87106
www.cnm.edu/depts/bit/programs/business/hit/
Prgm Dir: Mechel McKinney, BSB RHIA
Tel: 505 224-3905   *Fax:* 505 224-3850
E-mail: mmckinney@cnm.edu

San Juan College
Health Information Tech Prgm
4601 College Blvd
Farmington, NM 87402
http://sanjuancollege.edu/pages/2203.asp
Prgm Dir: Carroll Schnabel, RHIA
Tel: 505 566-3005   *Fax:* 505 566-3820
E-mail: schnabelc@sanjuancollege.edu

University of New Mexico - Gallup
Health Information Tech Prgm
200 College Dr
Gallup, NM 87301
Prgm Dir: Melody Brashear, RHIT
Tel: 505 863-7659   *Fax:* 505 863-7513
E-mail: mbrash@unm.edu

New York

Alfred State College - SUNY
Cosponsor: State University of New York
Health Information Tech Prgm
SUNY College of Technology at Alfred
10 Upper College Dr
Alfred, NY 14802
www.alfredstate.edu
Prgm Dir: Tracy Locke, MS RHIA
Tel: 607 587-3617   *Fax:* 607 587-3270
E-mail: locketf@alfredstate.edu

Broome Community College
Health Information Tech Prgm
Decker Health Science Bldg, PO Box 1017
Binghamton, NY 13902
www.sunybroome.edu
Prgm Dir: Jane A Hlopko, MA RHIA
Tel: 607 778-5063   *Fax:* 607 778-5467
E-mail: hlopko_j@sunybroome.edu

Suffolk County Community College - Grant Campus
Health Information Tech Prgm
Crooked Hill Rd
Brentwood, NY 11717
Prgm Dir: Diane P Fabian, MBA RHIA
Tel: 631 851-6342   *Fax:* 631 851-6807
E-mail: fabiand@sunysuffolk.edu

Suffolk County Community College - Grant Campus
Health Information Tech Prgm
Crooked Hill Rd
MA204
Brentwood, NY 11717
Prgm Dir: Diane Fabian, MBA RHIA
Tel: 631 851-6342   *Fax:* 631 851-6807
E-mail: fabiand@sunysuffolk.edu

Trocaire College
Health Information Tech Prgm
360 Choate Ave
Buffalo, NY 14220-2094
Prgm Dir: Laurie J Rivet, MBA
Tel: 716 827-2561   *Fax:* 716 828-6107
E-mail: rivetl@trocaire.edu

CUNY Borough of Manhattan Community Coll
Health Information Tech Prgm
199 Chambers St, N 749
New York, NY 10007
Prgm Dir: Lynda Carlson, MPH MS RHIT
Tel: 212 220-8339   *Fax:* 212 748-7465
E-mail: lcarlson@bmcc.cuny.edu

Monroe Community College
Health Information Tech Prgm
1000 E Henrietta Rd
Rochester, NY 14623
www.monroecc.edu
Prgm Dir: Sharon L Insero, RHIA
Tel: 585 292-2375   *Fax:* 585 292-3834
E-mail: sinsero@monroecc.edu

Molloy College
Health Information Tech Prgm
1000 Hempstead Ave
PO Box 5002
Rockville Centre, NY 11571-5002
Prgm Dir: Peter Micallef, MS RHIA CCS
Tel: 516 678-5000, Ext 6463   *Fax:* 516 256-2252
E-mail: ppmicallef@molloy.edu

Onondaga Community College
Health Information Tech Prgm
Rte 173
Syracuse, NY 13215
Prgm Dir: Judith Chrisman, MS RRA
Tel: 315 469-2102   *Fax:* 315 469-2180
E-mail: chrismaj@sunyocc.edu

Mohawk Valley Community College
Health Information Tech Prgm
1101 Sherman Dr
Utica, NY 13501
Prgm Dir: Sue Bice, MS RHIA
Tel: 315 792-5513   *Fax:* 315 731-5855
E-mail: sbice@mvcc.edu

Erie Community College - North Campus
Health Information Tech Prgm
6205 Main St
Williamsville, NY 14221-7095
Prgm Dir: Gail M Lauritsen, EdM RHIA
Tel: 716 851-5293   *Fax:* 716 851-1429
E-mail: lauritsen@ecc.edu

North Carolina

Central Piedmont Community College
Health Information Tech Prgm
PO Box 35009
Charlotte, NC 28235
Prgm Dir: Marty Long, MPH RHIA
Tel: 704 330-6187   *Fax:* 704 330-6131
E-mail: Marty.Long@cpcc.edu

Pitt Community College
Health Information Tech Prgm
PO Drawer 7007
Greenville, NC 27835-7007
Prgm Dir: Kay Gooding, MPH MA Ed RHIA
Tel: 252 493-7361   *Fax:* 252 321-4451
E-mail: kgooding@email.pittcc.edu

Catawba Valley Community College
Health Information Tech Prgm
2550 Hwy 70 SE
Hickory, NC 28602
Prgm Dir: Debra W Cook, MAEd RHIA
Tel: 704 327-7000, Ext 4342   *Fax:* 704 327-7276
E-mail: dcook@cvcc.edu

Davidson County Community College
Health Information Tech Prgm
PO Box 1287
Lexington, NC 27293-1287
Prgm Dir: Heather Kyles-Watson, RHIA
Tel: 336 249-8186, Ext 310   *Fax:* 336 249-9060
E-mail: hkwatson@davidsonccc.edu

McDowell Technical Community College
Health Information Tech Prgm
54 College Dr
Marion, NC 28752
www.mcdowelltech.cc.nc.us
Prgm Dir: Valerie Dobson, RHIA
Tel: 828 652-0699   *Fax:* 828 652-1014
E-mail: valeried@mcdowelltech.edu

Brunswick Community College
Health Information Tech Prgm
PO Box 30
50 College Rd NE
Supply, NC 28462
www.brunswickcc.edu
Prgm Dir: Polly Decker, RHIA
Tel: 910 755-7347   *Fax:* 910 755-7469
E-mail: deckerp@brunswickcc.edu

Southwestern Community College
Health Information Tech Prgm
447 College Dr
Sylva, NC 28779
www.southwest.cc.nc.us
Prgm Dir: Penny Wells, MA Ed RHIA
Tel: 828 586-4091, Ext 362   *Fax:* 828 586-3129
E-mail: pwells@southwesterncc.edu

Edgecombe Community College
Health Information Tech Prgm
2009 W Wilson St
Tarboro, NC 27886
Prgm Dir: Kim A Bell, RHIA
Tel: 252 823-5166, Ext 186   *Fax:* 252 985-2212
E-mail: bellk@edgecombe.edu

North Dakota

United Tribes Technical College
Health Information Tech Prgm
3315 University Dr
Bismarck, ND 58504
Prgm Dir: Karla Baxter, RHIA
Tel: 701 255-3285, Ext 1245   *Fax:* 701 530-0630
E-mail: kbaxter@uttc.edu

North Dakota State College of Science
Health Information Tech Prgm
800 N Sixth St
Wahpeton, ND 58076
www.ndscs.edu
Prgm Dir: Ken Kompelien, MA
Tel: 701 671-2297   *Fax:* 701 671-2587
E-mail: ken.kompelien@ndscs.edu

Ohio

Cincinnati State Tech & Comm College
Health Information Tech Prgm
3520 Central Pkwy
Cincinnati, OH 45223
Prgm Dir: Sherri Mallett, MEd RHIA
Tel: 513 569-1674   *Fax:* 513 569-4963
E-mail: sherri.mallett@cincinnatistate.edu

Cuyahoga Community College
Health Information Tech Prgm
Metro Campus, 2900 Community College Ave
Cleveland, OH 44115
Prgm Dir: Kathleen D Loflin, RHIA
Tel: 216 987-4456   *Fax:* 216 987-4386
E-mail: kathy.loflin@tri-c.edu

Columbus State Community College
Health Information Tech Prgm
550 E Spring St
Columbus, OH 43215
Prgm Dir: Lisa A Cerrato, MSBS RHIA
Tel: 614 287-2541   *Fax:* 614 287-5144
E-mail: lcerrato@cscc.edu

Sinclair Community College
Health Information Tech Prgm
444 W Third St
Dayton, OH 45402
www.sinclair.edu
Prgm Dir: Barbara Wallace, MBA RHIA CCS CCS-P
Tel: 937 512-2973   *Fax:* 937 512-2239
E-mail: barbara.wallace@sinclair.edu

Bowling Green State University - Firelands
Health Information Tech Prgm
One University Dr
Huron, OH 44839
www.firelands.bgsu.edu
Prgm Dir: Mona M Burke, MA RHIA
Tel: 419 433-5560, Ext 20860   *Fax:* 419 433-9696
E-mail: burkem@bgnet.bgsu.edu

Hocking College
Health Information Tech Prgm
3301 Hocking Pkwy
Nelsonville, OH 45764
Prgm Dir: Karen Wright, MHSA RHIA RHIT
Tel: 614 753-6433   *Fax:* 614 753-5105
E-mail: wright_k@hocking.edu

Stark State College of Technology
Health Information Tech Prgm
6200 Frank Ave NW
North Canton, OH 44720
Prgm Dir: Darlene S Horn, RHIA
Tel: 330 966-5458, Ext 4296   *Fax:* 330 966-6586
E-mail: dhorn@starkstate.edu

Mercy College of Northwest Ohio
Health Information Tech Prgm
2221 Madison Ave
Toledo, OH 43624-1198
Prgm Dir: Tammy Mathewson, RHIA CCS-P
Tel: 419 251-1452   *Fax:* 419 251-1730
E-mail: tammy.mathewson@mercycollege.edu

Owens Community College
Health Information Tech Prgm
Oregon Rd
PO Box 10,000
Toledo, OH 43699
www.owens.edu
Prgm Dir: Bonnie Hemp, MBA RHIA CPHQ
Tel: 567 661-7286   *Fax:* 567 661-7331
E-mail: bonnie_hemp@owens.edu

Professional Skills Institute
Health Information Tech Prgm
20 Arco Dr
Toledo, OH 43607
Prgm Dir: Cynthia Topel, BS RHIA
Tel: 419 531-9610
E-mail: ctopel@proskills.com

Oklahoma

Rose State College
Health Information Tech Prgm
6420 SE 15th St
Midwest City, OK 73110
www.rose.edu
Prgm Dir: Cecil D Brooks, RHIA CCS
Tel: 405 733-7578   *Fax:* 405 736-0338
E-mail: cbrooks@rose.edu

Tulsa Community College
Health Information Tech Prgm
Allied Health Div Metro Campus
909 S Boston Ave
Tulsa, OK 74119-2095
Prgm Dir: Sandra S Smith, MEd BS RHIA
Tel: 918 595-7201   *Fax:* 918 595-7091
E-mail: ssmith@tulsacc.edu

Oregon

Central Oregon Community College
Health Information Tech Prgm
2600 NW College Way
Bend, OR 97701
Prgm Dir: Beverlee Jackson, RHIT
Tel: 541 383-7736   *Fax:* 541 318-3785
E-mail: bjackson@cocc.edu

Portland Community College
Health Information Tech Prgm
12000 SW 49th Ave
Portland, OR 97219
Prgm Dir: Larry Clausen
Tel: 503 978-5665   *Fax:* 503 978-5257
E-mail: lclausen@pcc.edu

Pennsylvania

Gwynedd-Mercy College
Health Information Tech Prgm
1325 Sumneytown Pike
Gwynedd Valley, PA 19437
Prgm Dir: Christine Staropoli, MS RHIA CCS
Tel: 215 542-4660   *Fax:* 215 641-5559
E-mail: staropoli.c@gmc.edu

Harrisburg Area Community College
Health Information Tech Prgm
1641 Old Philadelphia Pike
Lancaster, PA 17602
Prgm Dir: Matthew Alfonso, RHIA
Tel: 717 358-2880   *Fax:* 717 358-2951
E-mail: malfonso@hacc.edu

Community College of Philadelphia
Health Information Tech Prgm
1700 Spring Garden St
Philadelphia, PA 19130
Prgm Dir: Joyce Garozzo, MS RHIA CCS
Tel: 215 751-8946   *Fax:* 215 751-8937
E-mail: jgarozzo@ccp.edu

Comm College of Allegheny County
Health Information Tech Prgm
808 Ridge Ave
Pittsburgh, PA 15212-6097
www.ccac.edu
Prgm Dir: JoAnn Avoli, MEd RHIA
Tel: 412 237-2614   *Fax:* 412 237-6579
E-mail: javoli@ccac.edu

Lehigh Carbon Community College
Health Information Tech Prgm
4525 Education Park Dr
Schnecksville, PA 18078-2598
Prgm Dir: George Peters, MS RHIA
Tel: 610 799-1596   *Fax:* 610 799-1527
E-mail: gpeters@lccc.edu

South Hills School of Business & Technology
Health Information Tech Prgm
480 Waupelani Dr
State College, PA 16801
www.southhills.edu
Prgm Dir: Kay Strigle, RHIA
Tel: 814 234-7755   *Fax:* 814 234-0926
E-mail: kstrigle@southhills.edu

Pennsylvania College of Technology
Health Information Tech Prgm
One College Ave
Williamsport, PA 17701
Prgm Dir: Daniel K Christopher, MBA RHIA
Tel: 570 326-3767, Ext 5774   *Fax:* 570 327-4529
E-mail: dchristo@pct.edu

Puerto Rico

Huertas Junior College
Health Information Tech Prgm
PO Box 8429
Caguas, PR 00726
Prgm Dir: Norma Rodriguez
Tel: 787 743-1242, Ext 266   *Fax:* 787 745-4815
E-mail: normadrodriguez@yahoo.com

Universidad del Este
Health Information Tech Prgm
PO Box 2010
Carolina, PR 00983
www.suagm.edu/une
Prgm Dir: Ada Lily Torres, RHIA MEd
Tel: 787 257-7373, Ext 3277   *Fax:* 787 257-8659
E-mail: altorres@mail.suagm.edu

Universidad Adventista de las Antillas
Health Information Tech Prgm
PO Box 118
Mayaguez, PR 00681-0118
Prgm Dir: Otoniel Cabrera
Tel: 787 834-9595, Ext 2320   *Fax:* 787 834-9597
E-mail: ocabrera@uaa.edu

Inter American University of Puerto Rico
Health Information Tech Prgm
Call Box 5100
San German, PR 00683
Prgm Dir: Magda Lopez, MS RHIA
Tel: 787 264-1912, Ext 7368   *Fax:* 787 892-6350
E-mail: maglopez@sg.inter.edu

South Carolina

Midlands Technical College
Health Information Tech Prgm
PO Box 2408
Columbia, SC 29202
www.midlandstech.edu
Prgm Dir: Natalie Sartori, RHIA
Tel: 803 822-3072   *Fax:* 803 822-3247
E-mail: sartorin@midlandstech.edu

Florence-Darlington Technical College
Health Information Tech Prgm
PO Box 100548
Florence, SC 29501-0548
Prgm Dir: Malissa Jackson, CCS RHIT
Tel: 843 661-8091   *Fax:* 843 292-0851
E-mail: Malissa.Jackson@fdtc.edu

Greenville Technical College
Health Information Tech Prgm
PO Box 5616
Greenville, SC 29606
Prgm Dir: Susan Walther, RHIA CCS
Tel: 864 848-2032   *Fax:* 864 848-2038
E-mail: susan.walther@gvltec.edu

South Dakota

Dakota State University
Health Information Tech Prgm
East Hall
Madison, SD 57042
www.dsu.edu
Prgm Dir: Dorine Bennett, MBA RHIA
Tel: 605 256-5137   *Fax:* 605 256-5060
E-mail: Dorine.Bennett@dsu.edu

Tennessee

Chattanooga State Technical Comm College
Health Information Tech Prgm
4501 Amnicola Hwy
Chattanooga, TN 37406-1097
Prgm Dir: Rose Scalise, RHIA CPHQ
Tel: 423 697-3381   *Fax:* 423 697-2586
E-mail: rose.scalise@chattanoogastate.edu

Dyersburg State Community College
Health Information Tech Prgm
1510 Lake Rd
Dyersburg, TN 38024
www.dscc.edu
Prgm Dir: Susan Osborne, MS RHIA CCS
Tel: 731 286-3294   *Fax:* 731 286-3271
E-mail: osborne@dscc.edu

Volunteer State Community College
Health Information Tech Prgm
1480 Nashville Pike
Gallatin, TN 37066-3188
Prgm Dir: Abby Cooper, BBA RHIA
Tel: 615 230-3337   *Fax:* 615 230-3251
E-mail: Abby.Cooper@volstate.edu

Roane State Community College
Health Information Tech Prgm
276 Patton Ln
Harriman, TN 37748-5011
www.roanestate.edu
Prgm Dir: Karen H Feltner, RHIT CCS
Tel: 865 354-3000, Ext 4327   *Fax:* 865 882-4535
E-mail: feltnerkh@roanestate.edu

Walters State Community College
Health Information Tech Prgm
500 S Davy Crockett Pkwy
Morristown, TN 37813-6899
Prgm Dir: Anita Gail Winkler, BS RHIA
Tel: 423 585-6990   *Fax:* 423 585-6955
E-mail: gail.winkler@ws.edu

Texas

Texas State Technical College - West Texas
Health Information Tech Prgm
650 E Hwy 80
Abilene, TX 79601
Prgm Dir: Martha Davis, RHIA
Tel: 325 734-3637   *Fax:* 325 670-9345
E-mail: martha.davis@abilene.tstc.edu

Lee College
Health Information Tech Prgm
PO Box 818
Baytown, TX 77522-0818
Prgm Dir: Ann Marice Ivey, MS RHIA CMT
Tel: 281 425-6569   *Fax:* 281 425-6585
E-mail: mivey@lee.edu

Lamar Institute of Technology
Health Information Tech Prgm
PO Box 10061
Beaumont, TX 77710
Prgm Dir: Debra Long, MS RHIA CCS
Tel: 409 839-2918   *Fax:* 409 880-8955
E-mail: debra.long@lit.edu

Panola College
Health Information Tech Prgm
1109 W Panola St
Carthage, TX 75633
Prgm Dir: Sandra Payne, RHIA
Tel: 903 693-1116   *Fax:* 903 693-1152
E-mail: spayne@panola.edu

Del Mar College
Health Information Tech Prgm
101 Baldwin Blvd
Corpus Christi, TX 78404-3897
Prgm Dir: Thomas Williams
Tel: 361 698-2330   *Fax:* 361 698-1172
E-mail: twilliams@delmar.edu

Dallas County Community College
Health Information Tech Prgm
4849 W Illinois Ave
Dallas, TX 75211
Prgm Dir: Cathy Beaty, RHIA
Tel: 214 860-8661
E-mail: cbeaty@dcccd.edu

El Paso Community College
Health Information Tech Prgm
PO Box 20500
El Paso, TX 79998
Prgm Dir: Jean A Garrison, RHIA
Tel: 915 831-4074   *Fax:* 915 831-4114
E-mail: JeanG@epcc.edu

Texas State Technical College - Harlingen
Health Information Tech Prgm
1902 N Loop 499
Harlingen, TX 78550-3697
www.harlingen.tstc.edu/healthinfo/
Prgm Dir: Deborah Woods, BBA RHIA
Tel: 956 364-4768   *Fax:* 956 364-5155
E-mail: dwoods@harlingen.tstc.edu

Houston Community College
Health Information Tech Prgm
Health Careers Education Div
1900 Pressler Dr
Houston, TX 77030
Prgm Dir: Carla Tyson, EdD MHA RHIA
Tel: 713 718-7347   *Fax:* 713 718-7521
E-mail: carla.tyson@hccs.edu

North Harris College
Health Information Tech Prgm
2700 W Thorne Dr
Houston, TX 77073-3499
www.northharriscollege.com
Prgm Dir: Jeanne Qualey, RHIA CCS
Tel: 281 765-7829   *Fax:* 281 618-1155
E-mail: jeanne.qualey@nhmccd.edu

San Jacinto College North
Health Information Tech Prgm
5800 Uvalde Rd
Houston, TX 77049-4599
Prgm Dir: James Steen, MBA BS RHIA
Tel: 281 459-7608   *Fax:* 281 459-7651
E-mail: james.steen@sjcd.edu

Tarrant County College - Northeast Campus
Health Information Tech Prgm
828 Harwood Rd
Hurst, TX 76054
Prgm Dir: DeeAnn Carver, RHIA
Tel: 817 515-6544   *Fax:* 817 515-6700
E-mail: deeann.carver@tccd.edu

DeVry University - Dallas
Health Information Tech Prgm
4800 Regent Blvd
Irving, TX 75063
www.dal.devry.edu
Prgm Dir: Barbara Odom-Wesley, PhD RHIA FAHIMA
Tel: 972 929-9322   *Fax:* 972 929-6778
E-mail: bodom-wesley@devry.edu

South Plains College
Health Information Tech Prgm
Reese Center
819 Gilbert Dr
Lubbock, TX 79416
Prgm Dir: Nancy Powell, BS RHIT
Tel: 806 885-3048, Ext 4644   *Fax:* 806 885-5608
E-mail: npowell@southplainscollege.edu

South Texas College
Health Information Tech Prgm
1101 E Vermont
McAllen, TX 78503
Prgm Dir: Irma Rodriguez, MEd RHIA CCS
Tel: 956 872-3170   *Fax:* 956 872-3180
E-mail: irmar@southtexascollege.edu

Midland College
Health Information Tech Prgm
3600 N Garfield
Midland, TX 79705
Prgm Dir: Melinda Teel, RHIA CCS
Tel: 915 685-5573   *Fax:* 915 685-4762
E-mail: mteel@midland.edu

Howard College
Health Information Tech Prgm
3501 N US Hwy 67
San Angelo, TX 76904
Prgm Dir: Sonja Davis, RHIA
Tel: 325 481-8300, Ext 236   *Fax:* 325 481-8321
E-mail: sdavis@howardcollege.edu

St Philip's College
Health Information Tech Prgm
1801 Martin Luther King Dr
San Antonio, TX 78203
Prgm Dir: Cheryl Spears, RHIA
Tel: 210 531-3456   *Fax:* 210 531-3459
E-mail: cspears@accd.edu

Tyler Junior College
Health Information Tech Prgm
PO Box 9020
Tyler, TX 75711
www.tjc.edu/hit
Prgm Dir: Charlotte Creason, RHIA
Tel: 903 510-2669   *Fax:* 903 597-6518
E-mail: ccre@tjc.edu

Vernon College
Health Information Tech Prgm
4105 Maplewood Ave
Vernon, TX 76308
Prgm Dir: Roxanne Hill, RHIA
Tel: 940 696-8752, Ext 3237   *Fax:* 940 696-3244
E-mail: rhill@vernoncollege.edu

McLennan Community College
Health Information Tech Prgm
1400 College Dr, AS 208
Waco, TX 76708
www.mclennan.edu
Prgm Dir: Lesley Weber, RHIA ALF
Tel: 254 299-8233   *Fax:* 254 299-8435
E-mail: lweber@mclennan.edu

Wharton County Junior College
Health Information Tech Prgm
911 Boling Hwy
Wharton, TX 77488
Prgm Dir: Mary W King, MS RHIA
Tel: 979 532-6363   *Fax:* 979 532-6489
E-mail: maryk@wcjc.edu

Utah

Weber State University
Health Information Tech Prgm
3911 University Circle
Ogden, UT 84408-3911
www.weber.edu
Prgm Dir: Patricia L Shaw, MEd RHIA
Tel: 801 626-7242   *Fax:* 801 626-6475
E-mail: pshaw@weber.edu

Virginia

Northern Virginia Community College
Health Information Tech Prgm
Medical Education Campus
6699 Springfield Center Dr
Springfield, VA 22150
www.nvcc.edu
Prgm Dir: Zakevia Green, MSHA RHIA
Tel: 703 822-6580   *Fax:* 703 822-6619
E-mail: dmunch@nvcc.edu

Tidewater Community College
Health Information Tech Prgm
1700 College Crescent
Virginia Beach, VA 23456
Prgm Dir: Gussie L Hammond, MS BS RHIA
Tel: 757 822-7262   *Fax:* 757 427-1338
E-mail: ghammond@tcc.edu

Washington

Shoreline Community College
Health Information Tech Prgm
16101 Greenwood Ave N
Seattle, WA 98133
www.shoreline.edu/hciprograms
Prgm Dir: Donna J Wilde, MPA RHIA
Tel: 206 543-4757   *Fax:* 206 533-5103
E-mail: dwilde@shoreline.edu

Spokane Community College
Health Information Tech Prgm
N 1810 Greene St, MS 2090
Spokane, WA 99217
Prgm Dir: Sharon Meyer, RHIT
Tel: 509 533-8852   *Fax:* 509 533-8621
E-mail: Smeyer@scc.spokane.edu

Tacoma Community College
Health Information Tech Prgm
6501 S 19th St
Tacoma, WA 98466-6100
Prgm Dir: Marion Miller, MBA RHIA CCS
Tel: 253 566-5227 *Fax:* 253 566-5273
E-mail: mmiller@tacomacc.edu

West Virginia

Fairmont State Univ
Cosponsor: Pierpont Comm & Tech College
Health Information Tech Prgm
Locust Ave
Fairmont, WV 26554
Prgm Dir: Vickie Findley, MPA RHIA
Tel: 304 367-4764 *Fax:* 304 367-4268
E-mail: vfindley@fairmontstate.edu

Marshall Community & Technical College
Health Information Tech Prgm
One John Marshall Dr
Huntington, WV 25755
Prgm Dir: Janet Smith, MS RHIA CCS
Tel: 304 696-6796
E-mail: smithjan@marshall.edu

Marshall University
Health Information Tech Prgm
One John Marshall Dr
Huntington, WV 25755
Prgm Dir: Janet Smith, RHIA
Tel: 304 696-6796 *Fax:* 304 696-3013
E-mail: smithjan@marshall.edu

West Virginia Northern Community College
Health Information Tech Prgm
1704 Market St
Wheeling, WV 26003
Prgm Dir: Korene Atkins, MA RHIA CCS CPC CPC-H
Tel: 304 233-5900, Ext 5559
E-mail: katkins@northern.wvnet.edu

Wisconsin

Chippewa Valley Technical College
Health Information Tech Prgm
620 W Clairemont Ave
Eau Claire, WI 54701
Prgm Dir: Margie Konik, MA RHIA
Tel: 715 858-1824 *Fax:* 715 833-6470
E-mail: mkonik@cvtc.edu

Northeast Wisconsin Technical College
Health Information Tech Prgm
2740 W Mason St, PO Box 19042
Green Bay, WI 54307-9042
Prgm Dir: Marilyn Toninato, BA RHIA
Tel: 920 498-5577 *Fax:* 920 498-5673
E-mail: marilyn.toninato@nwtc.edu

Western Technical College
Health Information Tech Prgm
304 N Sixth St, PO Box C-908
La Crosse, WI 54602-0908
http://learn.westerntc.edu/brownt
Prgm Dir: Tamra R Brown, ME RHIA
Tel: 608 785-9549 *Fax:* 608 785-9087
E-mail: brownt@westerntc.edu

Gateway Technical College
Health Information Tech Prgm
1001 S Main St
Racine, WI 53403
Prgm Dir: Cynthia Fickenscher, MBA RHIA CCA
Tel: 262 619-6396 *Fax:* 262 631-6811
E-mail: fickenscherc@gtc.edu

Moraine Park Technical College
Health Information Tech Prgm
2151 N Main St
West Bend, WI 53090
www.morainepark.edu
Prgm Dir: Gloria Madison, MS RHIA
Tel: 262 335-5730 *Fax:* 262 335-5708
E-mail: gmadison@morainepark.edu

Health Information Technician

Programs*	Class Capacity	Begins	Length (months)	Award	Res. Tuition	Non-res. Tuition	Stipend	Offers:‡ 1	2	3	4
Alaska											
University of Alaska Southeast (Sitka)	20	Sep Jan	15, 24	Cert, AAS	$120	$0		•			•
Arizona											
Phoenix College	50	Every semester	24	Cert, AAS	$1,950	$4,410		•		•	
Arkansas											
University of Arkansas for Medical Sciences (Little Rock)	25	Aug Jan	22	AS	$4,860	$12,330		•			
California											
Cypress College	100	Jun Aug Jan	24	Cert, AS	$20	$162		•			•
San Diego Mesa College	25	Aug	24	AS	$20	$160		•			
Santa Barbara City College	40	Aug	24	AS	$650	$5,500					•
Colorado											
Arapahoe Community College (Littleton)	60	Aug Jan	24	AAS	$4,900	$9,800					•
Florida											
Central Florida Community College (Ocala)	30	Fall term	24	Dipl, AA	$4,552	$16,487		•			•
Daytona Beach Community College	20	Aug	21	AAS	$69	$263					
Lake-Sumter Community College (Leesburg)	24	Aug Jan	24	AAS	$2,300	$6,292		•			
Miami Dade College	50	Aug	24	Dipl, AS	$4,154	$12,988		•			
Polk Community College (Winter Haven)	30	Aug	24	Dipl, AS, AAS	$66	$246		•			•
Santa Fe Community College (Gainesville)	24	Aug	24, 36	AS	$1,876	$7,084		•			
Georgia											
Darton College (Albany)	50	Aug	21	AS	$1,440	$3,944					•
Idaho											
Boise State University	27	Aug Jan	24	Dipl, AS	$5,146	$12,924					
Illinois											
College of DuPage (Glen Ellyn)	20	Aug	21	AAS	$3,090	$8,760	$103	•			
Danville Area Community College	30	Aug	20	Assoc	$2,000	$4,000					
Northwestern Business College (Chicago)	24	Sep Dec Mar Jun	18	AAS	$17,410	$17,410		•	•	•	
Oakton Community College (Des Plaines)	20	Aug Jan	21, 30	AAS	$2,460	$8,897					
Southern Illinois Collegiate Common Market (Herrin)	24	Aug	18	AS	$3,216	$11,078					
Southwestern Illinois College (Belleville)	20	Aug	22	AAS	$2,278	$5,896					
Indiana											
Vincennes University	24	Aug	19	AS	$4,543	$11,034					•

*Data are shown only for programs that completed the 2007 AMA Survey of Health Professions Education Programs.
‡Key to Offers: 1: Evening or weekend classes; 2: Non-English instruction; 3: Cultural competence instruction; 4: Distance education component.

Health Information Technician

Programs*	Class Capacity	Begins	Length (months)	Award	Res. Tuition	Non-res. Tuition	Stipend	Offers:‡ 1	2	3	4
Iowa											
Northeast Iowa Community College (Calmar)	20	Aug	24	AAS	$3,400	$3,400					
Scott Community College (Bettendorf)	20	Aug	14, 24	Dipl, AAS	$97	$135		•			•
Kansas											
Hutchinson Community College	16	Aug	22	AAS	$2,016	$3,296		•			•
Washburn University (Topeka)	20	Aug	12, 24	Cert, AS	$6,300	$14,292		•			•
Kentucky											
Jefferson Community and Technical College (Louisville)	20	Fall semester	24	AAS	$115	$0		•			
National College - Louisville	20	Dec Mar Jun Sep	24	AS	$5,760	$5,760		•			
Western Kentucky University (Bowling Green)	30	Aug	21	AS	$6,416	$15,470		•			•
Louisiana											
Delgado Community College (New Orleans)	20	Aug	22	AAS	$1,674	$4,284					
Maryland											
Montgomery College (Takoma Park)	25	Sep	21	AAS	$3,100	$7,996		•			•
Prince George's Community College (Largo)	20	Sep	24	AAS	$3,290	$8,855		•			•
Massachusetts											
Caritas Labour, College (Boston)	40	Sep Jan	48, 24	Dipl, Cert, AS	$500	$500		•		•	•
Michigan											
Davenport University - Grand Rapids (Fulton St)		Aug Jan May		AAS	$7,656	$7,656		•		•	
Ferris State University (Big Rapids)	30	Aug	24	AAS	$7,200	$14,640		•		•	
Schoolcraft College (Garden City)	30	Aug	24	AAS	$4,760	$7,004		•			
Minnesota											
College of St Catherine (Minneapolis)	20	Sep Feb	24	AAS	$14,000	$0		•			
Mississippi											
Hinds Community College (Jackson)	20	Aug	22	AAS	$1,660	$3,866					
Meridian Community College	15	Aug	18	AAS	$1,450	$2,740					
Missouri											
Metropolitan Community College - Penn Valley (Kansas City)	25	Aug	24	AS	$2,400	$3,700					
Ozarks Technical Community College (Springfield)		Aug	22	Cert, AAS	$3,088	$4,063		•			•
St Charles Community College (St Peters)	50	Aug	21	AS	$2,720	$4,012		•			•
Montana											
Montana State Univ - Great Falls Coll of Tech	25	Sep	23	AAS	$1,872	$4,654					•
Nebraska											
Central Community College (Hastings)		Aug	20	Dipl, Cert, AAS	$1,600	$2,336		•			
Nevada											
College of Southern Nevada (Las Vegas)	15	Sep	24	AAS	$1,917	$6,716		•		•	•
New Jersey											
Burlington County College (Pemberton)	20	Sep	21	AAS	$2,669	$3,104		•			
New Mexico											
Central New Mexico Community College (Albuquerque)	25	Jan	25	AAS				•			•
San Juan College (Farmington)	20	Aug Jan	24	AAS	$720	$1,040		•	•	•	•
University of New Mexico - Gallup	15	Sep	24	AAS	$1,170	$1,170		•			
New York											
Alfred State College - SUNY	27	Aug	20	AAS	$6,000	$6,000		•			•
Broome Community College (Binghamton)	24	Aug	20	AAS	$2,914	$5,828		•			•
Monroe Community College (Rochester)	33	Sep	18	AAS	$2,800	$5,600		•			
Suffolk County Comm Coll - Grant Campus (Brentwood)	24	Sep	24	AAS	$1,550	$3,100		•			
Suffolk County Comm Coll - Grant Campus (Brentwood)	28	Fall	30	AAS	$3,000	$0		•			
North Carolina											
Brunswick Community College (Supply)	20	Aug	21	Dipl, AAS	$1,533	$8,103					
McDowell Technical Community College (Marion)	25	Aug	21	Cert, AAS	$1,264	$6,154		•		•	•
Southwestern Community College (Sylva)	25	Aug	12, 21	Dipl, Cert, AAS	$664	$3,544					•
North Dakota											
North Dakota State College of Science (Wahpeton)	26	Aug	13, 22	Cert, AAS	$6,257	$8,697					•
Ohio											
Bowling Green State University - Firelands (Huron)	18	Aug	18	AAS	$4,212	$17,368		•	•	•	•
Owens Community College (Toledo)	25	Aug	24	Assoc	$2,784	$5,520		•			•
Sinclair Community College (Dayton)	30	Sep	22	AAS	$2,248	$3,369		•			
Oklahoma											
Rose State College (Midwest City)	15	Aug	12, 21	Cert, AAS	$2,481	$7,236					
Oregon											
Central Oregon Community College (Bend)	28	Sep	18	Cert, AAS	$63	$176		•			•
Portland Community College	35	Sep	18	AAS	$3,000	$8,500					•

*Data are shown only for programs that completed the 2007 AMA Survey of Health Professions Education Programs.
‡Key to Offers: 1: Evening or weekend classes; 2: Non-English instruction; 3: Cultural competence instruction; 4: Distance education component.

Health Information Technician

Programs*	Class Capacity	Begins	Length (months)	Award	Res. Tuition	Non-res. Tuition	Stipend	Offers:‡ 1	2	3	4
Pennsylvania											
Comm College of Allegheny County (Pittsburgh)	25	Aug	18	AS	$3,432	$9,169		•			
South Hills School of Business & Technology (State College)	25	Sep	20	AST	$11,050	$11,637					
Puerto Rico											
Universidad del Este (Carolina)	40	Aug	20	AS	$4,142	$4,142			•		
South Carolina											
Greenville Technical College	20	Aug	21	AS	$4,350	$8,850	$450	•		•	•
Midlands Technical College (Columbia)	18	Aug	12, 24	Cert, AS	$3,138	$9,504					
South Dakota											
Dakota State University (Madison)	30	Sep	24	AS	$2,767	$4,149					•
Tennessee											
Dyersburg State Community College	50	Aug	24	Cert, AAS	$2,481	$9,157					•
Roane State Community College (Harriman)	18	Aug	21	Cert, AAS	$2,230	$6,676		•			•
Texas											
DeVry University - Dallas (Irving)	25	Mar May Jul Sep Nov Jan	15	AAS, BS				•			•
Lamar Institute of Technology (Beaumont)	25	Aug	24	AAS	$2,000	$7,000					
McLennan Community College (Waco)	25	Aug	24	AAS	$4,464	$0		•			
North Harris College (Houston)	40	Aug	24	AAS	$1,344	$2,994		•			
South Plains College (Lubbock)	19	Aug	9, 20	Cert, AAS	$1,918	$2,581		•		•	
Texas State Technical College - Harlingen	25	Aug	24	AAS	$4,176	$11,664					
Tyler Junior College	20	Aug	24	AAS	$3,781	$6,395	$1,500				•
Utah											
Weber State University (Ogden)	20	Aug	24	AAS	$2,988	$10,495		•			•
Virginia											
Northern Virginia Community College (Springfield)	25	Aug	18	AAS	$86	$264		•			•
Washington											
Shoreline Community College (Seattle)	20	Sep	21	AAAS	$6,738	$13,864		•		•	•
West Virginia											
West Virginia Northern Community College (Wheeling)	14	Aug	24	AAS	$1,824	$5,808		•			
Wisconsin											
Chippewa Valley Technical College (Eau Claire)	18	Aug Jan	24	AS	$2,762	$17,117					
Moraine Park Technical College (West Bend)	20	Aug	24	AAS	$3,700	$10,100		•			•
Western Technical College (La Crosse)	16	Aug	20	AAS	$2,991	$15,551					•

*Data are shown only for programs that completed the 2007 AMA Survey of Health Professions Education Programs.
‡Key to Offers: 1: Evening or weekend classes; 2: Non-English instruction; 3: Cultural competence instruction; 4: Distance education component.

The kinesiotherapist is academically and clinically prepared to provide rehabilitation exercise and education under the prescription of a licensed physician in an appropriate setting. Kinesiotherapists are qualified to implement exercise programs designed to reverse or minimize debilitation and enhance the functional capacity of medically stable patients in a wellness, sub-acute, or extended care setting. The role of the kinesiotherapist demands intelligence, judgment, honesty, interpersonal skills, and the capacity to react to emergencies in a calm and reasoned manner. An attitude of respect for self and others, adherence to the concepts of privilege and confidentiality in communicating with patients, and a commitment to the patient's welfare are standard attributes. At a minimum, a kinesiotherapist is educated in areas of basic exercise science and clinical applications of rehabilitation exercise. Training is received in orthopedic, neurological, psychiatric, pediatric, cardiovascular- pulmonary, and geriatric practice settings.

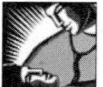

Career Description

Kinesiotherapy is the application of scientifically based exercise principles adapted to enhance the strength, endurance, and mobility of individuals with functional limitations or those requiring extended physical conditioning.

The kinesiotherapist is a health care professional competent in the administration of musculoskeletal, neurological, ergonomic, biomechanical, psychosocial, and task-specific functional tests and measures. The kinesiotherapist determines the appropriate evaluation tools and interventions necessary to establish, in collaboration with the client, a goal-specific treatment plan.

The intervention process includes the development and implementation of a treatment plan, assessment of progress toward goals, modification as necessary to achieve goals and outcomes, and client education. The foundation of clinician-client rapport is based on education, instruction, demonstration, and mentoring of therapeutic techniques and behaviors to restore, maintain, and improve overall functional abilities.

The *Scope of Practice for Kinesiotherapy* identities the job tasks that registered kinesiotherapists are qualified to perform. This document reflects the evaluation procedures and treatment interventions for medically stable individuals who need extended physical conditioning. The individual kinesiotherapist may obtain additional training and credentials in areas beyond the scope of practice. The *Standards of Practice for Registered Kinesiotherapists* serves as a guideline for practicing registered kinesiotherapists and provides a basis for assessment of kinesiotherapy practices.

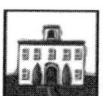

Employment Characteristics

Registered kinesiotherapists are employed in Department of Veterans Affairs Medical Centers, public and private hospitals, medical fitness facilities, rehabilitation facilities, learning disability centers, schools, colleges and universities, private practice, and as exercise consultants.

The types of treatments carried out by kinesiotherapists focus on but are not limited to
- Therapeutic exercise
- Ambulation training
- Geriatric rehabilitation
- Aquatic therapy
- Adapted fitness and conditioning
- Prosthetic/orthotic rehabilitation
- Psychiatric rehabilitation
- Driver training
- Adapted exercise for the home setting

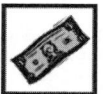

Salary

Depending on the particular job setting, the average projected starting salary for registered kinesiotherapists is $32,500 to $38,000 annually. The overall average is $48,000; upper-level salaries are in the range of $60,000. Refer to Section IV, Table 5 of this *Directory* for more information, or see www.ama-assn.org/go/hpsalary.

Educational Programs

Length. The kinesiotherapy program is 4 to 5 years. The total minimum requirements are 128 semester hours. Minimum requirements for years 1 and 2 are 59 semester hours and for years 3 and 4 are 67 semester hours.

Prerequisites. Applicants should have a high school diploma or equivalent and meet institutional entrance requirements.

Curriculum. The program has a comprehensive academic and clinical curriculum plan that fulfills or exceeds the minimum requirements for kinesiotherapy accreditation.

The curriculum plan includes an organized and sequential series of integrated learning experiences designed to achieve or exceed minimum competencies.

All academic and clinical courses are guided by written measurable behavioral objectives and use case-based, patient-centered, problem-solving activities.

The curriculum plan includes academic learning experiences, which lead to the attainment of all academic competencies listed in the *Minimum Core Competencies of Kinesiotherapists*.

Students must complete the following content areas:
- Human anatomy
- Human physiology
- Exercise physiology
- Kinesiology/biomechanics
- Therapeutic exercise/adapted physical education
- Growth and development
- Motor learning/control/performance
- General psychology
- Organization and administration
- Tests and measurements
- Research methods or statistics
- First aid and cardiopulmonary resuscitation
- Introduction to kinesiotherapy
- Pathophysiology
- Clinical neurology
- Rehabilitation procedures
- Patient assessment and management
- Therapeutic activities

Students are strongly encouraged to complete the following academic courses:
- Abnormal psychology or mental health
- Physiological psychology

- Exercise testing and prescription
- Gerontology
- Medical ethics
- Medical terminology
- Pharmacology
- Health/medical/functional outcomes management
- Health education
- Kinesiotherapy I and II

 **Inquiries**

Careers
American Kinesiotherapy Association
118 College Drive, #5142
Hattiesburg, MS 39406
601 266-5371
601 266-4445 Fax
E-mail: helen.fuller@usm.edu

Credentialing
Board of Registration for Kinesiotherapy
University of Toledo
2801 W Bancroft
Toledo, OH 43606-2434
419 530-2731
E-mail: dwoods@utnet.utoledo.edu

Program Accreditation
Commission on Accreditation of Allied Health Education Programs
(CAAHEP) in collaboration with:
Committee on Accreditation of Education Programs for
Kinesiotherapy
University of Southern Mississippi
118 College Drive, #5142
Hattiesburg, MS 39406
601 266-5371
601 266-4445 Fax
E-mail: jerry.purvis@usm.edu

Kinesiotherapist

California

California State University - Long Beach
Kinesiotherapy Prgm
1250 Bellflower Blvd
Long Beach, CA 90840
Prgm Dir: Janet M Fisher, PhD
Tel: 562 985-8481
E-mail: fisherja@csulb.edu

San Diego State University
Kinesiotherapy Prgm
5500 Campanile Dr
Department of Exercise & Nutritional Sciences
San Diego, CA 92182-7251
Prgm Dir: James A Yaggie, PhD RKT
Tel: 619 594-2392   *Fax:* 619 594-6553
E-mail: jyaggie@mail.sdsu.edu

Mississippi

University of Southern Mississippi
Kinesiotherapy Prgm
118 College Dr #5142
Hattiesburg, MS 39406-5142
www.usm.edu
Prgm Dir: Jerry W Purvis, MS RKT
Tel: 601 266-5371   *Fax:* 601 266-4445
E-mail: Jerry.Purvis@usm.edu

North Carolina

Shaw University
Kinesiotherapy Prgm
118 E South St
Raleigh, NC 27601
www.shawu.edu
Prgm Dir: Edwards Bennett, PhD
Tel: 919 546-8316   *Fax:* 919 743-4693
E-mail: bedwards@shawu.edu

Ohio

University of Toledo
Kinesiotherapy Prgm
2801 W Bancroft St
Toledo, OH 43606-3390
www.utoledo.edu
Prgm Dir: Leonard O Greninger, PhD RKT
Tel: 419 530-2953   *Fax:* 419 530-2477
E-mail: Leonard.Greninger@utoledo.edu

Virginia

Norfolk State University
Kinesiotherapy Prgm
700 Park Ave
Norfolk, VA 23504
Prgm Dir: Delano Tucker, PhD
Tel: 757 823-8703   *Fax:* 757 823-9412
E-mail: dtucker@nsu.edu

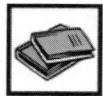

History

Massage has its roots in the far reaches of human history. Rubbing a sore muscle or stroking another person for comfort is a natural response. The first written records that refer to massage date back more than 4,000 years to China. In ancient Greece, Hippocrates, the father of modern medicine, wrote, "The physician must be experienced in many things, but most assuredly in rubbing."

Massage comes from both Western and Eastern traditions. Western traditions date back to ancient Greece and Rome. Modern Western massage owes a great deal to the work of Peter Henrik Ling, a 19th-century educator and athlete from Sweden. His approach, which combined hands-on techniques with active movements, became known as Swedish Massage, probably the most common therapeutic massage modality in the West.

Eastern traditions can be traced back to the folk medicine of China and the Ayurvedic medicine of India. Shiatsu, acupressure, reflexology, and many other contemporary techniques have their roots in these sources.

The incorporation of massage into health care was fairly well-established in the 19th century, but those connections decreased through most of the 20th century. A growing body of clinical research on the efficacy and value of massage as part of integrated health care, as well as a rapid acceptance and adoption of use of massage in recent years, has fueled a renewed collaboration between massage therapists and other health professionals.

Surveys of hospitals, conducted through the American Hospital Association, have shown a rapid increase in use of massage in the hospital setting. A consumer survey released in 2007 shows 38% of American adults have received a massage some time in their lives. Growth in the consumer acceptance of massage over the last 2 decades has been substantial.

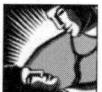

Career Description

Leading professional massage associations have defined massage as systems of structured palpation or movement of the soft tissue of the body, including holding, causing movement, and/or applying pressure to the body. Massage therapy is a profession in which the practitioner applies manual techniques (by use of hand or body), and may apply adjunctive therapies, with the intention of positively affecting the health and well-being of the client.

An increasing body of research shows massage reduces heart rate, can help lower blood pressure, increases blood circulation and lymph flow, relaxes muscles, improves range of motion, and increases endorphins. Recent studies indicate massage enhances the functioning of the immune system. Although therapeutic massage does not increase muscle strength, it can stimulate weak, inactive muscles and, thus, partially compensate for the lack of exercise and inactivity resulting from illness or injury. It also can hasten and lead to a more complete recovery from exercise or injury.

Some of the most common types of massage are Swedish massage, deep-tissue massage, Shiatsu-acupressure, neuromuscular, trigger point, and sports massage. Massage therapy can be strenuous work at times. Practitioners must use correct body mechanics to prevent injury and fatigue. If the therapist travels to give massage, they transport either a massage table or massage chair and all supplies necessary to give a massage. The profession requires good listening skills and the ability to make clients comfortable and relaxed. Massage therapists often adopt massage practice as a second or third career and many enjoy the freedom of part-time work and independent practice.

In addition to the actual massage, massage therapists market their practices, keep financial and client records, maintain supplies and equipment, educate their clients about massage and inform them of any physical irregularities they discover, and work with health insurance companies to receive fees. Practitioners take basic medical histories on clients and discuss with the client their current health. During massage, therapists pay close attention to how the client is responding and discuss levels of massage pressure with the client. They also must be aware of medical conditions that might contraindicate massage and advise clients when massage is not appropriate.

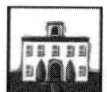

Employment Characteristics

Massage therapists work in many different environments. The vast majority work at least some of their hours in private practice, and many combine that practice with parttime work in hospitals, physician or chiropractor offices, nursing homes, pain clinics, resorts, cruise ships, shopping malls, airports, spas, and salons. Some travel to clients' homes or to business offices. Onsite chair massage has become a very popular form of massage because of its convenience of use in a variety of settings, such as corporate offices. Some therapists focus exclusively on massage for stress relief and relaxation, while others specialize in such modalities as pregnancy massage, massage to reduce lymphedema after cancer surgery, massage for pain relief, and sports massage, among other specialties. There has been a proliferation of massage modalities in recent years, and many therapists combine several to create unique offerings.

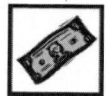

Salary

Earnings among massage therapists vary widely, depending on where the therapist practices, their level of experience, the number of client contact hours, and their ability to establish and sustain an independent business. Responsibilities in addition to massage include practice management, billing, marketing, etc.

While government statistics place annual earnings for massage therapists at about $30,000, these figures are based on an assumption therapists work strictly as employees who keep strenuous year-round schedules of 40 hours weekly in client massage. More complete industry surveys reflecting prevalent part-time and private-practice models, however, show practitioners having an average closer to 15 client contact hours weekly, earning them annual massage-related incomes between $15,000 to $19,000. Refer to Section IV, Table 5 of this *Directory* for more information, or see www.ama-assn.org/go/hpsalary.

Educational Programs

Minimum entry-level standards for massage therapy training vary greatly, based on state or local requirements, professional association standards, or insurance requirements. State regulatory requirements for massage practice range from a minimum of 500 in-class hours at a recognized massage schools—the most prevalent standard—to 1,000 in-class hours of massage training in accredited massage programs.

Massage therapy training programs and schools can voluntarily seek accreditation from seven accrediting agencies recognized by the US Department of Education. Only 30% of state-approved massage therapy training programs have received such accreditation. The Commission on Massage Therapy Accreditation (COMTA) is one of these agencies and is the only one dedicated solely to accreditation for massage therapy.

There are two major professional massage associations, Associated Bodywork & Massage Professionals and the American Massage Therapy Association. As a condition of membership, both require completion of a minimum number of classroom hours and state licensing in states where licensing has been enacted.

Licensure

Currently, 38 states and Washington, DC, regulate massage, and the trend is toward other states passing licensing regulation as well. Some states license massage therapists, while others have basic standards. Regulation of massage therapy by the states has increased dramatically in recent years, with 26 states having passed regulations between 1990 and 2008.

Entry Examination and Certification

Some states require passage of an exam before granting a license. In 2007, the Federation of State Massage Therapy Boards introduced the Massage and Bodywork Licensing Exam (MBLEx), which is designed to assess a massage therapist's readiness to practice safely and competently. Some states also accept for entry purposes a passing score on the test component involved in securing voluntary professional certification from the National Certification Board for Therapeutic Massage & Bodywork or the American Organization for Bodywork Therapies of Asia.

Inquiries

Massage Careers, Organizational Memberships
Associated Bodywork & Massage Professionals
1271 Sugarbush Drive
Evergreen, CO 80439-9766
800 458-2267
800 667-8260 Fax
E-mail: expectmore@abmp.com
www.abmp.com

American Massage Therapy Association
500 Davis Street, Suite 900
Evanston, IL 60201-4695
847 864-0123
847 864-1178 Fax
E-mail: info@amtamassage.org
www.amtamassage.org

Certification

Federation of State Massage Therapy Boards
7111 W 151st Street, Suite 356
Overland Park, KS 66223
888 703-7682
913 681-0391 Fax
E-mail: info@fsmtb.org
www.fsmtb.org

National Certification Board for Therapeutic Massage & Bodywork
8201 Greensboro Drive, Suite 300
McLean, VA 22102
800 296-0664
703 610-9015
703 610-9005 Fax
E-mail: info@ncbtmb.com
www.ncbtmb.com

Program Accreditation

Commission on Massage Therapy Accreditation
1007 Church Street, Suite 302
Evanston, IL 60201
847 869-5039
847 869-6739 Fax
E-mail: info@comta.org
www.comta.org

Massage Therapist

Alaska

University of Alaska Anchorage
Massage Therapy Prgm
3211 Providence Dr
Adm 216
Anchorage, AK 99508
Prgm Dir: Sally Mead
Tel: 907 786-6930   *Fax:* 907 272-4742
E-mail: afslm1@uaa.alaska.edu

Arizona

Desert Institute of the Healing Arts
Massage Therapy Prgm
140 E 4th St
Tucson, AZ 85705
Prgm Dir: Ginger Castle
Tel: 800 733-8098   *Fax:* 520 624-2996
E-mail: diha@azstarnet.com

California

Mueller College of Holistic Massage Therapies
Massage Therapy Prgm
4607 Park Blvd
San Diego, CA 92116-2630
Prgm Dir: Jeffrey Welsh, PhD MA RRT HHP
Tel: 619 291-9811   *Fax:* 619 543-1113
E-mail: paul@mueller.edu

Colorado

Massage Therapy Institute of Colorado
Massage Therapy Prgm
1441 York St, Ste 301
Denver, CO 80206
Prgm Dir: Mark Manton
Tel: 303 329-6345

Academy of Natural Therapy
Massage Therapy Prgm
123 Elm Ave
PO Box 237
Eaton, CO 80615
Prgm Dir: Elisha Newhouse
Tel: 970 352-1181
E-mail: newhouse@naturaltheraphy.com

Connecticut

Connecticut Center for Massage Therapy
Massage Therapy Prgm
1154 Poquonnock Rd
Groton, CT 06340
Prgm Dir: Linda Derick
Tel: 860 446-2299   *Fax:* 860 446-9410
E-mail: linda@ccmt.com

Connecticut Center for Massage Therapy
Massage Therapy Prgm
75 Kitts Ln
Newington, CT 06111
Prgm Dir: Linda Derick
Tel: 860 667-1886   *Fax:* 860 667-2175
E-mail: linda@ccmt.com

Connecticut Center for Massage Therapy
Massage Therapy Prgm
25 Sylvan Rd S
Westport, CT 06880
Prgm Dir: Linda Derick
Tel: 203 221-7325   *Fax:* 203 221-0144
E-mail: linda@ccmt.com

Delaware

National Massage Therapy Institute
Massage Therapy Prgm
1601 Concord Pike, Ste 82-84
Wilmington, DE 19803
Prgm Dir: Lisa Jakober
Tel: 302 436-4508
E-mail: lisa@studymassage.com

District of Columbia

Potomac Massage Training Institute
Massage Therapy Prgm
5028 Wisconsin Ave NW - LL
Washington, DC 20016-4118
www.pmti.org
Prgm Dir: Demara Stamler
Tel: 202 686-7046, Ext 115   *Fax:* 202 966-4579
E-mail: dstamler@pmti.org

Florida

Florida College of Natural Health
Massage Therapy Prgm
616 67th St Circle E
Bradenton, FL 34208
Prgm Dir: Kathryn Knox
Tel: 800 966-7117   *Fax:* 941 744-1242
E-mail: kknox@fcnh.com

Florida School of Massage
Massage Therapy Prgm
6421 SW 13th St
Gainesville, FL 32608
Prgm Dir: Paul Davenport
Tel: 352 378-7891
E-mail: info@floridaschoolofmassage.com

Florida College of Natural Health
Massage Therapy Prgm
2600 Lake Lucien Dr, Ste 140
Maitland, FL 32751
Prgm Dir: Diane Owens, PhD
Tel: 800 393-7337   *Fax:* 407 261-0342
E-mail: dowens@fcnh.com

Educating Hands School of Massage
Massage Therapy Prgm
120 SW 8th St
Miami, FL 33130-3513
Prgm Dir: Janet Gonzalez
Tel: 800 999-6991   *Fax:* 305 857-0298
E-mail: janet@educatinghands.com

Florida College of Natural Health
Massage Therapy Prgm
7925 NW 12th St, Ste 201
Miami, FL 33126
Prgm Dir: Debra Starr Cohen
Tel: 800 599-9599   *Fax:* 305 597-9110
E-mail: dstarr@fcnh.com

Florida College of Natural Health
Massage Therapy Prgm
2001 W Sample Rd, Ste 100
Pompano Beach, FL 33064
Prgm Dir: Sherry Parker
Tel: 800 541-9299   *Fax:* 954 975-9633
E-mail: sparker@fcnh.com

Sarasota School of Massage Therapy
Massage Therapy Prgm
1932 Ringling Blvd
Sarasota, FL 34236
www.sarasotaschoolofmassagetherapy.edu
Prgm Dir: Joe Lubow, BS LMT
Tel: 877 613-7768   *Fax:* 941 957-1049
E-mail: joe@sarasotaschoolofmassagetherapy.edu

Core Institute
Massage Therapy Prgm
223 W Carolina St
Tallahassee, FL 32301
Prgm Dir: Philip R Arcuri
Tel: 850 222-8673   *Fax:* 850 561-6160
E-mail: phil@coreinstitute.com

Illinois

Chicago School of Massage Therapy
Cosponsor: Cortiva Institute
Massage Therapy Prgm
17 N State St, 5th Fl
Chicago, IL 60602
Prgm Dir: Jason Scholte
Tel: 312 753-7900, Ext 7929   *Fax:* 312 753-7901
E-mail: jscholte@cortiva.com

Morton College
Massage Therapy Prgm
3801 S Central Ave
Cicero, IL 60804
www.morton.edu
Prgm Dir: Linda Moore
Tel: 708 656-2000, Ext 412
E-mail: Linda.Moore@morton.edu

Chicago School of Massage Therapy
Cosponsor: McHenry County College Satellite
Massage Therapy Prgm
100 S Main St
Crystal Lake, IL 60014
Prgm Dir: C Connie Love
Tel: 773 477-9444   *Fax:* 773 477-7256
E-mail: clove.cortiva@com

National University of Health Sciences
Massage Therapy Prgm
200 E Roosevelt Rd
Lombard, IL 60148
www.nuhs.edu
Prgm Dir: Randy Swenson, BS DC MHPE
Tel: 630 889-6545   *Fax:* 630 889-6635
E-mail: rswenson@nuhs.edu

Kishwaukee College
Massage Therapy Prgm
21193 Malta Rd
Malta, IL 60150-9699
Prgm Dir: Leslie Ciaccio, BFA CMT
Tel: 815 825-2086, Ext 259   *Fax:* 815 825-2072
E-mail: lciaccio@kishwaukeecollege.edu

Indiana

Alexandria School of Scientific Therapeutics
Massage Therapy Prgm
809 S Harrison
PO Box 287
Alexandria, IN 46001
Prgm Dir: Herbert Hobbs
Tel: 800 622-8756   *Fax:* 765 724-9156
E-mail: alexssin.edudir@insightbb.com

Iowa

Carlson College of Massage Therapy
Massage Therapy Prgm
11809 County Rd X-28
Anamosa, IA 52205
www.carlsoncollege.com
Prgm Dir: Wayne Pakulis, BA LMT NCTMB
Tel: 319 462-3402   *Fax:* 319 462-5990
E-mail: waynepakulis@carlsoncollege.com

Institute of Therapeutic Massage & Wellness
Massage Therapy Prgm
1730 Wilkes Ave
Davenport, IA 52804
Prgm Dir: Bonita Howes
Tel: 563 445-1055
E-mail: itwtraining@aol.com

Kansas

BMSI Institute
Massage Therapy Prgm
8665 W 96th St, Ste 300
Overland, KS 66212
www.bmsi.edu
Prgm Dir: Michael Pizzuto, NCBTMB
Tel: 913 649-3322   *Fax:* 913 649-1010
E-mail: michael@bmsi.edu

Louisiana

Blue Cliff College - Baton Rouge
Massage Therapy Prgm
6160 Perkins Rd, Ste 200
Baton Rouge, LA 70808-4191
Prgm Dir: Rose Steptoe
Tel: 225 757-3770   *Fax:* 225 757-7422
E-mail: roses@bluecliffcollege.com

Maine

New Hamp Inst for Therapeutic Arts
Massage Therapy Prgm
27 Sandy Creek Rd
Bridgton, ME 04009
Prgm Dir: Patrick Ian Cowan, PhD
Tel: 207 647-3794   *Fax:* 207 647-2954
E-mail: nhita@nhita.com

Downeast School of Massage
Massage Therapy Prgm
PO Box 24
99 Moose Meadow Ln
Waldoboro, ME 04572-0024
Prgm Dir: Nancy Dail, BA LMT NCTMB
Tel: 207 832-5531   *Fax:* 207 832-0504
E-mail: ndail@aol.com

Manitoba, Canada

Massage Therapy College of Manitoba
Massage Therapy Prgm
691 Wolseley Ave, 2nd Fl
Winnipeg, MB R3G 1C3
Prgm Dir: Garth Beddome
Tel: 204 772-8999   *Fax:* 204 772-5090
E-mail: mcollege@mts.net

Maryland

Allegany College of Maryland
Massage Therapy Prgm
12401 Willowbrook Rd
Cumberland, MD 21502
Prgm Dir: Paula Jilanis
Tel: 301 784-5191
E-mail: pjilanis@allegany.edu

Baltimore School of Massage
Massage Therapy Prgm
517 Progress Dr
Ste A-L
Linthicum, MD 21090
Prgm Dir: Richard Rynders
Tel: 410 636-7929   *Fax:* 410 636-7857
E-mail: richardr@bsom.com

Massachusetts

Stillpoint Program - Greenfield Comm Coll
Massage Therapy Prgm
270 Main St
Greenfield, MA 01301
Prgm Dir: Patricia A Wachter
Tel: 413 775-1634   *Fax:* 413 774-2285
E-mail: wachter@gcc.mass.edu

Springfield Technical Community College
Massage Therapy Prgm
Dept of Myofascial
One Amory Square
Springfield, MA 01105
Prgm Dir: Bernadette Della Bitta Nicholson
Tel: 413 755-4885
E-mail: Nicholson@stcc.edu

Cortiva Institute - Muscular Therapy Inst
Massage Therapy Prgm
103 Morse St
Watertown, MA 02472
Prgm Dir: Dianne Polseno
Tel: 617 668-1000
E-mail: katie475@aol.com

Michigan

Ann Arbor Institute of Massage Therapy
Massage Therapy Prgm
180 Jackson Plaza
Ste 100
Ann Arbor, MI 48103
www.aaimt.edu
Prgm Dir: Jocelyn Granger, NCBTMB
Tel: 734 677-4430, Ext 24   *Fax:* 734 677-4520
E-mail: jgranger@aaimt.edu

Lakewood School of Therapeutic Massage
Massage Therapy Prgm
1102 6th St
Port Huron, MI 48060
Prgm Dir: Nancy J Levitt, RN BSN
Tel: 810 987-3959
E-mail: lakewoodschool@sbcglobal.net

Minnesota

Northwestern Health Science University School of Massage Therapy
Massage Therapy Prgm
School of Massage Therapy
2501 W 84th St
Bloomington, MN 55431
www.nwhealth.edu
Prgm Dir: Dale Healey, BS DC
Tel: 952 888-4777, Ext 348   *Fax:* 952 888-6713
E-mail: dhealey@nwhealth.edu

Mississippi

Mississippi School of Therapeutic Massage
Massage Therapy Prgm
5140 Galaxie Dr
Jackson, MS 39206-4339
www.mstm.info
Prgm Dir: Sara Simpson, RMT Instructor NCBTMB
Tel: 601 362-3624   *Fax:* 601 362-3694
E-mail: mstmjxn@aol.com

Missouri

St Charles School of Massage Therapy
Massage Therapy Prgm
2440 Executive Dr
Ste 100
St Charles, MO 63303
Prgm Dir: Kathleen Crawford, LMT
Tel: 636 498-0777   *Fax:* 636 498-0708
E-mail: oasis@anet-stl.com

Montana

Health Works Institute
Massage Therapy Prgm
111 S Grand Annex 3
Bozeman, MT 59715
Prgm Dir: Ruth Marion
Tel: 406 582-1555   *Fax:* 406 522-0493
E-mail: director@healthworksinstitute.com

New Hampshire

New Hampshire Institute for Therapeutic Arts
Massage Therapy Prgm
153 Lowell Rd
Hudson, NH 03051
Prgm Dir: Janet Alexis
Tel: 603 882-3022   *Fax:* 603 598-9101
E-mail: janhita@aol.com

New Jersey

Institute for Therapeutic Massage - Browns Mills
Massage Therapy Prgm
200 Trenton Rd
Browns Mills, NJ 08015
Prgm Dir: Lisa Helbig
Tel: 973 839-6131
E-mail: joanne@massageprogram.com

National Massage Therapy Institute
Massage Therapy Prgm
6712 Washington Ave, Ste 302
Egg Harbor, NJ 08234
Prgm Dir: Lisa Jakober
Tel: 609 277-1599
E-mail: lisa@studymassage.com

Academy of Massage Therapy
Massage Therapy Prgm
321 Main St, 2nd Fl
Hackensack, NJ 07601
www.academyofmassage.com
Prgm Dir: Ron Beier
Tel: 888 268-7898   *Fax:* 201 568-5181
E-mail: info@academyofmassage.com

Institute for Therapeutic Massage - Morristown
Massage Therapy Prgm
95 Mount Kemble Ave
Morristown, NJ 07962
Prgm Dir: Lisa Helbig
Tel: 973 839-6131
E-mail: admissions@massageprogram.com

Institute for Therapeutic Massage - University of Medicine & Dentistry
Massage Therapy Prgm
150 Bergen St
Newark, NJ 07103
Prgm Dir: Lisa Helbig
Tel: 973 839-6131
E-mail: admissions@massageprogram.com

Omega Institute
Massage Therapy Prgm
7050 Rte 38 E
Pennsauken, NJ 08109
Prgm Dir: Therese Recchiuti
Tel: 856 663-4299, Ext 221   *Fax:* 856 661-9585
E-mail: trecchiuti@omegacareers.com

Cortiva Inst, Somerset Sch of Massage Therapy - Piscataway
Massage Therapy Prgm
180 Centennial Ave
Piscataway, NJ 08854
Prgm Dir: Adrienne Asta
Tel: 732 885-3400, Ext 29   *Fax:* 732 885-0440
E-mail: aasta@cortiva.com

Institute for Therapeutic Massage - Pompton Lakes
Massage Therapy Prgm
125 Wanaque Ave
Pompton Lakes, NJ 07442
Prgm Dir: Lisa Helbig
Tel: 973 839-6131
E-mail: admissions@massageprogram.com

Institute for Therapeutic Massage
Massage Therapy Prgm
99 Hwy 37 W
Toms River, NJ 08755
Prgm Dir: Angela Harris
Tel: 732 936-9111
E-mail: angela@massageprogram.com

National Massage Therapy Institute - Turnersville
Massage Therapy Prgm
108-L Greentree Rd and Black Horse Pike
Turnersville, NJ 08012
Prgm Dir: Lisa Jakober
Tel: 856 227-1754
E-mail: lisa@studymassage.com

Cortiva Inst, Somerset Sch of Massage Therapy - Wall Township
Massage Therapy Prgm
1985 Hwy 34
Wall Township, NJ 07719
Prgm Dir: Rhonda Brunelle
Tel: 732 282-0100   *Fax:* 732 282-1108
E-mail: rbrunelle@cortiva.com

Healing Hands Institute for Massage Therapy
Massage Therapy Prgm
41 Bergenline Ave
Westwood, NJ 07675
Prgm Dir: Eva Carey, NCMT MBA
Tel: 201 722-0099   *Fax:* 201 722-0690
E-mail: hhi@aol.com

New Mexico

Crystal Mountain Sch of Therapeutic Massage
Massage Therapy Prgm
4775 Indian School Rd NE
Ste 102
Albuquerque, NM 87110
Prgm Dir: Judy Gray, LMT RMTI BA
Tel: 505 872-2030
E-mail: info@crystalmtnmassage.com

North Carolina

Body Therapy Institute
Massage Therapy Prgm
300 Southwind Rd
Siler City, NC 27344
Prgm Dir: Rick Rosen, MA NC LMT
Tel: 919 663-3111, Ext 13   *Fax:* 919 663-0369
E-mail: rick@bti.edu

Nova Scotia, Canada

ICT Northumberland College
Massage Therapy Prgm
1888 Brunswick St, 5th Fl
Halifax, NS B3J 3J8
Prgm Dir: Florent Villeneuve
Tel: 416 762-4857, Ext 241   *Fax:* 416 762-5733
E-mail: florentv@ictschools.com

Ohio

Cincinnati School of Medical Massage
Massage Therapy Prgm
11250 Cornell Park Dr, Ste 203
Cincinnati, OH 45242
Prgm Dir: Pete Elsers
Tel: 513 469-6300
E-mail: tarmstrong@fuse.net

Dayton School of Medical Message
Massage Therapy Prgm
4457 Far Hills Ave
Dayton, OH 45429
Prgm Dir: Bill Tahy
Tel: 937 294-6994
E-mail: nikoleguirnalda@ameritech.net

Dayton School of Medical Message
Massage Therapy Prgm
Apollo Career Center
3325 Shawnee Rd
Lima, OH 45806
Prgm Dir: Bill Tahy
Tel: 888 860-4544
E-mail: nikoleguirnalda@ameritch.net

Cleveland Institute of Medical Massage
Massage Therapy Prgm
18334-D E Bagley Rd
Middleburg Heights, OH 44130
Prgm Dir: Karen Taylor
Tel: 440 243-8650
E-mail: ktaylorcimm@sbcglobal.net

Ontario, Canada

ICT Kikkawa College
Massage Therapy Prgm
2340 Dundas St W, Unit G-04
Toronto, ON M6P 4A9
Prgm Dir: Florent Villeneuve, BA RMT
Tel: 416 762-4857, Ext 241   *Fax:* 416 762-5733
E-mail: florentv@ictshools.com

Oregon

East-West Coll of the Healing Arts
Massage Therapy Prgm
525 NE Oregon St
Portland, OR 97232
www.eastwestcollege.com
Prgm Dir: David Slawson
Tel: 800 635-9141   *Fax:* 503 232-4392
E-mail: dslawson@eastwestcollege.com

Pennsylvania

Synergy Healting Arts Center & Massage School
Massage Therapy Prgm
13593 Monterey Ln
Blue Ridge Summit, PA 17214
Prgm Dir: Margie Schaeffer
Tel: 800 286-1931
E-mail: message@synergymessage.edu

Cortiva Inst - Penn School of Muscle Therapy
Massage Therapy Prgm
1173 Egypt Rd, PO Box 400
Oaks, PA 19456-0400
Prgm Dir: Joanne Slanga, BA MSLS MTS NCBTMB LMT
Tel: 610 666-9060, Ext 18   *Fax:* 610 666-9061
E-mail: psmt@psmt.com

National Massage Therapy Insitute
Massage Therapy Prgm
Division of PSB
10050 Roosevelt Blvd
Philadelphia, PA 19116
Prgm Dir: Lisa Jakober
Tel: 800 264-9835   *Fax:* 215 969-1368
E-mail: lisa@studymassage.com

Baltimore School of Massage
Massage Therapy Prgm
170 Red Rock Rd
York, PA 17402
Prgm Dir: Anita Perry-Strong
Tel: 717 268-1881   *Fax:* 717 268-1991
E-mail: anitas@steinerleisure.com

Rhode Island

Community College of Rhode Island
Massage Therapy Prgm
One John H Chafee Blvd
Newport, RI 02840
Prgm Dir: Regina Cobb
Tel: 401 851-1681
E-mail: rmcobb@ccri.edu

Tennessee

Roane State Community College
Massage Therapy Prgm
Somatic Massage Therapy Program
701 Briarcliff Ave
Oak Ridge, TN 37830
Prgm Dir: Paula Keefe
Tel: 865 481-2017
E-mail: KeefePK@roanestate.edu

Virginia

Virginia School of Massage
Massage Therapy Prgm
2008 Morton Dr
Charlottesville, VA 22903
Prgm Dir: Terri Leap
Tel: 888 599-2001   *Fax:* 804 293-4190
E-mail: virginia@vasom.com

National Massage Therapy Institute
Massage Therapy Prgm
803 W Broad St, Ste 110
Falls Church, VA 22046
Prgm Dir: Lisa Jakober
Tel: 703 237-3905
E-mail: lisa@studymassage.com

Cayce/Reilly School of Massotherapy
Massage Therapy Prgm
215 67th St
Virginia Beach, VA 23451
Prgm Dir: Nancy Hallingse-Smith
Tel: 757 457-7202   *Fax:* 757 428-0398
E-mail: nsmith@edgarcayce.org

Washington

Cortiva Inst - Brian Utting School of Massage
Massage Therapy Prgm
Massage Licensing Program
900 Thomas St
Seattle, WA 98109
www.cortiva.com/busm
Prgm Dir: Dina Boon
Tel: 206 292-8055   *Fax:* 206 292-0113
E-mail: dboon@cortiva.com

Cortiva Institute - Seattle
Massage Therapy Prgm
425 Pontius Ave N, Ste 100
Seattle, WA 98109
www.cortiva.com
Prgm Dir: Dina Boon, LMP
Tel: 206 282-1233, Ext 107   *Fax:* 206 282-9183
E-mail: dboon@cortiva.com

West Indies

Trinidad & Tobago Coll of Therapeutic Massage
Massage Therapy Prgm
68 Market St
Trinidad West Indies, WN
Prgm Dir: Marabella Gopaul Lands
Tel: 868 658-3907

West Virginia

Mountain State School of Massage
Massage Therapy Prgm
601 50th St
Charleston, WV 25304
Prgm Dir: Rob Rogers
Tel: 304 926-8822   *Fax:* 304 926-8837
E-mail: robrogers@mtnstmassage.com

Wisconsin

Blue Sky School of Professional Massage
Massage Therapy Prgm
220 American Blvd
De Pere, WI 54155
Prgm Dir: Robin Liebermann
Tel: 920 338-9500
E-mail: info@blueskyedu.org

Blue Sky School of Professional Massage
Massage Therapy Prgm
220 Oak St
Grafton, WI 53024
Prgm Dir: Vlad Timofeev
Tel: 262 376-1011
E-mail: info@blueskyedu.org

Blue Sky School of Professional Massage
Massage Therapy Prgm
2122 Luann Ln
Madison, WI 53713
Prgm Dir: Linda Orton
Tel: 608 270-5245
E-mail: info@blueskyedu.org

Lakeside School of Massage Therapy - Madison
Massage Therapy Prgm
6121 Odana Rd
Madison, WI 53219
Prgm Dir: Claude Gagnon
Tel: 414 372-4345, Ext 12   *Fax:* 414 372-5350
E-mail: claude@lakesideschoolmassage.org

Lakeside School of Massage Therapy - Milwaukee
Massage Therapy Prgm
1726 N 1st St, Ste 200
Milwaukee, WI 53212
Prgm Dir: Carole Ostendorf, PhD
Tel: 414 372-4345, Ext 14   *Fax:* 414 372-5350
E-mail: carole@lakeside.edu

Massage Therapist

Programs*	Class Capacity	Begins	Length (months)	Award	Res. Tuition	Non-res. Tuition	Stipend	Offers:‡ 1	2	3	4
Colorado											
Massage Therapy Institute of Colorado (Denver)	18			Cert	$7,900	$7,900		•			
District of Columbia											
Potomac Massage Training Institute (Washington)	80	Feb Aug	18	Cert	$8,190	$8,190		•		•	
Florida											
Sarasota School of Massage Therapy	22	Jan Apr Jun Sep	9, 18	Dipl	$8,325	$8,325		•			
Illinois											
Morton College (Cicero)	20	Aug	16	Cert, AAS	$3,700	$6,825		•		•	
National University of Health Sciences (Lombard)	60	Jan May Sep	12	Cert, AAS	$8,742	$8,742		•		•	
Iowa											
Carlson College of Massage Therapy (Anamosa)	46	Mar Sep (FT) Sep (PT)	6, 11	Dipl	$8,000	$8,000		•			
Kansas											
BMSI Institute (Overland)	48		6, 12	Cert	$9,100	$9,100		•			
Michigan											
Ann Arbor Institute of Massage Therapy	70	Sep Feb	12	Dipl	$7,800	$7,800		•			•
Minnesota											
Northwestern Health Science University School of Massage Therapy (Bloomington)	52	Sep Jan May	12, 16	Cert	$10,296	$10,296		•		•	•
Mississippi											
Mississippi School of Therapeutic Massage (Jackson)	12	3x/yr	8, 16	Cert	$9,000	$9,000		•			
New Jersey											
Academy of Massage Therapy (Hackensack)	20	4x/yr	8, 12	Cert	$14,200	$0		•	•	•	
Omega Institute (Pennsauken)	80+	4x/yr	5, 12	Cert	$7,500	$7,500		•			
Nova Scotia, Canada											
ICT Northumberland College (Halifax)	80	Sep Jan	20, 18	Dipl	$7,400	$7,400					
Ontario, Canada											
ICT Kikkawa College (Toronto)	60	Sep Jan	20, 18	Dipl	$7,500	$7,500					
Oregon											
East-West Coll of the Healing Arts (Portland)	18	Jan Apr Jul Oct	12, 18	Dipl	$193	$193		•			
Washington											
Cortiva Inst - Brian Utting School of Massage (Seattle)	80	Apr	12	Cert	$12,900	$12,900		•		•	
Cortiva Institute - Seattle	250	Jan Apr Jul Oct	9, 12	Dipl				•		•	

*Data are shown only for programs that completed the 2007 AMA Survey of Health Professions Education Programs.
‡Key to Offers: 1: Evening or weekend classes; 2: Non-English instruction; 3: Cultural competence instruction; 4: Distance education component.

Medical assisting is a multi-skilled allied health profession; practitioners work primarily in ambulatory settings such as medical offices and clinics. Medical assistants function as members of the health care delivery team and perform administrative and clinical procedures.

Career Description

Medical assistants work under the supervision of physicians in their offices or other medical settings. In accordance with respective state laws, they perform a broad range of administrative and clinical duties:

Administrative Duties
- Scheduling and receiving patients
- Preparing and maintaining medical records
- Performing basic secretarial skills and medical transcription
- Handling telephone calls and writing correspondence
- Serving as a liaison between the physician and other individuals
- Managing practice finances

Clinical Duties
- Asepsis and infection control
- Taking patient histories and vital signs
- Performing first aid and CPR
- Preparing patients for procedures
- Assisting the physician with examinations and treatments
- Collecting and processing specimens
- Performing selected diagnostic tests
- Preparing and administering medications as directed by the physician

Both administrative and clinical duties involve maintenance of equipment and supplies for the practice. A medical assistant who is sufficiently qualified by education and/or experience may be responsible for supervising personnel, developing and conducting public outreach programs to market the physician's professional services, and participating in the negotiation of leases and of equipment and supply contracts.

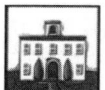

Employment Characteristics

More medical assistants are employed by practicing physicians than any other type of allied health personnel. Medical assistants are usually employed in physicians' offices and other ambulatory healthcare settings, where they perform a variety of administrative and clinical tasks to facilitate the work of the physician. The responsibilities of medical assistants vary, depending on whether they work in a clinic, hospital, large group practice, or small private office. With demand from more than 200,000 physicians, there are, and will probably continue to be, almost unlimited opportunities for formally educated medical assistants.

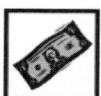

Salary

According to the American Association of Medical Assistants (AAMA), the average entry-level salary for Certified Medical Assistants (CMAs) in 2004 was $22,650. The average annual salary for full-time practitioners with a CMA was $27,951. Refer to Section IV, Table 5 of this *Directory* for more information, or see www.ama-assn.org/go/hpsalary.

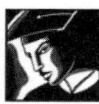

Educational Programs

Length. Programs grant an associates degree, certificate, or diploma.

Prerequisites. High school diploma or equivalent is usually required.

Curriculum. The curricula of accredited programs must ensure achievement of the *Entry-Level Competencies for the Medical Assistant.* The curriculum must include anatomy and physiology, medical terminology, medical law and ethics, psychology, communications (oral and written), medical assisting administrative procedures, and medical assisting clinical procedures. Programs must include an externship that provides practical experience in qualified physicians' offices, accredited hospitals, or other health care facilities.

Inquiries

Careers
American Association of Medical Assistants
20 North Wacker Drive, Suite 1575
Chicago, IL 60606-2903
800 228-2262
312 899-1500
www.aama-ntl.org

Certification/Registration
Director of Certification
American Association of Medical Assistants
20 North Wacker Drive, Suite 1575
Chicago, IL 60606-2903
312 424-3100

Program Accreditation
Commission on Accreditation of Allied Health Education Programs (CAAHEP) in collaboration with:
American Association of Medical Assistants Endowment
20 North Wacker Drive, Suite 1575
Chicago, IL 60606-2963
312 899-1500
312 899-1259 Fax
E-mail: accreditation@aama-ntl.org

Medical Assistant

Alabama

George C Wallace Community College
Medical Assistant Prgm
1141 Wallace Dr
Dothan, AL 36303
Tel: 334 556-2427, Ext 2427 *Fax:* 334 556-2231
E-mail: warwood@wallace.edu

Wallace State Community College
Medical Assistant Prgm
PO Box 2000
Hanceville, AL 35077-2000
Tel: 205 352-8321, Ext 256 *Fax:* 205 352-8320
E-mail: tracie.fuqua@wallacestate.edu

H Council Trenholm State Technical College
Medical Assistant Prgm
1225 Air Base Blvd, PO Box 9000
Montgomery, AL 36108-3105
www.trenholmtech.cc.al.us
Tel: 334 420-4483 *Fax:* 334 420-4335
E-mail: alove@trenholmtech.cc.al.us

South University
Medical Assistant Prgm
5355 Vaughn Rd
Montgomery, AL 36116-1120
Tel: 334 395-8800, Ext 8827 *Fax:* 334 395-8859
E-mail: lreynolds@southuniversity.edu

Alaska

University of Alaska Anchorage
Medical Assistant Prgm
Allied Health Sciences Building Rm 166
3211 Providence Dr
Anchorage, AK 99508-4630
www.uaa.alaska.edu/ctc/alliedhealth/ma
Tel: 907 786-6932 *Fax:* 907 786-6938
E-mail: afrjw@uaa.alaska.edu

University of Alaska - Fairbanks
Medical Assistant Prgm
PO Box 758040
Fairbanks, AK 99701-8040
Tel: 907 455-2887 *Fax:* 907 455-2865
E-mail: ffclb2@uaf.edu

Arizona

Kaplan College
Medical Assistant Prgm
13450 N Black Canyon Hwy, Ste 104
Phoenix, AZ 85029
Tel: 602 548-1955, Ext 214 *Fax:* 602 548-1956
E-mail: lmuniz@longtechnicalcollege.com

Arkansas

Arkansas Tech University
Medical Assistant Prgm
1311 N El Paso Ave, T5
Russellville, AR 72801
www.atu.edu
Tel: 479 498-6073 *Fax:* 479 964-0504
E-mail: pcox@atu.edu

California

Everest College - Alhambra
Medical Assistant Prgm
2215 Mission Rd
Alhambra, CA 91803
Tel: 626 979-4940, Ext 121 *Fax:* 626 979-4961
E-mail: rmarin@cci.edu

Everest College
Medical Assistant Prgm
511 N Brookhurst St, Ste 300
Anaheim, CA 92801
Tel: 714 953-6500, Ext 139 *Fax:* 714 953-4163
E-mail: jenlow@cci.edu

Western Career College - Antioch
Medical Assistant Prgm
2157 Country Hills Dr
Antioch, CA 94509
www.westercareercollege.edu
Tel: 925 522-7777, Ext 47120 *Fax:* 925 755-0079
E-mail: rmessiha@ant.westerncollege.com

Cabrillo College
Medical Assistant Prgm
6500 Soquel Dr
Aptos, CA 95003
Tel: 831 479-6438 *Fax:* 831 479-5054
E-mail: chjensen@cabrillo.edu

Western Career College - Citrus
Medical Assistant Prgm
7301 Greenback Ln, Ste A
Citrus Heights, CA 95621
Tel: 916 722-8200, Ext 45115
E-mail: sbravo@westerncollege.com

Heald College - Concord
Medical Assistant Prgm
5130 Commerical Circle
Concord, CA 94520
www.heald.edu
Tel: 925 288-5800, Ext 5824 *Fax:* 925 687-2428
E-mail: Ekbal_Fakhoury@heald.edu

Orange Coast College
Medical Assistant Prgm
2701 Fairview Rd
Costa Mesa, CA 92628-5005
Tel: 714 432-5658 *Fax:* 714 432-5534
E-mail: mwillis@mail.occ.cccd.edu

Western Career College - Emeryville Campus
Medical Assistant Prgm
6001 Shellmound St, Ste 145
Emeryville, CA 94608
Tel: 510 601-0133, Ext 27 *Fax:* 510 601-0793
E-mail: pdancy@emv.westerncollege.com

Heald College - Fresno
Medical Assistant Prgm
255 W Bullard Ave
Fresno, CA 93704
Tel: 559 437-4134 *Fax:* 559 438-6368
E-mail: jo_lynn_dowell@Heald.edu

Concorde Career College - Garden Grove
Medical Assistant Prgm
12951 Euclid St, Ste 101
Garden Grove, CA 92804
Tel: 714 620-1043 *Fax:* 714 530-8421
E-mail: sruiz@concorde.edu

Everest College - Gardena
Medical Assistant Prgm
1045 W Redondo Beach Blvd, Ste 275
Gardena, CA 90247
Tel: 310 527-7105 *Fax:* 310 527-7985
E-mail: jcrohn@cci.edu

Chabot College
Medical Assistant Prgm
25555 Hesperian Blvd
Hayward, CA 94545-5001
www.chabotcollege.edu
Tel: 510 723-7211 *Fax:* 510 782-9315
E-mail: medassistvallely@yahoo.com

Heald College - Hayward
Medical Assistant Prgm
25500 Industrial Blvd
Hayward, CA 94545
Tel: 510 259-7265
E-mail: pamela_stoker@heald.edu

Everest College - Los Angeles
Medical Assistant Prgm
3460 Wilshire Blvd, Ste 500
Los Angeles, CA 90010
Tel: 213 388-9950, Ext 123 *Fax:* 213 388-9907
E-mail: jandres@cci.edu

Heald College - San Jose
Medical Assistant Prgm
341 Great Mall Pkwy
Milpitas, CA 95035
www.heald.edu
Tel: 408 934-4900, Ext 127 *Fax:* 408 934-1006
E-mail: nelly_mangarova@heald.edu

Modesto Junior College
Medical Assistant Prgm
435 College Ave
Modesto, CA 95350-5800
www.mjc.edu
Tel: 209 575-6377 *Fax:* 209 575-6593
E-mail: buzbees@yosemite.cc.ca.us

Pasadena City College
Medical Assistant Prgm
1570 E Colorado Blvd
Pasadena, CA 91106-2003
www.pasadena.edu
Tel: 626 585-7431 *Fax:* 626 585-7977
E-mail: jynakano@pasadena.edu

Western Career College - Pleasant Hill
Medical Assistant Prgm
380 Civic Dr, Ste 300
Pleasant Hill, CA 94523
Tel: 925 609-6650 *Fax:* 925 609-6666
E-mail: rebeccab@westerncollege.com

Heald College - Rancho Cordova
Medical Assistant Prgm
2910 Prospect Park Dr
Rancho Cordova, CA 95670
www.heald.edu
Tel: 916 638-1616, Ext 2335 *Fax:* 916 853-7021
E-mail: Cynthia_Smith@heald.edu

Heald College - Roseville
Medical Assistant Prgm
7 Sierra Gate Plaza
Roseville, CA 95678
Tel: 916 780-4425 *Fax:* 916 789-8606
E-mail: gene_bryan@heald.edu

Cosumnes River Community College
Medical Assistant Prgm
8401 Center Pkwy
Sacramento, CA 95823-5704
www.crc.losrios.edu
Tel: 916 691-7296 *Fax:* 916 691-7146
E-mail: burnsc@crc.losrios.edu

Western Career College - Sacramento
Medical Assistant Prgm
8909 Folsom Blvd
Sacramento, CA 95826-3203
Tel: 916 361-5140 *Fax:* 916 361-6666
E-mail: dmalott@westerncollege.com

Heald College - Salinas
Medical Assistant Prgm
1450 N Main St
Salinas, CA 93906
www.heald.edu
Tel: 831 443-1700, Ext 141 *Fax:* 831 443-1050
E-mail: don_stanley@heald.edu

Concorde Career College - San Bernardino
Medical Assistant Prgm
201 E Airport Dr, Ste A
San Bernardino, CA 92408
Tel: 909 884-8891, Ext 336   *Fax:* 909 384-1768
E-mail: mkarimkani@concorde.edu

Everest College - San Bernardino
Medical Assistant Prgm
217 E Club Center Dr, Ste A
San Bernardino, CA 92408
www.cci.edu
Tel: 909 777-3300   *Fax:* 909 777-3550
E-mail: dorap@cci.edu

San Diego Mesa College
Medical Assistant Prgm
7250 Mesa College Dr
San Diego, CA 92111
Tel: 619 388-2267
E-mail: dtwyman@sdccd.edu

City College of San Francisco
Medical Assistant Prgm
1860 Hayes St
San Francisco, CA 94117
Tel: 415 561-1821   *Fax:* 415 561-1999
E-mail: drincon@ccsf.edu

Everest College - San Francisco
Medical Assistant Prgm
A Corinthian School
814 Mission St, 5th Fl
San Francisco, CA 94103-3038
www.everest-college.com
Tel: 415 777-2500, Ext 250   *Fax:* 415 495-3457
E-mail: jjeong@cci.edu

Heald College - San Francisco
Medical Assistant Prgm
350 Mission St
San Francisco, CA 94105
www.heald.edu
Tel: 415 808-3000, Ext 3037   *Fax:* 415 808-3006
E-mail: carol_qare@heald.edu

Everest College
Medical Assistant Prgm
1245 S Winchester, Ste 102
San Jose, CA 95128
Tel: 408 246-4171   *Fax:* 408 557-9855
E-mail: tkidane@cci.edu

Western Career College - San Jose
Medical Assistant Prgm
6201 San Ignacio Ave
San Jose, CA 95119
Tel: 408 360-0840, Ext 243   *Fax:* 408 360-0848
E-mail: cread@sj.westerncollege.com

Western Career College - San Leandro
Medical Assistant Prgm
15555 E 14th St, Ste 500
San Leandro, CA 94578
Tel: 510 276-3888, Ext 117   *Fax:* 510 276-3653
E-mail: ldianda@westerncollege.com

West Valley Community College District
Medical Assistant Prgm
14000 Fruitvale Ave
Saratoga, CA 95070
Tel: 408 741-4019   *Fax:* 408 741-2145
E-mail: jekr@comcast.net

Heald College - Stockton Campus
Medical Assistant Prgm
1605 E March Lane
Stockton, CA 95210
www.heald.edu
Tel: 209 473-5200, Ext 5229   *Fax:* 209 477-2739
E-mail: ruth_brown@heald.edu

Southern California Regional Occupational Ctr
Medical Assistant Prgm
2300 Crenshaw Blvd
Torrance, CA 90501
http://scroc.com
Tel: 310 224-4200, Ext 262   *Fax:* 310 782-1589
E-mail: rhecht@scroc.k12.ca.us

East San Gabriel Valley ROP
Medical Assistant Prgm
Technical Center
1501 W Del Norte St
West Covina, CA 91790
www.esgvrop.org
Tel: 626 962-5080, Ext 136   *Fax:* 626 472-5125
E-mail: khill@esgvrop.org

Colorado

Everest College
Medical Assistant Prgm
14280 E Jewell Ave, Ste 100
Aurora, CO 80012
Tel: 303 745-6244   *Fax:* 303 745-6245
E-mail: mplitzuweit@cci.edu

Everest College
Medical Assistant Prgm
1815 Jet Wing Dr
Colorado Springs, CO 80916-2300
Tel: 719 638-6580, Ext 139   *Fax:* 719 638-6818
E-mail: marmorin@cci.edu

Community College of Denver
Medical Assistant Prgm
Medical Office Technology-Comprehensive
    Medical Assistant
3240 Humboldt St
Denver, CO 80205
www.ccd.edu
Tel: 303 293-8737, Ext 214   *Fax:* 303 292-4315
E-mail: darla.ruff@ccd.edu

Everest College
Medical Assistant Prgm
9065 Grant St
North Campus-Thornton
Denver, CO 80229-4339
Tel: 303 457-2757, Ext 128   *Fax:* 303 457-4030
E-mail: SMcintire@cci.edu

Westwood College
Medical Assistant Prgm
Institute of Health Careers
7350 N Broadway
Denver, CO 80221
Tel: 800 992-5050, Ext 685   *Fax:* 303 426-1832
E-mail: chollander@westwood.edu

Red Rocks Community College
Medical Assistant Prgm
13300 Sixth Ave
Lakewood, CO 80228
Tel: 303 914-6625   *Fax:* 303 914-6626
E-mail: rita.stoffel@rrcc.edu

Arapahoe Community College
Medical Assistant Prgm
5900 S Santa Fe Dr
PO Box 9002
Littleton, CO 80160-9002
www.arapahoe.edu
Tel: 303 797-5898   *Fax:* 303 797-5842
E-mail: connie.nelsen@arapahoe.edu

Front Range Comm College
Medical Assistant Prgm
2121 Miller Dr
Longmont, CO 80501
www.frontrange.edu
Tel: 303 678-3833   *Fax:* 303 678-3856
E-mail: kari.williams@frontrange.edu

Connecticut

Branford Hall Career Institute
Medical Assistant Prgm
One Summit Pl
Branford, CT 06405
Tel: 203 488-2525   *Fax:* 203 488-2920
E-mail: nmaisonet@branfordhall.com

St Vincent's College
Medical Assistant Prgm
2800 Main St
Bridgeport, CT 06606
Tel: 203 576-5518   *Fax:* 203 581-6533
E-mail: hmulrenan@stvincentscollege.edu

Quinebaug Valley Community College
Medical Assistant Prgm
742 Upper Maple St
Danielson, CT 06239-1436
Tel: 860 774-1160, Ext 349   *Fax:* 860 774-7768
E-mail: cgoretti@qvcc.commnet.edu

Goodwin College
Medical Assistant Prgm
745 Burnside Ave
East Hartford, CT 06108
http://goodwin.edu
Tel: 860 727-6780   *Fax:* 860 282-4625
E-mail: dwilken@goodwin.edu

Stone Academy
Medical Assistant Prgm
1315 Dixwell Ave
Hamden, CT 06514
Tel: 203 288-7474   *Fax:* 203 288-8869
E-mail: kpiscitello@stoneacademy.com

Capital Community College
Medical Assistant Prgm
950 Main St
Hartford, CT 06103
Tel: 860 906-5156   *Fax:* 860 906-5148
E-mail: sperreira@ccc.commnet.edu

Lincoln Tech Institute
Medical Assistant Prgm
200 John Downey Dr
New Britain, CT 06051
Tel: 860 225-8641, Ext 45815   *Fax:* 860 224-2983
E-mail: epierpaoli@lincolntech.com

Ridley-Lowell Business & Technical Institute
Medical Assistant Prgm
470 Bank St
New London, CT 06320
Tel: 860 443-7441   *Fax:* 860 442-3096
E-mail: rrbg4@att.net

Norwalk Community College
Medical Assistant Prgm
188 Richards Ave
Norwalk, CT 06854-1655
www.ncc.commnet.edu
Tel: 203 857-6852   *Fax:* 203 857-3364
E-mail: lperlstein@ncc.commnet.edu

Briarwood College
Medical Assistant Prgm
2279 Mt Vernon Rd
Southington, CT 06489
Tel: 860 628-4751, Ext 178   *Fax:* 860 628-6444
E-mail: florese@briarwood.edu

Fox Institute of Business
Medical Assistant Prgm
99 South St
West Hartford, CT 06110-1922
Tel: 860 947-2299   *Fax:* 860 947-2290
E-mail: foxmedicalhead@yahoo.com

Porter and Chester Institute - Wethersfield
Medical Assistant Prgm
125 Silas Deane Hwy
Wethersfield, CT 06109
Tel: 860 529-2519   *Fax:* 860 563-2595
E-mail: kjuchniewicz@porterchester.com

Northwestern Connecticut Comm College
Medical Assistant Prgm
Park Place E
Winsted, CT 06098
www.nwcc.commnet.edu
Tel: 860 738-6308   *Fax:* 860 738-6439
E-mail: bberger@nwcc.commnet.edu

Delaware

Delaware Technical & Community College - Wilmington
Medical Assistant Prgm
333 Shipley St
Wilmington, DE 19801-2412
www.dtcc.edu/wilmington/ah
Tel: 302 657-5170   *Fax:* 302 577-6431
E-mail: valerie@dtcc.edu

Florida

Manatee Technical Institute
Medical Assistant Prgm
5520 Lakewood Ranch Blvd
Bradenton, FL 34211
Tel: 941 751-7900, Ext 2001
E-mail: cantrellm@manateeschools.net

Florida Metropolitan Univ - Pinellas Campus
Medical Assistant Prgm
2471 McMullen Booth Rd, Ste 200
Clearwater, FL 33759
http://FMU.edu
Tel: 727 725-2688, Ext 131   *Fax:* 727 796-3722
E-mail: bbruns@cci.edu

Brevard Community College
Medical Assistant Prgm
1519 Clearlake Rd
Cocoa, FL 32922-6503
http://brevardcc.edu
Tel: 321 433-7545   *Fax:* 321 634-3731
E-mail: hardyk@brevardcc.edu

McFatter Technical Center
Medical Assistant Prgm
6500 Nova Dr
Davie, FL 33317
www.mcfattertech.com
Tel: 754 321-5886   *Fax:* 754 321-5820
E-mail: peter.Doolin@browardschools.com

Daytona Beach Community College
Medical Assistant Prgm
1200 W International Speedway Blvd
Daytona Beach, FL 32120-2811
http://dbcc.edu
Tel: 386 506-3215   *Fax:* 386 506-3300
E-mail: fieldis@dbcc.edu

Keiser University - Daytona Beach
Medical Assistant Prgm
1800 Business Park Blvd
Daytona Beach, FL 32114
www.keiseruniversity.edu
Tel: 386 274-5060   *Fax:* 386 274-2725
E-mail: bmclarnan@keiseruniversity.edu

Broward Community College
Medical Assistant Prgm
3501 SW Davie Rd
Fort Lauderdale, FL 33314
www.broward.edu
Tel: 954 201-6906   *Fax:* 954 201-9037
E-mail: adelagua@broward.edu

International College
Medical Assistant Prgm
4501 Colonial Blvd
Fort Myers, FL 33912
Tel: 239 513-1122, Ext 6179   *Fax:* 239 513-9108
E-mail: charrison@internationalcollege.edu

Palm Beach Community College
Medical Assistant Prgm
4200 Congress Ave
Lake Worth, FL 33461
Tel: 561 357-1330   *Fax:* 561 868-3635
E-mail: kalfinb@pbcc.edu

Florida Metropolitan Univ - Lakeland Campus
Medical Assistant Prgm
995 E Memorial Blvd, Ste 110
Lakeland, FL 33801
Tel: 863 686-1444, Ext 110   *Fax:* 863 688-9881
E-mail: ssowers@cci.edu

Florida Metropolitan Univ - Melbourne Campus
Medical Assistant Prgm
2401 N Harbor City Blvd
Melbourne, FL 32935-6657
Tel: 321 253-2929   *Fax:* 321 255-2017
E-mail: jlesser@cci.edu

Robert Morgan Educational Center
Medical Assistant Prgm
18180 SW 122nd Ave
Miami, FL 33177
Tel: 305 253-9920, Ext 2207   *Fax:* 305 253-3023
E-mail: GarciaJudith@msn.com

Florida Career Institute
Medical Assistant Prgm
5925 Imperial Pkwy, Ste 200
Mulberry, FL 33860
Tel: 941 646-1400   *Fax:* 941 646-5236
E-mail: judys@marcogrp.com

Lorenzo Walker Institute of Technology
Medical Assistant Prgm
3702 Estey Ave
Naples, FL 34104
Tel: 239 377-0938   *Fax:* 239 377-0336
E-mail: amsalefa@collier.k12.fl.us

Community Technical & Adult Education Center
Medical Assistant Prgm
1014 SW Seventh Rd
Ocala, FL 34474
Tel: 352 671-7200
E-mail: gail.mcpadden@marion.k12.fl.us

Florida Metro Univ - North Orlando Campus
Medical Assistant Prgm
5421 Diplomat Cir
Orlando, FL 32810
Tel: 407 628-5870, Ext 142   *Fax:* 407 628-1344
E-mail: tbaker@cci.edu

Florida Metro Univ - Orlando College South
Medical Assistant Prgm
9200 South Park Center Loop
Orlando, FL 32819-8606
www.cci.edu
Tel: 407 851-2525, Ext 174   *Fax:* 407 851-1477
E-mail: Brmiller@cci.edu

Pensacola Junior College
Medical Assistant Prgm
Warrington Campus
5555 W Hwy 98
Pensacola, FL 32507
Tel: 850 484-2221   *Fax:* 850 454-2365
E-mail: DBrewer@pjc.edu

Indian River Community College
Medical Assistant Prgm
500 NW California Blvd
Port St Lucie, FL 34986
Tel: 772 336-6237   *Fax:* 772 336-6235
E-mail: tparrino@ircc.edu

Seminole Community College
Medical Assistant Prgm
100 Weldon Blvd
Sanford, FL 32773-6199
www.scc-fl.edu
Tel: 407 328-2016   *Fax:* 407 708-2402
E-mail: mautnera@scc-fl.edu

Sarasota County Technical Institute
Medical Assistant Prgm
4748 Beneva Rd
Sarasota, FL 34233-1758
Tel: 941 924-1365, Ext 382   *Fax:* 941 361-6886
E-mail: harlean_satin@srqit.sarasota.k12.fl.us
Notes: Currently inactive

First Coast Technical Institute
Medical Assistant Prgm
2980 Collins Ave
St Augustine, FL 32084
Tel: 904 829-1087   *Fax:* 904 829-1077
E-mail: oakleyd@fcti.org

Pinellas Tech Educ Ctr - St Petersburg
Medical Assistant Prgm
901 34th St S
St Petersburg, FL 33711-2209
www.myptec.org
Tel: 727 893-2500, Ext 1069   *Fax:* 727 323-6638
E-mail: kliegerd@pcsb.org

Lively Technical Center
Medical Assistant Prgm
500 Appleyard Dr
Tallahassee, FL 32304-2810
Tel: 850 487-7489   *Fax:* 850 487-7478
E-mail: stradeb@mail.lively.leon.k12.fl.us

Erwin Technical Center
Medical Assistant Prgm
2010 E Hillsborough Ave
Tampa, FL 33610-8299
Tel: 813 231-1800, Ext 1344   *Fax:* 813 231-1820
E-mail: waldbart_e@popmail.firn.edu

Florida Metro U - Tampa Coll - Hillsborough
Medical Assistant Prgm
3319 W Hillsborough Ave
Tampa, FL 33614-5801
Tel: 813 879-6000, Ext 122   *Fax:* 813 871-2483
E-mail: rcohen@cci.edu

Florida Metropolitan Univ - Tampa College
Medical Assistant Prgm
3924 Coconut Palm Dr
Tampa, FL 33619
Tel: 813 621-0041, Ext 68   *Fax:* 813 623-5769
E-mail: cconklin@cci.edu

South University
Medical Assistant Prgm
1760 N Congress Ave
West Palm Beach, FL 33409
www.southuniversity.edu
Tel: 561 697-9200, Ext 3370   *Fax:* 561 697-9944
E-mail: ccarpenter@southuniversity.edu

Central Florida College
Medical Assistant Prgm
1573 W Fairbanks Ave
Winter Park, FL 32789
Tel: 407 843-3984   *Fax:* 407 843-9828
E-mail: jphillips@centralfloridacollege.edu

Winter Park Tech
Medical Assistant Prgm
901 Webster Ave
Winter Park, FL 32789-3098
Tel: 407 622-2900, Ext 2228   *Fax:* 407 975-2435
E-mail: gioielm@ocps.net

Georgia

North Metro Technical College - Acworth
Medical Assistant Prgm
5198 Ross Rd
Acworth, GA 30102
Tel: 770 975-4107
E-mail: dcrane@northmetrotech.edu

Albany Technical College
Medical Assistant Prgm
1704 S Slappey Blvd
Albany, GA 31701
Tel: 229 430-3542   *Fax:* 229 430-2853
E-mail: cbenson@albanytech.edu

Atlanta Technical College
Medical Assistant Prgm
1560 Metropolitan Pkwy SW
Atlanta, GA 30310
www.atlantatech.edu
Tel: 404 225-4570   *Fax:* 404 758-8522
E-mail: chelms@atlantatech.edu

Augusta Technical College
Medical Assistant Prgm
3200 Augusta Tech Dr
Augusta, GA 30906
www.augustatech.edu
Tel: 706 771-4189   *Fax:* 706 771-4181
E-mail: lnagle@augustatech.edu

Savannah River College
Medical Assistant Prgm
2528 Centerwest Pkwy, Bldg A
Augusta, GA 30909
Tel: 706 738-5046, Ext 22   *Fax:* 706 736-3599
E-mail: kbarton@savannahrivercollege.edu

North Georgia Technical College - Blairsville Campus
Medical Assistant Prgm
434 Meeks Ave
Blairsville, GA 30512
Tel: 706 754-7784   *Fax:* 706 754-7777
E-mail: kivester@ngtcollege.org

North Georgia Technical College
Medical Assistant Prgm
PO Box 65
1500 Hwy 197 N
Clarkesville, GA 30523
Tel: 706 754-7784   *Fax:* 706 754-7777
E-mail: kivester@northgatech.edu

DeKalb Technical College
Medical Assistant Prgm
495 N Indian Creek Dr
Clarkston, GA 30021
Tel: 404 297-9522, Ext 1164   *Fax:* 404 294-4234
E-mail: rialsl@dekalbtech.edu

Columbus Technical College
Medical Assistant Prgm
928 Manchester Expwy
Columbus, GA 31904-6572
Tel: 706 649-1499   *Fax:* 706 641-5284
E-mail: bgaither@columbustech.org

Dalton State College
Medical Assistant Prgm
213 N College Dr
Dalton, GA 30720
Tel: 706 272-4559   *Fax:* 706 272-4563
E-mail: kearley@em.daltonstate.edu

East Central Technical College
Medical Assistant Prgm
706 W Baker Hwy
Douglas, GA 31533
www.eastcentraltech.edu
Tel: 912 389-4300, Ext 2214   *Fax:* 912 389-4308
E-mail: kanderson@eastcentraltech.edu

Heart of Georgia Technical College
Medical Assistant Prgm
560 Pinehill Rd
Dublin, GA 31021
www.heartofgatech.edu
Tel: 478 274-7885   *Fax:* 478 275-6642
E-mail: bgurr@heartofgatech.edu

Griffin Technical College
Medical Assistant Prgm
501 Varsity Rd
Griffin, GA 30223
Tel: 770 233-5498
E-mail: fjohnson@griffintech.edu

Appalachian Technical College
Medical Assistant Prgm
100 Campus Dr
Jasper, GA 30143
Tel: 706 692-4500, Ext 4576   *Fax:* 706 692-4433
E-mail: tjackson@appalachiantech.edu

West Georgia Technical College
Medical Assistant Prgm
303 Fort Dr
LaGrange, GA 30240
Tel: 706 837-4267   *Fax:* 706 845-4339
E-mail: egilbert@westgatech.edu

Gwinnett Technical College
Medical Assistant Prgm
5150 Sugarloaf Pkwy
Lawrenceville, GA 30043-5702
Tel: 678 226-6346   *Fax:* 770 962-1506
E-mail: mjones@gwinnetttech.edu

Chattahoochee Technical College
Medical Assistant Prgm
980 S Cobb Dr
Marietta, GA 30060-3300
Tel: 770 528-4590   *Fax:* 770 528-4584
E-mail: jadair@chattcollege.com

Clayton State University
Medical Assistant Prgm
2000 Clayton State University
Morrow, GA 30260
www.clayton.edu
Tel: 678 466-4609   *Fax:* 678 466-4669
E-mail: latanyayoung@clayton.edu

Moultrie Technical College
Medical Assistant Prgm
361 Industrial Dr
Moultrie, GA 31768
www.moultrietech.edu
Tel: 229 891-7000, Ext 4195   *Fax:* 229 217-4211
E-mail: rkern@moultrietech.edu

Lanier Technical College
Medical Assistant Prgm
2990 Landrum Education Dr
Oakwood, GA 30566
Tel: 770 531-6354   *Fax:* 770 531-6306
E-mail: ccelorio@laniertech.edu

Northwestern Technical College
Medical Assistant Prgm
265 Bicentennial Trail
Rock Spring, GA 30739
Tel: 706 764-3544   *Fax:* 706 764-3718
E-mail: msmith@northwesterntech.edu

Coosa Valley Technical College
Medical Assistant Prgm
One Maurice Culberson Dr
Rome, GA 30161
www.cvtcollege.org
Tel: 706 295-6479   *Fax:* 706 295-6894
E-mail: jstephenson@coosavalleytech.edu

Savannah Technical College
Medical Assistant Prgm
5717 White Bluff Rd
Savannah, GA 31405-5521
Tel: 912 443-5810   *Fax:* 912 443-5826
E-mail: jmuller@savannahtech.edu

South University
Medical Assistant Prgm
Educational Management Corporation
709 Mall Blvd
Savannah, GA 31406
Tel: 912 201-8051   *Fax:* 912 201-8070
E-mail: heissa@southuniversity.edu

Medix School
Medical Assistant Prgm
2108 Cobb Pkwy
Smyrna, GA 30080-7630
Tel: 770 980-0002   *Fax:* 770 980-0811
E-mail: afielden@edaff.com

Ogeechee Technical College
Medical Assistant Prgm
One Joe Kennedy Blvd
Statesboro, GA 30458-3199
www.ogeecheetech.edu
Tel: 912 486-7616   *Fax:* 912 486-7604
E-mail: mturner@ogeecheetech.edu

Swainsboro Technical College
Medical Assistant Prgm
346 Kite Rd
Swainsboro, GA 30401-5700
Tel: 478 289-2243   *Fax:* 478 289-2214
E-mail: kbrown@swainsborotech.edu

Southwest Georgia Technical College
Medical Assistant Prgm
15689 US Hwy 19 N
Thomasville, GA 31792
www.southwestgatech.edu
Tel: 229 225-5081   *Fax:* 229 225-5289
E-mail: ghatcher@southwestgatech.edu

Southeastern Technical College
Medical Assistant Prgm
3001 E First St
Vidalia, GA 30474
www.southeasterntech.edu
Tel: 912 538-3198   *Fax:* 912 538-3106
E-mail: droessler@southeasterntech.edu

West Central Technical College
Medical Assistant Prgm
176 Murphy Campus Blvd
Waco, GA 30182
www.westcentraltech.edu
Tel: 770 537-6051   *Fax:* 770 537-7992
E-mail: jshell@westcentraltech.edu

Guam

Guam Community College
Medical Assistant Prgm
PO Box 23069
GMF Barrigada, GU 96921
Tel: 671 735-5656   *Fax:* 671 734-2550
E-mail: bmafnas@guamcc.net

Hawaii

Heald College - Honolulu Campus
Medical Assistant Prgm
1500 Kapiolani Blvd
Honolulu, HI 96814
www.heald.edu
Tel: 808 682-5533   *Fax:* 808 955-6964
E-mail: perfecto_salvador@heald.edu

Kapi'olani Community College
Medical Assistant Prgm
4303 Diamond Head Rd
Honolulu, HI 96816-4496
Tel: 808 734-9240   *Fax:* 808 734-9126
E-mail: lynnh@hawaii.edu

Idaho

Eastern Idaho Technical College
Medical Assistant Prgm
1600 S 25th E
Idaho Falls, ID 83404-5788
Tel: 208 524-3000, Ext 3340   *Fax:* 208 524-3007
E-mail: cmills@eitc.edu

Lewis-Clark State College
Medical Assistant Prgm
500 8th Ave
Lewiston, ID 83501
Tel: 208 792-2466
E-mail: jawyatt@lcsc.edu

Idaho State University
Medical Assistant Prgm
Campus Box 8380
Pocatello, ID 83209-8380
Tel: 208 282-4317   *Fax:* 208 282-3975
E-mail: birdnorm@isu.edu

College of Southern Idaho
Medical Assistant Prgm
PO Box 1238
Twin Falls, ID 83303-1238
Tel: 208 732-6728, Ext 6728   *Fax:* 208 736-4743
E-mail: pglenn@csi.edu

Illinois

Robert Morris College - Aurora
Medical Assistant Prgm
905 Meridian Lake Dr
Aurora, IL 60504
Tel: 312 935-6805   *Fax:* 312 935-6060
E-mail: jdavis@robertmorris.edu

Southwestern Illinois College
Medical Assistant Prgm
2500 Carlyle Rd
Belleville, IL 62221
www.swic.edu
Tel: 618 235-2700, Ext 5332   *Fax:* 618 235-2052
E-mail: cheryl.hutchison@swic.edu

Robert Morris College - Bensenville
Medical Assistant Prgm
1000 Tower Ln
Bensenville, IL 60106
Tel: 312 935-6805   *Fax:* 312 935-6060
E-mail: jdavis@robertmorris.edu

Northwestern Business College - Southwest Campus
Medical Assistant Prgm
South Campus
7725 S Harlem Ave
Bridgeview, IL 60455
www.northwesternbc.edu
Tel: 773 777-4220, Ext 2344   *Fax:* 773 777-2861
E-mail: mcbrady@nwbc.edu

Everest College - Burr Ridge
Medical Assistant Prgm
6880 N Frontage Rd, Ste 400
Burr Ridge, IL 60527
Tel: 630 920-1102, Ext 114   *Fax:* 630 920-9012
E-mail: mpowell@cci.edu

Northwestern Business College
Medical Assistant Prgm
4811 N Milwaukee Ave
Chicago, IL 60630
www.northwesternbc.edu
Tel: 773 777-4220, Ext 2344
E-mail: mcbrady@nwbc.edu

Robert Morris College - Chicago
Medical Assistant Prgm
401 S State St
Chicago, IL 60605
www.robertmorris.edu
Tel: 312 935-6805   *Fax:* 312 935-6060
E-mail: jdavis@robertmorris.edu

Spanish Coalition for Jobs Inc
Medical Assistant Prgm
2011 W Pershing Rd
Chicago, IL 60609
www.scj.org
Tel: 773 247-0707, Ext 252   *Fax:* 773 247-4975
E-mail: bbenway@scj-usa.org

Westwood College
Medical Assistant Prgm
8501 W Higgins Rd
Chicago, IL 60631
Tel: 847 928-1710
E-mail: areaves@westwood.edu

Northwestern Business College
Medical Assistant Prgm
Naperville Campus
1809 N Mill St
Naperville, IL 60563
www.northwesternbc.edu
Tel: 773 777-4220, Ext 2344
E-mail: mcbrady@nwbc.edu

Everest College - North Aurora
Medical Assistant Prgm
150 S Lincolnway #100
North Aurora, IL 60542
Tel: 630 896-2140
E-mail: bgreenfield@cci.edu

Robert Morris College - Orland Park
Medical Assistant Prgm
43 Orland Square Dr
Orland Park, IL 60462
Tel: 312 935-6805   *Fax:* 312 935-6060
E-mail: jdavis@robertmorris.edu

Harper College
Medical Assistant Prgm
1200 W Algonquin Rd
Health Careers and Public Safety
Palatine, IL 60067-7398
Tel: 847 925-6444   *Fax:* 847 925-6047
E-mail: gkalesmi@harpercollege.edu

Moraine Valley Community College
Medical Assistant Prgm
10900 S 88th Ave
Palos Hills, IL 60465-0937
Tel: 708 974-5708
E-mail: o'malley-absalon@morainevalley.edu

Midstate College
Medical Assistant Prgm
411 W Northmoor Rd
Peoria, IL 61614-3558
Tel: 309 692-4092, Ext 2040   *Fax:* 309 692-3893
E-mail: jholly@midstate.edu

Robert Morris College - Peoria
Medical Assistant Prgm
1 Technology Plaza
211 Fulton St
Peoria, IL 61602
Tel: 217 726-1631   *Fax:* 217 793-4210
E-mail: fegan@warpnet.net

Rockford Business College
Medical Assistant Prgm
730 N Church
Rockford, IL 61103-6917
Tel: 815 965-8616   *Fax:* 815 965-0360
E-mail: rchurch@rbcsuccess.com

Everest College - Skokie
Medical Assistant Prgm
9811 Woods Dr, Ste 200
Skokie, IL 60077
Tel: 847 470-0277
E-mail: rtaha@cci.edu

South Suburban College
Medical Assistant Prgm
15800 S State St, Rm 4453
South Holland, IL 60473
Tel: 708 596-2000
E-mail: lcampbell@southsuburbancollege.edu

Midwest Technical Institute
Medical Assistant Prgm
2731 Farmer's Market Rd
Springfield, IL 62707
Tel: 217 735-3105, Ext 107   *Fax:* 217 735-1055
E-mail: banderson@midwesttech.edu

Robert Morris College - Springfield
Medical Assistant Prgm
3101 Montvale Dr
Springfield, IL 62704
Tel: 217 726-1631   *Fax:* 217 793-4210
E-mail: fegan@warpnet.net

Waubonsee Community College
Medical Assistant Prgm
Rte 47 at Waubonsee Dr
Sugar Grove, IL 60554
www.waubonsee.edu
Tel: 630 466-7900, Ext 2467   *Fax:* 630 466-2441
E-mail: jtoussaint@waubonsee.edu

Robert Morris College - Waukegan
Medical Assistant Prgm
1507 Waukegan Rd
Waukegan, IL 60085
Tel: 312 935-6805   *Fax:* 312 935-6060
E-mail: jdavis@robertmorris.edu

Indiana

Indiana Business College - Anderson
Medical Assistant Prgm
140 E 53rd St
Anderson, IN 46013
www.ibcschools.edu
Tel: 765 644-7514   *Fax:* 765 644-5724
E-mail: jacki.hill@ibcschools.edu

Ivy Tech Community College - Anderson
Medical Assistant Prgm
104 W 53rd St
Anderson, IN 46013
Tel: 765 643-7133   *Fax:* 765 643-3294
E-mail: nschulz@ivytech.edu

Indiana Business College - Columbus
Medical Assistant Prgm
2222 Poshard Dr
Columbus, IN 47203
Tel: 812 379-9000
E-mail: kim.bricker@ibcschools.edu

Ivy Tech Community College - Columbus
Medical Assistant Prgm
4475 Central Ave
Columbus, IN 47203-1868
www.ivytech.edu/columbus
Tel: 812 374-5163   *Fax:* 812 372-0311
E-mail: khawkins@ivytech.edu

Indiana Business College - Evansville
Medical Assistant Prgm
4601 Theater Dr
Evansville, IN 47715
www.ibcschools.edu
Tel: 812 476-6000   *Fax:* 812 471-8576
E-mail: brenda.emge@ibcschools.edu

Ivy Tech Community College - Evansville
Medical Assistant Prgm
3501 First Ave
Evansville, IN 47710-3319
www.ivytech.edu
Tel: 812 429-1381   *Fax:* 812 429-9805
E-mail: klutz@ivytech.edu

Brown Mackie College - Ft Wayne
Medical Assistant Prgm
3000 E Coliseum Blvd
Fort Wayne, IN 46805
Tel: 260 481-5060   *Fax:* 260 484-2678
E-mail: plucas@brownmackie.edu

Indiana Business College - Ft Wayne
Medical Assistant Prgm
6413 N Clinton St
Fort Wayne, IN 46825
Tel: 260 471-7667   *Fax:* 260 471-6918
E-mail: barb.bley@ibcschools.edu

International Business Coll - Ft Wayne
Medical Assistant Prgm
5699 Coventry Ln
Fort Wayne, IN 46804
Tel: 260 459-4541   *Fax:* 260 436-1896
E-mail: pneu@ibcfortwayne.edu

Ivy Tech Community College - Ft Wayne
Medical Assistant Prgm
3800 N Anthony Blvd
Fort Wayne, IN 46805-1430
www.ivytech.edu
Tel: 260 480-4163   *Fax:* 260 480-4149
E-mail: tgreen@ivytech.edu

**Davenport University - South Bend/
   Mishawaka**
Medical Assistant Prgm
7121 Grape Rd
Granger, IN 46530
Tel: 574 277-8447, Ext 237
E-mail: cindy.pavel@davenport.edu

Indiana Business College
Medical Assistant Prgm
550 E Washington St
Indianapolis, IN 46204
www.ibcschools.edu
Tel: 317 656-4768   *Fax:* 317 351-1871
E-mail: bonnie.crist@ibcschools.edu

International Business Coll - Indianapolis
Medical Assistant Prgm
7205 Shadeland Station
Indianapolis, IN 46256
Tel: 317 813-2304   *Fax:* 317 841-6419
E-mail: jmackey@ibcindianapolis.edu

Ivy Tech Community College
Medical Assistant Prgm
9301 E 59th St
PO Box 1763
Indianapolis, IN 46216
Tel: 317 921-4409   *Fax:* 317 921-4432
E-mail: landrews@ivytech.edu

Kaplan College
Medical Assistant Prgm
7302 Woodland Dr
Indianapolis, IN 46278-1736
Tel: 317 299-6001, Ext 341   *Fax:* 317 298-6342
E-mail: tburton714@sbcglobal.net

Ivy Tech Community College - Kokomo
Medical Assistant Prgm
700 E Firmin St
Kokomo, IN 46903
www.ivytech.edu
Tel: 765 457-0858, Ext 105   *Fax:* 765 457-1036
E-mail: pslusher@ivytech.edu

Indiana Business College - Lafayette
Medical Assistant Prgm
4705 Meijer Court
Lafayette, IN 47905
Tel: 765 447-9550   *Fax:* 765 447-0868
E-mail: susan.horn@ibcschools.edu

Ivy Tech Community College - Lafayette
Medical Assistant Prgm
3101 S Creasy Ln
PO Box 6299
Lafayette, IN 47903
Tel: 765 269-5206   *Fax:* 765 269-5248
E-mail: cbolinger14@ivytech.edu

Ivy Tech Community College - Lawrenceburg
Medical Assistant Prgm
50 Walnut St
Lawrenceburg, IN 47025
www.ivytech.edu
Tel: 812 537-4010, Ext 234   *Fax:* 812 537-0993
E-mail: tdisch@ivytech.edu

Ivy Tech Community College - Madison
Medical Assistant Prgm
590 Ivy Tech Dr
Madison, IN 47250
Tel: 812 273-0105, Ext 27   *Fax:* 812 265-4028
E-mail: agarner@ivytech.edu

Indiana Business College - Marion
Medical Assistant Prgm
830 N Miller Ave
Marion, IN 46952
Tel: 765 662-7497
E-mail: jean.heath@ibcschools.edu

Ivy Tech Community College - Marion
Medical Assistant Prgm
1015 E 3rd St
Marion, IN 46952
Tel: 765 662-9843, Ext 320   *Fax:* 765 664-4256
E-mail: lpruitt@ivytech.edu

Davenport University - Merrillville
Medical Assistant Prgm
8200 Georgia St
Merrillville, IN 46410
www.davenport.edu
Tel: 219 769-5556
E-mail: barbara.kunshek@davenport.edu

Ivy Tech Community College - Michigan City
Medical Assistant Prgm
3714 Franklin St
Michigan City, IN 46360-7311
Tel: 219 879-9137, Ext 230   *Fax:* 219 879-9157
E-mail: vpavlakovic@ivytech.edu

Indiana Business College - Muncie
Medical Assistant Prgm
411 W Riggin Rd
Muncie, IN 47303
Tel: 765 288-8681, Ext 117
E-mail: nicole.hall@ibcschools.edu

Ivy Tech Community College - Muncie
Medical Assistant Prgm
4301 S Cowan Rd
Muncie, IN 47302

Ivy Tech Community College - Richmond
Medical Assistant Prgm
2325 Chester Blvd
Richmond, IN 47374
Tel: 765 966-2656, Ext 375   *Fax:* 765 939-2641
E-mail: kplanken@ivytech.edu

Ivy Tech Community College - Sellersburg
Medical Assistant Prgm
8204 Hwy 311
Sellersburg, IN 47172
www.ivytech.edu/sellersburg
Tel: 812 246-3301, Ext 4198   *Fax:* 812 246-9905
E-mail: pburton@ivytech.edu

Brown Mackie College - South Bend
Medical Assistant Prgm
1030 E Jefferson Blvd
South Bend, IN 46617
Tel: 574 237-0774, Ext 6557   *Fax:* 574 237-3585
E-mail: sgerald@brownmackie.edu

Ivy Tech Community College - South Bend
Medical Assistant Prgm
220 Dean Johnson Blvd
South Bend, IN 46601
Tel: 574 289-7001, Ext 5719   *Fax:* 574 236-7166
E-mail: cpavel1@ivytech.edu

Indiana Business College - Terre Haute
Medical Assistant Prgm
1378 South State Rd 46
Terre Haute, IN 47803
http://ibcschools.edu
Tel: 812 877-2100
E-mail: ursula.cole@ibcschools.edu

Ivy Tech Community College - Terre Haute
Medical Assistant Prgm
8000 S Education Dr
Terre Haute, IN 47802-4845
www.goivytech.net
Tel: 800 377-4882, Ext 2245   *Fax:* 812 298-2245
E-mail: bschonbe@ivytech.edu

Iowa

Des Moines Area Community College
Medical Assistant Prgm
2006 Ankeny Blvd, Bldg 9
Ankeny, IA 50023
www.dmacc.edu
Tel: 515 964-6457   *Fax:* 515 964-6440
E-mail: dmvanderploeg@dmacc.edu

Kirkwood Community College
Medical Assistant Prgm
6301 Kirkwood Blvd SW, PO Box 2068
Cedar Rapids, IA 52406-2068
www.kirkwood.edu
Tel: 319 398-5564   *Fax:* 319 398-1293
E-mail: dawn.eitel@kirkwood.edu

Iowa Western Community College
Medical Assistant Prgm
2700 College Rd/PO Box 4C
Council Bluffs, IA 51502-3004
www.iwcc.edu
Tel: 712 325-3348   *Fax:* 712 325-3736
E-mail: knelson@iwcc.edu

Kaplan University, Davenport Campus
Medical Assistant Prgm
1801 E Kimberly Rd, Ste 1
Davenport, IA 52807
Tel: 563 441-2453   *Fax:* 563 355-1320
E-mail: ejackson@kucampus.edu

Mercy College of Health Sciences
Medical Assistant Prgm
928 6th Ave
Des Moines, IA 50309-1239
Tel: 515 643-6705
E-mail: janderson@mercydesmoines.org

Iowa Central Community College
Medical Assistant Prgm
330 Ave M
Fort Dodge, IA 50501
Tel: 515 576-7201, Ext 2308   *Fax:* 515 576-5656
E-mail: kruger@iowacentral.com

North Iowa Area Community College
Medical Assistant Prgm
500 College Dr
Mason City, IA 50401
Tel: 641 422-4146   *Fax:* 641 422-4115
E-mail: stockdeb@niacc.edu

Iowa Lakes Community College
Medical Assistant Prgm
1900 N Grand
Spencer, IA 51301-3881
Tel: 712 262-7141   *Fax:* 712 262-4047
E-mail: chartig@iowalakes.edu

Southeastern Community College
Medical Assistant Prgm
1500 W Agency Rd
West Burlington, IA 52655
www.scciowa.edu
Tel: 319 208-5213   *Fax:* 319 752-4957
E-mail: dshaffer@scciowa.edu

Kansas

Northwest Kansas Technical College
Medical Assistant Prgm
1209 Harrison St, PO Box 668
Goodland, KS 67735-0668
Tel: 785 890-2072   *Fax:* 785 899-5711
E-mail: klucas@mail.nwktc.org

Wichita Area Technical College
Medical Assistant Prgm
324 N Emporia St
Wichita, KS 67202-2512
www.watc.edu
Tel: 316 677-1377, Ext 71377   *Fax:* 316 677-1332
E-mail: bbuchholz@watc.edu

Kentucky

National College - Danville
Medical Assistant Prgm
115 E Lexington Ave
Danville, KY 40422
www.national-college.edu
Tel: 606 236-6991   *Fax:* 606 236-1063
E-mail: adenson@national-college.edu

National College - Florence
Medical Assistant Prgm
7627 Ewing Blvd
Florence, KY 41042
Tel: 859 525-6510, Ext 19   *Fax:* 859 525-8961
E-mail: eonan@national-college.edu

Henderson Community College
Medical Assistant Prgm
2660 S Green St
Henderson, KY 42420
www.hencc.kctcs.edu
Tel: 270 831-9722   *Fax:* 270 831-9718
E-mail: Randa.Hawa@kctcs.edu

Bluegrass Community and Technical College
Medical Assistant Prgm
308 Vo-Tech Rd
Lexington, KY 40511
Tel: 859 246-2400, Ext 2321   *Fax:* 859 246-2417
E-mail: joyce.combs@kctcs.edu

National College - Lexington
Medical Assistant Prgm
2376 Sir Barton Way
Lexington, KY 40508
www.national-college.edu
Tel: 859 253-0621   *Fax:* 859 233-3054
E-mail: jhart@ncbt.edu

Spencerian College
Medical Assistant Prgm
1575 Winchester Rd
Lexington, KY 40505
Tel: 859 223-9608
E-mail: kbertrand@facultyspencerian.edu

Sullivan University - Lexington
Medical Assistant Prgm
2355 Harrodsburg Rd
Lexington, KY 40504
Tel: 606 276-4357   *Fax:* 606 276-1153
E-mail: jferrari@faculty.sullivan.edu

Jefferson Community and Technical College
Medical Assistant Prgm
727 W Chestnut St
Louisville, KY 40203-2074
www.jefferson.kctcs.edu
Tel: 502 213-4233   *Fax:* 502 213-4502
E-mail: jannie.washington@kctcs.edu

National College - Louisville
Medical Assistant Prgm
4205 Dixie Hwy
Louisville, KY 40216-3801
http://national-college.edu
Tel: 502 447-7634   *Fax:* 502 447-7665
E-mail: cmiles@national-college.edu

Spencerian College
Medical Assistant Prgm
4627 Dixie Hwy
Louisville, KY 40216
Tel: 502 449-7879, Ext 221   *Fax:* 502 449-7869
E-mail: lwarren@spencerian.edu

Maysville Comm & Tech College
Medical Assistant Prgm
609 Viking Dr
Morehead, KY 40351
Tel: 606 783-1538, Ext 66363   *Fax:* 606 783-1538
E-mail: diana.reeder@kctcs.edu

West Kentucky Community & Technical College
Medical Assistant Prgm
Blandville Rd, PO Box 7408
Paducah, KY 42002-7408
Tel: 270 534-3480   *Fax:* 502 554-2695
E-mail: Vicki.Kirschner@kctcs.edu

National College - Pikeville
Medical Assistant Prgm
50 National College Blvd
Pikeville, KY 41501
www.national-college.edu
Tel: 606 478-7200   *Fax:* 606 478-7209
E-mail: rmwolford@national-college.edu

Eastern Kentucky University
Medical Assistant Prgm
Dizney 225
521 Lancaster Ave
Richmond, KY 40475-3135
www.eku.edu
Tel: 859 622-6334   *Fax:* 859 622-6333
E-mail: joy.renfro@eku.edu

National College - Richmond
Medical Assistant Prgm
125 S Killarney Ln
Richmond, KY 40475
www.national-college.edu
Tel: 859 623-8956   *Fax:* 859 624-5544
E-mail: pciolek@national-college.edu

Louisiana

Bossier Parish Community College
Medical Assistant Prgm
6220 E Texas St
Bossier City, LA 71111
www.bpcc.edu
Tel: 318 678-6382   *Fax:* 318 678-6199
E-mail: cwinter@bpcc.edu

Career Technical College
Medical Assistant Prgm
2319 Louisville Ave
Monroe, LA 71201
Tel: 318 323-2889   *Fax:* 318 323-3113
E-mail: rjackson@careertc.com

Maine

Beal College
Medical Assistant Prgm
99 Farm Rd
Bangor, ME 04401
www.bealcollege.edu
Tel: 207 947-4591   *Fax:* 207 947-0208
E-mail: bmarchelletta@bealcollege.edu

Kennebec Valley Community College
Medical Assistant Prgm
92 Western Ave
Fairfield, ME 04937-1367
Tel: 207 453-5005   *Fax:* 207 453-5197
E-mail: ahickman@kvcc.me.edu

Maryland

Anne Arundel Community College
Medical Assistant Prgm
101 College Pkwy
Arnold, MD 21012
Tel: 410 777-7366   *Fax:* 410 777-7099
E-mail: hmmclean@aacc.edu

Allegany College of Maryland
Medical Assistant Prgm
12401 Willowbrook Rd SE
Cumberland, MD 21502
www.allegany.edu
Tel: 301 784-5319   *Fax:* 301 784-5022
E-mail: phughes@allegany.edu

Kaplan College - Frederick
Medical Assistant Prgm
5301 Buckeystown Pike
Frederick, MD 21704
Tel: 301 682-4882   *Fax:* 301 682-5855
E-mail: knave@kaplan.edu

Kaplan College
Medical Assistant Prgm
18618 Crestwood Dr
Hagerstown, MD 21742
www.hagerstownbusinesscol.edu
Tel: 301 739-2670, Ext 146   *Fax:* 301 791-7661
E-mail: KNave@hagerstownbusinesscol.edu

Cecil Community College
Medical Assistant Prgm
1 Seahawk Dr
North East, MD 21901
Tel: 410 287-6060, Ext 707
E-mail: jpalaisa@cecilcc.edu

Medix School
Medical Assistant Prgm
700 York Rd
Towson, MD 21204
www.medixschool.edu
Tel: 410 337-5155   *Fax:* 410 337-5104
E-mail: cwirtz@edaff.com

Massachusetts

Clark University
Medical Assistant Prgm
725 Granite St
Braintree, MA 02184
Tel: 781 794-3400, Ext 2023   *Fax:* 781 794-3408
E-mail: mrivera@clarktrain.com

Massasoit Community College
Medical Assistant Prgm
900 Randolph St
Canton, MA 02021-1355
www.massasoit.mass.edu
Tel: 781 821-2222, Ext 2601   *Fax:* 781 575-9428
E-mail: LDente@massasoit.mass.edu

Porter and Chester Institute - Chicopee
Medical Assistant Prgm
134 Dulong Circle
Chicopee, MA 01022
Tel: 413 593-3162   *Fax:* 413 593-6439
E-mail: medicalassisting@porterchester-ch.com

North Shore Community College
Medical Assistant Prgm
One Ferncroft Rd
Danvers, MA 01923-0840
Tel: 978 762-4179   *Fax:* 978 762-4022
E-mail: msplaine@northshore.edu

Bristol Community College
Medical Assistant Prgm
777 Elsbree St
Fall River, MA 02719
Tel: 508 678-2811, Ext 2629   *Fax:* 508 730-3281
E-mail: lwright@bristol.mass.edu

Mt Wachusett Community College
Medical Assistant Prgm
444 Green St
Gardner, MA 01440-1000
Tel: 978 630-9357   *Fax:* 978 630-9555
E-mail: b_tatro@mwcc.mass.edu

Northern Essex Community College
Medical Assistant Prgm
45 Franklin St
Lawrence, MA 01841-1121
www.necc.mass.edu
Tel: 978 738-7512   *Fax:* 978 738-7450
E-mail: khudson@necc.mass.edu

Middlesex Community College - Lowell
Medical Assistant Prgm
33 Kearney Square
Lowell, MA 01852-1901
www.middlesex.mass.edu
Tel: 978 656-3024   *Fax:* 978 656-3078
E-mail: hunts@middlesex.mass.edu

Charles H McCann Technical School
Medical Assistant Prgm
70 Hodges Cross Rd
North Adams, MA 01247
www.mccanntech.org
Tel: 413 663-5383, Ext 182   *Fax:* 413 664-9424
E-mail: tleclair@mccanntech.org

Southeastern Technical Institute
Medical Assistant Prgm
250 Foundry St
South Easton, MA 02375
www.sersd.org
Tel: 508 230-1337   *Fax:* 508 230-1558
E-mail: mdualsky@sersd.org

Cape Cod Community College
Medical Assistant Prgm
2240 Lyanough Rd
West Barnstable, MA 02668-1599
Tel: 508 362-2131, Ext 4324
E-mail: bcolocino@capecod.edu

The Salter School
Medical Assistant Prgm
184 W Boylston
West Boylston, MA 01583
Tel: 508 853-1074, Ext 20   *Fax:* 508 853-1083
E-mail: ctravis@salterschool.com

Quinsigamond Community College
Medical Assistant Prgm
670 W Boylston St
Worcester, MA 01606-2031
www.qcc.mass.edu
Tel: 508 854-2738   *Fax:* 508 852-6943
E-mail: pfleming@qcc.mass.edu

Michigan

Alpena Community College
Medical Assistant Prgm
666 Johnson St
Alpena, MI 49707-1495
www.alpenacc.edu
Tel: 989 358-7321   *Fax:* 989 358-7561
E-mail: putkamec@alpenacc.edu

Baker College of Auburn Hills
Medical Assistant Prgm
1500 University Dr
Auburn Hills, MI 48326-2642
www.baker.edu
Tel: 248 276-8785   *Fax:* 248 276-8785
E-mail: zetta.mcclain@baker.edu

Davenport University - Battle Creek
Medical Assistant Prgm
200 Van Buren St W
Battle Creek Career Center
Battle Creek, MI 49017
www.davenport.edu
Tel: 269 968-6105
E-mail: marybeth.pieri@davenport.edu

Baker College of Cadillac
Medical Assistant Prgm
9600 E 13th St
Cadillac, MI 49601
www.baker.edu
Tel: 231 876-3116   *Fax:* 231 876-3445
E-mail: becky.rodenbaugh@baker.edu

Davenport University - Caro
Medical Assistant Prgm
1231 Cleaver Rd
Caro, MI 48723
www.davenport.edu
Tel: 989 673-5857
E-mail: lisa.bannerman@davenport.edu

Glen Oaks Community College
Medical Assistant Prgm
62249 Shimmel Rd
Centerville, MI 49032
Tel: 888 994-7818   *Fax:* 269 467-4114
E-mail: kganger@glenoaks.edu

Baker College of Clinton Township
Medical Assistant Prgm
34950 Little Mack Ave
Clinton Township, MI 48035-4701
Tel: 586 791-6610, Ext 2689   *Fax:* 586 791-6611
E-mail: elizabeth.hoffman@baker.edu

Macomb Community College
Medical Assistant Prgm
Health and Human Services
44575 Garfield Rd
Clinton Township, MI 48038-1139
www.macomb.edu
Tel: 586 286-2194   *Fax:* 586 286-2098
E-mail: austind@macomb.edu

Henry Ford Community College
Medical Assistant Prgm
5101 Evergreen Rd
Dearborn, MI 48128-1495
www.hfcc.edu
Tel: 313 845-9877   *Fax:* 313 317-6569
E-mail: rbodurka@hfcc.edu

Baker College of Flint
Medical Assistant Prgm
G 1050 W Bristol Rd
Flint, MI 48507
Tel: 810 766-4233   *Fax:* 810 766-2055
E-mail: denise.gruener@baker.edu

Schoolcraft College
Medical Assistant Prgm
1751 Radcliff St
Garden City, MI 48135-1197
www.schoolcraft.edu
Tel: 734 462-4770, Ext 6025   *Fax:* 734 462-4775
E-mail: prubio@schoolcraft.edu

Davenport University - Grand Rapids (Fulton St)
Medical Assistant Prgm
415 E Fulton St E
Grand Rapids, MI 49503
www.davenport.edu
Tel: 616 451-3511, Ext 1184   *Fax:* 616 732-1145
E-mail: suzanne.garman@davenport.edu

Mid Michigan Community College
Medical Assistant Prgm
1375 S Clare Ave
Harrison, MI 48625
www.midmich.edu
Tel: 989 386-6645   *Fax:* 989 386-6666
E-mail: cking@midmich.edu

Baker College of Jackson
Medical Assistant Prgm
2800 Springport Rd
Jackson, MI 49202-1255
Tel: 517 841-4527   *Fax:* 517 789-7331
E-mail: angela.marin@baker.edu

Jackson Community College
Medical Assistant Prgm
2111 Emmons Rd
Jackson, MI 49201
https://www.jccmi.edu
Tel: 517 796-8557   *Fax:* 517 768-7004
E-mail: dennerljeanm@jccmi.edu

Kalamazoo Valley Community College
Medical Assistant Prgm
PO Box 4070, 6767 West O Ave
Kalamazoo, MI 49003-4070
http://kvcc.edu
Tel: 269 488-4324   *Fax:* 269 488-4458
E-mail: mdey@kvcc.edu

Davenport University - Lansing
Medical Assistant Prgm
220 E Kalamazoo St
Lansing, MI 48933
www.davenport.edu
Tel: 517 484-2600, Ext 8212   *Fax:* 517 484-9719
E-mail: linda.spang@davenport.edu

Baker College of Muskegon
Medical Assistant Prgm
1903 Marquette Ave
Muskegon, MI 49442-1453
Tel: 231 777-5318   *Fax:* 231 777-5265
E-mail: cindy.gordon@baker.edu

Baker College of Owosso
Medical Assistant Prgm
1020 S Washington St
Owosso, MI 48867-4400
Tel: 989 729-3416, Ext 3417   *Fax:* 989 729-3415
E-mail: kristin.black@baker.edu

Montcalm Community College
Medical Assistant Prgm
2800 College Dr
Sidney, MI 48885
Tel: 989 328-2111   *Fax:* 989 328-2950
E-mail: bethm@montcalm.edu

National Institute of Technology
Medical Assistant Prgm
26111 Evergreen Rd, Ste 201
Southfield, MI 48076
Tel: 248 799-9933   *Fax:* 248 799-2912
E-mail: yharris@cci.edu

Carnegie Institute
Medical Assistant Prgm
550 Stephenson Hwy, Ste 100
Troy, MI 48083
www.carnegie-institute.com
Tel: 248 589-1078   *Fax:* 248 589-1631
E-mail: info@carnegie-institute.edu

Oakland Community College
Medical Assistant Prgm
7350 Cooley Lake Rd
Waterford, MI 48327
Tel: 248 942-3068
E-mail: kakittle@oaklandcc.edu

Minnesota

Anoka Technical College
Medical Assistant Prgm
1355 W Hwy 10
Anoka, MN 55303-1564
Tel: 763 576-4700, Ext 4844   *Fax:* 763 576-4715
E-mail: slehrke@anokatech.edu

Minnesota School of Business - Brooklyn Center
Medical Assistant Prgm
Brooklyn Center
5910 Shingle Creek Pkwy, Ste 200
Brooklyn Center, MN 55430
Tel: 763 566-7777   *Fax:* 763 566-7000

Herzing College
Medical Assistant Prgm
5700 W Broadway Ave
Crystal, MN 55428
Tel: 763 535-3000   *Fax:* 763 535-9205
E-mail: ncaselius@mpls.herzing.edu

Duluth Business University
Medical Assistant Prgm
4724 Mike Colalillo Dr
Duluth, MN 55807
www.dbumn.edu
Tel: 218 740-4348   *Fax:* 218 628-2127
E-mail: maryb@dbumn.edu

Lake Superior College
Medical Assistant Prgm
2101 Trinity Rd
Duluth, MN 55811
Tel: 218 733-5919   *Fax:* 218 723-4921
E-mail: l.fox@lsc.mnscu.edu

Argosy University - Twin Cities
Medical Assistant Prgm
1515 Central Parkway
Eagan, MN 55121
www.argosyu.edu
Tel: 651 846-3560   *Fax:* 651 994-0170
E-mail: penocson@argosyu.edu

Northland Community & Technical College
Medical Assistant Prgm
2022 Central Ave NE
East Grand Forks, MN 56721-2702
Tel: 218 773-3441, Ext 4632   *Fax:* 218 773-4502
E-mail: elizabeth.mcmahon@northlandcollege.edu

Globe University - Oakdale
Medical Assistant Prgm
Oakdale Center
7166 Tenth St N
Oakdale, MN 55128
Tel: 651 714-7343   *Fax:* 651 730-5151
E-mail: ssuddendorf@globecollege.edu

Minnesota School of Business - Richfield
Cosponsor: Globe College
Medical Assistant Prgm
1401 W 76th St, Ste 500
Richfield, MN 55423-3841
Tel: 612 861-2000   *Fax:* 612 861-5548
E-mail: sende@msbcollege.edu

Dakota County Technical College
Medical Assistant Prgm
1300 E 145th St
Rosemount, MN 55068-2999
Tel: 651 861-8355, Ext 355   *Fax:* 651 423-8210
E-mail: patrice.nadeau@dctc.edu

Minneapolis Business College
Medical Assistant Prgm
1711 W County Rd B
Roseville, MN 55113
www.minneapolisbusinesscollege.edu
Tel: 651 636-7406, Ext 124   *Fax:* 651 636-8185
E-mail: cziegler@minneapolisbusinesscollege.edu

Century College
Medical Assistant Prgm
3300 Century Ave N
White Bear Lake, MN 55110-1842
Tel: 651 773-1731   *Fax:* 651 779-5779
E-mail: michelle.blesi@century.mnscu.edu

Ridgewater College - Willmar Campus
Medical Assistant Prgm
2101 15th Ave NW, PO Box 1097
Willmar, MN 56201
www.ridgewater.edu
Tel: 320 222-7571   *Fax:* 320 222-5216
E-mail: julene.bredeson@ridgewater.edu

Minnesota West Comm & Tech College
Medical Assistant Prgm
1450 Collegeway
Worthington, MN 56187
www.mnwest.edu
Tel: 507 372-3400, Ext 3489   *Fax:* 507 372-5801
E-mail: lisa.smith@mnwest.edu

Mississippi

Northeast Mississippi Community College
Medical Assistant Prgm
Cunningham Blvd
Booneville, MS 38829
www.nemcc.edu
Tel: 662 720-7393, Ext 393   *Fax:* 662 728-1165
E-mail: kcroberson@nemcc.edu

Hinds Community College
Medical Assistant Prgm
3805 Hwy 80 E
Pearl, MS 39208-4295
www.hindscc.edu
Tel: 601 936-5582   *Fax:* 601 936-1828
E-mail: cmking@hindscc.edu

Missouri

Everest College - Springfield Campus
Medical Assistant Prgm
1010 W Sunshine St
Springfield, MO 65807-2446
www.springfield-college.com
Tel: 417 864-7220, Ext 122   *Fax:* 417 864-5697
E-mail: mteal@cci.edu

Montana

Montana State University - Billings
Medical Assistant Prgm
3803 Central Ave
Billings, MT 59102
Tel: 406 247-3000
E-mail: sfloyd@msubillings.edu

Montana State Univ - Great Falls Coll of Tech
Medical Assistant Prgm
2100 16th Ave S
Great Falls, MT 59406-6010
Tel: 406 771-4383   *Fax:* 406 771-4317
E-mail: cmyles@msugf.edu

Flathead Valley Community College
Medical Assistant Prgm
777 Grandview Dr
Kalispell, MT 59901-2622
Tel: 406 756-3918   *Fax:* 406 756-3815
E-mail: kwest@fvcc.edu

Nebraska

Central Community College
Medical Assistant Prgm
Hastings Campus, PO Box 1024
Hastings, NE 68902-1024
http://cccneb.edu
Tel: 402 461-2405   *Fax:* 402 460-2138
E-mail: mmckinney@cccneb.edu

Hamilton College
Medical Assistant Prgm
1821 K St
Lincoln, NE 68508
Tel: 402 474-5315   *Fax:* 402 474-5302
E-mail: mguthard@hamiltonlincoln.edu

Southeast Community College
Medical Assistant Prgm
8800 O St
Lincoln, NE 68520-1227
Tel: 402 437-2756   *Fax:* 402 437-2404
E-mail: jgoodwin@southeast.edu

Alegent Health
Medical Assistant Prgm
6901 N 72nd St
Omaha, NE 68122
Tel: 402 572-2676   *Fax:* 402 572-3486
E-mail: dwitters@alegent.org

Hamilton College - Omaha
Medical Assistant Prgm
3350 N 90th St
Omaha, NE 68134-4710
Tel: 402 572-8500, Ext 257   *Fax:* 402 573-1341
E-mail: kgargano@hcomaha.com

Nebraska Methodist College
Medical Assistant Prgm
720 N 87th St
Omaha, NE 68114
Tel: 402 354-7076   *Fax:* 402 354-7130
E-mail: marcia.franklin@methodistcollege.edu

Nevada

College of Southern Nevada
Medical Assistant Prgm
6375 W Charleston Blvd, W4K
Las Vegas, NV 89146-1124
Tel: 702 651-5659   *Fax:* 702 651-5501
E-mail: gail.silva@csn.edu

New Hampshire

New Hampshire Comm Tech Coll - Claremont
Medical Assistant Prgm
One College Dr
Claremont, NH 03743
Tel: 603 542-7744, Ext 2743   *Fax:* 603 543-1844
E-mail: lgould@nhctc.edu

Hesser College
Medical Assistant Prgm
3 Sundial Ave
Manchester, NH 03103-7230
Tel: 603 668-6660, Ext 2259   *Fax:* 603 621-8995
E-mail: bsalines@hesser.edu

New Hampshire Comm Tech College - Manchester
Medical Assistant Prgm
1066 Front St
Manchester, NH 03102-8528
www.manchester.nhctc.edu
Tel: 603 668-6706, Ext 231   *Fax:* 603 668-5354
E-mail: cfeldhousen@nhctc.edu

New Jersey

Somerset County Technology Institute
Medical Assistant Prgm
North Bridge and Vogt Dr
PO Box 6350
Bridgewater, NJ 08807-0350
Tel: 908 526-8900, Ext 7244   *Fax:* 908 526-9494
E-mail: jpurdy@scettc.org

Dover Business College - Clifton
Medical Assistant Prgm
600 Getty Ave
Clifton, NJ 07011
www.doverbusinesscollege.org
Tel: 973 546-0123   *Fax:* 973 546-0017
E-mail: eskuka@doverbusinesscollege.org

Dover Business College - Paramus
Medical Assistant Prgm
600 Getty Ave
Clifton, NJ 07011
Tel: 973 546-0123   *Fax:* 973 546-0017
E-mail: hk@doverbusinesscollege.org

Hudson County Community College
Medical Assistant Prgm
870 Bergen Ave
Jersey City, NJ 07306-4403
www.hccc.edu
Tel: 201 360-4279   *Fax:* 201 418-7800
E-mail: JBender@hccc.edu

Sussex County Community College
Medical Assistant Prgm
1 College Hill
Newton, NJ 07860
http://sussex.edu
Tel: 973 300-2172   *Fax:* 973 300-2303
E-mail: tmiserendino@sussex.edu

Bergen Community College
Medical Assistant Prgm
400 Paramus Rd
Paramus, NJ 07652
www.bergen.edu
Tel: 201 612-5490   *Fax:* 201 612-3876
E-mail: stoth@bergen.edu

Technical Institute of Camden County
Medical Assistant Prgm
343 Berlin-Cross Keys Rd
Sicklerville, NJ 08081-9707
Tel: 856 767-7002, Ext 5539   *Fax:* 856 767-6625
E-mail: jjackyra@yahoo.com

Berdan Institute
Medical Assistant Prgm
265 Rte 46 W
Totowa, NJ 07512
Tel: 973 256-3444   *Fax:* 973 256-0816
E-mail: ifigliolina@berdaninstitute.com

Mercer County Technical Schools
Medical Assistant Prgm
1070 Klockner Rd
Trenton, NJ 08619
www.mcts.edu
Tel: 609 587-7640   *Fax:* 609 587-3304
E-mail: GKenney@mcts.edu

Warren County Community College
Medical Assistant Prgm
475 Rte 57 W
Washington, NJ 07882-4343
www.warren.edu
Tel: 908 835-2430   *Fax:* 908 689-8032
E-mail: vandeursen@warren.edu

New Mexico

Eastern New Mexico University - Roswell
Medical Assistant Prgm
PO Box 6000
Roswell, NM 88202-6000
Tel: 505 624-7199   *Fax:* 505 624-7100
E-mail: Cheryl.Vineyard@roswell.enmu.edu

New York

Bryant & Stratton College - Albany
Medical Assistant Prgm
1259 Central Ave
Albany, NY 12205-5230
Tel: 518 437-1802   *Fax:* 518 437-1048
E-mail: al.nathu.maqsood@mail.bryantstratton.edu

Broome Community College
Medical Assistant Prgm
Decker Bldg/PO Box 1017
Binghamton, NY 13902-1017
www.sunybroome.edu
Tel: 607 778-5211   *Fax:* 607 778-5467
E-mail: wade_a@sunybroome.edu

Ridley-Lowell Business & Technical Institute
Medical Assistant Prgm
116 Front St
Binghamton, NY 13905
www.ridley.edu
Tel: 607 724-2941   *Fax:* 607 724-0799
E-mail: pamhurst@stny.rr.com

ASA Institute of Business & Computer Tech
Medical Assistant Prgm
81 Willoughby St
Brooklyn, NY 11201-5208
www.asa.edu
Tel: 718 534-0782   *Fax:* 718 522-5880
E-mail: rcollazo@asa.edu

Bryant & Stratton College - Buffalo
Medical Assistant Prgm
465 Main St, Ste 400
Buffalo, NY 14203-1795
www.bryantstratton.edu
Tel: 716 884-9120   *Fax:* 716 884-0091
E-mail: st.armstrong.johanna@mail.bryantstratton.edu

Trocaire College
Medical Assistant Prgm
360 Choate Ave
Buffalo, NY 14220-2094
Tel: 716 827-2475   *Fax:* 716 828-6107
E-mail: kopruckiv@trocaire.edu

Elmira Business Institute
Medical Assistant Prgm
303 N Main St
Elmira, NY 14901
Tel: 607 733-7177   *Fax:* 607 733-7178
E-mail: smcsain@ebi-college.com

Wood Tobe'-Coburn School
Medical Assistant Prgm
8 E 40th St
New York, NY 10016-0190
Tel: 212 886-9040, Ext 138   *Fax:* 212 686-9171
E-mail: lmcwtc@aol.com

Ridley-Lowell Business & Technical Institute
Medical Assistant Prgm
26 S Hamilton St
Poughkeepsie, NY 12601
Tel: 845 471-0330   *Fax:* 845 471-4990
E-mail: pcdirector@ridley.edu

Bryant & Stratton College - Rochester
Medical Assistant Prgm
Henrietta Campus, 1225 Jefferson Rd
Greece Campus, 150 Bellwood Dr
Rochester, NY 14623-3185
Tel: 585 292-5627, Ext 148   *Fax:* 585 292-6015
E-mail: kcparysek@bryantstratton.edu

Rochester Business Institute
Medical Assistant Prgm
1630 Portland Ave
Rochester, NY 14621
Tel: 585 266-0430   *Fax:* 585 338-2464
E-mail: mhodges@cci.edu

Niagara County Community College
Medical Assistant Prgm
3111 Saunders Settlement Rd
Sanborn, NY 14132
Tel: 716 614-6411   *Fax:* 716 614-6879
E-mail: spassane@niagaracc.suny.edu

Bryant & Stratton College - Syracuse
Medical Assistant Prgm
953 James St
Syracuse, NY 13203-2555
Tel: 315 472-6603   *Fax:* 315 474-4383
E-mail: sy.pearsall.cheryl@mail.bryantstratton.edu

Erie Community College - North Campus
Medical Assistant Prgm
6205 Main St
Williamsville, NY 14221
www.ecc.edu
Tel: 716 851-1553   *Fax:* 716 851-1429
E-mail: bermel@ecc.edu

North Carolina

Stanly Community College
Medical Assistant Prgm
141 College Dr
Albemarle, NC 28001
www.Stanly.edu
Tel: 704 991-0397 *Fax:* 704 991-0350
E-mail: robinssk@stanly.edu

South College - Asheville
Medical Assistant Prgm
29 Turtle Creek Dr
Asheville, NC 28803
Tel: 828 277-5521 *Fax:* 828 277-6151
E-mail: cgee@southcollegenc.com

Miller-Motte College
Medical Assistant Prgm
2205 Walnut St
Cary, NC 27518
Tel: 919 532-7171, Ext 7168 *Fax:* 919 532-7151
E-mail: droche@miller-motte.edu

Central Piedmont Community College
Medical Assistant Prgm
PO Box 35009
Charlotte, NC 28235-5009
Tel: 704 330-6797 *Fax:* 704 330-6131
E-mail: leesa.whicker@cpcc.edu

Guilford Technical Community College
Medical Assistant Prgm
7815 National Service Rd
Charlotte, NC 28262
Tel: 704 547-8600
E-mail: dwarden@brookstone.edu

King's College
Medical Assistant Prgm
322 Lamar Ave
Charlotte, NC 28204
www.kingscollegecharlotte.edu
Tel: 704 688-3620 *Fax:* 704 348-2029
E-mail: bgallucci@kingscollegecharlotte.edu

Haywood Community College
Medical Assistant Prgm
185 Freelander Dr
Clyde, NC 28721-9454
Tel: 828 627-4658 *Fax:* 828 627-4656
E-mail: skelly@haywood.edu

Cabarrus College of Health Sciences
Medical Assistant Prgm
401 Medical Park Dr
Concord, NC 28025
Tel: 704 783-1639 *Fax:* 704 783-1764
E-mail: SWilson@northeastmedical.org

Gaston College - Dallas
Medical Assistant Prgm
201 Hwy 321 S
Dallas, NC 28034-1499
www.gaston.edu
Tel: 704 922-6465 *Fax:* 704 922-2333
E-mail: bdjones@gaston.edu

Surry Community College
Medical Assistant Prgm
630 S Main St
Dobson, NC 27017-8432
Tel: 336 386-3256, Ext 3256 *Fax:* 336 386-3497
E-mail: gantt@surry.edu

College of The Albemarle
Medical Assistant Prgm
1208 N Road St
Elizabeth City, NC 27906
Tel: 252 335-0821, Ext 2307
E-mail: kcarrion@albermarle.edu

Wayne Community College
Medical Assistant Prgm
Caller Box 8002
Goldsboro, NC 27534-8002
Tel: 919 735-5151, Ext 753 *Fax:* 919 736-9425
E-mail: lbrown@waynecc.edu

Alamance Community College
Medical Assistant Prgm
PO Box 8000
Graham, NC 27253
www.alamance.cc.nc.us
Tel: 336 506-4213 *Fax:* 336 578-7047
E-mail: actonk@alamancecc.edu

Pamlico Community College
Medical Assistant Prgm
PO Box 185
Grantsboro, NC 28529-0185
Tel: 252 249-1851, Ext 3044 *Fax:* 252 249-2377
E-mail: dholadia@pamlicocc.edu

Pitt Community College
Medical Assistant Prgm
PO Drawer 7007, Hwy 11 S
Greenville, NC 27835-7007
www.pitt.cc.nc.us/
Tel: 252 493-7284 *Fax:* 252 321-4451
E-mail: mhemby@email.pittcc.edu

Richmond Community College
Medical Assistant Prgm
1042 W Hamlet Ave
Hamlet, NC 28345
Tel: 910 582-7000, Ext 7174
E-mail: denae@richmondcc.edu

Guilford Technical Community College
Medical Assistant Prgm
601 High Point Rd, PO Box 309
Jamestown, NC 27282-0309
Tel: 336 454-1126, Ext 2307 *Fax:* 336 454-2510
E-mail: kgcannon@gtcc.edu

James Sprunt Community College
Medical Assistant Prgm
PO Box 398
Hwy 11 S
Kenansville, NC 28349-0398
Tel: 910 296-2400 *Fax:* 910 296-1636
E-mail: gradyland2@earthlink.net

Lenoir Community College
Medical Assistant Prgm
PO Box 188
231 Hwy 58S
Kinston, NC 28502-0188
www.lenoircc.edu
Tel: 252 527-6223, Ext 815 *Fax:* 252 233-6893
E-mail: ljohnson@lenoircc.edu

Davidson County Community College
Medical Assistant Prgm
PO Box 1287
Lexington, NC 27293-1287
Tel: 336 249-8186, Ext 6721 *Fax:* 336 249-9060
E-mail: srohr@davidsonccc.edu

Central Carolina Community College - Harnett
Medical Assistant Prgm
1075 E Cornelius Harnett Blvd
Lillington, NC 27546
www.cccc.edu
Tel: 919 718-7325 *Fax:* 919 718-7477
E-mail: mfogarty@cccc.edu

Vance-Granville Community College
Medical Assistant Prgm
PO Box 777
8100 NC 56 Hwy W
Louisburg, NC 27549
Tel: 252 738-3607 *Fax:* 252 496-6604
E-mail: care@vgcc.edu

Mitchell Community College
Medical Assistant Prgm
219 N Academy St
Mooresville, NC 28115
www.mitchellcc.edu
Tel: 704 978-5424 *Fax:* 704 663-5239
E-mail: mmarks@mitchellcc.edu

Carteret Community College
Medical Assistant Prgm
3505 Arendell St
Morehead City, NC 28557
www.carteret.edu
Tel: 252 222-6168 *Fax:* 252 222-6074
E-mail: godettev@carteret.edu

Western Piedmont Community College
Medical Assistant Prgm
1001 Burkemont Ave
Morganton, NC 28655
www.wpcc.edu
Tel: 828 438-6130 *Fax:* 828 430-7183
E-mail: agiles@wpcc.edu

Tri-County Community College
Medical Assistant Prgm
4600 Hwy 64 East
Murphy, NC 28906
Tel: 704 837-6810 *Fax:* 704 837-3266
E-mail: khearl@tricountycc.edu

Central Carolina Community College - Chatham
Medical Assistant Prgm
764 West St
Pittsboro, NC 27312
Tel: 919 718-7281 *Fax:* 919 718-7477
E-mail: mfogarty@cccc.edu

South Piedmont Community College
Medical Assistant Prgm
PO Box 126
Polkton, NC 28135-0126
Tel: 704 290-5800, Ext 5825 *Fax:* 704 272-8904
E-mail: lstarnes@spcc.edu

Wake Technical Community College
Medical Assistant Prgm
9101 Fayetteville Rd
Raleigh, NC 27603-5656
www.waketech.edu
Tel: 919 250-4333 *Fax:* 919 250-4329
E-mail: caparker@waketech.edu

Johnston Community College
Medical Assistant Prgm
PO Box 2350
245 College Rd
Smithfield, NC 27577
Tel: 919 209-2140
E-mail: leer@johnstoncc.edu

Mayland Community College
Medical Assistant Prgm
PO Box 547
Spruce Pine, NC 28777
Tel: 828 765-7351, Ext 330
E-mail: dhorton@mayland.edu

Edgecombe Community College
Medical Assistant Prgm
2009 W Wilson St
Tarboro, NC 27886
Tel: 252 446-0436, Ext 353 *Fax:* 252 985-2212
E-mail: tolsond@edgecombe.edu

Montgomery Community College
Medical Assistant Prgm
1011 Page St
Troy, NC 27371
Tel: 910 576-6222, Ext 208 *Fax:* 910 576-3005
E-mail: cavinessc@montgomery.edu

Wilkes Community College
Medical Assistant Prgm
PO Box 120
1328 Collegiate Dr
Wilkesboro, NC 28697-0120
Tel: 910 838-6251   *Fax:* 910 838-6255
E-mail: mintonj@wilkescc.edu

Martin Commuity College
Medical Assistant Prgm
1161 Kehukee Park Rd
Williamston, NC 27892-8307
www.martin.cc.nc.us
Tel: 252 792-1521, Ext 292   *Fax:* 252 792-4425
E-mail: mflynn@martincc.edu

Miller-Motte College
Medical Assistant Prgm
5000 Market St
Wilmington, NC 28405
Tel: 910 392-4660, Ext 2015   *Fax:* 910 799-6224
E-mail: ggrady@miller-motte.com

Forsyth Technical Community College
Medical Assistant Prgm
2100 Silas Creek Pkwy
Winston-Salem, NC 27103
Tel: 336 734-7362   *Fax:* 336 734-7581
E-mail: ldurham@bit.forsythtech.edu

Ohio

Akron Institute
Medical Assistant Prgm
1600 S Arlington, Ste 100
Akron, OH 44306
Tel: 330 724-1600, Ext 15   *Fax:* 330 724-9688
E-mail: cgarman@akroninstitute.com

Brown Mackie College - Akron
Medical Assistant Prgm
755 White Pond Dr
Akron, OH 44320
www.brownmackie.edu
Tel: 330 869-3600, Ext 3619   *Fax:* 330 869-3650
E-mail: dtymcio@brownmackie.edu

University of Akron
Medical Assistant Prgm
Polsky 124C
Akron, OH 44325-3702
www.uakron.edu
Tel: 330 972-6515   *Fax:* 330 972-2016
E-mail: gibsonr@uakron.edu

Ashland County - West Holmes Career Center
Medical Assistant Prgm
1783 State Rte 60
Ashland, OH 44805-9377
www.acwhcc-jvs.k12.oh.us/
Tel: 419 289-3313, Ext 207   *Fax:* 419 289-3729
E-mail: awhj_Kleinsc@tccsa.net

Mahoning County Career & Technical Center
Medical Assistant Prgm
7300 N Palmyra Rd
Canfield, OH 44406-9710
www.mahoningctc.com
Tel: 330 729-4100, Ext 1953   *Fax:* 330 729-4150
E-mail: mjvs_ajs@access-k12.org

Canton City Schools
Medical Assistant Prgm
Adult Community Education Center
116 McKinley Ave NW Rm 206
Canton, OH 44702
Tel: 330 456-1092   *Fax:* 330 454-6767
E-mail: kjsdean@yahoo.com

Stark State College of Technology
Medical Assistant Prgm
6200 Frank Ave NW
Canton, OH 44720
www.starkstate.edu
Tel: 330 966-5458, Ext 4233   *Fax:* 330 966-6586
E-mail: gtodaro@starkstate.edu

Fairfield Career Center (EVSD)
Medical Assistant Prgm
4000 Columbus-Lancaster Rd
Carroll, OH 43112
Tel: 740 756-9245   *Fax:* 740 837-9447
E-mail: ttipton@efcts.us

RETS Tech Center
Medical Assistant Prgm
555 E Alex-Bell Rd
Centerville, OH 45459
Tel: 937 433-3410, Ext 218   *Fax:* 937 435-6516
E-mail: squinn@retstechcenter.com

Pickaway Ross Joint Vocational School
Medical Assistant Prgm
17273 St Rte 104 Bldg 4
Chillicothe, OH 45601
www.pickawayross.com
Tel: 740 642-1440, Ext 450   *Fax:* 740 642-1454
E-mail: faye.vermillion@pickawayross.com

Brown Mackie College - Cincinnati
Medical Assistant Prgm
1011 Glendale-Milford Rd
Cincinnati, OH 45215
Tel: 513 771-2424, Ext 1935   *Fax:* 513 771-3413
E-mail: lreddington@brownmackie.edu

Cincinnati State Tech & Comm College
Medical Assistant Prgm
3520 Central Pkwy
Cincinnati, OH 45223
Tel: 513 569-1571   *Fax:* 513 569-1659
E-mail: olivia.watts@cincinnatistate.edu

National College of Business and Technology - Cincinnati
Medical Assistant Prgm
6871 Steger Dr
Cincinnati, OH 45237
Tel: 513 761-1291
E-mail: gacameron@national-college.edu

University of Cincinnati
Cosponsor: Raymond Walters College
Medical Assistant Prgm
9555 Plainfield Rd
Cincinnati, OH 45236
Tel: 513 745-5664   *Fax:* 513 745-5771
E-mail: rachael.allstatter@uc.edu

Miami Valley Career Technology Center
Medical Assistant Prgm
6800 Hoke Rd
Clayton, OH 45315
www.mvctc.com
Tel: 937 854-6297   *Fax:* 937 837-5619
E-mail: apatton@mvctc.com

Cuyahoga Community College
Medical Assistant Prgm
Metro Campus
2900 Community College Ave
Cleveland, OH 44115
www.tri-c.edu
Tel: 216 987-4439   *Fax:* 216 987-4386
E-mail: Sherry.brewer@tri-c.edu

American School of Technology
Medical Assistant Prgm
2100 Morse Rd
Columbus, OH 43229
Tel: 614 436-4820   *Fax:* 614 436-4343
E-mail: bruble@ast.edu

Bradford School
Medical Assistant Prgm
2469 Stelzer Rd
Columbus, OH 43219
www.bradfordschoolcolumbus.edu
Tel: 614 416-6200, Ext 110   *Fax:* 614 416-6210
E-mail: arumich@bradfordschoolcolumbus.edu

Columbus State Community College
Medical Assistant Prgm
550 E Spring St
Columbus, OH 43216
www.cscc.edu
Tel: 614 287-3638   *Fax:* 614 287-5198
E-mail: fstout@cscc.edu

Ohio Institute of Health Careers - Columbus
Medical Assistant Prgm
1880 E Dublin-Granville Rd, Ste 100
Columbus, OH 43229
Tel: 614 891-5030, Ext 118   *Fax:* 614 891-5130
E-mail: mheller@ohioinstitueofhealthcareers.edu

Miami-Jacobs Career College
Medical Assistant Prgm
110 N Patterson Blvd
Dayton, OH 45402
Tel: 937 746-1830, Ext 207   *Fax:* 937 806-1027
E-mail: teresa.rivers@miamijacobs.edu

Ohio Institute of Photography & Technology
Medical Assistant Prgm
Division of Allied Health
2029 Edgefield Rd
Dayton, OH 45439
Tel: 937 294-6155, Ext 208   *Fax:* 937 294-2259
E-mail: ronda@oipt.com

Sinclair Community College
Medical Assistant Prgm
444 W Third St
Dayton, OH 45402-1421
Tel: 937 512-2973   *Fax:* 937 512-2239
E-mail: jennifer.barr@sinclair.edu

Ohio Valley College of Technology
Medical Assistant Prgm
16808 St Clair Ave, PO Box 7000
East Liverpool, OH 43920
Tel: 330 385-1070   *Fax:* 330 385-4606

Lorain County Community College
Medical Assistant Prgm
1005 N Abbe Rd
Elyria, OH 44035
www.lorainccc.edu
Tel: 440 366-4189   *Fax:* 440 366-4116
E-mail: cwatkins@lorainccc.edu

Ohio Institute of Health Careers - Elyria
Medical Assistant Prgm
631 Griswold Rd
Elyria, OH 44035
www.ohioinstituteofhealthcareers.edu
Tel: 440 324-2293   *Fax:* 440 324-2610
E-mail: rcatella@ohioinstituteofhealthcareers.edu

Portage Lakes Career Center
Medical Assistant Prgm
4401 Shriver Rd
PO Box 248
Green, OH 44232-0248
Tel: 330 896-8113   *Fax:* 330 896-8197
E-mail: pl_mcbride@portagelakescareercenter.org

Southern State Community College
Medical Assistant Prgm
100 Hobart Dr
Hillsboro, OH 45133-9487
Tel: 937 393-3431, Ext 2639   *Fax:* 937 393-9370
E-mail: cdeatley@sscc.edu

National College of Business and Technology - Kettering
Medical Assistant Prgm
1837 Woodman Center Dr
Kettering, OH 45429
Tel: 937 299-9450
E-mail: ghaines@national-college.edu

Lakeland Community College
Medical Assistant Prgm
7700 Clocktower Dr
Kirtland, OH 44094
http://lakelandcc.edu/ACADEMIC/SH/MedAsst/
    MedAsst.htm
Tel: 440 525-7428   *Fax:* 440 525-7433
E-mail: mmiller@lakelandcc.edu

Ohio University - Lancaster
Medical Assistant Prgm
1570 Granville Pike
Lancaster, OH 43130
Tel: 740 654-6711, Ext 276   *Fax:* 740 687-9497
E-mail: maxwell@ohio.edu

Apollo Career Center
Medical Assistant Prgm
3325 Shawnee Rd
Lima, OH 45806
www.apollocareercenter.com
Tel: 419 998-2971   *Fax:* 419 998-2994
E-mail: tara.shepherd@apollocc.org

Rhodes State College
Medical Assistant Prgm
4240 Campus Dr KH 109
Lima, OH 45804
www.rhodesstate.edu
Tel: 419 995-8016, Ext 8016   *Fax:* 419 995-8093
E-mail: kiel.d@rhodesstate.edu

University of Northwestern Ohio
Medical Assistant Prgm
1441 N Cable Rd
Lima, OH 45805
Tel: 419 227-3141   *Fax:* 419 229-6926
E-mail: jashelle@unoh.edu

Washington County Career Center
Medical Assistant Prgm
1750 Lancaster St
Marietta, OH 45750
Tel: 740 373-6283   *Fax:* 740 373-9026
E-mail: wks@1st.net

Marion Technical College
Medical Assistant Prgm
1467 Mt Vernon Ave
Marion, OH 43302-5694
www.mtc.edu
Tel: 614 389-4636, Ext 319   *Fax:* 614 389-6136
E-mail: smithp@mtc.edu

Stautzenberger College
Medical Assistant Prgm
1796 Indian Wood Cir
Maumee, OH 43537
Tel: 419 866-0261   *Fax:* 419 867-9821
E-mail: sahahn@stautzenberger.com

Medina County Career Center
Medical Assistant Prgm
1101 W Liberty St
Medina, OH 44256-9969
Tel: 330 725-8461, Ext 314   *Fax:* 330 725-3842
E-mail: mayes@mcjvsd.org

Polaris Career Center
Medical Assistant Prgm
7285 Old Oak Blvd
Middleburg Heights, OH 44130
www.polaris.edu
Tel: 440 891-7600, Ext 7635   *Fax:* 440 243-3952
E-mail: klazroff@polaris.edu

EHOVE Ghrist Adult Career Center
Medical Assistant Prgm
316 W Mason Rd
Milan, OH 44846
www.ehove.net
Tel: 419 499-4663, Ext 287   *Fax:* 419 499-5391
E-mail: jballard@ehove-jvs.k12.oh.us

Knox County Career Center
Medical Assistant Prgm
308 Martinsburg Rd
Mount Vernon, OH 43050-4298
www.knoxcc.org
Tel: 740 393-2933, Ext 102   *Fax:* 740 393-1659
E-mail: kimber.williams@yahoo.com

Hocking College
Medical Assistant Prgm
3301 Hocking Pkwy
Nelsonville, OH 45764-9582
Tel: 614 753-3591, Ext 6434   *Fax:* 614 753-6430
E-mail: west_k@hocking.edu

Lorain Cnty Joint Voc School - Adult Career
Medical Assistant Prgm
15181 State Route 58
Oberlin, OH 44074
Tel: 440 774-1051   *Fax:* 440 776-2070
E-mail: nsmith@leeca.org

Bryant & Stratton College - Parma
Medical Assistant Prgm
12955 Snow Rd
Parma, OH 44130
Tel: 216 265-3151   *Fax:* 216 265-0325
E-mail: pr.batheja.sheila@mail.bryantstratton.edu

Edison Community College
Medical Assistant Prgm
1973 Edison Dr
Piqua, OH 45356
Tel: 937 778-7994
E-mail: balters-spring@edisonohio.edu

Belmont Technical College
Medical Assistant Prgm
120 Fox-Shannon Pl
St Clairsville, OH 43950-9766
Tel: 740 695-9500, Ext 1171   *Fax:* 740 695-2247
E-mail: dfolmar@btc.edu

Jefferson Community College
Medical Assistant Prgm
4000 Sunset Blvd
Steubenville, OH 43952
www.jcc.edu
Tel: 740 264-5591, Ext 159   *Fax:* 740 264-1338
E-mail: rflohr@jcc.edu

Davis College
Medical Assistant Prgm
4747 Monroe St
Toledo, OH 43623-4389
www.daviscollege.edu
Tel: 419 473-2700, Ext 312   *Fax:* 419 473-2472
E-mail: rlazette@daviscollege.edu

Trumbull Career & Technical Center
Medical Assistant Prgm
528 Educational Hwy
Warren, OH 44483
www.tctcadulttraining.org
Tel: 330 847-0503, Ext 1620   *Fax:* 330 847-1177
E-mail: joan.bushey@neomin.org

Youngstown State University
Medical Assistant Prgm
Medical Assisting Technology Program
Dept of Health Professions
Youngstown, OH 44555-0001
www.ysu.edu
Tel: 330 742-1760   *Fax:* 330 742-2921
E-mail: klfeld@ysu.edu

Zane State College
Medical Assistant Prgm
1555 Newark Rd
Zanesville, OH 43701
Tel: 740 588-1270   *Fax:* 740 454-0035
E-mail: tberger@zanestate.edu

Oklahoma

Moore Norman Technology Center
Medical Assistant Prgm
PO Box 4701
Norman, OK 73070-4701
Tel: 405 364-5763, Ext 6524   *Fax:* 405 447-6289
E-mail: amcbride@mntechnology.com

Francis Tuttle Technology Center
Medical Assistant Prgm
12777 N Rockwell Ave
Oklahoma City, OK 73142-2789
www.francistuttle.com
Tel: 405 717-4142   *Fax:* 405 717-4789
E-mail: dwiggins@francistuttle.com

Metro Technology Centers
Medical Assistant Prgm
1720 Springlake Dr
Oklahoma City, OK 73111-5240
Tel: 405 605-4644   *Fax:* 405 424-9403
E-mail: pam.ashley@metrotech.org

Tulsa Community College
Medical Assistant Prgm
909 S Boston Ave
Tulsa, OK 74119-2095
www.tulsacc.edu
Tel: 918 595-7321   *Fax:* 918 595-7091
E-mail: jwood@tulsacc.edu

Oregon

Linn-Benton Community College
Medical Assistant Prgm
6500 SW Pacific Blvd
Albany, OR 97321-3755
http://linnbenton.edu
Tel: 541 917-4288   *Fax:* 541 917-4445
E-mail: rick.durling@linnbenton.edu

Central Oregon Community College
Medical Assistant Prgm
2600 NW College Way
Bend, OR 97701
www.cocc.edu
Tel: 541 383-7292   *Fax:* 541 318-3750
E-mail: lmatthews@cocc.edu

Lane Community College
Medical Assistant Prgm
4000 E 30th Ave
Eugene, OR 97405-0640
Tel: 541 463-5621   *Fax:* 541 463-4151
E-mail: meashintubbyd@lanecc.edu

Mt Hood Community College
Medical Assistant Prgm
26000 SE Stark St
Gresham, OR 97030
Tel: 503 491-7136   *Fax:* 503 491-7618
E-mail: bouldens@mhcc.edu

Clackamas Community College
Medical Assistant Prgm
19600 S Molalla Ave
Oregon City, OR 97045-8980
Tel: 503 657-6958, Ext 2910   *Fax:* 503 655-5153
E-mail: maureenm@clackamas.edu

Concorde Career Institute - Portland
Medical Assistant Prgm
1425 NE Irving St
Portland, OR 97232-4203
Tel: 503 281-4181, Ext 107   *Fax:* 503 281-6739
E-mail: wcampbell@concorde.edu

Everest College
Medical Assistant Prgm
425 SW Washington St
Portland, OR 97204
Tel: 503 222-3225   *Fax:* 503 241-3144
E-mail: Snewman@cci.edu

Heald College - Portland
Medical Assistant Prgm
625 SW Broadway, Ste 200
Portland, OR 97205
www.heald.edu
Tel: 503 229-0492   *Fax:* 503 229-0498
E-mail: tina_egeland@heald.edu

Portland Community College
Medical Assistant Prgm
12000 SW 49th Ave
705 N Killingsworth St
Portland, OR 97219-7132
Tel: 503 978-5664   *Fax:* 503 978-5257
E-mail: drigsbee@pcc.edu

Pennsylvania

Greater Altoona Career & Technology Center
Medical Assistant Prgm
1500 Fourth Ave
Altoona, PA 16602
Tel: 814 946-8469   *Fax:* 814 941-4690
E-mail: sybert5@verizon.net

Butler County Community College
Medical Assistant Prgm
PO Box 1203
College Dr
Butler, PA 16003-1203
http://bc3.edu
Tel: 724 287-8711, Ext 8373   *Fax:* 724 285-6047
E-mail: debby.proctor@bc3.edu

Mount Aloysius College
Medical Assistant Prgm
7373 Admiral Peary Hwy
Cresson, PA 16630-1999
Tel: 814 886-6322   *Fax:* 814 886-2978
E-mail: ckowalczyk@mtaloy.edu

Tri-State Business Institute
Medical Assistant Prgm
5757 W 26th St
Erie, PA 16506
Tel: 814 838-7673
E-mail: klucore@tsbi.edu

Harrisburg Area Community College
Medical Assistant Prgm
One HACC Dr, PC-333
Harrisburg, PA 17110
Tel: 717 221-1326   *Fax:* 717 909-4010
E-mail: jlbacon@hacc.edu

Thompson Institute
Medical Assistant Prgm
5650 Derry St
Harrisburg, PA 17111
Tel: 800 272-4632   *Fax:* 717 558-8560
E-mail: bsnyder@thompson.edu

YTI Career Institute
Medical Assistant Prgm
3050 Hempland Rd
Lancaster, PA 17602
Tel: 717 295-1100, Ext 1013   *Fax:* 717 295-1135
E-mail: cox_s@yti.edu

Delaware County Community College
Medical Assistant Prgm
Rte 252 and Media Line Rd
Media, PA 19063-1094
www.dccc.edu
Tel: 610 359-5289   *Fax:* 610 359-7350
E-mail: jdecaro@dccc.edu

Career Training Academy
Medical Assistant Prgm
950 Fifth Ave
New Kensington, PA 15068
Tel: 724 337-1000, Ext 12   *Fax:* 724 335-7140
E-mail: vp@careerta.com

Bucks County Community College
Medical Assistant Prgm
275 Swamp Rd
Newtown, PA 18940
Tel: 215 968-8341   *Fax:* 215 504-8509
E-mail: zieziula@bucks.edu

Community College of Philadelphia
Medical Assistant Prgm
1700 Spring Garden St
Philadelphia, PA 19130-3936
Tel: 215 751-8947   *Fax:* 215 751-8937
E-mail: drossi@ccp.edu

Thompson Institute
Medical Assistant Prgm
3010 Market St
Philadelphia, PA 19104
Tel: 215 594-4034   *Fax:* 215 594-4093
E-mail: ssuddendorf@thompson.edu

Bradford School - Pittsburgh
Medical Assistant Prgm
125 W Station Square Dr, Ste 129
Pittsburgh, PA 15219
www.bradfordpittsburgh.edu
Tel: 412 391-6366   *Fax:* 412 471-6714
E-mail: cboles@bradfordpittsburgh.edu

Everest Institute
Medical Assistant Prgm
100 Forbes Ave, Ste 1200
Pittsburgh, PA 15222
Tel: 412 261-4520, Ext 219   *Fax:* 412 261-4546
E-mail: mpopulo@cci.edu

Kaplan Career Institute - ICM Campus
Medical Assistant Prgm
10 Wood St
Pittsburgh, PA 15222
Tel: 412 261-2647, Ext 253   *Fax:* 412 261-6491
E-mail: lslack@icmschool.com

Central Pennsylvania Institute of Sci & Tech
Medical Assistant Prgm
540 N Harrison Rd
Pleasant Gap, PA 16823
Tel: 814 359-2793, Ext 308   *Fax:* 814 359-2599
E-mail: lbergam@cpi.edu

Montgomery County Community College
Medical Assistant Prgm
101 College Dr
Pottstown, PA 19464
www.mc3.edu
Tel: 610 718-1812   *Fax:* 610 718-1983
E-mail: kschreiner@mc3.edu

Lehigh Carbon Community College
Medical Assistant Prgm
4525 Education Park Dr
Schnecksville, PA 18078-2502
www.lccc.edu
Tel: 610 799-1516   *Fax:* 610 799-1527
E-mail: jehninger@lccc.edu

Central Pennsylvania College
Medical Assistant Prgm
College Hill and Valley Roads
Summerdale, PA 17093-0309
www.cenralpenn.edu
Tel: 717 728-2216   *Fax:* 717 732-5254
E-mail: nikkimarhefka@centralpenn.edu

Penn Commercial Inc
Medical Assistant Prgm
242 Oak Spring Rd
Washington, PA 15301
Tel: 724 222-5330, Ext 240   *Fax:* 724 222-4722
E-mail: bshingle@penncommerical.net

Comm College of Allegheny County
Medical Assistant Prgm
1750 Clairton Rd
West Mifflin, PA 15122
www.ccac.edu
Tel: 412 469-6324   *Fax:* 412 237-4521
E-mail: bgregg@ccac.edu

Berks Technical Institute
Medical Assistant Prgm
2205 Ridgewood Rd
Wyomissing, PA 19610
Tel: 610 372-1722, Ext 151   *Fax:* 610 376-4684
E-mail: cgarman@berkstech.com

Westmoreland County Community College
Medical Assistant Prgm
400 Armbrust Rd
Youngwood, PA 15697-1895
Tel: 724 925-4028   *Fax:* 724 925-4293
E-mail: mihalcinp@wccc-pa.edu

South Carolina

Aiken Technical College
Medical Assistant Prgm
PO Drawer 696
Aiken, SC 29802-0696
www.atc.edu
Tel: 803 593-9231, Ext 1654   *Fax:* 803 593-3106
E-mail: barnett@atc.edu

Forrest Junior College
Medical Assistant Prgm
601 E River St
Anderson, SC 29624-2498
Tel: 864 225-7653, Ext 310   *Fax:* 864 261-7471
E-mail: emilienelson@forrestcollege.com

Miller-Motte Technical College
Medical Assistant Prgm
8085 Rivers Ave
Charleston, SC 29406
Tel: 843 574-0101, Ext 43   *Fax:* 843 266-3424
E-mail: krodgers@miller-motte.net

Trident Technical College
Medical Assistant Prgm
7000 Rivers Ave
PO Box 118067
Charleston, SC 29423
www.tridenttech.edu
Tel: 843 574-6103   *Fax:* 843 574-6585
E-mail: deborah.white@tridenttech.edu

South University
Medical Assistant Prgm
9 Science Court
Columbia, SC 29203
Tel: 803 376-5163   *Fax:* 803 799-9083
E-mail: lschoenbeck@southuniversity.edu

Greenville Technical College
Medical Assistant Prgm
PO Box 5616
Greenville, SC 29606-5616
www.gvltec.edu
Tel: 864 250-8431   *Fax:* 864 250-8806
E-mail: Brenda.Owens@gvltec.edu

Piedmont Technical College
Medical Assistant Prgm
PO Box 1467
620 N Emerald Rd
Greenwood, SC 29648-1467
www.ptc.edu
Tel: 864 941-8526   *Fax:* 864 941-8684
E-mail: rumfelt.g@ptc.edu

Orangeburg Calhoun Technical College
Medical Assistant Prgm
3250 St Matthews Rd
Orangeburg, SC 29118
Tel: 803 535-1346, Ext 1346   *Fax:* 803 535-1350
E-mail: cheeks@octech.edu

Tri-County Technical College
Medical Assistant Prgm
Hwy 76, PO Box 587
Pendleton, SC 29670
Tel: 864 646-8361, Ext 1352   *Fax:* 864 646-1892
E-mail: kbathe@tctc.edu

Spartanburg Community College
Medical Assistant Prgm
PO Box 4386
Spartanburg, SC 29305-4386
www.sccsc.edu
Tel: 864 592-4791   *Fax:* 864 591-3881
E-mail: buchanand@sccsc.edu

Central Carolina Technical College
Medical Assistant Prgm
506 N Guignard Dr
Sumter, SC 29150
www.cctech.edu
Tel: 803 778-7809   *Fax:* 803 778-7868
E-mail: wheelermb@cctech.edu

Midlands Technical College
Medical Assistant Prgm
Airport Campus
1260 Lexington Dr
West Columbia, SC 29170
Tel: 803 822-3398   *Fax:* 803 822-3417
E-mail: rollisonl@midlandstech.edu

South Dakota

Presentation College
Medical Assistant Prgm
1500 N Main St
Aberdeen, SD 57401
Tel: 605 229-8544
E-mail: Mary.Gjernes@presentation.edu

Mitchell Technical Institute
Medical Assistant Prgm
821 N Capital
Michell, SD 57301
www.mitchelltech.edu
Tel: 605 995-3002   *Fax:* 605 996-3299
E-mail: cori.hoffman@mitchelltech.edu

Colorado Technical University
Medical Assistant Prgm
3901 W 59th St
Sioux Falls, SD 57108
Tel: 605 361-0200   *Fax:* 605 361-5954
E-mail: mcrissman@sf.coloradotech.edu

National American University - Sioux Falls Campus
Medical Assistant Prgm
2801 S Kiwanis Ave, Ste 100
Sioux Falls, SD 57105-0889
www.national.edu/sioux_falls.html
Tel: 605 336-4695   *Fax:* 605 336-4605
E-mail: cogdie@national.edu

Lake Area Technical Institute
Medical Assistant Prgm
230 11th St NE
PO Box 730
Watertown, SD 57201-0730
www.lakeareatech.edu
Tel: 800 657-4344, Ext 217   *Fax:* 605 882-5284
E-mail: lindahlk@lakeareatech.edu

Tennessee

National College of Business and Technology - Bristol
Medical Assistant Prgm
Tri-Cities Campus
1328 Hwy 11 W
Bristol, TN 37620
Tel: 423 878-4440   *Fax:* 423 793-1060
E-mail: shjesse@national-college.edu

Chattanooga State Technical Comm College
Medical Assistant Prgm
4501 Amnicola Hwy
Chattanooga, TN 37406
www.chattanoogastate.edu/Industrial_Technology/
intprog.asp
Tel: 423 697-4438   *Fax:* 423 697-3203
E-mail: alexis.jenkins@chattanoogastate.edu

Miller-Motte Technical College - Chattanooga
Medical Assistant Prgm
6020 Shallowford Rd
Chattanooga, TN 37421
www.miller-motte.com
Tel: 423 510-9675   *Fax:* 423 510-1985
E-mail: scross@miller-motte.com

Miller-Motte Technical College - Clarksville
Medical Assistant Prgm
1820 Business Park Dr
Clarksville, TN 37040-0415
Tel: 931 553-0071   *Fax:* 931 552-2916
E-mail: spigg@miller-motte.com

Cleveland State Community College
Medical Assistant Prgm
Office Systems Admin-Medical Ofc Asst
PO Box 3570
Cleveland, TN 37320-3570
Tel: 423 614-8702, Ext 702   *Fax:* 423 478-6258
E-mail: kkingsley@clevelandstatecc.edu

National College of Business and Technology - Knoxville
Medical Assistant Prgm
8415 Kingston Pike
Knoxville, TN 37919
www.national-college.edu
Tel: 865 539-2011
E-mail: repps@ncbt.edu

South College
Medical Assistant Prgm
3904 Lonas Dr
Knoxville, TN 37909
www.southcollegetn.edu
Tel: 865 251-1843   *Fax:* 865 584-9816
E-mail: afritz@southcollegetn.edu

Tennessee Technology Center - Knoxville
Medical Assistant Prgm
1100 Liberty St
Knoxville, TN 37919
Tel: 423 546-5567, Ext 145   *Fax:* 423 971-4474
E-mail: dwilliams@knoxville.tec.tn.us

Tennessee Technology Center - McMinnville
Medical Assistant Prgm
241 Vo-Tech Dr
McMinnville, TN 37110
Tel: 931 473-5587, Ext 248   *Fax:* 931 473-6380
E-mail: dwomack@mcminnville.tec.tn.us

Concorde Career College - Memphis
Medical Assistant Prgm
5100 Poplar Ave, Ste 132
Memphis, TN 38137
Tel: 901 761-9494, Ext 243   *Fax:* 901 761-3293
E-mail: aray@concordecareercolleges.com

Tennessee Technology Center - Memphis
Medical Assistant Prgm
550 Alabama Ave
Memphis, TN 38105
www.ttcmemphis.edu
Tel: 901 543-6186   *Fax:* 901 543-6126
E-mail: paul.holmes@ttcmemphis.edu

National College of Business and Technology - Nashville
Medical Assistant Prgm
3748 Nolensville Pike
Nashville, TN 37211
www.ncbt.edu
Tel: 615 333-3344   *Fax:* 615 333-3429
E-mail: asamuels@national-college.edu

Texas

Cisco Junior College
Medical Assistant Prgm
717 E Industrial Blvd
Abilene, TX 79602
http://http:www.cjc.edu
Tel: 325 794-4441   *Fax:* 254 442-2546
E-mail: kelly.meyer@cjc.edu

Cy-Fair College
Medical Assistant Prgm
9191 Barker Cypress Rd
Cypress, TX 77433
Tel: 281 290-5274
E-mail: gina.r.scott@nhmccd.edu

El Centro College
Medical Assistant Prgm
801 Main St
Dallas, TX 75202
www.elcentrocollege.edu
Tel: 214 860-2328   *Fax:* 214 860-2268
E-mail: pgm5704@dcccd.edu

Richland College
Medical Assistant Prgm
12800 Abrams Rd
Dallas, TX 75243-2199
www.richlandcollege.edu/hp
Tel: 972 238-6117   *Fax:* 972 761-6793
E-mail: shannony@dcccd.edu

Westwood College
Medical Assistant Prgm
8390 LBJ Freeway, Ste 100
Dallas, TX 75243
Tel: 214 570-0100
E-mail: mrougely@westwood.edu

Career Centers of Texas
Medical Assistant Prgm
8360 Burnham Rd, Ste 100
El Paso, TX 79907
Tel: 915 595-1935 *Fax:* 915 595-6619
E-mail: doe@cctep.com

Computer Career Center
Medical Assistant Prgm
6101 Montana Ave
El Paso, TX 79925-2021
Tel: 915 779-8031, Ext 11 *Fax:* 915 779-8097
E-mail: jbaird@computercareercenter.com

El Paso Community College
Medical Assistant Prgm
PO Box 20500
El Paso, TX 79998-0500
Tel: 915 831-4139 *Fax:* 915 831-4021
E-mail: CathyS@epcc.edu

Texas School of Business - Friendswood
Medical Assistant Prgm
3208 FM 528
Friendswood, TX 77546
Tel: 281 648-0880, Ext 3301 *Fax:* 281 648-0821
E-mail: bwilmore@tsb.edu

Texas State Technical College - Harlingen
Medical Assistant Prgm
1902 N Loop 499
Harlingen, TX 78550-3697
Tel: 956 364-4797 *Fax:* 956 364-5160
E-mail: jean.lashbrook@harlingen.tstc.edu

Bradford School
Medical Assistant Prgm
4669 SW Freeway, Ste 300
Houston, TX 77027
Tel: 713 629-8940 *Fax:* 713 629-0059
E-mail: scooper@bradfordschoolhouston.edu

Houston Community College
Medical Assistant Prgm
1900 Pressler, Ste 434
Houston, TX 77030-3717
Tel: 713 718-7361 *Fax:* 713 718-7521
E-mail: cynthia.lundgren@hccs.edu

San Jacinto College North
Medical Assistant Prgm
5800 Uvalde Rd
Houston, TX 77049-4599
www.sjcd.edu
Tel: 281 459-5410 *Fax:* 281 459-7640
E-mail: diana.houston@sjcd.edu

Texas School of Business - East Campus
Medical Assistant Prgm
12030 East Freeway
Houston, TX 77029
Tel: 713 455-8555
E-mail: ccook@tsb.edu

Texas School of Business - North Campus
Medical Assistant Prgm
711 E Airtex
Houston, TX 77073
Tel: 281 443-8900, Ext 224
E-mail: mlarose@tsb.edu

Texas School of Business - Southwest Campus
Medical Assistant Prgm
6363 Richmond Ave, Ste 400
Houston, TX 77057
Tel: 713 975-7527 *Fax:* 713 975-1857
E-mail: getinspirit@yahoo.com

Kilgore College
Medical Assistant Prgm
1100 Broadway
Kilgore, TX 75662-3299
www.kilgore.edu
Tel: 903 983-8147, Ext 147 *Fax:* 903 988-7596
E-mail: mwhite@kilgore.edu

Hallmark Institute of Technology
Medical Assistant Prgm
10401 IH - 10 West
San Antonio, TX 78230
www.hallmarkcollege.edu
Tel: 210 690-9000
E-mail: nlewis@hallmarkcollege.edu

San Antonio College
Medical Assistant Prgm
1300 San Pedro Ave
San Antonio, TX 78212
www.accd.edu/sac/alldhlth/medasst
Tel: 210 733-2437 *Fax:* 210 733-2429
E-mail: cstartzell@mail.accd.edu

San Antonio College of Med & Dental Assts - San Antonio
Medical Assistant Prgm
4205 San Pedro
San Antonio, TX 78212
Tel: 210 733-0777 *Fax:* 210 735-2431
E-mail: gdeleon@sac-mda.com

Utah

Davis Applied Technology College
Medical Assistant Prgm
550 East 300 South
Kaysville, UT 84037-2699
Tel: 801 593-2369 *Fax:* 801 593-2400
E-mail: gaiterrm@datc.tec.ut.us

Bridgerland Applied Technology College
Medical Assistant Prgm
1301 North 600 West
Logan, UT 84321
Tel: 435 750-3047
E-mail: mwright@batc.tec.ut.us

Stevens-Henager College
Medical Assistant Prgm
755 S Main St
Logan, UT 84321
www.stevenshenager.edu
Tel: 435 152-2772, Ext 5008 *Fax:* 435 755-7611
E-mail: nerickson_shclogan@yahoo.com

Ogden-Weber Applied Technology College
Medical Assistant Prgm
200 N Washington Blvd
Ogden, UT 84404-4089
www.owatc.edu
Tel: 801 627-8445 *Fax:* 801 395-3703
E-mail: andersoe@owatc.edu

Stevens-Henager College
Medical Assistant Prgm
PO Box 9428
Ogden, UT 84409
http://stevenshenager.edu
Tel: 801 394-7791, Ext 1044 *Fax:* 801 621-0853
E-mail: drmerida@email.com

AmeriTech College
Medical Assistant Prgm
1675 N Freedom Blvd Bldg 3
Provo, UT 84604
www.ameritech.edu
Tel: 801 377-2900, Ext 116 *Fax:* 801 375-3077
E-mail: broberts@ameritech.edu

Provo College
Medical Assistant Prgm
1450 W 820 N
Provo, UT 84601
Tel: 801 818-8912 *Fax:* 801 375-9728
E-mail: lesliee@provocollege.edu

Latter Day Saints Business College
Medical Assistant Prgm
95 North 300 West
Salt Lake City, UT 84101
Tel: 801 524-8131 *Fax:* 801 524-1900
E-mail: edith@ldsbc.edu

Salt Lake Community College
Medical Assistant Prgm
3491 Wights Fort Rd
West Jordan, UT 84088
www.slcc.edu
Tel: 801 957-4596 *Fax:* 801 957-6353
E-mail: jana.tucker@slcc.edu

Utah Career College
Medical Assistant Prgm
1902 West 7800 South
West Jordan, UT 84088
www.utahcollege.edu
Tel: 801 304-4224, Ext 131 *Fax:* 801 304-4229
E-mail: chammond@utahcollege.edu

Everest College
Medical Assistant Prgm
3280 West 3500 South
West Valley City, UT 84119
Tel: 801 840-4800, Ext 133 *Fax:* 801 969-0828
E-mail: migreen@cci.edu

Virginia

National College - Bluefield
Medical Assistant Prgm
PO Box 629
100 Logan St
Bluefield, VA 24605
www.national-college.edu
Tel: 276 326-3621, Ext 19 *Fax:* 276 322-5731
E-mail: carney@national-college.edu

National College - Charlottesville
Medical Assistant Prgm
1819 Emmet St
Charlottesville, VA 22903
www.national-college.edu
Tel: 434 295-0136 *Fax:* 434 979-8061
E-mail: lmliggan@national-college.edu

National College - Danville
Medical Assistant Prgm
336 Old Riverside Dr
Danville, VA 24541
www.national-college.edu
Tel: 434 793-6822 *Fax:* 434 793-3634
E-mail: gorr@national-college.edu

National College - Harrisonburg
Medical Assistant Prgm
1515 Country Club Rd
Harrisonburg, VA 22801
www.national-college.edu
Tel: 540 432-0943 *Fax:* 540 432-1133
E-mail: lbreeden@ncbt.edu

Miller-Motte Technical College
Medical Assistant Prgm
1011 Creekside Lane
Lynchburg, VA 24502
Tel: 434 239-5222, Ext 214 *Fax:* 434 239-1069
E-mail: deegzachau@yahoo.com

National College - Lynchburg
Medical Assistant Prgm
104 Candlewood Court
Lynchburg, VA 24502
www.national-college.edu
Tel: 434 239-3500 *Fax:* 434 239-3948
E-mail: scoleman@national-college.edu

National College - Martinsville
Medical Assistant Prgm
10 Church St
PO Box 232
Martinsville, VA 24114
Tel: 276 632-5621 *Fax:* 276 632-7915
E-mail: gdjenkins@national-college.edu

Medical Careers Institute
Medical Assistant Prgm
1001 Omni Blvd, Ste 200
Newport News, VA 23606
Tel: 757 873-2423, Ext 318 *Fax:* 757 873-2472
E-mail: rgohsman@medical.edu

Bryant & Stratton College - Richmond
Medical Assistant Prgm
8141 Hull Street Rd
Richmond, VA 23235-6411
Tel: 804 745-2444, Ext 328 *Fax:* 804 745-6884
E-mail: nabeaman@bryantstratton.edu

National College - Roanoke Valley
Medical Assistant Prgm
1813 E Main St
Salem, VA 24153
http://national-college.edu
Tel: 540 986-1800
E-mail: mjwilliams@national-college.edu

Bryant & Stratton College - Virginia Beach
Medical Assistant Prgm
301 Centre Pointe Dr
Virginia Beach, VA 23462
Tel: 757 499-7900 *Fax:* 757 499-9977
E-mail: cwmutts@bryantstratton.edu

Tidewater Community College
Medical Assistant Prgm
1700 College Crescent
Virginia Beach, VA 23453-1918
Tel: 757 822-7252 *Fax:* 757 427-1338
E-mail: kmcnamara@tcc.edu

Washington

Whatcom Community College
Medical Assistant Prgm
237 W Kellogg Rd
Bellingham, WA 98226-8033
Tel: 360 676-2170, Ext 3306 *Fax:* 360 752-6767
E-mail: bdahl@whatcom.ctc.edu

Everest College - Port Orchard
Medical Assistant Prgm
155 Washington Ave, Ste 200
Bremerton, WA 98337
Tel: 360 473-1120, Ext 133 *Fax:* 360 792-2404
E-mail: lcook@cci.edu

Olympic College
Medical Assistant Prgm
1600 Chester Ave
Bremerton, WA 98337-1699
Tel: 360 475-7741 *Fax:* 360 475-7491
E-mail: clieseke@olympic.edu

Highline Community College
Medical Assistant Prgm
PO Box 98000
Des Moines, WA 98198-9800
http://flightline.highline.edu/medassist
Tel: 206 878-3710, Ext 3493 *Fax:* 206 870-4850
E-mail: bcerna@highline.edu

Everest College - Everett
Medical Assistant Prgm
906 SE Everett Mall Way, Ste 600
Everett, WA 98208
Tel: 425 789-7960, Ext 7994 *Fax:* 425 789-7989
E-mail: lrickard@cci.edu

Everett Community College
Medical Assistant Prgm
2000 Tower St
Everett, WA 98201-1352
www.everettcc.edu
Tel: 425 388-9467 *Fax:* 425 388-9135
E-mail: eadolphsen@everettcc.edu

Lake Washington Technical College
Medical Assistant Prgm
11605 132nd Ave NE
Kirkland, WA 98034-8506
Tel: 425 739-8100, Ext 257 *Fax:* 425 739-8298
E-mail: marti.garrels@lwtc.edu

Clover Park Technical College
Medical Assistant Prgm
4500 Steilacoom Blvd SW
Lakewood, WA 98499
Tel: 253 589-5841 *Fax:* 253 589-5866
E-mail: michele.jones@cptc.edu

Lower Columbia College
Medical Assistant Prgm
1600 Maple St
Longview, WA 98632
www.lowercolumbia.edu
Tel: 360 442-2889 *Fax:* 360 442-2879
E-mail: jweyer@lcc.ctc.edu

Skagit Valley College
Medical Assistant Prgm
2405 E College Way
Mount Vernon, WA 98273
Tel: 360 416-7720 *Fax:* 360 416-7918
E-mail: jeanette.hemming@skagit.edu

South Puget Sound Community College
Medical Assistant Prgm
2011 Mottman Rd SW
Olympia, WA 98512-6218
www.spscc.ctc.edu
Tel: 360 596-5297 *Fax:* 360 664-0780
E-mail: sthunell@spscc.ctc.edu

Everest College - Renton
Medical Assistant Prgm
981 Powell Ave SW, Ste 200
Renton, WA 98055-2990
Tel: 425 255-3281 *Fax:* 425 255-9327
E-mail: tiedwards@cci.edu

Renton Technical College
Medical Assistant Prgm
3000 NE Fourth St
Renton, WA 98056
www.rtc.edu
Tel: 425 235-2352, Ext 5734 *Fax:* 425 235-5836
E-mail: pjeffcoat@rtc.edu

North Seattle Community College
Medical Assistant Prgm
9600 College Way N
Seattle, WA 98103-3599
www.northseattle.edu/health/medasst/
Tel: 206 527-5667 *Fax:* 206 527-3715
E-mail: mallen@sccd.ctc.edu

Seattle Vocational Institute
Medical Assistant Prgm
2120 S Jackson St
Seattle, WA 98144
Tel: 206 587-4921 *Fax:* 206 587-4939
E-mail: lzielinski@sccd.ctc.edu

Spokane Community College
Medical Assistant Prgm
1810 N Greene St
Spokane, WA 99217-5399
Tel: 509 533-8138 *Fax:* 509 533-8621
E-mail: cthomas@scc.spokane.edu

Clark College
Medical Assistant Prgm
1933 Fort Vancouver Way
Vancouver, WA 98663-3598
www.clark.edu
Tel: 360 992-2468 *Fax:* 360 992-2863
E-mail: jclausen@clark.edu

Everest College
Medical Assistant Prgm
120 NE 136th Ave, Ste 130
Vancouver, WA 98684
www.cci.edu
Tel: 360 254-3282 *Fax:* 360 254-3035
E-mail: pstoddard@cci.edu

Wenatchee Valley College
Medical Assistant Prgm
1300 Fifth Ave
Wenatchee, WA 98801
Tel: 509 682-6667 *Fax:* 509 682-6661
E-mail: seagle@wvcmail.ctc.edu

Yakima Valley Community College
Medical Assistant Prgm
PO Box 22520
Yakima, WA 98907
Tel: 509 574-4847
E-mail: smohsenian@yvcc.edu

West Virginia

Mountain State University
Medical Assistant Prgm
PO Box 9003
Beckley, WV 25802-9003
Tel: 304 929-1423 *Fax:* 304 929-1600
E-mail: fhash@mountainstate.edu

Benjamin Franklin Career & Technical Ed Ctr
Medical Assistant Prgm
500 28th St
Dunbar, WV 25064
Tel: 304 766-0369 *Fax:* 304 766-0371
E-mail: elongsworth@kcs.kana.k12.wv.us

Huntington Junior College
Medical Assistant Prgm
900 Fifth Ave
Huntington, WV 25701
www.huntingtonjuniorcollege.edu
Tel: 304 697-7550 *Fax:* 304 697-7554
E-mail: lwest@huntingtonjuniorcollege.edu

Marshall Community & Technical College
Medical Assistant Prgm
2000 7th Ave
Huntington, WV 25703-1527
Tel: 304 696-3008 *Fax:* 304 696-2396
E-mail: smithjan@marshall.edu

Wisconsin

Wisconsin Indianhead Technical College - Ashland Campus
Medical Assistant Prgm
2100 Beaser Ave
Ashland, WI 54806
www.witc.edu
Tel: 715 682-4591, Ext 3168 *Fax:* 715 682-8040
E-mail: carol.utpadel@witc.edu

Chippewa Valley Technical College
Medical Assistant Prgm
Health Education Center
620 W Clairemont Ave
Eau Claire, WI 54701
www.cvtc.edu
Tel: 715 833-6398   *Fax:* 715 833-6470
E-mail: bniedzwiecki@cvtc.edu

Gateway Technical College - Elkhorn
Medical Assistant Prgm
400 County Rd H
Elkhorn, WI 53121-2020
Tel: 262 741-8340   *Fax:* 262 741-8201
E-mail: Formanekr@gtc.edu

Southwest Wisconsin Technical College
Medical Assistant Prgm
1800 Bronson Blvd
Fennimore, WI 53809-9778
Tel: 608 822-3262, Ext 2163   *Fax:* 608 822-4018
E-mail: kanderson@swtc.edu

Moraine Park Technical College
Medical Assistant Prgm
235 N National Ave
Fond du Lac, WI 53936
www.morainepark.edu
Tel: 920 924-3276
E-mail: clace@morainepark.edu

Northeast Wisconsin Technical College
Medical Assistant Prgm
2740 W Mason St, PO Box 19042
Green Bay, WI 54307-9042
www.nwtc.edu
Tel: 920 498-5523   *Fax:* 920 491-2660
E-mail: karen.koenig@nwtc.edu

Lac Courte Oreills Ojibwa Community College
Medical Assistant Prgm
13466 W Trepania Rd
Hayward, WI 54843
Tel: 715 634-4790, Ext 172   *Fax:* 715 634-5049
E-mail: ljensen@lco.edu

Blackhawk Technical College
Medical Assistant Prgm
6004 Prairie Rd, PO Box 53547
Janesville, WI 53547
Tel: 608 743-4573   *Fax:* 608 743-4407
E-mail: hfranklin1@blackhawk.edu

Western Technical College
Medical Assistant Prgm
304 N Sixth St, PO Box C-908
La Crosse, WI 54602-0908
Tel: 608 785-9922   *Fax:* 608 785-9087
E-mail: lentzm@wwtc.edu

Madison Area Technical College
Medical Assistant Prgm
3550 Anderson St
Madison, WI 53791-9674
Tel: 608 264-6110   *Fax:* 608 246-6013
E-mail: ksellnow@matcmadison.edu

Mid-State Technical College - Marshfield
Medical Assistant Prgm
2600 W Fifth St
Marshfield, WI 54449
www.mstc.edu
Tel: 715 389-7024   *Fax:* 715 389-2864
E-mail: pam.alt@mstc.edu

Bryant & Stratton College - Milwaukee
Medical Assistant Prgm
310 W Wisconsin Ave
Ste 500 E
Milwaukee, WI 53203
www.bryantstratton.edu
Tel: 414 276-5200, Ext 244   *Fax:* 414 276-3930
E-mail: kmolewinski@bryantstratton.edu

Concordia University Wisconsin
Medical Assistant Prgm
1127 S 35th St
Milwaukee, WI 53215
Tel: 414 649-0795   *Fax:* 414 647-2545
E-mail: susan.lowrey@cuw.edu

Milwaukee Area Technical College
Medical Assistant Prgm
700 W State St
Milwaukee, WI 53233-1419
Tel: 414 297-6934   *Fax:* 414 297-6851
E-mail: bradfoga@matc.edu

Wisconsin Indianhead Technical College
Medical Assistant Prgm
1019 S Knowles Ave
New Richmond, WI 54017
www.witc.edu
Tel: 715 246-6561, Ext 4351   *Fax:* 715 246-2777
E-mail: loakley@witc.edu

Fox Valley Technical College
Medical Assistant Prgm
150 N Campbell Rd
Oshkosh, WI 54903-2217
www.fvtc.edu
Tel: 920 735-5774   *Fax:* 920 831-4314
E-mail: tuchschb@fvtc.edu

Waukesha County Technical College
Medical Assistant Prgm
800 Main St
Pewaukee, WI 53072-4601
Tel: 414 691-5563   *Fax:* 414 691-5451
E-mail: mblankenheim@wctc.edu

Gateway Technical College
Medical Assistant Prgm
1001 S Main St
Racine, WI 53403
http://gtc.edu
Tel: 262 619-6604   *Fax:* 262 619-6811
E-mail: andreuccil@gtc.edu

Nicolet Area Technical College
Medical Assistant Prgm
PO Box 518
Rhinelander, WI 54501-0518
Tel: 715 365-4539   *Fax:* 715 365-4603
E-mail: csdailey@nicoletcollege.edu

Mid-State Technical College - Stevens Point
Medical Assistant Prgm
933 Michigan Ave
Stevens Point, WI 54481-3141
www.mstc.edu
Tel: 715 389-7024   *Fax:* 715 342-3134
E-mail: pam.alt@mstc.edu

Wisconsin Indianhead Technical College - Superior
Medical Assistant Prgm
600 N 21st St
Superior, WI 54880
Tel: 715 394-6677, Ext 6324   *Fax:* 715 934-3771
E-mail: luci.gunderson@witc.edu

Northcentral Technical College
Medical Assistant Prgm
1000 W Campus Dr
Wausau, WI 54401
Tel: 715 675-3331, Ext 1367
E-mail: salmlittle@ntc.edu

Medical Assistant

Programs*	Class Capacity	Begins	Length (months)	Award	Res. Tuition	Non-res. Tuition	Stipend	Offers:‡ 1	2	3	4
Alabama											
George C Wallace Community College (Dothan)	24	Aug Jan May	24	AAS	$5,000	$10,000				•	
H Council Trenholm State Technical College (Montgomery)	30	Aug Jan May	18	Cert, AAT	$4,040	$5,080				•	
Alaska											
University of Alaska Anchorage	20	Sep Jan May	12, 24	Cert, AAS	$5,248	$17,507		•		•	
Arkansas											
Arkansas Tech University (Russellville)	10	Aug	24	AS	$3,576	$7,152			•	•	
California											
Chabot College (Hayward)	20	Aug	9	Cert, AA	$20	$175				•	
City College of San Francisco	30	Aug Jan	12, 18	Cert, AS	$800	$3,000		•		•	
Cosumnes River Community College (Sacramento)	25	Aug Jan	15	Cert, AS	$1,100	$6,200		•		•	•
East San Gabriel Valley ROP (West Covina)	15	Open	10	Cert	$1,500	$1,500					
Everest College - San Bernardino	24	Monthly	8	Dipl				•			
Everest College - San Francisco	24	Monthly	8, 10	Dipl	$13,386	$13,386		•		•	
Heald College - Concord	25	Every quarter	18	AAS	$10,275	$10,275	$10,500	•			
Heald College - Fresno	25	Quarterly	18	AAS	$10,800	$10,800		•		•	
Heald College - Hayward	25	Every quarter	18	AAS	$9,900	$0		•		•	

*Data are shown only for programs that completed the 2007 AMA Survey of Health Professions Education Programs.
‡Key to Offers: 1: Evening or weekend classes; 2: Non-English instruction; 3: Cultural competence instruction; 4: Distance education component.

Medical Assistant

Programs*	Class Capacity	Begins	Length (months)	Award	Res. Tuition	Non-res. Tuition	Stipend	1	2	3	4
Heald College - Rancho Cordova	25	Every quarter	18	AAS	$9,900	$0		•		•	
Heald College - Roseville	25	Quarterly	18	AAS	$9,900	$9,900		•		•	
Heald College - Salinas	24	Every quarter	18	AAS	$9,900	$0		•		•	
Heald College - San Francisco	25	Each quarter	18	AAS	$9,900	$9,900		•		•	
Heald College - San Jose (Milpitas)	25	Every quarter	18	AAS	$14,400	$14,400		•		•	
Heald College - Stockton Campus	25	Every quarter	18	AAS	$9,900	$0		•		•	
Modesto Junior College	25	Aug	7	Cert, AS	$512	$3,977				•	
Pasadena City College	20	Aug Sep	11	Cert	$760	$6,401		•			
Southern California Regional Occupational Ctr (Torrance)	75	Open	11	Cert	$700	$700				•	
Western Career College - Antioch	25	Every 3 wks	9, 17	Cert, AS	$26,761	$0		•			
Western Career College - Citrus (Citrus Heights)	30	Every 6 wks	8	Cert	$14,000	$14,000		•			
Western Career College - Pleasant Hill	72	Continuous	8	Cert	$14,160	$0		•			
Western Career College - Sacramento	384	Semi-monthly	10, 15	Cert	$12,917	$0		•			
Colorado											
Arapahoe Community College (Littleton)	50	Aug Jan	12, 24	Cert, AAS	$2,000	$9,000		•			•
Community College of Denver	24	Fall Spring	12	Cert	$3,730	$16,194				•	
Everest College (Aurora)	30	Monthly	8	Dipl	$10,500	$10,500		•		•	
Front Range Comm College (Longmont)	18	Aug Jan	10, 24	Cert, AAS	$3,853	$8,466					
Connecticut											
Goodwin College (East Hartford)	50	Every 8 wks	12, 16	Cert, AS	$13,600	$13,600		•		•	
Lincoln Tech Institute (New Britain)	30	Sep Mar Jun	15, 21	Dipl	$14,248	$14,270		•			•
Northwestern Connecticut Comm College (Winsted)	40	Sep Jan	16	Cert, AS	$2,828	$8,444		•		•	
Norwalk Community College	33	Sep	10	Cert	$3,544	$8,783				•	
Delaware											
Delaware Technical & Community College - Wilmington	18	Aug	12, 24	AAS	$2,070	$5,176		•		•	•
Florida											
Brevard Community College (Cocoa)	32	Open	12	Cert	$2,000	$5,265		•		•	•
Broward Community College (Fort Lauderdale)	18	Aug	10	Cert	$3,600	$7,000		•		•	
Central Florida College (Winter Park)	100	Every 10 wks	9, 14	Dipl, AS	$8,981	$0		•		•	
Daytona Beach Community College	48	Aug	10	Cert	$2,494	$9,964		•		•	
Florida Metro Univ - Orlando College South	400	Jan Apr Jul Oct	24	AS	$11,740	$11,740					•
Florida Metropolitan Univ - Pinellas Campus (Clearwater)	30	Quarterly	24	AS	$29,003	$29,003		•		•	
Indian River Community College (Port St Lucie)	25	Jan Aug	12	Cert	$1,560	$7,605				•	
Keiser University - Daytona Beach	20	Varies	16	AS	$17,460	$17,460				•	
Manatee Technical Institute (Bradenton)	20	Aug Oct Jan	11	Cert	$2,975	$9,605				•	
McFatter Technical Center (Davie)	34	Aug	11, 22	Cert	$2,435	$7,305		•		•	
Palm Beach Community College (Lake Worth)	15	Fall Spring	18	Cert	$2,500	$8,500				•	
Pensacola Junior College	25	Aug	12	Cert	$2,455	$9,628					
Pinellas Tech Educ Ctr - St Petersburg	50	5x/yr	13	Cert	$2,470	$9,282	$250			•	•
Seminole Community College (Sanford)	25	Aug	12	Cert	$2,639	$10,114		•		•	
South University (West Palm Beach)	100	Jan Apr Jun Sep	18	AS	$9,585	$9,585		•		•	•
Georgia											
Atlanta Technical College	25	Mar Oct Jan Apr	15	Dipl	$1,816	$3,304		•		•	•
Augusta Technical College	25	Mar Sep	15	Dipl	$1,870	$3,740		•	•	•	
Clayton State University (Morrow)	60	Aug Jan May	12, 24	Cert, AAS	$4,686	$16,209		•			
Coosa Valley Technical College (Rome)	20	Oct	15	Dipl	$1,008	$2,016					
East Central Technical College (Douglas)	35	Sep	15	Dipl	$2,553	$4,754				•	•
Griffin Technical College	18	Jan Apr Oct	15	Dipl	$1,480	$3,960		•		•	
Gwinnett Technical College (Lawrenceville)	20	Mar Sep	15	Dipl	$2,750	$4,610				•	•
Heart of Georgia Technical College (Dublin)	20	Oct Apr	12	Dipl	$2,232	$4,464				•	
Medix School (Smyrna)	175	Every 5 wks	10	Dipl	$11,702	$11,702		•		•	
Moultrie Technical College	30	2x/yr	15	Dipl	$1,248	$2,496			•	•	•
Northwestern Technical College (Rock Spring)	25	Jul	12	Dipl	$382	$382					•
Ogeechee Technical College (Statesboro)	40	Sep Apr	15	Dipl	$1,384	$2,768		•		•	•
Southeastern Technical College (Vidalia)	20	Apr Oct	15	Dipl	$2,136	$4,272		•		•	•
Southwest Georgia Technical College (Thomasville)	24	Jul	15, 18	Dipl, AAS	$1,488	$2,976		•		•	
West Central Technical College (Waco)	20	Jul	12	Dipl	$1,371	$2,487					
West Georgia Technical College (LaGrange)	15	Year-round	18	Dipl	$2,430	$4,860		•		•	
Hawaii											
Heald College - Honolulu Campus	24	Quarterly	18	AAS	$13,700	$13,700		•		•	
Illinois											
Everest College - North Aurora	24	1x/mo	8	Dipl				•	•	•	
Harper College (Palatine)	30	Aug Jan Jun	12, 24	Cert	$85	$255		•		•	•
Midstate College (Peoria)		Mar Jun Aug Nov	24	AAS	$10,000	$10,000		•		•	
Northwestern Business Coll (Chicago)	48	Sep Dec Mar Jun	18	AAS	$17,750	$17,750		•	•	•	•
Northwestern Business Coll (Naperville)	30	Sep Dec Mar Jun	18	AAS	$335	$335		•		•	•
Northwestern Business Coll - Southwest Campus (Bridgeview)	48	Sep Dec Mar Jun	18	AAS	$355	$355		•		•	•

*Data are shown only for programs that completed the 2007 AMA Survey of Health Professions Education Programs.
‡Key to Offers: 1: Evening or weekend classes; 2: Non-English instruction; 3: Cultural competence instruction; 4: Distance education component.

Medical Assistant

Programs*	Class Capacity	Begins	Length (months)	Award	Res. Tuition	Non-res. Tuition	Stipend	Offers:‡ 1	2	3	4
Robert Morris College - Chicago	120	Jul Sep Feb	10, 15	Dipl, AAS, BBA	$15,900	$15,900		•			
Rockford Business College	62	Mar Jun Sep Nov	24	Dipl, AAS	$6,445	$0		•		•	
Southwestern Illinois College (Belleville)	60	Aug Jan Jun	10, 24	Cert, AAS	$4,700	$7,800					
Spanish Coalition for Jobs Inc (Chicago)	20	Sep Jan Apr	10	Cert	$7,500	$7,500				•	
Waubonsee Community College (Sugar Grove)	12	Jun	14	Cert	$2,980	$8,515					•
Indiana											
Brown Mackie College - Ft Wayne (Fort Wayne)	25	Every 4 wks	24	Dipl, AAS	$8,112	$8,112		•			
Davenport University - Merrillville		Aug Jan May	24	Dipl, AAS	$7,656	$7,656				•	
Indiana Business College (Indianapolis)	20	Jan Apr Jun Sep	18	AAS	$12,360	$0		•	•	•	•
Indiana Business College - Anderson	90	Jan Apr Jun Sep	18	AS	$21,750	$0		•	•	•	•
Indiana Business College - Evansville	100	Jan Apr Jun Sep	18	AAS	$14,500	$14,500		•	•	•	
Indiana Business College - Ft Wayne (Fort Wayne)	20	Quarterly	18	AAS	$10,875	$10,875		•			•
Indiana Business College - Terre Haute	30	Quarterly	18	AAS	$9,660	$9,660		•		•	•
Ivy Tech Community College - Columbus	25	Aug Jan May	18, 24	Cert, TC, AAS	$4,029	$7,792		•		•	•
Ivy Tech Community College - Evansville	40	Aug	16, 21	Cert, AAS	$87	$178	$1,500	•	•	•	
Ivy Tech Community College - Ft Wayne (Fort Wayne)	900	Aug Jan May	18, 24	Dipl, Cert, AAS	$4,000	$5,100		•		•	
Ivy Tech Community College - Kokomo	150	Aug Jan May	18, 24	Cert, AAS, TC	$3,104	$6,316		•		•	
Ivy Tech Community College - Lawrenceburg	50	Aug Jan May	18, 24	Cert, TC, AAS	$2,000	$4,200		•		•	
Ivy Tech Community College - Muncie		May Aug Jan	12, 24	Cert, AAS	$3,949	$8,033		•			•
Ivy Tech Community College - Sellersburg	60	Aug Jan May	12, 24	Cert, TC, AAS	$3,158	$5,400		•		•	•
Ivy Tech Community College - South Bend	200	Aug Jan May	15, 20	Cert, TC, AAS	$3,200	$5,000		•			
Ivy Tech Community College - Terre Haute	30	Aug	12, 18	Cert, AAS	$4,029	$8,172		•		•	
Iowa											
Des Moines Area Community College (Ankeny)	36	Aug	11	Dipl	$4,800	$9,600		•		•	
Iowa Western Community College (Council Bluffs)	20	Aug	10	Dipl	$4,500	$6,750					
Kaplan University, Davenport Campus	25	Jul Oct Jan Apr	15, 18	Dipl, AAS	$12,960	$12,960		•			
Kirkwood Community College (Cedar Rapids)	39	Aug Jan May	12	AAS	$5,901	$11,803				•	
Southeastern Community College (West Burlington)	25	Aug	11	Dipl	$4,896	$5,472				•	
Kansas											
Wichita Area Technical College	30	Aug Jan	9	Cert, AAS	$3,118	$10,867				•	•
Kentucky											
Eastern Kentucky University (Richmond)	16	Aug Jan	22	AAS	$5,682	$15,382		•		•	
Henderson Community College	20	Aug	22	AAS	$2,760	$8,280				•	•
Jefferson Community and Technical College (Louisville)	20	Jan	16	Dipl, Cert	$6,197	$18,387					
National College - Danville	60	Mar Jun Sep Dec	24	AS	$6,624	$6,624		•		•	
National College - Florence	60	Mar Jun Sep Dec	24	AS	$8,544	$8,544		•			
National College - Lexington	60	Mar Jun Sep Dec	24	AS	$6,624	$6,624		•			
National College - Louisville	75	Dec Jan Mar Apr Jun Jul	24	AS	$6,624	$6,624		•			
National College - Pikeville	60	Mar Jun Sep Dec	24	AS	$7,104	$7,104		•			
National College - Richmond	60	Dec Mar Jun Sep	24	AS	$6,624	$6,624		•			
Louisiana											
Bossier Parish Community College (Bossier City)	20	Aug	16	AS	$1,720	$3,900		•		•	•
Maine											
Beal College (Bangor)	30	Bimonthly	24	AS	$5,940	$5,940		•			
Maryland											
Allegany College of Maryland (Cumberland)	20	Sep	24	AAS	$3,602	$7,324		•		•	•
Kaplan College (Hagerstown)		Oct Jan Apr Jul	9, 20	Cert, AAS	$22,264	$22,264		•		•	
Medix School (Towson)	485	Concurrent	10	Cert	$9,950	$0		•		•	
Massachusetts											
Charles H McCann Technical School (North Adams)	20	Sep	9	Cert	$2,500	$12,748					
Clark University (Braintree)	20	Monthly	9	Cert	$10,990	$10,990		•			
Massasoit Community College (Canton)	20	Sep	9	Cert	$4,447	$12,046		•			
Middlesex Community College - Lowell	24	Sep Jan	10, 22	Cert	$3,567	$9,541				•	
Northern Essex Community College (Lawrence)	30	Sep	10	Cert	$3,935	$4,540		•		•	•
Quinsigamond Community College (Worcester)	20	Sep	9	Cert	$4,370	$12,198		•		•	
Southeastern Technical Institute (South Easton)	24	Sep	10	Cert	$2,500	$3,500					
Michigan											
Alpena Community College	20	Aug	24	AAS	$2,200	$3,200		•			
Baker College of Auburn Hills	30	Sep	27	AAS	$16,275	$16,275		•			
Baker College of Cadillac	100	Sep Jan May	30	AAS	$7,625	$0		•			•
Baker College of Flint	75	Jan Mar Jun Sep	24	Cert, AAS	$6,680	$6,680		•		•	
Baker College of Owosso	36	Sep Jan Apr	24	Cert, AAS	$8,640	$8,640		•			
Carnegie Institute (Troy)	70	Jan Mar Jun Sep	12, 24	Dipl	$9,240	$9,240		•			
Davenport University - Battle Creek	30	Sep Jan May	18	Dipl, AAS	$7,656	$7,656		•		•	
Davenport University - Caro		Sep	36	Dipl, AAS	$7,176	$7,176		•		•	
Davenport University - Grand Rapids (Fulton St)		Sep Jan Mar	18	Dipl, AAS	$7,656	$7,656		•		•	

*Data are shown only for programs that completed the 2007 AMA Survey of Health Professions Education Programs.
‡Key to Offers: 1: Evening or weekend classes; 2: Non-English instruction; 3: Cultural competence instruction; 4: Distance education component.

Medical Assistant

Programs*	Class Capacity	Begins	Length (months)	Award	Res. Tuition	Non-res. Tuition	Stipend	Offers:‡ 1	2	3	4
Davenport University - Lansing	12	Jan May Aug	18	AS	$9,240	$9,240		•		•	•
Henry Ford Community College (Dearborn)	24	Aug Jan	10	Cert	$2,526	$4,500		•			
Jackson Community College	30	Aug Jan May	18	Cert	$2,400	$2,800		•		•	
Kalamazoo Valley Community College	40	Aug	12	Cert	$1,312	$2,368		•		•	
Macomb Community College (Clinton Township)		Aug Jan	12, 24	Cert, AAS	$3,710	$5,671		•		•	•
Mid Michigan Community College (Harrison)	25	Aug	24	AAS	$1,785	$2,970		•		•	
Schoolcraft College (Garden City)	30	Sep	12	Cert	$2,448	$3,600		•			
Minnesota											
Argosy University - Twin Cities (Eagan)	20	Sep Jan May Jul	18	AAS	$7,830	$7,830		•			•
Century College (White Bear Lake)	20	Aug Jan	14, 24	Dipl	$3,394	$6,443		•		•	•
Duluth Business University	45	Jan Apr Jul Oct	14, 24	Dipl, AAS				•		•	•
Herzing College (Crystal)	144	Jan Mar May Jul Sep Oct	14, 20	Dipl, AAS	$17,595	$17,959				•	•
Minneapolis Business College (Roseville)	120	Sep	10, 14	Dipl, AAS	$15,950	$15,950				•	
Minnesota West Comm & Tech College (Worthington)	30	Aug	12, 19	Dipl, AAS	$5,800	$11,000		•	•	•	•
Ridgewater College - Willmar Campus	40	Aug	14	Dipl	$7,300	$15,000				•	
Mississippi											
Hinds Community College (Pearl)	15	Aug	18	AAS	$1,660	$3,866		•		•	
Northeast Mississippi Community College (Booneville)	20	Aug	18	AAS	$915	$1,830					
Missouri											
Everest College - Springfield Campus	100	Jan Apr Jul Oct	24	AAS	$27,515	$27,515		•		•	•
Nebraska											
Alegent Health (Omaha)	20	Aug	12	Dipl	$6,000	$8,000				•	
Central Community College (Hastings)	30	Varies	12, 24	Dipl, AAS	$1,295	$1,903		•		•	
Southeast Community College (Lincoln)	25	Apr Oct	12	Dipl	$5,130	$5,915		•			•
New Hampshire											
New Hampshire Comm Tech Coll - Claremont	30	Sep	12, 4	Cert	$7,287	$10,649		•		•	
New Hampshire Comm Tech College - Manchester	32	Sep Jan	10, 18	Cert, AS	$5,248	$7,872		•		•	•
New Jersey											
Bergen Community College (Paramus)	35	Sep	24	AAS	$4,250	$8,500		•		•	
Dover Business College - Clifton	25	4x/yr	12	Dipl	$14,400	$14,400		•		•	
Dover Business College - Paramus (Clifton)	25	4x/yr	12	Dipl	$13,605	$13,605		•		•	
Hudson County Community College (Jersey City)	25	Sep Jan	24	AAS	$2,924	$5,848		•		•	
Mercer County Technical Schools (Trenton)	20	Aug	11	Dipl, Cert	$3,140	$3,140		•			
Sussex County Community College (Newton)	25	Fall Spring	10, 18	Cert, MA	$7,746	$7,746				•	•
Warren County Community College (Washington)	20	Aug Jan	7	Cert	$4,999	$4,999		•			
New Mexico											
Eastern New Mexico University - Roswell	30	Aug	12, 24	Cert, AS	$525	$2,160		•		•	•
New York											
ASA Institute of Business & Computer Tech (Brooklyn)	30	Feb Jun Oct	16	AOS	$16,920	$16,920		•		•	•
Broome Community College (Binghamton)	35	Aug	18	AAS	$3,058	$6,116				•	
Bryant & Stratton College - Buffalo		Jan May Sep	16	AOS	$18,675	$0		•		•	
Elmira Business Institute	100	Feb Jun Oct	16	AOS	$18,000	$18,000		•		•	
Erie Community College - North Campus (Williamsville)	60	Sep Jan	12, 21	Cert, AAS	$2,987	$5,974		•		•	
Niagara County Community College (Sanborn)	24	Sep Jan	24	AAS	$3,192	$4,788		•		•	
Ridley-Lowell Business & Technical Institute (Binghamton)	15	Sep Jan Apr	12	Dipl	$11,600	$11,600		•		•	
North Carolina											
Alamance Community College (Graham)	35	Aug	18	AAS	$280	$2,282		•		•	•
Carteret Community College (Morehead City)	25	Aug	12	Dipl	$1,731	$9,513					
Central Carolina Community College - Chatham (Pittsboro)	35	Aug	12, 18	Dipl, AAS	$1,896	$10,536					
Central Carolina Community College - Harnett (Lillington)	35	Aug	12, 18	Dipl, AAS	$1,896	$10,536					
Davidson County Community College (Lexington)	24	Aug	12, 21	Dipl, AAS	$1,800	$10,500				•	
Forsyth Technical Community College (Winston-Salem)	24	Aug	24	AAS	$1,382	$7,682				•	•
Gaston College - Dallas	45	Aug	21	AAS	$2,016	$11,198					
King's College (Charlotte)	120	Mar Jul Sep	10, 14	Dipl, AAS	$12,440	$12,440	$2,500			•	
Lenoir Community College (Kinston)	20	Aug	21	AAS	$1,724	$9,104		•		•	•
Martin Commuity College (Williamston)	24	Aug	12, 24	Dipl, AAS	$1,344	$7,465		•		•	•
Miller-Motte College (Cary)	40	Jan Feb Apr May Jul Aug	18	AAS	$13,440	$13,440		•		•	
Mitchell Community College (Mooresville)	20	Aug	12	Dipl, Cert, AAS	$1,700	$7,000				•	•
Pitt Community College (Greenville)	30	Aug Jan May	24	Cert, AAS	$1,461	$8,121				•	•
South College - Asheville	100	Jan Apr Jun Oct	24	AAS	$16,000	$16,000		•		•	
South Piedmont Community College (Polkton)	20	Aug	12, 21	Dipl, AAS	$3,564	$17,146				•	•
Stanly Community College (Albemarle)	34	Aug	12, 21	Dipl, Cert, AAS	$1,764	$9,212		•	•	•	•
Wake Technical Community College (Raleigh)	20	Aug Jan	12	Dipl	$1,768	$9,726				•	•
Western Piedmont Community College (Morganton)	25	Aug	12, 21	Dipl, Cert, AAS	$1,856	$10,316				•	

*Data are shown only for programs that completed the 2007 AMA Survey of Health Professions Education Programs.

‡Key to Offers: 1: Evening or weekend classes; 2: Non-English instruction; 3: Cultural competence instruction; 4: Distance education component.

Medical Assistant

Programs*	Class Capacity	Begins	Length (months)	Award	Res. Tuition	Non-res. Tuition	Stipend	1	2	3	4
Ohio											
American School of Technology (Columbus)	200	Jan Feb Mar May Jun Aug	12	Dipl	$8,600	$8,600		•			
Apollo Career Center (Lima)	24	Aug	10	Cert	$7,000	$7,000		•			
Ashland County - West Holmes Career Center	25	Sep	9	Cert	$6,250	$6,250					
Bradford School (Columbus)	100	Sep Mar	10, 14	Dipl, AAB	$12,960	$12,960					
Brown Mackie College - Akron	300	Monthly	24, 12	Dipl, AAS	$9,072	$0		•			
Brown Mackie College - Cincinnati	200	Monthly	12, 24	Dipl, AAS	$9,984	$0		•		•	
Columbus State Community College	28	Sep	12	Cert	$4,450	$11,000				•	
Cuyahoga Community College (Cleveland)	20	Aug	9, 18	Cert, AAS	$2,520	$6,400		•		•	•
Davis College (Toledo)	15	Aug Nov Feb May	24	AS	$9,786	$9,786		•			
EHOVE Ghrist Adult Career Center (Milan)	25	Sep	9	Cert	$4,600	$4,600					
Jefferson Community College (Steubenville)	25	Aug	12, 18	Cert, AAS	$3,600	$3,800		•		•	
Knox County Career Center (Mount Vernon)	20	Sep	10	Dipl	$7,395	$0				•	
Lakeland Community College (Kirtland)	24	Aug	12	Cert	$3,054	$3,169		•		•	•
Lorain County Community College (Elyria)	20	Aug	9, 24	Cert, AAS	$2,399	$2,889	$45				
Mahoning County Career & Technical Center (Canfield)	25	Sep	9	Cert	$4,950	$4,950				•	
Marion Technical College	15	Sep	12	Cert	$4,300	$0		•		•	•
Miami Valley Career Technology Center (Clayton)	24	Oct	9	Cert	$5,925	$5,925					
Miami-Jacobs Career College (Dayton)	25	Every 6 wks	24	AAS	$13,248	$0		•		•	
Ohio Institute of Health Careers - Elyria	45	Every 12 wks	11, 13	Dipl	$11,342	$11,342					
Ohio Valley College of Technology (East Liverpool)	30	Aug Oct Jan Feb May	16	AAB	$7,990	$7,990					
Pickaway Ross Joint Vocational School (Chillicothe)	18	Aug	10	Cert	$5,950	$5,950				•	
Polaris Career Center (Middleburg Heights)	25	Aug	9	Cert	$5,295	$0		•		•	
Portage Lakes Career Center (Green)	25	Sep	10	Cert	$6,800	$6,800		•		•	
Rhodes State College (Lima)	20	Fall quarter	24	AAS	$4,725	$8,162		•		•	•
Stark State College of Technology (Canton)	38	Aug	20	AAS	$4,445	$6,545		•		•	
Stautzenberger College (Maumee)	200	4x/yr	15, 24	Dipl, AAS	$12,240	$12,240					
Trumbull Career & Technical Center (Warren)	25	Aug Jan Feb	10, 16	Cert	$6,825	$6,825		•			
University of Akron	35	Aug	24	AAS	$3,288	$7,403		•			
Youngstown State University	65	Aug Jan May	24	AAS	$6,500	$9,000					
Oklahoma											
Francis Tuttle Technology Center (Oklahoma City)	15	Controlled Entry	10	Cert	$1,520	$1,520				•	
Moore Norman Technology Center	24	Aug Jan	10	Dipl	$1,060	$1,565				•	
Tulsa Community College	20	Jan Aug	11, 22	Cert, MA	$2,273	$6,005		•	•	•	•
Oregon											
Central Oregon Community College (Bend)	24	Sep	12	Cert	$3,717	$10,384		•			
Everest College (Portland)	30	Jan Feb Apr May Jul Oct	15, 18	Dipl, AAS				•		•	•
Heald College - Portland	25	Quarterly	12, 18	Dipl, AAS	$9,900	$0		•		•	
Linn-Benton Community College (Albany)	30	Open entry	18	Dipl, AAS	$2,475	$5,850		•		•	•
Portland Community College	24	Sep	10	Cert	$2,924	$8,385				•	
Pennsylvania											
Bradford School - Pittsburgh	75	Jul Sep	10, 14	Dipl, ASB	$13,640	$13,640				•	
Butler County Community College	35	Aug	10, 24	Cert, AS	$3,627	$6,474		•		•	•
Central Pennsylvania College (Summerdale)	35	Oct Jan Apr Jul	21	AA	$12,380	$12,380				•	
Comm College of Allegheny County (West Mifflin)	20	Aug	9, 15	Dipl	$2,400	$4,800		•		•	
Delaware County Community College (Media)	24	Sep	12, 24	Cert, AAS	$3,315	$6,630		•		•	
Greater Altoona Career & Technology Center	18	Aug	11	Dipl	$6,800	$6,800					
Lehigh Carbon Community College (Schnecksville)	24	Aug Jan	15	AAS	$2,850	$5,700		•			•
Montgomery County Community College (Pottstown)	20	Sep Jan	11	Cert	$97	$181				•	
Mount Aloysius College (Cresson)	30	Aug	24	AS	$15,390	$15,390		•		•	
South Carolina											
Aiken Technical College	30	Aug	12	Cert	$1,600	$4,500					
Central Carolina Technical College (Sumter)	24	May	12	Dipl	$4,050	$4,752					
Greenville Technical College	25	Mar Aug	18	Cert	$2,844	$2,844		•			
Miller-Motte Technical College (Charleston)	250	Jan Apr Jul Oct	18	AAS	$11,520	$11,520		•			
Piedmont Technical College (Greenwood)	20	Aug	12	Dipl	$4,110	$4,758				•	
Spartanburg Community College	20	Aug	12	Dipl	$4,641	$8,922				•	
Trident Technical College (Charleston)	30	May	12	Dipl	$4,671	$8,847		•			
South Dakota											
Colorado Technical University (Sioux Falls)		Oct Jan Apr Jul Aug	18	AS				•			•
Lake Area Technical Institute (Watertown)	30	Aug Jan	14, 18	Dipl, AAS	$4,385	$4,385		•			
Mitchell Technical Institute (Michell)	20	Aug	18	AAS	$5,106	$0					
National American University - Sioux Falls Campus	30	Jun Sep Dec Mar	24	AAS				•			•
Presentation College (Aberdeen)		Aug Jan	18	AS	$12,300	$12,300		•		•	•

*Data are shown only for programs that completed the 2007 AMA Survey of Health Professions Education Programs.

‡Key to Offers: 1: Evening or weekend classes; 2: Non-English instruction; 3: Cultural competence instruction; 4: Distance education component.

Medical Assistant

Programs*	Class Capacity	Begins	Length (months)	Award	Res. Tuition	Non-res. Tuition	Stipend	Offers:‡ 1	2	3	4
Tennessee											
Chattanooga State Technical Comm College	20	Aug	12	Dipl	$2,136	$2,136					
Miller-Motte Technical College - Chattanooga	40	Every 6 wks	24	AAS	$9,600	$9,600					
National College of Business and Technology - Bristol	60	Mar Jun Sep Dec	24	AS	$6,188	$6,188		•			
National College of Business and Technology - Knoxville	60	Mar Jun Sep Dec	24	AAS	$6,188	$6,188		•			
National College of Business and Technology - Nashville	25	Mar Jun Sep Dec	24	AS	$7,104	$7,104		•			
South College (Knoxville)	150	Jan Apr Jun Oct	21	AS	$16,000	$16,000		•		•	
Tennessee Technology Center - Memphis	25	May	12	Dipl	$2,169	$2,169					
Texas											
Cisco Junior College (Abilene)	20	Sep Jan Jun Jul	12, 24	Cert, AAS	$3,395	$3,701		•		•	•
Cy-Fair College (Cypress)	12	Aug	12	Cert	$1,780	$3,672					
El Centro College (Dallas)	52	Sep Jan	12	Cert	$1,521	$2,808			•	•	
Hallmark Institute of Technology (San Antonio)	350	Rolling admission	11	AAS	$17,610	$0					
Houston Community College	75	Aug Jan Jun	12	Cert	$3,500	$5,498		•		•	
Kilgore College	16	Aug	12, 21	Cert, AAS	$1,963	$3,690					
Richland College (Dallas)	60	Jan Sep (flex entry)	8, 15	Cert	$3,000	$3,000	$1,500	•	•	•	
San Antonio College	50	Jan Aug	13, 24	Cert, AAS	$1,929	$6,674		•		•	
San Jacinto College North (Houston)	50	Aug	12	Cert	$2,600	$3,000					•
Texas School of Business - North Campus (Houston)	30	Every 6 wks	7, 11	Dipl	$0	$11,400		•			
Utah											
AmeriTech College (Provo)	160	Every 5 wks	9	Dipl	$10,084	$10,084					
Ogden-Weber Applied Technology College	20	Year-round	12	Cert, AAT	$1,950	$0		•			
Salt Lake Community College (West Jordan)	90	Aug Jan May	12	Cert	$3,500	$9,900				•	•
Stevens-Henager College (Logan)	185	Monthly	20	AOS	$16,350	$16,350		•			•
Stevens-Henager College (Ogden)	60	Every 4 wks	15, 20	AOS	$14,200	$14,200		•			
Utah Career College (West Jordan)	16	Jan Apr Jul Oct	12, 18	Dipl, AAS	$16,120	$16,120		•		•	
Virginia											
Bryant & Stratton College - Richmond	20	Sep Jan May	20	AAS	$18,600	$18,600		•		•	
Miller-Motte Technical College (Lynchburg)	75	Jan Apr Jul Oct	18	Dipl, AOS	$200	$200		•			•
National College - Bluefield	60	Dec Mar Jun Sep	24	AS	$6,624	$6,624		•			
National College - Charlottesville	60	Mar Jun Sep Dec	24	AS	$6,624	$6,624		•			
National College - Danville	60	Mar Jun Sep Dec	24	AS	$7,104	$7,104		•			
National College - Harrisonburg	30	Mar Jun Sep Dec	24	AS	$7,776	$7,776		•			
National College - Lynchburg	60	Dec Mar Jun Sep	24	AS	$7,104	$7,104		•			
National College - Martinsville	60	Mar Jun Sep Dec	24	AS	$6,188	$6,188		•		•	
National College - Roanoke Valley (Salem)	60	Mar Jun Sep Dec	24	AAS	$6,624	$6,624		•			
Washington											
Clark College (Vancouver)	30	Sep	12	Cert, AAS	$3,964	$4,223				•	
Everest College (Vancouver)	30	Every 6 wks	15, 18	Dipl, AAS	$11,808	$11,808		•		•	
Everest College - Everett	270	Every 4 wks	8	Dipl	$12,291	$12,291		•			
Everest College - Port Orchard (Bremerton)	24	Every 4 wks	8	Dipl	$12,730	$0		•			
Everett Community College	Var	Continuous	15, 24	Cert, ATA	$4,458	$14,760		•		•	•
Highline Community College (Des Moines)	70	Quarterly	18	AAS	$2,664	$7,443		•		•	
Lake Washington Technical College (Kirkland)	30	Sep Apr	12, 15	Cert, AAS	$3,483	$3,483				•	
Lower Columbia College (Longview)	24	Sep	12	Cert	$3,526	$4,535					
North Seattle Community College	100	Sep Jan Mar Jun	12, 15	Cert, AAS	$3,350	$10,243		•		•	
Renton Technical College	26	Sep Jan	11	Cert	$3,490	$3,490					
South Puget Sound Community College (Olympia)	20	Sep	12, 24	Cert, ATA	$2,971	$3,164				•	
West Virginia											
Huntington Junior College	200	Sep Jan Apr Jun	18, 12	Dipl, AS	$7,800	$7,800		•			
Wisconsin											
Blackhawk Technical College (Janesville)	24	Aug	9	Dipl	$2,100	$13,825					
Bryant & Stratton College - Milwaukee	300	Varies	24	AS	$11,820	$0		•		•	
Chippewa Valley Technical College (Eau Claire)	24	Jan Aug	12	Dipl	$2,432	$18,984		•		•	•
Concordia University Wisconsin (Milwaukee)	30	Aug	9	Cert	$6,970	$6,970				•	
Fox Valley Technical College (Oshkosh)	24	Jan	9	Dipl	$3,073	$17,659		•		•	•
Gateway Technical College (Racine)	30	Aug Jan	10	Dipl	$1,760	$9,880					
Mid-State Technical College - Marshfield	12	Aug Jan	9	Dipl	$3,300	$3,300					
Mid-State Technical College - Stevens Point	12	Jan Aug	9	Dipl	$3,300	$3,300		•			
Moraine Park Technical College (Fond du Lac)	30	Aug	9	Dipl	$4,230	$20,007		•		•	•
Northeast Wisconsin Technical College (Green Bay)	56	Aug Jan	10	Dipl	$4,576	$0		•		•	•
Wisconsin Indianhead Technical College (New Richmond)	30	Aug Jan	9	Dipl	$3,672	$0		•		•	•
Wisconsin Indianhead Technical College - Ashland Campus	20	Aug	9	Dipl	$4,491	$19,976				•	

*Data are shown only for programs that completed the 2007 AMA Survey of Health Professions Education Programs.
‡Key to Offers: 1: Evening or weekend classes; 2: Non-English instruction; 3: Cultural competence instruction; 4: Distance education component.

Medical illustrators specialize in the visual transformation, display, and communication of scientific information. Their graduate level training in biomedical science, art, design, visual technology, education, and communication enables them to understand and visualize scientific data and concepts to teach the general public and professionals in the fields of health care, research, pharmaceuticals, biotechnology, and demonstrative evidence. Medical illustrations appear in medical textbooks, medical advertisements, professional journals, instructional animations, computer-assisted learning programs, scientific exhibits, lecture presentations, general magazines, and courtroom presentations. Depending on the intended use, medical illustrations can be highly realistic and anatomically precise or they can be thematic, interpretive, abstract, or even wildly conceptual. Although medical illustration is commonly seen in print and electronic media, medical illustrators also work in three dimensions, creating anatomical teaching models, models for simulated medical procedures, and prosthetic parts for patients.

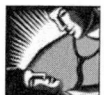

Career Description

Medical illustrators work closely with clients to interpret their needs and create visual solutions for them through effective problem solving. While some medical illustrators specialize in a single art medium or work primarily for one medical specialty, the majority handle an ever-changing variety of assignments from different clients, involving a variety of biomedical content, and requiring a variety of media solutions. In addition to design and production roles, medical illustrators may function as consultants, art directors, supervisors, and administrators within the field of biocommunications.

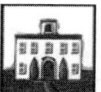

Employment Characteristics

Many medical illustrators are employed in medical schools and large medical centers that have teaching and research programs. Other medical artists are employed by hospitals, clinics, dental schools, or schools of veterinary medicine. Some institutional medical illustrators work alone, whereas, others are part of large multimedia departments. Other medical illustrators choose to target specific markets such as medical publishers, pharmaceutical companies, advertising agencies, animation studios, physicians, or attorneys. Some work independently on a freelance basis; others set up small companies designed to provide illustration services to various targeted markets.

The employment outlook for medical illustrators is good. This is in part due to the relatively few medical illustrators who graduate each year, and in part due to the growth in medical research that continually reveals new treatments and technologies that require medical illustrations. A growing demand by patients to better understand their own bodies and medical options has expanded the need for medical illustration aimed at the lay public. In addition, increased need for medical illustrations and models to educate juries during courtroom presentations has expanded the medical-legal subspecialty of medical illustration.

Salary

Earnings vary significantly according to 1) the experience and ability of the artist, 2) the type of work, and 3) the area of the country where one works. The average starting salary in an institutional setting for a graduate of an accredited program of medical illustration is around $45,000 a year plus fringe benefits. Experienced salaried illustrators usually earn about $53,000 a year. Administrators and faculty members generally earn somewhat more. Salaried illustrators often supplement their income with freelance work. Refer to Section IV, Table 5 of this *Directory* for more information, or see www.ama-assn.org/go/hpsalary.

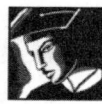

Educational Programs

Length. Accredited programs generally last 2 full years resulting in a master's degree.

Prerequisites. All current medical illustrator programs are at an advanced level and are based on a master's model. Although admission requirements to accredited programs vary, a bachelors degree with an emphasis on art and science is preferred. In addition, a portfolio of artwork and a personal interview are required.

Curriculum. While the area of emphasis may vary from program to program, the curriculum includes the following courses: an advanced course in human anatomy with dissection and courses in other biomedical sciences such as embryology, histology, neuroanatomy, cell biology, molecular biology, physiology, pathology, immunology, pharmacology, and genetics. Art and theory courses include anatomical drawing, illustration techniques in line, tone, and color (hand-rendered and computer-generated), surgical illustration, graphic design, computer graphics and multimedia, instructional design, motion media production, three-dimensional models and exhibits, management and business practices, and professional ethics.

Inquiries

Careers/Curriculum
Association of Medical Illustrators
PO Box 1897
Lawrence, KS 66044
866 393-4264
E-mail: hq@ami.org
www.ami.org

Program Accreditation
Commission on Accreditation of Allied Health Education Programs (CAAHEP) in collaboration with:
Accreditation Review Committee for the Medical Illustrator
c/o CAAHEP
1361 Park Street
Clearwater, FL 33756
727 210-2350

Medical Illustrator

Georgia

Medical College of Georgia
Medical Illustrator Prgm
Allied Hlth and Grad Studies -Ste CJ-1101
1120 15th St
Augusta, GA 30912-0300
www.mcg.edu/medart
Prgm Dir: Steven J Harrison, MS CMI FAMI FBPA
Tel: 706 721-3266   *Fax:* 706 721-7855
E-mail: sharriso@mcg.edu

Illinois

University of Illinois at Chicago
Medical Illustrator Prgm
Dept Biomed Visualization (MC-527)
College of Applied Health Sciences
Chicago, IL 60612
www.bhis.uic.edu
Prgm Dir: Scott Barrows, BS CMI FAMI
Tel: 312 996-8344   *Fax:* 312 996-8342
E-mail: sbarrows@uic.edu

Maryland

Johns Hopkins School of Medicine
Medical Illustrator Prgm
Dept of Art Applied to Med
1830 E Monument St, Ste 7000
Baltimore, MD 21205
Prgm Dir: Gary P Lees, MS CMI FAMI
Tel: 410 955-3213   *Fax:* 410 955-1085
E-mail: glees@jhmi.edu

Ontario, Canada

University of Toronto
Medical Illustrator Prgm
1 King's College Circle
Medical Sciences Bldg, Rm 2356
Toronto, ON M5S 1A8
www.bmc.med.utoronto.ca/BMC
Prgm Dir: Linda Wilson-Pauwels, AOCA BScAAM MEd
    EdD
Tel: 416 978-5357   *Fax:* 416 978-6891
E-mail: l.wilson.pauwels@utoronto.ca

Texas

Univ of Texas Southwestern Med Ctr
Medical Illustrator Prgm
Biomedical Communications Graduate Program
5323 Harry Hines Blvd
Dallas, TX 75235-8881
www.utsouthwestern.edu/graduateschool/
    biomedicalcommunications.html
Prgm Dir: Lewis E Calver, MS
Tel: 214 648-4699   *Fax:* 214 648-5353
E-mail: biocomm@utsouthwestern.edu

Medical Illustrator

Programs*	Class Capacity	Begins	Length (months)	Award	Res. Tuition	Non-res. Tuition	Stipend	Offers:‡ 1	2	3	4
Georgia											
Medical College of Georgia (Augusta)	8	Aug	21	MSMI	$7,645	$7,645				•	
Illinois											
University of Illinois at Chicago	15	Aug	21	MS	$7,790	$19,788					
Ontario, Canada											
University of Toronto	32	Sep	24	MSc, BMC	$7,006	$16,800					
Texas											
Univ of Texas Southwestern Med Ctr (Dallas)	7	May	24	Dipl, MA	$1,200	$7,800					

*Data are shown only for programs that completed the 2007 AMA Survey of Health Professions Education Programs.
‡Key to Offers: 1: Evening or weekend classes; 2: Non-English instruction; 3: Cultural competence instruction; 4: Distance education component.

Medical Librarian

Medical librarians are information professionals who specialize in health resources and provide medical information for physicians, allied health professionals, patients, consumers, students, and corporations. Using materials ranging from traditional print sources to electronic databases, medical librarians devise and use innovative strategies to assess and deliver information to their clients. Physicians often call upon medical librarians to provide life-saving information for patient care.

Career Description

Medical librarians help improve the quality of patient care by helping health care professionals stay abreast of new developments and treatments. Additionally, they find relevant health information for patients and consumers, serve as educators for students pursuing health care degrees, and provide training in the location and use of medical resources. Increasingly medical librarians use technology to design Web sites and distance education programs and to construct digital libraries. Others work for Internet companies and electronic publishers that index and organize information for the Web. Medical librarians also participate as members of research teams on university campuses and serve health care corporations, such as insurance and pharmaceutical companies, by providing information necessary for developing new products and services.

In administrative roles, medical librarians serve as directors, chief information officers, and deans or associate deans of information technology departments. Librarians ensure their informational mission is accomplished by providing leadership and strategic planning for their institutions, managing multimillion dollar budgets, pursuing grant funding, and developing marketing and public relations plans for their libraries.

Medical librarians work closely with support staff in the library to accomplish day-to-day tasks. Known as medical library assistants, these support staff provide critical operations support in all areas of the library, including circulation, serials management, acquisitions, interlibrary loan, cataloging, billing, and reference services. Some states have associations and special interest groups that support the educational needs of library support staff. Such organizations include the New York State Library Assistants' Association (NYSLAA) and the Metropolitan New York Library Council's Library Assistants, Support Staff and Associates special interest group. NYSLAA sponsors a Certificate of Achievement Program that recognizes library assistants for their contributions to libraries and the library profession.

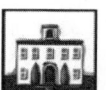

Employment Characteristics

Medical librarians and medical library assistants are employed anywhere health information is needed, including hospitals, academic medical centers, clinics, colleges, universities, professional schools, consumer health libraries, research centers, foundations, biotechnology centers, insurance companies, medical equipment manufacturers, pharmaceutical companies, publishers, and federal state and local government agencies.

Salary

Salaries vary according to the type and location of the institution, level of responsibility and technical skill, and length of employment. According to the Medical Library Association (MLA), the average starting salary for entry-level medical librarians was $40,832 in 2005. The overall average salary for experienced medical librarians was $57,982. Library directors can earn up to $158,600. Refer to Section IV, Table 5 of this *Directory* for more information, or see www.ama-assn.org/go/hpsalary.

Educational Programs

Length. Programs are 1 to 2 years and result in a master's degree.

Prerequisites. Medical librarians must have a master of library and information science degree from an American Library Association–accredited school. An undergraduate degree in any field is necessary for admission to a master's program. Undergraduate courses in biology, medical sciences, medical terminology, computer science, education, and management are helpful. Medical librarians may also apply for membership in the Academy of Health Information Professionals, a credentialing program for medical librarians sponsored by the Medical Library Association.

Curriculum. Programs leading to a master of library and information science degree include a wide variety of courses. All students take core courses in research, information resources, cataloging, and management and choose between tracks for public, school, academic, or special libraries. Upon choosing a track, the student and academic advisor select courses that reflect the student's career goals. Those wishing to focus on systems and technology will take a variety of technology courses in addition to the core and specialty track courses. Medical librarianship falls within the special library curriculum in many schools of library and information science. Medical library curriculum courses include resources for consumer health information, resources and services for health sciences information, medical informatics, and resources and services for special populations.

Inquiries

Careers/Credentialing

Medical Library Association
65 East Wacker Place, Suite 1900
Chicago, IL 60601-7246
312 419-9094
312 419-8950 Fax
E-mail: mlapd2@mlahq.org
www.mlanet.org/career

Library Assistants

New York State Library Assistants' Association
www.nyslaa.org

Metropolitan New York Library Council
Library Assistants, Support Staff and Associates
Vergie Savage-Branch
Cornell University Medical College Library
1300 York Avenue
New York, NY 10021
212 746-6091
www.metro.org/SIGs/lassa.html

Program Accreditation
American Library Association, Committee on Accreditation/Office
    for Accreditation
Karen O'Brien, Director
50 East Huron
Chicago, IL 60611
312 280-2434
E-mail: kobrien@ala.org

Medical Librarian

Alabama

University of Alabama
Medical Librarian Prgm
School of Library and Information Studies
Box 870252
Tuscaloosa, AL 35487-0252
Prgm Dir: Elizabeth Aversa, Dean
Tel: 205 348-4610   *Fax:* 205 348-3746
E-mail: info@slis.ua.edu

Alberta, Canada

University of Alberta
Medical Librarian Prgm
School for Library and information Studies
3-20 Rutherford S
Edmonton, AB T6G 2J4
Prgm Dir: Anna Altmann
Tel: 780 492-4578   *Fax:* 780 492-2430
E-mail: slis@ualberta.ca

Arizona

University of Arizona
Medical Librarian Prgm
School of Information Resources and Library Science
1515 E First St
Tucson, AZ 85719
Prgm Dir: Brooke E Sheldon, Dean
Tel: 520 621-3565   *Fax:* 520 621-3279
E-mail: sirls@u.arizona.edu

British Columbia, Canada

University of British Columbia
Medical Librarian Prgm
School of Library, Archival and Information Studies
Ste 301, 6190 Agronomy Rd
Vancouver, BC V6T 1Z3
Prgm Dir: Edie Rasmussen
Tel: 604 822-2404   *Fax:* 604 822-6006
E-mail: slais@interchange.ubc.ca

California

University of California - Los Angeles
Medical Librarian Prgm
Graduate School of Education and Information
Studies Bldg
Los Angeles, CA 90095-1520
Prgm Dir: Virginia A Walter, Chair
Tel: 310 825-8799   *Fax:* 310 206-3076
E-mail: vwalter@ucla.edu

San Jose State University
Medical Librarian Prgm
School of Library and Information Science
One Washington Square
San Jose, CA 95192-0029
Prgm Dir: Blanche Woolls
Tel: 408 924-2490   *Fax:* 408 924-2476
E-mail: office@slis.sjsu.edu

Connecticut

Southern Connecticut State University
Medical Librarian Prgm
Information and Library Sciences
501 Crescent St
New Haven, CT 06515
Prgm Dir: Edward Harris, Dean
Tel: 203 392-5781   *Fax:* 203 392-5780
E-mail: mckayl1@southernct.edu

District of Columbia

Catholic University of America
Medical Librarian Prgm
School of Library and Information Science
620 Michigan Ave NE
Washington, DC 20064
Prgm Dir: Martha Hale, Dean
Tel: 202 319-5085   *Fax:* 202 319-5574
E-mail: cua-slis@cua.edu

Florida

Florida State University
Medical Librarian Prgm
School of Information Studies
Shores Bldg
Tallahassee, FL 32306-2100
Prgm Dir: Jane B Robbins, Dean
Tel: 850 644-5775   *Fax:* 850 644-9763
E-mail: grad@lis.fsu.edu

University of South Florida
Medical Librarian Prgm
School of Library and Information Sciences
4202 E Fowler Ave
Tampa, FL 33620
Prgm Dir: Vicki Gregory
Tel: 813 974-3520   *Fax:* 813 974-6840
E-mail: lis@cas.usf.edu

Hawaii

University of Hawaii
Medical Librarian Prgm
Library and Information Science Program
2550 McCarthy Mall
Honolulu, HI 96822
Prgm Dir: Diane Nahl, Chair
Tel: 808 956-7321   *Fax:* 808 956-5835
E-mail: slis@hawaii.edu

Illinois

Univ of Illinois at Urbana-Champaign
Medical Librarian Prgm
Graduate School of Library and Information Science
501 E Daniel St
Champaign, IL 61820-6211
Prgm Dir: John Unsworth, Dean
Tel: 217 333-3280   *Fax:* 217 244-3302
E-mail: apply@alexia.lis.uiuc.edu

Dominican University
Medical Librarian Prgm
Graduate School of Library and Information Science
7900 W Division St
River Forest, IL 60305
Prgm Dir: Susan Roman, Dean
Tel: 708 524-6845   *Fax:* 708 524-6657
E-mail: gslis@dom.edu

Indiana

Indiana University - Indianapolis
Medical Librarian Prgm
School of Library and Information Science at
    Indianapolis
755 W Michigan St
Indianapolis, IN 46202
Prgm Dir: Katherine Schilling, MLS EdD AHIP
Tel: 317 278-2375   *Fax:* 317 278-1807
E-mail: katschil@iupui.edu

Iowa

University of Iowa
Medical Librarian Prgm
School of Library and Information Science
3087 Main Library
Iowa City, IA 52242-1420
Prgm Dir: David Eichmann
Tel: 319 335-5707   *Fax:* 319 335-5374
E-mail: slis@uiowa.edu

Kansas

Emporia State University
Medical Librarian Prgm
School of Library and Information Management
1200 Commerical, Campus Box 4025
Emporia, KS 66801
Prgm Dir: Diane Bailiff, Interim Dean
Tel: 620 341-5203   *Fax:* 620 641-5233
E-mail: kitselmc@emporia.edu

Kentucky

University of Kentucky
Medical Librarian Prgm
School of Library and Information Science
502 King Library
Lexington, KY 40506-0039
Prgm Dir: Timothy W Sineath
Tel: 859 257-8876   *Fax:* 859 257-4205
E-mail: salsman@uky.edu

Louisiana

Louisiana State University
Medical Librarian Prgm
School of Library and Information Science
267 Coates Hall
Baton Rouge, LA 70803
Prgm Dir: Beth Paskoff, Dean, PhD
Tel: 225 578-3158   *Fax:* 225 578-4581
E-mail: slis@lsu.edu

Maryland

University of Maryland
Medical Librarian Prgm
College of Information Studies
4105 Hornbake Bldg
College Park, MD 20742
Prgm Dir: Bruce Dearstyne, Dean
Tel: 301 405-2033   *Fax:* 301 314-9145
E-mail: lbscgrad@deans.umd.edu

Massachusetts

Simmons College
Medical Librarian Prgm
Graduate School of Library and Information Science
300 The Fenway
Boston, MA 02115
Prgm Dir: Michele Cloonan, Dean
Tel: 617 521-2800   *Fax:* 617 521-3192
E-mail: gslis@simmons.edu

Michigan

University of Michigan
Medical Librarian Prgm
School of Information
550 E University Ave, 304 W Hall Bldg
Ann Arbor, MI 48109-1092
Prgm Dir: John L King, Dean
Tel: 734 764-9376   *Fax:* 734 764-2475
E-mail: si.admissions@umich.edu

Wayne State University
Medical Librarian Prgm
Library and Information Science Program
106 Kresge Library
Detroit, MI 48202
Prgm Dir: Joseph J Mika, PhD MLS
Tel: 313 577-1825   *Fax:* 313 577-7563
E-mail: asklis@wayne.edu

Mississippi

University of Southern Mississippi
Medical Librarian Prgm
School of Library and Information Science
118 College Dr #5146
Hattiesburg, MS 39406-0001
Prgm Dir: M J Norton
Tel: 601 266-4228   *Fax:* 601 266-5774
E-mail: slis@usm.edu

Missouri

University of Missouri - Columbia
Medical Librarian Prgm
Information Science and Learning Technologies
303 Townsend Hall
Columbia, MO 65211
Prgm Dir: John Wedman, Dean
Tel: 573 882-4546   *Fax:* 573 884-0122
E-mail: sislt@missouri.edu

New Jersey

Rutgers University
Medical Librarian Prgm
Dept of Library and Information Science
4 Huntington St
New Brunswick, NJ 08901-1071
Prgm Dir: Nicholas J Belkin
Tel: 732 932-7500, Ext 1071   *Fax:* 732 932-2644
E-mail: scilsmls@scils.rutgers.edu

New York

SUNY at Albany
Medical Librarian Prgm
School of Inform Science and Policy Draper 113
135 Western Ave
Albany, NY 12222
Prgm Dir: Peter Bloniarz, Dean
Tel: 518 442-5110   *Fax:* 518 442-5367
E-mail: infosci@albany.edu

Long Island University - C W Post Campus
Medical Librarian Prgm
Palmer School of Library and Information Science
720 Northern Blvd
Brookville, NY 11548
Prgm Dir: Michael E D Koenig, Dean
Tel: 516 299-2866   *Fax:* 516 299-4168
E-mail: palmer@cwpost.liu.edu

University at Buffalo - SUNY
Medical Librarian Prgm
Library and Information Studies
534 Baldy Hall
Buffalo, NY 14260
Prgm Dir: Judith Robinson, Chair
Tel: 716 645-2412   *Fax:* 716 645-3775
E-mail: ub-lis@buffalo.edu

CUNY Queens College
Medical Librarian Prgm
Graduate School of Library and Information Studies
65-30 Kissena Blvd
Flushing, NY 11367-1597
Prgm Dir: Marianne Cooper
Tel: 718 997-3790   *Fax:* 718 997-3797
E-mail: gslis@qcunix1.qc.edu

St John's University
Medical Librarian Prgm
Division of Library and Information Science
8000 Utopia Pkwy
Jamaica, NY 11439
Prgm Dir: Sherry Vellucci
Tel: 718 990-6200   *Fax:* 718 990-2071
E-mail: libis@stjohns.edu

Pratt Institute
Medical Librarian Prgm
School of Information and Library Science
144 W 14th St, 6th Fl
New York, NY 10011
Prgm Dir: Marie Radford, Acting Dean
Tel: 212 647-7682   *Fax:* 212 367-2492
E-mail: infosils@pratt.edu

Syracuse University
Medical Librarian Prgm
School of Information Studies
4-206 Center for Science and Technology
Syracuse, NY 13244
Prgm Dir: Raymond Von Dran, Dean
Tel: 315 443-2911   *Fax:* 315 443-5673
E-mail: ist@syr.edu

North Carolina

University of North Carolina - Chapel Hill
Medical Librarian Prgm
School of Information and Library Science
100 Manning Hall, CB 3360
Chapel Hill, NC 27599-3360
Prgm Dir: Joanne Gard Marshall, Dean
Tel: 919 962-8366   *Fax:* 919 962-8071
E-mail: info@ils.unc.edu

North Carolina Central University
Medical Librarian Prgm
School of Library and Information Sciences
1800 Fayetteville St
Durham, NC 27707
Prgm Dir: Robert M Ballard, Dean
Tel: 919 530-6485   *Fax:* 919 530-6402
E-mail: lsis@nccu.edu

University of North Carolina - Greensboro
Medical Librarian Prgm
Dept of Library and Information Studies
349 Curry Bldg
Greensboro, NC 27401-6170
Prgm Dir: Lee Shiflett
Tel: 336 334-3477   *Fax:* 336 334-5060
E-mail: lis@uncg.edu

Nova Scotia, Canada

Dalhousie University
Medical Librarian Prgm
School of Library and Information Studies
3rd Fl, Killiam Library
Halifax, NS B3H 3J5
Prgm Dir: Fiona Black
Tel: 902 494-3656   *Fax:* 902 494-2451
E-mail: slis@dal.ca

Ohio

Kent State University
Medical Librarian Prgm
School of Library and Information Sciences
PO Box 5190
Kent, OH 44242-0001
Prgm Dir: Richard E Rubin
Tel: 330 672-2782   *Fax:* 330 672-7965
E-mail: inform@slis.kent.edu

Oklahoma

University of Oklahoma
Medical Librarian Prgm
School of Library and Information Studies
401 W Brooks, Rm 120
Norman, OK 73019-6032
Prgm Dir: Danny P Wallace
Tel: 405 325-3921   *Fax:* 405 325-7648
E-mail: slisinfo@ou.edu

Ontario, Canada

University of Western Ontario
Medical Librarian Prgm
Graduate Programs in Library and Information Science
255 Middlesex College
London, ON N6A 5B7
Prgm Dir: Catherine Ross, Dean
Tel: 519 661-4017   *Fax:* 519 661-3506
E-mail: mlisinfo@uwo.ca

University of Toronto
Medical Librarian Prgm
Master of Information Studies
Faculty of Information Studies
Toronto, ON M5S 3G6
Prgm Dir: Brian Cantwell Smith, Dean, PhD
Tel: 416 978-3202, Ext 1   *Fax:* 416 978-5762
E-mail: dean@fis.utoronto.ca

Pennsylvania

Clarion University of Pennsylvania
Medical Librarian Prgm
Department of Library Science
210 Carlson Library Bldg
Clarion, PA 16214
Prgm Dir: Andrea L Miller
Tel: 814 393-2271   *Fax:* 814 393-2150
E-mail: reed@clarion.edu

Drexel University
Medical Librarian Prgm
College of Information Science and Technology
3141 Chestnut St
Philadelphia, PA 19104-2875
Prgm Dir: David E Fenske, Dean
Tel: 215 895-2474   *Fax:* 215 895-2494
E-mail: info@cis.drexel.edu

University of Pittsburgh
Medical Librarian Prgm
Department of Library and Information Science
135 N Bellefield Ave
Pittsburgh, PA 15260
Prgm Dir: Ronald Larsen, Dean
Tel: 412 624-5142   *Fax:* 412 624-5231
E-mail: inquiry@mail.sis.pitt.edu

Puerto Rico

University of Puerto Rico
Medical Librarian Prgm
Information Science and Technologies
PO Box 210906
San Juan, PR 00031-1906
Prgm Dir: Consuelo Figueras
Tel: 787 763-6199   *Fax:* 787 764-2311
E-mail: egcti@rrpac.upr.clu.edu

Quebec, Canada

McGill University
Medical Librarian Prgm
Graduate School of Library and Information Studies
3459 McTavish St, MS 57-F
Montreal, QC H3A 1Y1
Prgm Dir: Jamshid Beheshti
Tel: 514 398-4204   *Fax:* 514 398-7193
E-mail: gslis@mcgill.ca

University de Montreal
Medical Librarian Prgm
Ecole de bibiotheconomie et des sciences de
l'information
CP 6128, succursale centre-ville
Montreal, QC H3C 3J7
Prgm Dir: Carol Couture
Tel: 514 343-6400   *Fax:* 514 343-5753
E-mail: ebsiinfo@ebsi.umontreal.ca

Rhode Island

University of Rhode Island
Medical Librarian Prgm
Graduate School of Library and Information Studies
Rodman Hall
Kingston, RI 02881
Prgm Dir: W Michael Havener
Tel: 401 874-2947   *Fax:* 401 874-4964
E-mail: gslis@etal.uri.edu

South Carolina

University of South Carolina
Medical Librarian Prgm
School of Library and Information Science
Davis College
Columbia, SC 29208
Prgm Dir: Daniel Barron
Tel: 803 777-3858   *Fax:* 803 777-7938
E-mail: ddbarron@gwm.sc.edu

Tennessee

University of Tennessee - Knoxville
Medical Librarian Prgm
School of Information Sciences
451 Communications Bldg
Knoxville, TN 37996-0341
Prgm Dir: Douglas Raber, Interim Dean
Tel: 865 974-2148   *Fax:* 865 974-4967
E-mail: sis@utk.edu

Texas

University of Texas at Austin
Medical Librarian Prgm
School of Information
1 University Station D7000
Austin, TX 78712-0390
Prgm Dir: Andrew Dillon, Dean
Tel: 512 471-3821   *Fax:* 512 471-3971
E-mail: info@ischool.utexas.edu

Texas Woman's University
Medical Librarian Prgm
School of Library and Information Studies
PO Box 425438
Denton, TX 76204-5438
Prgm Dir: Lynn Westbrook
Tel: 940 898-2602   *Fax:* 940 898-2611
E-mail: slis@twu.edu

University of North Texas
Medical Librarian Prgm
School of Library and Information Sciences
PO Box 311068
Denton, TX 76203-1068
Prgm Dir: Philip Turner, Dean
Tel: 940 565-2731   *Fax:* 940 565-3101
E-mail: slis@unt.edu

Washington

University of Washington
Medical Librarian Prgm
Information School
370 Mary Gates Hall
Seattle, WA 98195-2840
Prgm Dir: Harry Bruce, Dean, PhD
Tel: 206 685-9937   *Fax:* 206 616-3152
E-mail: mlis@u.washington.edu

Wisconsin

University of Wisconsin - Madison
Medical Librarian Prgm
Library and Information Studies
600 N Park St
Madison, WI 53706
Prgm Dir: Catherine Arnott Smith
Tel: 608 263-2900   *Fax:* 608 263-4849
E-mail: casmith24@wisc.edu

University of Wisconsin - Milwaukee
Medical Librarian Prgm
School of Information Studies
PO Box 413
Milwaukee, WI 53201
Prgm Dir: Thomas D Walker, Interim Dean
Tel: 414 229-4707   *Fax:* 414 229-6699
E-mail: info@sois.uwm.edu

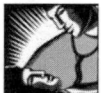

Career Description

Music therapists use music within a therapeutic relationship to address physical, emotional, cognitive, and social needs of individuals of all ages, improving quality of life for persons who are well and meeting the needs of children and adults with disabilities or illnesses. After assessing the strengths and needs of each client, qualified music therapists develop a treatment plan with goals and objectives and then provide the indicated treatment. Music therapists structure the use of both instrumental and vocal music strategies to facilitate changes that are non-musical in nature. They may improvise or compose music with clients, accompany and conduct group music experiences, provide instrument instruction, direct music and movement activities, or structure music listening opportunities. Music therapists provide services for children and adults with psychiatric disorders, developmental disabilities, speech and hearing impairments, physical disabilities, and neurological impairments, among others. Music therapy interventions can be designed to promote wellness, manage stress, alleviate pain, enhance memory, improve communication, and provide unique opportunities for interaction. Depending upon the needs of the clients involved, music therapy sessions are offered on an individual or group basis. Music therapists are usually members of an interdisciplinary team of health care professionals who work collaboratively to address clients' treatment needs.

Personal Qualifications

Music therapists should have a genuine interest in people and a desire to help others empower themselves. The essence of music therapy practice involves establishing caring and professional relationships with people of all ages and abilities. Empathy, patience, tact, a sense of humor, imagination, creativity, and an understanding of oneself are important characteristics for professionals in this field. People thinking about music therapy as a career must be accomplished musicians. They must be versatile and able to adjust to changing circumstances. Music therapists must express themselves well in speech and in writing. In addition, they must be able to work well with other health care providers.

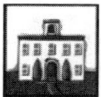

Employment Characteristics

Music therapists are employed in many different settings including general and psychiatric hospitals, mental health agencies, physical rehabilitation centers, nursing homes, public and private schools, substance abuse programs, forensic facilities, hospice programs, and day care facilities. Typically, full-time therapists work a standard 40-hour workweek. Some therapists prefer part-time work and choose to develop contracts with specific agencies, providing music therapy services for an hourly or contractual fee. In addition, a growing number of clinicians are choosing to start private practices in music therapy to benefit from opportunities provided through self-employment.

Salary

According to the American Music Therapy Association (AMTA), the overall average salary for full-time music therapists was $42,364 in 2004. Individual salaries can vary by population served, work setting, geographic location, years of experience, and level of graduate education completed. The income range reported in 2004 included salaries up to $200,000. Refer to Section IV, Table 5 of this *Directory* for more information, or see www.ama-assn.org/go/hpsalary.

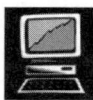

Future Outlook

As an increasing number of consumers seek non-invasive, alternative and complementary therapies as treatment options, the need for music therapists continues to rise. An increased need for music therapists in early intervention programs, special education settings, geriatric facilities, and community based services offers a variety of employment options. The next 10 years hold positive opportunities for the music therapy profession.

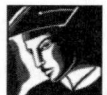

Educational Programs

Length. Those who wish to become music therapists must earn a bachelor's degree or higher in music therapy from one of over 70 AMTA-approved colleges and universities. Entry-level study requires academic coursework and 1,200 hours of clinical training, including a supervised internship.

Prerequisites. For entry into undergraduate programs, a high school diploma is required, along with demonstration of musicianship. Candidates for the masters degree must hold a baccalaureate degree or equivalent in music therapy (see "Certification" below) or be working concurrently toward fulfilling degree equivalency requirements.

Curriculum. The curriculum is designed to impart entry-level competencies in three main areas: musical foundations, clinical foundations, and music therapy foundations and principles. Graduate programs in music therapy examine, with greater breadth and depth, issues relevant to the clinical, professional, and academic preparation of music therapists, usually in combination with established methods of research inquiry.

Certification

At the completion of academic and clinical training, students are eligible to take the national examination administered by the Certification Board for Music Therapists (CBMT), an independent, non-profit certifying agency fully accredited by the National Commission for Certifying Agencies. After successful completion of the CBMT examination, graduates are issued the credential necessary for professional practice, Music Therapist-Board Certified (MT-BC). To demonstrate continued competence and to maintain this credential, music therapists are required to complete 100 hours of continuing music therapy education, or to retake and pass the CBMT examination within every 5-year recertification cycle.

Inquiries

Education and Careers

American Music Therapy Association (AMTA)
8455 Colesville Road, Suite 1000
Silver Spring, MD 20910
301 589-3300
301 589-5175 Fax
E-mail: info@musictherapy.org
www.musictherapy.org

Certification

Certification Board for Music Therapists (CBMT)
506 East Lancaster Avenue, Suite 102
Downingtown, PA 19335
800 765-2268 or 610 269-8900
610 269-9232 Fax
E-mail: info@cbmt.org
www.cbmt.org

Program Accreditation

National Association of Schools of Music (NASM)
11250 Roger Bacon Drive, Suite 21
Reston, VA 20190
703 437-0700
703 437-6312
E-mail: info@arts-accredit.org
http://nasm.arts-accredit.org

Music Therapist

Alabama

University of Alabama
Music Therapy Prgm
School of Music
PO Box 870366
Tuscaloosa, AL 35487-0366
Prgm Dir: Carol A Prickett, PhD MT-BC
Tel: 205 348-1432   *Fax:* 205 348-1675
E-mail: cpricket@music.ua.edu

Arizona

Arizona State University
Music Therapy Prgm
School of Music
PO Box 870405
Tempe, AZ 85287-0405
Prgm Dir: Barbara Crowe, MM MT-BC
Tel: 480 965-7413   *Fax:* 480 965-2659
E-mail: Barbara.J.Crowe@asu.edu

California

California State University - Northridge
Music Therapy Prgm
18111 Nordhoff St
Northridge, CA 91330
Prgm Dir: Ronald Borczon, MM RMT-BC
Tel: 818 677-3174
E-mail: rborczon@csun.edu

Chapman University
Music Therapy Prgm
School of Music
One University Dr
Orange, CA 92866
http://www1.chapman.edu/music/
Prgm Dir: David W Luce, PhD MT-BC
Tel: 714 532-6032   *Fax:* 714 744-7671
E-mail: luce@chapman.edu

University of the Pacific
Music Therapy Prgm
Conservatory of Music
3601 Pacific Ave
Stockton, CA 95211
Prgm Dir: Therese M West, PhD MT-BC FAMI
Tel: 209 946-2419   *Fax:* 209 946-2770
E-mail: twest@pacific.edu

Colorado

Colorado State University
Music Therapy Prgm
School of the Arts
Department of Music, Theatre and Dance
Fort Collins, CO 80523-1178
www.colostate.edu
Prgm Dir: William Davis, PhD RMT
Tel: 970 491-5888   *Fax:* 970 491-7541
E-mail: william.davis@colostate.edu

District of Columbia

Howard University
Music Therapy Prgm
College of Arts and Sciences, Music Dept
6th and Fairmont St NW
Washington, DC 20059
Prgm Dir: Donna Washington, MCAT RMT-BC
Tel: 202 806-7136   *Fax:* 202 806-9673
E-mail: dwashington@howard.edu

Florida

University of Miami
Music Therapy Prgm
Frost School of Music
PO Box 248165
Coral Gables, FL 33124
Prgm Dir: Shannon de l'Etoile, PhD MT-BC
Tel: 305 284-3943   *Fax:* 305 284-3901
E-mail: sdel@miami.edu

Florida State University
Music Therapy Prgm
College of Music
Tallahassee, FL 32306-1180
Prgm Dir: Jayne M Standley, PhD MT-BC
Tel: 850 644-4565   *Fax:* 850 644-6100
E-mail: jstandle@mailer.fsu.edu

Georgia

University of Georgia
Music Therapy Prgm
School of Music
Fine Arts Bldg
Athens, GA 30602-3153
Prgm Dir: Roy Kennedy
Tel: 706 542-2801   *Fax:* 706 542-0276
E-mail: rkennedy@uga.edu

Georgia College & State University
Music Therapy Prgm
Campus Box 067
Milledgeville, GA 31061
http://musictherapy.gcsu.edu
Prgm Dir: Chesley S Mercado, EdD MT-BC
Tel: 478 445-2645   *Fax:* 478 445-2645
E-mail: chesley.mercado@gcsu.edu

Illinois

Western Illinois University
Music Therapy Prgm
Music Dept
Macomb, IL 61455
Prgm Dir: Bruce A Prueter, MS MT-BC
Tel: 309 298-1187   *Fax:* 309 298-1968
E-mail: BA-Prueter@wiu.edu

Illinois State University
Music Therapy Prgm
5660 School of Music
Normal, IL 61790-5660
Prgm Dir: Marie Di Giammarino, EdD MT-BC
Tel: 309 438-8198   *Fax:* 309 438-8318
E-mail: mdigiam@ilstu.edu

Indiana

University of Evansville
Music Therapy Prgm
Dept of Music
1800 Lincoln Ave
Evansville, IN 47722
http://music.evansville.edu
Prgm Dir: Mary Ellen Wylie, PhD MT-BC
Tel: 812 488-2754   *Fax:* 812 488-2101
E-mail: mw26@evansville.edu

Indiana Univ - Purdue Univ Ft Wayne
Music Therapy Prgm
2101 Coliseum Blvd E
Fort Wayne, IN 46805-1499
www.ipfw.edu/academics/programs/undergraduate/m/
    music-therapy/
Prgm Dir: Nancy Jackson, MMT MT-BC
Tel: 260 481-6716   *Fax:* 260 481-5422
E-mail: jacksonn@ipfw.edu

Indiana Univ-Purdue U-Indianapolis
Music Therapy Prgm
IU School of Music at IUPUI
535 W Michigan St, IT 379
Indianapolis, IN 46202
www.music.iupui.edu
Prgm Dir: Debra Burns, PhD MT-BC
Tel: 317 278-2014
E-mail: desburns@iupui.edu

St Mary of the Woods College
Music Therapy Prgm
Dept of Performing and Visual Arts
St Mary of the Woods, IN 47876
Prgm Dir: Tracy Richardson, MS MT BC
Tel: 812 535-5154   *Fax:* 812 535-5177
E-mail: trichard@smwc.edu

Iowa

University of Iowa
Music Therapy Prgm
School of Music
Voxman Music Bldg
Iowa City, IA 52242
Prgm Dir: Kate Gfeller, PhD RMT
Tel: 319 335-1657   *Fax:* 319 335-2637
E-mail: kay-gfeller@uiowa.edu

Wartburg College
Music Therapy Prgm
Music Department, 100 Wartburg Blvd
Waverly, IA 50677
Prgm Dir: Marjorie O'Konski, MME MT-BC
Tel: 319 352-8401   *Fax:* 319 352-8501
E-mail: marj.okonski@wartburg.edu

Kansas

University of Kansas
Music Therapy Prgm
Art, Music Ed and Music Therapy
311 Bailey Hall
Lawrence, KS 66045
Prgm Dir: Cynthia Colwell, PhD MT-BC
Tel: 785 864-4784   *Fax:* 785 864-9640
E-mail: ccolwell@ku.edu

Kentucky

University of Louisville
Music Therapy Prgm
School of Music
Louisville, KY 40292
www.louisville.edu/music/therapy
Prgm Dir: Barbara L Wheeler, PhD MT-BC
Tel: 502 852-2316   *Fax:* 502 852-0520
E-mail: barbara.wheeler@louisville.edu

Louisiana

Loyola University New Orleans
Music Therapy Prgm
College of Music
6363 St Charles Ave
New Orleans, LA 70118
Prgm Dir: Victoria Vega, MMT MT-BC
Tel: 504 865-2142   *Fax:* 504 865-2852
E-mail: vpvega@loyno.edu

Massachusetts

Berklee College of Music
Music Therapy Prgm
Chair, Music Therapy Dept
1140 Boylston St
Boston, MA 02215-3693
Prgm Dir: Suzanne B Hanser, EdD MT-BC
Tel: 617 747-2639   *Fax:* 617 747-2605
E-mail: shanser@berklee.edu

Lesley University
Music Therapy Prgm
Expressive Therapics Division
29 Everett St
Cambridge, MA 02138
www.lesley.edu
Prgm Dir: Michele Forinash, DA LMHC MT-BC
Tel: 617 349-8166   *Fax:* 617 349-8431
E-mail: mforinas@lesley.edu

Anna Maria College
Music Therapy Prgm
Dept of Music, Box 45
Paxton, MA 01612-1198
Prgm Dir: Lisa Summer, MCAT MT-BC
Tel: 508 849-3454
E-mail: lsummer@annamaria.edu

Michigan

Michigan State University
Music Therapy Prgm
School of Music
East Lansing, MI 48824-1043
Prgm Dir: Fredrick Tims, PhD MT BC
Tel: 517 432-2613   *Fax:* 517 432-2880
E-mail: tims@msu.edu

Western Michigan University
Music Therapy Prgm
School of Music
1903 W Michigan Ave
Kalamazoo, MI 49008-3834
www.wmich.edu/musictherapy
Prgm Dir: Brian Wilson, MM MT-BC
Tel: 269 387-4724   *Fax:* 269 387-1113
E-mail: brian.wilson@wmich.edu

Eastern Michigan University
Music Therapy Prgm
Dept of Music and Dance
N101 Alexander Bldg
Ypsilanti, MI 48197
Prgm Dir: Michael G McGuire, MM MT-BC
Tel: 734 487-0292   *Fax:* 734 487-6939
E-mail: michael.mcguire@emich.edu

Minnesota

Augsburg College
Music Therapy Prgm
2211 Riverside Ave
Minneapolis, MN 55454
Prgm Dir: Roberta Kagin, MME MT-BC
Tel: 612 330-1273   *Fax:* 612 330-1264
E-mail: kagin@augsburg.edu

University of Minnesota - Minneapolis
Music Therapy Prgm
School of Music
2106 4th St S
Minneapolis, MN 55455
Prgm Dir: Annie Heiderscheit, PhD MT-BC FAMI NMT
Tel: 612 624-7512
E-mail: heide007@umn.edu

Mississippi

Mississippi University for Women
Music Therapy Prgm
Department of Music and Theatre W-70
1100 College St
Columbus, MS 39701
Prgm Dir: Carmen Osburn, MA MT-BC
Tel: 662 241-7897
E-mail: cosburn@muw.edu

William Carey College
Music Therapy Prgm
498 Tuscan Ave
Hattiesburg, MS 39401
Prgm Dir: Paul D Cotton, PhD RMT
Tel: 601 318-6416   *Fax:* 601 582-6414
E-mail: paul.cotten@wmcarey.edu

Missouri

University of Missouri - Kansas City
Music Therapy Prgm
Conservatory of Music, 316 Grant Hall
4949 Cherry
Kansas City, MO 64110-2229
Prgm Dir: Robert Groene, PhD MT-BC
Tel: 816 235-2920   *Fax:* 816 235-5864
E-mail: groener@umkc.edu

Drury University
Music Therapy Prgm
900 N Benton Ave
Springfield, MO 65802
Prgm Dir: Michael Cassity, PhD MT-BC
Tel: 417 873-7370   *Fax:* 417 873-7898
E-mail: mcassity@drury.edu

Maryville University
Music Therapy Prgm
650 Maryville University Dr
St Louis, MO 63141
Prgm Dir: Cynthia A Briggs, MM PsyD MT-BC
Tel: 314 589-9441   *Fax:* 314 529-9039
E-mail: cbriggs@maryville.edu

New Jersey

Montclair State University
Music Therapy Prgm
Music Dept
Upper Montclair, NJ 07043
Prgm Dir: Karen Goodman, PhD MT-BC
Tel: 973 655-7583
E-mail: goodmank@mail.montclair.edu

New York

SUNY Fredonia
Music Therapy Prgm
School of Music
Mason Hall
Fredonia, NY 14063
www.fredonia.edu/som/musTherapy.asp
Prgm Dir: Joni Milgram-Luterman, PhD MT-BC LCAT
Tel: 716 673-4648   *Fax:* 716 673-3154
E-mail: joni.milgram-luterman@fredonia.edu

SUNY at New Paltz
Music Therapy Prgm
Music Dept
1 Hawk Dr
New Paltz, NY 12561
Prgm Dir: Mary Boyle, EdD LCAT MT-BC
Tel: 845 257-2709   *Fax:* 845 257-3121
E-mail: boylem@newpaltz.edu

New York University
Music Therapy Prgm
35 W 4th St
New York, NY 10012
Prgm Dir: Barbara Hesser, MA CMT
Tel: 212 998-5452
E-mail: barbara.hesser@nyu.edu

Nazareth College of Rochester
Music Therapy Prgm
4245 East Ave
Rochester, NY 14618
Prgm Dir: Bryan C Hunter, PhD MT-BC
Tel: 716 389-2702   *Fax:* 716 586-2452
E-mail: bhunter7@naz.edu

North Carolina

Appalachian State University
Music Therapy Prgm
Hayes School of Music
813 River St
Boone, NC 28608
www.music.appstate.edu
Prgm Dir: Cathy McKinney, PhD MT-BC FAMI LCAT
Tel: 828 262-6444   *Fax:* 828 262-6446
E-mail: mckinnych@appstate.edu

Queens University of Charlotte
Music Therapy Prgm
Music Dept
1900 Selwyn Ave
Charlotte, NC 28274-0001
Prgm Dir: Frances McClain, PhD MT-BC
Tel: 704 337-2570   *Fax:* 704 337-2356
E-mail: mcclainf@queens.edu

East Carolina University
Music Therapy Prgm
212 AJ Fletcher Music Center
Greenville, NC 27858
Prgm Dir: Barbara Cobb Memory, PhD RMT-BC
Tel: 252 328-6343
E-mail: memoryb@mail.ecu.edu

North Dakota

University of North Dakota
Music Therapy Prgm
3350 Campus Rd, Stop 7125
HFA Building, Rm 110
Grand Forks, ND 58202
www.undmusic.org
Prgm Dir: Therese Costes, MT-BC MA MSW
Tel: 701 777-2828
E-mail: therese_costes@und.nodak.edu

Ohio

Ohio University
Music Therapy Prgm
School of Music
440 Music Bldg
Athens, OH 45701
www.ohio.edu
Prgm Dir: Anita Louise Steele, MT
Tel: 740 593-4249   *Fax:* 740 593-1429
E-mail: steelea@ohio.edu

Baldwin-Wallace College
Music Therapy Prgm
Cleveland Consortium
275 Eastland Rd
Berea, OH 44017
Prgm Dir: Lalene Kay
Tel: 740 593-4249
E-mail: lkay@bw.edu

University of Dayton
Music Therapy Prgm
Music Dept
300 College Park Ave
Dayton, OH 45469-0290
Prgm Dir: Susan Gardstrom, PhD MT-BC
Tel: 937 229-3908   *Fax:* 937 229-3916
E-mail: SGardstrom@udayton.edu

College of Wooster
Cosponsor: Cleveland Music Therapy Consortium
Music Therapy Prgm
Dept of Music
Wooster, OH 44691
Prgm Dir: Lalene DyShere Kay, MM MT-BC
Tel: 330 263-2419
E-mail: lkay@wooster.edu

Oklahoma

Southwestern Oklahoma State University
Music Therapy Prgm
Music Therapy Division
100 Campus Dr
Weatherford, OK 73096
www.swosu.edu/music/therapy
Prgm Dir: ChihChen Sophia Lee, PhD MT-BC
Tel: 580 774-3218   *Fax:* 580 774-3714
E-mail: sophia.lee@swosu.edu

Ontario, Canada

University of Windsor
Music Therapy Prgm
School of Music
Windsor, ON N9B 3P4
www.uwindsor.ca/music
Prgm Dir: Sandia Curtis, PhD MT-BC MTA
Tel: 519 253-3000, Ext 2796   *Fax:* 519 971-3614
E-mail: scurtis@uwindsor.ca

Oregon

Marylhurst University
Music Therapy Prgm
17600 Pacific Hwy (Hwy 43)
Marylhurst, OR 97036-0261
Prgm Dir: Christine Korb, MM MT-BC
Tel: 800 634-9982, Ext 3361   *Fax:* 503 636-9526
E-mail: ckorb@marylhurst.edu

Pennsylvania

Elizabethtown College
Music Therapy Prgm
Dept of Fine and Performing Arts
One Alpha Dr
Elizabethtown, PA 17022-2298
Prgm Dir: Gene Ann Behrens, PhD MT-BC
Tel: 717 361-1991   *Fax:* 717 361-1187
E-mail: behrenga@etown.edu

Immaculata University
Music Therapy Prgm
Dept of Music
Box 703
Immaculata, PA 19345
Prgm Dir: Brian Abrams, PhD MT-BC LPC LCAT FAMI
Tel: 610 647-4400, Ext 3490   *Fax:* 610 251-1668
E-mail: babrams@immaculata.edu

Mansfield University
Music Therapy Prgm
Dept of Music
Mansfield, PA 16933
Prgm Dir: Ellen Timmerman, MA MT-BC
Tel: 570 662-4717, Ext 4717   *Fax:* 570 662-4114
E-mail: etimmerm@mnsfld.edu

Drexel University
Music Therapy Prgm
245 N 15th St, MS 905
Philadelphia, PA 19102-1192
Prgm Dir: Paul Nolan, MCAT LPC MT-BC
Tel: 215 762-6927   *Fax:* 215 762-6933
E-mail: paul.nolan@drexel.edu

Temple University
Music Therapy Prgm
Boyer College of Music and Dance 012-00
Philadelphia, PA 19122
www.temple.edu/musictherapy
Prgm Dir: Kenneth Bruscia, PhD MT-BC
Tel: 215 204-8314   *Fax:* 215 204-4957
E-mail: kbruscia@temple.edu

Duquesne University
Music Therapy Prgm
Mary Pappert School of Music
600 Forbes Ave
Pittsburgh, PA 15282
www.duq.edu
Prgm Dir: Donna Marie Beck, PhD FAMI MT-BC
Tel: 412 396-6080, Ext 6086   *Fax:* 412 396-5479
E-mail: beckd@duq.edu

Marywood University
Music Therapy Prgm
2300 Adams Ave
Scranton, PA 18509
Prgm Dir: Mariam Pfeifer, MA MT-BC
Tel: 717 348-6211, Ext 2527   *Fax:* 717 961-4768
E-mail: pfeifer@marywood.edu

Slippery Rock University of Pennsylvania
Music Therapy Prgm
SRU Dept of Music
Slippery Rock, PA 16057
Prgm Dir: Sue Shuttleworth, EdD MT-BC
Tel: 724 738-2447   *Fax:* 724 738-4469
E-mail: sue.shuttleworth@sru.edu

South Carolina

Charleston Southern University
Music Therapy Prgm
9200 University Blvd, PO Box 118087
Charleston, SC 29423-8087
www.csuniv.edu
Prgm Dir: April Malone, MM MT-BC
Tel: 843 863-7969   *Fax:* 843 863-7042
E-mail: amalone@csuniv.edu

Texas

West Texas A&M University
Music Therapy Prgm
Dept of Music
WTAMU Box 60879
Canyon, TX 79016-0001
Prgm Dir: Edward Kahler, PhD MT-BC
Tel: 806 651-2822   *Fax:* 806 651-2958
E-mail: ekahler@mail.wtamu.edu

Southern Methodist University
Music Therapy Prgm
Meadows School of the Arts
Div of Music Therapy
Dallas, TX 75275
Prgm Dir: Robert Krout, EdD MT-BC
Tel: 214 768-3175   *Fax:* 214 768-4669
E-mail: rkrout@smu.edu

Texas Woman's University
Music Therapy Prgm
PO Box 425768
TWU Station
Denton, TX 76204
Prgm Dir: Nancy Hadsell, PhD MT-BC
Tel: 940 898-2514   *Fax:* 940 898-2494
E-mail: nhadsell@twu.edu

Sam Houston State University
Music Therapy Prgm
School of Music, Box 2208, SHSU
Huntsville, TX 77341
Prgm Dir: Karen Miller, MM MT-BC NMT
Tel: 936 294-1376   *Fax:* 936 294-3765
E-mail: musictherapy@shsu.edu

University of the Incarnate Word
Music Therapy Prgm
4301 Broadway Ave
PO Box 65
San Antonio, TX 78209
Prgm Dir: Janice Dvorkin, DPsy ACMT
Tel: 210 829-3856   *Fax:* 210 829-3880
E-mail: dvorkin@uiwtx.edu

Utah

Utah State University
Music Therapy Prgm
4015 Old Main Hill, Department of Music
Logan, UT 84322
Prgm Dir: Maureen Hearns, MEd MT-BC
Tel: 435 797-3009   *Fax:* 435 797-1862
E-mail: mhearns@cc.usu.edu

Virginia

Radford University
Music Therapy Prgm
Dept of Music
Radford, VA 24142
Prgm Dir: James E Borling, MM MT-BC
Tel: 540 831-5177   *Fax:* 540 831-6133
E-mail: jborling@radford.edu

Shenandoah University
Music Therapy Prgm
1460 University Dr
Winchester, VA 22601-5195
Prgm Dir: Michael J Rohrbacher, PhD RMT-BC
Tel: 540 665-4560   *Fax:* 540 665-5402
E-mail: Mrohrbac@su.edu

Wisconsin

University of Wisconsin - Eau Claire
Music Therapy Prgm
Dept of Public Health Professions
College of Nursing and Health Sciences
Eau Claire, WI 54702-4004
Prgm Dir: Lee Anna Rasar, MT-BC WMTR NMT
Tel: 715 836-4260   *Fax:* 715 836-3952
E-mail: rasarla@uwec.edu

Alverno College
Music Therapy Prgm
3401 S 39th St, PO Box 3439222
Milwaukee, WI 53234-3922
www.alverno.edu
Prgm Dir: Diane Knight, MS MT-BC
Tel: 414 382-6135   *Fax:* 414 382-6954
E-mail: diane.knight@alverno.edu

Music Therapist

Programs*	Class Capacity	Begins	Length (months)	Award	Res. Tuition	Non-res. Tuition	Stipend	Offers:‡ 1	2	3	4
California											
Chapman University (Orange)	25	Sep Feb	54	Dipl, BM	$29,900	$0				•	
Colorado											
Colorado State University (Fort Collins)	100	Aug	38	BM, MM	$5,500	$15,000					
District of Columbia											
Howard University (Washington)	15	Aug	48	BMT	$12,172	$12,172					
Florida											
University of Miami (Coral Gables)	50	Aug	24, 54	BM, MM	$20,034	$20,034				•	
Georgia											
Georgia College & State University (Milledgeville)	50	Aug	54	BMT, MMT	$1,379	$2,815				•	
Indiana											
Indiana Univ - Purdue Univ Ft Wayne (Fort Wayne)	15	Aug	54	BS	$4,300	$9,800		•		•	
Indiana Univ-Purdue U-Indianapolis	12		36	MS				•			•
University of Evansville	40	Aug	54	BMMT	$26,000	$0				•	
Kentucky											
University of Louisville	28	Aug	54	BM	$6,940	$17,734				•	
Massachusetts											
Lesley University (Cambridge)	20	Sep	24	MA, PhD				•		•	•
Michigan											
Western Michigan University (Kalamazoo)	20	Sep	38	BM	$5,262	$13,248		•			
Mississippi											
Mississippi University for Women (Columbus)	25	Aug Jan		BM	$4,000	$9,000					
Missouri											
Drury University (Springfield)	27			BMT	$15,174	$15,174					
New York											
SUNY at New Paltz	30	Aug 23	54	BS, MS	$4,200	$8,400		•		•	
SUNY Fredonia		Aug	54	BS	$2,770	$5,900		•		•	
North Carolina											
Appalachian State University (Boone)	18	Aug Jan	54	BM, MMT	$4,416	$14,158				•	
Queens University of Charlotte	40	Aug	60	BM	$19,450	$0		•			
North Dakota											
University of North Dakota (Grand Forks)	25	Fall	48	BM	$5,792	$13,786				•	
Ohio											
Ohio University (Athens)	50	Sep	46, 24	Dipl, BM, MM	$15,840	$15,840				•	
Oklahoma											
Southwestern Oklahoma State University (Weatherford)	20	Aug	48	Cert, BM	$115	$265	$45,373			•	•
Ontario, Canada											
University of Windsor		Sep	6, 48	BA	$4,778	$12,687				•	
Pennsylvania											
Duquesne University (Pittsburgh)	15	Aug Jan	48	Dipl, Cert, BSMT	$17,223	$24,223		•		•	
Mansfield University	40	Aug Jan	54	BM	$5,178	$12,954					
Temple University (Philadelphia)	80	Sep Jan	54, 24	BMT, MMT	$6,200	$11,530		•		•	•
South Carolina											
Charleston Southern University		Aug Jan	54	BA	$17,620	$0					
Texas											
West Texas A&M University (Canyon)		Aug Jan May	54	Dipl, BMus						•	
Wisconsin											
Alverno College (Milwaukee)	45	Aug Jan	48	Dipl, Cert, BM	$8,000	$8,000					

*Data are shown only for programs that completed the 2007 AMA Survey of Health Professions Education Programs.
‡Key to Offers: 1: Evening or weekend classes; 2: Non-English instruction; 3: Cultural competence instruction; 4: Distance education component.

Nuclear medicine is the medical specialty that utilizes the nuclear properties of radioactive and stable nuclides to make diagnostic evaluations of the anatomic or physiologic conditions of the body and to provide therapy with unsealed radioactive sources. The skills of the nuclear medicine technologist complement those of the nuclear medicine physician and of other professionals in the field.

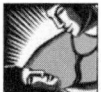

Career Description

Nuclear medicine technologists perform a number of tasks in the areas of patient care, technical skills, and administration. When caring for patients, they acquire adequate knowledge of the patients' medical histories to understand and relate to their illnesses and pending diagnostic procedures for therapy, instruct patients before and during procedures, evaluate the satisfactory preparation of patients before commencing a procedure, and recognize emergency patient conditions and initiate life-saving first aid when appropriate.

Nuclear medicine technologists apply their knowledge of radiation physics and safety regulations to limit radiation exposure, prepare and administer radiopharmaceuticals, use radiation detection devices and other kinds of laboratory equipment that measure the quantity and distribution of radionuclides deposited in the patient or in a patient specimen, perform in vivo and in vitro diagnostic procedures, use quality control techniques as part of a quality assurance program covering all procedures and products in the laboratory, and participate in research activities.

Administrative functions may include supervising other nuclear medicine technologists, students, laboratory assistants, and other personnel; participating in procuring supplies and equipment; documenting laboratory operations; participating in departmental inspections conducted by various licensing, regulatory, and accrediting agencies; and participating in scheduling patient examinations.

Employment Characteristics

Opportunities in nuclear medicine technology may be found in major medical centers, smaller hospitals, and independent imaging centers. Opportunities also are available for obtaining positions in clinical research, education, and administration.

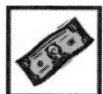

Salary

Salaries vary depending on the employer and geographic location. According to a 2007 survey from the American Society of Radiologic Technologists, the overall average salary is$69,083, although salaries vary by geographic location. Refer to Section IV, Table 5 of this *Directory* for more information, or see www.ama-assn.org/go/hpsalary.

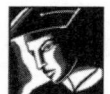

Educational Programs

Length. The professional portion of the programs is 1 to 2 years. Institutions offering accredited programs may provide an integrated educational sequence leading to an associate or baccalaureate degree over a period of 2 or 4 years.

Prerequisites. Applicants for admission must have graduated from high school or the equivalent and have acquired postsecondary competencies in human anatomy and physiology, physics, algebra, medical terminology, computer applications, oral and written communications, and general chemistry.

Curriculum. The curriculum includes:
- Patient care
- Statistics
- Nuclear medicine physics and radiation physics
- Radiation biology
- Radiation safety and protection
- Radionuclide chemistry and radiopharmacy
- Nuclear instrumentation
- Positron emission tomography (PET)
- Computer applications for nuclear medicine
- Diagnostic nuclear medicine imaging and nonimaging in vivo and in vitro procedures
- Immunology as related to nuclear medicine
- Radionuclide therapy
- Quality control and quality assurance

Inquiries

Careers/Curriculum
American Society of Radiologic Technologists
15000 Central Avenue SE
Albuquerque, NM 87123
www.asrt.org

Society of Nuclear Medicine—Technologist Section
1850 Samuel Morse Drive
Reston, VA 22090-5316
703 708-9000
www.snm.org

Certification/Registration
Nuclear Medicine Technology Certification Board
3558 Habersham at Northlake, Building I
Tucker, GA 30084
404 315-1739
www.nmtcb.org

American Registry of Radiologic Technologists
1255 Northland Drive
Mendota Heights, MN 55120
www.arrt.org

Program Accreditation
Joint Review Committee on Educational Programs in Nuclear Medicine Technology (JRCNMT)
2000 West Danforth Road, Suite 130, #203
Edmond, OK 73003
405 285-0546
405 285-0579 Fax
E-mail: jrcnmt@coxinet.net
www.jrcnmt.org

Nuclear Medicine Technologist

Alabama

University of Alabama at Birmingham
Nuclear Medicine Technology Prgm
RMSB 441
1530 Third Ave S
Birmingham, AL 35294-1212
www.uab.edu/NMTProgram
Prgm Dir: Norman Bolus, MPH CNMT
Tel: 205 934-4168 *Fax:* 205 975-7302
E-mail: bolusn@uab.edu

Arizona

GateWay Community College
Nuclear Medicine Technology Prgm
108 N 40th St
Phoenix, AZ 85034
www.gatewaycc.edu
Prgm Dir: Jeanne Dial, CNMT
Tel: 602 286-8512 *Fax:* 602 286-8480
E-mail: dial@gatewaycc.edu

Arkansas

Baptist Health Schools Little Rock
Nuclear Medicine Technology Prgm
11900 Colonel Glenn Rd, Ste 1000
Little Rock, AR 72210-2820
http://baptist-health.com
Prgm Dir: Sharon S Ward, MA CNMT RT(N) ASCP(N)
Tel: 501 202-7447 *Fax:* 501 202-7712
E-mail: sharon.ward@baptist-health.org

University of Arkansas for Medical Sciences
Nuclear Medicine Technology Prgm
4301 W Markham St #714
Little Rock, AR 72205
www.uams.edu/chrp/nuclearmedicine
Prgm Dir: Paul Thaxton, MAT CNMT ARRT(N)
Tel: 501 686-6848 *Fax:* 501 526-7975
E-mail: thaxtonpauld@uams.edu

California

VA Palo Alto Health Care System
Nuclear Medicine Technology Prgm
3801 Miranda Ave
Nuclear Medicine (115)
Palo Alto, CA 94304
www.palo-alto.med.va.gov/nucmed
Prgm Dir: Kent Hutchings, MS CNMT
Tel: 650 493-5000, Ext 64135 *Fax:* 650 849-1279
E-mail: kent.hutchings@med.va.gov

Kaiser Permanente Sch of Allied Hlth Sciences
Nuclear Medicine Technology Prgm
938 Marina Way S
Richmond, CA 94804
www.kpsahs.org
Prgm Dir: Linda Bogner, BS CNMT
Tel: 510 231-5053 *Fax:* 510 231-5001
E-mail: Linda.Bogner@kp.org

LA County Harbor UCLA Medical Center
Nuclear Medicine Technology Prgm
1000 W Carson St, Rm B-108
Torrance, CA 90509
Prgm Dir: Huyen Le Pham, BS CNMT
Tel: 310 222-2842 *Fax:* 310 328-7288
E-mail: hlepham@humc.edu

Connecticut

Gateway Community College
Nuclear Medicine Technology Prgm
88 Bassett Rd
North Haven, CT 06473
www.gwcc.commnet.edu/academics.aspx?id=258
Prgm Dir: Kathleen Murphy, MS CNMT ARRT(N) NCT
Tel: 203 285-2381 *Fax:* 203 285-2400
E-mail: kmurphy@gwcc.commnet.edu

Delaware

Delaware Technical & Community College - Wilmington
Nuclear Medicine Technology Prgm
333 Shipley St
Wilmington, DE 19801
www.dtcc.edu/wilmington/ah/
Prgm Dir: LaRay A Fox, MEd CNMT
Tel: 302 765-4590 *Fax:* 302 765-4599
E-mail: lfox@christianacare.org

Florida

Santa Fe Community College
Nuclear Medicine Technology Prgm
3000 NW 83rd St
Health Sciences West Bldg
Gainesville, FL 32606-6200
http://inst.sfcc.edu/~health/nucmed/
Prgm Dir: Stelio N Marchionno, BS RT(N) CNMT
Tel: 352 395-5673 *Fax:* 352 395-5711
E-mail: stelio.marchionno@sfcc.edu

St Vincent's Medical Center
Nuclear Medicine Technology Prgm
Medical Sciences Education Department
1800 Barrs St
Jacksonville, FL 32204
Prgm Dir: LeRoy Stecker, MBA RT(N) CNMT
Tel: 904 308-8484 *Fax:* 904 308-5109
E-mail: lstec001@stvincentshealth.com

Jackson Mem Medical Center
Nuclear Medicine Technology Prgm
1611 NW 12th Ave, Central Building #250
Miami, FL 33136
Prgm Dir: Sharon S Halula, BS CNMT
Tel: 305 585-6345 *Fax:* 305 585-8538
E-mail: shalula@jhsmiami.org

Florida Hospital College of Health Sciences
Nuclear Medicine Technology Prgm
671 Winyah Dr
Orlando, FL 32803
www.fhchs.edu
Prgm Dir: Joseph Hawkins, BS CNMT
Tel: 407 303-9380
E-mail: joe_hawkins@fhchs.edu

Hillsborough Community College
Nuclear Medicine Technology Prgm
PO Box 30030
Tampa, FL 33630-3030
www.hccfl.edu
Prgm Dir: Larry Gibson, RT(N) CNMT
Tel: 813 253-7418 *Fax:* 813 253-7491
E-mail: lgibson@hccfl.edu

Georgia

Medical College of Georgia
Nuclear Medicine Technology Prgm
Department of Biomedical and Radiological Technologies
987 St Sebastian Way
Augusta, GA 30912-0600
www.mcg.edu/SAH/brt/NMed.htm
Prgm Dir: Mary Anne Owen, MHE RT(N)
Tel: 706 721-3691 *Fax:* 706 721-8293
E-mail: mowen@mail.mcg.edu

Coosa Valley Technical College
Nuclear Medicine Technology Prgm
One Maurice Culberson Dr
Rome, GA 30161
www.coosavalleytech.edu
Prgm Dir: Karen Fluharty, CNMT RT(N) NCT
Tel: 706 295-6883 *Fax:* 706 295-6894
E-mail: kfluharty@coosavalleytech.edu

Armstrong Atlantic State University
Nuclear Medicine Technology Prgm
11935 Abercorn St
Savannah, GA 31419-1997
Prgm Dir: Rochelle Bornett Lee, MBA RT(N)
Tel: 912 920-6564 *Fax:* 912 921-5838
E-mail: rochelle.lee@armstrong.edu

Middle Georgia Technical College
Nuclear Medicine Technology Prgm
80 Cohen Walker Dr
Warner Robins, GA 31088
www.middlegatech.edu
Prgm Dir: Patricia Melnick, MEd BSRT(R) (M)
Tel: 478 988-6800, Ext 4047 *Fax:* 478 988-6875
E-mail: pmelnick@middlegatech.edu

Illinois

Northwestern Memorial Hospital
Nuclear Medicine Technology Prgm
Sch of Nuclear Med Tech, Galter 8th Fl, Rm 128
251 E Huron St
Chicago, IL 60611-2908
www.nmh.org/nmh/forhealthcareprofessionals/sdnmt.htm
Prgm Dir: Nancy McDonald, BS CNMT
Tel: 312 926-1777 *Fax:* 312 926-8118
E-mail: nmcdonal@nmh.org

College of DuPage
Nuclear Medicine Technology Prgm
425 Fawell Blvd
Glen Ellyn, IL 60137-6599
https://www.cod.edu
Prgm Dir: Joanne M Metler, MS CNMT PET
Tel: 630 942-3065 *Fax:* 630 858-5409
E-mail: metler@cod.edu

Edward Hines Jr VA Hospital
Nuclear Medicine Technology Prgm
Fifth Ave and Roosevelt Rd
Hines, IL 60141-5000
www.gammaquality.com/snmt
Prgm Dir: Gary Eastman, CNMT
Tel: 708 202-8387, Ext 21976 *Fax:* 708 202-2390
E-mail: gary.eastman@med.va.gov

Triton College
Nuclear Medicine Technology Prgm
2000 N Fifth Ave
River Grove, IL 60171-1995
Prgm Dir: Susan Campos, MEd BA CNMT
Tel: 708 456-0300, Ext 3655 *Fax:* 708 583-3336
E-mail: scampos2@triton.edu

Indiana

Indiana University
Nuclear Medicine Technology Prgm
School of Medicine
541 Clinical Dr CL-120
Indianapolis, IN 46202-5111
www.indyrad.iupui.edu/radweb
Prgm Dir: Judith Kosegi, MS RT(R)(N) CNMT
Tel: 317 274-7431   *Fax:* 317 274-4074
E-mail: jkosegi@iupui.edu

Iowa

Mercy College of Health Sciences
Nuclear Medicine Technology Prgm
928 6th Ave
Des Moines, IA 50309
Prgm Dir: Robert J Loch, BS CNMT
Tel: 515 643-6679
E-mail: rloch@mercydesmoines.org

University of Iowa Hospitals & Clinics
Nuclear Medicine Technology Prgm
Dept of Radiology
200 Hawkins Drive
Iowa City, IA 52242-1009
http://radiology.uiowa.edu/RadTech/
    NucMedTechProgram/NMTech1.htm
Prgm Dir: Anthony W Knight, MBA CNMT RT(N)
Tel: 319 356-2954   *Fax:* 319 384-6389
E-mail: anthony-knight@uiowa.edu

Kansas

University of Kansas Medical Center
Nuclear Medicine Technology Prgm
3901 Rainbow Blvd
Kansas City, KS 66160-7234
www.rad.kumc.edu/nucmed/
Prgm Dir: Tina R Crain, MS CNMT RT(R)(N)(QM)
Tel: 913 588-6858   *Fax:* 913 588-8393
E-mail: tcrain@kumc.edu

Kentucky

Jefferson Community and Technical College
Nuclear Medicine Technology Prgm
Allied Health Div
109 E Broadway
Louisville, KY 40202
Prgm Dir: Cybil Nielsen, MBA CNMT
Tel: 502 629-3683   *Fax:* 502 629-2088
E-mail: cnielsen0001@kctcs.edu

Louisiana

Delgado Community College
Nuclear Medicine Technology Prgm
615 City Park Ave
New Orleans, LA 70119-4399
Prgm Dir: Steve Trichell, BS RT(N)
Tel: 504 671-6232   *Fax:* 504 483-4609
E-mail: strich@dcc.edu

Maine

Central Maine Medical Center
Nuclear Medicine Technology Prgm
300 Main St
Lewiston, ME 04240-0305
www.cmmc.org
Prgm Dir: Heather D Poulin, BS CNMT RTNM CDT
Tel: 207 795-5956   *Fax:* 207 795-2476
E-mail: PoulinHe@cmhc.org

Maryland

Johns Hopkins Hospital
Nuclear Medicine Technology Prgm
600 N Wolfe St
Radiology Admin B-179
Baltimore, MD 21287-1010
www.jhmi.edu
Prgm Dir: Pamela Vorce, BS CNMT MBA
Tel: 410 528-8299   *Fax:* 410 528-8308
E-mail: pvorce1@jhmi.edu

Prince George's Community College
Nuclear Medicine Technology Prgm
301 Largo Rd
Lanham Hall 323
Largo, MD 20774-2199
Prgm Dir: Nancy Meman, BS CNMT RT(N)
Tel: 301 341-3026   *Fax:* 301 386-7528
E-mail: nmeman@pgcc.edu

Massachusetts

Mass College of Pharmacy & Health Sciences
Nuclear Medicine Technology Prgm
179 Longwood Ave
Boston, MA 02115-5896
www.mcphs.edu/MCPHSWeb
Prgm Dir: Frances K Keech, RT(N) MBA
Tel: 617 732-2928   *Fax:* 617 732-2075
E-mail: frances.keech@.mcphs.edu

Salem State College
Cosponsor: North Shore Medical Center, Salem
Nuclear Medicine Technology Prgm
352 Lafayette St
Salem, MA 01970-5353
Prgm Dir: T Ware, PhD
Tel: 978 542-6236   *Fax:* 978 542-6863
E-mail: tware@salemstate.edu

Springfield Technical Community College
Nuclear Medicine Technology Prgm
One Armory Sq
PO Box 9000
Springfield, MA 01102-9000
www.stcc.edu
Prgm Dir: Richard T Serino, MEd CNMT
Tel: 413 755-4871   *Fax:* 413 755-6312
E-mail: rserino@stcc.edu

UMass Memorial Medical Center
Cosponsor: Worcester State College
Nuclear Medicine Technology Prgm
55 Lake Ave N
Worcester, MA 01655-0243
www.umassmed.edu/nuclear_med/NMT
Prgm Dir: Peter H Simkin, MD
Tel: 508 856-4253   *Fax:* 508 856-6867
E-mail: simkinp@ummhc.org

Michigan

Ferris State University
Nuclear Medicine Technology Prgm
200 Ferris Dr/VFS 405A
Big Rapids, MI 49307-9989
Prgm Dir: Sheila MacEachron, CNMT
Tel: 231 591-2319   *Fax:* 231 591-3788
E-mail: maceacs@ferris.edu

William Beaumont Hospital
Nuclear Medicine Technology Prgm
3601 W 13 Mile Rd
Royal Oak, MI 48073-6769
Prgm Dir: Mary Premo, BA CNMT RT(N)
Tel: 248 898-4125   *Fax:* 248 898-0487
E-mail: mpremo@beaumont.edu

Minnesota

Mayo School of Health Sciences
Nuclear Medicine Technology Prgm
School of Health Sciences
200 First St SW
Rochester, MN 55905
http://mayo.edu/mshs
Prgm Dir: Nancy Hockert, BS CNMT
Tel: 507 284-3245   *Fax:* 507 284-2818
E-mail: hockert.nancy@mayo.edu

St Mary's University of Minnesota
Nuclear Medicine Technology Prgm
700 Terrace Hts #10
Winona, MN 55987
Prgm Dir: Jeanne Minnerath, PhD
Tel: 507 457-1770   *Fax:* 507 494-6035
E-mail: jminnera@smumn.edu

Mississippi

University of Mississippi Medical Center
Nuclear Medicine Technology Prgm
2500 N State St
Jackson, MS 39216-4505
Prgm Dir: John Vanderslice Jr, MS RT(R)(N) CNMT
Tel: 601 984-2585   *Fax:* 601 984-4986
E-mail: jvanderslice@radiology.umsmed.edu

Missouri

University of Missouri - Columbia
Nuclear Medicine Technology Prgm
605 Lewis Hall
Columbia, MO 65211-4230
www.umshp.org/shpsite/shp_home.htm
Prgm Dir: Glen Heggie, RTNMEdD FCAMRT
Tel: 573 884-7843   *Fax:* 573 884-1490
E-mail: heggieg@health.missouri.edu

Research Medical Center
Nuclear Medicine Technology Prgm
2316 E Meyer Blvd
Kansas City, MO 64132-1199
www.researchmedicalcenter.com
Prgm Dir: Charlotte Ament, MA BS CNMT
Tel: 816 276-4068   *Fax:* 816 276-3138
E-mail: Charlotte.Ament@hcamidwest.com

Saint Louis University
Nuclear Medicine Technology Prgm
Doisy College of Health Sciences
3437 Caroline St
St Louis, MO 63104-1395
Prgm Dir: William Hubble, MA CNMT RT (R)(N)(CT)
Tel: 314 577-8526   *Fax:* 314 577-8503
E-mail: hubblewl@slu.edu

Nebraska

University of Nebraska Medical Center
Nuclear Medicine Technology Prgm
984545 Nebraska Medical Center
Omaha, NE 68198-4545
www.unmc.edu/alliedhealth/rste
Prgm Dir: Marcia Hess Smith, BS CNMT
Tel: 402 559-7224   *Fax:* 402 559-4667
E-mail: mhesssmith@unmc.edu

Nevada

University of Nevada - Las Vegas
Nuclear Medicine Technology Prgm
4505 Maryland Pkwy, 3037
Las Vegas, NV 89154-3037
www.unlv.edu
Prgm Dir: Joanie MacDonald, MS RT(N)
Tel: 702 895-3136   *Fax:* 702 895-4819
E-mail: joan.macdonald@unlv.edu

New Jersey

Muhlenberg Regional Medical Center
Nuclear Medicine Technology Prgm
Park Ave and Randolph Rd
Harold B and Dorothy A Snyder Schools
Plainfield, NJ 07061
Prgm Dir: Maunesh C Soni, MS MHA CNMT
Tel: 908 668-2770   *Fax:* 908 226-4568
E-mail: msoni@solarishs.org

Univ of Medicine & Dent of New Jersey
Nuclear Medicine Technology Prgm
School of Health Related Professions
1776 Raritan Rd, Rm 538
Scotch Plains, NJ 07076
http://shrp.umdnj.edu/admissions/brochures_pdf/
   12066_nuclear.pdf
Prgm Dir: Michael Teters, MS RT(N) DABR
Tel: 908 889-2449   *Fax:* 908 889-2487
E-mail: tetersms@umdnj.edu

Gloucester County College
Nuclear Medicine Technology Prgm
1400 Tanyard Rd
Sewell, NJ 08080
Prgm Dir: Laura J Sharkey, BS CNMT
Tel: 856 415-2196   *Fax:* 856 464-8463
E-mail: lsharkey@gccnj.edu

New York

Bronx Community College
Nuclear Medicine Technology Prgm
University Ave and W 181st St
Bronx, NY 10453
Prgm Dir: Sherman Heller, PhD
Tel: 718 920-5012   *Fax:* 718 920-2629
E-mail: sheller@montefiore.org

University at Buffalo - SUNY
Nuclear Medicine Technology Prgm
105 Parker Hall, 3435 Main St
Buffalo, NY 14214-3007
www.buffalo.edu
Prgm Dir: Elpida S Crawford, MS CNMT
Tel: 716 838-5889, Ext 115   *Fax:* 716 838-4918
E-mail: esc@buffalo.edu

Institute of Allied Medical Professions
Nuclear Medicine Technology Prgm
405 Park Ave, Ste 501
New York, NY 10022-4405
Prgm Dir: John W Hart, CNMT RT(N)
Tel: 212 758-1410   *Fax:* 212 758-1424
E-mail: john.hart@msnyuhealth.org

St Vincent's Hospital Manhattan SVCMC
Nuclear Medicine Technology Prgm
170 West 12 St
New York, NY 10011
www.nucmedicine.com
Prgm Dir: Samy Sadek, PhD
Tel: 212 604-8716   *Fax:* 212 604-8714
E-mail: samy@nucmedicine.com

Molloy College
Nuclear Medicine Technology Prgm
1000 Hempstead Ave
PO Box 5002
Rockville Centre, NY 11571-5002
Prgm Dir: Marc Fischer, MBA CNMT ARRT
Tel: 516 678-5000, Ext 6887   *Fax:* 516 256-2252
E-mail: mfischer@molloy.edu

North Carolina

University of North Carolina Hospitals
Nuclear Medicine Technology Prgm
101 Manning Dr
CB 7510 Radiology-Nuclear Medcine
Chapel Hill, NC 27514
www.unchealthcare.org/site/nuclear_medicine
Prgm Dir: Gregory S Beavers, MBA CNMT RT(N)
Tel: 919 843-2963   *Fax:* 919 843-0591
E-mail: gbeavers@unch.unc.edu

Caldwell Comm College & Tech Institute
Nuclear Medicine Technology Prgm
2855 Hickory Blvd
Hudson, NC 28638-2397
www.cccti.edu
Prgm Dir: Jimmy L Council, RT(N) CNMT MBA
Tel: 828 726-2370   *Fax:* 828 726-2489
E-mail: jcouncil@cccti.edu

Forsyth Technical Community College
Nuclear Medicine Technology Prgm
2100 Silas Creek Pkwy
Winston-Salem, NC 27103
Prgm Dir: Donald G Harkness, MEd CNMT
Tel: 336 734-7187   *Fax:* 336 734-7444
E-mail: dharkness@forsyth.cc.nc.us

Ohio

Aultman Hospital
Nuclear Medicine Technology Prgm
2600 Sixth St SW
Canton, OH 44710-1799
www.aultman.com
Prgm Dir: Cheryl Beitzel, BS CNMT RT(N)
Tel: 330 363-2335   *Fax:* 330 580-6651
E-mail: cbeitzel@aultman.org

University of Cincinnati College of Allied Health Sciences
Nuclear Medicine Technology Prgm
Advanced Medical Imaging Technology Program
3202 Goodman St
Cincinnati, OH 45267
Prgm Dir: Alan Vespie, MEd CNMT RT(N)
Tel: 513 558-2018   *Fax:* 513 558-6002
E-mail: alan.vespie@uc.edu

Ohio State University Medical Center
Nuclear Medicine Technology Prgm
212 E Doan Hall
410 W 10th Ave
Columbus, OH 43210-1228
http://radiology.osu.edu/tech/nuc_med/
   nuc_tech_home.htm
Prgm Dir: Stacey R Copley, BS CNMT RT(N)
Tel: 614 293-3131   *Fax:* 614 293-2529
E-mail: stacey.copley@osumc.edu

University of Findlay
Nuclear Medicine Technology Prgm
Nuclear Medicine Institute
1000 N Main St
Findlay, OH 45840-3695
www.findlay.edu/academics/colleges/cohp
Prgm Dir: Richard States, MBA CNMT RT(N)
Tel: 419 434-5328   *Fax:* 419 434-4168
E-mail: states@findlay.edu

Cuyahoga Community College
Nuclear Medicine Technology Prgm
11000 Pleasant Valley Rd
Parma, OH 44130
www.tri-c.edu/NMED
Prgm Dir: David Frazee, MS CRA CNMT
Tel: 216 987-5298   *Fax:* 216 987-5066
E-mail: david.frazee@tri-c.edu

Kent State University - Salem Campus
Nuclear Medicine Technology Prgm
2491 State Route 45 S
Salem, OH 44460
www.salem.kent.edu
Prgm Dir: Janet Long, RT(RN) CNMT
Tel: 330 337-4261   *Fax:* 330 337-4122
E-mail: jlong1@kent.edu

St Elizabeth Health Center
Nuclear Medicine Technology Prgm
1044 Belmont Ave
Youngstown, OH 44501-1790
Prgm Dir: Richard M Blanco, RT(N) CNMT
Tel: 330 480-3266   *Fax:* 330 480-2624
E-mail: rick_blanco@hmis.org

Oklahoma

Univ of Oklahoma Health Sciences Center
Nuclear Medicine Technology Prgm
PO Box 26901
CHB-451
Oklahoma City, OK 73190-0901
Prgm Dir: Vesper Grantham, MEd CNMT RT(N)
Tel: 405 271-6477   *Fax:* 405 271-1424
E-mail: vesper-grantham@ouhsc.edu

Pennsylvania

Cedar Crest College
Nuclear Medicine Technology Prgm
100 College Dr
Allentown, PA 18104-6196
www.cedarcrest.edu
Prgm Dir: Brian S Misanko, PhD
Tel: 610 606-4611   *Fax:* 610 606-4616
E-mail: bsmisank@cedarcrest.edu

Lancaster Gen Coll of Nursing & Hlth Sciences
Nuclear Medicine Technology Prgm
410 N Lime St
Lancaster, PA 17602
www.LancasterGeneralCollege.edu
Prgm Dir: Penni A Longenecker, MEd CNMT RT(N)
Tel: 717 544-5668   *Fax:* 717 544-5970
E-mail: pelongen@lancastergeneralcollege.edu

Jameson Health System
Nuclear Medicine Technology Prgm
South Campus
1000 S Mercer St
New Castle, PA 16101
Prgm Dir: Robert Ondo, BS CNMT
Tel: 724 656-4123, Ext 4123   *Fax:* 724 656-4165
E-mail: rondo@jamesonhealth.org

Comm College of Allegheny County
Nuclear Medicine Technology Prgm
808 Ridge Ave
Pittsburgh, PA 15212-6097
Prgm Dir: Carl Mazzetti, BS CNMT
Tel: 412 237-2751   *Fax:* 412 237-4521
E-mail: cmazzett@ccac.edu

Wyoming Valley Health Care System
Nuclear Medicine Technology Prgm
575 N River St
Wilkes-Barre, PA 18764
Prgm Dir: Cindy Turchin, MBA RT(R)(N) CNMT
Tel: 570 552-1706   *Fax:* 570 552-1758
E-mail: cturchin@wvhcs.org

Abington Memorial Hospital
Nuclear Medicine Technology Prgm
2500 Maryland Rd, Ste 214
Willow Grove, PA 19090
www.amh.org
Prgm Dir: Nancy R Butterworth, MS RT(R)(N) CNMT
Tel: 215 481-5421   *Fax:* 215 481-5490
E-mail: nbutterworth@amh.org

Puerto Rico

University of Puerto Rico
Nuclear Medicine Technology Prgm
GPO Box 365067
San Juan, PR 00936-5067
http://cprsweb.rcm.upr.edu
Prgm Dir: Miriam Espada, MPH CNMT
Tel: 787 758-2525, Ext 4607 *Fax:* 787 764-1760
E-mail: miriamespada@cprs.rcm.upr.edu

Rhode Island

Rhode Island Hospital
Nuclear Medicine Technology Prgm
School of Nuclear Medicine Technology
3 Davol Square, Bldg A, Box 162
Providence, RI 02903
www.lifespan.org
Prgm Dir: Pamela C Maisano, ARRT (R) (N) CNMT
Tel: 401 528-8531, Ext 229 *Fax:* 401 457-0219
E-mail: pmaisano@lifespan.org

South Carolina

Midlands Technical College
Nuclear Medicine Technology Prgm
PO Box 2408
Columbia, SC 29202
Prgm Dir: Ray Wiegner, BSRT(R)(N)
Tel: 803 822-3483 *Fax:* 803 822-3417
E-mail: wiegnerr@midlandstech.edu

South Dakota

Southeast Technical Institute
Nuclear Medicine Technology Prgm
2320 Career Ave
Sioux Falls, SD 57107
www.southeasttech.com
Prgm Dir: Doug Warner, CNMT
Tel: 605 367-7625 *Fax:* 605 367-5724
E-mail: doug.warner@southeasttech.com

Tennessee

Chattanooga State Technical Comm College
Nuclear Medicine Technology Prgm
4501 Amnicola Hwy
Chattanooga, TN 37406-1097
www.chattanoogastate.edu/Allied_Health/nuclear.asp
Prgm Dir: Leesa Ross, MA CNMT PET RT(N)
Tel: 423 697-3331 *Fax:* 423 697-3324
E-mail: Leesa.Ross@ChattanoogaState.edu

South College
Nuclear Medicine Technology Prgm
3904 Lonas Dr
Knoxville, TN 37909
Prgm Dir: Lisa Satterfield, RT(R)(M)
Tel: 865 251-1887 *Fax:* 865 584-9816
E-mail: lsatterfield@southcollegetn.edu

Univ of Tennessee Medical Ctr at Knoxville
Nuclear Medicine Technology Prgm
Nuclear Medicine Department
Knoxville, TN 37920-6999
www.utmedicalcenter.org/radiology
Prgm Dir: Glenn Hathaway, BS CNMT
Tel: 865 305-9726 *Fax:* 865 305-9074
E-mail: ghathawa@utmck.edu

Baptist College of Health Sciences
Nuclear Medicine Technology Prgm
1003 Monroe Ave
Memphis, TN 38104
www.bchs.edu
Prgm Dir: Kathy Thompson Hunt, MS CNMT
Tel: 901 572-2642 *Fax:* 901 572-2750
E-mail: kathy.thompson@bchs.edu

Methodist University Hospital
Nuclear Medicine Technology Prgm
School of Nuclear Medicine Technology
1265 Union Ave
Memphis, TN 38104
http://methodisthealth.org
Prgm Dir: Nancy A Clifton, RT(R)(N)CNMT
Tel: 901 516-8521 *Fax:* 901 516-2870
E-mail: cliftonn@methodisthealth.org

Vanderbilt University Medical Center
Nuclear Medicine Technology Prgm
Rad Dept 21st and Garland
CCC-1124 MCN
Nashville, TN 37232-2675
www.mc.vanderbilt.edu/radiology
Prgm Dir: James A Patton, PhD
Tel: 615 322-0508 *Fax:* 615 322-3764
E-mail: jim.patton@vanderbilt.edu

Texas

Amarillo College
Nuclear Medicine Technology Prgm
PO Box 447
Amarillo, TX 79178
www.actx.edu
Prgm Dir: Mark Rowh, BS RT(R) CNMT
Tel: 806 354-6071 *Fax:* 806 354-6076
E-mail: rowh-me@actx.edu

Del Mar College
Nuclear Medicine Technology Prgm
101 Baldwin Blvd
Corpus Christi, TX 78404
Prgm Dir: Tonya Pigulski, CNMT
Tel: 361 698-2830 *Fax:* 361 698-2811
E-mail: tpigulski@delmar.edu

Baylor University Med Center
Nuclear Medicine Technology Prgm
3500 Gaston Ave
Dallas, TX 75246
www.baylorhealth.edu/RAHS
Prgm Dir: Amy J Hatch, BA CNMT RT(N)
Tel: 214 820-1420 *Fax:* 214 820-1421
E-mail: AmyHa@baylorhealth.edu

Galveston College
Nuclear Medicine Technology Prgm
4015 Ave Q
Galveston, TX 77550-2782
www.gc.edu
Prgm Dir: Bobby R Brown, BS CNMT
Tel: 409 944-1491 *Fax:* 409 944-1511
E-mail: bbrown@gc.edu

Houston Community College
Nuclear Medicine Technology Prgm
1900 Pressler
Houston, TX 77030
www.hccs.edu/discipline/nmtt/nmtt.html
Prgm Dir: Glenn Smith, BS CNMT NCT
Tel: 713 718-7354 *Fax:* 713 718-7608
E-mail: glenn.smith@hccs.edu

University of the Incarnate Word
Nuclear Medicine Technology Prgm
4301 Broadway St
San Antonio, TX 78209-6397
Prgm Dir: Norma Green, MBA RT(N)
Tel: 210 829-3991 *Fax:* 210 829-3174
E-mail: green@uiwtx.edu

Utah

University of Utah Health Science Center
Nuclear Medicine Technology Prgm
30 North 1900 East #1A971
Salt Lake City, UT 84132-2140
www.uuhsc.utah.edu/rad/nuctech.html
Prgm Dir: Delynn Strate, CNMT
Tel: 801 585-2326 *Fax:* 801 581-2403
E-mail: dstrate@hsc.utah.edu

Vermont

University of Vermont
Nuclear Medicine Technology Prgm
302 Rowell Bldg
Burlington, VT 05405
www.uvm.edu/cnhs
Prgm Dir: Louis M Izzo, MS CNMT
Tel: 802 656-3811 *Fax:* 802 656-2191
E-mail: louis.izzo@uvm.edu

Virginia

Old Dominion University
Nuclear Medicine Technology Prgm
2118 Technology Building
Norfolk, VA 23529-0287
http://hs.odu.edu/medlab/academics/nmed/
Prgm Dir: Scott R Sechrist, EdD CNMT ARRT(N)
Tel: 757 683-3589 *Fax:* 757 683-5028
E-mail: ssechris@odu.edu

Naval School of Health Sciences
Nuclear Medicine Technology Prgm
1001 Holcomb Rd
Portsmouth, VA 23708-5200
Prgm Dir: Edward Eck, BS CNMT RT(R)(QM)(CT)
Tel: 757 953-5050 *Fax:* 757 953-7380
E-mail: eeck@hsp.med.navy.mil

Virginia Commonwealth University
Nuclear Medicine Technology Prgm
701 W Grace St
Box 843057
Richmond, VA 23284-3057
www.sahp.vcu.edu/radsci
Prgm Dir: Mark Crosthwaite, MEd CNMT
Tel: 804 828-9104 *Fax:* 804 828-5778
E-mail: mhcrosthwaite@vcu.edu

Washington

Bellevue Community College
Nuclear Medicine Technology Prgm
3000 Landerholm Circle SE
Radiation and Imaging Sciences, B243
Bellevue, WA 98007-6484
www.bellevuecollege.edu/nucmed
Prgm Dir: Jennifer L Prekeges, MS CNMT
Tel: 425 564-2475 *Fax:* 425 564-4193
E-mail: jprekege@bcc.ctc.edu

West Virginia

West Virginia State Comm & Tech College
Nuclear Medicine Technology Prgm
PO Box 1000
221 Cole Complex
Institute, WV 25112-1000
www.wvstateu.edu
Prgm Dir: John Gaskins, RBA CNMT
Tel: 304 766-3202 *Fax:* 304 766-5243
E-mail: gaskinsj@wvsctc.edu

West Virginia University Hospitals

Nuclear Medicine Technology Prgm
Medical Ctr Dr, PO Box 8062
Morgantown, WV 26506-8062
Prgm Dir: Kelsie J Kittle, BS RT(R)(N) CNMT
Tel: 304 598-4000, Ext 73179   *Fax:* 304 598-4348
E-mail: kittlek@wvuh.com

Wheeling Jesuit University

Nuclear Medicine Technology Prgm
316 Washington Ave
Wheeling, WV 26003-6295
Prgm Dir: Robert George, PhD CNMT RT(N)
Tel: 304 243-2387   *Fax:* 304 243-2608
E-mail: rfgeorge@wju.edu

Wisconsin

Gundersen Lutheran Medical Foundation

Nuclear Medicine Technology Prgm
Gundersen Lutheran Medical Center
1900 South Ave C03-003
La Crosse, WI 54601
Prgm Dir: Robyn Loeffelholz, CNMT
Tel: 608 775-5074   *Fax:* 608 775-5973
E-mail: rrloeffe@gundluth.org
Notes: Currently inactive

St Joseph's Hospital

Cosponsor: University of Wisconsin - La Crosse
Nuclear Medicine Technology Prgm
611 St Joseph Ave
Marshfield, WI 54449
Prgm Dir: Carlyn M Johnson, BS CNMT
Tel: 715 387-7787   *Fax:* 715 387-7775
E-mail: johnsoca@stjosephs-marshfield.org

Aurora St Luke's Medical Center

Nuclear Medicine Technology Prgm
2900 W Oklahoma Ave
Milwaukee, WI 53201-2901
www.aurorahealthcare.org
Prgm Dir: Kerry Michell, BS CNMT
Tel: 414 649-6418   *Fax:* 414 649-5118
E-mail: kerry.michell@aurora.org

Froedtert Memorial Lutheran Hospital

Nuclear Medicine Technology Prgm
9200 W Wisconsin Ave
Milwaukee, WI 53226-3596
www.froedtert.com
Prgm Dir: Frank G Steffel, BS CNMT
Tel: 414 805-2071   *Fax:* 414 771-3460
E-mail: fsteffel@fmlh.edu

PROGRAMS

Nuclear Medicine Technologist

Programs*	Class Capacity	Begins	Length (months)	Award	Res. Tuition	Non-res. Tuition	Stipend	Offers:‡ 1	2	3	4
Alabama											
University of Alabama at Birmingham	15	Aug	16	Cert, BS	$9,280	$23,200				•	
Arizona											
GateWay Community College (Phoenix)	25	Aug	21, 18	Cert, AAS	$2,350	$10,500				•	
Arkansas											
Baptist Health Schools Little Rock	9	Jul	12	Cert	$4,590	$4,590				•	
University of Arkansas for Medical Sciences (Little Rock)	67	Aug	12	BS	$6,981	$16,029				•	•
California											
Kaiser Permanente Sch of Allied Hlth Sciences (Richmond)	40	Oct	18	Cert	$9,000	$9,000					
VA Palo Alto Health Care System	14	Jul	12	Cert						•	•
Connecticut											
Gateway Community College (North Haven)	31	Sep	22	Cert, AS	$3,728	$9,874				•	•
Delaware											
Delaware Technical & Community College - Wilmington	10	May	24	AAS	$3,104	$7,764		•			
Florida											
Florida Hospital College of Health Sciences (Orlando)	29	May Aug	15, 24	Cert, AS	$9,750	$9,750				•	
Hillsborough Community College (Tampa)	20	Aug	24	AAS	$2,480	$9,040				•	
Jackson Mem Medical Center (Miami)	12	Jul	15	Cert	$10,000	$10,000				•	
Santa Fe Community College (Gainesville)		Aug	22	Cert, AS	$6,394	$20,321				•	
St Vincent's Medical Center (Jacksonville)	8	Jan May Sep	12	Cert	$4,000	$4,000				•	
Georgia											
Armstrong Atlantic State University (Savannah)	10	Jun	24	BS	$2,734	$9,702					
Coosa Valley Technical College (Rome)	14	Sep	12	Cert	$1,888	$3,200					
Medical College of Georgia (Augusta)	31	Aug	12, 21	Cert, BS	$6,336	$22,920		•		•	
Middle Georgia Technical College (Warner Robins)	10	Staggered	12	Cert	$2,478	$4,956		•		•	
Illinois											
College of DuPage (Glen Ellyn)	22	Jun	15	Cert	$4,200	$10,250				•	•
Edward Hines Jr VA Hospital	8	Jul	12	Cert, BS							
Northwestern Memorial Hospital (Chicago)	12	Sep	12, 48	Cert, BS	$5,000	$5,000				•	
Indiana											
Indiana University (Indianapolis)	7	Jun	22	BS	$6,739	$19,797				•	
Iowa											
Mercy College of Health Sciences (Des Moines)	9	Aug	12	Cert	$19,350	$19,350					
University of Iowa Hospitals & Clinics (Iowa City)	10	Aug	12	Cert, BS	$6,720	$23,186				•	
Kansas											
University of Kansas Medical Center (Kansas City)	6	Sep	12	Cert	$3,600	$3,600					
Kentucky											
Jefferson Community and Technical College (Louisville)	16	Aug	21, 12	AS	$2,352	$7,056				•	
Louisiana											
Delgado Community College (New Orleans)	6	Aug	12	Cert	$2,230	$6,150				•	

*Data are shown only for programs that completed the 2007 AMA Survey of Health Professions Education Programs.
‡Key to Offers: 1: Evening or weekend classes; 2: Non-English instruction; 3: Cultural competence instruction; 4: Distance education component.

Programs*	Class Capacity	Begins	Length (months)	Award	Res. Tuition	Non-res. Tuition	Stipend	Offers:‡ 1	2	3	4
Maine											
Central Maine Medical Center (Lewiston)	7	Aug	12	Cert	$6,000	$6,000				•	
Maryland											
Johns Hopkins Hospital (Baltimore)	15	Jun	14	Cert	$6,750	$6,750				•	
Prince George's Community College (Largo)	13	Jan	18	Cert, AAS	$3,600	$8,400					
Massachusetts											
Mass College of Pharmacy & Health Sciences (Boston)	25	Sep	32, 20	BS	$31,000	$31,000				•	
Springfield Technical Community College	18	Sep	24	AS	$3,927	$10,892		•			•
UMass Memorial Medical Center (Worcester)	8	Jun	12, 48	Cert, BS	$5,079	$14,000				•	
Michigan											
Ferris State University (Big Rapids)	40	Aug	21, 39	AAS	$8,700	$15,900				•	
William Beaumont Hospital (Royal Oak)	10	Sep	14	Cert	$3,000	$3,000				•	
Minnesota											
Mayo School of Health Sciences (Rochester)	10	Sep	12	Cert, BA/BS	$6,500	$7,000					
St Mary's University of Minnesota (Winona)	8	Sep	48	Dipl, Cert, BA	$21,918	$21,918					
Mississippi											
University of Mississippi Medical Center (Jackson)	10	Jul	12	Cert							
Missouri											
Research Medical Center (Kansas City)	9	Sep	12	Cert	$3,600	$3,600				•	
Saint Louis University (St Louis)	12	Sep	12, 49	Cert, BS	$30,040	$30,040					
University of Missouri - Columbia	12	Aug	24	Cert, BHS	$8,170	$18,116				•	
Nebraska											
University of Nebraska Medical Center (Omaha)	12	Aug	21, 12	BS	$6,340	$18,820				•	
Nevada											
University of Nevada - Las Vegas	18	Aug	48	BS	$2,121	$7,117		•		•	
New Jersey											
Gloucester County College (Sewell)	24	Sep	21	AAS	$6,000	$8,044		•		•	
Muhlenberg Regional Medical Center (Plainfield)	17	Jan	12	Dipl, Cert, AS	$22,000	$22,000				•	
Univ of Medicine & Dent of New Jersey (Scotch Plains)	15	Sep	15	Dipl, Cert, BS	$10,000	$14,000				•	
New York											
Institute of Allied Medical Professions (New York)	27	Oct Apr	12	Cert	$30,000	$30,000		•		•	
Molloy College (Rockville Centre)	46	Sep	22	AAS	$16,000	$16,000					
St Vincent's Hospital Manhattan SVCMC (New York)	6	Oct	12	Cert	$12,000	$12,000					
University at Buffalo - SUNY	15	Aug	18	Dipl, BS	$6,129	$12,389				•	
North Carolina											
Caldwell Comm College & Tech Institute (Hudson)	15	Aug	21	AAS	$2,016	$11,196					
Forsyth Technical Community College (Winston-Salem)	12/	Aug Sep	20	AAS	$1,580	$8,780				•	
University of North Carolina Hospitals (Chapel Hill)	10	Aug	12	Cert							
Ohio											
Aultman Hospital (Canton)	6	Jul	12	Cert	$7,500	$7,500					
Cuyahoga Community College (Parma)	15	Aug	22	AAS	$5,890	$14,250		•		•	
Kent State University - Salem Campus	14	Aug	12	Dipl, BS	$7,911	$19,059					
Ohio State University Medical Center (Columbus)	10	Last wk of Jun	12	Cert	$6,000	$6,000				•	
St Elizabeth Health Center (Youngstown)	11	Jul	24	Cert	$6,000	$6,000					
University of Findlay	56	Aug Jan	12, 48	Cert, AS, BS	$14,550	$14,550				•	
Oklahoma											
Univ of Oklahoma Health Sciences Center (Oklahoma City)	11	Aug	48	BS	$8,200	$12,800				•	
Pennsylvania											
Abington Memorial Hospital (Willow Grove)	5	Sep	12	Cert	$9,000	$9,000				•	
Cedar Crest College (Allentown)	8	Jun	12, 48	Cert, BS	$11,920	$0		•			
Jameson Health System (New Castle)	2	Jul	12	Cert	$3,600	$3,600				•	
Lancaster Gen Coll of Nursing & Hlth Sciences	35	Aug	12	Cert	$14,000	$14,000				•	
Puerto Rico											
University of Puerto Rico (San Juan)	10	Aug	12	BS	$1,700	$3,200			•	•	
Rhode Island											
Rhode Island Hospital (Providence)	10	Jul	15	Cert	$6,500	$6,500				•	
South Carolina											
Midlands Technical College (Columbia)	30	Aug	12	Cert	$4,104	$12,312					
South Dakota											
Southeast Technical Institute (Sioux Falls)	41	Aug	24	AAS	$17,584	$17,584		•		•	
Tennessee											
Baptist College of Health Sciences (Memphis)	23	Sep	36	BHS	$10,070	$10,070		•		•	•
Chattanooga State Technical Comm College	26	Aug	12	Cert	$4,000	$13,000				•	
Methodist University Hospital (Memphis)	4-6	Aug	15	Cert	$4,500	$4,500					
Univ of Tennessee Medical Ctr at Knoxville	7	Aug	12	Cert, BS	$4,000	$4,000					

*Data are shown only for programs that completed the 2007 AMA Survey of Health Professions Education Programs.
‡Key to Offers: 1: Evening or weekend classes; 2: Non-English instruction; 3: Cultural competence instruction; 4: Distance education component.

Nuclear Medicine Technologist

Programs*	Class Capacity	Begins	Length (months)	Award	Res. Tuition	Non-res. Tuition	Stipend	Offers:‡ 1	2	3	4
Vanderbilt University Medical Center (Nashville)	8	Aug	12	Cert	$1,900	$0					
Texas											
Amarillo College	16	Aug	24	AAS	$1,750	$3,250				•	
Baylor University Med Center (Dallas)	9	Aug	20	Cert	$4,500	$4,500					
Del Mar College (Corpus Christi)	8	Aug	21	AS							
Galveston College	12	Aug	23	Dipl, AAS	$1,812	$2,867					•
Houston Community College	44	Aug	18, 24	Cert, AAS	$1,967	$4,631				•	
Utah											
University of Utah Health Science Center (Salt Lake City)	7	Jul	12	Cert	$4,000	$4,000				•	
Vermont											
University of Vermont (Burlington)	8	Sep	48	BS	$9,832	$24,816				•	
Virginia											
Naval School of Health Sciences (Portsmouth)	28	Jan Jul	12	Cert							
Old Dominion University (Norfolk)	12	Aug	22	BSNMT	$6,330	$17,550				•	
Virginia Commonwealth University (Richmond)	10	Aug	33	BS	$6,142	$18,680				•	
Washington											
Bellevue Community College	10	Sep	18	Assoc	$6,000	$6,000				•	•
West Virginia											
West Virginia State Comm & Tech College (Institute)	16	May	24	AAS	$2,766	$7,718		•		•	
West Virginia University Hospitals (Morgantown)	4	Jul	12	Cert	$2,000	$2,000					
Wheeling Jesuit University	25	Aug	48	BS	$21,000	$0		•	•	•	•
Wisconsin											
Aurora St Luke's Medical Center (Milwaukee)	7	Jun	12	BS	$3,600	$5,400					
Froedtert Memorial Lutheran Hospital (Milwaukee)	6	Sep	12	Cert, BS	$2,500	$2,500					
Gundersen Lutheran Medical Foundation (La Crosse)	2	Sep	12	Cert, BS	$7,555	$15,200				•	
St Joseph's Hospital (Marshfield)	6	Aug	12	Cert	$5,000	$12,000					

*Data are shown only for programs that completed the 2007 AMA Survey of Health Professions Education Programs.
‡Key to Offers: 1: Evening or weekend classes; 2: Non-English instruction; 3: Cultural competence instruction; 4: Distance education component.

PROGRAMS

Career Description

Nursing is the largest health care occupation, with 2.4 million Registered Nurses (RNs) in the nation's workforce. RNs provide a variety of essential care services that include treating patients, educating patients and the public about various medical conditions, and providing advice and emotional support to patients' family members. RNs record patients' medical histories and symptoms, help to perform diagnostic tests and analyze results, operate medical machinery, administer treatment and medications, and help with patient follow-up and rehabilitation. RNs teach patients and their families how to manage illness or injury, including post-treatment home care needs, diet and exercise programs, and self-administration of medication and physical therapy. Some RNs also are educated to provide grief counseling to family members of critically ill patients. RNs work to promote general health by educating the public on various warning signs and symptoms of disease and where to go for help. RNs also might run health screening or immunization clinics, blood drives, and public seminars on various conditions.

RNs can specialize in one or more patient care specialties. The most common specialties can be divided into roughly four categories—by work setting or type of treatment; disease, ailment, or condition; organ or body system type; or population. RNs may combine specialties from more than one area—for example, pediatric oncology or cardiac emergency—depending on personal interest and employer needs.

RNs may specialize by work setting or by type of care provided:
- *Ambulatory care nurses* treat patients with a variety of illnesses and injuries on an outpatient basis, either in physicians' offices or in clinics or through electronic telehealth media
- *Critical care nurses* work in critical or intensive care hospital units and provide care to patients with cardiovascular, respiratory, or pulmonary failure
- *Emergency or trauma, nurses* work in hospital emergency departments and treat patients with life-threatening conditions caused by accidents, heart attacks, and strokes
- *Holistic nurses* provide care such as acupuncture, massage and aroma therapy, and biofeedback, which are meant to treat patients' mental and spiritual health in addition to their physical health
- *Home health care nurses* provide at-home care for patients who are recovering from surgery, accidents, and childbirth
- *Hospice and palliative care nurses* provide care for, and help ease the pain of, terminally ill patients outside of hospitals
- *Infusion nurses* administer medications, fluids, and blood to patients through injections into patients' veins
- *Long- term care nurses* provide medical services on a recurring basis to patients with chronic physical or mental disorders
- *Medical-surgical nurses* provide basic medical care to a variety of patients in all health settings
- *Occupational health nurses* provide treatment for job-related injuries and illnesses and help employers to detect workplace hazards and implement health and safety standards
- *Perianesthesia nurses* provide preoperative and postoperative care to patients undergoing anesthesia during surgery
- *Perioperative nurses* assist surgeons by selecting and handling instruments, controlling bleeding, and suturing incisions
- *Psychiatric nurses* treat patients with personality and mood disorders
- *Radiologic nurses* provide care to patients undergoing diagnostic radiation procedures such as ultrasounds and magnetic resonance imaging
- *Rehabilitation nurses* care for patients with temporary and permanent disabilities
- *Transplant nurses* care for both transplant recipients and living donors and monitor signs of organ rejection

RNs specializing in a particular disease, ailment, or condition are employed in virtually all work settings, including hospitals, physicians' offices, outpatient treatment facilities, home health care agencies, and private practices. These specialties include:
- Addictions
- Developmental disabilities
- Diabetes management
- Genetics
- HIV/AIDS
- Oncology
- Wound, ostomy, and continence

RNs specializing in treatment of a particular organ or body system usually are employed in specialty physicians' offices or outpatient care facilities, although some are employed in hospital specialty or critical care units. These specialties include:
- Cardiology and vascular medicine
- Dermatology
- Gastroenterology
- Gynecology
- Nephrology
- Neuroscience
- Ophthalmology
- Orthopedics
- Otorhinolaryngology
- Respiratory disorders
- Urology

Finally, RNs may specialize by providing preventive and acute care in all health care settings to various segments of the population, including newborns (neonatology), children and adolescents (pediatrics), adults, and the elderly (gerontology or geriatrics). RNs also may provide basic health care to patients in correctional facilities, schools, summer camps, and the military.

Most RNs work as staff nurses, providing critical health care services along with physicians, surgeons, and other health care practitioners. Some RNs, however, choose to become advanced practice nurses, who often are considered primary health care practitioners and work independently or in collaboration with physicians. These would include:
- Clinical nurse specialists
- Nurse anesthetists
- Nurse midwives
- Nurse practitioners

Some nurses pursue careers that require little or no direct patient contact, although most of these positions still require an active RN license:
- Case managers
- Forensics nurses

- Infection control nurses
- Legal nurse consultants
- Nurse administrators
- Nurse educators
- Nurse informaticists

RNs also may work as health care consultants, public policy advisors, pharmaceutical and medical supply researchers and salespersons, and medical writers and editors.

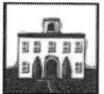

Employment Characteristics

Most RNs work in well-lighted, comfortable health care facilities. Home health and public health nurses travel to patients' homes, schools, community centers, and other sites. RNs may spend considerable time walking and standing. Patients in hospitals and nursing care facilities require 24-hour care; consequently, nurses in these institutions may work nights, weekends, and holidays. RNs also may be on call—available to work on short notice. Nurses who work in office settings are more likely to work regular business hours. About 23 percent of RNs worked part time in 2004, and 7 percent held more than one job.

Nursing has its hazards, especially in hospitals, nursing care facilities, and clinics, where nurses may care for individuals with infectious diseases. RNs must observe rigid, standardized guidelines to guard against disease and other dangers, such as those posed by radiation, accidental needle sticks, chemicals used to sterilize instruments, and anesthetics. In addition, they are vulnerable to back injury when moving patients, shocks from electrical equipment, and hazards posed by compressed gases. RNs who work with critically ill patients also may suffer emotional strain from observing patient suffering and from close personal contact with patients' families.

About three out of five nursing jobs in 2004 were in hospitals, in inpatient and outpatient departments. Other nurses worked in physicians' offices, nursing care facilities, home health care services, employment services, government agencies, and outpatient care centers. The remainder worked mostly in social assistance agencies and educational services, both public and private.

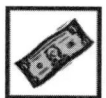

Salary

Median annual earnings of registered nurses were $52,330 in May 2004. The middle 50 percent earned between $43,370 and $63,360. The lowest 10 percent earned less than $37,300, and the highest 10 percent earned more than $74,760. Median annual earnings in the industries employing the largest numbers of registered nurses in May 2004 were as follows:

- Employment services $63,170
- General medical and surgical hospitals $53,450
- Home health care services $48,990
- Offices of physicians $48,250
- Nursing care facilities $48,220

Many employers offer flexible work schedules, child care, educational benefits, and bonuses. Advanced practice nurses and those holding positions requiring master's or doctoral preparation often earn annual salaries exceeding $100,000.

For more information on RN salaries, see www.ama-assn.org/go/hpsalary.

Employment Outlook

Job opportunities for RNs in all specialties are expected to be excellent. Employment of registered nurses is expected to grow much faster than average for all occupations through 2014, and, because the occupation is very large, many new jobs will result. In fact, registered nurses are projected to create the second largest number of new jobs among all occupations. Thousands of job openings also will result from the need to replace experienced nurses who leave the occupation through retirement, especially as the median age of the registered nurse population continues to rise.

Much faster-than-average growth will be driven by technological advances in patient care, which permit a greater number of health problems to be treated, and by an increasing emphasis on preventive care. In addition, the number of older people, who are much more likely than younger people to need nursing care, is projected to grow rapidly.

Employers in some parts of the country and in certain employment settings are reporting difficulty in attracting and retaining an adequate number of RNs, primarily because of an aging RN workforce and a lack of younger workers to fill positions. Enrollments in nursing programs at all levels have increased more rapidly in the past couple of years as students seek jobs with stable employment. Many qualified applicants are being turned away, however, because of a shortage of nursing faculty to teach classes. The need for nursing faculty will only increase as more instructors near retirement. Many employers also are relying on foreign-educated nurses to fill open positions.

Even though employment opportunities for all nursing specialties are expected to be excellent, they can vary by employment setting. For example, employment is expected to grow more slowly in hospitals—which comprise health care's largest industry—than in most other health care settings. While the intensity of nursing care is likely to increase, requiring more nurses per patient, the number of inpatients (those who remain in the hospital for more than 24 hours) is not likely to grow significantly. Patients are being discharged earlier, and more procedures are being done on an outpatient basis, both inside and outside hospitals. Rapid growth is expected in hospital outpatient facilities, such as those providing same-day surgery, rehabilitation, and chemotherapy.

Despite the slower employment growth in hospitals, job opportunities should still be excellent because of the relatively high turnover of hospital nurses. RNs working in hospitals frequently work overtime and night and weekend shifts and also treat seriously ill and injured patients, all of which can contribute to stress and burnout. Hospital departments in which these working conditions occur most frequently—critical care units, emergency departments, and operating rooms—generally will have more job openings than other departments.

To attract and retain qualified nurses, hospitals may offer signing bonuses, family-friendly work schedules, or subsidized training. In addition, a growing number of hospitals are experimenting with voluntary online bidding to fill open shifts, at premium wages. This can decrease the amount of mandatory overtime that nurses are required to work.

More and more sophisticated procedures, once performed only in hospitals, are being performed in physicians' offices and in outpatient care centers, such as freestanding ambulatory surgical and emergency centers. Accordingly, employment is expected to grow much faster than average in these places as health care in general expands. However, RNs may face greater competition for these positions because they generally offer regular working hours and more comfortable working environments.

Employment in nursing care facilities is expected to grow faster than average because of increases in the number of elderly, many of whom require long-term care. In addition, the financial pressure on hospitals to discharge patients as soon as possible should produce more admissions to nursing care facilities. Job growth also is expected in units that provide specialized long-term rehabilitation for stroke and head injury patients, as well as units that treat Alzheimer's victims.

Employment in home health care is expected to increase rapidly in response to the growing number of older persons with functional disabilities, consumer preference for care in the home, and technological advances that make it possible to bring increasingly complex treatments into the home. The type of care demanded will require nurses who are able to perform complex procedures.

Generally, RNs with at least a bachelor's degree will have better job prospects than those without a bachelor's. In addition, all four advanced practice specialties—clinical nurse specialists, nurse practitioners, midwives, and anesthetists—will be in high demand, particularly in medically underserved areas such as inner cities and rural areas. Relative to physicians, these RNs increasingly serve as lower-cost primary care providers.

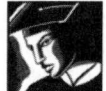

Educational Programs

Award, Length. The three major educational paths to registered nursing are 1) a bachelor's of science degree in nursing (BSN), 2) an associate degree in nursing (ADN), and 3) a diploma. BSN programs, offered by colleges and universities, take about 4 years to complete, ADN programs, offered by community and junior colleges, take about 2 to 3 years to complete, and diploma programs, administered in hospitals, last about 3 years.

Many RNs with an ADN or diploma later enter bachelor's programs to prepare for a broader scope of nursing practice, through an RN-to-BSN program. Similarly, accelerated master's degree programs in nursing also are available. These RN-to-MSN programs combine 1 year of an accelerated BSN program with 2 years of graduate study. In addition, accelerated BSN programs, lasting 12 to 18 months, are available for individuals who have a bachelor's or higher degree in another field and who are interested in moving quickly into nursing.

A bachelor's degree often is necessary for advanced clinical and administrative positions and is a prerequisite for admission to graduate nursing programs in research, consulting, and teaching, and all four advanced practice nursing specialties—clinical nurse specialists, nurse anesthetists, nurse midwives, and nurse practitioners. Individuals who complete a bachelor's receive more education in areas such as communication, leadership, and critical thinking, all of which are becoming more important as nursing care becomes more complex. Additionally, bachelor's degree programs offer more clinical experience in nonhospital settings.

Prerequisites. High school students considering a nursing career should take science, mathematics, and communications courses. Nurses should be caring, sympathetic, responsible, and detail oriented. They must be able to direct or supervise others, correctly assess patients' conditions, and determine when consultation is required. They need emotional stability to cope with human suffering, emergencies, and other stresses.

Curriculum. All nursing education programs include classroom instruction and supervised clinical experience in hospitals and other health care facilities. Students take courses in anatomy, physiology, microbiology, chemistry, nutrition, psychology and other behavioral sciences, and nursing. Coursework also includes the liberal arts for ADN and BSN students.

Supervised clinical experience is provided in hospital departments such as pediatrics, psychiatry, maternity, and surgery. A growing number of programs include clinical experience in nursing care facilities, public health departments, home health agencies, and ambulatory clinics.

Advanced Training. All four advanced practice nursing specialties currently require at least a master's degree, and the profession is moving toward doctoral preparation for these roles. Most programs last about 2 years and require a BSN degree for admission; some programs require at least 1 to 2 years of clinical experience as an RN. Upon completion of a program, most advanced practice nurses become nationally certified in their area of specialty. In some states, certification in a specialty is required in order to practice that specialty.

Licensure, Certification, Registration

In all states and the District of Columbia, students must graduate from an approved nursing program and pass a national licensing examination, known as the National Council Licensure Examination (NCLEX-RN), to obtain a nursing license. Nurses may be licensed in more than one state, either by examination or by the endorsement of a license issued by another state. Currently 22 states participate in the Nurse Licensure Compact Agreement, which allows nurses to practice in member states without recertifying. All states require periodic renewal of licenses, which may involve continuing education.

Inquiries

Education, Careers, Resources
American Association of Colleges of Nursing
One Dupont Circle NW, Suite 530
Washington, DC 20036
www.aacn.nche.edu

American Nurses Association
8515 Georgia Avenue, Suite 400
Silver Spring, MD 20910
www.nursingworld.org

National League for Nursing
61 Broadway
New York, NY 10006
www.nln.org

Licensure
National Council of State Boards of Nursing
111 East Wacker Drive, Suite 2900
Chicago, IL 60611
www.ncsbn.org

Program Accreditation
(*Note:* The programs listed in this Directory are those accredited at the baccalaureate level by the following organization.)

Commission on Collegiate Nursing Education
American Association of Colleges of Nursing
One Dupont Circle NW, Suite 530
Washington, DC 20036
www.aacn.nche.edu

National League for Nursing Accrediting Commission
61 Broadway
New York, NY 10006
www.nlnac.org

Note: Adapted in part from the Bureau of Labor Statistics, U.S. Department of Labor, *Occupational Outlook Handbook*, 2006-07 Edition, Registered Nurses, on the Internet at www.bls.gov/oco/ocos083.htm (visited October 10, 2007).

Nurse

Alabama

Auburn University
Nursing Prgm
Auburn University, AL 36849
www.nursing.auburn.edu

Samford University
Nursing Prgm
Birmingham, AL 35229
www.samford.edu

University of Alabama at Birmingham
Nursing Prgm
Birmingham, AL 35294
www.uab.edu

University of North Alabama
Nursing Prgm
College of Nursing and Allied Health
Florence, AL 35632

Univ of Alabama at Birmingham - Huntsville
Nursing Prgm
Huntsville, AL 35899
onlinenurse.nb.uah.edu

Jacksonville State University
Nursing Prgm
Jacksonville, AL 36265
www.jsu.edu/depart/nursing

Spring Hill College
Nursing Prgm
Division of Nursing
Mobile, AL 36608

University of Mobile
Nursing Prgm
Mobile, AL 36613
www.umobile.edu

University of South Alabama
Nursing Prgm
Mobile, AL 36688
www.usouthal.edu

Auburn University Montgomery
Nursing Prgm
Montgomery, AL 36124
www.aum.edu

University of Alabama
Nursing Prgm
Tuscaloosa, AL 35487
www.ua.edu

Arizona

Northern Arizona University
Nursing Prgm
Flagstaff, AZ 86011
www.nau.edu/~hp/dept/nurse

Arizona State University
Nursing Prgm
Phoenix, AZ 85004
www.asu.edu

Grand Canyon University
Nursing Prgm
Phoenix, AZ 85017
www.gcu.edu/scon

University of Phoenix
Nursing Prgm
Phoenix, AZ 85040
www.universityof phoenix-online.com

Phoenix College
Nursing Prgm
Tucson, AZ 85721
www.nursing.arizona.edu

Arkansas

Henderson State University
Nursing Prgm
Arkadelphia, AR 71999
www.hsu.edu

University of Central Arkansas
Nursing Prgm
Conway, AR 72035
www.uca.edu/chas/nursing.html

University of Arkansas
Nursing Prgm
Fayetteville, AR 72701
nurs.uark.edu

University of Arkansas for Medical Sciences
Nursing Prgm
Little Rock, AR 72701
nursing.uams.edu

California

Humboldt State University
Nursing Prgm
Arcata, CA 95521
www.humboldt.edu

Azusa Pacific University
Nursing Prgm
Azusa, CA 91702
www.apu.edu

California State University - Bakersfield
Nursing Prgm
Department of Nursing
Bakersfield, CA 93311

California State University - Dominguez Hills
Nursing Prgm
Carson, CA 90747
www.csudh.edu

California State University - Chico
Nursing Prgm
Chico, CA 95929
www.csuchico.edu/nurs

California State University - Fresno
Nursing Prgm
Fresno, CA 93740
www.csufresno.edu/nursing

California State University - Fullerton
Nursing Prgm
Fullerton, CA 92834
http://nursing.fullerton.edu

National University
Nursing Prgm
Department of Nursing
La Jolla, CA 92037

Loma Linda University
Nursing Prgm
Loma Linda, CA 92350
www.llu.edu

California State University - Long Beach
Nursing Prgm
Long Beach, CA 90840
www.csulb.edu/~nursing

Mount St Mary's College
Nursing Prgm
Los Angeles, CA 90049
www.msmc.la.edu

University of California - Los Angeles
Nursing Prgm
Los Angeles, CA 90095
www.nursing.ucla.edu

California State University - Northridge
Nursing Prgm
Northridge, CA 91330
www.csun.edu

Holy Names University
Nursing Prgm
Department of Nursing
Oakland, CA 94619

Samuel Merritt College
Nursing Prgm
Oakland, CA 94609
www.samuelmerritt.edu

California State University - Sacramento
Nursing Prgm
Sacramento, CA 95819
www.hhs.csus.edu/NRS

California State University - San Bernardino
Nursing Prgm
San Bernardino, CA 92407
www.csusb.edu

Point Loma Nazarene University
Nursing Prgm
San Diego, CA 92106
www.ptloma.edu/nursing

San Diego State University
Nursing Prgm
San Diego, CA 92182
www.sdsu.edu

Univ of California San Diego Med Ctr
Nursing Prgm
San Diego, CA 92110
www.acusd.edu

San Francisco State University
Nursing Prgm
San Francisco, CA 94132
www.nursing.sfsu.edu

University of California - San Francisco
Nursing Prgm
San Francisco, CA 94117
www.usfca.edu/nursing

San Jose State University
Nursing Prgm
San Jose, CA 95192
www.sjsu.edu/nursing

Dominican University of California
Nursing Prgm
San Rafael, CA 94901
www.dominican.edu

California State University - Stanislaus
Nursing Prgm
Turlock, CA 95382

Colorado

Adams State College
Nursing Prgm
Alamosa, CO 81102
www2.adams.edu/academics/bs-nursing/bs-nursing.php

University of Colorado at Colorado Springs
Nursing Prgm
Colorado Springs, CO 80917
www.web.uccs.edu/bethel

Regis University
Nursing Prgm
Denver, CO 80221
www.regis.edu

University of Colorado at Denver
Nursing Prgm
Denver, CO 80262
www2.uchsc.edu/son

Mesa State College
Nursing Prgm
Grand Junction, CO 81501
www.mesastate.edu

University of Northern Colorado
Nursing Prgm
Greeley, CO 80639
www.univnorthco.edu/nurses/son.html

Connecticut

Western Connecticut State University
Nursing Prgm
Danbury, CT 06810
wcsu.edu

Fairfield University
Nursing Prgm
Fairfield, CT 06824
www.fairfield.edu

Sacred Heart University
Nursing Prgm
Fairfield, CT 06825
www.sacredheart.edu

Central Connecticut State University
Nursing Prgm
Department of Nursing
New Britain, CT 06050

Southern Connecticut State University
Nursing Prgm
New Haven, CT 06515
www.scsu.ctstateu.edu

Southern Connecticut State University
Nursing Prgm
Storrs, CT 06269
www.nursing.uconn.edu

Saint Joseph College
Nursing Prgm
West Hartford, CT 06117
www.sjc.edu

University of Hartford
Nursing Prgm
West Hartford, CT 06117
www.hartford.edu

Delaware

Delaware State University
Nursing Prgm
Dover, DE 19901
www.desu.edu/colleges/chpp/nursing

Wilmington College
Nursing Prgm
New Castle, DE 19720
www.wilmcoll.edu

University of Delaware
Nursing Prgm
Newark, DE 19716
www.udel.edu/health

District of Columbia

Catholic University of America
Nursing Prgm
Washington, DC 20065
http://nursing.cua.edu

Georgetown University Medical Center
Nursing Prgm
Washington, DC 20057
www.georgetown.edu

Howard University
Nursing Prgm
Washington, DC 20059
www.cpnahs.howard.edu

Florida

Florida Atlantic University
Nursing Prgm
Boca Raton, FL 33431
www.fau.edu/nursing

University of Miami
Nursing Prgm
Coral Gables, FL 33146
www.miami.edu/nur

Nova Southeastern University
Nursing Prgm
Fort Lauderdale, FL 33328
www.nova.edu/nursing

Florida Gulf Coast University
Nursing Prgm
Fort Myers, FL 33965
www.fgcu.edu/chp/nursing

University of Florida
Nursing Prgm
Gainesville, FL 32610
www.nursing.ufl.edu

Jacksonville University
Nursing Prgm
School of Nursing
Jacksonville, FL 32211

University of North Florida
Nursing Prgm
Jacksonville, FL 32224
www.unf.edu/coh

Florida Southern College
Nursing Prgm
Lakeland, FL 33801
www.flsouthern.edu

Barry University
Nursing Prgm
Miami Shores, FL 33161
www.barry.edu/nursing

University of Central Florida
Nursing Prgm
Orlando, FL 32816
www.cohpa.ucf.edu/nursing

University of West Florida
Nursing Prgm
Pensacola, FL 32514
www.uwf.edu/nursing

St Petersburg College
Nursing Prgm
Pinellas Park, FL 33781
www.spcollege.edu

Florida State University
Nursing Prgm
Tallahassee, FL 32306
www.fsu.edu

University of South Florida
Nursing Prgm
Tampa, FL 33612
http://hsc.usf.edu/

Palm Beach Atlantic University
Nursing Prgm
West Palm Beach, FL 33416
www.pba.edu

South University
Nursing Prgm
West Palm Beach, FL 33409
www.southuniversity.edu

Georgia

Emory University
Nursing Prgm
Atlanta, GA 30322
www.nursing.emory.edu

Georgia State University
Nursing Prgm
Atlanta, GA 30303
www.gsu.edu

Mercer University
Nursing Prgm
Atlanta, GA 30341
www.mercer.edu

Medical College of Georgia
Nursing Prgm
Augusta, GA 30912
www.mcg.edu/son/

University of West Georgia
Nursing Prgm
Carrollton, GA 30118
www.westga.edu

Brenau University
Nursing Prgm
Gainesville, GA 30501
www.brenau.edu

Kennesaw State University
Nursing Prgm
Kennesaw, GA 30144
www.kennesaw.edu

Clayton State University
Nursing Prgm
Morrow, GA 30260
http://healthsci.clayton.edu

Armstrong Atlantic State University
Nursing Prgm
Savannah, GA 31419
www.don.armstrong.edu

Georgia Southern University
Nursing Prgm
Statesboro, GA 30458
www.georgiasouthern.edu

Valdosta State University
Nursing Prgm
Valdosta, GA 31698
www.valdosta.edu/nursing

Hawaii

University of Hawaii
Nursing Prgm
Honolulu, HI 96822
www.nursing.hawaii.edu

Idaho

Lewis-Clark State College
Nursing Prgm
Division of Nursing and Health Sciences
Lewiston, ID 83501

Northwest Nazarene University
Nursing Prgm
Nampa, ID 83686
www.nnu.edu/nursing

Idaho State University
Nursing Prgm
Pocatello, ID 83209
www.isu.edu/departments/nursing

Illinois

Aurora University
Nursing Prgm
Aurora, IL 60506
www.aurora.edu/nursing

Illinois Wesleyan University
Nursing Prgm
School of Nursing
Bloomington, IL 61702

Olivet Nazarene University
Nursing Prgm
Bourbonnais, IL 60914
www.olivet.edu

DePaul University
Nursing Prgm
Department of Nursing
Chicago, IL 60614

Kaplan University
Nursing Prgm
School of Nursing and Health Care
Chicago, IL 60607

Loyola University of Chicago
Nursing Prgm
Chicago, IL 60626
www.luc.edu/schools/nursing

North Park University
Nursing Prgm
Chicago, IL 60625
www.northpark.edu

Rush University
Nursing Prgm
Chicago, IL 60612
www.rush.edu/rushu/nursing.html

Saint Xavier University
Nursing Prgm
Chicago, IL 60655
www.sxu.edu

University of Illinois at Chicago
Nursing Prgm
Chicago, IL 60612
www.uic.edu

Lakeview College of Nursing
Nursing Prgm
Danville, IL 61832

Millikin University
Nursing Prgm
Decatur, IL 62522
www.millikin.edu

Northern Illinois University
Nursing Prgm
Dekalb, IL 60115
www.niu.edu

Southern Illinois University
Nursing Prgm
Edwardsville, IL 62026
www.siue.edu

Elmhurst College
Nursing Prgm
Deicke Center for Nursing Education
Elmhurst, IL 60126

MacMurray College
Nursing Prgm
Department of Nursing
Jacksonville, IL 62650

University of St Francis
Nursing Prgm
College of Nursing and Allied Health
Joliet, IL 60435

Illinois State University
Nursing Prgm
Normal, IL 61790
www.mcn.ilstu.edu

West Suburban College of Nursing
Nursing Prgm
Oak Park, IL 60302

Trinity Christian College
Nursing Prgm
Department of Nursing
Palos Heights, IL 60463

Blessing Hospital
Nursing Prgm
Rieman Collge of Nursing
Quincy, IL 62305

Trinity College of Nursing & Health Sciences
Nursing Prgm
Rock Island, IL 61201
www.trinitycollegequ.edu

OSF St Anthony Medical Center
Nursing Prgm
Rockford, IL 61108
www.sacn.edu

Lewis University
Nursing Prgm
College of Nursing and Health Professions
Romeoville, IL 60446

Indiana

Anderson University
Nursing Prgm
Anderson, IN 46012
www.anderson.edu

University of Southern Indiana
Nursing Prgm
Evansville, IN 47712
http://heath_p.usi.edu

University of Saint Francis
Nursing Prgm
Fort Wayne, IN 46808
www.sf.edu/nursing

Indiana University Northwest
Nursing Prgm
Gary, IN 46408
www.iun.indiana.edu

Goshen College
Nursing Prgm
Department of Nursing
Goshen, IN 46526

Indiana University
Nursing Prgm
Indianapolis, IN 46202
nursing.iupui.edu

Marian College
Nursing Prgm
Indianapolis, IN 46222
www.marian.edu

University of Indianapolis
Nursing Prgm
Indianapolis, IN 46227
www.uindy.edu

Indiana University - Kokomo
Nursing Prgm
Kokomo, IN 46904
www.iuk.indiana/edu.iuk/iuk_nursing.html

Indiana Wesleyan University
Nursing Prgm
Division of Nursing Education
Marion, IN 46953

Ball State University
Nursing Prgm
Muncie, IN 47306
www.bsu.edu/nursing

Indiana University Southeast
Nursing Prgm
Division of Nursing
New Albany, IN 47150

Indiana University South Bend
Nursing Prgm
South Bend, IN 46634
www.iusb.edu/~nursing

Valparaiso University
Nursing Prgm
College of Nursing
Valparaiso, IN 46383

Purdue University
Nursing Prgm
West Lafayette, IN 47907
www.nursing.purdue.edu

Iowa

Coe College
Nursing Prgm
Cedar Rapids, IA 52402
www.coe.edu

Mount Mercy College
Nursing Prgm
Department of Nursing
Cedar Rapids, IA 52402

St Ambrose University
Nursing Prgm
Davenport, IA 52803
web.sau.edu/nursing

Luther College
Nursing Prgm
Decorah, IA 52101
www.luther.edu/learning/dept/nursing.html

Grand View College
Nursing Prgm
Division of Nursing
Des Moines, IA 50316

Mercy College of Health Sciences
Nursing Prgm
Des Moines, IA 50309
www.mchs.edu

Clarke College
Nursing Prgm
Dubuque, IA 52001
www.clarke.edu

University of Iowa
Nursing Prgm
Iowa City, IA 52242
www.nursing.uiowa.edu

Dordt College
Nursing Prgm
Nursing Department
Sioux Center, IA 51250

Allen College
Nursing Prgm
Waterloo, IA 50703
www.allencollege.edu

Kansas

Fort Hays State University
Nursing Prgm
Hays, KS 67601
www.fhsu.edu

University of Kansas
Nursing Prgm
Kansas City, KS 66160
www.kumc.edu/son

Bethel College
Nursing Prgm
North Newton, KS 67117
www.bethelks.edu

Mid-America Nazarene University
Nursing Prgm
Olathe, KS 66062
www.mnu.edu

Pittsburg State University
Nursing Prgm
Pittsburg, KS 66762
www.pittstate.edu/nurs

Baker University
Nursing Prgm
School of Nursing
Topeka, KS 66604

Washburn University
Nursing Prgm
Topeka, KS 66621
www.washburn.edu/sonu/

Newman University
Nursing Prgm
Wichita, KS 67213
www.newman.edu

Tabor College
Nursing Prgm
Wichita, KS 67205
www.tabor.edu

Wichita State University
Nursing Prgm
Wichita, KS 67260
www.wichita.edu/nurs

Southwestern College
Nursing Prgm
Department of Nursing
Winfield, KS 67156

Kentucky

Berea College
Nursing Prgm
Berea, KY 40404
www.berea.edu

Western Kentucky University
Nursing Prgm
Bowling Green, KY 42101
www.wku.edu

Kentucky Christian University
Nursing Prgm
School of Nursing
Grayson, KY 41143

University of Kentucky
Nursing Prgm
Lexington, KY 40536
www.uky.edu

Bellarmine University
Nursing Prgm
Louisville, KY 40205
www.bellarmine.edu/lansing

Spalding University
Nursing Prgm
School of Nursing
Louisville, KY 40203

University of Louisville
Nursing Prgm
Louisville, KY 40202
www.louisville.edu/nursing

Morehead State University
Nursing Prgm
Morehead, KY 40351
www.moreheadstate.edu

Murray State University
Nursing Prgm
Murray, KY 42071
www.murraystate.edu/nursing

Eastern Kentucky University
Nursing Prgm
Richmond, KY 40475
www.eku.edu

Louisiana

Southern Univ and A&M College
Nursing Prgm
School of Nursing
Baton Rouge, LA 70813

University of Louisiana at Monroe
Nursing Prgm
Monroe, LA 71209
www.ulm.edu/nursing

Louisiana State Univ Health Sciences Center
Nursing Prgm
New Orleans, LA 70112
www.lsumc.edu

Louisiana College
Nursing Prgm
Pineville, LA 71359
www.lacollege.edu

Northwestern State University
Nursing Prgm
Shreveport, LA 71101
www.nsula.edu

Nicholls State University
Nursing Prgm
Thibodaux, LA 70310
www.nicholls.edu

Maine

Husson College
Nursing Prgm
Bangor, ME 04401
www.husson.edu

University of Maine Fort Kent
Nursing Prgm
Division of Nursing
Fort Kent, ME 04743

University of Maine - Orono
Nursing Prgm
Orono, ME 04469
www.umaine.edu/nursing

University of Southern Maine
Nursing Prgm
Portland, ME 04104
www.usm.maine.edu/conhp

Saint Joseph's College of Maine
Nursing Prgm
Department of Nursing
Standish, ME 04084

Maryland

Johns Hopkins University
Nursing Prgm
School of Nursing
Baltimore, MD 21205

Salisbury University
Nursing Prgm
Salisbury, MD 21801
www.salisbury.edu

Towson University
Nursing Prgm
Towson, MD 21252
www.towson.edu

Massachusetts

University of Massachusetts - Amherst
Nursing Prgm
Amherst, MA 01003
www.umass.edu

Emmanuel College
Nursing Prgm
Department of Nursing
Boston, MA 02115

Mass College of Pharmacy & Health Sciences
Nursing Prgm
School of Nursing
Boston, MA 02115

Northeastern University
Nursing Prgm
Boston, MA 02115
www.bouve.neu.edu/programs/nursing/

Simmons College
Nursing Prgm
Boston, MA 02115
www.simmons.edu

University of Massachusetts - Boston
Nursing Prgm
Boston, MA 02125
www.cnhs.umb.edu

Boston College
Nursing Prgm
William F Connell School of Nursing
Chestnut Hill, MA 02467

Elms College
Nursing Prgm
Department of Nursing
Chicopee, MA 01013

Fitchburg State College
Nursing Prgm
Fitchburg, MA 01420
www.fsc.edu

University of Massachusetts - Lowell
Nursing Prgm
Lowell, MA 01854
www.uml.edu/college/she

Curry College
Nursing Prgm
Division of Nursing
Milton, MA 02186

Salem State College
Nursing Prgm
Salem, MA 01970
www.salemstate.edu

Michigan

University of Michigan
Nursing Prgm
Ann Arbor, MI 48109
www.nursing.umich.edu

University of Detroit Mercy
Nursing Prgm
Detroit, MI 48219
www.udmercy.edu

Wayne State University
Nursing Prgm
Detroit, MI 48202
www.wayne.edu

Michigan State University
Nursing Prgm
East Lansing, MI 48824
nursing.msu.edu

University of Michigan - Flint
Nursing Prgm
Flint, MI 48502
www.umflint.edu/nursing

Calvin College
Nursing Prgm
Department of Nursing
Grand Rapids, MI 49546

Grand Valley State University
Nursing Prgm
Grand Rapids, MI 49503
www.gvsu.edu/kcon

Finlandia University
Nursing Prgm
Hancock, MI 49930
www.finlandia.edu

Hope College
Nursing Prgm
Holland, MI 49423
www.hope.edu/academic/nursing

Western Michigan University
Nursing Prgm
Kalamazoo, MI 49008
www.wmich.edu/hhs/nursing/

Madonna University
Nursing Prgm
Livonia, MI 48150
www.madonna.edu

Northern Michigan University
Nursing Prgm
Marquette, MI 49855
www.nmu.edu

Oakland University
Nursing Prgm
Rochester, MI 48309
www.oakland.edu

Spring Arbor University
Nursing Prgm
BSN Program
Spring Arbor, MI 49283

Saginaw Valley State University
Nursing Prgm
University Center, MI 48710
www.svsu.edu

Eastern Michigan University
Nursing Prgm
Ypsilanti, MI 48197
www.emich.edu

Minnesota

Bemidji State University
Nursing Prgm
Department of Nursing
Bemidji, MN 56601

College of St Scholastica
Nursing Prgm
Duluth, MN 55811
www.css.edu

Minnesota State University - Mankato
Nursing Prgm
Mankato, MN 56001
www.mnsu.edu

Augsburg College
Nursing Prgm
Minneapolis, MN 55454
www.augsburg.edu

University of Minnesota - Minneapolis
Nursing Prgm
Minneapolis, MN 55455
www.nurs.umn.edu

Concordia College - Moorhead
Nursing Prgm
Moorhead, MN 56562
www.cord.edu/dept/splash/nursing

Minnesota State University - Moorhead
Nursing Prgm
Moorhead, MN 56563
www.mnstate.edu/nursing

Minnesota Intercollegiate Nursing Consortium
Nursing Prgm
Northfield, MN 55057

St Cloud State University
Nursing Prgm
St Cloud, MN 56303
www.stcloudstate.edu

College of St Benedict/St John's University
Nursing Prgm
St Joseph, MN 56374
www.csbsju.edu/nursing

Bethel University
Nursing Prgm
St Paul, MN 55112
www.bethel.edu

Metropolitan State University
Nursing Prgm
School of Nursing
St Paul, MN 55106

Winona State University
Nursing Prgm
Winona, MN 55987
www.winona.edu/nursing

Mississippi

Delta State University
Nursing Prgm
Cleveland, MS 38733
www.deltast.edu

Mississippi University for Women
Nursing Prgm
Columbus, MS 39701
www.muw.edu/nursing

University of Southern Mississippi
Nursing Prgm
Hattiesburg, MS 39406
www.nursing.usm.edu

University of Mississippi Medical Center
Nursing Prgm
Jackson, MS 39216
son.umc.edu

Missouri

Southeast Missouri State University
Nursing Prgm
Cape Girardeau, MO 63701
www2.semo.edu/nursing

University of Missouri - Columbia
Nursing Prgm
Columbia, MO 65211
www.hsc.missouri.edu/son/docs/sonhome.html

Central Methodist University
Nursing Prgm
Fayette, MO 65248
www.centralmethodist.edu

Graceland University
Nursing Prgm
Independence, MO 64050
www.graceland.edu

Avila University
Nursing Prgm
Kansas City, MO 64145
www.avila.edu

Saint Luke's Hospital
Nursing Prgm
Kansas City, MO 64111
www.saint-lukes.org/about/slc

University of Missouri - Kansas City
Nursing Prgm
Kansas City, MO 64108
www.umkc.edu

Truman State University
Nursing Prgm
Kirksville, MO 63501
www.truman.edu

William Jewell College
Nursing Prgm
Department of Nursing
Liberty, MO 64068

Cox College of Nursing and Health Services
Nursing Prgm
Springfield, MO 65802

Missouri State University
Nursing Prgm
Springfield, MO 65897
www.smsu.edu/nursing

Missouri Western State University
Nursing Prgm
St Joseph, MO 64507
mwsc.edu/~nursing

Barnes-Jewish Coll of Nursing/Allied Health
Nursing Prgm
St Louis, MO 63110
www.barnesjewishcollege.edu

Maryville University
Nursing Prgm
St Louis, MO 63141
www.maryville.edu

Saint Louis University
Nursing Prgm
St Louis, MO 63104
www.slu.edu/colleges/nr

University of Missouri - St Louis
Nursing Prgm
St Louis, MO 63121
www.umsl.edu/divisions/nursing

University of Central Missouri
Nursing Prgm
Warrensburg, MO 64093
www.cmsu.edu

Montana

Montana State University
Nursing Prgm
Bozeman, MT 59717
www.montana.edu

Carroll College
Nursing Prgm
Helena, MT 59625
www.carroll.edu

Nebraska

Union College
Nursing Prgm
Lincoln, NE 68506
www.ucollege.edu

Creighton University
Nursing Prgm
Omaha, NE 68178
www.creighton.edu

Nebraska Methodist College
Nursing Prgm
Omaha, NE 68114
www.methodistcollege.edu

University of Nebraska Medical Center
Nursing Prgm
Omaha, NE 68198
www.unmc.edu/nursing

Nevada

Nevada State College
Nursing Prgm
School of Nursing
Henderson, NV 89002

Touro University - Nevada
Nursing Prgm
Henderson, NV 89014
www.tu.edu/nursing/

University of Nevada - Reno
Nursing Prgm
Reno, NV 89557
www.unr.edu/osn

New Hampshire

University of New Hampshire
Nursing Prgm
Durham, NH 03824
www.unh.edu/nursing/

Saint Anselm College
Nursing Prgm
Department of Nursing
Manchester, NH 03102

Colby-Sawyer College
Nursing Prgm
New London, NH 03257
www.colby-sawyer.edu

New Jersey

Bloomfield College
Nursing Prgm
Division of Nursing
Bloomfield, NJ 07003

SUNJ Rutgers Camden and UMDNJ
Nursing Prgm
Camden, NJ 08102
www.camden.rutgers.edu

College of New Jersey
Nursing Prgm
Ewing, NJ 08628
www.tcnj.edu

Saint Peter's College
Nursing Prgm
School of Nursing
Jersey City, NJ 07306

Felician College
Nursing Prgm
Lodi, NJ 07644
www.felician.edu

Rutgers - SUNJ
Nursing Prgm
College of Nursing
Newark, NJ 07102

Richard Stockton College of New Jersey
Nursing Prgm
Pomona, NJ 08240
www.stockton.edu

Seton Hall University
Nursing Prgm
South Orange, NJ 07079
nursing.shu.edu

Fairleigh Dickinson University
Nursing Prgm
Teaneck, NJ 07666
www.fdu.edu

William Paterson Univ of New Jersey
Nursing Prgm
Wayne, NJ 07470
www.wpunj.edu

Monmouth University
Nursing Prgm
Majorie K Unterberg School of Nursing and Health
Studies
West Long Beach, NJ 07764

New Mexico

University of New Mexico
Nursing Prgm
Albuquerque, NM 87131
http://hsc.unm.edu/consg

New Mexico State University
Nursing Prgm
Las Cruces, NM 88003
www.nmsu.edu/~nursing

New York

Binghamton University
Nursing Prgm
Decker School of Nursing
Binghamton, NY 13902

SUNY Brockport
Nursing Prgm
Brockport, NY 14420
www.brockport.edu

CUNY Herbert H Lehman College
Nursing Prgm
Bronx, NY 10468
www.lehman.cuny.edu

Long Island University
Nursing Prgm
Brooklyn, NY 11201
www.liu.edu

SUNY Downstate Medical Center
Nursing Prgm
Brooklyn, NY 11203
www.downstate.edu

St Francis College
Nursing Prgm
Department of Nursing
Brooklyn Heights, NY 11201

Long Island University
Nursing Prgm
Brookville, NY 11548
www.liu.edu

D'Youville College
Nursing Prgm
Buffalo, NY 14201
www.dyc.edu

University at Buffalo - SUNY
Nursing Prgm
Buffalo, NY 14214
nursing.buffalo.edu

Mercy College
Nursing Prgm
Dobbs Ferry, NY 10522
www.mercy.edu

Adelphi University
Nursing Prgm
Garden City, NY 11530
www.adephi.edu

SUNY at New Paltz
Nursing Prgm
New Paltz, NY 12561
www.newpaltz.edu

College of New Rochelle
Nursing Prgm
New Rochelle, NY 10805
www.cnr.edu

Columbia University
Nursing Prgm
New York, NY 10032
www.nursing.hs.columbia.edu

CUNY Hunter College
Nursing Prgm
New York, NY 10010
www.hunter.cuny.edu

New York University
Nursing Prgm
New York, NY 10003
www.nyu.edu/education/nursing

Mt St Mary College
Nursing Prgm
Division of Nursing
Newburgh, NY 12550

Hartwick College
Nursing Prgm
Department of Nursing
Oneonta, NY 13820

Dominican College
Nursing Prgm
Orangeburg, NY 10962
www.dc.edu

SUNY College at Plattsburgh
Nursing Prgm
Plattsburgh, NY 12901
www.plattsburgh.edu

Pace University
Nursing Prgm
Lienhard School of Nursing
Pleasantville, NY 10570

College of Mount St Viencent
Nursing Prgm
Department of Nursing
Riverdale, NY 10471

Nazareth College of Rochester
Nursing Prgm
Rochester, NY 14618
www.naz.edu

St John Fisher College
Nursing Prgm
Wegman's School of Nursing
Rochester, NY 14618

Molloy College
Nursing Prgm
Rockville Centre, NY 11571
www.molloy.edu

SUNY at Stony Brook
Nursing Prgm
Stony Brook, NY 11794
www.uhmc.sunysb.edu

Le Moyne College
Nursing Prgm
Syracuse, NY 13214
www.lemoyne.edu/nursing

SUNY Upstate Medical University
Nursing Prgm
Syracuse, NY 13210
www.upstate

The Sage Colleges
Nursing Prgm
Troy, NY 12180
www.sage.edu

SUNY Institute of Tech - Utica/Rome
Nursing Prgm
Utica, NY 13504
www.sunyit.edu

North Carolina

Lees-McRae College
Nursing Prgm
Banner Elk, NC 28604

University of North Carolina
Nursing Prgm
Chapel Hill, NC 27599
www.unc.edu/depts/nursing

Queens University of Charlotte
Nursing Prgm
Charlotte, NC 28274
www.queens.edu/nursing/

Univ of North Carolina at Charlotte
Nursing Prgm
Charlotte, NC 28223
www.uncc.edu

Cabarrus College of Health Sciences
Nursing Prgm
Concord, NC 28025
www.cabarruscollege.edu

Western Carolina University
Nursing Prgm
Cullowhee, NC 28723
www.wcu.edu

Duke University
Nursing Prgm
Durham, NC 27710
son3mc.duke.edu

Fayetteville State University
Nursing Prgm
Department of Nursing
Fayetteville, NC 28301

University of North Carolina - Greensboro
Nursing Prgm
Greensboro, NC 27402
www.uncg.edu

Lenoir-Rhyne College
Nursing Prgm
Hickory, NC 28601
www.lrc.edu

University of North Carolina Pembroke
Nursing Prgm
Department of Nursing
Pembroke, NC 28372

Fayetteville State University
Nursing Prgm
Wilmington, NC 28403
www.uncwil.edu

Winston-Salem State University
Nursing Prgm
Division of Nursing
Winston-Salem, NC 27110

North Dakota

Medcenter One
Nursing Prgm
Bismarck, ND 58501
www.medcenterone.com/college/nursing.htm

University of Mary
Nursing Prgm
Bismarck, ND 58504
www.umary.edu

North Dakota State University
Nursing Prgm
Fargo, ND 58105
nursing.ndsu.nodak.edu

University of North Dakota
Nursing Prgm
Grand Forks, ND 58202
www.und.nodak.edu/dept/nursing

Ohio

University of Akron
Nursing Prgm
Akron, OH 44325
www.uakron.edu

Ashland University
Nursing Prgm
Ashland, OH 44805
www.ashland.edu

Ohio University
Nursing Prgm
Athens, OH 45701
www.ohiou.edu

Malone College
Nursing Prgm
School of Nursing
Canton, OH 44709

Cedarville University
Nursing Prgm
Cedarville, OH 45314
www.cedarville.edu

University of Cincinnati
Nursing Prgm
Cincinnati, OH 45221
www.uc.edu

Xavier University
Nursing Prgm
Cincinnati, OH 45207
www.xu.edu

Cleveland State University
Nursing Prgm
Cleveland, OH 44115
www.scuohio.edu

Capital University
Nursing Prgm
Columbus, OH 43209
www.capital.edu

Chamberlain College of Nursing
Nursing Prgm
Columbus, OH 43209

Ohio State University
Nursing Prgm
Columbus, OH 43210
www.acs.ohio-state.edu

Wright State University
Nursing Prgm
Dayton, OH 45435
www.wright.edu

Kent State University
Nursing Prgm
Kent, OH 44242
www.kent.edu/nursing/nursing.html

Medcentral College
Nursing Prgm
Mansfield, OH 44903

Ursuline College
Nursing Prgm
Pepper Pike, OH 44124
www.ursuline.edu

Lourdes College
Nursing Prgm
Sylvania, OH 43560
www.lourdes.edu

Mercy College of Northwest Ohio
Nursing Prgm
Toledo, OH 43624
www.mercycollege.edu

University of Toledo Consortium
Nursing Prgm
Toledo, OH 43614

Urbana University
Nursing Prgm
Urbana, OH 43078
www.urbana.edu

Otterbein College
Nursing Prgm
Westerville, OH 43081
www.otterbein.edu/nursing

Oklahoma

Oklahoma Wesleyan University
Nursing Prgm
Division of Nursing
Bartlesville, OK 74006

Southern Nazarene University
Nursing Prgm
Bethany, OK 73008
www.snu.edu

Oral Roberts University
Nursing Prgm
Anna Vaughn School of Nursing
Tulsa, OK 74171

Oregon

Linfield College
Nursing Prgm
Portland, OR 97210
www.linfield.edu

Oregon Health & Science University
Nursing Prgm
Portland, OR 97239
www.ohsu.edu/son

University of Portland
Nursing Prgm
School of Nursing
Portland, OR 97203

Pennsylvania

Moravian College
Nursing Prgm
St Luke's Hospital School of Nursing
Bethlehem, PA 18018

Bloomsburg University
Nursing Prgm
Bloomsburg, PA 17815
www.bloomu.edu

California University of Pennsylvania
Nursing Prgm
California, PA 15419
www.cup.edu

Widener University
Nursing Prgm
Chester, PA 19013
www.widener.edu

Misericordia Unversity
Nursing Prgm
Dallas, PA 18612
www.miseri.edu

Edinboro University of Pennsylvania
Nursing Prgm
Edinboro, PA 16444
www.edinboro.edu

Gannon University
Nursing Prgm
Erie, PA 16541
www.gannon.edu

Messiah College
Nursing Prgm
Grantham, PA 17027
www.messiah.edu

Immaculata University
Nursing Prgm
Immaculata, PA 19345
www.immaculata.edu

Indiana University of Pennsylvania
Nursing Prgm
Indiana, PA 15705
www.iup.edu

St Francis University
Nursing Prgm
Loretto, PA 15940
www.francis.edu/nursing/nursinghome.shtml

Robert Morris College/Allegheny Gen Hosp
Nursing Prgm
Moon Township, PA 15108
www.rmu.edu

Drexel University
Nursing Prgm
Philadelphia, PA 19102
www.drexel.edu

Holy Family University
Nursing Prgm
Philadelphia, PA 19114
www.holyfamily.edu

La Salle University
Nursing Prgm
Philadelphia, PA 19141
www.lasalle.edu

Temple University
Nursing Prgm
Philadelphia, PA 19140
www.temple.edu

Thomas Jefferson University
Nursing Prgm
Philadelphia, PA 19107
tju.edu/chp

University of Pennsylvania
Nursing Prgm
School of Nursing
Philadelphia, PA 19104

Carlow University
Nursing Prgm
School of Nursing
Pittsburgh, PA 15213

Duquesne University
Nursing Prgm
Pittsburgh, PA 15282
www.nursing.duq.edu

University of Pittsburgh
Nursing Prgm
Pittsburgh, PA 15261
www.pitt.edu/~nursing

Alvernia College
Nursing Prgm
Reading, PA 19607
www.alvernia.edu

University of Scranton
Nursing Prgm
Scranton, PA 18510
www.scranton.edu

Eastern University
Nursing Prgm
St Davids, PA 19087
www.eastern.edu

Penn State University
Nursing Prgm
University Park, PA 16802
www.psu.edu

Villanova University
Nursing Prgm
College of Nursing
Villanova, PA 19085

Waynesburg College
Nursing Prgm
Waynesburg, PA 15370
www.waynesburg.edu

West Chester University
Nursing Prgm
West Chester, PA 19383
www.wcupa.edu

Wilkes University
Nursing Prgm
Department of Nursing
Wilkes-Barre, PA 18766

York College of Pennsylvania
Nursing Prgm
York, PA 17405
www.ycp.edu

Puerto Rico

Universidad Del Turabo
Nursing Prgm
School of Health Sciences
Gurabo, PR 00778

University of Puerto Rico
Nursing Prgm
San Juan, PR 00936
www.upr.edu

Rhode Island

University of Rhode Island
Nursing Prgm
Kingston, RI 02881
www.uri.edu

South Carolina

Medical University of South Carolina
Nursing Prgm
Charleston, SC 29425
www.musc.edu/nursing

Clemson University
Nursing Prgm
Clemson, SC 29634
www.clemson.edu

University of South Carolina
Nursing Prgm
Columbia, SC 29208
www.sc.edu/nursing/index.htm

South Carolina State University
Nursing Prgm
Orangeburg, SC 29117
www.scsu.edu

University of South Carolina Upstate
Nursing Prgm
Mary Black School of Medicine
Spartanburg, SC 29303

South Dakota

South Dakota State University
Nursing Prgm
Brookings, SD 57007
www3.sdstate.edu/academics/collegeofnursing/

Augustana College
Nursing Prgm
Sioux Falls, SD 57197
www.augie.edu

Mt Marty College
Nursing Prgm
Yankton, SD 57078
www.mtmc.edu

Tennessee

King College
Nursing Prgm
School of Nursing
Bristol, TN 37620

University of Tennessee - Chattanooga
Nursing Prgm
Chattanooga, TN 37403
www.utc.edu

Tennessee Technological University
Nursing Prgm
Cookeville, TN 38505
www.tntech.edu/nursing

Union University
Nursing Prgm
Jackson, TN 38305
www.uu.edu/academcis/son

Carson-Newman College
Nursing Prgm
Jefferson City, TN 37760
www.cn.edu

East Tennessee State University
Nursing Prgm
Johnson City, TN 37614
www.etsu.edu/nursing

Tennessee Wesleyan College
Nursing Prgm
Fort Sanders Nursing Department
Knoxville, TN 37932

University of Tennessee - Knoxville
Nursing Prgm
Knoxville, TN 37996
nightingale.com.utk.edu

Baptist College of Health Sciences
Nursing Prgm
Memphis, TN 38104
www.bchs.edu

University of Memphis
Nursing Prgm
Memphis, TN 38152
nursing.memphis.edu

University of Tennessee Health Science Ctr
Nursing Prgm
Memphis, TN 38163
www.utmem.edu/nursing

Milligan College
Nursing Prgm
Milligan College, TN 37682
www.milligan.edu

Middle Tennessee State University
Nursing Prgm
Murfreesboro, TN 37132
www.mtsu.edu/~nursing

Belmont University
Nursing Prgm
Nashville, TN 37212

Texas

Patty Hanks Shelton School of Nursing
Nursing Prgm
Abilene, TX 79601

University of Texas at Arlington
Nursing Prgm
Arlington, TX 76019
www.uta.edu

University of Texas at Austin
Nursing Prgm
Austin, TX 78701
www.utexas.edu/nursing

University of Mary Hardin-Baylor
Nursing Prgm
Belton, TX 76513
www.umhb.edu

West Texas A&M University
Nursing Prgm
Canyon, TX 79016
www.wtamu.edu

Texas A&M University - Corpus Christi
Nursing Prgm
Corpus Christi, TX 78412
www.tamucc.edu

Baylor University
Nursing Prgm
Dallas, TX 75246
www.baylor.edu/nursing

Texas Woman's University
Nursing Prgm
Denton, TX 76204
www.twu.edu

Univ of Texas - Pan American
Nursing Prgm
Edinburg, TX 78540
www.panam.edu/dept/nursing

University of Texas at El Paso
Nursing Prgm
El Paso, TX 79902
www.utep.edu

Texas Christian University
Nursing Prgm
Fort Worth, TX 76129
www.tcu.edu

University of Texas Medical Branch
Nursing Prgm
Galveston, TX 77555
www.utmb.edu

Prairie View A&M University
Nursing Prgm
Houston, TX 77030
www.pvamu.edu

Univ of Texas Hlth Sci Ctr at Houston
Nursing Prgm
Houston, TX 77030
son.uth.tmc.edu

Texas Tech University
Nursing Prgm
Lubbock, TX 79430
www.ttuhsc.edu/son

East Texas Baptist University
Nursing Prgm
Marshall, TX 75670
www.etbu.edu

Univ of Texas Hlth Sci Ctr at San Antonio
Nursing Prgm
San Antonio, TX 78229
www.uthscsa.edu

University of the Incarnate Word
Nursing Prgm
San Antonio, TX 78209
www.uiw.edu

Tarleton State University
Nursing Prgm
Stephenville, TX 76402
www.tarleton.edu/~nursing

Texas A&M University Texarkana
Nursing Prgm
RN-BSN Program
Texarkana, TX 75501

University of Texas at Tyler
Nursing Prgm
Tyler, TX 75799
www.uttyler.edu

Midwestern State University
Nursing Prgm
Wichita Falls, TX 76308
www.mwsu.edu

Utah

Southern Utah University
Nursing Prgm
Cedar City, UT 84720
www.suu.edu/sci/nursing

Brigham Young University
Nursing Prgm
Provo, UT 84602
www.byu.edu

University of Utah
Nursing Prgm
Salt Lake City, UT 84112
www.nurs.utah.edu

Westminster College
Nursing Prgm
School of Nursing and Health Sciences
Salt Lake City, UT 84105

Vermont

University of Vermont
Nursing Prgm
Burlington, VT 05405
www.uvm.edu

Virginia

Marymount University
Nursing Prgm
Arlington, VA 22207
www.marymount.edu

University of Virginia
Nursing Prgm
Charlottesville, VA 22903
www.nursing.virginia.edu

George Mason University
Nursing Prgm
Fairfax, VA 22030
http://chhs.gmu.edu/

Hampton University
Nursing Prgm
Hampton, VA 23668
www.hamptonu.edu

Eastern Mennonite University
Nursing Prgm
Department of Nursing
Harrisonburg, VA 22802

James Madison University
Nursing Prgm
Harrisonburg, VA 22807
www.nursing.jmu.edu

Liberty University
Nursing Prgm
Lynchburg, VA 24502
www.liberty.edu

Lynchburg College
Nursing Prgm
Lynchburg, VA 24501
www.lynchburg.edu

Old Dominion University
Nursing Prgm
Norfolk, VA 23529
www.odu.edu

Radford University
Nursing Prgm
Radford, VA 24142
www.runet.edu

Jefferson College of Health Sciences
Nursing Prgm
Roanoke, VA 24031
www.jchs.edu

Shenandoah University
Nursing Prgm
Winchester, VA 22601
www.su.edu/nursing

University of Virginia - Wise
Nursing Prgm
Department of Nursing
Wise, VA 24293

Washington

Northwest University
Nursing Prgm
Mark and Huldah Buntain School of Nursing
Kirkland, WA 98033

Seattle Pacific University
Nursing Prgm
Seattle, WA 98119
www.spu.edu

Seattle University
Nursing Prgm
Seattle, WA 98122
www.seattleu.edu/nurs

University of Washington
Nursing Prgm
Seattle, WA 98195
www.son.washington.edu

Gonzaga University
Nursing Prgm
Department of Nursing
Spokane, WA 99258

Washington State University
Nursing Prgm
Spokane, WA 99224
www.nursing.wsu.edu

Pacific Lutheran University
Nursing Prgm
School of Nursing
Tacoma, WA 98447

West Virginia

Bluefield State College
Nursing Prgm
Bluefield, WV 24701
www.bluefield.wvnet.edu

Fairmont State Univ
Nursing Prgm
Fairmont, WV 26554
www.fscwv.edu

West Virginia University
Nursing Prgm
Morgantown, WV 26506
www.hsc.wvuledu/son

West Liberty State College
Nursing Prgm
West Liberty, WV 26074
www.westliberty.edu

Wheeling Jesuit University
Nursing Prgm
Wheeling, WV 26003
www.wju.edu

Wisconsin

University of Wisconsin - Eau Claire
Nursing Prgm
Eau Claire, WI 54701
www.uwec.edu/academics/nurs

Marian College
Nursing Prgm
School of Nursing
Fond du Lac, WI 54935

Bellin Health Hosp/Bellin Health Systems Inc
Nursing Prgm
Green Bay, WI 54305

University of Wisconsin - Green Bay
Nursing Prgm
Green Bay, WI 54311
www.uwgb.edu

Viterbo College
Nursing Prgm
LaCrosse, WI 54601
www.viterbo.edu

Edgewood College
Nursing Prgm
Department of Nursing
Madison, WI 53711

University of Wisconsin - Madison
Nursing Prgm
Madison, WI 53792
www.son.wisc.edu

Concordia University Wisconsin
Nursing Prgm
Mequon, WI 53097
www.cuw.edu

Alverno College
Nursing Prgm
Milwaukee, WI 53234
www.alverno.edu

Cardinal Stritch University
Nursing Prgm
College of Nursing
Milwaukee, WI 53217

Marquette University
Nursing Prgm
Milwaukee, WI 53201
www.mu.edu

Milwaukee School of Engineering
Nursing Prgm
Milwaukee, WI 53202
www.msoe.edu

University of Wisconsin - Milwaukee
Nursing Prgm
Milwaukee, WI 53201
www.uwm.edu

University of Wisconsin - Oshkosh
Nursing Prgm
Oshkosh, WI 54901
www.uwosh.edu/home_pages/colleges/con

Carroll College
Nursing Prgm
Waukesha, WI 53186
www.cc.edu

Wyoming

University of Wyoming
Nursing Prgm
Laramie, WY 82071
www.uwyo.edu/nursing

Occupational Therapy

Includes:
- Occupational therapist
- Occupational therapy assistant

Occupational Therapist

The practice of occupational therapy means the therapeutic use of everyday life activities (occupations) with clients (individuals, organizations, or populations) for the purpose of participation in roles and situations in home, school, workplace, community, and other settings. Occupational therapy services are provided for the purpose of promoting health and wellness and to those who have or are at risk for developing an illness, injury, disease, disorder, condition, impairment, disability, activity limitation, or participation restriction. Occupational therapy addresses the physical, cognitive, psychosocial, sensory, and other aspects of performance in a variety of contexts to support engagement in everyday life activities that affect health, well-being, and quality of life.

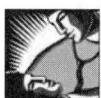

Career Description

Occupational therapy services are based on evaluation and assessment methods, including the use of skilled observation and the administration and interpretation of standardized or nonstandardized tests and measurements to identify areas for occupational therapy services.

The practice of occupational therapy includes:

A. Methods or strategies selected to direct the process of interventions, such as:
   1. Establishing, remediating, or restoring a skill or ability that has not yet developed or is impaired.
   2. Compensating, modifying, or adapting activity or environment to enhance performance.
   3. Maintaining and enhancing capabilities without which performance in everyday life activities would decline.
   4. Health promotion and wellness to enable or enhance performance in everyday life activities.
   5. Preventing barriers to performance, including disabilities.

B. Evaluation of factors affecting activities of daily living (ADL), instrumental activities of daily living (IADL), education, work, play, leisure, and social participation, including:
   1. Client factors, including body functions (such as neuromuscular, sensory, visual, perceptual, cognitive) and body structures (such as cardiovascular, digestive, integumentary, and genitourinary systems).
   2. Habits, routines, roles, and behavior patterns.
   3. Cultural, physical, environmental, social, and spiritual contexts and activity demands that affect performance.
   4. Performance skills, including motor, process, and communication/interaction skills.

C. Interventions and procedures to promote or enhance safety and performance in activities of daily living (ADL), instrumental activities of daily living (IADL), education, work, play, leisure, and social participation, including:
   1. Therapeutic use of occupations, exercises, and activities.
   2. Training in self-care, self-management, home management, and community/work reintegration.

3. Development, remediation, or compensation of physical, cognitive, neuromuscular, sensory functions and behavioral skills.
4. Therapeutic use of self, including one's personality, insights, perceptions, and judgments, as part of the therapeutic process.
5. Education and training of individuals, including family members, caregivers, and others.
6. Care coordination, case management, and transition services.
7. Consultative services to groups, programs, organizations, or communities.
8. Modification of environments (home, work, school, or community) and adaptation of processes, including the application of ergonomic principles.
9. Assessment, design, fabrication, application, fitting, and training in assistive technology, adaptive devices, and orthotic devices, and training in the use of prosthetic devices.
10. Assessment, recommendation, and training in techniques to enhance functional mobility, including wheelchair management.
11. Driver rehabilitation and community mobility.
12. Management of feeding, eating, and swallowing to enable eating and feeding performance.
13. Application of physical agent modalities, and use of a range of specific therapeutic procedures (such as wound care management; techniques to enhance sensory, perceptual, and cognitive processing; and manual therapy techniques) to enhance performance skills.

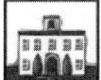

Employment Characteristics

The wide range of clients (individuals, organizations, and populations) served by occupational therapists is located in a variety of settings, such as hospitals, clinics, rehabilitation facilities, long-term care facilities, extended care facilities, private practices, schools, camps, the clients' own homes, and community agencies. Occupational therapists both receive referrals from and make referrals to the appropriate health, educational, or medical specialists.

Salary

AOTA studies conducted in 2006 indicate that the average entry-level salary for occupational therapists is $46,334. Refer to Section IV, Table 5 of this *Directory* for more information, or see www.ama-assn.org/go/hpsalary.

Educational Programs

Length. Programs at the combined baccalaureate/master's level entail 4 to 5 years of college or university preparation.

Postbaccalaureate programs leading to a master's degree are generally 2 to 2 ½ years and programs leading to a doctoral degree are generally 2 to 3 years. Following completion of all educational requirements, individuals take a national certification examination. All states also regulate the practice of occupational therapy.

Prerequisites. Prerequisites vary among programs. A baccalaureate degree is a prerequisite for most master's and doctorallevel occupational therapy programs. A strong foundation of liberal arts and biological, physical, social, and behavioral sciences may be prerequisite to, or concurrent with, the professional education of the program curriculum.

Curriculum. Curricula of accredited occupational therapy programs are required to include a broad foundation in the liberal arts and sciences, basic tenets of occupational therapy, occupational therapy theoretical perspectives, the process of screening and evaluation, the process of formulation and implementation of an intervention plan, context of service delivery, management of occupational therapy services, use of research, professional ethics, values, and responsibilities, and 24 weeks of fieldwork education. Doctoral-level programs have additional experiential requirements.

Licensure, Registration, Certification

All states, Puerto Rico, Guam, and the District of Columbia regulate the practice of occupational therapy. To obtain a license, applicants must graduate from an accredited educational program and pass a national certification examination. Those who pass the exam are awarded the title "Occupational Therapist Registered (OTR)." Some states have additional requirements for therapists who work in schools or early intervention programs. These requirements may include education-related classes, an education practice certificate, or early intervention certification requirements.

Occupational Therapy Assistant

Under the supervision of and in collaboration with an occupational therapist, the occupational therapy assistant provides services to clients focusing on participation in selected activities to restore, reinforce, and enhance performance; facilitate learning of those skills and functions essential for adaptation and participation; diminish or correct pathology; and promote and maintain health and wellness. A fundamental concern is the development and maintenance of the skill and capacity throughout the lifespan to perform with satisfaction to self and others meaningful tasks and roles essential to social participation and to the mastery of self and the environment. Under the supervision of and in partnership with the occupational therapist, the occupational therapy assistant participates in the development of adaptive skills and performance capacity and is concerned with factors that promote, influence, or enhance performance, as well as those that serve as barriers or impediments to the individual's occupational performance. The occupational therapy assistant provides service to those clients whose abilities to perform meaningful activities of living are threatened or impaired by:

- Developmental deficits
- The aging process
- Poverty and cultural differences
- Physical injury or illness
- Psychological or social disability

Career Description

A contemporary entry-level occupational therapy assistant must:

- Have acquired an educational foundation in the liberal arts and sciences, including a focus on issues related to diversity
- Be educated as a generalist, with a broad exposure to the delivery models and systems utilized in settings where occupational

therapy is currently practiced and where it is emerging as a service

- Have achieved entry-level competence through a combination of academic and fieldwork education
- Be prepared to work under the supervision of and in cooperation with the occupational therapist
- Be prepared to articulate and apply occupational therapy principles, intervention approaches and rationales, and expected outcomes as these relate to occupational performance of the client
- Be prepared to be a lifelong learner and keep current with best practice
- Uphold the ethical standards, values, and attitudes of the occupational therapy profession

Employment Characteristics

Occupational therapy assistants assist in the planning and implementation of treatment of a diverse population in a variety of settings, such as nursing homes, hospitals and clinics, rehabilitation facilities, long-term care facilities, extended care facilities, sheltered workshops, schools and camps, private homes, and community agencies.

Salary

AOTA studies conducted in 2006 indicate that the average entry-level salary for occupational therapy assistants is approximately $33,000. Refer to Section IV, Table 5 of this *Directory* for more information, or see www.ama-assn.org/go/hpsalary.

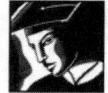

Educational Programs

Length. Education may be acquired in either a 2-year associate degree program or a 1- to 2-year certificate program. These technical-level education programs are located in 2-year and 4-year colleges and universities, and postsecondary vocational/technical schools and institutions and include academic and fieldwork components, as do the professional level programs. Following completion of all educational requirements, individuals take a national certification examination. Many states also regulate the practice of occupational therapy assistants.

Prerequisites. High school diploma or equivalent. A foundation of liberal arts and biological, physical, social, and behavioral sciences may be prerequisite to, or concurrent with, the technical education of the program curriculum.

Curriculum. Curricula of accredited occupational therapy assistant programs are required to include a broad foundation of the liberal arts and sciences, basic tenets of occupational therapy, the process of screening and evaluation, the process of intervention and implementation, context of service delivery, assistance in the management of occupational therapy services, use of professional literature, professional ethics, values, and responsibilities, and 16 weeks of fieldwork education.

Inquiries

Careers Education

American Occupational Therapy Association
4720 Montgomery Lane
PO Box 31220
Bethesda, MD 20824-1220
301 652-2682
www.aota.org

Certification
National Board for Certification in Occupational Therapy (NBCOT)
800 S Frederick Avenue, Suite 200
Gaithersburg, MD 20877-4150
301 990-7979
www.nbcot.org

Program Accreditation
Accreditation Council for Occupational Therapy Education
4720 Montgomery Lane, PO Box 31220
Bethesda, MD 20824-1220
301 652-2682
301 652-1417 Fax
www.aota.org

Occupational Therapist

Alabama

University of Alabama at Birmingham
Occupational Therapy Prgm
School of Health Professions
1530 3rd Ave S - RMSB 354
Birmingham, AL 35294-1212
Prgm Dir: Penelope Moyers, EdD OTR/L FAOTA
Tel: 205 934-9229   *Fax:* 205 975-7787
E-mail: pmoyers@uab.edu

University of South Alabama
Occupational Therapy Prgm
Department of Occupational Therapy
1504 Springhill Ave, Rm 5108
Mobile, AL 36604-3273
www.southalabama.edu
Prgm Dir: Rebecca I Estes, PhD OTR ATP
Tel: 251 434-3939   *Fax:* 251 434-3934
E-mail: riestes@usouthal.edu

Alabama State University
Occupational Therapy Prgm
915 S Jackson St
PO Box 271
Montgomery, AL 36101-0271
www.alasu.edu
Prgm Dir: Angela T Davis, EdD OTR/L
Tel: 334 229-5612   *Fax:* 334 229-5882
E-mail: adavis@alasu.edu

Tuskegee University
Occupational Therapy Prgm
Basil O'Connor Hall
Tuskegee, AL 36088-1696
www.tuskegee.edu/ot
Prgm Dir: Gwendolyn Gray, PhC MA OTR/L
Tel: 334 727-8695   *Fax:* 334 727-8259
E-mail: grayg@tuskegee.edu

Arizona

Midwestern University - Glendale Campus
Occupational Therapy Prgm
19555 N 59th Ave
Glendale, AZ 85308-6814
www.midwestern.edu
Prgm Dir: Christine Merchant, MA OTR/L
Tel: 623 572-3630   *Fax:* 623 572-3635
E-mail: cmerch@midwestern.edu

AT Still University of Health Sciences
Occupational Therapy Prgm
5850 E Still Circle
Mesa, AZ 85206-3618
Prgm Dir: Bernadette Mineo, PhD OTR/L
Tel: 480 219-6071   *Fax:* 480 219-6100
E-mail: bmineo@atsu.edu

Arkansas

University of Central Arkansas
Occupational Therapy Prgm
201 Donaghey Ave HSC, Ste 300
Box 5001
Conway, AR 72035-0001
www.uca.edu
Prgm Dir: Linda D Musselman, PhD OTR FAOTA
Tel: 501 450-3192   *Fax:* 501 450-3622
E-mail: LindaS@mail.uca.edu

California

California State University - Dominguez Hills
Occupational Therapy Prgm
1000 E Victoria Blvd
Carson, CA 90747-0005
www.csudh.edu/hhs/dhs/ot
Prgm Dir: Claudia G Peyton, PhD OTR/L FAOTA
Tel: 310 243-3067, Ext 3067   *Fax:* 310 516-3542
E-mail: cpeyton@csudh.edu

Loma Linda University
Occupational Therapy Prgm
Sch of Allied Health Professions
Nichol Hall Rm A901
Loma Linda, CA 92350-0001
www.llu.edu
Prgm Dir: Liane Hewitt, DrPH OTR/L
Tel: 909 558-4628, Ext 47327   *Fax:* 909 558-0239
E-mail: lhewitt@llu.edu

University of Southern California
Occupational Therapy Prgm
1540 Alcazar, CHP 133
Los Angeles, CA 90089-9003
www.usc.edu/ot
Prgm Dir: Florence A Clark, PhD OTR/L FAOTA
Tel: 323 442-2850   *Fax:* 323 442-1540
E-mail: fclark@usc.edu

Samuel Merritt College
Occupational Therapy Prgm
450 30th St, 4th Fl
Oakland, CA 94609-3108
Prgm Dir: Kate Hayner, EdD OTR/L
Tel: 510 869-6511, Ext 4780   *Fax:* 510 869-6951
E-mail: khayner@samuelmerritt.edu

San Jose State University
Occupational Therapy Prgm
Coll of Applied Sciences and Arts
One Washington Square
San Jose, CA 95192-0059
www.sjsu.edu/ot
Prgm Dir: Marti Southam, PhD OTR/l FAOTA
Tel: 408 924-3072   *Fax:* 408 924-3088
E-mail: msoutham@casa.sjsu.edu

Dominican University of California
Occupational Therapy Prgm
50 Acacia Ave
San Rafael, CA 94901-2298
Prgm Dir: Ruth Ramsey, EdDOTR/L
Tel: 415 257-1393   *Fax:* 415 458-3774
E-mail: rramsey@dominican.edu

Colorado

Colorado State University
Occupational Therapy Prgm
219 Occupational Therapy Bldg
Fort Collins, CO 80523-1573
www.ot.cahs.colostate.edu
Prgm Dir: Karen Spencer, PhD OTR
Tel: 970 491-5016   *Fax:* 970 491-6290
E-mail: kspencer@cahs.colostate.edu

Connecticut

Sacred Heart University
Occupational Therapy Prgm
5151 Park Ave
Fairfield, CT 06825-1000
Prgm Dir: Jody Bortone, EdD OTR/L
Tel: 203 396-8023   *Fax:* 203 396-8206
E-mail: BortoneJ@sacredheart.edu

Quinnipiac University
Occupational Therapy Prgm
Sch of Health Sciences
275 Mt Carmel Ave
Hamden, CT 06518-0569
Prgm Dir: Kimberly D Hartmann, PhD OTR/L FAOTA
Tel: 203 582-8679   *Fax:* 203 582-8706
E-mail: hartmann@quinnipiac.edu

District of Columbia

Howard University
Occupational Therapy Prgm
Division of Allied Health Sciences
Sixth and Bryant Sts NW
Washington, DC 20059-0001
Prgm Dir: Felecia M Banks, PhD OTR/L
Tel: 202 806-7617   *Fax:* 202 462-5248
E-mail: fbanks@howard.edu

Florida

Nova Southeastern University
Occupational Therapy Prgm
Occupational Therapy Department
Health Profs Div, Coll of Allied Health and Nursing
Fort Lauderdale, FL 33328-2018
www.nova.edu/ot
Prgm Dir: Sandra Dunbar, DPA OTR/L
Tel: 954 262-1243   *Fax:* 954 262-2290
E-mail: sdunbar@nova.edu

Florida Gulf Coast University
Occupational Therapy Prgm
10501 FGCU Blvd South
Fort Myers, FL 33965-6565
www.fgcu.edu/chp/ot
Prgm Dir: Linda Martin, PhD OTR/L FAOTA
Tel: 239 590-7556   *Fax:* 239 590-7460
E-mail: lmartin@fgcu.edu

University of Florida
Occupational Therapy Prgm
101 S Newell Dr
PO Box 100164 HSC
Gainesville, FL 32610-0164
www.ot.phhp.ufl.edu
Prgm Dir: Joanne Jackson Foss, PhD OTR
Tel: 352 273-6135   *Fax:* 352 846-6042
E-mail: jfoss@phhp.ufl.edu

Florida International University
Occupational Therapy Prgm
University Park Campus, HLS 237
Miami, FL 33199
www.ot.fiu.edu
Prgm Dir: Alma R Abdel-Moty, DrOT MS OTR
Tel: 305 348-3092   *Fax:* 305 348-1240
E-mail: abdela@fiu.edu

Barry University
Occupational Therapy Prgm
11300 NE 2nd Ave
Miami Shores, FL 33161-6695
www.barry.edu
Prgm Dir: Douglas M Mitchell, PhD OTR/L
Tel: 305 899-3210   *Fax:* 305 899-2958
E-mail: dmitchell@mail.barry.edu

Univ of St Augustine for Health Sciences
Occupational Therapy Prgm
1 University Blvd
St Augustine, FL 32086-5783
Prgm Dir: Karen S Howell, PhD OTR/L FAOTA
Tel: 904 826-0084, Ext 222   *Fax:* 904 827-0069
E-mail: khowell@usa.edu

Florida A&M University
Occupational Therapy Prgm
Lewis-Beck Building
Rm 318
Tallahassee, FL 32307-3500
www.famu.edu
Prgm Dir: Rosalie J Miller, PhD OTR FAOTA
Tel: 850 561-2014   *Fax:* 850 561-2457
E-mail: rosalie.miller@famu.edu

Georgia

Medical College of Georgia
Occupational Therapy Prgm
School of Allied Health, EF 102
1120 Fifteenth St EC2312
Augusta, GA 30912-0700
www.mcg.edu/sahs/ot
Prgm Dir: Kathy P Bradley, EdD OTR/L FAOTA
Tel: 706 721-3641   *Fax:* 706 721-9718
E-mail: kbradley@mcg.edu

Brenau University
Occupational Therapy Prgm
500 Washington SE
Gainesville, GA 30501
Prgm Dir: Sara Jane Brayman, PhD OTR/L FAOTA
Tel: 770 534-6139, Ext 6139   *Fax:* 770 534-6186
E-mail: sbrayman@brenau.edu

Idaho

Idaho State University
Occupational Therapy Prgm
Campus Box 8045
Pocatello, ID 83209-8045
Prgm Dir: Aaron Eakman, PhD OTR/L
Tel: 208 282-3758   *Fax:* 208 282-4962
E-mail: eakmaar@isu.edu

Illinois

Chicago State University
Occupational Therapy Prgm
9501 S King Dr, Library, Rm 132
Chicago, IL 60628-1598
Prgm Dir: Leslie K Roundtree, OTR/L DHS
Tel: 773 995-2525   *Fax:* 773 995-2839
E-mail: l-roundtree@csu.edu

Rush University
Occupational Therapy Prgm
600 S Paulina, Ste 1010
Chicago, IL 60612-3833
www.rushu.rush.edu/occuth
Prgm Dir: Clare Giuffrida, PhD OTR/L FAOTA
Tel: 312 942-7138   *Fax:* 312 942-6989
E-mail: Clare_Giuffrida@rush.edu

University of Illinois at Chicago
Occupational Therapy Prgm
1919 W Taylor St M/C 811
Chicago, IL 60612-7250
www.ahs.uic.edu/ot/
Prgm Dir: Brent Braveman, PhD OTR/L FAOTA
Tel: 312 355-2656   *Fax:* 312 413-0256
E-mail: bbravema@uic.edu

Midwestern University
Occupational Therapy Prgm
College of Health Sciences
555 31st St
Downers Grove, IL 60515-1235
www.midwestern.edu
Prgm Dir: Kimberly A Bryze, PhD OTR/L
Tel: 630 515-7226   *Fax:* 630 515-7418
E-mail: kbryze@midwestern.edu

Governors State University
Occupational Therapy Prgm
College of Health Professions
University Park, IL 60466-0975
Prgm Dir: Elizabeth Cada, EdD OTR/L FAOTA
Tel: 708 534-7295   *Fax:* 708 534-1647
E-mail: b-cada@govst.edu

Indiana

University of Southern Indiana
Occupational Therapy Prgm
8600 University Blvd/HP
Evansville, IN 47712-3534
Prgm Dir: Barbara J Williams, DrOT OTR
Tel: 812 465-1179   *Fax:* 812 465-7092
E-mail: bjwilliams4@usi.edu

Indiana University
Occupational Therapy Prgm
School of Health and Rehabilitation Sciences
1140 W Michigan St, Coleman Hall 311
Indianapolis, IN 46202-5119
Prgm Dir: Thomas F Fisher, PhD OTR FAOTA
Tel: 317 274-8006   *Fax:* 317 274-2150
E-mail: tffisher@iupui.edu

University of Indianapolis
Occupational Therapy Prgm
1400 E Hanna Ave
Indianapolis, IN 46227-3697
ot.uindy.edu
Prgm Dir: Kate DeCleene, OTD MS OTR
Tel: 317 788-4908   *Fax:* 317 788-3542
E-mail: decleenek@uindy.edu

Iowa

St Ambrose University
Occupational Therapy Prgm
518 W Locust
Davenport, IA 52803-2898
www.sau.edu
Prgm Dir: Phyllis Wenthe, MEd OTR/L
Tel: 563 333-6276   *Fax:* 563 333-6410
E-mail: WenthePhyllisJ@sau.edu

Kansas

University of Kansas Medical Center
Occupational Therapy Prgm
3033 Robinson, Mail Stop 2003
3901 Rainbow Blvd
Kansas City, KS 66160-7602
www.kumc.edu/SAH/OTEd
Prgm Dir: Winnie Dunn, PhD OTR FAOTA
Tel: 913 588-7195   *Fax:* 913 588-4568
E-mail: wdunn@kumc.edu

Kentucky

Spalding University
Occupational Therapy Prgm
851 S Fourth St
Louisville, KY 40203-2188
Prgm Dir: Laura S Strickland, EdD OTR/L
Tel: 502 585-7125   *Fax:* 502 585-7104
E-mail: lstrickland@spalding.edu

Eastern Kentucky University
Occupational Therapy Prgm
Department of Occupational Therapy
Dizney 103
Richmond, KY 40475-3135
Prgm Dir: Colleen M Schneck, ScD OTR/L FAOTA
Tel: 859 622-6328   *Fax:* 859 622-1601
E-mail: Colleen.Schneck@eku.edu

Louisiana

Louisiana State Univ Health Sciences Center
Occupational Therapy Prgm
Sch of Allied Health Professions
1900 Gravier St
New Orleans, LA 70112
http://alliedhealth.lsuhsc.edu/OccupationalTherapy/
Prgm Dir: Eve Taylor, PhD LOTR
Tel: 504 568-4302   *Fax:* 504 568-4306
E-mail: taylor@lsuhsc.edu

Louisiana State U Hlth Sci Ctr - Shreveport
Occupational Therapy Prgm
1501 Kings Hwy
Shreveport, LA 71130-3932
Prgm Dir: Lucinda Murray, MHS LOTR
Tel: 318 813-2951   *Fax:* 318 861-2957
E-mail: lmurra@lsuhsc.edu

Maine

Husson College
Occupational Therapy Prgm
1 College Circle
3rd Floor Commons
Bangor, ME 04401-2999
http://health.husson.edu/ot/
Prgm Dir: Lynn Gitlow, PhD OTR/L ATP
Tel: 207 973-1074   *Fax:* 207 973-1061
E-mail: gitlowl@husson.edu

University of New England
Occupational Therapy Prgm
11 Hills Beach Rd
Biddeford, ME 04005-9599
Prgm Dir: Regula Robnett, PhD OTR/L
Tel: 207 221-4102   *Fax:* 207 602-5963
E-mail: rrobnett@une.edu

University of Southern Maine -
    Lewiston/Auburn
Occupational Therapy Prgm
51 Westminster St
Lewiston, ME 04240-3534
www.usm.maine.edu/lac/ot
Prgm Dir: Roxie M Black, PhD OTR/L FAOTA
Tel: 207 753-6515   *Fax:* 207 753-6555
E-mail: rblack@usm.maine.edu

Maryland

Towson University
Occupational Therapy Prgm
8000 York Rd
Towson, MD 21252-0001
www.towson.edu/ot
Prgm Dir: S Maggie Reitz, PhD OTR/L FAOTA
Tel: 410 704-3499   *Fax:* 410 704-2322
E-mail: mreitz@towson.edu

Massachusetts

Boston University/Sargent College
Occupational Therapy Prgm
Health and Rehabilitation Sciences
635 Commonwealth Ave
Boston, MA 02215-1605
www.bu.edu/sargent
Prgm Dir: Wendy Coster, PhD OTR/L FAOTA
Tel: 617 353-2000, Ext 2727   *Fax:* 617 353-2926
E-mail: wjcoster@bu.edu

Bay Path College
Occupational Therapy Prgm
588 Longmeadow St
Longmeadow, MA 01106-2212
www.baypath.edu
Prgm Dir: Karen Sladyk, PhD OTR/L FAOTA
Tel: 413 565-1450   *Fax:* 413 565-1102
E-mail: ksladyk@baypath.edu

Tufts University
Occupational Therapy Prgm
Department of Occupational Therapy
26 Winthrop St
Medford, MA 02155-7084
www.ase.tufts.edu/bsot
Prgm Dir: Linda Tickle-Degnen, PhD OTR/L FAOTA
Tel: 617 627-5863   *Fax:* 617 627-3722
E-mail: Linda.Tickle_Degnen@tufts.edu

Salem State College
Occupational Therapy Prgm
352 Lafayette St
Salem, MA 01970-5353
www.salemstate.edu
Prgm Dir: Jeramie S Silveira, MS OTR/L
Tel: 978 542-6694   *Fax:* 978 542-6818
E-mail: jeramie.silveira@salemstate.edu

American International College
Occupational Therapy Prgm
1000 State St
Springfield, MA 01109-3189
Prgm Dir: Cathy A Dow-Royer, MA OTR CHT
Tel: 413 205-3262   *Fax:* 413 205-3957
E-mail: cathy.dow-royer@aic.edu

Springfield College
Occupational Therapy Prgm
263 Alden St
Springfield, MA 01109-3797
Prgm Dir: Katherine M Post, PhD OTR/L FAOTA
Tel: 413 748-3785   *Fax:* 413 748-3796
E-mail: kpost@spfldcol.edu

Worcester State College
Occupational Therapy Prgm
486 Chandler St
Worcester, MA 01602-2597
Prgm Dir: Joanne Gallagher, EdD OTR/L
Tel: 508 929-8783   *Fax:* 508 929-8178
E-mail: Joanne.Gallagher@worcester.edu

Michigan

Wayne State University
Occupational Therapy Prgm
Eugene Applebaum College of Pharmacy and Health
    Sciences
259 Mack Ave
Detroit, MI 48202-3489
www.wayne.edu
Prgm Dir: Joseph M Pellerito, Jr, MS OTR
Tel: 313 577-1435   *Fax:* 313 577-5822
E-mail: pellerito@wayne.edu

Baker College Center of Graduate Studies
Occupational Therapy Prgm
1116 W Bristol Rd
Flint, MI 48507-5508
www.baker.edu
Prgm Dir: JoAnne Crain, PhD OTR
Tel: 810 766-4298   *Fax:* 810 766-2003
E-mail: joanne.crain@baker.edu

Grand Valley State University
Occupational Therapy Prgm
School of Health Professions
301 Michigan St NE, Ste 200
Grand Rapids, MI 49503-3314
Prgm Dir: Nancy J Powell, PhD OTR FAOTA
Tel: 616 331-3356   *Fax:* 616 895-3350
E-mail: powellna@gvsu.edu

Western Michigan University
Occupational Therapy Prgm
1903 W Michigan Ave
Kalamazoo, MI 49008-5333
www.wmich.edu/hhs/ot
Prgm Dir: Cindee Quake-Rapp, PhD OTR
Tel: 269 387-7263   *Fax:* 269 387-7262
E-mail: cindee.quake-rapp@wmich.edu

Saginaw Valley State University
Occupational Therapy Prgm
Brown Hall 232
7400 Bay Rd
University Center, MI 48710-0001
Prgm Dir: Janet Nagayda, OTD MS OTR
Tel: 989 964-7353   *Fax:* 989 964-7325
E-mail: jnagayda@svsu.edu

Eastern Michigan University
Occupational Therapy Prgm
School of Health Sciences
315 Marshall Hall
Ypsilanti, MI 48197-2239
www.emich.edu
Prgm Dir: Judith A Olson, PhD OTR
Tel: 734 487-2280   *Fax:* 734 487-4095
E-mail: judy.olson@emich.edu

Minnesota

College of St Scholastica
Occupational Therapy Prgm
1200 Kenwood Ave
Duluth, MN 55811-4199
www.css.edu
Prgm Dir: Carolyn Dorfman, PhD OTR/L
Tel: 218 723-6697   *Fax:* 218 723-6472
E-mail: cdorfman@css.edu

University of Minnesota - Minneapolis
Occupational Therapy Prgm
MMC 368
420 Delaware St SE
Minneapolis, MN 55455-0392
www.ot.umn.edu
Prgm Dir: Peggy Martin, MS OTR/L
Tel: 612 626-4358   *Fax:* 612 625-7192
E-mail: marti370@umn.edu

College of St Catherine - St Paul
Occupational Therapy Prgm
2004 Randolph Ave, Mail 4092
St Paul, MN 55105-1794
Prgm Dir: Mary Lou Henderson, MS OTR/L FAOTA
Tel: 612 690-6622   *Fax:* 612 690-8804
E-mail: mlhenderson@stkate.edu

Mississippi

University of Mississippi Medical Center
Occupational Therapy Prgm
2500 N State St
Jackson, MS 39216-4505
www.shrp.umsmed.edu
Prgm Dir: Bette A Groat, MA OTR/L
Tel: 601 984-6350   *Fax:* 601 815-1717
E-mail: bgroat@shrp.umsmed.edu

Missouri

University of Missouri - Columbia
Occupational Therapy Prgm
407 Lewis Hall
Columbia, MO 65211-4240
Prgm Dir: Guy L McCormack, Phd OTR/L FAOTA
Tel: 573 882-4183   *Fax:* 573 884-2610
E-mail: mccormackg@health.missouri.edu

Rockhurst University
Occupational Therapy Prgm
1100 Rockhurst Rd
Kansas City, MO 64110-2561
Prgm Dir: Kris M Vacek, OTD OTR/L
Tel: 816 501-4819   *Fax:* 816 501-4643
E-mail: kris.vacek@rockhurst.edu

Maryville University
Occupational Therapy Prgm
650 Maryville University Dr
St Louis, MO 63141
Prgm Dir: Paula C Bohr, PhD OTR/L FAOTA
Tel: 314 529-9682   *Fax:* 314 529-9191
E-mail: pbohr@maryville.edu

Saint Louis University
Occupational Therapy Prgm
Doisy College of Health Sciences
3437 Caroline St, Rm 2020
St Louis, MO 63104-1111
Prgm Dir: Karen Barney, PhD OTR/L FAOTA
Tel: 314 977-8514   *Fax:* 314 977-5414
E-mail: barneykf@slu.edu

Washington University
Occupational Therapy Prgm
School of Medicine, 4444 Forest Park Ave
Campus Box 8505
St Louis, MO 63108
www.ot.wustl.edu
Prgm Dir: M Carolyn Baum, PhD OTR/L FAOTA
Tel: 314 286-1600   *Fax:* 314 286-1601
E-mail: baumc@msnotes.wustl.edu

Nebraska

College of Saint Mary
Occupational Therapy Prgm
7000 Mercy Rd
Omaha, NE 68106-2606
Prgm Dir: Kristin Haas, OTD OTR/L
Tel: 402 384-5281   *Fax:* 402 399-2654
E-mail: khaas@csm.edu

Creighton University
Occupational Therapy Prgm
School of Pharmacy and Health Professions
2500 California Plaza
Omaha, NE 68178-0259
http://ot.creigton.edu
Prgm Dir: Brenda M Coppard, PhD OTR/L
Tel: 402 280-5932   *Fax:* 402 280-5692
E-mail: bcoppard@creighton.edu

Nevada

Touro University - Nevada
Occupational Therapy Prgm
874 American Pacific Dr
Henderson, NV 89014
www.tu.edu
Prgm Dir: Karen Picus, EdD OTR/L
Tel: 702 777-1811   *Fax:* 702 777-1825
E-mail: kpicus@touro.edu

New Hampshire

University of New Hampshire
Occupational Therapy Prgm
Sch of Health and Human Services
Hewitt Hall, 4 Library Way
Durham, NH 03824-3563
Prgm Dir: Shelley Mulligan, PhD OTR/L
Tel: 603 862-3528   *Fax:* 603 862-0778
E-mail: shelleym@cisunix.unh.edu

New Jersey

Richard Stockton College of New Jersey
Occupational Therapy Prgm
PO Box 195
Jim Leeds Rd
Pomona, NJ 08240-0195
www.stockton.edu
Prgm Dir: Victoria Schindler, PhD OTR/L BCMH FAOTA
Tel: 609 652-4687   *Fax:* 609 652-4858
E-mail: victoria.schindler@stockton.edu

Seton Hall University
Occupational Therapy Prgm
School of Graduate Medical Education
McQuaid Hall
South Orange, NJ 07079-2689
www.shu.edu/academics/gradmed/
   ms-occupational-therapy/
Prgm Dir: Ruth Segal, PhD OTR
Tel: 973 275-2443   *Fax:* 973 275-2370
E-mail: segalrut@shu.edu

Kean University
Occupational Therapy Prgm
1000 Morris Ave
PO Box 411
Union, NJ 07083-9982
www.kean.edu/~ot
Prgm Dir: Laurie Knis-Matthews, PhD
Tel: 908 737-3380   *Fax:* 908 737-3377
E-mail: lknis@kean.edu

New Mexico

University of New Mexico
Occupational Therapy Prgm
School of Medicine
Health Science & Service Bldg Rm 215 MSC09 5240
Albuquerque, NM 87131-0001
Prgm Dir: L Diane Parham, PhD OTR/L FAOTA
Tel: 505 272-8454   *Fax:* 505 272-3583
E-mail: diparham@salud.unm.edu

New York

Touro College - Bay Shore
Occupational Therapy Prgm
1700 Union Blvd
Bay Shore, NY 11706
www.touro.edu
Prgm Dir: Vera-Jean Clark-Brown, MS OTR/L
Tel: 631 665-1600, Ext 231   *Fax:* 631 665-6084
E-mail: vjclark-brown@touro.edu

Long Island University - Brooklyn Campus
Occupational Therapy Prgm
One University Plaza
Brooklyn, NY 11201-5372
www.brooklyn.liu.edu/health/bsmsoccthe.html
Prgm Dir: Ann Burkhardt, OTD OTR/L FAOTA
Tel: 718 780-4332   *Fax:* 718 780-4535
E-mail: ann.burkhardt@liu.edu

SUNY Downstate Medical Center
Occupational Therapy Prgm
Coll of Health Related Professions
450 Clarkson Ave Box 81
Brooklyn, NY 11203-2098
Prgm Dir: Joyce Sabari, PhD OTR BCN FAOTA
Tel: 718 270-7731   *Fax:* 718 270-7464
E-mail: joyce.sabari@downstate.edu

D'Youville College
Occupational Therapy Prgm
One D'Youville Sq, 320 Porter Ave
Buffalo, NY 14201-1084
www.dyc.edu
Prgm Dir: Merlene C Gingher, EdD OT
Tel: 716 829-7830   *Fax:* 716 829-8137
E-mail: gingherm@dyc.edu

University at Buffalo - SUNY
Occupational Therapy Prgm
515 Stockton Kimball Tower
3435 Main St
Buffalo, NY 14214-3079
http://phhp.buffalo.edu/rs/ot/
Prgm Dir: Susan M Nochajski, PhD OTR
Tel: 716 829-6942   *Fax:* 716 829-3217
E-mail: nochajsk@buffalo.edu

Mercy College
Occupational Therapy Prgm
555 Broadway
Dobbs Ferry, NY 10522-1134
Prgm Dir: Joan Toglia, PhD OTR
Tel: 914 674-7815   *Fax:* 914 674-7840
E-mail: jtoglia@mercy.edu

Ithaca College
Occupational Therapy Prgm
206 Smiddy Hall
Ithaca, NY 14850
Prgm Dir: Carol White Dennis, ScD OTR/L
Tel: 607 274-1057   *Fax:* 607 274-3055
E-mail: cdennis@ithaca.edu

CUNY York College
Occupational Therapy Prgm
94-20 Guy R Brewer Blvd
Jamaica, NY 11451-9902
Prgm Dir: Andrea Krauss, DSW OTR/L BCP
Tel: 718 262-2727   *Fax:* 718 262-2767
E-mail: akrauss@york.cuny.edu

Keuka College
Occupational Therapy Prgm
141 Central Ave
Keuka Park, NY 14478
www.keuka.edu
Prgm Dir: Vickie Smith, EdD MBA OTR/L
Tel: 315 279-5666   *Fax:* 315 279-5439
E-mail: vlsmith@mail.keuka.edu

Columbia University
Occupational Therapy Prgm
Neurological Institute 8th Fl
710 W 168th St
New York, NY 10032-2603
www.columbiaot.org
Prgm Dir: Janet Falk-Kessler, EdD OTR FAOTA
Tel: 212 305-5267   *Fax:* 212 305-4569
E-mail: jf6@columbia.edu

New York University
Occupational Therapy Prgm
Steinhardt School of Culture, Education and Human
   Develpment
35 W 4th St, 11th Fl
New York, NY 10012-1172
www.steinhardt.nyu.edu/ot/
Prgm Dir: Jane Bear-Lehman, PhD OTR FAOTA
Tel: 212 998-5825   *Fax:* 212 995-4044
E-mail: jbl285@nyu.edu

Touro College - Manhattan
Occupational Therapy Prgm
27-33 W 23rd St
New York, NY 10010
www.touro.edu
Prgm Dir: Vera-Jean Clark-Brown, MS OTR/L
Tel: 212 463-0400, Ext 691   *Fax:* 631 665-6084
E-mail: vjclark-brown@touro.edu

New York Institute of Technology
Occupational Therapy Prgm
Department of Occupational Therapy
PO Box 8000
Old Westbury, NY 11568-8000
www.nyit.edu
Prgm Dir: Hermine Plotnick, MA OTR/L
Tel: 516 686-3865   *Fax:* 516 686-3795
E-mail: hplotnic@nyit.edu

Dominican College
Occupational Therapy Prgm
470 Western Hwy
Orangeburg, NY 10962-1299
www.dc.edu
Prgm Dir: Sandra F Countee, PhD OTR/L
Tel: 845 359-7800, Ext 6039   *Fax:* 845 398-4893
E-mail: sandra.countee@dc.edu

Stony Brook University
Occupational Therapy Prgm
Sch of Health Tech and Management
Div of Rehabilitation Sciences
Stony Brook, NY 11794-8201
Prgm Dir: Donna Costa, DHS OTR/L
Tel: 631 444-8126   *Fax:* 631 444-6305
E-mail: Donna.Costa@stonybrook.edu

The Sage Colleges
Occupational Therapy Prgm
45 Ferry St
Troy, NY 12180-4115
www.sage.edu/ot
Prgm Dir: Wendy Krupnick, PhD OTR/L
Tel: 518 244-2267   *Fax:* 518 244-4524
E-mail: krupnw@sage.edu

Utica College
Occupational Therapy Prgm
1600 Burrstone Rd
Utica, NY 13502-4892
Prgm Dir: Saly C Townsend, PhD OTR
Tel: 315 792-3239   *Fax:* 315 792-3248
E-mail: stownsend@utica.edu

North Carolina

University of North Carolina - Chapel Hill
Occupational Therapy Prgm
Ste 2050 Bondurant Hall, 301A S Columbia St
CB #7122
Chapel Hill, NC 27599-7120
Prgm Dir: Virginia A Dickie, PhD OTR/L FAOTA
Tel: 919 843-4465   *Fax:* 919 966-9007
E-mail: vdickie@med.unc.edu

East Carolina University
Occupational Therapy Prgm
School of Allied Hlth Sciences
3305 Health Sciences Building
Greenville, NC 27858-4353
www.ecu.edu/ot
Prgm Dir: Leonard G Trujillo, PhD OTR/L
Tel: 252 477-6195   *Fax:* 252 477-6990
E-mail: trujillol@ecu.edu

Lenoir-Rhyne College
Occupational Therapy Prgm
Box 7547
Hickory, NC 28603-7547
Prgm Dir: Toni S Oakes, EdD OTR/L
Tel: 828 328-7366   *Fax:* 828 328-7364
E-mail: oakest@lrc.edu

Winston-Salem State University
Occupational Therapy Prgm
School of Health Sciences
601 Martin Luther King Jr Dr
Winston-Salem, NC 27110-0003
www.wssu.edu
Prgm Dir: Dorothy Bethea, EdD OTR/L
Tel: 336 750-3177, Ext 3172   *Fax:* 336 750-3173
E-mail: betheadp@wssu.edu

North Dakota

University of Mary
Occupational Therapy Prgm
7500 University Dr
Bismarck, ND 58504-9652
Prgm Dir: Janeene Sibla, OTD MS OTR/L
Tel: 701 255-7500, Ext 8212   *Fax:* 701 255-7687
E-mail: jsibla@umary.edu

University of North Dakota
Occupational Therapy Prgm
Box 7126
Grand Forks, ND 58202-7126
Prgm Dir: Janet S Jedlicka, PhD OTR/L
Tel: 701 777-2209   *Fax:* 701 777-2212
E-mail: jjedlicka@medicine.nodak.edu

Ohio

Xavier University
Occupational Therapy Prgm
3800 Victory Pkwy
Cincinnati, OH 45207-7341
www.xavier.edu/ot_grad
Prgm Dir: Carol Scheerer, EdD OTR/L
Tel: 513 745-3310   *Fax:* 513 745-3261
E-mail: scheerer@xavier.edu

Cleveland State University
Occupational Therapy Prgm
2121 Euclid Ave
Health Sciences (HS) 101
Cleveland, OH 44115-2440
http://sciences.csuohio.edu/departments/health/
Prgm Dir: Glenn Goodman, PhD OTR/L
Tel: 216 687-2493   *Fax:* 216 687-9316
E-mail: g.goodman@csuohio.edu

Ohio State University
Occupational Therapy Prgm
453 West 10th St
406 Atwell Hall
Columbus, OH 43210-1234
www.amp.osu.edu/ot
Prgm Dir: Jane Case-Smith, EdD OTR/L FAOTA
Tel: 614 292-0357   *Fax:* 614 292-0210
E-mail: jane.case-smith@osumc.edu

University of Findlay College of Health Professions
Occupational Therapy Prgm
1000 N Main St
Findlay, OH 45840-3695
www.findlay.edu
Prgm Dir: Cynthia Goodwin, MS OTR/L
Tel: 419 434-4083   *Fax:* 419 434-4083
E-mail: goodwin@findlay.edu

Shawnee State University
Occupational Therapy Prgm
940 Second St
Portsmouth, OH 45662-4303
Prgm Dir: Debra S Scurlock, MOT OTR/L
Tel: 740 351-3272   *Fax:* 740 351-3354
E-mail: DScurlock@Shawnee.edu

University of Toledo
Occupational Therapy Prgm
3000 Arlington Ave
Mail Stop 1027
Toledo, OH 43614-2598
http://hsc.utoledo.edu/healthsciences/ot
Prgm Dir: Julie J Thomas, PhD OTR/L FAOTA
Tel: 419 383-5068   *Fax:* 419 383-5880
E-mail: JulieJ.Thomas@UToledo.edu

Oklahoma

Univ of Oklahoma Health Sciences Center
Occupational Therapy Prgm
801 NE 13th St
Oklahoma City, OK 73104-2512
Prgm Dir: Cyndy Robinson, MS OTR/L
Tel: 405 271-2411, Ext 47139   *Fax:* 405 271-2432
E-mail: cyndy-robinson@ouhsc.edu

Univ of Oklahoma Health Sciences Center - Tulsa
Cosponsor: Univ of Oklahoma at Schusterman
Occupational Therapy Prgm
4502 E 41st St
Tulsa, OK 74135-5072
Prgm Dir: Cyndy Robinson, MS OTR/L
Tel: 405 271-2131, Ext 47139   *Fax:* 405 271-2432
E-mail: cyndy-robinson@ouhsc.edu

Oregon

Pacific University
Occupational Therapy Prgm
222 SE 8th Ave, Ste 363
Hillsboro, OR 97123
www.pacificu.edu/ot/
Prgm Dir: John A White, Jr, PhD OTR
Tel: 503 352-7360, Ext 7360   *Fax:* 503 352-7360
E-mail: whiteja@pacificu.edu

Pennsylvania

Misericordia Unversity
Occupational Therapy Prgm
Division of Health Sciences
301 Lake St
Dallas, PA 18612-1098
Prgm Dir: Grace S Fisher, EdD OTR/L
Tel: 570 674-8015   *Fax:* 570 674-3052
E-mail: gfisher@misericordia.edu

Elizabethtown College
Occupational Therapy Prgm
One Alpha Dr
Elizabethtown, PA 17022-2298
Prgm Dir: Nancy Carlson, PhD OTR/L
Tel: 717 361-1995   *Fax:* 717 361-1176
E-mail: carlsona@etown.edu

Gannon University
Occupational Therapy Prgm
109 University Square
Erie, PA 16541-0001
Prgm Dir: Jeffrey L Boss, MS OTR/L
Tel: 814 871-5670   *Fax:* 814 871-7759
E-mail: boss001@gannon.edu

St Francis University
Occupational Therapy Prgm
PO Box 600
Loretto, PA 15940-0600
www.francis.edu
Prgm Dir: Donald E Walkovich, DHSc MS OTR/L
Tel: 814 472-3899   *Fax:* 814 472-3950
E-mail: dwalkovich@francis.edu

Philadelphia University
Occupational Therapy Prgm
School House Ln and Henry Ave
Philadelphia, PA 19144-5497
www.philau.edu/ot
Prgm Dir: Catherine Verrier Piersol, MS OTR/L
Tel: 215 951-2911   *Fax:* 215 951-2526
E-mail: piersolc@philau.edu

Temple University
Occupational Therapy Prgm
College of Health Professions
3307 N Broad St
Philadelphia, PA 19140-5101
www.temple.edu/ot
Prgm Dir: Moya Kinnealey, PhD OTR/L FAOTA
Tel: 215 707-4881   *Fax:* 215 707-7656
E-mail: moya.kinnealey@temple.edu

Thomas Jefferson University
Occupational Therapy Prgm
Jefferson College of Health Professions
130 S 9th St, Rm 810, Edison Bldg
Philadelphia, PA 19107-5233
Prgm Dir: Janice P Burke, PhD OTR/L FAOTA
Tel: 215 503-9606   *Fax:* 215 503-3499
E-mail: janice.burke@jefferson.edu

University of the Sciences in Philadelphia
Occupational Therapy Prgm
600 S 43rd St, Box 24
Philadelphia, PA 19104-4495
Prgm Dir: Paula Kramer, PhD OTR/L FAOTA
Tel: 215 596-8767   *Fax:* 215 596-8690
E-mail: p.kramer@usip.edu

Chatham University

Occupational Therapy Prgm
Woodland Rd
Pittsburgh, PA 15232-2826
www.chatham.edu/ot
Prgm Dir: Joyce Salls, OTD OTR/L
Tel: 412 365-1177   *Fax:* 412 365-1213
E-mail: salls@chatham.edu

Duquesne University

Occupational Therapy Prgm
Department of Occupational Therapy
Rangos School of Health Sciences Bldg/Rm 234, 600
    Forbes Ave
Pittsburgh, PA 15282-0020
www.healthsciences.duq.edu/ot/othome.html
Prgm Dir: Patricia Crist, PhD OTR/L FAOTA
Tel: 412 396-5945   *Fax:* 412 396-4343
E-mail: crist@duq.edu

University of Pittsburgh

Occupational Therapy Prgm
Sch of Health and Rehab Sciences
5012 Forbes Tower
Pittsburgh, PA 15260
www.shrs.pitt.edu/CMS/Departments/OT.asp
Prgm Dir: Joan C Rogers, PhD OTR/L FAOTA
Tel: 412 383-6621   *Fax:* 412 383-6613
E-mail: jcr@pitt.edu

Alvernia College

Occupational Therapy Prgm
400 St Bernardine St
Reading, PA 19607-1799
www.alvernia.edu
Prgm Dir: Karen Ann Cameron, PhD OTD OTR/L
Tel: 610 796-8386   *Fax:* 610 796-8378
E-mail: karen.cameron@alvernia.edu

University of Scranton

Occupational Therapy Prgm
Leahy Hall
800 Linden St
Scranton, PA 18510-4501
Prgm Dir: Marlene J Morgan, EdD OTR/L
Tel: 570 941-4125   *Fax:* 570 941-4380
E-mail: morganm8@Scranton.edu

Puerto Rico

University of Puerto Rico

Occupational Therapy Prgm
Medical Sciences Campus-SHP
PO Box 365067
San Juan, PR 00936-5067
cprsweb.rcm.upr.edu
Prgm Dir: Dyhalma Irizarry, PhD OTR/L FAOTA
Tel: 787 758-2525, Ext 4200   *Fax:* 787 282-8174
E-mail: dyhalmairizarry@cprs.rcm.upr.edu

South Carolina

Medical University of South Carolina

Occupational Therapy Prgm
151B Rutledge Ave
PO Box 2507965
Charleston, SC 29425
Prgm Dir: Maralynne D Mitcham, PhD OTR/L FAOTA
Tel: 843 792-9734   *Fax:* 843 792-0710
E-mail: mitchamm@musc.edu

South Dakota

University of South Dakota

Occupational Therapy Prgm
414 E Clark St
Vermillion, SD 57069-2390
Prgm Dir: Barbara Brockevelt, PhD OTR/L
Tel: 605 677-5601   *Fax:* 605 677-6581
E-mail: barb.brockevelt@usd.edu

Tennessee

University of Tennessee - Chattanooga

Occupational Therapy Prgm
615 McCallie Ave, Dept 3103
Chattanooga, TN 37403
Prgm Dir: Susan S McDonald, MA OTR/L BCP
Tel: 423 425-2358   *Fax:* 423 425-2380
E-mail: susan-mcdonald@utc.edu

University of Tennessee Health Science Ctr

Occupational Therapy Prgm
College of Allied Health Sciences
930 Madison Ave, Ste 601
Memphis, TN 38163-0002
www.utmem.edu/occ_therapy/home.html
Prgm Dir: Ann Nolen, PsyD OTR
Tel: 901 448-9393   *Fax:* 901 448-7545
E-mail: anolen@utmem.edu

Milligan College

Occupational Therapy Prgm
PO Box 130
Milligan College, TN 37682
www.milligan.edu/msot/
Prgm Dir: Jeff Snodgrass, PhD MPH OTR
Tel: 423 975-8010   *Fax:* 423 975-8019
E-mail: jsnodgrass@milligan.edu

Belmont University

Occupational Therapy Prgm
1900 Belmont Blvd
Nashville, TN 37212-3757
www.belmont.edu/ot
Prgm Dir: Ruth Ford, EdD MSBS OTR/L
Tel: 615 460-6708   *Fax:* 615 460-6475
E-mail: fordr@mail.belmont.edu

Tennessee State University

Occupational Therapy Prgm
College of Health Sciences
3500 John A Merritt Blvd
Nashville, TN 37209-1561
www.tnstate.edu/ot
Prgm Dir: Larry Snyder, PhD OTR/L
Tel: 615 963-5891   *Fax:* 615 963-5956
E-mail: lsnyder@tnstate.edu

Texas

Texas Woman's University - Dallas

Occupational Therapy Prgm
1810 Inwood Rd
Dallas, TX 76204-5648
Prgm Dir: Sally Schultz, PhD OTR FAOTA
Tel: 940 898-2801   *Fax:* 940 898-2806
E-mail: SSchultz@twu.edu

Texas Woman's University - Denton

Occupational Therapy Prgm
Box 425648 TWU Station
Denton, TX 76204-5648
www.twu.edu/ot
Prgm Dir: Sally Schultz, PhD OTR LPC
Tel: 940 898-2801   *Fax:* 940 898-2806
E-mail: sschultz@twu.edu
Notes: Two satellite programs (Dallas and Houston)

Univ of Texas - Pan American

Occupational Therapy Prgm
1201 W University Dr
Edinburg, TX 78541-2999
Prgm Dir: Angela E Scoggin, PhD OTR FAOTA
Tel: 956 381-2475   *Fax:* 956 381-2476
E-mail: ascoggin@utpa.edu

University of Texas at El Paso

Occupational Therapy Prgm
1101 N Campbell St
El Paso, TX 79902-4299
Prgm Dir: Karen P Funk, OTD OTR
Tel: 915 747-8226   *Fax:* 915 747-8211
E-mail: kfunk@utep.edu

University of Texas Medical Branch

Occupational Therapy Prgm
301 University Blvd
Galveston, TX 77555-1142
Prgm Dir: Gretchen V M Stone, PhD OTR FAOTA
Tel: 409 747-1628   *Fax:* 409 747-1615
E-mail: grstone@utmb.edu

Texas Woman's University - Houston

Occupational Therapy Prgm
1130 John Freeman Blvd
Houston, TX 77030-2897
Prgm Dir: Sally Schultz, PhD OTR FAOTA
E-mail: SSchultz@twu.edu

Texas Tech Univ Health Sciences Center

Occupational Therapy Prgm
3601 4th St, Stop 6220
Lubbock, TX 79430-6220
www.ttuhsc.edu
Prgm Dir: Dawndra Scott, PhD OTR
Tel: 806 743-3240   *Fax:* 806 743-6005
E-mail: Dawndra.Scott@ttuhsc.edu

Univ of Texas Hlth Sci Ctr at San Antonio

Occupational Therapy Prgm
Department of Occupational Therapy
7703 Floyd Curl Dr
San Antonio, TX 78229-3900
www.uthscsa.edu/ot2/
Prgm Dir: Karin J Barnes, PhD OTR
Tel: 210 567-8890   *Fax:* 210 567-8893
E-mail: barnesk@uthscsa.edu
Notes: Currently inactive

Utah

University of Utah

Occupational Therapy Prgm
520 Wakara Way
Salt Lake City, UT 84108-1290
https://www.health.utah.edu/octh
Prgm Dir: JoAnne Wright, PhD OTR/L CLVT
Tel: 801 585-9135   *Fax:* 801 585-1001
E-mail: jwright@hsc.utah.edu

Virginia

James Madison University

Occupational Therapy Prgm
Department of Health Sciences
Coll of Integrated Sci & Tech, MSC 4301
Harrisonburg, VA 22807-0001
Prgm Dir: Jeffrey D Loveland, OTD MS OTR/L
Tel: 540 568-8170   *Fax:* 540 568-3336
E-mail: lovelajd@jmu.edu

Virginia Commonwealth Univ/Health System

Occupational Therapy Prgm
PO Box 980008
1000 E Marshall St
Richmond, VA 23298-0008
www.sahp.vcu.edu/occu/
Prgm Dir: Shelly J Lane, PhD OTR/L FAOTA
Tel: 804 828-2219   *Fax:* 804 828-0782
E-mail: sjlane@vcu.edu

Jefferson College of Health Sciences
Occupational Therapy Prgm
920 S Jefferson St
Roanoke, va 24016
Prgm Dir: David A Haynes, MBA OTR/L
Tel: 540 985-4020   *Fax:* 540 985-9773
E-mail: dhaynes@jchs.edu

Shenandoah University
Occupational Therapy Prgm
333 W Cork St, 5th Fl
Ste 510
Winchester, VA 22601-5195
www.su.edu/ot/
Prgm Dir: Deborah Marr, ScD OTR/L
Tel: 540 678-4312   *Fax:* 540 665-5564
E-mail: dmarr@su.edu

Washington

University of Washington
Occupational Therapy Prgm
Department of Rehabilitation Medicine
Box 356490
Seattle, WA 98195-6490
http://depts.washington.edu/rehab/ot/
Prgm Dir: Elizabeth M Kanny, PhD OTR/L FAOTA
Tel: 206 598-5393   *Fax:* 206 685-3244
E-mail: ekanny@u.washington.edu

Eastern Washington University
Occupational Therapy Prgm
310 N Riverpoint Blvd
Box R
Spokane, WA 99004
www.ewu.edu/ot
Prgm Dir: Greg Wintz, PhD OTR/L
Tel: 509 368-6562   *Fax:* 509 368-6561
E-mail: gwintz@mail.ewu.edu

University of Puget Sound
Occupational Therapy Prgm
School of Occupational Therapy
1500 N Warner St #1070
Tacoma, WA 98416-1070
www.ups.edu/ot
Prgm Dir: George Tomlin, PhD OTR/L
Tel: 253 879-3522   *Fax:* 253 879-2933
E-mail: tomlin@ups.edu

West Virginia

West Virginia University
Occupational Therapy Prgm
School of Medicine, Robert C Byrd Health Sciences Center
PO Box 9139
Morgantown, WV 26506-9139
www.hsc.wvu.edu/som/ot
Prgm Dir: Randy P McCombie, PhD OTR/L
Tel: 304 293-8828   *Fax:* 304 293-7105
E-mail: rmccombie@hsc.wvu.edu

Wisconsin

University of Wisconsin - La Crosse
Occupational Therapy Prgm
4031 Health Science Ctr
1725 State St
La Crosse, WI 54601-9959
www.uwlax.edu/ot
Prgm Dir: Peggy Denton, PhD OTR FAOTA
Tel: 608 785-5059   *Fax:* 608 785-6647
E-mail: denton.pegg@uwlax.edu

University of Wisconsin - Madison
Occupational Therapy Prgm
1300 University Ave, 2110 MSC
Madison, WI 53706-1532
www.soemadison.wisc.edu/kinesiology/
Prgm Dir: Mary Schneider, PhD OTR/L
Tel: 608 262-2936   *Fax:* 608 262-1639
E-mail: schneider@education.wisc.edu

Concordia University Wisconsin
Occupational Therapy Prgm
12800 N Lake Shore Dr
Mequon, WI 53092-2402
Prgm Dir: Linda Samuel, PhD OTR
Tel: 262 243-4469   *Fax:* 262 243-4506
E-mail: linda.samuel@cuw.edu

Mount Mary College
Occupational Therapy Prgm
2900 N Menomonee River Pkwy
Milwaukee, WI 53222-4597
Prgm Dir: Jane Olson, PhD OTR
Tel: 414 256-1246   *Fax:* 414 256-0194
E-mail: olsonj@mtmary.edu

University of Wisconsin - Milwaukee
Occupational Therapy Prgm
College of Health Sciences
PO Box 413
Milwaukee, WI 53201-0413
www.uwm.edu/CHS
Prgm Dir: Phyllis King, PhD OT FAOTA
Tel: 414 229-5616   *Fax:* 414 229-5100
E-mail: pking@uwm.edu

Wyoming

University of North Dakota at Casper College
Occupational Therapy Prgm
125 College Dr
Casper, WY 82601-9958
Prgm Dir: Janet S Jedlicka, PhD OTR/L
Tel: 701 777-2217   *Fax:* 701 777-2212
E-mail: jjedlicka@medicine.nodak.edu

Occupational Therapist

Programs*	Class Capacity	Begins	Length (months)	Award	Res. Tuition	Non-res. Tuition	Stipend	Offers:‡ 1	2	3	4
Alabama											
Alabama State University (Montgomery)	5	Jun	30	MS	$2,004	$4,008				•	
Tuskegee University	20+	Aug	24	MS	$13,520	$13,520				•	•
University of South Alabama (Mobile)	25	Aug	27	MS	$5,960	$11,920				•	
Arizona											
Midwestern University - Glendale Campus	35	Aug Sep	27	MOT	$25,436	$25,436				•	
Arkansas											
University of Central Arkansas (Conway)	48	May	37	MS	$6,205	$11,035				•	
California											
California State University - Dominguez Hills (Carson)	48	Jan	27	MSOT	$3,301	$12,832		•		•	
Loma Linda University	30	Jun	33	MOT	$19,720	$19,720				•	
San Jose State University	40	Aug	36, 25	BS, MS	$2,900	$0				•	•
University of Southern California (Los Angeles)	110	Jun	18, 27	BS, MA	$44,692	$44,692				•	
Colorado											
Colorado State University (Fort Collins)	40	Aug	24	Dipl, MS	$6,208	$17,764				•	
Florida											
Barry University (Miami Shores)	25	Aug	30	MS	$765	$0		•		•	
Florida A&M University (Tallahassee)	25	Aug	33	MS	$2,383	$8,591				•	
Florida Gulf Coast University (Fort Myers)	24	Aug	23	MS	$239	$892				•	
Florida International University (Miami)	70	Aug	39, 27	BS/MS, MS	$3,043	$16,252				•	
Nova Southeastern University (Fort Lauderdale)	45	Jun	28	MOT, OTD Ph	$17,735	$19,880				•	
University of Florida (Gainesville)	45	May Aug	15, 18	MOT	$7,170	$23,880				•	
Georgia											
Brenau University (Gainesville)	32	Aug	33	BS, MS	$24,990	$24,990				•	

*Data are shown only for programs that completed the 2007 AMA Survey of Health Professions Education Programs.
‡Key to Offers: 1: Evening or weekend classes; 2: Non-English instruction; 3: Cultural competence instruction; 4: Distance education component.

Occupational Therapist

Programs*	Class Capacity	Begins	Length (months)	Award	Res. Tuition	Non-res. Tuition	Stipend	Offers:‡ 1	2	3	4
Medical College of Georgia (Augusta)	40	Aug	28, 36	MHS	$9,990	$16,122			•	•	
Illinois											
Midwestern University (Downers Grove)	35	Sep	27	MOT	$25,000	$27,000				•	
Rush University (Chicago)	25	Jun	27	MS	$21,000	$21,000				•	
University of Illinois at Chicago	30	Aug	24, 48	Dipl, MS	$17,000	$31,846					
Indiana											
University of Indianapolis	51	Aug	30	MOT	$21,785	$21,785				•	
University of Southern Indiana (Evansville)	30	Aug	32, 12	Dipl, BS, MS	$5,446	$13,342				•	
Iowa											
St Ambrose University (Davenport)	30	Sep	29	MOT	$21,500	$0					
Kansas											
University of Kansas Medical Center (Kansas City)	32	Jun	36, 45	Dipl, MOT, OTD	$6,256	$15,183					•
Louisiana											
Louisiana State U Hlth Sci Ctr - Shreveport	20	Summer	27	MOT	$5,121	$8,246				•	
Louisiana State Univ Health Sciences Center (New Orleans)	30	Jan	27	MOT	$4,018	$7,143				•	
Maine											
Husson College (Bangor)	24	Sep Jan	46	MSOT	$15,000	$0		•		•	
University of New England (Biddeford)	42	Sep	60	MSOT, MSPPOT	$24,440	$24,440				•	
University of Southern Maine - Lewiston/Auburn	24	Sep	27	MOT	$200	$560				•	
Maryland											
Towson University	40	Sep	37, 30	BS/MS, MS	$7,234	$17,174		•		•	
Massachusetts											
Bay Path College (Longmeadow)	40	Aug	24	BS, MOT	$18,000	$0				•	
Boston University/Sargent College	50	Sep	66, 30	BSMSOT, MSOT	$34,930	$34,930				•	
Salem State College	20	Jun	48, 72	BS, BS/MS				•		•	•
Tufts University (Medford)	45	Sep Jan	21	MS MA	$25,254	$25,254				•	
Worcester State College	40	Sep	48, 12	BSOS, MOT	$4,123	$10,203				•	
Michigan											
Baker College Center of Graduate Studies (Flint)	50	Apr Sep	46	MOT	$8,840	$8,840				•	
Eastern Michigan University (Ypsilanti)	45	Sep	30	MOT, MS	$8,172	$16,104		•		•	
Wayne State University (Detroit)	30	Sep	30, 16	Dipl, MOT	$14,668	$31,257		•		•	
Western Michigan University (Kalamazoo)	64	Sep Jan	28	BS/MS	$4,657	$10,109		•		•	
Minnesota											
College of St Scholastica (Duluth)	32	Sep	28	MA	$24,840	$24,840				•	
University of Minnesota - Minneapolis	37	Sep	24	MOT	$13,643	$24,053				•	•
Mississippi											
University of Mississippi Medical Center (Jackson)	38	May	36	MOT	$6,905	$15,850				•	
Missouri											
Maryville University (St Louis)	35	Aug	48	MOT	$18,600	$18,600				•	
Washington University (St Louis)	60	Aug	28, 40	MSOT, OTD	$20,515	$20,515				•	
Nebraska											
Creighton University (Omaha)	45	Aug	40	OTD	$17,600	$0				•	
Nevada											
Touro University - Nevada (Henderson)	34	Jul 9	24	MS	$22,000	$22,000				•	
New Hampshire											
University of New Hampshire (Durham)	60	Sep	58, 21	Dipl, BS/MS, MS	$9,778	$21,498					
New Jersey											
Kean University (Union)	30	Sep	26	MS	$11,108	$13,508		•		•	
Richard Stockton College of New Jersey (Pomona)	20	Sep	30	MSOT	$16,000	$19,000				•	
Seton Hall University (South Orange)	30	Sep	36	MSOT	$23,128	$23,128				•	
New York											
Columbia University (New York)	45	Sep	24, 36	MS	$30,112	$0				•	
D'Youville College (Buffalo)	215	Aug	44, 26	BS/MS, MS	$17,600	$17,600				•	
Dominican College (Orangeburg)	32	Sep	24, 36	BS/MS	$8,775	$0		•			
Keuka College (Keuka Park)	30	Sep	36, 12	BS, MS	$18,850	$18,850				•	
Long Island University - Brooklyn Campus	30	Sep	36	BS/MS	$729	$0				•	
New York Institute of Technology (Old Westbury)	40	May	33, 66	BS/MS, MS	$20,000	$20,000				•	
New York University	50	Sep	30, 48	MS							
The Sage Colleges (Troy)	24	Aug	27	MS	$670	$670	$6,000			•	
Touro College - Bay Shore	30	Sep	34	BS HS, MSOT	$19,500	$19,500				•	
Touro College - Manhattan (New York)	35	Jan	34	BS HS, MSOT	$19,500	$19,500				•	
University at Buffalo - SUNY	40	May	60, 24	BS/MS, MS	$5,861	$11,811				•	
North Carolina											
East Carolina University (Greenville)	20	Aug	28	MS	$1,000	$4,453					
Winston-Salem State University	30	Aug	24	BSOT, MSOT	$4,909	$9,204		•		•	

*Data are shown only for programs that completed the 2007 AMA Survey of Health Professions Education Programs.
‡Key to Offers: 1: Evening or weekend classes; 2: Non-English instruction; 3: Cultural competence instruction; 4: Distance education component.

Programs*	Class Capacity	Begins	Length (months)	Award	Res. Tuition	Non-res. Tuition	Stipend	Offers:‡ 1	2	3	4
North Dakota											
University of Mary (Bismarck)	30	Sep	40	MS	$12,000	$12,000				•	
University of North Dakota (Grand Forks)	36	May	32	MOT	$10,080	$13,698				•	
Ohio											
Cleveland State University	30	Aug	28	MOT	$17,130	$32,535				•	
Ohio State University (Columbus)	40	Jun	27	MOT	$10,050	$23,403					
University of Findlay College of Health Professions	32	Sep	65, 36	BS/MOT	$19,000	$0		•		•	
University of Toledo	20	Aug	32	OTD	$13,104	$24,852		•		•	
Xavier University (Cincinnati)	30	Aug	33	MOT	$24,660	$24,660				•	
Oregon											
Pacific University (Hillsboro)	31	Aug	31	Dipl, MOT	$21,952	$21,952			•	•	
Pennsylvania											
Alvernia College (Reading)	30	Aug	60	MSOT, BS/MSO	$16,200	$0		•			
Chatham University (Pittsburgh)	44	Aug	22, 16	MOT, OTD	$21,500	$21,500					•
Duquesne University (Pittsburgh)	30	Jan	25, 53	BS, MS	$24,462	$0				•	
Gannon University (Erie)	45	Aug	60, 36	MS	$15,000	$15,000					
Philadelphia University	30	Sep	28	Dipl, MS	$23,000	$23,000		•		•	•
St Francis University (Loretto)	40	Jun	60	MOT							
Temple University (Philadelphia)	35	Jul	24, 36	MOT	$17,848	$24,742				•	
University of Pittsburgh	40	Jun	22	MOT	$20,410	$26,512				•	
Puerto Rico											
University of Puerto Rico (San Juan)	16	Aug	27	MS	$4,010	$4,810			•	•	
South Dakota											
University of South Dakota (Vermillion)	26	Aug	28, 40	MS	$8,658	$25,525		•		•	
Tennessee											
Belmont University (Nashville)	32	Aug	33, 23	OTD, MSOT	$22,740	$22,740		•		•	•
Milligan College	30	Aug	28	MSOT	$16,000	$16,000					
Tennessee State University (Nashville)	30	Aug	26	MOT	$5,868	$15,568		•		•	
University of Tennessee - Chattanooga	10	Aug	26	MOT	$4,000	$5,563					
University of Tennessee Health Science Ctr (Memphis)	30	Jan	27	MOT	$5,169	$17,106					
Texas											
Texas Tech Univ Health Sciences Center (Lubbock)	35	May	30	MOT	$8,500	$20,000				•	
Texas Woman's University - Denton	35	Sep	27, 46	MOT	$13,464	$23,520		•			•
Univ of Texas Hlth Sci Ctr at San Antonio	35	Jun	33	MOT	$1,428	$10,416				•	
Utah											
University of Utah (Salt Lake City)	28	Aug	33	MOT	$13,000	$25,700				•	
Virginia											
James Madison University (Harrisonburg)	20	Jun	30	Dipl, MOT	$8,960	$25,472				•	
Shenandoah University (Winchester)	26	Aug	30, 54	MS	$640	$640				•	•
Virginia Commonwealth Univ/Health System (Richmond)	40	Jun	30, 24	MSOT, MS	$13,326	$26,598					
Washington											
Eastern Washington University (Spokane)	30	Summer	27	BS/MOT, MOT	$8,297	$16,583				•	
University of Puget Sound (Tacoma)	40	Sep	28	MSOT, MOT	$29,000	$29,000				•	
University of Washington (Seattle)	25	Sep	27	Dipl, MOT	$12,092	$27,856				•	
West Virginia											
West Virginia University (Morgantown)	30	Jul	30	Dipl, MOT	$5,356	$16,800		•		•	•
Wisconsin											
University of Wisconsin - La Crosse	24	May	30	MS	$5,049	$17,045				•	
University of Wisconsin - Madison	25	Jun	30, 48	MS OT, MS TS	$8,320	$23,590					
University of Wisconsin - Milwaukee	36	Sep	36	MS	$5,835	$18,587		•		•	•
Wyoming											
University of North Dakota at Casper College	14	May	32	Masters	$12,251	$12,251				•	

*Data are shown only for programs that completed the 2007 AMA Survey of Health Professions Education Programs.
‡Key to Offers: 1: Evening or weekend classes; 2: Non-English instruction; 3: Cultural competence instruction; 4: Distance education component.

Occupational Therapy Assistant

Alabama

Wallace State Community College - Faulkner
Occupational Therapy Asst Prgm
Bay Minette, AL 36507
Prgm Dir: Tammy R Gipson, OTR/L
Tel: 256 352-8334
E-mail: tammy.gipson@wallacestate.edu

Wallace State Community College
Occupational Therapy Asst Prgm
PO Box 2000
Hanceville, AL 35077-2000
Prgm Dir: Tammy R Gipson, OTR/L
Tel: 256 352-8333   *Fax:* 256 352-8183
E-mail: tammy.gipson@wallacestate.edu

Arkansas

South Arkansas Community College
Occupational Therapy Asst Prgm
PO Box 7010
300 S West Ave
El Dorado, AR 71731-7010
Prgm Dir: Sandra Pugh, OTD OTR/L
Tel: 870 862-8131, Ext 227   *Fax:* 870 864-7104
E-mail: spugh@southark.edu

Baptist Health Schools Little Rock
Cosponsor: Pulaski Technical College
Occupational Therapy Asst Prgm
11900 Colonel Glenn Rd
Little Rock, AR 72210-2820
Prgm Dir: Karen L James, MS OTR/L
Tel: 501 202-7243   *Fax:* 501 202-7712
E-mail: karen.james@baptist-health.org

California

Grossmont College
Occupational Therapy Asst Prgm
8800 Grossmont College Dr
El Cajon, CA 92020-1799
Prgm Dir: Christine Vicino, BA COTA
Tel: 619 644-7305   *Fax:* 619 644-7961
E-mail: Christi.Vicino@gcccd.edu

Loma Linda University
Occupational Therapy Asst Prgm
Sch of Allied Health Professions
SAHP-Nichol Hall, Rm A912
Loma Linda, CA 92350-0001
www.llu.edu
Prgm Dir: Karen Pendleton, MA OTR/L
Tel: 909 558-4628   *Fax:* 909 558-0239
E-mail: kpendleton@llu.edu
Notes: Currently inactive

Sacramento City College
Occupational Therapy Asst Prgm
Allied Health Dept
3835 Freeport Blvd
Sacramento, CA 95822-1386
Prgm Dir: Susan M Hussey, MS OTR/L
Tel: 916 558-2297   *Fax:* 916 558-2392
E-mail: husseys@scc.losrios.edu

Santa Ana College
Occupational Therapy Asst Prgm
1530 W 17th St
Santa Ana, CA 92706-3398
Prgm Dir: Michelle Parolise, MBA OTR/L
Tel: 714 564-6833   *Fax:* 714 564-6158
E-mail: parolise_michelle@sac.edu

Colorado

Pueblo Community College
Occupational Therapy Asst Prgm
900 W Orman Ave
Pueblo, CO 81004-1499
Prgm Dir: Tricia Vigil, OTR MBA
Tel: 719 549-3268   *Fax:* 719 549-3381
E-mail: tricia.vigil@pueblocc.edu

Connecticut

Housatonic Community College
Occupational Therapy Asst Prgm
900 Lafayette Blvd
Bridgeport, CT 06604-4704
Prgm Dir: Michele M Reed, MS Ed OTR/L
Tel: 203 332-5214   *Fax:* 203 332-5123
E-mail: mreed@hcc.commnet.edu

Manchester Community College
Occupational Therapy Asst Prgm
PO Box 1046
Great Path MS 17
Manchester, CT 06045-1046
Prgm Dir: Martha Nieman, MS OTR/L
Tel: 860 512-2717   *Fax:* 860 512-2621
E-mail: MNieman@mcc.commnet.edu

Briarwood College
Occupational Therapy Asst Prgm
2279 Mt Vernon Rd
Southington, CT 06489
Prgm Dir: Katherine Krivanec, MA COTA/L
Tel: 860 628-4751, Ext 174   *Fax:* 860 628-6444
E-mail: krivaneck@briarwood.edu

Delaware

Delaware Technical & Community College - Owens Campus
Occupational Therapy Asst Prgm
Owens Campus, PO Box 610
Georgetown, DE 19947-0610
Prgm Dir: Bobbi Butch, MS OTR/L
Tel: 302 855-5932   *Fax:* 302 858-5460
E-mail: bbutch@dtcc.edu

Delaware Technical & Community College - Wilmington
Occupational Therapy Asst Prgm
333 Shipley St
Wilmington, DE 19801-2499
Prgm Dir: Jan Gorecki, MS OTR/L
Tel: 302 888-5298   *Fax:* 302 577-6431
E-mail: jgorecki@dtcc.edu

Florida

Manatee Community College
Occupational Therapy Asst Prgm
5840 26th St W
Bldg 28
Bradenton, FL 34207-7046
www.mccfl.edu/pages/1.asp
Prgm Dir: Debra Chasanoff, MEd OTR/L
Tel: 941 752-5346   *Fax:* 941 727-8304
E-mail: chasand@mccfl.edu

Daytona Beach Community College
Occupational Therapy Asst Prgm
1200 International Speedway Blvd
Daytona Beach, FL 32120-2811
www.dbcc.edu
Prgm Dir: Mary Beth Craig-Oatley, EdM OT/L
Tel: 386 506-3624   *Fax:* 368 506-3300
E-mail: craigom@dbcc.edu

Keiser University
Occupational Therapy Asst Prgm
1500 NW 49th St
Fort Lauderdale, FL 33309
www.keiseruniversity.edu
Prgm Dir: Arlene Kinney, MEd OT/L
Tel: 954 776-4456, Ext 331   *Fax:* 954 776-5157
E-mail: arlenek@keiseruniversity.edu

Keiser University - Melbourne Campus
Occupational Therapy Asst Prgm
900 S Babcock St
Melbourne, FL 32901
Prgm Dir: Rene Nyberg, COTA/L
Tel: 321 409-4800   *Fax:* 321 725-3766
E-mail: rnyberg@keisercollege.edu

Florida Hospital College of Health Sciences
Occupational Therapy Asst Prgm
671 Winyah Dr
Orlando, FL 32803-1235
www.fhchs.edu
Prgm Dir: Tia Hughes, MBA OTR/L
Tel: 407 303-7747, Ext 9855   *Fax:* 407 303-7820
E-mail: tia_hughes@fhchs.edu

Polk Community College
Occupational Therapy Asst Prgm
999 Avenue H NE
Winter Haven, FL 33881-4299
Prgm Dir: Saritza Guzman-Sardina, MEd OTR/L
Tel: 863 297-1010, Ext 5753   *Fax:* 863 297-1047
E-mail: sguzman-sardina@polk.edu

Georgia

Darton College
Occupational Therapy Asst Prgm
2400 Gillionville Rd
Albany, GA 31707-3098
www.darton.edu
Prgm Dir: Stacey R Cowart, MS OTR/L
Tel: 229 317-6908   *Fax:* 229 317-6682
E-mail: stacey.cowart@darton.edu

Augusta Technical College
Occupational Therapy Asst Prgm
3200 Augusta Tech Dr
1400 Building
Augusta, GA 30906-3399
Prgm Dir: Cindy L Loar, MHS OTR/L PTA
Tel: 706 771-4188   *Fax:* 706 771-4181
E-mail: cloar@augustatech.edu

Middle Georgia College
Occupational Therapy Asst Prgm
1100 Second St SE
Cochran, GA 31014-1599
Prgm Dir: Heather Copan, MHE OTR/L
Tel: 478 934-3402   *Fax:* 478 934-3461
E-mail: hcopan@mgc.edu

Northwestern Technical College
Occupational Therapy Asst Prgm
PO Box 569
265 Bicentennial Trail
Rock Spring, GA 30739
www.northwesterntech.edu
Prgm Dir: Lisa Carruth, MSEd OTR/L
Tel: 706 764-3846   *Fax:* 706 764-3718
E-mail: lcarruth@northwesterntech.edu

Hawaii

Kapi'olani Community College
Occupational Therapy Asst Prgm
Health Sciences Dept
4303 Diamond Head Rd, Kauila 210C
Honolulu, HI 96816-4421
Prgm Dir: Shelley Boling, OTR
Tel: 808 734-9229   *Fax:* 808 734-9126
E-mail: boling@hawaii.edu

Illinois

Parkland College
Occupational Therapy Asst Prgm
2400 W Bradley Ave
Champaign, IL 61821-1899
Prgm Dir: Rebecca R Bahnke, MHS OTR/L
Tel: 217 351-2394   *Fax:* 217 373-3830
E-mail: rbahnke@parkland.edu

Wright College
Occupational Therapy Asst Prgm
4300 N Narragansett Ave
Chicago, IL 60634-1591
Prgm Dir: Joyce Wandel, MS OTR/L
Tel: 773 481-8875   *Fax:* 773 481-8892
E-mail: jwandel@ccc.edu

Lewis & Clark Community College
Occupational Therapy Asst Prgm
5800 Godfrey Rd
Godfrey, IL 62035-2466
Prgm Dir: Linda L Orr, MPA OTR/L
Tel: 618 468-4416   *Fax:* 618 468-7811
E-mail: lorr@lc.edu

Southern Illinois Collegiate Common Market
Occupational Therapy Asst Prgm
3213 S Park Ave
Herrin, IL 62948
Prgm Dir: Verlinda Henshaw, OTD OTR/L
Tel: 618 942-6902   *Fax:* 618 942-6658
E-mail: teachota@siccm.com

Illinois Central College
Occupational Therapy Asst Prgm
201 SW Adams St
Peoria, IL 61635-0001
Prgm Dir: Donna Augustyn-Sloan, MS OTR/L
Tel: 309 999-4674   *Fax:* 309 673-9626
E-mail: das@icc.edu

South Suburban College
Occupational Therapy Asst Prgm
15800 S State St
South Holland, IL 60473-1262
Prgm Dir: Cathy M Mistovich, MS OTR/L
Tel: 708 596-2000, Ext 2473   *Fax:* 708 210-5792
E-mail: CMistovich@southsuburbancollege.edu

Lincoln Land Community College
Occupational Therapy Asst Prgm
5250 Shepherd Rd
PO Box 19256
Springfield, IL 62794-9256
www.llcc.edu
Prgm Dir: Ruth J Bixby, OTR/L
Tel: 217 786-2872   *Fax:* 217 786-2824
E-mail: ruth.bixby@llcc.edu

Indiana

University of Southern Indiana
Occupational Therapy Asst Prgm
College of Nursing and Health Professions
8600 University Blvd, HP 2068
Evansville, IN 47712-3534
Prgm Dir: Susan G Ahmad, MS OTR/L
Tel: 812 465-1140   *Fax:* 812 465-7092
E-mail: sahmad@usi.edu

Brown Mackie College
Occupational Therapy Asst Prgm
Fort Wayne Campus
3000 E Coliseum Blvd
Fort Wayne, IN 46802
Prgm Dir: LaNiece Clark, COTA
Tel: 260 484-4400   *Fax:* 260 484-2678
E-mail: laclark@brownmackie.edu

Brown Mackie College
Occupational Therapy Asst Prgm
1030 E Jefferson Blvd
South Bend, IN 46617-3123
Prgm Dir: Michelle Sheperd, MEd OTR
Tel: 574 237-0774   *Fax:* 574 237-3585
E-mail: msheperd@brownmackie.edu

Iowa

Kirkwood Community College
Occupational Therapy Asst Prgm
6301 Kirkwood Blvd SW, PO Box 2068
Cedar Rapids, IA 52406-9973
Prgm Dir: Nichelle Miedema, MPA OTR/L
Tel: 319 398-5566, Ext 4941   *Fax:* 319 398-1293
E-mail: ncline@kirkwood.edu

Kansas

Newman University
Occupational Therapy Asst Prgm
3100 McCormick Ave
Wichita, KS 67213-2097
www.newmanu.edu
Prgm Dir: Clint Stucky, MS MSEd OTR
Tel: 316 942-4291, Ext 2349   *Fax:* 316 942-4483
E-mail: stuckyc@newmanu.edu

Kentucky

Jefferson Community and Technical College
Occupational Therapy Asst Prgm
109 E Broadway St
Louisville, KY 40202-2005
Prgm Dir: Carolyn Thornsberry, OTR/L CLT
Tel: 502 213-2342   *Fax:* 502 213-2343
E-mail: carolyn.thornsberry@kctcs.edu

Madisonville Community College
Occupational Therapy Asst Prgm
750 N Laffoon St
Madisonville, KY 42431-1636
Prgm Dir: Helen M Grothem, MS OTR/L
Tel: 270 824-1742   *Fax:* 270 824-1879
E-mail: helen.grothem@kctcs.edu

Louisiana

University of Louisiana at Monroe
Occupational Therapy Asst Prgm
College of Health Sciences
700 University Ave, Rm 111 Caldwell Hall
Monroe, LA 71209-0430
Prgm Dir: Donna Eichhorn, MEd LOTR
Tel: 318 342-1613   *Fax:* 318 342-5584
E-mail: eichhorn@ulm.edu

Delgado Community College
Occupational Therapy Asst Prgm
City Park Campus
615 City Park Ave
New Orleans, LA 70119-4399
Prgm Dir: Linda Kelly, MA LOTR
Tel: 504 485-2372   *Fax:* 504 483-4609
E-mail: lkelly@dcc.edu

Maine

Kennebec Valley Community College
Occupational Therapy Asst Prgm
92 Western Ave
Fairfield, ME 04937-1367
Prgm Dir: Diane Sauter-Davis, MA OTR/L
Tel: 207 453-5172   *Fax:* 207 453-5194
E-mail: dsauter@kvcc.me.edu

Maryland

Community College of Baltimore County - Catonsville
Occupational Therapy Asst Prgm
800 S Rolling Rd
Catonsville, MD 21228-9987
www.ccbcmd.edu
Prgm Dir: Judith Blum, MS OTR/L
Tel: 410 455-4482   *Fax:* 410 719-6501
E-mail: jblum@ccbcmd.edu

Allegany College of Maryland
Occupational Therapy Asst Prgm
12401 Willowbrook Rd SE
Cumberland, MD 21502-2596
www.allegany.edu
Prgm Dir: Rae Ann Smith, MEd OTR/L
Tel: 301 784-5536   *Fax:* 301 784-5015
E-mail: rasmith@allegany.edu

Massachusetts

North Shore Community College
Occupational Therapy Asst Prgm
One Ferncroft Rd, PO Box 3340
Danvers, MA 01923-0840
www.northshore.edu
Prgm Dir: Maureen S Nardella, MS OTR/L
Tel: 978 762-4176   *Fax:* 978 762-4022
E-mail: mnardell@northshore.edu

Bristol Community College
Occupational Therapy Asst Prgm
777 Elsbree St
Fall River, MA 02720-9960
www.BristolCommunityCollege.edu
Prgm Dir: Johanna Duponte, EdD OTR/L
Tel: 508 678-2811, Ext 2325   *Fax:* 508 730-3281
E-mail: jduponte@bristol.mass.edu

Springfield Technical Community College
Occupational Therapy Asst Prgm
One Armory Sq, Ste 1
PO Box 9000
Springfield, MA 01102-9000
www.stcc.edu
Prgm Dir: Marianne Joyce, MA OTR/L
Tel: 413 755-4881   *Fax:* 413 755-4764
E-mail: mjoyce@stcc.edu

Quinsigamond Community College
Occupational Therapy Asst Prgm
670 W Boylston St
Worcester, MA 01606
www.qcc.mass.edu
Prgm Dir: Brenda Marshall, MA OTR/L
Tel: 508 854-4546   *Fax:* 508 852-6943
E-mail: brendam@qcc.mass.edu

Michigan

Wayne County Community College District
Occupational Therapy Asst Prgm
1001 W Fort St
Detroit, MI 48226-9975
Prgm Dir: Lettie Redley, MS OTR CHSA
Tel: 313 496-2692   *Fax:* 313 496-8723
E-mail: lredley1@wcccd.edu

Mott Community College - Southern Lakes Branch Campus
Occupational Therapy Asst Prgm
2100 W Thompson Rd
Fenton, MI 48430-9798
www.mcc.edu
Prgm Dir: Wendy Blair Early, MS OTR
Tel: 810 762-5018   *Fax:* 810 750-8588
E-mail: wearly@mcc.edu

Grand Rapids Community College
Occupational Therapy Asst Prgm
143 Bostwick St NE
Grand Rapids, MI 49503-3295
Prgm Dir: Karen Walker, MA OTR
Tel: 616 234-4236   *Fax:* 616 234-4317
E-mail: kwalker@grcc.edu

Baker College of Muskegon
Occupational Therapy Asst Prgm
1903 Marquette Ave
Muskegon, MI 49442-1490
Prgm Dir: Matthew Mekkes, MS OTR
Tel: 231 777-5289   *Fax:* 231 777-5291
E-mail: matthew.mekkes@baker.edu

Macomb Community College
Occupational Therapy Asst Prgm
14500 E Twelve Mile Rd
Warren, MI 48088
Prgm Dir: Phyllis Clements, MA OTR
Tel: 586 286-2097   *Fax:* 586 286-2098
E-mail: clementsp@macomb.edu

Minnesota

Anoka Technical College
Occupational Therapy Asst Prgm
1355 W Hwy 10
Anoka, MN 55303-1590
Prgm Dir: Marietta Cosky Saxon, MEd OTR/L
Tel: 763 576-4935   *Fax:* 763 576-4715
E-mail: msaxon@anokatech.edu

Northland Community & Technical College
Occupational Therapy Asst Prgm
2022 Central Ave NE
East Grand Forks, MN 56721-2702
www.northlandcollege.edu
Prgm Dir: Cassie Hilts, MOT OTR/L
Tel: 218 773-3441   *Fax:* 218 773-4502
E-mail: cassie.hilts@northlandcollege.edu

College of St Catherine - Minneapolis
Occupational Therapy Asst Prgm
601 25th Ave S
Minneapolis, MN 55454-1494
www.stkate.edu/ota
Prgm Dir: Marianne F Christiansen, MA OTR/L FAOTA
Tel: 651 690-7772   *Fax:* 651 690-7849
E-mail: mfchristiansen@stkate.edu

Mississippi

Itawamba Community College
Occupational Therapy Asst Prgm
602 W Hill St
Fulton, MS 38843
Prgm Dir: Suzanne Chittom, MS OTR/L
Tel: 662 862-8344   *Fax:* 662 862-8350
E-mail: jschittom@iccms.edu

Pearl River Community College
Occupational Therapy Asst Prgm
5448 US Hwy 49 S
Hattiesburg, MS 39401-7806
Prgm Dir: Tim Pulver, OTR/L
Tel: 601 554-5541   *Fax:* 601 554-5511
E-mail: tpulver@prcc.edu

Holmes Community College
Occupational Therapy Asst Prgm
Ridgeland Campus
412 W Ridgeland Ave
Ridgeland, MS 39157
www.holmescc.edu
Prgm Dir: Sherry Hager, MOTR/L
Tel: 601 605-3337   *Fax:* 601 605-3410
E-mail: shager@holmescc.edu

Missouri

Sanford-Brown College - Hazelwood Campus
Occupational Therapy Asst Prgm
75 Village Square
Hazelwood, MO 63042
Prgm Dir: William C Gielow, Jr, MS OTR/L
Tel: 314 687-2991, Ext 2991   *Fax:* 314 731-0550
E-mail: wgielow@sbc-Hazelwood.com

Metropolitan Community College - Penn Valley
Occupational Therapy Asst Prgm
3201 SW Trafficway
Kansas City, MO 64111-2764
www.mcckc.edu
Prgm Dir: Amber Jenkins, MLS OTR/L
Tel: 816 759-4235   *Fax:* 816 759-4553
E-mail: amber.jenkins@mcckc.edu

Ozarks Technical Community College
Occupational Therapy Asst Prgm
1001 E Chestnut Expressway
Springfield, MO 65802-3625
Prgm Dir: Becky Jenkins, OTR/L
Tel: 417 447-8855   *Fax:* 417 447-8806
E-mail: jenkinsr@otc.edu

St Louis Community College - Meramec
Occupational Therapy Asst Prgm
11333 Big Bend Blvd
St Louis, MO 63122-5799
www.stlcc.edu
Prgm Dir: Nancy M Klein, MS OTR/L
Tel: 314 984-7364   *Fax:* 314 984-7250
E-mail: nklein@stlcc.edu

St Charles Community College
Occupational Therapy Asst Prgm
4601 Mid Rivers Mall Dr
PO Box 76975
St Peters, MO 63376-0975
www.stchas.edu
Prgm Dir: Francesca Woods, MA OTR/L
Tel: 636 922-8638   *Fax:* 636 922-8478
E-mail: fwoods@stchas.edu

Nevada

College of Southern Nevada
Occupational Therapy Asst Prgm
West Charleston Campus
6375 W Charleston Blvd, WCL
Las Vegas, NV 89146-1139
Prgm Dir: Christine R Privott, PhD OTR/L
Tel: 702 651-7411   *Fax:* 702 651-5506
E-mail: christine.privott@csn.edu

New Hampshire

New Hampshire Comm Tech Coll - Claremont
Occupational Therapy Asst Prgm
One College Dr
Claremont, NH 03743-9707
Prgm Dir: Jennifer J Saylor, MEd OTR/L
Tel: 603 542-7744, Ext 2525   *Fax:* 603 542-1844
E-mail: jsaylor@nhctc.edu

New Mexico

Eastern New Mexico University - Roswell
Occupational Therapy Asst Prgm
Div of Health
52 University Blvd, PO Box 6000
Roswell, NM 88202-6000
Prgm Dir: Pat Herrera, OTR/L
Tel: 505 624-7267   *Fax:* 505 624-7257
E-mail: Pat.Herrera@roswell.enmu.edu

Western New Mexico University
Occupational Therapy Asst Prgm
PO Box 680
Silver City, NM 88062-0680
Prgm Dir: Gwen Cassel, MOT OTR/L
Tel: 505 574-5171   *Fax:* 505 574-5150
E-mail: casselg@wnmu.edu

New York

Maria College
Occupational Therapy Asst Prgm
700 New Scotland Ave
Albany, NY 12208-1798
www.mariacollege.edu
Prgm Dir: Sandra C Jung, OTR/L
Tel: 518 438-3111, Ext 257   *Fax:* 518 453-1366
E-mail: sandyj@mariacollege.edu

Genesee Community College
Occupational Therapy Asst Prgm
One College Rd
Batavia, NY 14020-9704
www.genesee.edu
Prgm Dir: Mary K Hartman, MS OTR/L
Tel: 585 345-6838   *Fax:* 585 343-0433
E-mail: mkhartman@genesee.edu

Suffolk County Community College - Grant Campus
Occupational Therapy Asst Prgm
Michael J Campus
Crooked Hill Rd - MA 308
Brentwood, NY 11717-1092
www.sunysuffolk.edu
Prgm Dir: Lisa E Hubbs, MS OTR/L
Tel: 631 851-6335   *Fax:* 631 851-6854
E-mail: hubbsl@sunysuffolk.edu

SUNY at Canton
Occupational Therapy Asst Prgm
34 Cornell Dr
Canton, NY 13617-1096
Prgm Dir: Cindy Hammecker, MS OTR/L
Tel: 315 379-3863   *Fax:* 315 386-7959
E-mail: hammeckc@canton.edu

Mercy College
Occupational Therapy Asst Prgm
555 Broadway
Dobbs Ferry, NY 10522-1134
Prgm Dir: Christine Sullivan, MS OTR/L
Tel: 914 674-7831   *Fax:* 914 674-7840
E-mail: csullivan@mercy.edu

Jamestown Community College
Occupational Therapy Asst Prgm
525 Falconer St
PO Box 20
Jamestown, NY 14701-0020
Prgm Dir: Heather L Panczykowski, MS OTR/L
Tel: 716 665-5220, Ext 1162   *Fax:* 716 661-3168
E-mail: HeatherPanczykowski@mail.sunyjcc.edu

LaGuardia Community College
Occupational Therapy Asst Prgm
31-10 Thomson Ave
Long Island City, NY 11101-3083
www.lagcc.cuny.edu
Prgm Dir: Naomi S Greenberg, PhD OTR/L
Tel: 718 482-5777   *Fax:* 718 609-2052
E-mail: ngreenbe@lagcc.cuny.edu

Orange County Community College
Occupational Therapy Asst Prgm
115 South St
Middletown, NY 10940-6404
Prgm Dir: Florence Hannes, MS OTR FAOTA
Tel: 845 341-4323   *Fax:* 845 341-4799
E-mail: fhannes@sunyorange.edu

Touro College
Occupational Therapy Asst Prgm
Main Campus
27-33 W 23rd St
New York, NY 10010-4202
www.touro.edu/shs
Prgm Dir: Rivka Molinsky, MA OTR/L
Tel: 212 463-0400, Ext 518   *Fax:* 212 989-2054
E-mail: rmolinsky@touro.edu

Rockland Community College
Occupational Therapy Asst Prgm
145 College Rd
Suffern, NY 10901-3699
Prgm Dir: Ellen Spergel, MS OTR
Tel: 845 574-4312   *Fax:* 845 574-4594
E-mail: espergel@sunyrockland.edu

Erie Community College - North Campus
Occupational Therapy Asst Prgm
6205 Main St
Williamsville, NY 14221-7095
Prgm Dir: Betsy Jones, MSEd OTR/L
Tel: 716 851-1320   *Fax:* 716 851-1267
E-mail: jones@ecc.edu

North Carolina

Cabarrus College of Health Sciences
Occupational Therapy Asst Prgm
401 Medical Park Dr
Concord, NC 28025-2405
Prgm Dir: Nancy S Green, MHA OTR/L
Tel: 704 783-3599, Ext 3599   *Fax:* 704 783-2077
E-mail: ngreen@cabarruscollege.edu

Durham Technical Community College
Occupational Therapy Asst Prgm
1637 Lawson St
Durham, NC 27703-5023
www.durhamtech.edu
Prgm Dir: Sue Cheng, MS OTR/L
Tel: 919 686-3717   *Fax:* 919 686-3705
E-mail: chengs@durhamtech.edu

Pitt Community College
Occupational Therapy Asst Prgm
PO Drawer 7007
Greenville, NC 27835-7007
www.pittcc.edu
Prgm Dir: Wendy Perrini, MS OTR/L CHT
Tel: 252 493-7458   *Fax:* 252 321-4451
E-mail: wperrini@email.pittcc.edu

Cape Fear Community College
Occupational Therapy Asst Prgm
411 N Front St
Wilmington, NC 28401-3993
http://cfcc.edu
Prgm Dir: Deborah A Amini, MEd OTR/L CHT
Tel: 910 362-7096   *Fax:* 910 362-7087
E-mail: damini@cfcc.edu

North Dakota

North Dakota State College of Science
Occupational Therapy Asst Prgm
Mayme Green Allied Health Facility
800 6th St N
Wahpeton, ND 58076-0002
Prgm Dir: Sr Carolita Mauer, MA OTR/L
Tel: 701 671-2982, Ext 2982   *Fax:* 701 671-2570
E-mail: carolita.mauer@ndscs.edu

Ohio

Kent State University - Ashtabula Campus
Occupational Therapy Asst Prgm
Ashtabula, OH 44004
Prgm Dir: Harrett Bynum, MS OTR/L
Tel: 440 964-3322
E-mail: hbynum@kent.edu

Stark State College of Technology
Occupational Therapy Asst Prgm
6200 Frank Ave NW
Canton, OH 44720
www.starkstate.edu
Prgm Dir: Doris Huston, MA OTR/L
Tel: 330 966-5458, Ext 4200   *Fax:* 330 966-6586
E-mail: dhuston@starkstate.edu

Cincinnati State Tech & Comm College
Occupational Therapy Asst Prgm
3520 Central Pkwy
Cincinnati, OH 45223-2690
www.cincinnatistate.edu
Prgm Dir: Claudia J Miller, MHS OTR/L
Tel: 513 569-1598   *Fax:* 513 487-1598
E-mail: claudia.miller@cincinnatistate.edu

Cuyahoga Community College
Occupational Therapy Asst Prgm
2900 Community College Ave
Cleveland, OH 44115-3196
www.tri-c.edu/otat
Prgm Dir: Hector L Merced, MS OTR/L
Tel: 216 987-4498   *Fax:* 216 987-4386
E-mail: hector.merced@tri-c.edu

Sinclair Community College
Occupational Therapy Asst Prgm
444 W Third St
Dayton, OH 45402-1460
www.sinclair.edu
Prgm Dir: S Kay Ashworth, MAT OTR/L
Tel: 937 512-5178   *Fax:* 937 512-5170
E-mail: kay.ashworth@sinclair.edu

Kent State University - East Liverpool Campus
Occupational Therapy Asst Prgm
East Liverpool Campus, 400 E Fourth St
East Liverpool, OH 43920-3497
www.eliv.kent.edu
Prgm Dir: Harriett Bynum, MS OTR/L
Tel: 330 382-7426   *Fax:* 330 382-7564
E-mail: hbynum@kent.edu

Rhodes State College
Occupational Therapy Asst Prgm
4240 Campus Dr
Lima, OH 45804-3597
Prgm Dir: Ann Best, OTR/L CEES
Tel: 419 995-8080   *Fax:* 419 995-8093
E-mail: Best.A@rhodesstate.edu

Shawnee State University
Occupational Therapy Asst Prgm
940 Second St
Portsmouth, OH 45662-4303
www.shawnee.edu
Prgm Dir: Melinda Sissel, MOT OTR
Tel: 740 351-3389   *Fax:* 740 351-2354
E-mail: msissel@shawnee.edu

Owens Community College
Occupational Therapy Asst Prgm
Toledo Campus Oregon Rd
PO Box 10,000
Toledo, OH 43699-1947
Prgm Dir: Barbara Sequine, BIS COTA/L
Tel: 567 661-7415   *Fax:* 567 661-2634
E-mail: barbara_seguine@owens.edu

Zane State College
Occupational Therapy Asst Prgm
1555 Newark Rd
Zanesville, OH 43701-2694
www.zanestate.edu
Prgm Dir: Mary Arnold, MA OTR/L
Tel: 740 588-1313   *Fax:* 740 588-1332
E-mail: marnold@zanestate.edu

Oklahoma

SW Oklahoma St Univ/Caddo Kiowa Tech Ctr
Occupational Therapy Asst Prgm
PO Box 190
Fort Cobb, OK 73038
Prgm Dir: Sherri Robertson, OTR/L
Tel: 405 643-5511, Ext 310   *Fax:* 405 643-2144
E-mail: srobertson@caddokiowa.com

Oklahoma City Community College
Occupational Therapy Asst Prgm
Health Professions Division
7777 S May Ave
Oklahoma City, OK 73159-4444
Prgm Dir: Thomas Kraft, MEd OTR/L
Tel: 405 682-1611, Ext 7227   *Fax:* 405 682-7826
E-mail: tkraft@occc.edu

Tulsa Community College
Occupational Therapy Asst Prgm
Metro Campus, Allied Hlth Services Div
909 S Boston Ave
Tulsa, OK 74119-2095
Prgm Dir: Gary Braswell, MS OTR/L
Tel: 918 595-7319   *Fax:* 918 535-7091
E-mail: gbraswel@tulsacc.edu

Pennsylvania

Mount Aloysius College
Occupational Therapy Asst Prgm
7373 Admiral Peary Hwy
Cresson, PA 16630-1999
Prgm Dir: Kristina Knott, MA OTR/L
Tel: 814 886-6355   *Fax:* 814 886-4278
E-mail: kknott@mtaloy.edu

Penn State University - DuBois
Occupational Therapy Asst Prgm
College Place
DuBois, PA 15801-3199
Prgm Dir: LuAnn Demi, MS OTR/L
Tel: 814 375-4748   *Fax:* 814 375-4784
E-mail: ldb4@psu.edu

Comm College of Allegheny County
Occupational Therapy Asst Prgm
Boyce Campus
595 Beatty Rd
Monroeville, PA 15146-1395
Prgm Dir: Lillian Briola, MOT OTR/L
Tel: 724 325-6751   *Fax:* 724 325-6701
E-mail: lbriola@ccac.edu

Penn State University - Mont Alto Campus
Occupational Therapy Asst Prgm
Mont Alto Campus
Campus Dr
Mont Alto, PA 17237-9703
www.ma.psu/OTA
Prgm Dir: Dorothy Rockwell, MS OT/L BCP
Tel: 717 749-6165   *Fax:* 717 749-6166
E-mail: dld14@psu.edu
Notes: Satellite programs in Reading, PA

Kaplan Career Institute - ICM Campus
Occupational Therapy Asst Prgm
10 Wood St
Pittsburgh, PA 15222-1977
Prgm Dir: John Sciulli
Tel: 412 261-2647, Ext 254   *Fax:* 412 261-6491
E-mail: jsciulli@kaplan.edu

Penn State University - Berks
Occupational Therapy Asst Prgm
PO Box 7009
Tulpehoeken Rd
Reading, PA 19610-6009
Prgm Dir: Tamera K Humbert, DEd OTR/L
Tel: 610 396-6179   *Fax:* 610 396-6024
E-mail: tkh110@psu.edu

Lehigh Carbon Community College
Occupational Therapy Asst Prgm
4525 Education Park Dr
Schnecksville, PA 18078-2598
www.lccc.edu
Prgm Dir: Cindy Rifenburg, MS OTR/L
Tel: 610 799-1548   *Fax:* 610 799-1527
E-mail: crifenburg@lccc.edu

Pennsylvania College of Technology
Occupational Therapy Asst Prgm
One College Ave
Williamsport, PA 17701-5799
www.pct.edu/catalog/majors/oc.shtml
Prgm Dir: Barbara J Natell, MSEd OTR/L
Tel: 570 321-5549   *Fax:* 570 327-4509
E-mail: bnatell@pct.edu

Puerto Rico

University of Puerto Rico at Humacao
Occupational Therapy Asst Prgm
CUH Postal Station 100, Carr 908
Humacao, PR 00791-4300
www.uprh.edu
Prgm Dir: Carlos A Galiano, MC MS OTR/L CPL
Tel: 787 850-9392   *Fax:* 787 850-9434
E-mail: ca_galiano@webmail.uprh.edu

Rhode Island

Community College of Rhode Island
Occupational Therapy Asst Prgm
Newport County Campus
One John H Chafee Blvd
Newport, RI 02840
www.ccri.edu
Prgm Dir: Michael A Nardone, MS OTR/L
Tel: 401 851-1667   *Fax:* 401 851-1671
E-mail: mnardone1@ccri.edu

New England Institute of Technology
Occupational Therapy Asst Prgm
2500 Post Rd
Warwick, RI 02886-2251
www.neit.edu
Prgm Dir: Nancy R Dooley, PhD OTR/L
Tel: 401 739-5000, Ext 3400   *Fax:* 401 732-9792
E-mail: ndooley@neit.edu

South Carolina

Trident Technical College
Occupational Therapy Asst Prgm
PO Box 118067
Charleston, SC 29423-8067
Prgm Dir: Mary Ellen Hiebert, MHS OTR/L
Tel: 843 574-6563   *Fax:* 843 574-6585
E-mail: maryellen.hiebert@tridenttech.edu

Greenville Technical College
Occupational Therapy Asst Prgm
Greer Campus
506 S Pleasantburg Dr, PO Box 5616
Greenville, SC 29606-5616
Prgm Dir: Jennifer Coyne, COTA/L
Tel: 864 848-2040   *Fax:* 864 848-2038
E-mail: jennifer.coyne@gvltec.edu

South Dakota

Lake Area Technical Institute
Occupational Therapy Asst Prgm
230 11th St NE
Watertown, SD 57201-0730
Prgm Dir: Julie Kalahar, MS OTR/L
Tel: 605 882-5284, Ext 371   *Fax:* 605 882-6299
E-mail: kalaharj@lakeareatech.edu

Tennessee

Roane State Community College
Occupational Therapy Asst Prgm
276 Patton Ln
Harriman, TN 37748-5011
Prgm Dir: Jeremy Keough, MSOT OTR/L
Tel: 865 481-2000, Ext 2108   *Fax:* 865 481-2019
E-mail: keoughjl@roanestate.edu

Nashville State Community College
Occupational Therapy Asst Prgm
120 White Bridge Rd, Ste W-60
Nashville, TN 37209
Prgm Dir: Donna Whitehouse, MHA OTR
Tel: 615 353-3382   *Fax:* 615 353-3608
E-mail: donna.whitehouse@nscc.edu

Texas

Amarillo College
Occupational Therapy Asst Prgm
PO Box 447
Amarillo, TX 79178-0001
www.actx.edu/occup_therapy
Prgm Dir: Sheree Hilliard Talkington, MA OTR
Tel: 806 354-6079   *Fax:* 806 354-6076
E-mail: talkington-sl@actx.edu

Austin Community College
Occupational Therapy Asst Prgm
Eastview Campus
3401 Webberville Rd
Austin, TX 78702
www.austincc.edu/health/ota
Prgm Dir: Carolyn O Cantu, MS OTR
Tel: 512 223-5934   *Fax:* 512 223-5897
E-mail: ccantu2@austincc.edu

Panola College
Occupational Therapy Asst Prgm
1109 W Panola St
Carthage, TX 75633-2397
Prgm Dir: Cheri Lambert, OTR
Tel: 903 694-4025   *Fax:* 903 694-4010
E-mail: clambert@panola.edu

Del Mar College
Occupational Therapy Asst Prgm
Dept of Allied Health
101 Baldwin and Ayers Sts
Corpus Christi, TX 78404-3897
Prgm Dir: Abel Villarreal, MOT OTR
Tel: 512 698-1845   *Fax:* 512 698-1849
E-mail: avillar@delmar.edu

Navarro College
Occupational Therapy Asst Prgm
3200 W Seventh Ave
Corsicana, TX 75110-4818
www.navarrocollege.edu
Prgm Dir: Anita Lane, MEd OTR
Tel: 903 875-7583   *Fax:* 903 875-7577
E-mail: anita.lane@navarrocollege.edu

US Army Medical Dept Center & School
Occupational Therapy Asst Prgm
Academy of Health Sciences
3151 Scott Rd, Ste 1230
Fort Sam Houston, TX 78234-6138
Prgm Dir: CDR Kimberly A Farland, MA OTR/L CHT
Tel: 210 221-3694   *Fax:* 210 221-4447
E-mail: kimberly.farland@cen.amedd.army.mil

Houston Community College
Occupational Therapy Asst Prgm
Coleman College for Health Sciences
1900 Pressler Dr
Houston, TX 77030-3717
www.hccs.edu
Prgm Dir: Linda Williams, MA OTR/L
Tel: 713 718-7392, Ext 87392   *Fax:* 713 718-6495
E-mail: linda.williams@hccs.edu

Kingwood College - NHMCCD
Occupational Therapy Asst Prgm
20000 Kingwood Dr
Kingwood, TX 77339-3801
Prgm Dir: Alma Watson, MOT OTR
Tel: 281 312-1464   *Fax:* 281 312-1490
E-mail: alma.r.watson@nhmccd.edu

Laredo Community College
Occupational Therapy Asst Prgm
West End Washington St
Laredo, TX 78040-4395
www.laredo.edu
Prgm Dir: Terri Gonzalez, MA OTR RMT
Tel: 956 721-5460   *Fax:* 956 721-5431
E-mail: trgon@laredo.edu

South Texas College
Occupational Therapy Asst Prgm
Nursing/Allied Health Division
1101 S Vermont, PO Box 9701
McAllen, TX 78501-9701
www.southtexascollege.edu/nah/program%20ota.htm
Prgm Dir: Espy J Brattin, MEd OTR
Tel: 956 872-3149   *Fax:* 956 872-3163
E-mail: ebrattin@southtexascollege.edu

St Philip's College
Occupational Therapy Asst Prgm
1801 Martin Luther King Dr
San Antonio, TX 78203-2098
www.accd.edu/spc
Prgm Dir: Jana Cragg, MA OTR
Tel: 210 531-3421   *Fax:* 210 531-3459
E-mail: jcragg@mail.accd.edu

Tomball College - NHMCCD
Occupational Therapy Asst Prgm
30555 Tomball Pkwy
Tomball, TX 77375-4036
Prgm Dir: Terra Ruppert, PhD OTR
Tel: 281 357-3733   *Fax:* 281 351-3384
E-mail: terra.ruppert@nhmccd.edu

Utah

Salt Lake Community College
Occupational Therapy Asst Prgm
Mail Code: JC
3491 W Wights Fort Rd
West Jordan, UT 84088
Prgm Dir: Brenda K Lyman, OTR/L
Tel: 801 957-4394   *Fax:* 801 957-2762
E-mail: brenda.lyman@slcc.edu

Virginia

Southwest Virginia Community College
Occupational Therapy Asst Prgm
PO Box SVCC
Richlands, VA 24641-1101
www.sw.edu/msht/healthtech/htprograms.htm
Prgm Dir: Annette Looney, OTR/L
Tel: 276 935-7748   *Fax:* 276 935-2019
E-mail: annette.looney@sw.edu

Jefferson College of Health Sciences
Occupational Therapy Asst Prgm
PO Box 13186
920 S Jefferson St
Roanoke, VA 24031-3186
www.jchs.edu
Prgm Dir: Viki Neurauter, MOT OTR/L
Tel: 540 224-4453   *Fax:* 540 985-9773
E-mail: vbneurauter@jchs.edu

Tidewater Community College
Occupational Therapy Asst Prgm
Virginia Beach Campus
1700 College Crescent
Virginia Beach, VA 23456-1918
Prgm Dir: William M Marcil, PhD OTR/L FAOTA
Tel: 757 822-7330   *Fax:* 757 427-1338
E-mail: wmarcil@tcc.edu

Washington

Green River Community College
Occupational Therapy Asst Prgm
12401 SE 320th St
Auburn, WA 98092-3622
www.greenriver.edu
Prgm Dir: S Noel Hepler, MS OTR/L
Tel: 253 833-9111, Ext 4341   *Fax:* 253 288-3413
E-mail: nhepler@greenriver.edu

West Virginia

Mountain State University
Occupational Therapy Asst Prgm
PO Box AG
Beckley, WV 25802-2830
Prgm Dir: Kay Blose, MOT OTR/L
Tel: 304 929-1362   *Fax:* 304 929-1617
E-mail: kblose@mountainstate.edu

Wisconsin

Fox Valley Technical College
Occupational Therapy Asst Prgm
1825 N Bluemound Dr, PO Box 2277
Appleton, WI 54912-2277
www.fvtc.edu
Prgm Dir: Patricia Holz, MS OT
Tel: 920 735-4843   *Fax:* 920 831-4314
E-mail: holz@fvtc.edu

Wisconsin Indianhead Technical College - Ashland Campus
Occupational Therapy Asst Prgm
2100 Beaser Ave
Ashland, WI 54806-3699
Prgm Dir: Mari Jo Ulrich, MA OTR
Tel: 715 682-4591, Ext 3167   *Fax:* 715 682-8040
E-mail: marijo.ulrich@witc.edu

Western Technical College
Occupational Therapy Asst Prgm
304 N Sixth St, PO Box C-908
La Crosse, WI 54602-0908
www.westerntc.edu
Prgm Dir: Doreen M Olson, MS OTR
Tel: 608 789-4757   *Fax:* 608 785-9299
E-mail: OlsonD@westerntc.edu

Madison Area Technical College
Occupational Therapy Asst Prgm
211 N Carroll St
Madison, WI 53703-2285
www.matcmadison.edu
Prgm Dir: Karen Romanowski, MS OTR
Tel: 608 258-2312   *Fax:* 608 258-2480
E-mail: kromanowski@matcmadison.edu

Milwaukee Area Technical College
Occupational Therapy Asst Prgm
700 W State St
Milwaukee, WI 53233-1443
Prgm Dir: Susan Heitman, MS OTR
Tel: 414 297-7158   *Fax:* 414 297-6851
E-mail: heitmasm@matc.edu

Wyoming

Casper College
Occupational Therapy Asst Prgm
125 College Dr
Casper, WY 82601-9958
www.caspercollege.edu
Prgm Dir: Marla Wonser, MSOT OTR/L
Tel: 307 268-2867   *Fax:* 307 268-3034
E-mail: mwonser@caspercollege.edu

Occupational Therapy Assistant

Programs*	Class Capacity	Begins	Length (months)	Award	Res. Tuition	Non-res. Tuition	Stipend	Offers:‡ 1	2	3	4
California											
Loma Linda University	60	Sep	15	Dipl, AA	$20,000	$20,000				•	
Sacramento City College	30	Jan	24	AS	$432	$3,696		•		•	
Santa Ana College	40	Jan Aug	24	AS	$20	$158		•		•	•
Colorado											
Pueblo Community College	20	Aug	22	AAS	$4,888	$11,044				•	
Connecticut											
Briarwood College (Southington)	35	Sep Jan	24	AAS	$16,400	$16,400					
Housatonic Community College (Bridgeport)	18	Sep	24, 36	AS	$1,176	$3,528		•			
Delaware											
Delaware Tech & Comm Coll - Owens Campus (Georgetown)	16	Aug	22	AAS	$2,190	$5,475				•	
Florida											
Daytona Beach Community College	24	Aug	22	AAS	$2,083	$7,904				•	
Florida Hospital College of Health Sciences (Orlando)	24	Aug	24	Dipl, AS	$10,000	$10,000				•	
Keiser University (Fort Lauderdale)	24	May Aug Jan	24	Dipl, AS						•	
Manatee Community College (Bradenton)	24	Fall semester	20	AS/AAS	$69	$256					
					Per credit hour						
Georgia											
Darton College (Albany)	22	Aug	24	AS	$4,037	$16,148		•		•	
Northwestern Technical College (Rock Spring)	20	Jul	24	AAS	$1,872	$1,872					
Hawaii											
Kapi'olani Community College (Honolulu)	16	Aug	24	Dipl, AS	$63	$256				•	
Illinois											
Lewis & Clark Community College (Godfrey)	26	Jan	24	AAS	$80	$284				•	
Lincoln Land Community College (Springfield)	16	Jan	24	AAS	$2,448	$4,896				•	
South Suburban College (South Holland)	24	Jun	18	AAS	$1,792	$6,160				•	

*Data are shown only for programs that completed the 2007 AMA Survey of Health Professions Education Programs.
‡Key to Offers: 1: Evening or weekend classes; 2: Non-English instruction; 3: Cultural competence instruction; 4: Distance education component.

Occupational Therapy Assistant

Programs*	Class Capacity	Begins	Length (months)	Award	Res. Tuition	Non-res. Tuition	Stipend	1	2	3	4
Indiana											
Brown Mackie College (South Bend)	24	Feb Jul	24	AAS	$7,488	$7,488				•	
Iowa											
Kirkwood Community College (Cedar Rapids)	24	Aug	22	AAS	$1,059	$2,118				•	
Kansas											
Newman University (Wichita)	30	Jan	13	AS	$18,000	$18,000				•	
Kentucky											
Jefferson Community and Technical College (Louisville)	20	Spring Jan	24	AAS	$109	$327				•	
Louisiana											
University of Louisiana at Monroe	30	Jul	25	AS	$4,050	$10,002				•	
Maryland											
Allegany College of Maryland (Cumberland)	16	Aug	28	AAS	$2,304	$4,992				•	
Community College of Baltimore County - Catonsville	40	Sep	24	Dipl, AAS	$2,481	$2,740				•	
Massachusetts											
Bristol Community College (Fall River)	20	Sep	24	AS	$123	$329				•	
North Shore Community College (Danvers)	36	Sep	14, 18	AS	$4,000	$12,000				•	
Quinsigamond Community College (Worcester)	15	Sep	21	AS	$129	$335		•		•	•
Springfield Technical Community College	12	Sep	18	AS	$812	$7,865				•	
Michigan											
Baker College of Muskegon	20	Sep	28	AAS	$6,480	$6,480					
Grand Rapids Community College	30	Aug	18	AAAS	$2,385	$4,710		•		•	
Mott Community College - Southern Lakes Branch Campus (Fenton)	15	Sep	24	Dipl, AAS	$2,053	$3,950				•	
Wayne County Community College District (Detroit)	30	Jun	18	AAS	$1,564	$1,988		•		•	•
Minnesota											
College of St Catherine - Minneapolis	21	Sep	18	AAS	$14,000	$14,000				•	
Northland Community & Technical College (East Grand Forks)	24	Jan	21	AAS	$144	$144				•	
Mississippi											
Holmes Community College (Ridgeland)	20	Aug	24	AAS	$2,136	$2,550				•	
Itawamba Community College (Fulton)	12	Jan		AAS						•	
Missouri											
Metropolitan Community College - Penn Valley (Kansas City)	20	Aug	22	AAS	$5,840	$13,870					
St Charles Community College (St Peters)	20	Aug 21	20	AAS	$65	$95				•	
St Louis Community College - Meramec	24	Aug	21	AAS	$2,592	$3,776				•	
Nevada											
College of Southern Nevada (Las Vegas)	12	Sep	24	AAS	$2,555	$4,155		•		•	•
New Mexico											
Eastern New Mexico University - Roswell	25	Aug	18	Dipl, AS	$1,051	$4,320				•	•
Western New Mexico University (Silver City)	20	Aug	24	AS	$3,072	$11,736				•	
New York											
Genesee Community College (Batavia)	32	Aug Jan	18	AAS	$3,200	$3,600		•		•	•
LaGuardia Community College (Long Island City)	40	Sep Mar	24, 36	AS	$2,800	$4,560		•		•	
Maria College (Albany)	46	Late Aug	18, 32	AAS	$8,000	$8,000		•		•	
Suffolk County Comm Coll - Grant Campus (Brentwood)	24	Aug Sep	21	AAS	$3,100	$5,780				•	
Touro College (New York)	30	Sep	24	AAS	$10,000	$10,000				•	
North Carolina											
Cape Fear Community College (Wilmington)	24	Aug	21	AAS	$400	$2,500				•	
Durham Technical Community College	24	May	24, 36	AAS	$2,050	$11,200				•	
Pitt Community College (Greenville)	24	Jan	24	AAS	$1,264	$7,024				•	
Ohio											
Cincinnati State Tech & Comm College	30	Sep	24	AAS	$8,954	$17,908				•	
Cuyahoga Community College (Cleveland)	24	Aug	24	AAS	$2,859	$3,780				•	
Kent State University - East Liverpool Campus	45	Aug	21	AAS	$4,770	$12,202				•	
Shawnee State University (Portsmouth)	24	Sep	21	AAS	$5,830	$9,970					
Sinclair Community College (Dayton)	30	Sep	22	AAS	$2,475	$4,042				•	
Stark State College of Technology (Canton)	30	Aug Jan	18	AAS	$3,800	$4,977				•	•
Zane State College (Zanesville)	25	Sep	25	AAS	$4,104	$8,208		•		•	•
Oklahoma											
Oklahoma City Community College	20	Aug	20	AAS	$78	$208		•			
Pennsylvania											
Lehigh Carbon Community College (Schnecksville)	30	Sep	24	AAS	$2,400	$4,800		•		•	
Penn State University - Mont Alto Campus	30	Aug Jan	24	AS	$5,188	$11,240				•	
Pennsylvania College of Technology (Williamsport)	32	Aug	22	AAS	$10,620	$13,350				•	

*Data are shown only for programs that completed the 2007 AMA Survey of Health Professions Education Programs.

‡Key to Offers: 1: Evening or weekend classes; 2: Non-English instruction; 3: Cultural competence instruction; 4: Distance education component.

Occupational Therapy Assistant

Programs*	Class Capacity	Begins	Length (months)	Award	Res. Tuition	Non-res. Tuition	Stipend	Offers:‡ 1	2	3	4
Puerto Rico											
University of Puerto Rico at Humacao	35	Aug	24	Dipl, AS	$1,900	$4,300			•	•	
Rhode Island											
Community College of Rhode Island (Newport)	24	Sep	15	AAS	$3,550	$7,470		•		•	
New England Institute of Technology (Warwick)	25	Jul Jan	18	AS	$14,000	$14,000					
Tennessee											
Roane State Community College (Harriman)	25	Aug	20	AAS	$2,485	$6,414				•	
Texas											
Amarillo College	15	Fall	22	AAS	$1,350	$2,950				•	•
Austin Community College	20	Aug	24	AAS	$1,568	$3,700					
Del Mar College (Corpus Christi)	20	Sep	18	AAS	$1,000	$0					
Houston Community College	20	Aug	12	Cert, AAS					•	•	
Laredo Community College	12	Sep	24	AAS	$1,400	$3,150		•		•	•
Navarro College (Corsicana)	30	Aug	30	AAS	$1,450	$2,450				•	
South Texas College (McAllen)	15	Sep	24	AAS	$1,639	$2,139				•	
St Philip's College (San Antonio)	24	Aug	24	AAS	$2,184	$3,288					
Utah											
Salt Lake Community College (West Jordan)	24	Fall	24	AAS	$1,201	$3,759				•	•
Virginia											
Jefferson College of Health Sciences (Roanoke)	30	Aug	22	AAS	$21,750	$21,750				•	•
Southwest Virginia Community College (Richlands)	24	Aug	22	Dipl	$2,776	$8,731				•	
Washington											
Green River Community College (Auburn)	32	Sep	22	AAS	$2,893	$3,318				•	
Wisconsin											
Fox Valley Technical College (Appleton)	32	Aug	24	AAS	$3,609	$16,269					
Madison Area Technical College	25	Aug	22	AA	$3,930	$17,200				•	
Western Technical College (La Crosse)	20	Aug	20	AAS	$3,221	$16,747		•		•	•
Wyoming											
Casper College	24	Aug	26	AS	$1,582	$4,440				•	•

*Data are shown only for programs that completed the 2007 AMA Survey of Health Professions Education Programs.
‡Key to Offers: 1: Evening or weekend classes; 2: Non-English instruction; 3: Cultural competence instruction; 4: Distance education component.

Ophthalmic Dispensing Optician

Ophthalmic dispensing opticians adapt and fit corrective eyewear, including eyeglasses and contact lenses, as prescribed by an ophthalmologist or optometrist. They help customers select appropriate frames, then prepare work orders for ophthalmic laboratory technicians, who grind and insert lenses into frames. The dispensing optician then adjusts the finished eyewear to fit customer needs.

Career Description

The ophthalmic dispensing optician combines an understanding of the human eye and vision with customer service skills to order the production of corrective eyewear, aid the patient/customer in selecting appropriate, aesthetically pleasing frames, and adjust the frames to fit the customer's face.

Chief duties of the dispensing optician:
- Analyze and interpret prescriptions
- Communicate effectively with patient/customer
- Determine facial and eye measurements
- Identify the human eye structure, function, and pathology
- Assist the customer in selecting appropriate frames and lenses by assessing individual patient needs
- Use an ophthalmologist's or optometrist's prescription to prepare work orders for the ophthalmic laboratory technician
- Deliver prescription eyewear/vision aids and instruct customers in use and care
- Maintain patient/customer records and address complaints
- Provide follow-up services, including eyewear adjustment, repair, and replacement
- Explain theory of refraction
- Identify procedures associated with dispensing artificial eyes and low vision aids, when appropriate
- Adapt, dispense, and fit contact lenses
- Assist in various business duties, including frame and lens inventory, supply and equipment maintenance, and patient insurance/claim forms submission and record keeping
- Apply rules for equipment safety

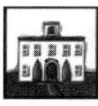

Employment Characteristics

Dispensing opticians work 40-hour weeks in retail stores, some of which may offer one-stop eye examinations, frames, and on-the-spot lens grinding and fitting, or are self-employed in other optical field areas, such as sales/marketing. Other dispensing opticians provide their eye care services in conjunction with ODs and MDs at eye care centers.

Employment Outlook

As the baby boomers reach middle age and the percentage of middle-aged and elderly people increases, so will these individuals' need for corrective eyewear. Eyewear as fashion—more and more people today now own two or more pairs of eyeglasses for different occasions—also translates into strong future demand for ophthalmic dispensing opticians, as do the many new vision products, available in plastic and glass, tinted lenses, multifocal extended-wear, and disposable contact lenses.

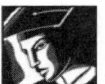

Educational Programs

Length. Ophthalmic dispensing optician degree programs require 2 years of study.

Prerequisites. A high school diploma or its equivalent is generally required for entrance into a program. Ophthalmic dispensing optician students should be familiar with the principles of physics, biology, algebra, and geometry.

Curriculum. Ophthalmic dispensing opticianry educational programs include instruction in geometrical optics; ophthalmic optics; anatomy of the eye; and the use of optical instruments, machinery, and tools.

Inquiries

Careers

American Board of Opticianry
6506 Loisdale Road, #209
Springfield, VA 22150
703 719-5800
www.abo-ncle.org

National Academy of Opticianry
8401 Corporate Drive, Suite 605
Landover, MD 20785
301 577-4828
www.nao.org

National Federation of Opticianry Schools
1238 Robinson Point Road
Mountain Home, AR 72653
870 492-6623
www.nfos.org

Opticians Association of America
441 Carlisle Drive
Herndon VA 20170
703 437 8780
www.oaa.org

Program Accreditation

Commission on Opticianry Accreditation (COA)
PO Box 4342
Chapel Hill, NC 27515
703 468 0566
E-mail: Ellen@COAccreditation.com
www.COAccreditation.com

Ophthalmic Dispensing Optician

Connecticut

Middlesex Community College
Ophthalmic Dispensing Optician Prgm
Ophthalmic Design and Dispensing
100 Training Hill Rd
Middletown, CT 06457
www.mxcc.commnet.edu
Prgm Dir: Raymond P Dennis, MA
Tel: 860 343-5845 *Fax:* 860 343-5874
E-mail: rdennis@mxcc.commnet.edu

Florida

Miami Dade College
Ophthalmic Dispensing Optician Prgm
Vision Care Technology/Opticianry
950 NW 20th St
Miami, FL 33127
Prgm Dir: Jerry Brown
Tel: 305 237-4267 *Fax:* 305 237-4278
E-mail: jerry.brown@mdc.edu

Hillsborough Community College
Ophthalmic Dispensing Optician Prgm
4001 Tampa Bay Blvd
Tampa, FL 33630
Prgm Dir: William Underwood
Tel: 813 253-7430 *Fax:* 813 253-7379
E-mail: bunderwood@hcc.cc.fl.us

Georgia

DeKalb Technical College
Ophthalmic Dispensing Optician Prgm
495 N Indian Creek Dr
Clarkston, GA 30021
Prgm Dir: Thomas Schulz
Tel: 404 297-9522, Ext 207 *Fax:* 404 294-4234
E-mail: schulzt@dekalbtech.edu

Ogeechee Technical College
Ophthalmic Dispensing Optician Prgm
One Joe Kennedy Blvd
Statesboro, GA 30458
Prgm Dir: Deborah Deloach
Tel: 912 486-7404 *Fax:* 912 486-7604
E-mail: ddeloach@ogeecheetech.edu

Nevada

College of Southern Nevada
Ophthalmic Dispensing Optician Prgm
6375 W Charleston Blvd
Las Vegas, NV 89146
Prgm Dir: Scott Helkaa
Tel: 702 651-5834 *Fax:* 702 651-5762
E-mail: scott.helkaa@csn.edu

New Jersey

Camden County College
Ophthalmic Dispensing Optician Prgm
PO Box 200, College Dr
Blackwood, NJ 08012
Prgm Dir: Raymond DiDonato
Tel: 856 374-5058 *Fax:* 856 227-4107
E-mail: rdidonato@camdencc.edu

Essex County College
Ophthalmic Dispensing Optician Prgm
303 University Ave
Newark, NJ 07102
Prgm Dir: Richard Palumbo
Tel: 973 877-3367 *Fax:* 973 877-1920
E-mail: palumbo@essex.edu

Raritan Valley Community College
Ophthalmic Dispensing Optician Prgm
Ophthalmic Science Program
PO Box 3300
Somerville, NJ 08876
www.raritanval.edu
Prgm Dir: Brian Thomas, MA ABOM
Tel: 908 526-1200, Ext 8277 *Fax:* 908 725-2831
E-mail: bthomas@raritanval.edu

New Mexico

Southwestern Indian Polytechnic Institute
Ophthalmic Dispensing Optician Prgm
Optical Technology
9169 Coors Rd NW
Albuquerque, NM 87184
Prgm Dir: Samuel Henderson
Tel: 505 346-7736 *Fax:* 505 346-2343
E-mail: shenders@sipi.bia.edu

New York

New York City College of Technology
Ophthalmic Dispensing Optician Prgm
Department of Vision Care Technology
300 Jay St
Brooklyn, NY 11201
Prgm Dir: Robert Russo, MA
Tel: 718 260-5298 *Fax:* 718 254-8521
E-mail: rrusso@citytech.cuny.edu

Interboro Institute
Ophthalmic Dispensing Optician Prgm
450 W 56th St
New York, NY 10019
Prgm Dir: Jayne H Weinberger
Tel: 212 399-0091 *Fax:* 212 765-5772
E-mail: Jweinberger@interboro.edu

Erie Community College - North Campus
Ophthalmic Dispensing Optician Prgm
6205 Main St
Williamsville, NY 14221-7095
Prgm Dir: John F Godert
Tel: 716 851-1570 *Fax:* 716 851-1429
E-mail: godert@ecc.edu

North Carolina

Durham Technical Community College
Ophthalmic Dispensing Optician Prgm
1637 Lawson St
Durham, NC 27703
Prgm Dir: Michael Szczerbiak
Tel: 919 686-3485 *Fax:* 919 686-3737
E-mail: szczerbiakm@durhamtech.edu

Tennessee

Roane State Community College
Ophthalmic Dispensing Optician Prgm
Opticianry
276 Patton Ln
Harriman, TN 37748
Prgm Dir: Michael Goggin, ABOC NCLC MS
Tel: 865 354-3000, Ext 4319 *Fax:* 865 882-4535
E-mail: goggin_mt@roanestate.edu

Texas

El Paso Community College
Ophthalmic Dispensing Optician Prgm
Ophthalmic Technology
PO Box 20500
El Paso, TX 79998
Prgm Dir: Jose Baca, BS
Tel: 915 831-4075 *Fax:* 915 831-4114
E-mail: mannyb@epcc.edu

Tyler Junior College
Ophthalmic Dispensing Optician Prgm
Vision Care Technology
PO Box 902
Tyler, TX 75711-9020
Prgm Dir: Steve Robbins, ABOC NCLC
Tel: 903 510-2961 *Fax:* 903 510-4928
E-mail: srob@tjc.edu

Virginia

J Sargeant Reynolds Community College
Ophthalmic Dispensing Optician Prgm
Opticianry Department
PO Box 85622
Richmond, VA 23285-5622
Prgm Dir: Kristina Ostrom, ABO-AC FCLSA
Tel: 804 523-5415 *Fax:* 804 786-5298
E-mail: kostrom@reynolds.edu

Tri-Service Optician School (TOPS)
Ophthalmic Dispensing Optician Prgm
160 Main Rd, Ste 350 Naval Weapons Station
Yorktown, VA 23691-9984
Prgm Dir: SFC Stephens
Tel: 757 887-7148 *Fax:* 757 887-4078

Washington

Seattle Central Community College
Ophthalmic Dispensing Optician Prgm
1701 Broadway
Seattle, WA 98122
Prgm Dir: Gary Clayton
Tel: 206 344-4321 *Fax:* 206 344-4316
E-mail: gclayt@sccd.ctc.edu

Wisconsin

Milwaukee Area Technical College
Ophthalmic Dispensing Optician Prgm
Opticianry Science
700 W State St
Milwaukee, WI 53233-1443
Prgm Dir: Laurie Zielinski, ABOC NCLC
Tel: 414 297-7425 *Fax:* 414 297-6851
E-mail: zielinsl@matc.edu

Ophthalmic Dispensing Optician

Programs*	Class Capacity	Begins	Length (months)	Award	Res. Tuition	Non-res. Tuition	Stipend	Offers:‡ 1	2	3	4
Connecticut											
Middlesex Community College (Middletown)	24	Sep	20	AS	$2,672	$7,976					
New Jersey											
Raritan Valley Community College (Somerville)	50	Aug Jan	24	Cert, AAS	$1,260	$1,260		•		•	•
New York											
New York City College of Technology (Brooklyn)	90	Sep Jan	21	AAS	$3,200	$6,800		•			
Virginia											
Tri-Service Optician School (TOPS) (Yorktown)	30	Quarterly	6	Cert							
Wisconsin											
Milwaukee Area Technical College	16	Fall semester	12	Dipl	$3,992	$0				•	

*Data are shown only for programs that completed the 2007 AMA Survey of Health Professions Education Programs.
‡Key to Offers: 1: Evening or weekend classes; 2: Non-English instruction; 3: Cultural competence instruction; 4: Distance education component.

Ophthalmic Professions

Includes:
- Ophthalmic assistant
- Ophthalmic medical technician/technologist

The ophthalmic assistant, ophthalmic technician, and ophthalmic medical technologist are skilled professionals, qualified by didactic and clinical ophthalmic training, who perform ophthalmic procedures under the direction or supervision of a licensed ophthalmologist who is responsible for the performance of the ophthalmic assistant, ophthalmic technician, and ophthalmic medical technologist.

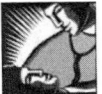

Career Description

The functions of the ophthalmic technician and ophthalmic medical technologist are to assist the ophthalmologist by performing delegable tasks, collecting data, administering treatment ordered by an ophthalmologist, and supervising patients.

The following are duties and tasks that may be delegated by an ophthalmologist, as applicable by state law, to ophthalmic assistants, ophthalmic technicians, and ophthalmic medical technologists.

Ophthalmic Assistants, Ophthalmic Technicians, and Ophthalmic Medical Technologists

1. Obtaining a medical history
2. Performing lensometry
3. Obtaining anatomical and functional ocular measurements of the eye, such as axial length
4. Obtaining functional measurements of the eye, such as visual acuity
5. Testing ocular functions, such as visual fields
6. Administering topical ophthalmic and oral medications
7. Instructing the patient (in personal care and the use of contact lenses)
8. Caring for and maintaining ophthalmic instruments
9. Caring for, maintaining, and sterilizing surgical instruments
10. Adjusting and making minor repairs on spectacles
11. Such other tasks as may be delegated consistent with sound medical practice (eg, use of computerized ophthalmic equipment)

Ophthalmic Technicians and Ophthalmic Medical Technologists

The ophthalmic technician and medical technologist will be expected to perform the duties listed above, at a higher level of expertise. The ophthalmic medical technologist will be expected to exercise considerable clinical skill in the performance of those delegated tasks. The ophthalmic technician and medical technologist may be expected to perform the following additional duties:

12. Performing diagnostic tests
13. Maintaining ophthalmic office equipment
14. Assisting in ophthalmic surgery in the office or hospital
15. Obtaining optical measurements including A-scan
16. Assisting in the fitting of contact lenses
17. Refractometry

Ophthalmic Medical Technologists

The ophthalmic medical technologist will be expected to perform the duties listed above at a higher level of expertise and exercise considerable clinical skill in the performance of those delegated tasks. They may be expected to perform the following additional duties:

18. Performing ophthalmic clinical photography and fluorescein angiography of the eye
19. Administering advanced ocular motility and binocular function tests
20. Performing ocular electrophysiological procedures
21. Performing advanced microbiological procedures
22. Providing supervision and instruction of other ophthalmic personnel and patients
23. Demonstrating advanced general medical knowledge

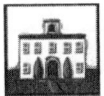

Employment Characteristics

Ophthalmic assistants and ophthalmic medical technicians and technologists are employed primarily by ophthalmologists, medical institutions, clinics, hospitals, ambulatory surgery centers, or physician groups, in which they may be assigned to an ophthalmologist responsible for their supervision and performance. They may be involved with the patients of an ophthalmologist in any setting for which the ophthalmologist is responsible.

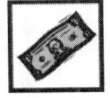

Salary

Salaries vary depending on employer and geographic location. Entry-level salaries range from $21,500 for ophthalmic assistants to $39,000 for ophthalmic technicians and $45,000 for ophthalmic medical technologists. Refer to Section IV, Table 5 of this *Directory* for more information, or see www.ama-assn.org/go/hpsalary.

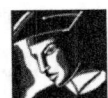

Educational Programs

Length. Programs are generally less than 1 year for assistants, 1 year for technicians and 2 years for technologists.

Prerequisites. High school diploma or equivalent for assistants and technicians and two years of undergraduate study for technologists.

Curriculum. Instruction should follow a planned outline, which includes courses in human anatomy and physiology, medical terminology, medical laws and ethics, psychology, ocular anatomy and physiology, ophthalmic optics, microbiology, ophthalmic pharmacology and toxicology, ocular motility, and diseases of the eye. The curriculum also includes diagnostic and treatment procedures, including visual field testing, contact lenses, ophthalmic surgery, and the care and maintenance of ophthalmic instruments and equipment. For technicians and medical technologists, students must also have supervised clinical experience, during which they have opportunities to apply theory to practice through correlated and supervised instruction in clinical practice areas.

Inquiries

Careers and Certification

Inquiries regarding careers, continuing education, and certification criteria should be addressed to:

Joint Commission on Allied Health Personnel in Ophthalmology
   (JCAHPO)
2025 Woodlane Drive
St Paul, MN 55125-2998
651 731-2944 or 800 284-3937
E-mail: jcahpo@jcahpo.org

Association of Technical Personnel in Ophthalmology (ATPO)
2025 Woodlane Drive
St Paul, MN 55125-2998
651 731-7233 or 800 482-4858
E-mail: ATPOmembership@jcahpo.org

Program Accreditation

Commission on Accreditation of Ophthalmic Medical Programs
   (CoA-OMP)
2025 Woodlane Drive
St Paul, MN 55125-2998
651 731-2944
651 731-0410 Fax
E-mail: CoA-OMP@jcahpo.org

Ophthalmic Assistant

California

Jules Stein Eye Institute, UCLA
Ophthalmic Assistant Prgm
100 Stein Plaza 3-223
Los Angeles, CA 90095
Prgm Dir: Bobbi E Ballenberg, COMT
Tel: 310 794-5603   *Fax:* 310 206-8015
E-mail: ballenberg@jsei.ucla.edu

Louisiana

Delgado Community College
Ophthalmic Assistant Prgm
Allied Health Division
615 City Park Ave, Bldg 4
New Orleans, LA 70119-4399
Prgm Dir: Francesa Langlow, BS COA
Tel: 504 483-4003   *Fax:* 504 483-4609
E-mail: fmorel@dcc.edu

Massachusetts

Holyoke Community College
Ophthalmic Assistant Prgm
303 Homestead Ave
Holyoke, MA 01040
Prgm Dir: Mary Farrell
Tel: 413 552-2288   *Fax:* 413 552-2045
E-mail: mfarrell@hcc.mass.edu

North Carolina

Caldwell Comm College & Tech Institute
Ophthalmic Assistant Prgm
2855 Hickory Blvd
Hudson, NC 28638
Prgm Dir: Barbara T Harris, PA-C MBA COA
Tel: 828 726-2356   *Fax:* 828 726-2489
E-mail: bharris@cccti.edu

Washington

Renton Technical College
Ophthalmic Assistant Prgm
3000 NE Fourth St
Renton, WA 98056
Prgm Dir: Larry Bovard
Tel: 425 235-2352, Ext 7926   *Fax:* 425 235-5836
E-mail: lbovard@rtc.edu

Ophthalmic Medical Technician/Technologist

Arkansas

University of Arkansas for Medical Sciences
Ophthalmic Med Technologist Prgm
4301 W Markham St #523
Little Rock, AR 72205-7199
www.uams.edu/chrp/omt
Prgm Dir: Suzanne Hansen, BA BS COMT
Tel: 501 526-5880   *Fax:* 501 686-6798
E-mail: hansensuzannej@uams.edu

Colorado

Pima Medical Institute - Denver
Ophthalmic Med Technician Prgm
1701 W 72nd Ave
Denver, CO 80221
Prgm Dir: Wendy Stanton, COT
Tel: 303 426-1800   *Fax:* 303 430-4048
E-mail: wstanton@pmi.edu

District of Columbia

Georgetown University Medical Center
Ophthalmic Med Technician Prgm
Center for Sight
3800 Reservoir Rd NW, LL PHC
Washington, DC 20007
Prgm Dir: Ella Rosamont-Morgan, BS COMT
Tel: 202 444-4862   *Fax:* 202 444-4978
E-mail: emm47@georgetown.edu

Florida

University of Florida
Ophthalmic Med Technologist Prgm
PO Box 100393, JHMHC
Gainesville, FL 32610
www.eye.ufl.edu/optkprog.htm
Prgm Dir: Diana J Shamis, MHSE CO COMT
Tel: 352 265-7080, Ext 87945   *Fax:* 352 265-7081
E-mail: dshamis@ufl.edu
Notes: Currently inactive

Georgia

Emory University
Ophthalmic Med Technologist Prgm
1365-B Clifton Rd NE, Rm B-4628
Atlanta, GA 30322
www.eyecenter.emory.edu/
   masters_medical_science.htm
Prgm Dir: Paul M Larson, MMSc MBA COMT COE
Tel: 404 778-4305   *Fax:* 404 778-5128
E-mail: plarson@emory.edu

Illinois

Triton College
Ophthalmic Med Technician Prgm
2000 N Fifth Ave
River Grove, IL 60171
Prgm Dir: Debra Baker, COMT MA
Tel: 708 456-0300, Ext 3442   *Fax:* 708 583-3121
E-mail: dbaker1@triton.edu

Louisiana

Louisiana State Univ Health Sciences Center
Ophthalmic Med Technologist Prgm
2020 Gravier St, Ste B
New Orleans, LA 70112
www.lsuhsc.edu
Prgm Dir: Robin Cooper, COMT ROUB
Tel: 504 412-1200, Ext 1213 *Fax:* 504 412-1243
E-mail: rcoope@lsuhsc.edu
Notes: Currently inactive

Minnesota

Regions Hospital
Ophthalmic Med Technician Prgm
640 Jackson St
St Paul, MN 55101
www.RegionsHospital.com
Prgm Dir: Kristine Fey, COMT
Tel: 651 254-3000 *Fax:* 651 254-2256
E-mail: Kristine.A.Fey@HealthPartners.com

Regions Hospital
Ophthalmic Med Technologist Prgm
640 Jackson St
St Paul, MN 55101
www.regionshospital.com
Prgm Dir: Kristine A Fey, COMT
Tel: 651 254-3000 *Fax:* 651 254-2256
E-mail: Kristine.A.Fey@HealthPartners.com

New Jersey

Camden County College
Ophthalmic Med Technologist Prgm
PO Box 200 College Dr
Blackwood, NJ 08012
Prgm Dir: Ray Didonato
Tel: 856 374-5058
E-mail: rdidonato@camdencc.edu

North Carolina

Duke University Medical Center
Ophthalmic Med Technician Prgm
2351 Erwin Rd, Eye Center Box 3802
Durham, NC 27710
Prgm Dir: Ray Fligman, COT ROUB FCLSA
Tel: 919 684-6261 *Fax:* 919 684-6844
E-mail: ray.fligman@duke.edu

Ontario, Canada

University of Ottawa
Ophthalmic Med Technologist Prgm
The Ottawa Hospital
General Campus, 501 Smyth Rd
Ottawa, ON K1H 8L6
Prgm Dir: Carla Barbery, BSc COMT
Tel: 613 737-8362 *Fax:* 613 737-8836
E-mail: cbarbery@ottawahospital.on.ca

Oregon

Portland Community College
Ophthalmic Med Technician Prgm
Cascade Campus, Jackson Hall 208B
705 N Killingsworth St
Portland, OR 97217
www.pcc.edu/omt
Prgm Dir: Joanne M Harris, COT
Tel: 503 978-5666 *Fax:* 503 978-5257
E-mail: jmharris@pcc.edu

Puerto Rico

University of Puerto Rico
Ophthalmic Med Technician Prgm
PO Box 365067
San Juan, PR 00936-5067
Prgm Dir: Mercedes Rivera, OMP MAEd
Tel: 787 758-2525, Ext 1935 *Fax:* 787 758-3488
E-mail: mercedesrivera@cprs.rcm.upr.edu

Tennessee

Volunteer State Community College
Ophthalmic Med Technician Prgm
1480 Nashville Pike
Annex Building 400, Rm 104a
Gallatin, TN 37066
www.volstate.edu
Prgm Dir: Kathleen Moore, COMT AAS
Tel: 615 230-3723 *Fax:* 615 230-3251
E-mail: Kathleen.Moore@volstate.edu

Virginia

Old Dominion University
Cosponsor: Eastern Virginia Medical School
Ophthalmic Med Technologist Prgm
Lions Center for Sight
600 Gresham Dr
Norfolk, VA 23507
Prgm Dir: Lori Williams, BS COMT
Tel: 757 388-3747 *Fax:* 757 388-2109
E-mail: optech@evms.edu

Ophthalmic Medical Technician/Technologist

Programs*	Class Capacity	Begins	Length (months)	Award	Res. Tuition	Non-res. Tuition	Stipend	Offers:‡ 1	2	3	4
Arkansas											
University of Arkansas for Medical Sciences (Little Rock)	8	Aug	24	BS	$5,780	$13,974					
Florida											
University of Florida (Gainesville)	6	Jul	24	Cert	$2,000	$2,000				•	
Georgia											
Emory University (Atlanta)	15	Jun	24	MMSc	$16,300	$16,300					
Louisiana											
Louisiana State Univ Health Sciences Center (New Orleans)	4	May	24	BS	$3,418	$7,766					
Minnesota											
Regions Hospital (St Paul)	9	Sep	21	Cert	$7,400	$7,400				•	
Regions Hospital (St Paul)	9	Sep	21	Cert	$7,400	$7,400				•	
Oregon											
Portland Community College	30	Sep	21	AAS	$3,149	$8,930					•
Tennessee											
Volunteer State Community College (Gallatin)	15	Aug	12	AAS	$3,600	$13,000				•	•

*Data are shown only for programs that completed the 2007 AMA Survey of Health Professions Education Programs.
‡Key to Offers: 1: Evening or weekend classes; 2: Non-English instruction; 3: Cultural competence instruction; 4: Distance education component.

Optometrist

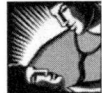

Career Description

Doctors of optometry (ODs) are the primary health care professionals for the eye. Optometrists examine, diagnose, treat, and manage diseases, injuries, and disorders of the visual system, the eye, and associated structures as well as identify related systemic conditions affecting the eye.

Doctors of optometry prescribe medications, low vision rehabilitation, vision therapy, spectacle lenses, and contact lenses and perform certain surgical procedures.

Optometrists counsel their patients regarding surgical and nonsurgical options that meet their visual needs related to their occupations, avocations, and lifestyles.

An optometrist has completed preprofessional undergraduate education in a college or university and 4 years of professional education at a college of optometry, leading to the doctor of optometry (OD) degree. Some optometrists complete an optional residency in a specific area of practice.

Optometrists are eye health care professionals state-licensed to diagnose and treat diseases and disorders of the eye and visual system.

Employment Characteristics

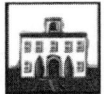

Most optometrists are in general practice. Some specialize in work with the elderly, children, or partially sighted persons who need specialized visual devices. Others develop and implement ways to protect workers' eyes from on-the-job strain or injury. Some specialize in contact lenses, low vision, sports vision, or vision therapy. A few teach optometry, perform research, or consult.

Most optometrists are private practitioners who also handle the business aspects of running an office, such as developing a patient base, hiring employees, keeping paper and electronic records, and ordering equipment and supplies. Optometrists who operate franchise optical stores also may have some of these duties.

Optometrists work in places—usually their own offices—that are clean, well lighted, and comfortable. Most full-time optometrists work about 40 hours a week. Many work weekends and evenings to suit the needs of patients, and are increasingly available for emergency calls as well

Salary

According to the 2007 American Optometric Association Economic Survey, median annual earnings of employed optometrists in 2006 was $105,000, which includes non-cash benefits and retirement contributions. The median net income of all self-employed ODs was $140,000 and varied by practice type as follows:

Self-employed optometrists median net annual income, 2006:
- Solo practice $115,000
- Partnership or group practice (2-person) $149,000
- Partnership or group practice (3-5 person) $141,000
- Partnership or group practice (6 or more) $92,500
- Optical franchisee or lessee $90,000
- Independent contractor $94,000

Salaried optometrists tend to earn more initially than do optometrists who set up their own practices. In the long run, however, those in private practice usually earn more.

For more information, see www.ama-assn.org/go/hpsalary.

Employment Outlook

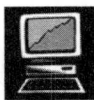

Employment of optometrists is expected to grow faster than average for all occupations through 2014, in response to the vision care needs of a growing and aging population. As baby boomers age, they will be more likely to visit optometrists and ophthalmologists because of the onset of vision problems in middle age, including those resulting from the extensive use of computers. The demand for optometric services also will increase because of growth in the oldest age group, with its increased likelihood of cataracts, glaucoma, diabetes, and hypertension. Greater recognition of the importance of vision care, along with rising personal incomes and growth in employee vision care plans, also will spur job growth.

Employment of optometrists would grow more rapidly were it not for anticipated productivity gains that will allow each optometrist to see more patients. These expected gains stem from greater use of optometric assistants and other support personnel, who will reduce the amount of time optometrists need with each patient. Also, laser surgery that can correct some vision problems is available, and although optometrists still will be needed to provide preoperative and postoperative care for laser surgery patients, patients who successfully undergo this surgery may not require optometrists to prescribe glasses or contacts for several years.

In addition to growth, the need to replace optometrists who retire or leave the occupation for another reason will create employment opportunities.

Educational Programs

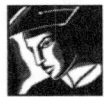

Award, Length. The Doctor of Optometry (OD) degree requires the completion of a 4-year program at an accredited school or college of optometry.

Prerequisites. Each optometry school has slightly different admission requirements. Some schools or colleges require a 4-year undergraduate degree, and many others strongly recommend it. All require at least 3 years of undergraduate study at an accredited college or university. Most optometry students hold a bachelor's or higher degree.

Admission requirements for most schools include general courses in biology, physics, and chemistry, in addition to organic chemistry, biochemistry, biology, microbiology (all with labs), calculus, statistics, English, psychology, social sciences, and other humanities. Because a strong background in science is important, many applicants to optometry school major in a science such as biology or chemistry, while other applicants major in another subject and take many science courses offering laboratory experience. Applicants must take the Optometry Admissions Test (OAT), which is designed to measure general academic ability and comprehension of scientific information.

Admission to optometry school is competitive. Applicants are encouraged to take the examination well in advance of intended enrollment. Most applicants take the test after their sophomore or junior year after taking courses in biology, general and organic chemistry, and physics. Some applicants are accepted to optometry school after 3 years of college and complete their bachelor's degree while attending optometry school.

Most schools also consider an applicant's exposure to optometry, such as becoming acquainted with at least one optometrist, as being of vital importance. Generally, schools and colleges of optometry admit students who have demonstrated strong academic commitment and who exhibit the potential to excel in deductive reasoning, interpersonal communication, and empathy.

Curriculum. Optometry programs include courses in the basic health sciences (anatomy, physiology, pathology, biochemistry, pharmacology, and public health), optics, and the vision sciences, as well as laboratory and clinical training in diagnosing and treating eye disease.

Residency and Advanced Training. Optometrists wishing to teach or conduct research may study for a master's or PhD degree in areas emphasizing the visual and ocular system. One-year postgraduate clinical residency programs are available for optometrists who wish to obtain advanced clinical competence, although residency training is not required to be licensed as an optometrist. Areas for residency programs include the following:

- Primary eye care
- Cornea and contact lenses
- Geriatric optometry
- Pediatric optometry
- Low vision rehabilitation
- Vision therapy and rehabilitation
- Ocular disease
- Refractive and ocular surgery
- Community health optometry

Licensure, Certification, Registration

All states and the District of Columbia require that optometrists be licensed. Applicants for a license must have a Doctor of Optometry degree from an accredited optometry school and must pass both a written national board examination and a national or state clinical board examination. The written and clinical examinations of the National Board of Examiners in Optometry usually are taken during the student's academic career. Many states also require applicants to pass an examination on relevant state laws. Licenses are renewed every 1 to 3 years, with continuing education credits required for renewal in all states.

Inquiries

Education, Careers, Resources
American Optometric Association, Career Guidance Materials
243 North Lindbergh Blvd, Floor 1
St Louis, MO 63141-7881
800 365-2219
www.aoa.org

Association of Schools and Colleges of Optometry
6110 Executive Blvd, Suite 420
Rockville, MD 20852
301 231-5944
www.opted.org
Licensure Exam

National Board of Examiners in Optometry
200 S College Street, #1920
Charlotte, NC 28202
www.optometry.org

Program Accreditation
Accreditation Council on Optometric Education, American
  Optometric Association
243 North Lindbergh Blvd
St Louis, MO 63141-7881
800 365-2219
www.theacoe.org
E-mail: ACOE@aoa.org

Note: Adapted in part from the Bureau of Labor Statistics, US Department of Labor, *Occupational Outlook Handbook*, 2006-07 Edition, Optometrists, on the Internet at www.bls.gov/oco/ocos073.htm (visited August 27, 2007).

Optometrist

Alabama

University of Alabama at Birmingham
Optometry Prgm
School of Optometry
1716 University Blvd
Birmingham, AL 35294
www.uab.edu

California

University of California - Berkeley
Optometry Prgm
School of Optometry
350 Minor Hall MC 2020
Berkeley, CA 94720
spectacle.berkeley.edu

Southern California College of Optometry
Optometry Prgm
2575 Yorba Linda Blvd
Fullerton, CA 92831
www.scco.edu

Florida

Nova Southeastern University
Optometry Prgm
College of Optometry
3200 S University Dr
Fort Lauderdale, FL 33328
www.nova.edu

Illinois

Illinois College of Optometry
Optometry Prgm
3241 S Michigan Ave
Chicago, IL 60616

Indiana

Indiana University - Bloomington
Optometry Prgm
School of Optometry
800 E Atwater
Bloomington, IN 47405
www.opt.indiana.edu

Massachusetts

New England College of Optometry
Optometry Prgm
424 Beacon St
Boston, MA 02115
www.neco.edu

Michigan

Ferris State University
Optometry Prgm
College of Optometry
1310 Cramer Circle
Big Rapids, MI 49307

Missouri

University of Missouri - St Louis
Optometry Prgm
College of Optometry
8001 Natural Bridge Rd
St Louis, MO 63121
umsl.edu/divisions/optometry

New York

SUNY - State College of Optometry
Optometry Prgm
33 W 42nd St
New York, NY 10036-8003
www.sunyopt.edu

Ohio

Ohio State University
Optometry Prgm
College of Optometry
338 W 10th Ave
Columbus, OH 43210
www.optometry.osu.edu

Oklahoma

Northeastern State University
Optometry Prgm
Oklahoma College of Optometry
1001 N Grand Ave
Tahlequah, OK 74464
http://arapaho.nsuok.edu/~optometry

Ontario, Canada

University of Waterloo
Optometry Prgm
School of Optometry
Waterloo, ON N2L 3G1
www.optometry.uwaterloo.ca

Oregon

Pacific University
Optometry Prgm
College of Optometry
2043 College Way
Forest Grove, OR 97116
www.opt.pacificu.edu

Pennsylvania

Pennsylvania College of Optometry
Optometry Prgm
Elkins Park Campus
8360 Old York Rd
Elkins Park, PA 19027
www.pco.edu

Puerto Rico

Inter American University of Puerto Rico
Optometry Prgm
School of Optometry
118 Eleanor Roosevelt St
Hato Rey, PR 00919
www.optonet.inter.edu

Quebec, Canada

University de Montreal
Optometry Prgm
Ecole d'Optometrie
3744 Jean-Brillant, Ste 260-7
Montreal, QC H3T 1P1
www.opto.umontreal.ca

Tennessee

Southern College of Optometry
Optometry Prgm
1245 Madison Ave
Memphis, TN 38104
www.sco.edu

Texas

University of Houston
Optometry Prgm
College of Optometry
505 J Davis Armistead Bldg
Houston, TX 77204
www.opt.uh.edu

Optometric Technician

Indiana

Indiana University - Bloomington
Optometric Technician Prgm
School of Optometry
800 E Atwater Ave
Bloomington, IN 47405

Texas

US Army Medical Dept Center & School
Optometric Technician Prgm
Acadmey of Health Sciences
Fort Sam Houston, TX 78234

US Air Force
Optometric Technician Prgm
383d Training Squadron/XUFG
939 Missile Rd
Sheppard AFB, TX 76311

Washington

Spokane Community College
Optometric Technician Prgm
1810 N Greene St
Spokane, WA 99217

Wisconsin

Madison Area Technical College
Optometric Technician Prgm
3550 Anderson St
Madison, WI 53704

Orthoptist

Career Description

Orthoptics involves the evaluation and treatment of disorders of vision, eye movements, and eye alignment in children and adults. The orthoptist performs a series of diagnostic tests and measurements on patients with visual disorders, including lazy eye, strabismus (misaligned eyes), and double vision. Through interpretation of testing procedures and clinical evaluation, the orthoptist helps the ophthalmologist design a treatment plan, which may involve treatment by the orthoptist, surgical treatment by the ophthalmologist, or some combination of the two.

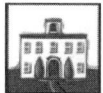

Employment Characteristics

The orthoptist is the liaison between an ophthalmologist and the patient, assisting in the explanation and execution of the treatment. Orthoptists work in a variety of professional settings:

- As a consultant, the orthoptist may travel to several offices or clinics to see patients or work as a professional advisor to vision-related community agencies.
- An orthoptist may serve as a director of state or local vision screening programs.
- Academic opportunities also exist for individuals who want to offer clinical expertise and instruction to orthoptic students, medical students, and resident physicians. Orthoptists may also participate in clinical research and in the presentation and publication of scientific papers.

Orthoptists possess diagnostic ability, technical understanding, and therapeutic skills. In addition, orthoptists should be able to work well with young children, who make up a large portion of orthoptic patients. It is not uncommon for these young patients to have physical, mental, or emotional disabilities.

Salary

Orthoptists receive compensation at the high end of that earned by other health professionals, including physical therapists and physician assistants. Refer to Section IV, Table 5 of this *Directory* for more information, or see www.ama-assn.org/go/hpsalary.

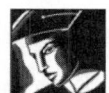

Educational Programs

Length. Orthoptist programs require 2 years of post-graduate study.

Prerequisites. A baccalaureate degree is required; however, exceptions are considered on an individual basis. The Graduate Record Examination is not required.

Curriculum. Lectures, textbooks, journal publications, and proceedings from scientific ophthalmology symposia and conferences form the basis of the didactic teaching. Primary subject areas include anatomy, neuroanatomy, physiology, pharmacology, ophthalmic optics, diagnostic testing and measurement, orthoptic treatment, systemic disease and ocular motor disorders, principles of surgery, and basic ophthalmic examination techniques, as well as genetics, child development, learning disabilities, clinical research methods, and medical writing. In most programs, preparation and presentation of scientific papers are usually required during the second year of education.

Programs are typically structured around an 8-hour day. On average, an orthoptic student will evaluate more than 1,500 patients and observe many more during the course of study. Extensive clinical experience is part of every program.

Inquiries

Inquiries regarding a career in orthoptics, certification, and program accreditation (brochures about the profession are available upon request):

Leslie France, CO, Executive Director
American Orthoptic Council
3914 Nakoma Rd
Madison, WI 53711
608 233-5383
608 263-4247 Fax (attn: Leslie)
E-mail: lwfranceco@att.net
www.orthoptics.org

American Association of Certified Orthoptists
Ron Biernacki, CO, President
E-mail: Ronald.j.biernacki@vanderbilt.edu
www.orthoptics.org

Orthoptist

British Columbia, Canada

British Columbia's Children's Hospital
Orthoptist Prgm
Dept of Ophthamology A135E
4480 Oak St
Vancouver, BC V6H 3N1
Prgm Dir: Christy Giligson, OC(C)
Tel: 604 875-2326   *Fax:* 604 875-3561
E-mail: cgiligson@cw.bc.ca

California

Childrens Hospital Los Angeles
Orthoptist Prgm
4650 Sunset Blvd
Los Angeles, CA 90027
Prgm Dir: Paula Edelman, CO
Tel: 323 361-5697   *Fax:* 323 361-9080
E-mail: pedelman@chla.usc.edu

Florida

University of Florida
Orthoptist Prgm
Box 100393, JHMHC
Gainesville, FL 32610
www.eye.ufl.edu/optkprog.htm
Prgm Dir: Diana Shamis, CO COMT MHSE
Tel: 352 265-0860   *Fax:* 352 265-7081
E-mail: dshamis@ufl.edu
Notes: Currently inactive

Iowa

University of Iowa Hospitals & Clinics
Orthoptist Prgm
Dept of Opthalmology
200 Hawkins Dr
Iowa City, IA 52242
http://webeye.ophth.uiowa.edu/dept/orthoptc/
   orthop.htm
Prgm Dir: Pamela Kutschke, BS CO
Tel: 319 356-3863   *Fax:* 319 384-9831
E-mail: Pamela-kutschke@uiowa.edu

Maryland

Greater Baltimore Medical Center
Orthoptist Prgm
Department of Ophthalmology
PPW Ste 505
Baltimore, MD 21204
Prgm Dir: Cheryl McCarus, CO COMT
Tel: 443 849-8097   *Fax:* 443 849-2648
E-mail: cmccarus@gbmc.org

Michigan

W K Kellogg Eye Center
Orthoptist Prgm
1000 Wall St
Ann Arbor, MI 48105
Prgm Dir: Bruce A Furr, CO
Tel: 734 764-7558   *Fax:* 734 763-7114
E-mail: bfurr@umich.edu

Minnesota

Park Nicollet Orthoptic Fellowship
Orthoptist Prgm
3900 Park Nicollet Blvd
Minneapolis, MN 55416
www.parknicollet.com
Prgm Dir: Lisa Rovick, CO COMT
Tel: 952 993-3737   *Fax:* 952 993-0288
E-mail: rovicl@parknicollet.com

University of Minnesota - Minneapolis
Orthoptist Prgm
Dept of Ophthalmology
516 Delaware St SE
Minneapolis, MN 55455
Prgm Dir: Kimberly Merrill, CO
Tel: 612 625-4400   *Fax:* 612 626-3119
E-mail: kmerrill@umphysicians.umn.edu

New York

University at Buffalo - SUNY
Cosponsor: Ross Eye Institute Orthoptic Program
Orthoptist Prgm
Dept of Ophthalmology
Ira G Ross Eye Institute
Buffalo, NY 14209
www.smbs.buffalo.edu/ophthalmology
Prgm Dir: Kyle Arnoldi, COMT CO
Tel: 716 881-7900
E-mail: kylea@buffalo.edu

New York Eye & Ear Infirmary
Orthoptist Prgm
Allied Health School in Ophthalmology
310 E 14th St
New York, NY 10003
Prgm Dir: Sara Shippman
Tel: 212 979-4375   *Fax:* 212 979-4564
E-mail: sshippman@nyee.edu

Nova Scotia, Canada

IWK Grace Health Centre
Cosponsor: Dalhousie University
Orthoptist Prgm
Clinical Vision Science Program
5850 University Ave, PO Box 9700
Halifax, NS B3K 6R8
Prgm Dir: Karen McMain, OC(C) COMT
Tel: 902 470-8959   *Fax:* 902 470-7207
E-mail: karen.mcmain@iwk.nshealth.ca

Oklahoma

Orthoptic Teaching Program of Tulsa
Orthoptist Prgm
6606 S Yale, Ste 110
Tulsa, OK 74136
Prgm Dir: Amy G McCarthy, CO COT
Tel: 918 481-2781   *Fax:* 918 481-2785
E-mail: amccarthy@pediatriceyeassociates.com

Ontario, Canada

Hospital for Sick Children
Orthoptist Prgm
555 University Ave, Rm M109
Toronto, ON M5G 1X8
Prgm Dir: Jennifer Schofield, OC(C) COMT
Tel: 416 813-5798   *Fax:* 416 813-7040
E-mail: jennifer.schofield@sickkids.ca

Saskatchewan, Canada

Orthoptic Clinic Eye Care Centre
Orthoptist Prgm
701 Queen St
Saskatoon, SK S7K 5T6
www.orthoptics.ca
Prgm Dir: Ronna Hjertaas, OC(C) COT
Tel: 306 655-8058   *Fax:* 306 655-8119
E-mail: ronna.hjertaas@saskatoonhealthregion.ca

Wisconsin

University of Wisconsin Hospital and Clinics
Orthoptist Prgm
Dept of Ophthalmology and Visual Services
2880 University Ave, Rm 223
Madison, WI 53705-9030
Prgm Dir: Jacqueline Shimko, BGS CO
Tel: 608 263-7189   *Fax:* 608 263-4247
E-mail: jw.shimko@hosp.wisc.edu

Orthotist and Prosthetist

Orthotics and prosthetics are applied physical disciplines that address neuromuscular and structural skeletal problems in the human body with a treatment process that includes evaluation and transfer of forces using orthoses and prostheses to achieve optimum function, prevent further disability, and provide cosmesis.

The orthotist and prosthetist work directly with the physician and representatives of other allied health professions in the rehabilitation of the physically challenged. The orthotist designs and fits devices, known as orthoses, to provide care to patients who have disabling conditions of the limbs and spine. The prosthetist designs and fits devices, known as prostheses, for patients who have partial or total absence of a limb.

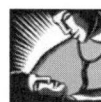

Career Description

The role of the orthotist and prosthetist includes, but may not be limited to, five major domains: clinical assessment, patient management, technical implementation, practice management, and professional responsibility.

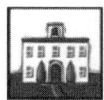

Employment Characteristics

Orthotists and prosthetists typically provide their services in one or more of the following settings: private facilities, hospitals and clinics, colleges and universities, and medical schools.

Salary

According to the National Commission on Orthotic and Prosthetic Education, the salary for board-certified orthotists and prosthetists averages between $42,000 and $60,000. Refer to Section IV, Table 5 of this *Directory* for more information, or see www.ama-assn.org/go/hpsalary.

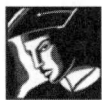

Educational Programs

Length. Orthotic and/or prosthetic education occurs in two forms: baccalaureate degree and certificate programs. Degree programs are based on a standard 4-year curriculum, and certificate courses range from 6 months to 1 year for one discipline to 18 months to 2 years for both disciplines.

Prerequisites. Applicants for the 4-year baccalaureate degree programs should have a high school diploma or equivalent and meet institutional entrance requirements. Applicants for postbaccalaureate programs should have a baccalaureate degree that includes appropriate coursework in biology, chemistry, physics, psychology, algebra, human anatomy, and physiology, as well as any other specified by the institution.

Curriculum. The professional curriculum includes formal instruction in biomechanics gait analysis/pathomechanics, kinesiology, pathology, materials science, research methods, diagnostic imaging techniques, measurement, impression taking, model rectification, diagnostic fitting, definitive fitting, postoperative management, external power, static and dynamic alignment of sockets related to various amputation levels, and fitting and alignment of orthoses for lower limb, upper limb, and spine with various

systems to be included. The curriculum also includes a clinical experience.

Inquiries

Careers

National Commission on Orthotic and Prosthetic Education
330 John Carlyle Street, Suite 200
Alexandria, VA 22314
703 836-7114
703 836-0838 Fax
E-mail: info@ncope.org
www.ncope.org

American Academy of Orthotists and Prosthetists
526 King Street, Suite 200
Alexandria, VA 22314
703 836-0788
703 836-0737 Fax
www.oandp.org

American Orthotic & Prosthetic Association
330 John Carlyle Street, Suite 200
Alexandria, VA 22314
571 431-0876
www.aopanet.org

Certification

American Board for Certification in Orthotics & Prosthetics, Inc
330 John Carlyle Street, Suite 200
Alexandria, VA 22314
703 836-7114
www.abcop.org

Program Accreditation

Commission on Accreditation of Allied Health Education Programs (CAAHEP) in collaboration with:
National Commission on Orthotic and Prosthetic Education
330 John Carlyle Street, Suite 200
Alexandria, VA 22314
703 836-7114
703 836-0838 Fax
E-mail: info@ncope.org
www.ncope.org

Orthotist/Prosthetist

California

California State University - Dominguez Hills
Orthotist/Prosthetist Prgm
1000 E Victoria Blvd
Carson, CA 90747
Prgm Dir: Scott Hornbeak, MBA CPO
Tel: 949 643-5374   *Fax:* 949 643-5337
E-mail: shornbeak@csudh.edu

Connecticut

Hanger Orthopedic Group
Orthotist/Prosthetist Prgm
Newington Certificate Program in Orthotics &
Prosthetics
181 Patricia M Genova Dr
Newington, CT 06111-1500
www.ncpschool.com
Prgm Dir: Robert Lin, CPO FAAOP
Tel: 860 667-5361   *Fax:* 860 666-5386
E-mail: blin@hanger.com

Georgia

Georgia Institute of Technology
Orthotist/Prosthetist Prgm
School of Applied Physiology
281 Ferst Dr
Atlanta, GA 30332-0356
www.ap.gatech.edu/mspo
Prgm Dir: Robert J Gregor, PhD
Tel: 404 894-3986   *Fax:* 404 894-9982
E-mail: robert.gregor@ap.gatech.edu

Illinois

Northwestern University
Orthotist/Prosthetist Prgm
345 E Superior St, Rm 1712
Chicago, IL 60611-4496
Prgm Dir: Michael Brncick, MEd CPO
Tel: 312 238-8006   *Fax:* 312 238-1186
E-mail: m-brncick@northwestern.edu

Michigan

Eastern Michigan University
Cosponsor: University of Michigan Orthotic-Prosthetic
Center
Orthotist/Prosthetist Prgm
318 Porter Bldg
Ypsilanti, MI 48197
Prgm Dir: Robert Rhodes, MPA CO
Tel: 734 487-7120, Ext 2724
E-mail: rrhodes4@emich.edu

Minnesota

Century College
Orthotist/Prosthetist Prgm
3300 Century Ave N
White Bear Lake, MN 55110
Prgm Dir: Edward Haddon, MEd CO
Tel: 651 779-5777   *Fax:* 651 779-3343
E-mail: e.haddon@century.mnscu.edu

Texas

Univ of Texas Southwestern Med Ctr
Orthotist/Prosthetist Prgm
5323 Harry Hines Blvd, Ste V5.400
Dallas, TX 75390-9091
www.utsouthwestern.edu/po
Prgm Dir: Susan Kapp, BS MEd CPO
Tel: 214 648-1580   *Fax:* 214 645-8258
E-mail: susan.kapp@utsouthwestern.edu

Washington

University of Washington
Orthotist/Prosthetist Prgm
1959 NE Pacific St
Box 356490
Seattle, WA 98195-6490
www.depts.washington.edu/rehab/po
Prgm Dir: Ann Yamane, BS CO LO
Tel: 206 616-8586   *Fax:* 206 685-3244
E-mail: pando96@u.washington.edu

Orthotist/Prosthetist

Programs*	Class Capacity	Begins	Length (months)	Award	Res. Tuition	Non-res. Tuition	Stipend	Offers:‡ 1	2	3	4
Connecticut											
Hanger Orthopedic Group (Newington)	60	Sep	9	Cert	$21,068	$21,068					•
Georgia											
Georgia Institute of Technology (Atlanta)	10	Aug	24	MSPO	$4,816	$20,170				•	
Michigan											
Eastern Michigan University (Ypsilanti)	18	Fall	21	Cert, MSOP	$5,908	$11,364		•			•
Texas											
Univ of Texas Southwestern Med Ctr (Dallas)	15	May	24	BS	$3,998	$13,493				•	
Washington											
University of Washington (Seattle)	24	Sep	20	BS	$5,985	$21,285					

*Data are shown only for programs that completed the 2007 AMA Survey of Health Professions Education Programs.
‡Key to Offers: 1: Evening or weekend classes; 2: Non-English instruction; 3: Cultural competence instruction; 4: Distance education component.

Perfusionist

A perfusionist is a skilled person, qualified by academic and clinical education, who operates extracorporeal circulation equipment during any medical situation where it is necessary to support or temporarily replace the patient's circulatory or respiratory function. The perfusionist is knowledgeable concerning the variety of equipment available to perform extracorporeal circulation functions and is responsible, in consultation with the physician, for selecting the appropriate equipment and techniques to be used.

Career Description

A perfusionist is a skilled allied health professional, trained and educated specifically as a member of an open-heart, surgical team responsible for the selection, setup, and operation of a mechanical device commonly referred to as the heart-lung machine.

During open heart surgery, when the patient's heart is immobilized and cannot function in a normal fashion while the operation is being performed, the patient's blood is diverted and circulated outside the body through the heart-lung machine and returned again to the patient. In effect, the machine assumes the function of both the heart and lungs.

The perfusionist is responsible for operating the machine during surgery, monitoring the altered circulatory process closely, taking appropriate corrective action when abnormal situations arise, and keeping both the surgeon and anesthesiologist fully informed.

In addition to the operation of the heart-lung machine during surgery, perfusionists often function in supportive roles for other medical specialties in operating mechanical devices to assist in the conservation of blood and blood products during surgery, and provide extended, long-term support of patients' circulation outside of the operating room environment.

Employment Characteristics

Perfusionists primarily work in the operating room during cardiac surgery procedures and may be employed by the hospital, by surgeons, or as employees of a contract independent group practice. The majority of procedures are performed during regular weekly work hours. As critical members of the clinical teams, perfusionists are required to take call and be available for emergency procedures, which can occur at any time. The call schedule is dependant on the number of perfusionists employed by the institution.

Salary

Perfusionists are well compensated for their services. According to the American Society of Extra-Corporeal Technology (AmSECT), the average base salary range for practicing perfusionists is as follows:

- Recently graduated perfusionist: $60,000-$75,000
- Perfusionist with 2 to 5 years experience: $70,000-$90,000
- Perfusionist with 6 to 10 years experience: $80,000-$100,000
- Perfusionist managers: over $100,000

Refer to Section IV, Table 5 of this *Directory* for more information, or see www.ama-assn.org/go/hpsalary.

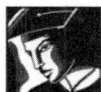

Educational Programs

Length. Programs are generally 1 to 4 years, depending on the program design, objectives, prerequisites, and student qualifications. Certificate programs require that applicants have a bachelor's degree.

Prerequisites. Prerequisites vary depending on the length and design of the program. Most programs require college-level science and mathematics. A background in medical technology, respiratory therapy, or nursing is suggested for some programs.

Curriculum. Curricula of accredited programs include courses covering heart-lung bypass for adult, pediatric, and infant patients undergoing heart surgery; long-term supportive extracorporeal circulation; monitoring of the patient undergoing extracorporeal circulation; autotransfusion; and special applications of the technology. Curricula include clinical experience that incorporates and requires performance of an adequate number and variety of circulation procedures.

Inquiries

Careers

American Society of Extra-Corporeal Technology (AmSECT)
National Office
2209 Dickens Road
Richmond, VA 23230-2005
www.amsect.org

American Academy of Cardiovascular Perfusion
PO Box 3596
Allentown, PA 18106-0596
610 395-4853
E-mail: officeAACP@aol.com
www.theaacp.com

Certification

American Board of Cardiovascular Perfusion
207 N 25th Avenue
Hattiesburg, MS 39401
601 582-2227
www.abcp.org

Program Accreditation

Commission on Accreditation of Allied Health Education Programs (CAAHEP) in collaboration with:
Accreditation Committee - Perfusion Education
6654 S Sycamore Street
Littleton, CO 80120
303 738-0770
303 738-3223 Fax
E-mail: ac-pe@msn.com
www.ac-pe.org

Perfusionist

Arizona

Midwestern University - Glendale Campus
Perfusion Prgm
19555 N 59th Ave
Glendale, AZ 85308
Prgm Dir: Jon W Austin
Tel: 623 572-3616   *Fax:* 623 572-3227
E-mail: jausti@midwestern.edu

University of Arizona College of Medicine
Perfusion Prgm
College of Medicine
1501 N Campbell Ave
Tucson, AZ 85724
www.perfusion.arizona.edu
Prgm Dir: Douglas F Larson, PhD CCP
Tel: 520 626-6339   *Fax:* 520 626-4042
E-mail: dflarson@u.arizona.edu

Connecticut

Quinnipiac University
Perfusion Prgm
275 Mt Carmel Ave
Hamden, CT 06518
www.quinnipiac.edu/x810.xml
Prgm Dir: Michael J Smith, PhD RRT CCP LP
Tel: 203 582-3427   *Fax:* 203 582-8706
E-mail: michael.smith@quinnipiac.edu

District of Columbia

Walter Reed Army Medical Center
Perfusion Prgm
6900 Georgia Ave NW
Bldg 2, Rm 4655
Washington, DC 20307-5001
Prgm Dir: James M Ogletree, MMS PA-C CCP
Tel: 202 782-3607   *Fax:* 202 782-8253
E-mail: james.ogletree@na.amedd.army.mil

Florida

Barry University
Perfusion Prgm
11300 NE 2nd Ave
Miami Shores, FL 33161
Prgm Dir: Jason L Freed, MS
Tel: 800 756-6000, Ext 3214   *Fax:* 305 899-3183
E-mail: jfreed@mail.barry.edu

Illinois

Rush University
Perfusion Prgm
600 S Paulina Ave
Chicago, IL 60612
www.rush.edu
Prgm Dir: Robin Sutton, MS LP (CCP)
Tel: 312 942-2305   *Fax:* 312 563-2984
E-mail: robin_g_sutton@rush.edu

Iowa

University of Iowa Hospitals & Clinics
Perfusion Prgm
200 Hawkins Dr, 1601 JCP
Iowa City, IA 52242-1086
www.healthcare.uiowa.edu/programs/perfusion/
Prgm Dir: Scott Niles, BA CCP
Tel: 319 356-8496   *Fax:* 319 353-7174
E-mail: scott-niles@uiowa.edu

Nebraska

University of Nebraska Medical Center
Perfusion Prgm
985155 Nebraska Medical Center
Omaha, NE 68198-5155
Prgm Dir: David W Holt, MA CCT NRABT
Tel: 402 559-7227   *Fax:* 402 559-6455
E-mail: dwholt@unmc.edu

New Jersey

Cooper University Hospital
Perfusion Prgm
One Cooper Plaza
310 Sarah Cooper Bldg
Camden, NJ 08103
Prgm Dir: Brian Schwartz, BA CCP RN BSN
Tel: 856 342-3277   *Fax:* 856 968-8529
E-mail: schwartz-brian@cooperhealth.edu

New York

North Shore University Hospital
Cosponsor: LIU CW Post
Perfusion Prgm
School of Cardiovascular Perfusion
225 Community Dr South Entrance
Great Neck, NY 11021
Prgm Dir: Richard Chan, BS CCP
Tel: 516 918-4356   *Fax:* 516 466-3780
E-mail: ehiscvp@aol.com

SUNY Upstate Medical University
Perfusion Prgm
750 E Adams St
Syracuse, NY 13210
http://perfusion.upstate.edu
Prgm Dir: Bruce Searles, BS CCP
Tel: 315 464-6933   *Fax:* 315 464-6914
E-mail: Searlesb@upstate.edu

Ohio

Christ Hospital
Perfusion Prgm
2139 Auburn Ave
Cincinnati, OH 45219
www.health-alliance.com/christ/perfusion_science.html
Prgm Dir: Craig Warmuth, MEd CCP
Tel: 513 585-1106   *Fax:* 513 585-3241
E-mail: warmutcr@healthall.com

Cleveland Clinic Foundation
Perfusion Prgm
School of Cardiovacular Perfusion
9500 Euclid Ave/G-33
Cleveland, OH 44195-5130
www.clevelandclinic.org/heartcenter/perfusion
Prgm Dir: Robert Farrow, CCP
Tel: 216 444-9215   *Fax:* 216 445-2725
E-mail: farrowr@ccf.org

Ohio State University
Perfusion Prgm
Circulation Technology Division, 152 Atwell Hall
1583 Perry St
Columbus, OH 43210
Prgm Dir: Jeffrey B Riley, MHPE CCT
Tel: 614 292-7261, Ext 2#   *Fax:* 614 292-0210
E-mail: riley.267@osu.edu

Pennsylvania

Drexel University
Perfusion Prgm
College of Nursing and Health Professions
Cardiovascular Perfusion Techology Prgm
Philadelphia, PA 19102-1192
Prgm Dir: William J D'Andrea, MS CCP
Tel: 215 762-7895   *Fax:* 215 762-1164
E-mail: william.j.dandrea@drexel.edu

UPMC Presbyterian Shadyside
Perfusion Prgm
5230 Centre Ave
Pittsburgh, PA 15232
Prgm Dir: Robert Rush, CCP
Tel: 412 623-2482   *Fax:* 412 623-1091
E-mail: schoolperf@upmc.edu

South Carolina

Medical University of South Carolina
Perfusion Prgm
College of Health Professions
151 B Rutledge Ave
Charleston, SC 29425
Prgm Dir: Joseph J Sistino, CCP
Tel: 843 792-2298   *Fax:* 843 792-4417
E-mail: sistinoj@musc.edu

Tennessee

Vanderbilt University Medical Center
Perfusion Prgm
2986 TVC
Nashville, TN 37232-5734
Prgm Dir: James J Ramsey, LCP CCP JD
Tel: 615 343-9195   *Fax:* 615 333-0742
E-mail: james.ramsey@vanderbilt.edu

Texas

Texas Heart Institute
Perfusion Prgm
PO Box 20345
Mail Code 1 - 224
Houston, TX 77225
Prgm Dir: Terry Crane, BS CCP LP
Tel: 832 355-4026   *Fax:* 832 355-8677

Wisconsin

Milwaukee School of Engineering
Perfusion Prgm
1025 N Broadway St
Milwaukee, WI 53202-3109
www.msoe.edu
Prgm Dir: Ron Gerrits, PhD
Tel: 414 277-7561   *Fax:* 414 277-7465
E-mail: gerrits@msoe.edu

Perfusionist

Programs*	Class Capacity	Begins	Length (months)	Award	Res. Tuition	Non-res. Tuition	Stipend	Offers:‡ 1	2	3	4
Arizona											
University of Arizona College of Medicine (Tucson)	4	Aug	22	Cert, MS	$4,764	$14,970					
Connecticut											
Quinnipiac University (Hamden)	12	Aug	21	MHS	$20,000	$20,000					
Illinois											
Rush University (Chicago)	10	Sep	21	BS, MS	$26,588	$26,588					
Iowa											
University of Iowa Hospitals & Clinics (Iowa City)	5	Aug	20	Cert	$7,340	$18,358					
New York											
North Shore University Hospital (Great Neck)	11	Sep	24	Cert, MS	$20,500	$20,500		•			
SUNY Upstate Medical University (Syracuse)	6	Aug	21	BS	$8,500	$20,750					
Ohio											
Christ Hospital(Cincinnati)	6	Sep	21	Cert	$16,000	$16,000					
Cleveland Clinic Foundation	8	Jan	18	Cert	$25,000	$25,000				•	
Texas											
Texas Heart Institute(Houston)	8	Jan Jul	12	Cert	$18,000	$18,000					
Wisconsin											
Milwaukee School of Engineering	8	Sep	21	MSP	$20,000	$20,000					

*Data are shown only for programs that completed the 2007 AMA Survey of Health Professions Education Programs.
‡Key to Offers: 1: Evening or weekend classes; 2: Non-English instruction; 3: Cultural competence instruction; 4: Distance education component.

PROGRAMS

Pharmacists play a vital role in the health care system through the medicine and information they provide. Although responsibilities vary among the different areas of pharmacy practice, the bottom line is that pharmacists help patients get well. Pharmacists are drug experts ultimately concerned about their patients' health and wellness.

The number of people requiring health care services has steadily increased, and this trend will likely continue. Due to many of society's changing social and health issues, pharmacists will face new challenges, including:

- Increases in average life span and the increased incidence of chronic diseases
- Increased complexity, number, and sophistication of medications and related products and devices
- Increased emphasis on primary and preventive health services, home health care, and long-term care
- Concerns about improving patients' access to health care while controlling costs and assuring quality

Career Description

Pharmacists distribute drugs prescribed by physicians and other health practitioners and provide information to patients about medications and their use. They advise physicians and other health practitioners on the selection, dosages, interactions, and side effects of medications. Pharmacists also monitor the health and progress of patients in response to drug therapy to ensure the safe and effective use of medication. Pharmacists must understand the use, clinical effects, and composition of drugs, including their chemical, biological, and physical properties. Compounding—the actual mixing of ingredients to form powders, tablets, capsules, ointments, and solutions—is a small part of a pharmacist's practice, because most medicines are produced by pharmaceutical companies in a standard dosage and drug delivery form.

About 61 percent of the nation's 230,000 pharmacists work in a community setting, such as a retail drugstore; about one quarter work in a health care facility, such as a hospital, nursing home, mental health institution, or neighborhood health clinic.

Pharmacists in community and retail pharmacies counsel patients and answer questions about prescription drugs, including questions regarding possible side effects or interactions among various drugs. They provide information about over-the-counter drugs and make recommendations after talking with the patient. They also may give advice about the patient's diet, exercise, or stress management or about durable medical equipment and home health care supplies. In addition, they also may complete third-party insurance forms and other paperwork. Those who own or manage community pharmacies may sell non-health-related merchandise, hire and supervise personnel, and oversee the general operation of the pharmacy. Some community pharmacists provide specialized services to help patients manage conditions such as diabetes, asthma, smoking cessation, or high blood pressure. Some community pharmacists also are trained to administer vaccinations.

Pharmacists in health care facilities dispense medications and advise the medical staff on the selection and effects of drugs. They may make sterile solutions to be administered intravenously. They also assess, plan, and monitor drug programs or regimens. Pharmacists counsel hospitalized patients on the use of drugs and on their use at home when the patients are discharged. Pharmacists also may evaluate drug-use patterns and outcomes for patients in hospitals or managed care organizations.

Pharmacists who work in home health care monitor drug therapy and prepare infusions—solutions that are injected into patients—and other medications for use in the home.

Some pharmacists specialize in specific drug therapy areas, such as intravenous nutrition support, oncology (cancer), nuclear pharmacy (used for chemotherapy), geriatric pharmacy, and psychopharmacotherapy (the treatment of mental disorders by means of drugs).

Most pharmacists keep confidential computerized records of patients' drug therapies to prevent harmful drug interactions. Pharmacists are responsible for the accuracy of every prescription that is filled, but they often rely upon pharmacy technicians and pharmacy aides to assist them in the dispensing process. Thus, the pharmacist may delegate prescription-filling and administrative tasks and supervise their completion. Pharmacists also frequently oversee pharmacy students serving as interns in preparation for graduation and licensure.

Increasingly, pharmacists are pursuing nontraditional pharmacy work. Some are involved in research for pharmaceutical manufacturers, developing new drugs and therapies and testing their effects on people. Others work in marketing or sales, providing expertise to clients on a drug's use, effectiveness, and possible side effects. Some pharmacists work for health insurance companies, developing pharmacy benefit packages and carrying out cost-benefit analyses on certain drugs. Other pharmacists work for the government, public health care services, the armed services, and pharmacy associations. Finally, some pharmacists are employed full time or part time as college faculty, teaching classes and performing research in a wide range of areas.

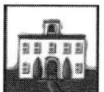

Employment Characteristics

Pharmacists work in clean, well-lighted, and well-ventilated areas. Many pharmacists spend most of their workday on their feet. When working with sterile or dangerous pharmaceutical products, pharmacists wear gloves and masks and work with other special protective equipment. Many community and hospital pharmacies are open for extended hours or around the clock, so pharmacists may work nights, weekends, and holidays. Consultant pharmacists may travel to nursing homes or other facilities to monitor patients' drug therapy.

About 21 percent of pharmacists worked part time in 2004. Most full-time salaried pharmacists worked approximately 40 hours a week. Some, including many self-employed pharmacists, worked more than 50 hours a week.

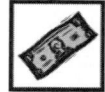

Salary

According to a 2006 survey by *Drug Topics* magazine, the median annual earning of pharmacists was $94,927 in 2006, as compared to $89,723 in 2004, $82,607 in 2002, $78,624 in 2000, and $64,980 in 1999. Retail pharmacists averaged $92,291, while institutional pharmacists earned an average of $97,545.

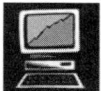

Employment Outlook

A shortfall of as many as 157,000 pharmacists is predicted by 2020, according to the findings of a conference sponsored by the Pharmacy Manpower Project, as detailed in *Professionally Determined Need for Pharmacy Services in 2020*. Similarly, a December 2000 report of the Health Resources and Services Administration of the Department of Health and Human Services, *The Pharmacy Workforce: A Study of the Supply and Demand for Pharmacists*, which concludes that the increasing demand for pharmacists' services is outpacing the current and possibly future pharmacist supply.

Accordingly, very good employment opportunities are expected for pharmacists through 2014 because the number of job openings created by employment growth and the need to replace pharmacists who leave the occupation or retire are expected to exceed the number of degrees granted in pharmacy. Enrollments in pharmacy programs are rising as more students are attracted by high salaries and good job prospects. Despite this increase in enrollments, job openings should still be more numerous than those seeking employment.

Employment of pharmacists is expected to grow faster than the average for all occupations through the year 2014, because of the increasing demand for pharmaceuticals, particularly from the growing elderly population. The increasing numbers of middle-aged and elderly people—who use more prescription drugs than younger people—will continue to spur demand for pharmacists in all employment settings. Other factors likely to increase the demand for pharmacists include scientific advances that will make more drug products available, new developments in genome research and medication distribution systems, increasingly sophisticated consumers seeking more information about drugs, and coverage of prescription drugs by a greater number of health insurance plans and Medicare.

Community pharmacies are taking steps to manage an increasing volume of prescriptions. Automation of drug dispensing and greater employment of pharmacy technicians and pharmacy aides will help these establishments to dispense more prescriptions.

With its emphasis on cost control, managed care encourages the use of lower cost prescription drug distributors, such as mail-order firms and online pharmacies, for purchases of certain medications. Prescriptions ordered through the mail and via the Internet are filled in a central location and shipped to the patient at a lower cost. Mail-order and online pharmacies typically use automated technology to dispense medication and employ fewer pharmacists. If the utilization of mail-order pharmacies increases rapidly, job growth among pharmacists could be limited.

Employment of pharmacists will not grow as fast in hospitals as in other industries, because hospitals are reducing inpatient stays, downsizing, and consolidating departments. The number of outpatient surgeries is increasing, so more patients are being discharged and purchasing their medications through retail, supermarket, or mail-order pharmacies, rather than through hospitals. An aging population means that more pharmacy services will be required in nursing homes, assisted-living facilities, and home care settings. The most rapid job growth among pharmacists is expected in these 3 settings.

New opportunities are emerging for pharmacists in managed care organizations where they analyze trends and patterns in medication use, and in pharmacoeconomics—the cost and benefit analysis of different drug therapies. Opportunities also are emerging for pharmacists trained in research and disease management—the development of new methods for curing and controlling diseases. Pharmacists also are finding jobs in research and development and in sales and marketing for pharmaceutical manufacturing firms. New breakthroughs in biotechnology will increase the potential for drugs to treat diseases and expand the opportunities for pharmacists to conduct research and sell medications. In addition, pharmacists are finding employment opportunities in pharmacy informatics, which uses information technology to improve patient care.

Job opportunities for pharmacists in patient care will arise as cost-conscious insurers and health systems continue to emphasize the role of pharmacists in primary and preventive health care. Health insurance companies realize that the expense of using medication to treat diseases and various health conditions often is considerably less than the costs for patients whose conditions go untreated. Pharmacists also can reduce the expenses resulting from unexpected complications due to allergic reactions or interactions among medications.

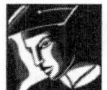

Educational Programs

Award, Length. The Doctor of Pharmacy (PharmD) degree requires at least 2 years of specific preprofessional (undergraduate) course work followed by 4 academic years (or 3 calendar years) of professional study. The PharmD degree has replaced the Bachelor of Pharmacy (BPharm) degree, which is no longer being awarded.

Prerequisites. Pharmacy colleges and schools may accept students directly from high school for both the prepharmacy and pharmacy curriculum, or after completion of the college course prerequisites. The majority of students enter a pharmacy program with 3 or more years of college experience. Entry requirements usually include courses in mathematics and natural sciences, such as chemistry, biology, and physics, as well as courses in the humanities and social sciences. Approximately two thirds of all colleges require applicants to take the Pharmacy College Admissions Test (PCAT).

Prospective pharmacists should have scientific aptitude, good communication skills, and a desire to help others. They also must be conscientious and pay close attention to detail, because the decisions they make affect human lives, and possess high ethical and professional standards. Other character traits of successful pharmacists include curiosity and desire and willingness to learn. Most importantly, pharmacists must enjoy working with people, be comfortable meeting them, and be willing to serve them in a variety of circumstances.

Curriculum. Pharmacy students learn about all aspects of drug therapy as well as how to communicate with patients and other health care providers about drug information and patient care. Other courses focus on professional ethics, public health, and developing and managing medication distribution systems. In addition to classroom instruction, students in PharmD programs spend about one fourth of their time learning in a variety of pharmacy practice settings under the supervision of licensed pharmacists.

Advanced Training. For individuals who want more laboratory and research experience, many colleges of pharmacy offer an MS or PhD degree after completion of the PharmD degree. Many master's and PhD degree holders do research for drug companies or teach at universities.

Other options for pharmacy graduates who are interested in further training include 1-year or 2-year residency programs or fellowships. Pharmacy residencies are postgraduate training programs in pharmacy practice and usually require the completion of a research study. There currently are more than 700 residency programs nationwide. Pharmacy fellowships are highly individualized programs that are designed to prepare participants to work in a specialized area of pharmacy, such as clinical practice or research laboratories. Some pharmacists who run their own pharmacy obtain a master's degree in business administration (MBA). Others may obtain a degree in public administration or public health.

Areas of graduate study include pharmaceutics and pharmaceutical chemistry (physical and chemical properties of drugs and dosage forms), pharmacology (effects of drugs on the body), toxicology and pharmacy administration.

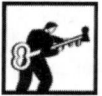

Licensure, Certification, Registration

A license to practice pharmacy is required in all states, the District of Columbia, and all US territories. To obtain a license, the prospective pharmacist must graduate from a college of pharmacy accredited by the Accreditation Council for Pharmacy Education (ACPE) and pass an examination. All states require the North American Pharmacist Licensure Exam (NAPLEX), which tests pharmacy skills and knowledge, and 43 states and the District of Columbia require the Multistate Pharmacy Jurisprudence Exam (MPJE), which tests pharmacy law. Both exams are administered by the National Association of Boards of Pharmacy. Pharmacists in the eight states that do not require the MJPE must pass a state-specific exam that is similar to the MJPE. In addition to the NAPLEX and MPJE, some states require additional exams unique to their state. All states except California currently grant a license without extensive reexamination to qualified pharmacists who already are licensed by another state. In Florida, reexamination is not required if a pharmacist has passed the NAPLEX and MPJE within 12 years of applying for a license transfer. Many pharmacists are licensed to practice in more than one state. Most states require continuing education for license renewal.

Inquiries

Education, Careers, Resources
American Association of Colleges of Pharmacy
1426 Prince Street
Alexandria, VA 22314
703 739-2330, x1024
www.aacp.org

American Society of Health-System Pharmacists
7272 Wisconsin Avenue
Bethesda, MD 20814
www.ashp.org

American Pharmacists Association
2215 Constitution Avenue NW
Washington, DC 20037-2985
www.aphanet.org

Licensure
National Association of Boards of Pharmacy
1600 Feehanville Drive
Mount Prospect, IL 60056
www.nabp.net

Program Accreditation
Accreditation Council for Pharmacy Education
20 N Clark Street, Suite 2500
Chicago, IL 60602
www.acpe-accredit.org

Note: Adapted in part from the Bureau of Labor Statistics, US Department of Labor, *Occupational Outlook Handbook*, 2006-07 Edition, Pharmacists, on the Internet at www.bls.gov/oco/ocos079.htm (visited October 12, 2007).

Pharmacist

Alabama

Auburn University
Pharmacy Prgm
School of Pharmacy
217 Walker Bldg
Auburn University, AL 36849-5501
www.pharmacy.auburn.edu
Tel: 334 844-8348   *Fax:* 334 844-8353

Samford University
Pharmacy Prgm
School of Pharmacy
800 Lakeshore Dr
Birmingham, AL 35229
www.samford.edu/schools/pharmacy.html
Tel: 205 726-2820   *Fax:* 205 726-2759

Arizona

Midwestern University - Glendale Campus
Pharmacy Prgm
College of Pharmacy
19555 N 59th Ave
Glendale, AZ 85308
www.midwestern.edu/pages/cpg.html
Tel: 623 572-3500   *Fax:* 623 752-3510

University of Arizona
Pharmacy Prgm
College of Pharmacy
PO Box 210207
Tucson, AZ 85721
www.pharmacy.arizona.edu
Tel: 520 626-1427   *Fax:* 520 626-4063

Arkansas

University of Arkansas for Medical Sciences
Pharmacy Prgm
College of Pharmacy
4301 W Markham St
Little Rock, AR 72205
www.uams.edu/cop
Tel: 501 686-5557   *Fax:* 501 686-8315

California

University of California - San Diego
Pharmacy Prgm
9500 Gilman Dr, MC-0657
La Jolla, CA 92093-0657
www.ucsd.edu
Tel: 858 534-1366   *Fax:* 858 534-8248

Loma Linda University
Pharmacy Prgm
School of Pharmacy
West Hall 1316
Loma Linda, CA 92350
www.llu.edu
Tel: 909 558-7442   *Fax:* 909 558-7973

University of Southern California
Pharmacy Prgm
School of Pharmacy
1985 Zonal Ave
Los Angeles, CA 90089-9121
www.usc.edu/schools/pharmacy
Tel: 323 442-1369   *Fax:* 323 442-1681

Western Univ of Health Sciences
Pharmacy Prgm
College of Pharmacy
309 E Second St
Pomona, CA 91766-1854
www.westernu.edu
Tel: 909 469-5581   *Fax:* 909 469-5539

University of California - San Francisco
Pharmacy Prgm
San Francisco School of Pharmacy
521 Parnassus Ave Rm C-156
San Francisco, CA 94143-0622
www.pharmacy.ucsf.edu
Tel: 415 476-1225   *Fax:* 415 476-6632

University of the Pacific
Pharmacy Prgm
Thomas J Long School of Pharmacy and Health Sciences
3601 Pacific Ave
Stockton, CA 95211
www.pacific.edu/pharmacy/
Tel: 209 946-2561   *Fax:* 209 946-2410

Touro University Mare Island
Pharmacy Prgm
California College of Pharmacy
1310 Johnson Lane
Vallejo, CA 94592
www.tu.edu/indexca.php
Tel: 707 638-5221   *Fax:* 707 632-5266

Colorado

University of Colorado at Denver
Pharmacy Prgm
Health Sciences Center School of Pharmacy
C-238 4200 E Ninth Ave
Denver, CO 80262
www.uchsc.edu
Tel: 303 315-5055   *Fax:* 303 315-6281

Connecticut

University of Connecticut
Pharmacy Prgm
School of Pharmacy
69 N Eagleville Rd Unit 3092
Storrs, CT 06269-3092
www.pharmacy.uconn.edu
Tel: 860 486-2129   *Fax:* 860 486-1553

District of Columbia

Howard University
Pharmacy Prgm
College of Pharmacy, Nursing, and
   Allied Health Sciences
School of Pharmacy
Washington, DC 20059
Tel: 202 806-5431   *Fax:* 202 234-1375

Florida

Nova Southeastern University
Pharmacy Prgm
College of Pharmacy
3200 S University Dr
Fort Lauderdale, FL 33328
http://pharmacy.nova.edu/
Tel: 954 262-1304   *Fax:* 954 262-3995

University of Florida
Pharmacy Prgm
College of Pharmacy
Box 100484
Gainesville, FL 32610
www.cop.ufl.edu
Tel: 352 392-9714   *Fax:* 352 392-3480

Florida A&M University
Pharmacy Prgm
College of Pharmacy and Pharmaceutical Sciences
New Pharmacy Bldg, Rm 333
Tallahassee, FL 32307
www.famu.edu
Tel: 850 599-3301   *Fax:* 850 599-3347

Palm Beach Atlantic University
Pharmacy Prgm
Lloyd L Gregory School of Pharmacy
900 S Olive Ave
West Palm Beach, FL 33401
www.pba.edu
Tel: 561 803-2700   *Fax:* 561 803-2703

Georgia

University of Georgia
Pharmacy Prgm
College of Pharmacy
Athens, GA 30602-2351
www.rx.uga.edu
Tel: 706 542-1914   *Fax:* 706 542-5269

Mercer University
Pharmacy Prgm
College of Pharmacy and Health Sciences
3001 Mercer University Dr
Atlanta, GA 30341-4155
www.mercer.edu/pharmacy
Tel: 678 547-6304   *Fax:* 678 547-6315

South University
Pharmacy Prgm
School of Pharmacy
709 Mall Blvd
Savannah, GA 31406
www.southuniversity.edu
Tel: 912 201-8120   *Fax:* 912 201-8154

Idaho

Idaho State University
Pharmacy Prgm
College of Pharmacy
PO Box 8288
Pocatello, ID 83209
www.pharmacy.isu.edu/live/
Tel: 208 282-2175   *Fax:* 208 282-4482

Illinois

University of Illinois at Chicago
Pharmacy Prgm
College of Pharmacy
833 S Wood St
Chicago, IL 60612
www.uic.edu/pharmacy/
Tel: 312 996-7240   *Fax:* 312 996-3272

Midwestern University
Pharmacy Prgm
Chicago College of Pharmacy
555 31st St
Downers Grove, IL 60515
www.midwestern.edu/pages/ccp.html
Tel: 630 971-6417   *Fax:* 630 971-6097

Southern Illinois University
Pharmacy Prgm
Edwardsville School of Pharmacy
Campus Box 2000
Edwardsville, IL 62026-2000
www.siue.edu/pharmacy/
Tel: 618 650-5150   *Fax:* 618 650-5152

Indiana

Butler University/Clarian Health
Pharmacy Prgm
College of Pharmacy and Health Sciences
4600 Sunset Ave
Indianapolis, IN 46208
www.butler.edu/academics/aca_pharmacy.asp
Tel: 317 940-9735   *Fax:* 317 940-6172

Purdue University
Pharmacy Prgm
School of Pharmacy and Pharmaceutical Sciences
575 Stadium Mall Dr
West Lafayette, IN 47907
www.pharmacy.purdue.edu
Tel: 765 494-1368   *Fax:* 765 494-7880

Iowa

Drake University
Pharmacy Prgm
College of Pharmacy and Health Sciences
2507 University Ave
Des Moines, IA 50311
www.pharmacy.drake.edu
Tel: 515 271-1814   *Fax:* 515 271-4171

University of Iowa
Pharmacy Prgm
College of Pharmacy
115 S Grand Ave
Iowa City, IA 52242
www.pharmacy.uiowa.edu
Tel: 319 335-8794   *Fax:* 319 353-5594

Kansas

University of Kansas
Pharmacy Prgm
School of Pharmacy
1251 Wescoe Hall Dr
Lawrence, KS 66045-7582
www.ku.edu
Tel: 785 864-3591   *Fax:* 785 864-5265

Kentucky

University of Kentucky
Pharmacy Prgm
College of Pharmacy
725 Rose St, Ste 327
Lexington, KY 40536
www.mc.uky.edu/pharmacy/
Tel: 859 323-7601   *Fax:* 859 257-2128

Lebanon

Lebanese American Univ School of Pharmacy
Pharmacy Prgm
PO Box 36
Byblos, Lebanon, LE
www.lau.edu.lb/
Tel: 961 954-7254   *Fax:* 961 954-7256

Louisiana

University of Louisiana at Monroe
Pharmacy Prgm
College of Pharmacy
700 University Ave
Monroe, LA 71209
www.ulm.edu
Tel: 318 342-1600   *Fax:* 318 342-1606

Xavier Univ of Louisiana College of Pharmacy
Pharmacy Prgm
1 Drexel Dr
New Orleans, LA 70125
www.xula.edu/pharmacy
Tel: 504 520-7421   *Fax:* 504 520-7930

Maryland

University of Maryland Baltimore County
Pharmacy Prgm
School of Pharmacy
20 N Pine St, Rm 730
Baltimore, MD 21201
www.pharmacy.umaryland.edu
Tel: 410 706-7651   *Fax:* 410 706-4012

Massachusetts

Mass College of Pharmacy & Health Sciences
Pharmacy Prgm
School of Pharmacy-Boston
179 Longwood Ave
Boston, MA 02115
www.mcphs.edu
Tel: 617 732-2781   *Fax:* 617 735-1082

Northeastern University
Pharmacy Prgm
Bouve College of Health Sciences School of Pharmacy
360 Huntington Ave, 206 Mugar
Boston, MA 02115
www.bouve.neu.edu/pharmacy
Tel: 617 373-3380   *Fax:* 617 373-7655

Mass College of Pharmacy & Health Sciences
Pharmacy Prgm
School of Pharmacy-Worcester
19 Foster St
Worcester, MA 01608
www.mcphs.edu
Tel: 508 890-8855, Ext 1911   *Fax:* 508 890-8515

Michigan

University of Michigan
Pharmacy Prgm
College of Pharmacy
428 Church St
Ann Arbor, MI 48109-1065
www.umich.edu/~pharmacy/
Tel: 734 764-7144   *Fax:* 734 763-2022

Ferris State University
Pharmacy Prgm
College of Pharmacy
220 Ferris Dr
Big Rapids, MI 49307
www.pharmacy.ferris.edu
Tel: 231 591-2254   *Fax:* 231 591-3829

Wayne State University
Pharmacy Prgm
Eugene Applebaum College of Pharmacy and
    Health Sciences
259 Mack Ave, Ste 2620
Detroit, MI 48201
www.cphs.wayne.edu
Tel: 313 577-1574   *Fax:* 313 577-0457

Minnesota

University of Minnesota - Minneapolis
Pharmacy Prgm
College of Pharmacy
308 Harvard St SE
Minneapolis, MN 55455
www.pharmacy.umn.edu
Tel: 612 624-1900   *Fax:* 612 624-2974

Mississippi

University of Mississippi
Pharmacy Prgm
School of Pharmacy
PO Box 1848
University, MS 38677
www.olemiss.edu/depts/pharm_school
Tel: 662 915-7265   *Fax:* 662 915-5118

Missouri

University of Missouri - Kansas City
Pharmacy Prgm
School of Pharmacy
5100 Rockhill Rd
Kansas City, MO 64110
www.umkc.edu/pharmacy
Tel: 816 235-1609   *Fax:* 816 235-5190

St Louis College of Pharmacy
Pharmacy Prgm
4588 Parkview Place
St Louis, MO 63110
www.stlcop.edu
Tel: 314 446-8341   *Fax:* 314 446-8304

Montana

University of Montana
Pharmacy Prgm
College of Health Professions and Biomedical Sciences
Skaggs School of Pharmacy
Missoula, MT 59812
www.health.umt.edu
Tel: 406 243-4621   *Fax:* 406 243-4209

Nebraska

Creighton University
Pharmacy Prgm
Medical Center School of Pharmacy and
    Health Professions
2500 California Plaza
Omaha, NE 68178
www.spahp.creighton.edu
Tel: 402 280-2950   *Fax:* 402 280-5738

University of Nebraska Medical Center
Pharmacy Prgm
College of Pharmacy
986000 Nebraska Medical Center
Omaha, NE 68198
www.unmc.edu/pharmacy/
Tel: 402 559-4333   *Fax:* 402 559-5060

Nevada

University of Southern Nevada
Pharmacy Prgm
College of Phamacy
11 Sunset Way
Henderson, NV 89014
www.usn.edu
Tel: 708 990-4433, Ext 2017   *Fax:* 702 990-4435

New Jersey

Rutgers University
Pharmacy Prgm
New Jersey Ernest Mario School of Pharmacy
William Levin Hall
Piscataway, NJ 08854
pharmacy.rutgers.edu
Tel: 732 445-2675   *Fax:* 732 445-5767

New Mexico

University of New Mexico
Pharmacy Prgm
College of Pharmacy
1 University of New Mexico
Albuquerque, NM 87131
www.hsc.unm.edu
Tel: 505 272-0906   *Fax:* 505 272-6749

New York

Albany College of Pharmacy
Pharmacy Prgm
106 New Scotland Ave
Albany, NY 12208
www.acp.edu
Tel: 518 445-7212   *Fax:* 518 445-7294

University at Buffalo - SUNY
Pharmacy Prgm
School of Pharmacy and Pharmaceutical Sciences
126 Cooke Hall
Amherst, NY 14260
www.pharmacy.buffalo.edu
Tel: 716 645-2823   *Fax:* 716 645-3688

Long Island University
Pharmacy Prgm
Arnold & Marie Schwartz College of Pharmacy &
    Health Science
75 DeKalb Ave
Brooklyn, NY 11201
www.liu.edu
Tel: 718 488-1004   *Fax:* 718 488-0628

St John's University
Pharmacy Prgm
College of Pharmacy and Allied Health Professions
8000 Utopia Pkwy
Jamaica, NY 11439
new.stjohns.edu/academics/graduate/pharmacy
Tel: 718 990-6411   *Fax:* 718 990-1871

North Carolina

Campbell University
Pharmacy Prgm
School of Pharmacy
PO Box 1090
Buies Creek, NC 27506
www.campbell.edu/pharmacy
Tel: 910 893-1685   *Fax:* 910 893-1943

University of North Carolina Hospitals
Pharmacy Prgm
School of Pharmacy
Beard Hall CB #7360
Chapel Hill, NC 27599
www.pharmacy.unc.edu
Tel: 919 966-1122   *Fax:* 919 966-6919

Wingate University
Pharmacy Prgm
School of Pharmacy
315 E Wilson St
Wingate, NC 28174
www.wingate.edu
Tel: 704 233-8015   *Fax:* 704 233-8332

North Dakota

North Dakota State University
Pharmacy Prgm
College of Pharmacy, Nursing and Allied Sciences
123 Sudro Hall
Fargo, ND 58105
www.ndsu.edu/pharmacy
Tel: 701 231-7609   *Fax:* 701 231-7606

Ohio

Ohio Northern University
Pharmacy Prgm
College of Pharmacy
Ada, OH 45810
www.onu.edu/pharmacy
Tel: 419 772-2277   *Fax:* 419 772-2720

University of Cincinnati
Pharmacy Prgm
College of Pharmacy
PO Box 670004
Cincinnati, OH 45267-0004
www.pharmacy.uc.edu
Tel: 513 558-3326   *Fax:* 513 558-4372

Ohio State University
Pharmacy Prgm
College of Pharmacy
500 W 12th Ave
Columbus, OH 43210
www.onu.edu/pharmacy
Tel: 614 292-5711   *Fax:* 614 292-3113

University of Findlay
Pharmacy Prgm
College of Pharmacy
1000 N Main St
Findlay, OH 45840
www.findlay.edu/academics/colleges/cohp/
    academicprograms/schoolofpharm/
Tel: 419 434-5327   *Fax:* 419 434-6977

Northeastern Ohio Univ College of Medicine
Pharmacy Prgm
College of Pharmacy
4209 State Rte 44
Rootstown, OH 44272
www.neoucom.edu/pharmd
Tel: 330 325-6461   *Fax:* 330 325-5930

University of Toledo
Pharmacy Prgm
College of Pharmacy
2801 W Bancroft St
Toledo, OH 43606-3390
www.utpharmacy.org
Tel: 419 530-1931   *Fax:* 419 530-1907

Oklahoma

University of Oklahoma
Pharmacy Prgm
College of Pharmacy
1110 N Stonewall, Rm 133
Oklahoma City, OK 73190
www.oupharmacy.com
Tel: 405 271-6485   *Fax:* 405 271-3830

Southwestern Oklahoma State University
Pharmacy Prgm
School of Pharmacy
100 Campus Dr
Weatherford, OK 73096
www.swosu.edu/pharmacy
Tel: 580 774-3105   *Fax:* 580 774-7020

Oregon

Oregon State University
Pharmacy Prgm
College of Pharmacy
203 Pharmacy Bldg
Corvallis, OR 97331
pharmacy.oregonstate.edu
Tel: 541 737-3424   *Fax:* 541 737-3999

Pacific University
Pharmacy Prgm
School of Pharmacy
2043 College Way
Forest Grove, OR 97116
www.pacificu.edu/pharmd/
Tel: 503 352-3123   *Fax:* 503 352-3158

Pennsylvania

Lake Erie Coll of Osteopathic Medicine - Erie
Pharmacy Prgm
School of Pharmacy
1858 W Grandview Blvd
Erie, PA 16509
Tel: 814 866-8409   *Fax:* 814 866-8450

Temple University
Pharmacy Prgm
School of Pharmacy
3307 N Broad St
Philadelphia, PA 19140
www.temple.edu/pharmacy/
Tel: 215 707-4990   *Fax:* 215 707-3678

University of the Sciences in Philadelphia
Pharmacy Prgm
Philadelphia College of Pharmacy
600 S 43rd St
Philadelphia, PA 19104
www.usip.edu
Tel: 215 596-8805   *Fax:* 215 596-8977

Duquesne University
Pharmacy Prgm
Mylan School of Pharmacy
306 Bayer Learning Center
Pittsburgh, PA 15282
www.pharmacy.duq.edu
Tel: 412 396-6377   *Fax:* 412 396-1810

University of Pittsburgh
Pharmacy Prgm
School of Pharmacy
1104 Salk Hall
Pittsburgh, PA 15261
www.pharmacy.pitt.edu
Tel: 412 624-3270   *Fax:* 412 648-1086

**Nesbitt Coll of Pharm & Nursing Sch of Pharm
    - Wilkes University**
Pharmacy Prgm
Wilkes-Barre, PA 18766
www.wilkes.edu/pages/390.asp
Tel: 570 408-4280   *Fax:* 570 408-7828

Puerto Rico

University of Puerto Rico
Pharmacy Prgm
Medical Sciences Campus School of Pharmacy
PO Box 365067
San Juan, PR 00936
www.upr.clu.edu
Tel: 787 758-2525   *Fax:* 787 751-5680

Rhode Island

University of Rhode Island
Pharmacy Prgm
College of Pharmacy
41 Lower College Rd
Kingston, RI 02881
www.uri.edu/
Tel: 401 874-2761   *Fax:* 401 874-2181

South Carolina

Medical University of South Carolina
Pharmacy Prgm
College of Pharmacy
280 Calhoun St
Charleston, SC 29425
www.musc.edu/pharmacy/
Tel: 843 792-8450   *Fax:* 843 792-9081

South Carolina College of Pharmacy
Pharmacy Prgm
280 Calhoun St
PO Box 250141
Charleston, SC 29425
sccp.sc.edu
Tel: 843 792-8450   *Fax:* 843 792-9081

University of South Carolina
Pharmacy Prgm
College of Pharmacy
Columbia, SC 29208
www.pharm.sc.edu
Tel: 803 777-4151   *Fax:* 803 777-4945

South Dakota

South Dakota State University
Pharmacy Prgm
Box 2202C
1 Administration Lane
Brookings, SD 57007
www.sdstate.edu
Tel: 605 688-6197   *Fax:* 605 688-6232

Tennessee

East Tennessee State University
Pharmacy Prgm
College of Pharmacy
PO Box 70414
Johnson City, TN 37614
www.etsu.edu/pharamcy
Tel: 423 439-6300

University of Tennessee Health Science Ctr
Pharmacy Prgm
College of Pharmacy
847 Monroe Ave, Ste 226
Memphis, TN 38163
pharmacy.utmem.edu
Tel: 901 448-6036   *Fax:* 901 448-7053

Texas

Texas Tech Univ Health Sciences Center
Pharmacy Prgm
School of Pharmacy
1300 S Coulter
Amarillo, TX 79106
www.ttuhsc.edu/sop/
Tel: 806 354-5463   *Fax:* 806 356-4613

University of Texas at Austin
Pharmacy Prgm
College of Pharmacy
1 University Station A1900
Austin, TX 78712
www.utexas.edu/pharmacy/
Tel: 512 471-1737   *Fax:* 512 417-8783

Texas Southern University
Pharmacy Prgm
College of Pharmacy and Health Sciences
3100 Celburne St
Houston, TX 77004
www.tsu.edu
Tel: 713 313-4277   *Fax:* 713 313-1091

University of Houston
Pharmacy Prgm
College of Pharmacy
141 Sciences & Research Bldg 2
Houston, TX 77204
www.uh.edu/pharmacy/
Tel: 713 743-1253   *Fax:* 713 743-5678

Texas A&M University
Pharmacy Prgm
Health Science Center Irma Lerma Rangel
College of Pharmacy
Kingsville, TX 78363
pharmacy.tamhsc.edu
Tel: 361 593-4271   *Fax:* 361 593-4233

University of the Incarnate Word
Pharmacy Prgm
Feik School of Pharmacy
4301 Broadway CPO 99
San Antonio, TX 78209
www.uiw.edu/pharmacy
Tel: 801 581-6731   *Fax:* 801 581-3716

Utah

University of Utah
Pharmacy Prgm
College of Pharmacy
30 South 2000 East
Salt Lake City, UT 84112
www.pharmacy.utah.edu
Tel: 801 581-6731   *Fax:* 801 581-3716

Virginia

University of Appalachia College of Pharmacy
Pharmacy Prgm
PO Box 2858
Grundy, VA 824614
www.uacp.org
Tel: 276 935-4277   *Fax:* 276 935-4279

Hampton University
Pharmacy Prgm
School of Pharmacy
Hampton, VA 23668
www.hamptonu.edu
Tel: 757 727-5071   *Fax:* 757 727-5840

Virginia Commonwealth Univ/Health System
Pharmacy Prgm
School of Pharmacy
410 N 12th St
Richmond, VA 23298
www.pharmacy.vcu.edu
Tel: 804 828-3006   *Fax:* 804 287-0002

Shenandoah University
Pharmacy Prgm
Bernard J Dunn School of Pharmacy
1460 University Dr
Winchester, VA 22601
www.su.edu/academic/pharmacy.asp
Tel: 540 665-1282   *Fax:* 540 665-1283

Washington

Washington State University
Pharmacy Prgm
College of Pharmacy
PO Box 646510
Pullman, WA 99164
www.pharmacy.wsu.edu
Tel: 509 335-4750   *Fax:* 509 335-2530

University of Washington
Pharmacy Prgm
School of Pharmacy
H364 Health Sciences
Seattle, WA 98195
http://depts.washington.edu/pha/
Tel: 206 543-2030   *Fax:* 206 685-9297

West Virginia

University of Charleston
Pharmacy Prgm
School of Pharmacy
2300 MacCorkle Ave SE
Charleston, WV 25304
www.ucwv.edu
Tel: 304 357-4858   *Fax:* 304 357-4868

West Virginia University
Pharmacy Prgm
School of Pharmacy
PO Box 9500
Morgantown, WV 26506
www.hsc.wvu.edu/sop
Tel: 304 293-5101   *Fax:* 304 293-5483

Wisconsin

University of Wisconsin - Madison
Pharmacy Prgm
School of Pharmacy
777 Highland Ave
Madison, WI 53705
www.wisc.edu
Tel: 608 262-1414   *Fax:* 608 262-3397

Wyoming

University of Wyoming
Pharmacy Prgm
School of Pharmacy
1000 E University Ave
Laramie, WY 82071
www.uwyo.edu/pharmacy/
Tel: 307 766-6120   *Fax:* 307 766-2953

Pharmacy Technician

Pharmacy technicians assist licensed pharmacists by performing duties that do not require the professional skills and judgment of a licensed pharmacist and assisting in those duties that require the expertise of a pharmacist. Pharmacy technicians are employed in every practice setting where pharmacy is practiced, including institutional, community, home care, long-term care, mail order, and managed care pharmacies. Technicians are also employed in education, research, and the pharmaceutical industry.

Technicians may be trained on the job or by completing a formal program. Some formal training programs meet the program accreditation standards established by the American Society of Health-System Pharmacists.

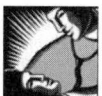

Career Description

According to the 1991-1994 Scope of Pharmacy Practice Project, pharmacy technicians spend their time in the following ways:

- 26%—collect, organize, and evaluate information to assist pharmacists in serving patients
- 21%—develop and manage medication distribution and control systems; about half of this time is spent preparing, dispensing, distributing, and administering medications
- 7%—provide drug information and education

These percentages, however, may vary widely for many reasons, including the wide range of training and qualifications of pharmacists, the use of technicians as directed by a given supervisory pharmacist, and variations in state pharmacy practice laws.

The ASHP Accreditation Standard for Pharmacy Technician Training Programs specifies that graduates of programs should be able to perform the following functions (among others):

- Assist the pharmacist in collecting, organizing, and evaluating information for direct patient care, drug use review, and departmental management
- Receive and screen prescription medication orders for completeness and accuracy
- Use pharmaceutical and medical terms, abbreviations, and symbols appropriately
- Prepare and distribute medications in a variety of health system settings
- Perform arithmetical calculations required for usual dosage determinations and solutions preparation
- Use knowledge of general chemical and physical properties of drugs in manufacturing and packaging operations
- Use knowledge of proper aseptic technique and packaging in the preparation of medications
- Collect payment and/or initiate billing for pharmacy services and goods
- Purchase pharmaceuticals, devices, and supplies according to an established plan in a variety of health systems
- Control medication, equipment, and device inventory according to an established plan in a variety of health systems
- Maintain pharmacy equipment in preparing, storing, and distributing investigational drug products
- Assist the pharmacist in monitoring the practice site and/or service area for compliance with federal, state, and local laws, regulations, and professional standards
- Assist the pharmacist in preparing, storing, and distributing investigational drug products

- Assist the pharmacist in the monitoring of drug therapy
- Assist the pharmacist in identifying patients who desire counseling on the use of medications, equipment, and devices
- Understand the use and side effects of prescription and nonprescription drugs used to treat common disease states
- Appreciate the need to adapt the delivery of pharmacy services for the culturally diverse
- Maintain confidentiality of patient information
- Communicate clearly orally and in writing
- Use computers to perform pharmacy functions
- Demonstrate ethical conduct in all activities related to the delivery of pharmacy services

Employment Characteristics

Pharmacy technicians typically provide their services in one or more of the following settings: health systems, community pharmacies, chain pharmacies, and home care pharmacies.

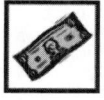

Salary

Salary for entry-level pharmacy technicians in 2002 was $19,000; overall average was $27,000; those in the upper ranges earned $35,000. Refer to Section IV, Table 5 of this *Directory* for more information, or see www.ama-assn.org/go/hpsalary.

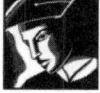

Educational Programs

Length. Programs are generally 15 weeks or longer and consist of a minimum of 600 hours of training (contact) time. Graduates generally receive a certificate or AS degree.

Prerequisites. Applicants should have a high school diploma or equivalent and meet institutional entrance requirements.

Curriculum. The professional curriculum includes formal instruction in didactic, practical, and laboratory areas of pharmacy practice. The curriculum consists of various aspects of pharmacy technician training pertinent to contemporary pharmacy practice. Courses include pharmacy mathematics/calculations, pharmacy for pharmacy technicians, sterile products, pharmaceutical care delivery systems, computer systems for pharmacy, and payment for pharmacy services.

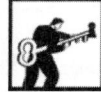

Certification

After completing their training, technicians may become a Certified Pharmacy Technician (CPhT) by successfully taking the national certification examination offered by the Pharmacy Technician Certification Board.

Inquiries

Careers

American Association of Pharmacy Technicians (AAPT)
PO Box 1447
Greensboro, NC 27402
877 368-4771
336 333-9068 Fax
www.pharmacytechnician.com

National Pharmacy Technician Association
3707 FM 1960 RD W, Suite 460
Houston, TX 77068
281 866-7900 or 888 247-8700
281 895-7320 Fax
www.pharmacytechnician.org

Certification

Pharmacy Technician Certification Board
1100 15th Street NW, Suite 730
Washington, DC 20005-1707
800 363-8012
202 429-7596 Fax
www.ptcb.org

Program Accreditation

American Society of Health System-Pharmacists
Accreditation Services Division
7272 Wisconsin Avenue
Bethesda, MD 20814
301 664-8720
301 664-8872 Fax
E-mail: llifshin@ashp.org
www.ashp.org

Pharmacy Technician

Alabama

George C Wallace Community College
Pharmacy Technician Prgm
801 Main St NW
PO Box 2000
Hanceville, AL 35077
Prgm Dir: Brandon Brooks
Tel: 256 352-8023   *Fax:* 256 352-8382
E-mail: brandon.brooks@wallacestate.edu

Arizona

Pima Community College
Pharmacy Technician Prgm
8181 E Irvington Rd
Tucson, AZ 85709-4000
Prgm Dir: Michael Heller
Tel: 520 206-7850   *Fax:* 520 206-7803
E-mail: mheller@email.arizona.edu

California

North Orange County Community College
Pharmacy Technician Prgm
Continuing Education
1830 W Romneya Dr
Anaheim, CA 92801
www.nocccd.cc.ca.us
Prgm Dir: Martha Gutierrez
Tel: 714 808-4668   *Fax:* 714 808-4659
E-mail: mgutierrez@sce.cc.ca.us

Western Career College - Antioch
Pharmacy Technician Prgm
2157 Country Hills Dr
Antioch, CA 94509
Prgm Dir: Krissy Raynor
Tel: 925 522-7777   *Fax:* 925 522-0097
E-mail: kraynor@ant.westerncollege.com

Western Career College - Citrus
Pharmacy Technician Prgm
7301 Greenback Ln, Ste A
Citrus Heights, CA 95621
Prgm Dir: Kari Roberts
Tel: 916 722-8200   *Fax:* 916 722-6883
E-mail: kroberts@westerncollege.com

Western Career College - Emeryville
Pharmacy Technician Prgm
1400 65th St
Emeryville, CA 94608
Prgm Dir: David A Jesitus, RPh
Tel: 510 601-0133   *Fax:* 510 601-0793
E-mail: mangeles@emv.westerncollege.com

North-West College - Glendale
Pharmacy Technician Prgm
124 S Glendale Ave
Glendale, CA 91205
Prgm Dir: Marsha Fuerst
Tel: 626 960-5046   *Fax:* 626 966-5949
E-mail: marshaf@marshaf@northwestcollege.com

American University of Health Sciences
Pharmacy Technician Prgm
3501 Atlantic Ave
Long Beach, CA 90807
www.auhs.edu
Prgm Dir: Jeanetta Mastron, CPhT BS Chem Voc Cert
   CBest Lev IIT Cred
Tel: 562 988-2278   *Fax:* 562 988-1791
E-mail: jmastron@auhs.edu

American Career College
Pharmacy Technician Prgm
4021 Rosewood Ave 101
Los Angeles, CA 90004
Prgm Dir: Dolores Salazar
Tel: 323 906-2211   *Fax:* 323 666-3519
E-mail: dsalazar@americancareer.com

Charles R Drew Univ of Med & Science
Pharmacy Technician Prgm
1731 E 120th St
Los Angeles, CA 90059
Prgm Dir: Gail Orum Alexander, PharmD
Tel: 323 563-4815   *Fax:* 323 563-4827
E-mail: gailorum@cdrewu.edu

Cerritos College
Pharmacy Technician Prgm
11110 E Alondra Blvd
Norwalk, CA 90650
www.cerritos.edu/ho
Prgm Dir: Hal Malkin, CPhT
Tel: 562 860-2451, Ext 3517   *Fax:* 562 947-4228
E-mail: hmalkin@Cerritos.edu

Foothill Community College
Pharmacy Technician Prgm
Middlefield Campus
4000 Middlefield Rd, Ste I
Palo Alto, CA 94303-4739
www.foothill.edu
Prgm Dir: Leonis A Osterdock, RPh
Tel: 650 949-6970   *Fax:* 650 949-6979
E-mail: osterdockleonis@foothill.edu

North-West College - Pasadena
Pharmacy Technician Prgm
530 East Union
Pasadena, CA 91101
Prgm Dir: Marsha Fuerst
Tel: 626 960-5046
E-mail: marshaf@northwestcollege.com

Western Career College - Pleasant Hill
Pharmacy Technician Prgm
380 Civic Dr, Ste 300
Pleasant Hill, CA 94523
Prgm Dir: Diana Evanson
Tel: 925 405-0632   *Fax:* 925 609-6666
E-mail: devanson@westerncollege.com

North-West College - Pomona
Pharmacy Technician Prgm
134 W Holt Ave
Pomona, CA 91768
Prgm Dir: Marsha Fuerst
Tel: 909 623-1552
E-mail: marshaf@northwestcollege.com

Charles A Jones Skills & Business Ed Center
Pharmacy Technician Prgm
5451 Lemon Hill Ave
Sacramento, CA 95824-1529
Prgm Dir: Sandra B Thi Huynh
Tel: 916 433-2600, Ext 1400   *Fax:* 916 433-2640
E-mail: sandrahu@sac-city.k12.ca.us

Western Career College - Sacramento
Pharmacy Technician Prgm
8909 Folsom Blvd
Sacramento, CA 95826
Prgm Dir: Michele Wootton, RPhT BA
Tel: 916 361-1660, Ext 41112   *Fax:* 916 361-6666
E-mail: mwootton@westerncollege.com

Western Career College - San Jose
Pharmacy Technician Prgm
6201 San Ignacio Ave
San Jose, CA 95119
Prgm Dir: Grigoriy Gertsvolf, CPhT
Tel: 408 360-0840, Ext 42143   *Fax:* 408 360-0848
E-mail: ggertsvolf@sj.westerncollege.com

Western Career College - San Leandro
Pharmacy Technician Prgm
170 Bayfair Mall
San Leandro, CA 94578
Prgm Dir: Marlene Lamnin, BS
Tel: 510 276-3888, Ext 123
E-mail: mlamnin@westerncollege.com

Santa Ana College
Pharmacy Technician Prgm
1530 W 17th St
Santa Ana, CA 92706
Prgm Dir: Gail B Askew, PharmD FCSHP
Tel: 714 564-6622   *Fax:* 714 564-6158
E-mail: askew_gail@sac.edu

Western Career College - Stockton
Pharmacy Technician Prgm
1313 W Robinhood Dr, Ste B
Stockton, CA 95207
Prgm Dir: Cindy Turner, CPhT
Tel: 209 956-1240, Ext 44120   *Fax:* 209 956-1244
E-mail: cturner@westerncollege.com

North-West College - West Covina
Pharmacy Technician Prgm
2121 Garvey Ave N
West Covina, CA 91790
Prgm Dir: Marsha Fuerst
Tel: 626 870-4113
E-mail: marshaf@northwestcollege.com

Colorado

Arapahoe Community College
Pharmacy Technician Prgm
5900 S Santa Fe Dr
Littleton, CO 80160-9002
Prgm Dir: Sue Treitz, BSN MA
Tel: 303 797-5962   *Fax:* 303 797-5842
E-mail: sue.treitz@arapahoe.edu

Front Range Comm College
Pharmacy Technician Prgm
Westminster Campus
3645 W 112th Ave
Westminster, CO 80030
Prgm Dir: Linda Calvert, CPhT BS
Tel: 303 404-5393   *Fax:* 303 404-2178
E-mail: Linda.Calvert@frontrange.edu

Florida

McFatter Technical Center
Pharmacy Technician Prgm
6500 Nova Dr
Davie, FL 33317
Prgm Dir: William J Shaheen, PharmD RPh
Tel: 754 321-5741   *Fax:* 754 321-5820
E-mail: william.shaheen@browardschools.com

Lake City Community College
Pharmacy Technician Prgm
149 SE College Place
Lake City, FL 32025-8703
Prgm Dir: Patricia Smith, CPhT
Tel: 386 754-4239   *Fax:* 386 754-4739
E-mail: smithp@lakecitycc.edu

**Florida Metropolitan Univ - Melbourne
Campus**
Pharmacy Technician Prgm
2401 N Harbor City Blvd
Melbourne, FL 32935
Prgm Dir: Karen Jenkins, MD MPH
Tel: 321 259-3211   *Fax:* 321 259-9797
E-mail: kjenkins@cci.edu

Pinellas Tech Educ Ctr - St Petersburg
Pharmacy Technician Prgm
901 34th St S
St Petersburg, FL 33711
www.myptec.org
Prgm Dir: Jeannie Pappas, CPhT
Tel: 813 893-2500, Ext 1131   *Fax:* 813 323-6653
E-mail: mcdaniel-pappasd@pcsb.org

Henry W Brewster Technical Center
Pharmacy Technician Prgm
2222 N Tampa St
Tampa, FL 33602
www.brewster.edu
Prgm Dir: Douglas J Botting, RPh CPh
Tel: 813 276-5448, Ext 393   *Fax:* 813 276-5756
E-mail: douglas.botting@sdhc.k12.fl.us

Georgia

Ogeechee Technical College
Pharmacy Technician Prgm
1 Joe Kennedy Blvd
Statesboro, GA 30458
Prgm Dir: Shelly P Jones, CPhT
Tel: 912 486-7620   *Fax:* 912 486-7604
E-mail: sjones@ogeecheetech.edu

Southwest Georgia Technical College
Pharmacy Technician Prgm
15689 US Hwy 19 N
Thomasville, GA 31799
Prgm Dir: Kathleen G Allen, BS RPh
Tel: 912 225-5093   *Fax:* 912 225-5289
E-mail: kallen@southwestgatech.edu

Valdosta Technical College
Pharmacy Technician Prgm
4089 Val Tech Rd
Valdosta, GA 31602
Prgm Dir: Frank Barnett, CPhT
Tel: 229 259-5581   *Fax:* 229 259-5567
E-mail: fbarnett@valdostatech.edu

Southeastern Technical College
Pharmacy Technician Prgm
3001 E First St
Vidalia, GA 30474
Prgm Dir: Karen Davis, CPhT
Tel: 912 538-3192   *Fax:* 912 538-3106
E-mail: kdavis@southeasterntech.edu

Illinois

Malcolm X College
Pharmacy Technician Prgm
1900 W Van Buren St, Ste 3524
Chicago, IL 60612-3145
www.ccc.edu
Prgm Dir: Ronald D Grimmette, M Ad Ed BS Pharm
Tel: 312 850-7385   *Fax:* 312 850-7453
E-mail: rgrimmette@ccc.edu

Blessing Hospital
Pharmacy Technician Prgm
Broadway and 14th St
Quincy, IL 62301
Prgm Dir: Patty Loeffler, RN BSN
Tel: 217 223-8400, Ext 4832   *Fax:* 217 223-6003
E-mail: ploeffler@blessinghospital.com

South Suburban College
Pharmacy Technician Prgm
15800 S State St
South Holland, IL 60473
Prgm Dir: Jan Keresztes, PharmD
Tel: 708 596-2000, Ext 2432   *Fax:* 708 210-5792
E-mail: jkeresztes@southsuburbancollege.edu

Indiana

Clarian Health Partners Inc
Pharmacy Technician Prgm
Clarian Health Education Center
Rm 506- Wile Hall, PO Box 1367
Indianapolis, IN 46206-1397
www.clarian.org
Prgm Dir: Mary E Mohr, RPh MS
Tel: 317 962-0919   *Fax:* 317 962-3483
E-mail: mmohr@clarian.org

Louisiana

Louisiana State University - Alexandria
Pharmacy Technician Prgm
8100 Hwy 71 S
Alexandria, LA 71302
Prgm Dir: David J Nassif, PharmD
Tel: 318 473-6533   *Fax:* 318 473-6567
E-mail: dnassif@lsua.edu

Bossier Parish Community College
Pharmacy Technician Prgm
6220 E Texas St
Science and Allied Health Division
Bossier City, LA 71111
www.bpcc.edu
Prgm Dir: Terri Mundy, RPh
Tel: 318 678-6215   *Fax:* 318 678-6199
E-mail: tmundy@bpcc.edu

Delgado Community College
Pharmacy Technician Prgm
Allied Health Div
615 City Park Ave
New Orleans, LA 70119
Prgm Dir: Anne LaVance, BS CPhT
Tel: 504 671-6237   *Fax:* 504 483-4609
E-mail: alavan@dcc.edu

Maryland

Anne Arundel Community College
Pharmacy Technician Prgm
101 College Pkwy
Florestano 306B
Arnold, MD 21012
Prgm Dir: Stephanie Smith-Baker
Tel: 410 777-7497   *Fax:* 410 777-7099
E-mail: sesmithbaker@aacc.edu

Massachusetts

Holyoke Community College
Pharmacy Technician Prgm
303 Homestead Ave
Holyoke, MA 01040-1099
Prgm Dir: Sharon Wetherby, BS Pharm MBA JD
Tel: 413 552-2263   *Fax:* 413 552-2045
E-mail: swetherby@hcc.mass.edu

Michigan

Washtenaw Community College
Pharmacy Technician Prgm
4800 E Huron River Dr
PO Box D-1
Ann Arbor, MI 48106
Prgm Dir: Dina Cheiman
Tel: 734 973-3418   *Fax:* 734 677-5078
E-mail: dcheiman@wccnet.edu

Henry Ford Community College
Pharmacy Technician Prgm
5101 Evergreen, HCEC Bldg
Dearborn, MI 48128-1495
Prgm Dir: Scott McCall, RPh
Tel: 313 845-9877
E-mail: mccalls@oakwood.org

Wayne County Community College District
Pharmacy Technician Prgm
801 W Fort St
Detroit, MI 48226
Prgm Dir: William Matthew, BS Pharm
Tel: 313 496-2686, Ext 2686   *Fax:* 313 961-9648
E-mail: wmatthe1@wcccd.edu

Minnesota

Northland Community & Technical College
Pharmacy Technician Prgm
2022 Central Ave NE
PO Box 111
East Grand Forks, MN 56721
Prgm Dir: Joe Farrell, RPh
Tel: 218 773-4790   *Fax:* 218 773-4502
E-mail: jfarrell@altru.org

Minnesota State Comm & Tech Coll -
Moorhead
Pharmacy Technician Prgm
405 SW Colfax, PO Box 566
Wadena, MN 56482-0566
Prgm Dir: Mary L Stende Mille, BS RPh
Tel: 218 773-7881
E-mail: mary.stende@minnesota.edu

Century College
Pharmacy Technician Prgm
3300 Century Ave N
White Bear Lake, MN 55110
Prgm Dir: Raymond K Vellenga
Tel: 651 779-5780   *Fax:* 651 779-5780
E-mail: ray.vellenga@century.edu

Mississippi

Jones County Junior College
Pharmacy Technician Prgm
900 S Court St
Ellisville, MS 39437
www.jcjc.edu/depts/pharmacy
Prgm Dir: Marsha M Sanders, RPh
Tel: 601 477-4230   *Fax:* 601 477-4152
E-mail: marsha.sanders@jcjc.edu

Montana

Univ of Montana-Missoula - College of Tech
Pharmacy Technician Prgm
909 S Avenue W
Missoula, MT 59801
www.cte.umt.edu
Prgm Dir: Mary McHugh, PharmD
Tel: 406 243-7813   *Fax:* 406 243-7899
E-mail: mary.mchugh@mso.umt.edu

North Carolina

Durham Technical Community College
Pharmacy Technician Prgm
1637 Lawson St
Durham, NC 27703
Prgm Dir: Joe Anne Griffith, BS RPh
Tel: 919 686-3686   *Fax:* 919 686-3705
E-mail: griffithj@durhamtech.edu

North Dakota

North Dakota State College of Science
Pharmacy Technician Prgm
800 6th St N
Wahpeton, ND 58076-0002
Prgm Dir: Kenneth Strandberg, MBA RPh
Tel: 701 671-2114   *Fax:* 701 671-2570
E-mail: Kenneth.Strandberg@ndsu.edu

Ohio

Collins Career Center
Pharmacy Technician Prgm
11627 State Route 243
Chesapeake, OH 45619
Prgm Dir: Linda Stiller
Tel: 740 532-7405
E-mail: lstiller@collins-cc.edu

Cuyahoga Community College
Pharmacy Technician Prgm
East Campus, Health Careers and Sciences
4250 Richmond Rd
Cleveland, OH 44122
Prgm Dir: MaryAnn Stuhan, RPh
Tel: 216 987-2381
E-mail: maryann.stuhan@tri-c.edu

Pennsylvania

Great Lakes Institute of Technology
Pharmacy Technician Prgm
5100 Peach St
Erie, PA 16509
www.glit.edu
Prgm Dir: Jeffrey A Baird, MBA CPhT
Tel: 814 864-6666, Ext 236   *Fax:* 814 868-1717
E-mail: jeffb@glit.edu

Western School of Health & Business -
Monroeville
Pharmacy Technician Prgm
1 Monroeville Center, Ste 250
Monroeville, PA 15146
Prgm Dir: G Scott Butler
Tel: 412 373-9038, Ext 271   *Fax:* 412 373-2544
E-mail: sbutler@western-school.com

Bidwell Training Center
Pharmacy Technician Prgm
1650 Metropolitan St
Pittsburgh, PA 15233
Prgm Dir: Dolores R Sewchok
Tel: 412 323-4000, Ext 215   *Fax:* 412 322-6539
E-mail: dsewchok@mcg-btc.org

Comm College of Allegheny County -
South Campus
Pharmacy Technician Prgm
1750 Clairton Rd, Rte 885
West Mifflin, PA 15122
Prgm Dir: Jane Coughanour, MT(ASCP) MEd
Tel: 412 469-6280
E-mail: jcoughanour@ccac.edu

South Carolina

Trident Technical College
Pharmacy Technician Prgm
7000 Rivers Ave
PO Box 118067
Charleston, SC 29423-8067
Prgm Dir: Karen Snipe, CPhT MAEd
Tel: 843 574-6481   *Fax:* 843 574-6585
E-mail: karen.snipe@tridenttech.edu

Midlands Technical College
Pharmacy Technician Prgm
PO Box 2408
Columbia, SC 29202
Prgm Dir: Kevin J Eisenhour, MSN RN CPhT
Tel: 803 822-3591   *Fax:* 803 822-3417
E-mail: eisenhourk@midlandstech.edu

Greenville Technical College
Pharmacy Technician Prgm
PO Box 5616
Greenville, SC 29606-5616
Prgm Dir: Lori J Stepp, CPhT
Tel: 864 848-2981   *Fax:* 864 848-2038
E-mail: lori.stepp@gvltec.edu

Spartanburg Community College
Pharmacy Technician Prgm
PO Box 4386
Spartanburg, SC 29305
Prgm Dir: Julia B Sherwood, CPht
Tel: 864 592-4870   *Fax:* 864 592-4881
E-mail: SherwoodJ@stcsc.edu

South Dakota

Western Dakota Technical Institute
Pharmacy Technician Prgm
800 Mickelson Dr
Rapid City, SD 57703
Prgm Dir: Gerald M McGraw, PA-C BS MPAS MBA
Tel: 605 394-2909   *Fax:* 605 394-1789
E-mail: jerry.mcgraw@wdt.edu

Tennessee

Chattanooga State Technical Comm College
Pharmacy Technician Prgm
4501 Amnicola Hwy
Chattanooga, TN 37406
Prgm Dir: Nancy V Watts
Tel: 423 697-2568   *Fax:* 423 697-2595
E-mail: nancy.watts@chattanoogastate.edu

Tennessee Technology Center - Jackson
Pharmacy Technician Prgm
2468 Technology Center Dr
Jackson, TN 38301
www.jackson.tec.tn.us
Prgm Dir: Darlene Redd, CPhT
Tel: 731 424-0691, Ext 115   *Fax:* 731 424-0807
E-mail: Darlene.Redd@TTCJackson.edu

Concorde Career College - Memphis
Pharmacy Technician Prgm
5100 Poplar Ave, Ste 132
Memphis, TN 38137
Prgm Dir: Sunethra Guy, CPht BA
Tel: 901 761-9494, Ext 216   *Fax:* 901 761-3293
E-mail: sguy@concorde.edu

Tennessee Technology Center - Memphis
Pharmacy Technician Prgm
550 Alabama Ave
Memphis, TN 38105-3604
Prgm Dir: Olivia Bowden
Tel: 901 543-6100   *Fax:* 901 543-6197
E-mail: Olivia.Bowden@ttcmemphis.edu

Walters State Community College
Pharmacy Technician Prgm
500 S Davy Crockett Pkwy
Morristown, TN 37813-6899
Prgm Dir: Kimberly Brown, CPhT
Tel: 423 318-2757   *Fax:* 423 585-6955
E-mail: kimberly.brown@ws.edu

Tennessee Technology Center - Murfreesboro
Pharmacy Technician Prgm
1303 Old Fort Pkwy
Murfreesboro, TN 37129
Prgm Dir: Jill Frost, BS CPhT
Tel: 615 898-8010, Ext 127   *Fax:* 615 893-4194
E-mail: jfrost@ttcmurfreesboro.edu

Tennessee Technology Center - Nashville
Pharmacy Technician Prgm
100 White Bridge Rd
Nashville, TN 37209
Prgm Dir: Daniel H Leffler, RPh
Tel: 615 284-4076
E-mail: dan.leffler@baptisthospital.com

Texas

Austin Community College
Pharmacy Technician Prgm
3401 Webberville Rd
Austin, TX 78702
Prgm Dir: Zachary D Corbell, PharmD RPh
Tel: 512 223-5948   *Fax:* 512 223-5895
E-mail: zcorbell@austincc.edu

Richland College
Pharmacy Technician Prgm
12800 Abrams Rd
Dallas, TX 75243-2199
www.richlandcollege.edu/hp
Prgm Dir: LiAnne Webster, RPhT CPhT
Tel: 972 238-6038   *Fax:* 972 761-6793
E-mail: liannewebster@dcccd.edu

El Paso Community College
Pharmacy Technician Prgm
PO Box 20500
El Paso, TX 79998
Prgm Dir: Nader Rassaei, MA(MHA) MD
Tel: 915 831-8836   *Fax:* 915 831-8861
E-mail: nrassaei@epcc.edu

US Army Medical Dept Center & School
Pharmacy Technician Prgm
Attn: MCCS-HCP (Pharmacy Branch)
3151 Scott Rd
Fort Sam Houston, TX 78234-6137
Prgm Dir: LTC Marc Caouette, PharmD MS
Tel: 210 221-8820   *Fax:* 210 221-6559
E-mail: marc.caouette@amedd.army.mil

University of Texas Medical Branch
Pharmacy Technician Prgm
Department of Pharmacy
301 Unversity Blvd
Galveston, TX 77555-0701
Prgm Dir: Madeline F Jensen, BSEd MSc
Tel: 409 772-6981   *Fax:* 409 747-9919
E-mail: mfjensen@utmb.edu

North Harris College
Pharmacy Technician Prgm
2700 W W Thorne Blvd
Houston, TX 77073
www.northharriscollege.com
Prgm Dir: Nancy L Lim, RPh PhD
Tel: 281 618-5727   *Fax:* 281 618-5756
E-mail: nancy.l.lim@nhmccd.edu

San Jacinto College North
Pharmacy Technician Prgm
5800 Uvalde Rd
Houston, TX 77049
www.sanjac.edu/PharmacyTech
Prgm Dir: Donald Becker, BA CPhT
Tel: 281 998-6150, Ext 7453   *Fax:* 281 459-7662
E-mail: donald.becker@sjcd.edu

San Jacinto College South
Pharmacy Technician Prgm
13735 Beamer Rd
Houston, TX 77089
Prgm Dir: Alexander C Okwonna, PharmD RPh
Tel: 281 929-4702   *Fax:* 281 922-3487
E-mail: Alexander.Okwonna@sjcd.edu

Angelina College
Pharmacy Technician Prgm
3500 S First (Hwy 595)
PO Box 1768
Lufkin, TX 75902-1768
www.angelina.edu
Prgm Dir: Elaine Young, MEd CPhT
Tel: 936 633-5433   *Fax:* 936 633-5241
E-mail: eyoung@angelina.edu

South Texas College
Pharmacy Technician Prgm
PO Box 9701
McAllen, TX 78502-9701
Prgm Dir: Theresa M Langlass-Garza, PharmD BCPS
Tel: 956 872-3024   *Fax:* 956 872-3138
E-mail: tmgarza@southtexascollege.edu

Lamar State College - Orange
Pharmacy Technician Prgm
410 Front St
Orange, TX 77630
Prgm Dir: Randy G Ford
Tel: 409 882-3035   *Fax:* 409 882-5000
E-mail: randy.ford@lsco.edu

Northwest Vista College
Pharmacy Technician Prgm
3535 N Ellison Dr
San Antonio, TX 78251
Prgm Dir: Christie E Martin
Tel: 210 348-2418   *Fax:* 210 348-2264
E-mail: cmartin@accd.edu

USAF School of Health Care Sciences
Pharmacy Technician Prgm
382d Training Squadron
917 Missile Rd, Ste 3
Sheppard AFB, TX 76311
Prgm Dir: Jeffrey E Eertmoed, PharmD BCPS MAJ BSC
Tel: 940 676-3847   *Fax:* 940 676-3850
E-mail: Jeff.Eertmoed@sheppard.af.mil

Weatherford College
Pharmacy Technician Prgm
225 College Park Dr
Weatherford, TX 76086
Prgm Dir: James Austin, RN BSN CPhT
Tel: 817 594-5471, Ext 229   *Fax:* 817 598-6455
E-mail: austin@wc.edu

Vernon College
Pharmacy Technician Prgm
4105 Maplewood Dr
Wichita Falls, TX 76308
www.vernoncollege.edu
Prgm Dir: Katrina Brasuell, BS CPhT
Tel: 940 696-8752, Ext 3231   *Fax:* 940 689-9129
E-mail: kbrasuell@vernoncollege.edu

Virginia

Naval School of Health Sciences
Pharmacy Technician Prgm
1001 Holcomb Rd
Portsmouth, VA 23708-5200
Prgm Dir: Christopher G Lynch, PharmD LCDR MSC
Tel: 757 953-6413   *Fax:* 757 953-5033
E-mail: christopher.lynch@med.navy.mil

Washington

Renton Technical College
Pharmacy Technician Prgm
3000 NE Fourth St
Renton, WA 98056
Prgm Dir: Cheryl Dedmon
Tel: 425 235-2495   *Fax:* 425 235-7832
E-mail: cdedmon@rtc.edu

Spokane Community College
Pharmacy Technician Prgm
N 1810 Greene St, MS 2090
Spokane, WA 99217-5399
www.scc.spokane.edu/fac/stschritter
Prgm Dir: Sandi Tschritter, CPhT BA
Tel: 509 533-8199   *Fax:* 509 533-8621
E-mail: stschritter@scc.spokane.edu

St Joseph Medical Center
Pharmacy Technician Prgm
1717 South J St
PO Box 2197
Tacoma, WA 98401-2197
Prgm Dir: Ronald L Broekemeier, MS RPh
Tel: 253 591-6692   *Fax:* 253 207-4949
E-mail: ronbroekemeier@fhshealth.org

West Virginia

Carver Career Center
Pharmacy Technician Prgm
4799 Midland Dr
Charleston, WV 25306
http://boe.kana.k12.wv.us/carver/
Prgm Dir: Janie L March, CPhT BS
Tel: 304 348-1965, Ext 132   *Fax:* 304 348-1938
E-mail: jmarchcpht@yahoo.com

Pharmacy Technician

Programs*	Class Capacity	Begins	Length (months)	Award	Res. Tuition	Non-res. Tuition	Stipend	Offers:‡ 1	2	3	4
California											
American University of Health Sciences (Long Beach)	20	Open	7, 11	Cert, BS CRA	$12,250	$0		•			
Cerritos College (Norwalk)	70	Aug Jan	24, 18	Cert, AA	$20	$160		•		•	•
Foothill Community College (Palo Alto)	35	Sep	9	Cert, AS	$1,500	$5,400					•
North Orange County Community College (Anaheim)	40	Jan Apr Jul Sep	18	Cert				•		•	
Western Career College - Sacramento	32	Every 6 wks	16	AAS	$18,224	$0		•		•	
Western Career College - San Jose	24	8x/yr	12, 18	Dipl, Cert, AS	$19,000	$19,000				•	
Western Career College - San Leandro	35	Every 6 wks		AAS	$16,535	$0					
Western Career College - Stockton	28	Every 3 wks	15, 12	Dipl, AS	$23,789	$0		•		•	
Florida											
Henry W Brewster Technical Center (Tampa)	25	Aug 20	12	Dipl, Cert	$1,911	$1,911					
Lake City Community College	25	Aug	12	Dipl	$2,578	$9,635					•
McFatter Technical Center (Davie)	24	Aug	10	Cert	$2,274	$6,822					

*Data are shown only for programs that completed the 2007 AMA Survey of Health Professions Education Programs.
‡Key to Offers: 1: Evening or weekend classes; 2: Non-English instruction; 3: Cultural competence instruction; 4: Distance education component.

Programs*	Class Capacity	Begins	Length (months)	Award	Res. Tuition	Non-res. Tuition	Stipend	Offers:‡ 1	2	3	4
Pinellas Tech Educ Ctr - St Petersburg	25	Every Term	11	Cert	$2,005	$7,140				•	•
Georgia											
Southeastern Technical College (Vidalia)	24	Fall Spring	15	Dipl	$2,265	$0			•	•	
Illinois											
Malcolm X College (Chicago)	25	Aug	9	Cert	$2,400	$9,636				•	
Indiana											
Clarian Health Partners Inc (Indianapolis)	18	Aug	9	Cert	$2,300	$2,300		•		•	
Louisiana											
Bossier Parish Community College (Bossier City)	16	Aug Jan	12	Dipl, Cert, AAS	$1,800	$0				•	
Delgado Community College (New Orleans)	24	Summer Fall	11, 9	Cert, CTS	$2,000	$5,000					
Michigan											
Wayne County Community College District (Detroit)	24	Jan Sep	8	Cert, AS	$2,484	$3,026			•	•	
Mississippi											
Jones County Junior College (Ellisville)	20	Aug	21	AAS	$1,400	$0					
Montana											
Univ of Montana-Missoula - College of Tech	15	Sep	10	Cert							
Pennsylvania											
Comm College of Allegheny County - South Campus (West Mifflin)	30	Aug	12	Cert, AS	$96	$110		•		•	
Great Lakes Institute of Technology (Erie)	25	Quarterly	8	Dipl	$9,610	$0					
South Dakota											
Western Dakota Technical Institute (Rapid City)	30	Aug	11	Dipl	$3,200	$0		•			
Tennessee											
Tennessee Technology Center - Jackson	20	Sep	12	Dipl	$2,038	$0					
Texas											
Angelina College (Lufkin)	20	Fall	9	Cert	$1,047	$1,546					
Austin Community College	30	Aug Jan	9	Cert	$2,002	$3,898		•			•
El Paso Community College	14	Aug Jan	8, 24	Cert, CC, AAS	$2,700	$0				•	
North Harris College (Houston)	25	Fall Spring	9, 12	Cert, AAS	$1,400	$0		•			
Richland College (Dallas)	54	Jan May Aug	10	Cert	$3,015	$3,015		•		•	•
San Jacinto College North (Houston)	40	Aug Jan	12	Cert	$1,945	$2,704		•			
University of Texas Medical Branch (Galveston)	10	Jan Sep	9	Cert	$2,500	$2,500					
US Army Medical Dept Center & School (Fort Sam Houston)	50	5x/yr	5	Cert							
Vernon College (Wichita Falls)	30	Fall	8	Cert	$2,052	$2,640					
Washington											
Spokane Community College	25	Sep	9	Cert	$870	$1,337				•	
West Virginia											
Carver Career Center (Charleston)	15	Aug Jan	6	Cert	$850	$0		•			

*Data are shown only for programs that completed the 2007 AMA Survey of Health Professions Education Programs.
‡Key to Offers: 1: Evening or weekend classes; 2: Non-English instruction; 3: Cultural competence instruction; 4: Distance education component.

Physical Therapy

Includes:
- Physical therapist
- Physical therapist assistant

Physical Therapist

The physical therapist provides services to many different kinds of patients/clients, from those recovering from accidents or illness and people with disabilities to world-class athletes. Physical therapists help improve patients' strength and mobility, relieve pain, and prevent or limit permanent physical disabilities. Physical therapists take a personal and direct approach to meeting an individual's health goals, working closely with the patient and other health care practitioners. They provide the patient and the patient's family with instruction and home programs to ensure that healing continues after direct patient care has ended.

Physical therapists also work to keep people well and safe from injury, emphasizing the importance of fitness and conditioning and showing people how to avoid injuries at work or play. Physical therapy promotes optimal physical performance and enables health-conscious people to increase their overall fitness level and muscular strength and endurance.

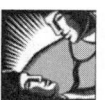

Career Description

The physical therapist is able to evaluate a patient's
- Aerobic capacity and endurance
- Joint motion
- Muscle strength and endurance
- Posture
- Pain
- Functional ability
- Muscle tone and reflexes
- Appearance and stability of walking
- Need and use of braces and artificial limbs
- Function of the heart and lungs
- Integrity of sensation and perception
- Integrity and health of skin
- Performance of activities required in daily living
- Developmental activities

Physical therapy techniques include:
- Therapeutic exercise
- Mobilization/manipulation and range-of-motion exercises
- Cardiovascular endurance training
- Relaxation exercises
- Therapeutic massage
- Biofeedback
- Training in activities of daily living
- Wound debridement
- Pulmonary physical therapy
- Ambulation training

Modalities, including traction, ultrasound, diathermy, electrotherapy, cryotherapy, hydrotherapy, and laser therapy, also can be applied during the treatment program.

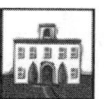

Employment Characteristics

Physical therapists work in hospitals as well as
- Private physical therapy offices
- Community health centers
- Corporate or industrial health centers
- Sports facilities
- Research institutions
- Rehabilitation centers
- Nursing homes
- Home health agencies
- Schools
- Pediatric centers
- Colleges and universities

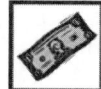

Salary

Average annual income for physical therapists is approximately $70,000, depending on geographic location and practice setting. Physical therapists have the potential to earn more than $100,000 annually. Refer to Section IV, Table 5 of this *Directory* for more information, or see www.ama-assn.org/go/hpsalary.

Employment Outlook

Career opportunities in the field of physical therapy will increase as the "baby boom" generation ages and more patients begin to require treatment for arthritis, stroke, heart disease, and other conditions common to older people. In addition, with the nation's increasing participation in sports and fitness activities, more physical therapists will be needed to treat and help prevent knee, leg, back, shoulder, and other musculoskeletal injuries.

Opportunities also exist for physical therapists from minority groups, who are in great demand but short supply in all aspects of the profession. When physical therapists and their clients share a common language and similar background, the effectiveness of treatment is enhanced.

Educational Programs

Length. All physical therapist education programs culminate in a post-baccalaureate degree. As of July 1, 2006, almost 77% of accredited programs offer the Doctor of Physical Therapy (DPT) degree; all but two of the remaining programs have indicated their intent to convert to offer the DPT in the future.

Prerequisites. Candidates should have a high overall grade point average (GPA) and a high GPA in prerequisite coursework. Volunteer experience as a physical therapy aide, letters of recommendation from physical therapists or science teachers, and excellent writing and interpersonal skills are also highly valued.

Curriculum. Educational programs include basic and clinical medical science courses and emphasize the theory and practice of physical therapy. The curriculum includes opportunities to apply and integrate theory through extensive clinical education and a variety of practice settings.

Licensure, Certification, and Registration

After graduating from an accredited education program, physical therapist candidates must pass a state-administered national exam. Other requirements for physical therapy practice vary from state to state according to physical therapy practice acts or state regulations that govern physical therapy. For more information, contact the state licensing boards.

Physical Therapist Assistant

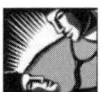

Career Description

Physical therapist assistants work under the supervision of a physical therapist. Their duties include assisting the physical therapist by providing selected interventions within the plan of care, training patients in exercises and activities of daily living, conducting treatments, using special equipment, administering modalities and other treatment procedures, and reporting to the physical therapist on the patient's responses.

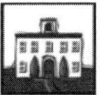

Employment Characteristics

Physical therapist assistants work in
- Hospitals
- Private physical therapy offices
- Community health centers
- Corporate or industrial health centers
- Sports facilities
- Research institutions
- Rehabilitation centers
- Nursing homes
- Home health agencies
- Schools
- Pediatric centers
- Colleges and universities

Salary

The median income for a physical therapist assistant is $26,000; PTAs employed in the southern and western regions of the nation generally earn higher salaries. Refer to Section IV, Table 5 of this *Directory* for more information, or see www.ama-assn.org/go/hpsalary.

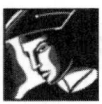

Educational Programs

Length. These associate's degree programs—usually offered in a community or junior college—are 2 years long.

Prerequisites. Successful completion of high school courses in social sciences, biology, mathematics, physics, English, and chemistry is encouraged but not required.

Curriculum. The curriculum includes 1 year of general education and 1 year of technical courses and clinical experience.

Inquiries

Careers, Education, and Certification
American Physical Therapy Association
1111 North Fairfax Street
Alexandria, VA 22314-1488
703 684-2782 or 800 999-2782
703 684-7343 Fax
www.apta.org

Program Accreditation
Commission on Accreditation in Physical Therapy Education
Mary Jane Harris, MS PT, Director of Accreditation
1111 North Fairfax Street
Alexandria, VA 22314
703 684-2782
www.apta.org/capte

Physical Therapist

Alabama

University of Alabama at Birmingham
Physical Therapy Prgm
Department of Physical Therapy RMSB 360X
1530 3rd Ave S
Birmingham, AL 35294-1212
Prgm Dir: Sharon Shaw, DrPH
Tel: 205 934-3566   *Fax:* 205 975-7787
E-mail: sshaw@uab.edu

University of South Alabama
Physical Therapy Prgm
Dept of Physical Therapy
1504 Springhill Ave, Rm 1214
Mobile, AL 36604
Prgm Dir: Dennis Fell, MD PT
Tel: 251 434-3575   *Fax:* 251 434-3822
E-mail: dfell@jaguar1.usouthal.edu

Alabama State University
Physical Therapy Prgm
PO Box 271
915 S Jackson St
Montgomery, AL 36101-0271
Prgm Dir: Senobia Crawford, PT PhD
Tel: 334 229-4707   *Fax:* 334 229-4945
E-mail: asupt@alasu.edu

Arizona

Northern Arizona University
Physical Therapy Prgm
CU Box 15105
Flagstaff, AZ 86011
Prgm Dir: Mark Cornwall, PhD PT CPed
Tel: 520 523-4092   *Fax:* 520 523-9289
E-mail: mark.cornwall@nau.edu

AT Still University of Health Sciences
Cosponsor: Arizona School of Health Sciences
Physical Therapy Prgm
5850 E Still Circle
Mesa, AZ 85206
Prgm Dir: Suzanne Robben Brown, PT MPH
Tel: 480 219-6061   *Fax:* 480 219-6100
E-mail: sbrown@atsu.edu

Arkansas

University of Central Arkansas
Physical Therapy Prgm
Dept of Physical Therapy
201 Donaghey, PTC 300
Conway, AR 72035-0001
Prgm Dir: Nancy Reese, PT PhD
Tel: 501 450-5548   *Fax:* 501 450-5822
E-mail: nancyr@uca.edu

Arkansas State University
Physical Therapy Prgm
PO Box 910
State University, AR 72467-0910
Prgm Dir: Jim W Farris, PT PhD
Tel: 870 972-3591   *Fax:* 870 972-3652
E-mail: jfarris@astate.edu

California

Azusa Pacific University
Physical Therapy Prgm
901 E Alosta Ave
Azusa, CA 91702-7000
Prgm Dir: Michael Laymon, DPTSc PT OCS
Tel: 626 815-5020   *Fax:* 626 815-5017
E-mail: mlaymon@apu.edu

California State University - Fresno
Physical Therapy Prgm
2345 E San Ramon Ave, MS-MH29
Fresno, CA 93740-8031
Prgm Dir: Peggy Trueblood, PhD PT
Tel: 559 278-3008   *Fax:* 559 278-3635
E-mail: peggyt@csufresno.edu

Loma Linda University
Physical Therapy Prgm
Dept of Physical Therapy
School of Allied Health Professions
Loma Linda, CA 92350
Prgm Dir: Larry Chinnock, EdD PT
Tel: 909 558-4632   *Fax:* 909 558-0459
E-mail: lchinnock@sahp.llu.edu

California State University - Long Beach
Physical Therapy Prgm
College of Health and Human Services
1250 Bellflower Blvd
Long Beach, CA 90840
Prgm Dir: Kay Cerny, PhD PT
Tel: 562 985-4956, Ext 54956   *Fax:* 562 985-4069
E-mail: kcerny@csulb.edu

Mount St Mary's College
Physical Therapy Prgm
Dept of Physical Therapy
10 Chester Place
Los Angeles, CA 90007-2598
Prgm Dir: Deborah Lowe, PT PhD
Tel: 213 477-2601   *Fax:* 213 477-2609
E-mail: dlowe@msmc.la.edu

University of Southern California
Physical Therapy Prgm
Biokinesiology and Physical Therapy
1540 E Alcazar St, CHP 155
Los Angeles, CA 90089
Prgm Dir: James Gordon, EdD PT FAPTA
Tel: 323 442-2900   *Fax:* 323 442-1515
E-mail: jamesgor@usc.edu

California State University - Northridge
Physical Therapy Prgm
Department of Physical Therapy
18111 Nordhoff St
Northridge, CA 91330-8411
Prgm Dir: Janna Beling, PT PhD
Tel: 818 677-2203, Ext 7445   *Fax:* 818 677-7411
E-mail: janna.beling@csun.edu

Samuel Merritt College
Physical Therapy Prgm
450 30th St
Oakland, CA 94609
Prgm Dir: Terrence Nordstrom, PT MA
Tel: 510 869-6649   *Fax:* 510 869-6282
E-mail: tnordstrom@samuelmerritt.edu

Chapman University
Physical Therapy Prgm
Department of Physical Therapy
One University Dr
Orange, CA 92866
Prgm Dir: Venita Lovelace-Chandler, PT PhD PCS
Tel: 714 744-7625   *Fax:* 714 744-7621
E-mail: lovelacech@chapman.edu

Western Univ of Health Sciences
Physical Therapy Prgm
Department of Physical Therapy Education
309 E Second St
Pomona, CA 91766-1854
Prgm Dir: Georgeanne Vlad, PT MA
Tel: 909 469-5295   *Fax:* 909 469-5692
E-mail: gvlad@westernu.edu

California State University - Sacramento
Physical Therapy Prgm
College of Health and Human Services
6000 J St
Sacramento, CA 95819-6020
Prgm Dir: Susan M McGinty, EdD MS PT
Tel: 916 278-6426, Ext 85056   *Fax:* 916 278-5053
E-mail: mcgintys@csus.edu

University of California - San Francisco
Cosponsor: San Francisco State Univ
Physical Therapy Prgm
1318 7th Ave
San Francisco, CA 94143-0736
Prgm Dir: Nancy Byl, PhD PT
Tel: 415 476-6650   *Fax:* 415 502-0323
E-mail: byl@itsa.ucsf.edu

University of the Pacific
Physical Therapy Prgm
Dept of Physical Therapy
3601 Pacific Ave
Stockton, CA 95211
Prgm Dir: Cathy Peterson, PT EdD
Tel: 209 946-2886   *Fax:* 209 946-2367
E-mail: cpeterson@pacific.edu

Colorado

Regis University
Physical Therapy Prgm
3333 Regis Blvd G-9
Denver, CO 80221-1099
Prgm Dir: Barbara A Tschoepe, PT PhD
Tel: 303 458-4152   *Fax:* 303 964-5474
E-mail: btschoep@regis.edu

U of Colorado (Denver) Health Sciences Center
Physical Therapy Prgm
4200 E 9th Ave, Mailstop C244
Denver, CO 80262
Prgm Dir: Margaret Schenkman, PT PhD
Tel: 303 372-9375   *Fax:* 303 372-9016
E-mail: margaret.schenkman@uchsc.edu

Connecticut

Sacred Heart University
Physical Therapy Prgm
5151 Park Ave
Fairfield, CT 06825-1000
Prgm Dir: Michael J Emery, PT EdD
Tel: 203 365-7656   *Fax:* 203 365-4723
E-mail: emerym@sacredheart.edu

Quinnipiac University
Physical Therapy Prgm
School of Health Sciences
Mt Carmel Ave
Hamden, CT 06518
Prgm Dir: Donald Kowalsky, PT EdD
Tel: 203 582-8200   *Fax:* 203 582-8706
E-mail: donald.kowalsky@quinnipiac.edu

University of Connecticut
Physical Therapy Prgm
School of Allied Health Professions
358 Mansfield Rd, Unit 2101
Storrs, CT 06269-2101
Prgm Dir: Scott Hasson, EdD PT
Tel: 860 486-0019   *Fax:* 860 486-1588
E-mail: scott.hasson@uconn.edu

University of Hartford
Physical Therapy Prgm
200 Bloomfield Ave
West Hartford, CT 06117-1599
Prgm Dir: Catherine M E Certo, PT ScD FAPTA
Tel: 860 768-5367   *Fax:* 860 768-4558
E-mail: certo@hartford.edu

Delaware

University of Delaware
Physical Therapy Prgm
Dept of Physical Therapy
301 McKinly Laboratory
Newark, DE 19716
Prgm Dir: Stuart A Binder-Macleod, PhD PT FAPTA
Tel: 302 831-8046   *Fax:* 302 831-4234
E-mail: sbinder@udel.edu

District of Columbia

George Washington University
Physical Therapy Prgm
School of Medicine and Health Sciences
900 23rd St NW, Ste 6145
Washington, DC 20037
Prgm Dir: Margaret M Plack, PT
Tel: 202 994-7763   *Fax:* 202 994-8400
E-mail: hspmxp@gwumc.edu

Howard University
Physical Therapy Prgm
Coll of Pharmacy, Nursing and Allied Health
6th and Bryant Sts NW
Washington, DC 20059
Prgm Dir: Steven Chesbro, PT EdD MHS GCS
Tel: 202 806-7613   *Fax:* 202 462-6194
E-mail: schesbro@howard.edu

Florida

University of Miami
Physical Therapy Prgm
School of Medicine
5915 Ponce de Leon Blvd, 5th Fl
Coral Gables, FL 33146
Prgm Dir: Sherrill H Hayes, PhD PT
Tel: 305 284-4535   *Fax:* 305 284-6128
E-mail: shayes@miami.edu

Nova Southeastern University
Physical Therapy Prgm
Health Professions Division
3200 S University Dr
Fort Lauderdale, FL 33328
Prgm Dir: Stanley Wilson, PT EdD CEAS
Tel: 954 262-1100, Ext 1662   *Fax:* 954 262-1783
E-mail: swilson@nova.edu

Florida Gulf Coast University
Physical Therapy Prgm
10501 FGCU Blvd South
Fort Myers, FL 33965-6565
Prgm Dir: Ellen Kroog Williamson, PT MS
Tel: 941 590-7530   *Fax:* 941 590-7474
E-mail: ekwill@fgcu.edu

University of Florida
Physical Therapy Prgm
Dept of Physical Therapy
Box 100154 HSC
Gainesville, FL 32610-0154
Prgm Dir: Krista Vandenborne, PhD PT
Tel: 352 273-6085   *Fax:* 352 273-6109
E-mail: kvandenb@phhp.ufl.edu

University of North Florida
Physical Therapy Prgm
College of Health
4567 St Johns Bluff Rd S
Jacksonville, FL 32224
Prgm Dir: John P Cummings, PT EdD OCS FAAOMPT
Tel: 904 620-2841   *Fax:* 904 620-2848
E-mail: jcumming@unf.edu

Florida International University
Physical Therapy Prgm
Dept of Physical Therapy, College of Nursing
  Health Sciences
11200 SW 8th St
Miami, FL 33199
Prgm Dir: Helen Z Cornely, PT EdD
Tel: 305 348-1968   *Fax:* 305 348-1979
E-mail: cornelyh@fiu.edu

University of Central Florida
Physical Therapy Prgm
HPA-1, Ste 256
Orlando, FL 32816-2205
Prgm Dir: Gerald Smith, PhD PT
Tel: 407 882-0094   *Fax:* 407 823-3464
E-mail: ptinfo@mail.ucf.edu

Univ of St Augustine for Health Sciences
Physical Therapy Prgm
1 University Blvd
St Augustine, FL 32086-5783
Prgm Dir: Gerard C Gorniak, PT PhD
Tel: 904 826-0084   *Fax:* 904 826-0085
E-mail: ggorniak@usa.edu

Florida A&M University
Physical Therapy Prgm
School of Allied Health Sciences
Rm 223 Ware-Rhaney Bldg
Tallahassee, FL 32307-3500
Prgm Dir: Eric Toran, PhD
Tel: 850 599-3820   *Fax:* 850 561-2457
E-mail: eric.toran@famu.edu

University of South Florida
Physical Therapy Prgm
12901 Bruce B Downs Blvd, MDC 77
Tampa, FL 33612
Prgm Dir: William S Quillen, PT PhD SCS FACSM
Tel: 813 974-8870   *Fax:* 813 974-8915
E-mail: wquillen@hsc.usf.edu

Georgia

Emory University
Physical Therapy Prgm
1441 Clifton Rd NE, Ste 180
Atlanta, GA 30322
Prgm Dir: Susan J Herdman, PT PhD FAPTA
Tel: 404 712-5660   *Fax:* 404 712-4130
E-mail: sherdma@emory.edu

Georgia State University
Physical Therapy Prgm
Division of Physical Therapy
PO Box 4019
Atlanta, GA 30302-4019
Prgm Dir: Leslie Taylor, PhD PT
Tel: 404 651-3092   *Fax:* 404 651-1584
E-mail: ltaylorl@gsu.edu

Medical College of Georgia
Physical Therapy Prgm
Dept of Physical Therapy
Augusta, GA 30912-0800
Prgm Dir: Douglas R Keskula, PT PhD ATC
Tel: 706 721-2141   *Fax:* 706 721-3209
E-mail: dkeskula@mcg.edu

North Georgia College & State University
Physical Therapy Prgm
Barnes Hall Rm A-8
Dahlonega, GA 30597
Prgm Dir: Robert J Laird, PhD PT
Tel: 706 864-1422   *Fax:* 706 864-1493
E-mail: rlaird@ngcsu.edu

Armstrong Atlantic State University
Physical Therapy Prgm
11935 Abercorn St
Savannah, GA 31419-1997
Prgm Dir: David A Lake, PhD PT
Tel: 912 921-2327   *Fax:* 912 921-5838
E-mail: lakedavi@mail.armstrong.edu

Idaho

Idaho State University
Physical Therapy Prgm
Dept of Physical and Occupational Therapy
Kasiska College of Health Professions, Box 8045
Pocatello, ID 83209
Prgm Dir: Alexander G Urfer, PhD PT
Tel: 208 282-4095, Ext 4459   *Fax:* 208 282-4962
E-mail: urfealex@isu.edu

Illinois

Northwestern University
Physical Therapy Prgm
Feinberg School of Medicine
645 N Michigan Ave, Ste 1100
Chicago, IL 60611-2814
Prgm Dir: Julius P A Dewald, PhD PT
Tel: 312 908-8160   *Fax:* 312 908-0741
E-mail: j-dewald@northwestern.edu

University of Illinois at Chicago
Physical Therapy Prgm
College of Applied Health Sciences
1919 W Taylor St, M/C 898
Chicago, IL 60612
Prgm Dir: Suzann Campbell, PT PhD FAPTA
Tel: 312 996-1502   *Fax:* 312 996-4583
E-mail: skc@uic.edu

Northern Illinois University
Physical Therapy Prgm
School of Allied Health Professions
DeKalb, IL 60115
Prgm Dir: M J Blaschak, PhD PT
Tel: 815 753-1383   *Fax:* 815 753-0720
E-mail: mblascha@niu.edu

Midwestern University
Physical Therapy Prgm
College of Health Sciences
555 31st St
Downers Grove, IL 60515
Prgm Dir: Donna Cech, PT MS PCS
Tel: 630 515-7221   *Fax:* 630 515-7224
E-mail: dcechx@midwestern.edu

Rosalind Franklin Univ of Medicine & Science
Physical Therapy Prgm
College of Health Professions
3333 Green Bay Rd
North Chicago, IL 60064
Prgm Dir: Dale Schuit, PhD PT
Tel: 847 578-3307   *Fax:* 847 578-8816
E-mail: Dale.Schuit@rosalindfranklin.edu

Bradley University
Physical Therapy Prgm
Dept of Physical Therapy and Health Science
1501 W Bradley Ave
Peoria, IL 61625
Prgm Dir: Mary Jo Mays, PhD PT
Tel: 309 677-3489   *Fax:* 309 677-3445
E-mail: jun@bumail.bradley.edu

Governors State University
Physical Therapy Prgm
1 University Parkway
University Park, IL 60466
Prgm Dir: Russell E Carter, PT EdD
Tel: 708 534-3147   *Fax:* 708 534-1647
E-mail: r-carter@govst.edu

Indiana

University of Evansville
Physical Therapy Prgm
1800 Lincoln Ave
Evansville, IN 47722
Prgm Dir: Mary Kessler, MHS PT
Tel: 812 488-2345   *Fax:* 812 488-2717
E-mail: mk43@evansville.edu

Indiana University
Physical Therapy Prgm
1140 W Michigan St, CF 326
Indianapolis, IN 46202-5119
Prgm Dir: Lisa Riolo, PhD PT
Tel: 317 278-1875   *Fax:* 317 278-1876
E-mail: lriolo@iupui.edu

University of Indianapolis
Physical Therapy Prgm
Krannert School of Physical Therapy
1400 E Hanna Ave
Indianapolis, IN 46227-3697
Prgm Dir: Christopher Petrosino, PhD PT
Tel: 317 788-2182   *Fax:* 317 788-3542
E-mail: cpetrosino@uindy.edu

Iowa

St Ambrose University
Physical Therapy Prgm
518 W Locust
Davenport, IA 52803
Prgm Dir: Sandra L Cassady, PT PhD FAACVPR
Tel: 563 333-6403   *Fax:* 563 333-6410
E-mail: pt@sau.edu

Des Moines University
Physical Therapy Prgm
College of Health Sciences
3200 Grand Ave
Des Moines, IA 50312
Prgm Dir: Traci Bush, MSPT OTR/L
Tel: 515 271-1634   *Fax:* 515 271-7078
E-mail: traci.bush@dmu.edu

Clarke College
Physical Therapy Prgm
1550 Clarke Dr
Dubuque, IA 52001-3198
Prgm Dir: Andrew Priest, PT EdD
Tel: 563 588-6382   *Fax:* 563 584-8684
E-mail: andrew.priest@clarke.edu

University of Iowa
Physical Therapy Prgm
Carver College of Medicine
1-252 Medical Education Bldg
Iowa City, IA 52242-1190
Prgm Dir: David H Nielsen, PhD PT
Tel: 319 335-9791   *Fax:* 319 335-9707
E-mail: david-nielsen@uiowa.edu

Kansas

University of Kansas Medical Center
Physical Therapy Prgm
3056 Robinson Hall
3901 Rainbow Blvd
Kansas City, KS 66160-7601
Prgm Dir: Lisa Stehno-Bittel, PhD PT
Tel: 913 588-6799   *Fax:* 913 588-4568
E-mail: ptadmissions@kumc.edu

Wichita State University
Physical Therapy Prgm
College of Health Professions
Ahlberg Hall, 1845 N Fairmont
Wichita, KS 67260-0043
Prgm Dir: Camilla Wilson, PhD
Tel: 316 978-3604   *Fax:* 316 978-3025
E-mail: Camilla.Wilson@wichita.edu

Kentucky

University of Kentucky
Physical Therapy Prgm
900 S Limestone Ave, CHS Bldg, Rm 204
Lexington, KY 40536-0200
Prgm Dir: Anne L Harrison, PT PhD
Tel: 859 323-1100, Ext 80596   *Fax:* 859 323-6003
E-mail: alharr01@uky.edu

Bellarmine University
Physical Therapy Prgm
Lansing School of Nursing and Health Science
2001 Newburg Rd
Louisville, KY 40205
Prgm Dir: Mark R Wiegand, PhD PT
Tel: 502 452-8368   *Fax:* 502 452-8429
E-mail: mwiegand@bellarmine.edu

Louisiana

Louisiana State Univ Health Sciences Center
Physical Therapy Prgm
1900 Gravier St
New Orleans, LA 70112
Prgm Dir: Elizabeth Weiss, PhD PT
Tel: 504 568-4288   *Fax:* 504 568-6552
E-mail: eweiss@lsuhsc.edu

Louisiana State U Hlth Sci Ctr - Shreveport
Physical Therapy Prgm
School of Allied Health Professions
1501 Kings Hwy, PO Box 33932
Shreveport, LA 71130-3932
Prgm Dir: Joseph McCulloch, PT PhD
Tel: 318 675-6820   *Fax:* 318 675-4208
E-mail: jmcclo@lsuhsc.edu

Maine

Husson College
Physical Therapy Prgm
1 College Circle
Bangor, ME 04401
Prgm Dir: Suzanne P Gordon, PT MA
Tel: 207 941-7101   *Fax:* 207 941-7883
E-mail: gordons@husson.edu

University of New England
Physical Therapy Prgm
Dept of Physical Therapy
716 Stevens Ave
Portland, ME 04103
Prgm Dir: Michael Sheldon, PT MS
Tel: 207 221-4591   *Fax:* 207 523-1910
E-mail: msheldon@une.edu

Maryland

University of Maryland - Baltimore
Physical Therapy Prgm
School of Medicine
Department of Physical Therapy and Rehabilitation
    Science
Baltimore, MD 21201
Prgm Dir: Mary Rodgers, PT PhD
Tel: 410 706-7720, Ext 5658   *Fax:* 410 706-6387
E-mail: mrodgers@umaryland.edu

University of Maryland Eastern Shore
Physical Therapy Prgm
Dept of Physical Therapy
Hazel Hall Rm 2093
Princess Anne, MD 21853
Prgm Dir: Raymond L Blakely, PhD PT
Tel: 410 651-6360   *Fax:* 410 651-6259
E-mail: rlblakely@umes.edu

Massachusetts

Boston University
Physical Therapy Prgm
Sargent Coll of Hlth and Rehab Sciences
635 Commonwealth Ave
Boston, MA 02215
Prgm Dir: Diane Dalton
Tel: 617 353-2720   *Fax:* 617 353-9463
E-mail: ddalton@bu.edu

MGH Institute of Health Professions
Physical Therapy Prgm
Charlestown Navy Yard
36 1st Ave
Boston, MA 02129
Prgm Dir: Leslie G Portney, DPT PhD FAPTA
Tel: 617 726-8009   *Fax:* 617 724-6321
E-mail: lportney@mghihp.edu

Northeastern University
Physical Therapy Prgm
360 Huntington Ave
Rm 6 Robinson Hall
Boston, MA 02115
Prgm Dir: Meredith H Harris, EdD PT
Tel: 617 373-5980   *Fax:* 617 373-3161
E-mail: m.harris@neu.edu

Simmons College
Physical Therapy Prgm
School for Health Studies
300 The Fenway
Boston, MA 02115
Prgm Dir: Shelley Goodgold, PT ScD
Tel: 617 521-2635   *Fax:* 617 521-3032
E-mail: goodgold@simmons.edu

University of Massachusetts - Lowell
Physical Therapy Prgm
Weed Hall, 3 Solomont Way Ste 5
Lowell, MA 01854-5124
Prgm Dir: Susan B O'Sullivan, EdD PT
Tel: 978 934-4412   *Fax:* 978 934-3006
E-mail: Susan_Osullivan@uml.edu

American International College
Physical Therapy Prgm
1000 State St
Springfield, MA 01109-983
Prgm Dir: Edward Swanson, PT PhD MEd MBA
Tel: 413 205-3320   *Fax:* 413 788-9961
E-mail: eswanson@acad.aic.edu

Springfield College
Physical Therapy Prgm
Dept of Physical Therapy
263 Alden St
Springfield, MA 01109
Prgm Dir: David Miller, PT PhD
Tel: 413 748-3590   *Fax:* 413 748-3371
E-mail: dmilller@spfldcol.edu

Michigan

Andrews University
Physical Therapy Prgm
Dept of Physical Therapy
Berrien Springs, MI 49104-0420
Prgm Dir: Wayne L Perry, PT MBA PhD
Tel: 269 471-6033   *Fax:* 269 471-2866
E-mail: perryw@andrews.edu

Wayne State University
Physical Therapy Prgm
2248 EACPHS
Detroit, MI 48202
Prgm Dir: Thomas Birk, PT PhD
Tel: 313 577-1432   *Fax:* 313 577-8685
E-mail: ae7647@wayne.edu

University of Michigan - Flint
Physical Therapy Prgm
School of Health Professions and Studies
303 E Kearsley St
Flint, MI 48502-2186
Prgm Dir: Donna Fry, PhD PT
Tel: 810 762-3373   *Fax:* 810 766-6668
E-mail: donnafry@umflint.edu

Grand Valley State University
Physical Therapy Prgm
301 Michigan St NE, Ste 200
Grand Rapids, MI 49503
Prgm Dir: John Peck, PhD PT
Tel: 616 331-2898   *Fax:* 616 331-5999
E-mail: peckj@gvsu.edu

Central Michigan University
Physical Therapy Prgm
1220 Health Professions Building
Mount Pleasant, MI 48859
Prgm Dir: Herman Triezenberg, PhD PT
Tel: 989 774-2347   *Fax:* 989 774-2908
E-mail: triez1hl@cmich.edu

Oakland University
Physical Therapy Prgm
School of Health Sciences
Rochester, MI 48309-4401
Prgm Dir: Kristine A Thompson, PT PhD
Tel: 248 370-4041   *Fax:* 248 370-4287
E-mail: kathomps@oakland.edu

Minnesota

College of St Scholastica
Physical Therapy Prgm
Graduate Studies Adm Asst
1200 Kenwood Ave
Duluth, MN 55811
Prgm Dir: Denise Wise, PT PhD
Tel: 218 723-6523   *Fax:* 218 723-6472
E-mail: dwise@css.edu

College of St Catherine - Minneapolis
Physical Therapy Prgm
601 25th Ave S
Minneapolis, MN 55454
Prgm Dir: Cort J Cieminski, PT MS ATC CSCS
Tel: 651 690-7884   *Fax:* 651 690-7876
E-mail: cjcieminski@stkate.edu

University of Minnesota - Minneapolis
Physical Therapy Prgm
Box 388
420 Delaware St SE
Minneapolis, MN 55455
Prgm Dir: James R Carey, PhD PT
Tel: 612 626-2746   *Fax:* 612 625-4274
E-mail: carey007@umn.edu

Mayo School of Health Sciences
Physical Therapy Prgm
200 First St SW
Rochester, MN 55905
Prgm Dir: John Hollman, PT PhD
Tel: 507 284-2054   *Fax:* 507 284-0656
E-mail: hollman.john@mayo.edu

Mississippi

University of Mississippi Medical Center
Physical Therapy Prgm
School of Health Related Professions
2500 N State St
Jackson, MS 39216-4505
Prgm Dir: Neva F Greenwald, PT MSPH
Tel: 601 984-6330   *Fax:* 601 984-6344
E-mail: ngreenwald@shrp.umsmed.edu

Missouri

Southwest Baptist University
Physical Therapy Prgm
1600 University Ave
Bolivar, MO 65613-2496
Prgm Dir: Steven G Lesh, PT PhD SCS ATC
Tel: 417 328-1672   *Fax:* 417 328-1658
E-mail: slesh@sbuniv.edu

University of Missouri - Columbia
Physical Therapy Prgm
School of Health Professions
106 Lewis Hall
Columbia, MO 65211
Prgm Dir: Marian A Minor, PhD PT
Tel: 573 882-7103   *Fax:* 573 884-8369
E-mail: minorm@health.missouri.edu

Rockhurst University
Physical Therapy Prgm
1100 Rockhurst Rd
Kansas City, MO 64110
Prgm Dir: Brian McKiernan, PT PhD
Tel: 816 501-4059   *Fax:* 816 501-4643
E-mail: brian.mckiernan@rockhurst.edu

Missouri State University
Physical Therapy Prgm
901 S National Ave
Springfield, MO 65804-0089
Prgm Dir: Akinniran Oladehin, PhD
Tel: 417 836-6179   *Fax:* 417 836-6229
E-mail: aoladehin@missouristate.edu

Maryville University
Physical Therapy Prgm
650 Maryville University Dr
St Louis, MO 63141
Prgm Dir: Judy Woehrle, PT PhD OCS
Tel: 314 529-9514   *Fax:* 314 529-9495
E-mail: jwoehrle@maryville.edu

Saint Louis University
Physical Therapy Prgm
Health Sciences Center
3437 Caroline St
St Louis, MO 63104-1111
Prgm Dir: Irma S Ruebling, MA PT
Tel: 314 577-8505   *Fax:* 314 577-8513
E-mail: ruebling@slu.edu

Washington University
Physical Therapy Prgm
School of Medicine, Campus Box 8502
4444 Forest Park Blvd, Ste 1101
St Louis, MO 63108
Prgm Dir: Susan S Deusinger, PT PhD FAPTA
Tel: 314 286-1407   *Fax:* 314 286-1410
E-mail: deusingers@msnotes.wustl.edu

Montana

University of Montana
Physical Therapy Prgm
School of Physical Therapy and Rehabilitation Science
Skaggs Bldg 135
Missoula, MT 59812
Prgm Dir: Reed Humphrey, PT PhD
Tel: 406 243-2417   *Fax:* 406 243-2795
E-mail: reed.humphrey@umontana.edu

Nebraska

Creighton University
Physical Therapy Prgm
School of Pharmacy and Health Professions
2500 California Plaza
Omaha, NE 68178
Prgm Dir: Robert Sandstrom, PhD PT
Tel: 402 280-4325   *Fax:* 402 280-5692
E-mail: rsandstr@creighton.edu

University of Nebraska Medical Center
Physical Therapy Prgm
984420 Nebraska Medical Center
Omaha, NE 68198-4420
Prgm Dir: Patricia A Hageman, PhD PT
Tel: 402 559-4259   *Fax:* 402 559-8626
E-mail: phageman@unmc.edu

Nevada

University of Nevada - Las Vegas
Physical Therapy Prgm
4505 Maryland Pkwy
Box 453029
Las Vegas, NV 89154-3029
Prgm Dir: J Wesley McWhorter, PT PhD
Tel: 702 895-3003   *Fax:* 702 895-4883
E-mail: james.mcwhorter@unlv.edu

New Hampshire

Franklin Pierce College
Physical Therapy Prgm
5 Chenell Dr
Concord, NH 03301
Prgm Dir: Jane Walter Venzke, PT EdD FAPTA
Tel: 603 899-4361
E-mail: venzkej@fpc.edu

New Jersey

Univ of Medicine & Dent of New Jersey
Physical Therapy Prgm
65 Bergen St, SSB 319
PO Box 1709
Newark, NJ 07101-1709
Prgm Dir: Alma S Merians, PhD PT
Tel: 973 972-7820   *Fax:* 973 972-3717
E-mail: merians@umdnj.edu

Richard Stockton College of New Jersey
Physical Therapy Prgm
Jim Leeds Rd
Pomona, NJ 08240
Prgm Dir: Bess Kathrins, PT MS
Tel: 609 652-4501   *Fax:* 609 652-4858
E-mail: bkathrins@stockton.edu

Seton Hall University
Physical Therapy Prgm
400 S Orange Ave
South Orange, NJ 07079-2689
Prgm Dir: Marc Campolo, PT PhD SCS
Tel: 973 275-2800   *Fax:* 973 275-2370
E-mail: campolma@shu.edu

SUNJ Rutgers Camden and UMDNJ
Physical Therapy Prgm
Primary Care Center, Ste 2105
40 E Laurel Rd
Stratford, NJ 08084
Prgm Dir: Marie Koval Nardone, PT EdD
Tel: 856 566-6456   *Fax:* 856 566-6458
E-mail: mptgradm@umdnj.edu

New Mexico

University of New Mexico
Physical Therapy Prgm
Health Sciences Center
1 University of New Mexico
Albuquerque, NM 87131-0001
Prgm Dir: Susan Queen, PT PhD
Tel: 505 272-5756   *Fax:* 505 272-8079
E-mail: squeen@salud.unm.edu

New York

Daemen College
Physical Therapy Prgm
4380 Main St
Amherst, NY 14226-3592
Prgm Dir: Sharon L Held, PT DPT MS PCS
Tel: 716 839-8344   *Fax:* 716 839-8537
E-mail: sheld@daemen.edu

Long Island University - Brooklyn Campus
Physical Therapy Prgm
Zeckendorf Health Sciences Center
One University Plaza
Brooklyn, NY 11201-5372
Prgm Dir: Stacy Jaffee Gropack, PT PhD
Tel: 718 488-1682   *Fax:* 718 780-4002
E-mail: rgabriel@liu.edu

SUNY Downstate Medical Center
Physical Therapy Prgm
450 Clarkson Ave, Box 16
Brooklyn, NY 11203-2098
Prgm Dir: Joanne S Katz, PhD PT
Tel: 718 270-7720   *Fax:* 718 270-7439
E-mail: jkatz@downstate.edu

D'Youville College
Physical Therapy Prgm
One D'Youville Sq
320 Porter Ave
Buffalo, NY 14201-1084
Prgm Dir: Lynn Rivers, PT PhD
Tel: 716 829-7702   *Fax:* 716 829-8137
E-mail: riversl@dyc.edu

University at Buffalo - SUNY
Physical Therapy Prgm
Department of Rehabilitation Science
515 Kimball Tower, 3435 Main St
Buffalo, NY 14214-3079
Prgm Dir: Louise Gilchrist, PhD PT
Tel: 716 829-3141, Ext 191   *Fax:* 716 829-3217
E-mail: lag@buffalo.edu

Mercy College
Physical Therapy Prgm
555 Broadway
Dobbs Ferry, NY 10522
Prgm Dir: Claudia B Fenderson, EdD PT
Tel: 914 674-7823   *Fax:* 914 674-7840
E-mail: cfenderson@mercy.edu

Ithaca College
Physical Therapy Prgm
Dept of Physical Therapy
335 Smiddy Hall
Ithaca, NY 14850-7183
Prgm Dir: Michael A Pagliarulo, PT EdD
Tel: 607 274-3716   *Fax:* 607 274-1137
E-mail: pags@ithaca.edu

Columbia University
Physical Therapy Prgm
710 W 168th St, 8th Fl
New York, NY 10032
Prgm Dir: Risa Granick, EdD MPA PT
Tel: 212 305-6907 *Fax:* 212 305-4569
E-mail: rg2135@columbia.edu

CUNY Hunter College
Physical Therapy Prgm
425 E 25th St
New York, NY 10010
Prgm Dir: Gary Krasilovsky, PhD PT
Tel: 212 481-7556 *Fax:* 212 481-8618
E-mail: gkrasilo@hunter.cuny.edu

New York University
Physical Therapy Prgm
380 2nd Ave, 4th Fl
New York, NY 10010
Prgm Dir: Wen Ling, PT
Tel: 212 998-9400, Ext 9415 *Fax:* 212 995-4190
E-mail: wen.ling@nyu.edu

Touro College
Physical Therapy Prgm
27 W 23rd St, 6th Fl
New York, NY 10010-4202
Prgm Dir: Christopher Kevin Wong, PT MS OCS
Tel: 212 463-0400, Ext 606 *Fax:* 631 665-4986
E-mail: ckwong@touro.edu

New York Institute of Technology
Physical Therapy Prgm
Northern Blvd
Box 8000
Old Westbury, NY 11568-8000
Prgm Dir: Karen Friel, PT DHS
Tel: 516 686-7696 *Fax:* 516 686-7699
E-mail: kfriel@nyit.edu

Dominican College
Physical Therapy Prgm
470 Western Hwy
Orangeburg, NY 10962-1299
Prgm Dir: Michael Gallucci, PT EdD
Tel: 845 398-4800 *Fax:* 845 398-4892
E-mail: michael.gallucci@dc.edu

Clarkson University
Physical Therapy Prgm
PO Box 5880
Potsdam, NY 13699-5880
Prgm Dir: Scott D Minor, PT PhD
Tel: 315 268-3786 *Fax:* 315 268-1539
E-mail: sminor@clarkson.edu

Nazareth College of Rochester
Physical Therapy Prgm
4245 East Ave
Rochester, NY 14618-3790
Prgm Dir: Jennifer Collins, PT MPA EdD
Tel: 585 389-2900 *Fax:* 585 389-2908
E-mail: jcollin9@naz.edu

CUNY College of Staten Island
Physical Therapy Prgm
2800 Victory Blvd
Staten Island, NY 10314
Prgm Dir: Jeffrey Rothman, EdD PT
Tel: 718 982-3153 *Fax:* 718 982-2984
E-mail: rothmanj@mail.csi.cuny.edu

Stony Brook University
Physical Therapy Prgm
Sch of Health Tech and Management
Health Sciences Center
Stony Brook, NY 11794-8201
Prgm Dir: Richard W Johnson, MA PT
Tel: 516 444-3250 *Fax:* 516 444-7621
E-mail: richard.johnson@stonybrook.edu

SUNY Upstate Medical University
Physical Therapy Prgm
College of Health Professions
750 E Adams St
Syracuse, NY 13210
Prgm Dir: Susan Miller, DPT OCS
Tel: 315 464-6881 *Fax:* 315 464-6887
E-mail: millers@upstate.edu

The Sage Colleges
Physical Therapy Prgm
Sage Graduate School, Dept of Physical Therapy
45 Ferry St
Troy, NY 12180
Prgm Dir: Marjane Selleck, PT MS PCS
Tel: 518 244-2060 *Fax:* 518 244-4524
E-mail: sellem@sage.edu

Utica College
Physical Therapy Prgm
Health and Human Studies Division
1600 Burrstone Rd
Utica, NY 13502-4892
Prgm Dir: Dale Scalise-Smith, PT PhD
Tel: 315 792-3059 *Fax:* 315 792-3248
E-mail: dscalise-smith@utica.edu

New York Medical College
Physical Therapy Prgm
Rm 302, School of Public Health
Valhalla, NY 10595
Prgm Dir: Michael Majsak, PT EdD
Tel: 914 594-4917 *Fax:* 914 594-4292
E-mail: michael_majsak@nymc.edu

North Carolina

University of North Carolina - Chapel Hill
Physical Therapy Prgm
Div of Physical Therapy
Medical School Wing E, CB 7135
Chapel Hill, NC 27599-7135
Prgm Dir: Rick Segal, PT PhD
Tel: 919 966-4708 *Fax:* 919 966-3678
E-mail: rsegal@med.unc.edu

Western Carolina University
Physical Therapy Prgm
312 Moore Bldg
Cullowhee, NC 28723-9646
Prgm Dir: Karen Y Lunnen, PT EdD
Tel: 828 227-2191 *Fax:* 828 227-7071
E-mail: klunnen@email.wcu.edu

Duke University Medical Center
Physical Therapy Prgm
PO Box 3965
Durham, NC 27710
Prgm Dir: Jan K Richardson, PhD PT OCS
Tel: 919 684-6020 *Fax:* 919 684-1846
E-mail: richa052@mc.duke.edu

Elon University
Cosponsor: Alamance Regional Medical Center
Physical Therapy Prgm
Campus Box 2085
Elon, NC 27244-2010
Prgm Dir: Elizabeth Rogers, PT EdD
Tel: 336 278-6350 *Fax:* 336 278-6414
E-mail: rogers@elon.edu

East Carolina University
Physical Therapy Prgm
Dept of Physical Therapy
School of Allied Health Sciences
Greenville, NC 27858-4353
Prgm Dir: Denis Brunt, EdD PT
Tel: 252 744-3238 *Fax:* 252 744-6240
E-mail: bruntd@ecu.edu

Winston-Salem State University
Physical Therapy Prgm
601 Martin Luther King Jr Dr
Winston-Salem, NC 27110
Prgm Dir: Robert J Cowie, PhD
Tel: 336 750-2190 *Fax:* 336 750-2192
E-mail: cowierj@wssu.edu

North Dakota

University of Mary
Physical Therapy Prgm
7500 University Dr
Bismarck, ND 58504-9652
Prgm Dir: Jodi Roller, PT EdD DPT
Tel: 701 355-8183 *Fax:* 701 255-7687
E-mail: rollerj@umary.edu

University of North Dakota
Physical Therapy Prgm
School of Medicine
PO Box 9037, 501 N Columbia Rd
Grand Forks, ND 58202-9037
Prgm Dir: Thomas M Mohr, PhD PT
Tel: 701 777-2831 *Fax:* 701 777-4199
E-mail: tommohr@medicine.nodak.edu

Ohio

Ohio University
Physical Therapy Prgm
School of Physical Therapy
W290 Grover Center
Athens, OH 45701
Prgm Dir: Averell S Overby, DrPH PT
Tel: 740 593-2624 *Fax:* 740 593-0293
E-mail: overbya@ohio.edu

College of Mt St Joseph
Physical Therapy Prgm
5701 Delhi Rd
Cincinnati, OH 45233-1672
Prgm Dir: Mary Romanello, PT PhD ATC SCS
Tel: 513 244-4890 *Fax:* 513 451-2547
E-mail: Mary_Romanello@mail.msj.edu

University of Cincinnati
Physical Therapy Prgm
College of Allied Health Science
PO Box 670394
Cincinnati, OH 45267-0394
Prgm Dir: Lizanne Mulligan, PhD PT PCS
Tel: 513 558-7482 *Fax:* 513 587-7474
E-mail: mulligea@uc.edu

Cleveland State University
Physical Therapy Prgm
Dept of Health Sciences HS 122
2121 Euclid Ave
Cleveland, OH 44115-2407
Prgm Dir: Ann Karas Reinthal, PT PhD
Tel: 216 687-3554 *Fax:* 216 687-9316
E-mail: a.karas@csuohio.edu

Ohio State University
Physical Therapy Prgm
516 Atwell Hall
453 West 10th Ave
Columbus, OH 43210
Prgm Dir: Deborah Givens Heiss, PT PhD DPT OCS
Tel: 614 292-5921 *Fax:* 614 292-0210
E-mail: heiss.8@osu.edu

University of Dayton
Physical Therapy Prgm
300 College Park
Dayton, OH 45469-1210
Prgm Dir: Philip Anloague, PT DHSc OCS MTC
Tel: 937 229-3250 *Fax:* 937 229-4224
E-mail: anloague@udayton.edu

University of Findlay
Physical Therapy Prgm
1000 North Main St
Findlay, OH 45840
Prgm Dir: Robert M Frampton, DHCE PT
Tel: 419 434-4863   *Fax:* 419 434-4336
E-mail: frampton@findlay.edu

Walsh University
Physical Therapy Prgm
2020 East Maple St
North Canton, OH 44720-3396
Prgm Dir: Susan A Bemis, PT EdD
Tel: 330 490-7370   *Fax:* 330 490-7371
E-mail: sbemis@walsh.edu

University of Toledo
Physical Therapy Prgm
4416 Collier Bldg
3015 Arlington Ave
Toledo, OH 43614
Prgm Dir: Clayton F Holmes, EdD PT
Tel: 419 383-3518   *Fax:* 419 383-5880
E-mail: cholmes@meduohio.edu

Youngstown State University
Physical Therapy Prgm
B080 Cushwa Hall
Youngstown, OH 44555-2558
Prgm Dir: Nancy Landgraff, PT PhD
Tel: 330 941-2558   *Fax:* 330 941-1898
E-mail: nlandgraff@ysu.edu

Oklahoma

Langston University
Physical Therapy Prgm
School of Physical Therapy
PO Box 1500
Langston, OK 73050
Prgm Dir: Milagros Jorge, PT EdD
Tel: 405 466-3411   *Fax:* 405 466-2915
E-mail: mjorge@lunet.edu

Univ of Oklahoma Health Sciences Center
Physical Therapy Prgm
College of Allied Health, Rm 235
PO Box 26901
Oklahoma City, OK 73190
Prgm Dir: Martha J Ferretti, MPH PT
Tel: 405 271-2131   *Fax:* 405 271-2432
E-mail: martha-ferretti@ouhsc.edu

Ontario, Canada

University of Western Ontario
Physical Therapy Prgm
Faculty of Health Sciences
Elborn College, Rm 1588
London, ON N6G 1H1
Prgm Dir: Tom Overend, PT PhD
Tel: 519 661-3360   *Fax:* 519 661-3866
E-mail: toverend@uwo.ca

University of Toronto
Physical Therapy Prgm
160 - 500 University Ave, 8th Fl
Toronto, ON M5G 1V7
Prgm Dir: Katherine Berg, PhD PT
Tel: 416 978-0173   *Fax:* 416 946-8562
E-mail: pt.chair@utoronto.ca

Oregon

Pacific University
Physical Therapy Prgm
School of Physical Therapy
222 SE 8th Ave, Ste 333
Hillsboro, OR 97123
Prgm Dir: Richard Rutt, PT PhD
Tel: 503 352-2846   *Fax:* 503 352-2995
E-mail: ruttra@pacificu.edu

Pennsylvania

Lebanon Valley College
Physical Therapy Prgm
101 N College Ave
Annville, PA 17003-0501
Prgm Dir: Stan M Dacko, PT PhD
Tel: 717 867-6840   *Fax:* 717 867-6365
E-mail: dacko@lvc.edu

Neumann College
Physical Therapy Prgm
Division of Nursing and Health Sciences
1 Neumann Dr
Aston, PA 19014-1298
Prgm Dir: Robert E Post, PT PhD
Tel: 610 361-5233   *Fax:* 610 361-5290
E-mail: postr@neumann.edu

Widener University
Physical Therapy Prgm
One University Plaza
Chester, PA 19013
Prgm Dir: Robin L Dole, PT EdD PCS
Tel: 610 499-1277   *Fax:* 610 499-1231
E-mail: rldole@widener.edu

Misericordia Unversity
Physical Therapy Prgm
301 Lake St
Dallas, PA 18612-1098
Prgm Dir: Susan Barker, PhD PT
Tel: 570 674-6422   *Fax:* 570 674-3052
E-mail: sbarker@misericordia.edu

Gannon University
Physical Therapy Prgm
Coll of Sciences, Engineering and Health
109 University Square
Erie, PA 16541-0001
Prgm Dir: Kristine S Legters, PT DSc NCS
Tel: 814 871-5639   *Fax:* 814 871-5662
E-mail: legters001@gannon.edu

Arcadia University
Physical Therapy Prgm
Dept of Physical Therapy
450 S Easton Rd
Glenside, PA 19038-3295
Prgm Dir: Rebecca L Craik, PhD PT
Tel: 215 572-2143   *Fax:* 215 572-2157
E-mail: admiss@arcadia.edu

St Francis University
Physical Therapy Prgm
PO Box 600
Loretto, PA 15940-0600
Prgm Dir: Michael Arnall, PT MS MBA
Tel: 814 472-3123   *Fax:* 814 472-3140
E-mail: marnall@francis.edu

Drexel University
Physical Therapy Prgm
Physical Therapy and Rehabilitation Sciences
Mail Stop 502, 245 N 15th St
Philadelphia, PA 19102
Prgm Dir: Susan S Smith, PT PhD
Tel: 215 762-1758   *Fax:* 215 762-3886
E-mail: sue.smith@drexel.edu

Temple University
Physical Therapy Prgm
College of Health Professions
3307 N Broad St
Philadelphia, PA 19140
Prgm Dir: Kim Nixon-Cave, PT PhD PCS
Tel: 215 707-4815   *Fax:* 215 707-7500
E-mail: deptpt@temple.edu

Thomas Jefferson University
Physical Therapy Prgm
College of Health Professions
130 S Ninth St, Ste 830 Edison
Philadelphia, PA 19107-5233
Prgm Dir: Penny Kroll, PT PhD
Tel: 215 503-8061   *Fax:* 215 503-3499
E-mail: penny.kroll@jefferson.edu

University of the Sciences in Philadelphia
Physical Therapy Prgm
600 S 43rd St
Philadelphia, PA 19104
Prgm Dir: Marc Campolo, PT PhD
Tel: 215 596-8849   *Fax:* 215 895-3121
E-mail: m.campol@usip.edu

Chatham University
Physical Therapy Prgm
114 Dilworth Hall
Woodland Rd
Pittsburgh, PA 15232-2826
Prgm Dir: Patricia Downey, PT PhD OCS
Tel: 412 365-1409   *Fax:* 412 365-1213
E-mail: downey@chatham.edu

Duquesne University
Physical Therapy Prgm
School of Health Sciences
139 Health Sciences Bldg
Pittsburgh, PA 15282
Prgm Dir: F Richard Clemente, PT PhD
Tel: 412 396-5541   *Fax:* 412 396-4399
E-mail: clemente@duq.edu

University of Pittsburgh
Physical Therapy Prgm
School of Health and Rehab Sciences
4019 Forbes Tower
Pittsburgh, PA 15260
Prgm Dir: Anthony Delitto, PT PhD FAPTA
Tel: 412 383-6630, Ext 1   *Fax:* 412 383-6629
E-mail: mizakd@upmc.edu

University of Scranton
Physical Therapy Prgm
800 Linden St
Scranton, PA 18510-4586
Prgm Dir: John P Sanko, PT EdD
Tel: 570 941-7934   *Fax:* 570 941-7940
E-mail: sankoj1@scranton.edu

Slippery Rock University of Pennsylvania
Physical Therapy Prgm
Graduate School of Physical Therapy
PT Building
Slippery Rock, PA 16057
Prgm Dir: Carol Martin-Elkins, PT PhD
Tel: 724 738-2080, Ext 2916   *Fax:* 724 738-2113
E-mail: carol.martin-elkins@sru.edu

Puerto Rico

University of Puerto Rico
Physical Therapy Prgm
Medical Sciences Campus
PO Box 365067
San Juan, PR 00936-5067
Prgm Dir: Annlee Burch, EdD MPH MSPT
Tel: 787 758-2525, Ext 4202   *Fax:* 787 753-7262
E-mail: annleeburch@cprs.rcm.upr.edu

Rhode Island

University of Rhode Island
Physical Therapy Prgm
Independence Square II
25 West Independence Way
Kingston, RI 02881-0180
Prgm Dir: Beth Marcoux, PhD PT
Tel: 401 874-5001   *Fax:* 401 874-5630
E-mail: bmarcoux@mail.uri.edu

South Carolina

Medical University of South Carolina
Physical Therapy Prgm
Dept of Rehabilitation Sciences
PO Box 250965
Charleston, SC 29425
Prgm Dir: Kathleen A Cegles, PT DEd
Tel: 843 792-2023   *Fax:* 843 792-0710
E-mail: cegles@musc.edu

University of South Carolina
Physical Therapy Prgm
School of Public Health
Columbia, SC 29208
Prgm Dir: Bruce A McClenaghan, MPT PED
Tel: 803 777-5267   *Fax:* 803 777-8422
E-mail: bmcclena@gwm.sc.edu

South Dakota

University of South Dakota
Physical Therapy Prgm
Dept of Physical Therapy
414 E Clark St
Vermillion, SD 57069
Prgm Dir: Lana R Svien, PT PhD
Tel: 605 677-5917   *Fax:* 605 677-6529
E-mail: lsvien@usd.edu

Tennessee

University of Tennessee - Chattanooga
Physical Therapy Prgm
615 McCallie Ave
Chattanooga, TN 37403
Prgm Dir: Cathie Smith, PT PhD PCS
Tel: 423 425-5259   *Fax:* 423 425-2215
E-mail: Cathie-Smith@utc.edu

East Tennessee State University
Physical Therapy Prgm
Box 70624
Johnson City, TN 37614
Prgm Dir: David A Arnall, PT PhD FACSM ES
Tel: 423 439-8275   *Fax:* 423 439-8077
E-mail: arnall@etsu.edu

University of Tennessee Health Science Ctr
Physical Therapy Prgm
930 Madison Ave
Ste 640
Memphis, TN 38163
Prgm Dir: Barbara H Connolly, PT EdD FAPTA
Tel: 901 448-5888   *Fax:* 901 448-7545
E-mail: bconnolly@utmem.edu

Belmont University
Physical Therapy Prgm
1900 Belmont Blvd
Nashville, TN 37212-3757
Prgm Dir: John S Halle, PT PhD ECS
Tel: 615 460-6727   *Fax:* 615 460-6729
E-mail: hallej@mail.belmont.edu

Tennessee State University
Physical Therapy Prgm
3500 John A Merritt Blvd, Box 9564
Nashville, TN 37209
Prgm Dir: Rosalyn Pitt, EdD PT
Tel: 615 963-5881   *Fax:* 615 963-5935
E-mail: rpitt@tnstate.edu

Texas

Hardin-Simmons University
Physical Therapy Prgm
2200 Hickory St
Box 16065 HSU Station
Abilene, TX 79698-6065
Prgm Dir: Janelle O'Connell, PhD PT ATC-L
Tel: 325 670-5860   *Fax:* 325 670-5868
E-mail: joconnel@hsutx.edu

Univ of Texas Southwestern Med Ctr
Physical Therapy Prgm
Southwestern Allied Health Sciences Sch
5323 Harry Hines Blvd
Dallas, TX 75390-8876
Prgm Dir: Patricia Winchester, PT PhD
Tel: 214 648-1551   *Fax:* 214 648-1511
E-mail: patricia.winchester@utsouthwestern.edu

University of Texas at El Paso
Physical Therapy Prgm
1101 N Campbell
El Paso, TX 79902-0581
Prgm Dir: J A Ryberg, PT MA
Tel: 915 747-8210   *Fax:* 915 747-8211
E-mail: jaryberg@utep.edu

Interservice
Cosponsor: Baylor University
Physical Therapy Prgm
3151 Scott Rd, Ste 1230
Fort Sam Houston, TX 78234-6138
Prgm Dir: Lt Col Josef H Moore, PT PhD SCS
Tel: 210 221-8410   *Fax:* 210 221-7585
E-mail: Cynthia.quiroz@cen.amedd.army.mil

University of Texas Medical Branch
Physical Therapy Prgm
School of Allied Health Sciences
301 University Blvd
Galveston, TX 77555-1144
Prgm Dir: Elizabeth Protas, PT PhD FACSM
Tel: 409 772-3068   *Fax:* 409 747-1613
E-mail: ejprotas@utmb.edu

Texas Woman's University
Physical Therapy Prgm
School of Physical Therapy
6700 Fannin St
Houston, TX 77030
Prgm Dir: Sharon Olson, PhD PT
Tel: 713 794-2090   *Fax:* 713 794-2071
E-mail: solson@mail.twu.edu

Texas Tech Univ Health Sciences Center
Physical Therapy Prgm
3601 Fourth St
Lubbock, TX 79430
Prgm Dir: Kerry K Gilbert, PT ScD
Tel: 806 743-3223   *Fax:* 806 743-1262
E-mail: kerry.gilbert@ttuhsc.edu

Angelo State University
Physical Therapy Prgm
2601 West Ave N
ASU Station #10923
San Angelo, TX 76909-0923
Prgm Dir: Shelly Weise, PT EdD
Tel: 325 942-2545   *Fax:* 325 942-2548
E-mail: shelly.weise@angelo.edu

Univ of Texas Hlth Sci Ctr at San Antonio
Physical Therapy Prgm
7703 Floyd Curl Dr
MSC 6247
San Antonio, TX 78229-3900
Prgm Dir: Giovanni DeDomenico, PhD
Tel: 210 567-8750   *Fax:* 210 567-8774
E-mail: dedomenico@uthscsa.edu

Texas State University - San Marcos
Physical Therapy Prgm
Health Science Center
601 University Dr
San Marcos, TX 78666
Prgm Dir: Barbara Sanders, PhD PT SCS
Tel: 512 245-8351   *Fax:* 512 245-8736
E-mail: bs04@txstate.edu

United Kingdom

Robert Gordon University
Physical Therapy Prgm
Faculty of Health and Social Care
Garthdee Rd
Garthdee Aberdeen, UK AB10 7QG
Prgm Dir: Alasdair MacSween, BSc (Hons) PhD MCSP
E-mail: a.macsween@rgu.ac.uk

Utah

University of Utah
Physical Therapy Prgm
Div of Physical Therapy
520 Wakara Way
Salt Lake City, UT 84108-1290
Prgm Dir: R Scott Ward, PhD PT
Tel: 801 581-4895   *Fax:* 801 585-5629
E-mail: scott.ward@hsc.utah.edu

Vermont

University of Vermont
Physical Therapy Prgm
College of Nursing and Health Sciences
305 Rowell Bldg, 106 Carrigan Dr
Burlington, VT 05405-0068
Prgm Dir: Diane U Jette, PT DSc
Tel: 802 656-3252   *Fax:* 802 656-6586
E-mail: diane.jette@uvm.edu

Virginia

Marymount University
Physical Therapy Prgm
2807 N Glebe Rd
Arlington, VA 22207-4299
Prgm Dir: Rita Wong, PT EdD
Tel: 703 284-5982   *Fax:* 703 284-5981
E-mail: rita.wong@marymount.edu

Hampton University
Physical Therapy Prgm
Department of Physical Therapy
Phenix Hall Rm 216
Hampton, VA 23668
Prgm Dir: Marilyn G Randolph, PT PhD
Tel: 757 727-5260   *Fax:* 757 728-6546
E-mail: marilys.randolph@hamptonu.edu

Old Dominion University
Physical Therapy Prgm
School of Physical Therapy
129 Wm B Spong Jr Hall
Norfolk, VA 23529-0288
Prgm Dir: George Maihafer, PhD PT
Tel: 757 683-4519   *Fax:* 757 683-4410
E-mail: gmaihafe@odu.edu

Virginia Commonwealth Univ/Health System
Physical Therapy Prgm
Medical College of Virginia Campus
Box 980224
Richmond, VA 23298-0224
Prgm Dir: Thomas P Mayhew, PhD PT
Tel: 804 828-0234   *Fax:* 804 828-8111
E-mail: tmayhew@vcu.edu

Shenandoah University
Physical Therapy Prgm
333 W Cork St
Winchester, VA 22601
Prgm Dir: Rose Schmieg, PT DHSc ATC OCS
Tel: 540 665-5520   *Fax:* 540 665-5530
E-mail: rschmieg@su.edu

Washington

University of Washington
Physical Therapy Prgm
Physical Therapy CC-902, Rehab Medicine
1959 NE Pacific St, Box 356490
Seattle, WA 98195-6490
Prgm Dir: Mark R Guthrie, PhD PT
Tel: 206 598-5340   *Fax:* 206 685-3244
E-mail: mguthrie@u.washington.edu

Eastern Washington University
Physical Therapy Prgm
310 N Riverpoint Blvd
Box T, Rm 270
Spokane, WA 99202-0002
Prgm Dir: Byron Russell, PhD
Tel: 509 368-6608   *Fax:* 509 368-6623
E-mail: byron.russell@mail.ewu.edu

University of Puget Sound
Physical Therapy Prgm
1500 N Warner
CMB 1070
Tacoma, WA 98416
Prgm Dir: Kathie Hummel-Berry, PhD PT
Tel: 253 879-3281   *Fax:* 253 879-2933
E-mail: hummel@ups.edu

West Virginia

West Virginia University
Physical Therapy Prgm
School of Medicine, Robert C Byrd Health Sciences
   Center
PO Box 9226
Morgantown, WV 26506-9226
Prgm Dir: MaryBeth Mandich, PhD PT
Tel: 304 293-1320   *Fax:* 304 293-7105
E-mail: mmandich@hsc.wvu.edu

Wheeling Jesuit University
Physical Therapy Prgm
316 Washington Ave
Wheeling, WV 26003
Prgm Dir: Luis G Vargas, PT PhD ATRIC
Tel: 304 243-2432, Ext 2291   *Fax:* 304 243-2042
E-mail: lvargas@wju.edu

Wisconsin

University of Wisconsin - La Crosse
Physical Therapy Prgm
4033 Health Science Ctr
1725 State St
La Crosse, WI 54601
Prgm Dir: Michele Thorman, PT MBA
Tel: 608 785-8475   *Fax:* 608 785-8460
E-mail: thorman.mich@uwlax.edu

University of Wisconsin - Madison
Physical Therapy Prgm
5173 Medical Sciences Center
1300 University Ave
Madison, WI 53706-1532
Prgm Dir: Lisa Steinkamp, PT MS MBA
Tel: 608 263-7131   *Fax:* 608 262-7809
E-mail: steinkam@surgery.wisc.edu

Concordia University Wisconsin
Physical Therapy Prgm
12800 N Lake Shore Dr
Mequon, WI 53092-7699
Prgm Dir: Ruth Gresley, PhD RN
Tel: 262 243-4280   *Fax:* 262 243-4506
E-mail: ruth.gresley@cuw.edu

Marquette University
Physical Therapy Prgm
PO Box 1881
Milwaukee, WI 53201-1881
Prgm Dir: Lawrence G Pan, PhD PT
Tel: 414 288-7194   *Fax:* 414 288-5987
E-mail: lawrence.pan@marquette.edu

Carroll College
Physical Therapy Prgm
100 N East Ave
Waukesha, WI 53186
Prgm Dir: Jane F Hopp, PT PhD
Tel: 262 524-7294   *Fax:* 262 524-7690
E-mail: jhopp@cc.edu

Alabama

Jefferson State Community College
Physical Therapist Assistant Prgm
Center for Health and Biological Sciences
4600 Valleydale Rd
Birmingham, AL 35242
Prgm Dir: Glenn Ross, MSPT
Tel: 205 520-5995   *Fax:* 205 520-5992
E-mail: gross@jeffstateonline.com

George C Wallace Community College
Physical Therapist Assistant Prgm
1141 Wallace Dr
Dothan, AL 36303
Prgm Dir: Priscilla Tucker, PT
Tel: 334 556-2213   *Fax:* 334 983-3600
E-mail: ptucker@wallace.edu

Wallace State Community College
Physical Therapist Assistant Prgm
PO Box 2000
Hanceville, AL 35077-2000
Prgm Dir: Alina C Adams, PT
Tel: 256 352-8332   *Fax:* 256 352-8320
E-mail: alina.adams@wallacestate.edu

Bishop State Community College
Physical Therapist Assistant Prgm
1365 Martin Luther King Ave
Mobile, AL 36603-5362
Prgm Dir: Pam Wehner, PT MS
Tel: 334 405-4441   *Fax:* 334 405-4442
E-mail: pwehner@bishop.edu

South University
Physical Therapist Assistant Prgm
5355 Vaughn Rd
Montgomery, AL 36116-1120
Prgm Dir: Joanne Rice, PT DPT
Tel: 334 395-8800   *Fax:* 334 834-9559
E-mail: jrice@southuniversity.edu

Arizona

GateWay Community College
Physical Therapist Assistant Prgm
108 N 40th St
Phoenix, AZ 85034
Prgm Dir: Peter Zawicki, MS PT
Tel: 602 286-8476   *Fax:* 602 286-8478
E-mail: peter.zawicki@gwmail.maricopa.edu

Arkansas

NorthWest Arkansas Community College
Physical Therapist Assistant Prgm
One College Dr
Bentonville, AR 72712-5091
Prgm Dir: Deanna Fletcher, MPH PT
Tel: 479 619-4153   *Fax:* 479 619-4254
E-mail: dfletche@nwacc.edu

South Arkansas Community College
Physical Therapist Assistant Prgm
300 West Ave
PO Box 7010
El Dorado, AR 71730
Prgm Dir: Jennifer Parks, PT
Tel: 870 862-8131, Ext 189   *Fax:* 870 864-7104
E-mail: jparks@southark.edu

Arkansas State University
Physical Therapist Assistant Prgm
Department of Health Professions
PO Box 910
State University, AR 72467
Prgm Dir: Becky Keith, BSPT
Tel: 870 972-3591   *Fax:* 870 972-3652
E-mail: beckeith@astate.edu

California

Loma Linda University
Physical Therapist Assistant Prgm
School of Allied Health Professions
Nichol Hall Rm 1911
Loma Linda, CA 92350
Prgm Dir: Jeannine Mendes, MPT
Tel: 909 558-4634   *Fax:* 909 558-0466
E-mail: jmendes@llu.edu

Ohlone College
Physical Therapist Assistant Prgm
Ohlone Community College Dist
Newark Ohlone Center, 35753 Cedar Blvd
Newark, CA 94560
Prgm Dir: Sheryl S Einfalt, MPT
Tel: 510 979-7482   *Fax:* 510 742-2315
E-mail: cthoel@ohlone.edu

Cerritos College
Physical Therapist Assistant Prgm
Health Occupations Div
11110 Alondra Blvd
Norwalk, CA 90650
Prgm Dir: Marijean Piorkowski, MS PT DPT
Tel: 562 860-2451, Ext 2580   *Fax:* 562 467-5077
E-mail: piorkowski@cerritos.edu

Sonoma College
Physical Therapist Assistant Prgm
1304 Southpoint Blvd, Ste 280
Petaluma, CA 94954
Prgm Dir: I Scott Thompson, MPT
Tel: 707 283-0800, Ext 106   *Fax:* 707 283-0808
E-mail: sthompson@sonomacollege.edu

Sacramento City College
Physical Therapist Assistant Prgm
Science and Allied Health
3835 Freeport Blvd
Sacramento, CA 95822
Prgm Dir: Elizabeth Chape, PT PhD
Tel: 916 558-2298   *Fax:* 916 558-2392
E-mail: chapee@scc.losrios.edu

San Diego Mesa College
Physical Therapist Assistant Prgm
7250 Mesa College Dr
San Diego, CA 92111-4998
Prgm Dir: Laura Crandall, PT MS OCS
Tel: 619 388-2839   *Fax:* 619 388-2677
E-mail: lcrandal@sdccd.edu

Colorado

Morgan Community College
Physical Therapist Assistant Prgm
17800 Rd 20
Fort Morgan, CO 80701
Prgm Dir: Carol J Leach, PT MHA PhD CHES
Tel: 970 542-3225   *Fax:* 970 867-3082
E-mail: carol.leach@morgancc.edu

Arapahoe Community College
Physical Therapist Assistant Prgm
2500 W College Dr, PO Box 9002
Littleton, CO 80160-9002
Prgm Dir: Paula Provence, MEd PT
Tel: 303 797-5897   *Fax:* 303 797-5935
E-mail: paula.provence@arapahoe.edu

Pueblo Community College
Physical Therapist Assistant Prgm
900 W Orman Ave
Pueblo, CO 81004
Prgm Dir: Lucinda (Cindy) Mihelich, PT MEd
Tel: 719 549-3433   *Fax:* 719 549-3381
E-mail: Cindy.Mihelich@pueblocc.edu

Connecticut

Naugatuck Valley Community College
Physical Therapist Assistant Prgm
750 Chase Pkwy
Waterbury, CT 06708
Prgm Dir: Cynthia M Lacouture, PT MA
Tel: 203 596-2157   *Fax:* 203 575-8146
E-mail: clacouture@nvcc.commnet.edu

Delaware

**Delaware Technical & Community College -
Owens Campus**
Physical Therapist Assistant Prgm
PO Box 610
Georgetown, DE 19947
Prgm Dir: Joanne Howell, PT
Tel: 302 855-5933   *Fax:* 302 858-5460
E-mail: jhowell@college.dtcc.edu

**Delaware Technical & Community College -
Wilmington**
Physical Therapist Assistant Prgm
333 Shipley St
Wilmington, DE 19801
Prgm Dir: Douglas P Huisenga, MPT ATC
Tel: 302 888-5292   *Fax:* 302 577-6431
E-mail: DHuisenga@Christianacare.org

Florida

Manatee Community College
Physical Therapist Assistant Prgm
5840 26th St W
Bradenton, FL 34207
Prgm Dir: Janice L Pollock, PT MHS
Tel: 941 752-5340   *Fax:* 941 727-8304
E-mail: pollocj@mccfl.edu

Broward Community College
Physical Therapist Assistant Prgm
Ctr for Health Science Education ll
1000 Coconut Creek Blvd
Coconut Creek, FL 33066
Prgm Dir: Susan Edelstein, PT MEd
Tel: 954 201-2086   *Fax:* 954 201-2348
E-mail: Sedelste@broward.edu

Daytona Beach Community College
Physical Therapist Assistant Prgm
1200 International Speedway Blvd
Daytona Beach, FL 32120-2811
Prgm Dir: Ruth A Freeman, PT MEd
Tel: 386 506-3752   *Fax:* 386 506-3300
E-mail: freemar@dbcc.edu

Keiser University
Physical Therapist Assistant Prgm
1500 NW 49th St
Fort Lauderdale, FL 33309
Prgm Dir: Joseph Vibert, PT MBA
Tel: 954 776-4456, Ext 520   *Fax:* 954 351-4046
E-mail: jvibert@keiseruniversity.edu

Indian River Community College
Physical Therapist Assistant Prgm
3209 Virginia Ave
Fort Pierce, FL 34981-5596
Prgm Dir: Leila J Darress, PT MS
Tel: 561 462-4477   *Fax:* 561 462-4900
E-mail: ldarress@ircc.edu

Florida Community College - Jacksonville
Physical Therapist Assistant Prgm
4501 Capper Rd
Jacksonville, FL 32218-4499
Prgm Dir: Gloria J Young, PT EdD
Tel: 904 766-5574   *Fax:* 904 766-5573
E-mail: gyoung@fccj.edu

Lake City Community College
Physical Therapist Assistant Prgm
149 SE College Place
Lake City, FL 32025
Prgm Dir: Olga Dreeben, PhD PT
Tel: 386 754-4358, Ext 4358   *Fax:* 386 754-4858
E-mail: dreebeno@lakecitycc.edu

Miami Dade College
Physical Therapist Assistant Prgm
MDCC Medical Campus
950 NW 20th St
Miami, FL 33127
Prgm Dir: Kenneth Lee, PT MA
Tel: 305 237-4141   *Fax:* 305 237-4116
E-mail: kenneth.lee@mdc.edu

Central Florida Community College
Physical Therapist Assistant Prgm
PO Box 1388
Ocala, FL 34478-1388
Prgm Dir: Jean M McCauley, MHSA PT
Tel: 352 854-2322, Ext 1442   *Fax:* 352 237-0510
E-mail: mccaulej@cfcc.cc.fl.us

Gulf Coast Community College
Physical Therapist Assistant Prgm
5230 W US Hwy 98
Panama City, FL 32401-1041
Prgm Dir: Laura (Holly) Gunning, PT MHS EdD
Tel: 850 913-3312   *Fax:* 850 747-3246
E-mail: lgunning@gulfcoast.edu

Seminole Community College
Physical Therapist Assistant Prgm
100 Weldon Blvd
Sanford, FL 32773-6199
Prgm Dir: Carol A Clayton, PT PhD
Tel: 407 708-2234   *Fax:* 407 708-2319
E-mail: claytonc@scc-fl.edu

St Petersburg College
Physical Therapist Assistant Prgm
PO Box 13489
St Petersburg, FL 33733
Prgm Dir: Rebecca Kramer, MPT
Tel: 813 341-3614   *Fax:* 813 341-3744
E-mail: kramer.rebecca@spcollege.edu

Pensacola Junior College
Physical Therapist Assistant Prgm
Warrington Campus
5555 W Hwy 98
Warrington, FL 32507
Prgm Dir: Cena Harmon, PT DPT
Tel: 850 484-2373   *Fax:* 850 484-2364
E-mail: charmon@pjc.edu

South University
Physical Therapist Assistant Prgm
West Palm Beach Campus
1760 N Congress Ave
West Palm Beach, FL 33409
Prgm Dir: Kenneth Amsler, PhD PT CQAUR
Tel: 561 697-9200   *Fax:* 561 697-9944
E-mail: kamsler@southuniversity.edu

Polk Community College
Physical Therapist Assistant Prgm
999 Avenue H NE
Winter Haven, FL 33881
Prgm Dir: Nelson Marquez, PT EdD
Tel: 863 297-1010, Ext 5751   *Fax:* 863 297-1036
E-mail: nmarquez@polk.edu

Georgia

Darton College
Physical Therapist Assistant Prgm
2400 Gillionville Rd
Albany, GA 31707
Prgm Dir: Kerri Johnson, MPT
Tel: 912 430-6904   *Fax:* 912 430-6910
E-mail: johnsonk@darton.edu

Athens Technical College
Physical Therapist Assistant Prgm
800 US Hwy 29 N
Athens, GA 30601-1500
Prgm Dir: Ellen P O'Keefe, PT DPT
Tel: 706 355-5055   *Fax:* 706 425-3104
E-mail: eokeefe@athenstech.edu

Gwinnett Technical College
Physical Therapist Assistant Prgm
5150 Sugarloaf Pkwy
Lawrenceville, GA 30043
Prgm Dir: Patricia Ann Balzer, PT MAHCE
Tel: 678 226-6635, Ext 6635   *Fax:* 770 962-7985
E-mail: pbalzer@GwinnettTech.edu

South University
Physical Therapist Assistant Prgm
709 Mall Blvd
Savannah, GA 31406
Prgm Dir: Kenneth R Amsler, PT PhD CQAUR
Tel: 561 697-9200   *Fax:* 561 697-9944
E-mail: kamsler@southuniversity.edu

Hawaii

Kapi'olani Community College
Physical Therapist Assistant Prgm
4303 Diamond Head Rd
Health Sciences Dept Kauila 122
Honolulu, HI 96816
Prgm Dir: Jill Wakabayashi, PTA MPH
Tel: 808 734-9398   *Fax:* 808 734-9126
E-mail: jwakabay@hawaii.edu

Idaho

Idaho State University
Physical Therapist Assistant Prgm
College of Technology
Campus Box 8380
Pocatello, ID 83209-8380
Prgm Dir: Jason B Shaw, MPT DA
Tel: 208 282-4815   *Fax:* 208 282-3975
E-mail: shawjaso@isu.edu

Illinois

Southwestern Illinois College
Physical Therapist Assistant Prgm
2500 Carlyle Rd
Belleville, IL 62221
Prgm Dir: Kim Snyder, PTA MEd ACCE
Tel: 618 235-2700, Ext 5390   *Fax:* 618 235-2052
E-mail: kim.snyder@swic.edu

Southern Illinois University Carbondale
Physical Therapist Assistant Prgm
SIU Clinical Ctr, 4602
Carbondale, IL 62901-4602
Prgm Dir: Janet L Rogers, PhD PTA
Tel: 618 453-6143   *Fax:* 618 453-6126
E-mail: jrogers@siu.edu

Kaskaskia College
Physical Therapist Assistant Prgm
27210 College Rd
Centralia, IL 62801
Prgm Dir: Keith Shaw, PT
Tel: 618 532-5931   *Fax:* 618 532-5948
E-mail: kshaw@kaskaskia.edu

Morton College
Physical Therapist Assistant Prgm
3801 S Central Ave
Cicero, IL 60804
Prgm Dir: Kelly Hawthorne
Tel: 708 656-8000, Ext 291   *Fax:* 708 656-8031
E-mail: Kelly.Hawthorn@morton.edu

Oakton Community College
Physical Therapist Assistant Prgm
1600 E Golf Rd
Des Plaines, IL 60016
Prgm Dir: Mary DeNotto, MSPT
Tel: 847 635-1857   *Fax:* 847 635-1764
E-mail: maryd@oakton.edu

Lake Land College
Physical Therapist Assistant Prgm
LLC Kluthe Center
1204 Network Center Dr
Effingham, IL 62401
Prgm Dir: Martha T Mioux, MHS PT
Tel: 217 540-3551   *Fax:* 217 540-3599
E-mail: mmioux@lakeland.cc.il.us

College of DuPage
Physical Therapist Assistant Prgm
IC 1028, 425 Fawell Blvd
Glen Ellyn, IL 60137-6599
Prgm Dir: Donald Schmidt, PT MS
Tel: 630 942-4076   *Fax:* 630 858-5409
E-mail: schmidt@cdnet.cod.edu

Black Hawk College
Physical Therapist Assistant Prgm
6600 34th Ave
Moline, IL 61265-5899
Prgm Dir: Larry Gillund, MS PT
Tel: 309 796-1311, Ext 5393   *Fax:* 309 796-5357
E-mail: gillundl@bhc.edu

Illinois Central College
Physical Therapist Assistant Prgm
201 SW Adams St
Peoria, IL 61635-0001
Prgm Dir: Julie A Feeny, PT MS
Tel: 309 999-4648   *Fax:* 309 673-9626
E-mail: jfeeny@icc.edu

Indiana

University of Evansville
Physical Therapist Assistant Prgm
1800 Lincoln Ave
Evansville, IN 47722
Prgm Dir: Barbara Hahn, MA PT
Tel: 812 479-2571   *Fax:* 812 479-2717
E-mail: bh38@evansville.edu

University of Saint Francis
Physical Therapist Assistant Prgm
2701 Spring St
Fort Wayne, IN 46808
Prgm Dir: Mary Kay Solon, PT MS
Tel: 260 434-7662   *Fax:* 260 434-7585
E-mail: mksolon@sf.edu

Ivy Tech Community College
Physical Therapist Assistant Prgm
1440 E 35th Ave
Gary, IN 46409
Prgm Dir: James Dye, DPT
Tel: 219 981-4430   *Fax:* 219 981-4821
E-mail: jdye@ivytech.edu

University of Indianapolis
Physical Therapist Assistant Prgm
Krannert School of Physical Therapy
1400 E Hanna Ave
Indianapolis, IN 46227-3697
Prgm Dir: William Staples, PT DPT GSC
Tel: 317 788-3500   *Fax:* 317 788-3542
E-mail: stapleswh@uindy.edu

Ivy Tech Community College - Muncie
Physical Therapist Assistant Prgm
4301 S Cowan Rd
Muncie, IN 47302
Prgm Dir: Mark Wise, PT MA
Tel: 765 289-2291, Ext 1404   *Fax:* 765 289-2292
E-mail: mwise@ivytech.edu

Brown Mackie College
Physical Therapist Assistant Prgm
1030 E Jefferson Blvd
South Bend, IN 46617
Prgm Dir: Shirley D Mapes, PT MS MBA
Tel: 574 237-0774   *Fax:* 574 237-3585
E-mail: smapes@amedcts.com

Vincennes University
Physical Therapist Assistant Prgm
Health Occupations Dept
Vincennes, IN 47591
Prgm Dir: Mark F Goodrich, PT MS ATC/L
Tel: 812 888-4416   *Fax:* 812 888-4550
E-mail: mgoodrich@vinu.edu

Iowa

Kirkwood Community College
Physical Therapist Assistant Prgm
6301 Kirkwood Blvd SW
Cedar Rapids, IA 52406
Prgm Dir: Maggie Thomas, MA PT
Tel: 319 398-5566   *Fax:* 319 398-1293
E-mail: maggie.thomas@kirkwood.edu

North Iowa Area Community College
Physical Therapist Assistant Prgm
500 College Dr
Mason, IA 50401
Prgm Dir: Carol Patnode, MA PTA
Tel: 515 422-4339   *Fax:* 515 422-4115
E-mail: patnocar@niacc.edu

Indian Hills Community College
Physical Therapist Assistant Prgm
Health Occupations Division
Ottumwa Campus, 525 Grandview
Ottumwa, IA 52501
Prgm Dir: Debi Fritz, MS PT
Tel: 641 683-5271   *Fax:* 641 683-5254
E-mail: dfritz@indianhills.edu

Western Iowa Tech Community College
Physical Therapist Assistant Prgm
4647 Stone Ave, PO Box 5199
Sioux City, IA 51102-5199
Prgm Dir: Barbara-Anne Huculak, EdD PT
Tel: 712 274-6400, Ext 1321   *Fax:* 712 274-6412
E-mail: huculab@witcc.edu

Kansas

Colby Community College
Physical Therapist Assistant Prgm
1255 South Range
Colby, KS 67701
Prgm Dir: Patricia A Erickson, PT DPT
Tel: 785 460-4797   *Fax:* 785 460-4788
E-mail: pate@colbycc.edu

Kansas City Kansas Community College
Physical Therapist Assistant Prgm
PO Box 12951
7250 State Ave
Kansas City, KS 66112-9978
Prgm Dir: Wanda Gattshall-Peresic, PT DPT
Tel: 913 288-7331   *Fax:* 913 288-7649
E-mail: wandag@toto.net

Washburn University
Physical Therapist Assistant Prgm
School of Applied Studies
1700 SW College Ave
Topeka, KS 66621
Prgm Dir: Lori Khan, PT DPT MS
Tel: 785 231-1010, Ext 1406   *Fax:* 785 231-1027
E-mail: lori.khan@washburn.edu

Kentucky

Hazard Community & Technical College
Cosponsor: Southeast Kentucky Community &
   Technical College
Physical Therapist Assistant Prgm
One Community College Dr
Hazard, KY 41701-2402
Prgm Dir: Tracy L Bowling, PT
Tel: 606 487-3379   *Fax:* 606 439-1600
E-mail: tracy.bowling@kctcs.edu

Jefferson Community and Technical College
Physical Therapist Assistant Prgm
109 E Broadway St
Louisville, KY 40202-2005
Prgm Dir: Peri Jacobson, PT MBA
Tel: 502 213-2193   *Fax:* 502 213-2491
E-mail: peri.jacobson@kctcs.edu

Madisonville Community College
Physical Therapist Assistant Prgm
750 N Laffoon St
Madisonville, KY 42431-9185
Prgm Dir: Angie Moser, PT
Tel: 270 824-7552, Ext 164   *Fax:* 270 824-7069
E-mail: angie.moser@kctcs.edu

West Kentucky Community & Technical College
Physical Therapist Assistant Prgm
PO Box 7380
Paducah, KY 42002-7380
Prgm Dir: Peggy R Block, MHS PT
Tel: 502 554-6274   *Fax:* 502 554-6227
E-mail: peggy.block@kctcs.edu

Somerset Community College
Physical Therapist Assistant Prgm
808 Monticello St
Somerset, KY 42501
Prgm Dir: Ronald L Meade, DPT
Tel: 606 451-6823   *Fax:* 606 676-3684
E-mail: ron.meade@kctcs.edu

Louisiana

Our Lady of the Lake College
Physical Therapist Assistant Prgm
7443 Picardy Ave
Baton Rouge, LA 70808
Prgm Dir: Kitty Krieg, PT MHS
Tel: 225 768-1702   *Fax:* 225 765-5838
E-mail: kkrieg@ololcollege.edu

Bossier Parish Community College
Physical Therapist Assistant Prgm
6220 E Texas St
Bossier City, LA 71111
Prgm Dir: Laura Bryant, PT MEd
Tel: 318 752-0885, Ext 6079   *Fax:* 318 752-0887
E-mail: lbryant@bpcc.edu

Delgado Community College
Physical Therapist Assistant Prgm
615 City Park Ave
New Orleans, LA 70119-4399
Prgm Dir: Susan M Welsh, PhD PT
Tel: 504 483-4207   *Fax:* 504 483-4609
E-mail: swelsh@dcc.edu

Maine

Kennebec Valley Community College
Physical Therapist Assistant Prgm
92 Western Ave
Fairfield, ME 04937-1367
Prgm Dir: Nancy Chandler, PT MPH
Tel: 207 453-5147   *Fax:* 207 453-5194
E-mail: nchandler@kvcc.me.edu

Maryland

Chesapeake Area Consortium for Higher Educ
Physical Therapist Assistant Prgm
101 College Pkwy
Arnold, MD 21012
Prgm Dir: David Thomas, PT MGA
Tel: 410 777-7039   *Fax:* 410 777-7099
E-mail: dcthomas@aacc.edu

Baltimore City Community College
Physical Therapist Assistant Prgm
Nursing Bldg Rm 302
2901 Liberty Heights Ave
Baltimore, MD 21215
Prgm Dir: Nijole D Kaltreider, PT MEd
Tel: 410 462-7727   *Fax:* 410 462-7734
E-mail: NKaltreider@bccc.edu

Allegany College of Maryland
Physical Therapist Assistant Prgm
12401 Willowbrook Rd SE
Cumberland, MD 21502-2596
Prgm Dir: Scott Love, PT DPT
Tel: 301 784-5535   *Fax:* 301 784-5015
E-mail: slove@allegany.edu

Montgomery College
Physical Therapist Assistant Prgm
7600 Takoma Ave
Takoma Park, MD 20912
Prgm Dir: LaVerne E Tuckson, MEd PT
Tel: 301 562-5520   *Fax:* 301 650-1446
E-mail: laverne.tuckson@montgomerycollege.edu

Carroll Community College
Physical Therapist Assistant Prgm
1601 Washington Rd
Westminster, MD 21157
Prgm Dir: Sharon Main, BS PT MBA
Tel: 410 386-8259   *Fax:* 410 386-8255
E-mail: smain@carrollcc.edu

Massachusetts

Bay State College
Physical Therapist Assistant Prgm
122 Commonwealth Ave
Boston, MA 02116
Prgm Dir: George B Coggeshall, MS PT
Tel: 617 217-9423   *Fax:* 617 375-0197
E-mail: gcoggeshall@baystate.edu

North Shore Community College
Physical Therapist Assistant Prgm
One Ferncroft Rd
Danvers, MA 01923-4093
Prgm Dir: Mary Meng-Rivas, PT MPH
Tel: 978 762-4000, Ext 4165   *Fax:* 978 762-4022
E-mail: mmengriv@northshore.edu

Massachusetts Bay Community College
Physical Therapist Assistant Prgm
19 Flagg Dr
Framingham, MA 01702
Prgm Dir: Brenda Carroll, MS PT
Tel: 508 270-4000   *Fax:* 508 270-4131
E-mail: bcarroll@massbay.edu

Mt Wachusett Community College
Physical Therapist Assistant Prgm
444 Green St
Gardner, MA 01440-1000
Prgm Dir: Jacqueline Shakar, MS PTAT
Tel: 978 632-6600, Ext 287   *Fax:* 978 632-6155
E-mail: j_shakar@mwcc.mass.edu

Berkshire Community College
Physical Therapist Assistant Prgm
1350 West St
Pittsfield, MA 01201-5786
Prgm Dir: Michele E Darroch, PT MEd
Tel: 413 499-4660, Ext 313   *Fax:* 413 447-7840
E-mail: mdarroch@berkshirecc.edu

Springfield Technical Community College
Physical Therapist Assistant Prgm
One Armory Sq, Ste 1
PO Box 9000
Springfield, MA 01102
Prgm Dir: Linda C Desmarais, PT DPT MPH
Tel: 413 775-4844   *Fax:* 413 755-6312
E-mail: ldesmarais@stcc.edu

Becker College
Physical Therapist Assistant Prgm
61 Sever St
Worcester, MA 01615-0071
Prgm Dir: Elizabeth V Fuller, MS PT EdD
Tel: 508 791-9241, Ext 362   *Fax:* 508 831-5213
E-mail: efuller@beckercollege.edu

Michigan

Kellogg Community College
Physical Therapist Assistant Prgm
450 North Ave
Battle Creek, MI 49017
Prgm Dir: Kathy A Mann, PT MA
Tel: 269 965-3931, Ext 2313   *Fax:* 269 565-2059
E-mail: mannk@kellogg.edu

Macomb Community College
Physical Therapist Assistant Prgm
44575 Garfield Rd
Clinton Township, MI 48038-1139
Prgm Dir: Carol Plisner, PT MA
Tel: 586 286-2097   *Fax:* 586 286-2098
E-mail: plisnerc@macomb.edu

Henry Ford Community College
Cosponsor: Oakwood Healthcare System, Inc
Physical Therapist Assistant Prgm
5101 Evergreen Rd
Dearborn, MI 48128
Prgm Dir: Cynthia M Scheuer, PT MS
Tel: 313 845-9877   *Fax:* 313 317-6569
E-mail: cscheuer@hfcc.edu

Mott Community College - Southern Lakes Branch Campus
Physical Therapist Assistant Prgm
2100 W Thompson Rd
Fenton, MI 48430
Prgm Dir: Kathleen Vielhaber, PT
Tel: 810 762-5021   *Fax:* 810 750-8588
E-mail: kvielhab@mcc.edu

Baker College of Flint
Physical Therapist Assistant Prgm
1050 W Bristol Rd
Flint, MI 48507-5508
Prgm Dir: Elaine Murphy, PhD
Tel: 810 766-4193   *Fax:* 810 766-2055
E-mail: elaine.murphy@baker.edu

Finlandia University
Physical Therapist Assistant Prgm
601 Quincy St
Hancock, MI 49930-1882
Prgm Dir: Cameron T Williams, PT MS
Tel: 906 487-7308   *Fax:* 906 487-7552
E-mail: cam.williams@finlandia.edu

Baker College of Muskegon
Physical Therapist Assistant Prgm
1903 Marquette Ave
Muskegon, MI 49442
Prgm Dir: Peter A Schaub, MS PT
Tel: 231 777-8800   *Fax:* 231 777-5265
E-mail: pete.schaub@baker.edu

Delta College
Physical Therapist Assistant Prgm
Rm P-172
University Center, MI 48710
Prgm Dir: A Michael Spitz, MSA BS PTA CSCS
Tel: 989 686-9478   *Fax:* 989 686-8736
E-mail: amspitz@delta.edu

Minnesota

Anoka Ramsey Community College
Physical Therapist Assistant Prgm
11200 Mississippi Blvd NW
Coon Rapids, MN 55433
Prgm Dir: Lisa Lentner, MS PT
Tel: 763 427-2600   *Fax:* 763 422-3341
E-mail: lisa.lentner@anokaramsey.edu

Lake Superior College
Physical Therapist Assistant Prgm
2101 Trinity Rd
Duluth, MN 55811
Prgm Dir: Jane Worley, MS PT
Tel: 218 733-7632   *Fax:* 218 723-4921
E-mail: j.worley@lsc.edu

College of St Catherine - Minneapolis
Physical Therapist Assistant Prgm
601 25th Ave S
Minneapolis, MN 55454
Prgm Dir: Susan R Nelson, MS PT
Tel: 612 690-7822   *Fax:* 612 690-7876
E-mail: srnelson@stkate.edu

Mississippi

Itawamba Community College
Physical Therapist Assistant Prgm
Dept of Applied Science and Technology
602 W Hill St
Fulton, MS 38843
Prgm Dir: Thomas W Hester, MS PT
Tel: 601 862-8342   *Fax:* 601 862-8350
E-mail: twhester@iccms.edu

Pearl River Community College - Hattiesburg
Physical Therapist Assistant Prgm
5448 US Hwy 49 S
Hattiesburg, MS 39401
Prgm Dir: Patricia R Crowson, PT MS
Tel: 601 554-5486   *Fax:* 601 554-5553
E-mail: pcrowson@prcc.edu

Hinds Community College
Physical Therapist Assistant Prgm
Nursing Applied Health Center
1750 Chadwick Dr
Jackson, MS 39204-3490
Prgm Dir: Lisa G Latham, PT
Tel: 601 371-3512   *Fax:* 601 371-3529
E-mail: lglatham@hindscc.edu

Meridian Community College
Physical Therapist Assistant Prgm
910 Hwy 19 N
Meridian, MS 39307-5890
Prgm Dir: Kimberly T Ennis, PT MHS
Tel: 601 484-8613   *Fax:* 601 484-8743
E-mail: kennis@meridiancc.edu

Missouri

Linn State Technical College
Physical Therapist Assistant Prgm
Capital Region Medical Center
Southwest Campus, 1432 Southwest Blvd
Jefferson City, MO 65101
Prgm Dir: Marlene Medin, PT MEd
Tel: 573 632-5625   *Fax:* 573 632-5623
E-mail: marlene.medin@linnstate.edu

Metropolitan Community College - Penn Valley
Physical Therapist Assistant Prgm
3201 SW Trafficway
Kansas City, MO 64111-2764
Prgm Dir: Gwen Robertson, MA PT
Tel: 816 759-4241   *Fax:* 816 759-4553
E-mail: Gwen.Robertson@mcckc.edu

Ozarks Technical Community College
Physical Therapist Assistant Prgm
1001 E Chestnut Expressway
Springfield, MO 65802
Prgm Dir: Rebecca McKnight, PT MS
Tel: 417 447-8838   *Fax:* 417 447-8806
E-mail: mcknighr@otc.edu

Missouri Western State University
Physical Therapist Assistant Prgm
4525 Downs Dr, JGM 304
St Joseph, MO 64507-2294
Prgm Dir: Maureen Raffensperger, PT OCS MS
Tel: 816 271-4251   *Fax:* 816 271-4168
E-mail: raffen@missouriwestern.edu

St Louis Community College - Meramec
Physical Therapist Assistant Prgm
11333 Big Bend Blvd
St Louis, MO 63122
Prgm Dir: Julie A High, MS PT
Tel: 314 984-7385   *Fax:* 314 984-7250
E-mail: jhigh@stlcc.edu

Nebraska

Northeast Community College
Physical Therapist Assistant Prgm
801 E Benjamin Ave, PO Box 469
Norfolk, NE 68702-0469
Prgm Dir: Jodie Aller, MPT
Tel: 402 844-7326, Ext 7326   *Fax:* 402 844-7390
E-mail: jodie@northeastcollege.com

Clarkson College
Physical Therapist Assistant Prgm
101 S 42nd St
Omaha, NE 68131-2739
Prgm Dir: Victoria Trost, DPT
Tel: 402 552-6178   *Fax:* 402 552-6019
E-mail: trost@clarksoncollege.edu

Nevada

College of Southern Nevada
Physical Therapist Assistant Prgm
6375 W Charleston Blvd
Las Vegas, NV 89146
Prgm Dir: Joseph D Cracraft, PhD PT
Tel: 702 651-5588   *Fax:* 702 651-5506
E-mail: joe.cracraft@ccsn.edu

New Hampshire

New Hampshire Comm Tech Coll - Claremont
Physical Therapist Assistant Prgm
One College Dr
Claremont, NH 03743-9707
Prgm Dir: Laurel Clute, PT MS
Tel: 603 542-7744, Ext 2554   *Fax:* 603 543-1844
E-mail: lclute@nhctc.edu

Hesser College
Physical Therapist Assistant Prgm
3 Sundial Ave
Manchester, NH 03103
Prgm Dir: Paula A Hould, PT
Tel: 603 668-6660, Ext 2113   *Fax:* 603 624-2836
E-mail: phould@hesser.edu

New Jersey

Essex County College
Physical Therapist Assistant Prgm
303 University Ave
Newark, NJ 07102
Prgm Dir: Christine M Stutz-Doyle, MA PT
Tel: 973 877-3456   *Fax:* 973 877-1930
E-mail: stutz@essex.edu

Bergen Community College
Physical Therapist Assistant Prgm
400 Paramus Rd, Rm S 336
Paramus, NJ 07652-1595
Prgm Dir: Kenneth H Mailly, PT
Tel: 201 612-5319   *Fax:* 201 612-3876
E-mail: kmailly@bergen.edu

Union County College
Physical Therapist Assistant Prgm
Plainfield Campus
232 E Second St
Plainfield, NJ 07060
Prgm Dir: Beth J Rothman, MS PT MEd
Tel: 908 412-3582   *Fax:* 908 754-2798
E-mail: rothman@ucc.edu

Mercer County Community College
Physical Therapist Assistant Prgm
1200 Old Trenton Rd, PO Box B
Trenton, NJ 08690
Prgm Dir: Barbara J Behrens, PTA MS
Tel: 609 570-3385   *Fax:* 609 570-3831
E-mail: behrensb@mccc.edu

New Mexico

San Juan College
Physical Therapist Assistant Prgm
4601 College Blvd
Farmington, NM 87402-4699
Prgm Dir: Wendy Bircher, PT EdD
Tel: 505 566-3407   *Fax:* 505 566-3767
E-mail: bircherw@sanjuancollege.edu

New York

Genesee Community College
Physical Therapist Assistant Prgm
One College Rd
Batavia, NY 14020-9704
Prgm Dir: Peggy Kerr, MS PT
Tel: 585 343-0055, Ext 6366   *Fax:* 585 343-0433
E-mail: pckerr@genesee.edu

Broome Community College
Physical Therapist Assistant Prgm
PO Box 1017
Decker Health Science Bldg 217C
Binghamton, NY 13902
Prgm Dir: Denise Abrams, PT MA
Tel: 607 778-5211   *Fax:* 607 778-5345
E-mail: abrams_d@sunybroome.edu

Kingsborough Comm Coll/The City Univ of NY
Physical Therapist Assistant Prgm
2001 Oriental Blvd
Brooklyn, NY 11235-2398
Prgm Dir: Steven B Skinner, PT MS EdD
Tel: 718 368-4818   *Fax:* 718 368-4873
E-mail: sskinner@kbcc.cuny.edu

Villa Maria College of Buffalo
Physical Therapist Assistant Prgm
240 Pine Ridge Rd
Buffalo, NY 14225
Prgm Dir: James J Kelley, PT EMMDS
Tel: 716 961-1835   *Fax:* 716 896-0705
E-mail: jkelley@villa.edu

SUNY at Canton
Physical Therapist Assistant Prgm
34 Cornell Dr
Canton, NY 13617-1096
Prgm Dir: Deborah S Molnar
Tel: 315 386-7394   *Fax:* 315 386-7959
E-mail: molnard@canton.edu

Nassau Community College
Physical Therapist Assistant Prgm
One Education Dr
Garden City, NY 11530
Prgm Dir: Laura Gilkes, PT MA
Tel: 516 572-9640   *Fax:* 516 572-7565
E-mail: gilkesl@ncc.edu

Herkimer County Community College
Physical Therapist Assistant Prgm
100 Reservoir Rd
Herkimer, NY 13350
Prgm Dir: Catherine E DeLorme, PT MS
Tel: 315 866-0300, Ext 8340   *Fax:* 315 866-7523
E-mail: delormece@herkimer.edu

LaGuardia Community College
Physical Therapist Assistant Prgm
31-10 Thomson Ave E 300 R
Long Island City, NY 11101
Prgm Dir: Debra Engel, PT DPT MS
Tel: 718 482-5780   *Fax:* 718 609-2052
E-mail: dengel@lagcc.cuny.edu

Orange County Community College
Physical Therapist Assistant Prgm
115 South St
Middletown, NY 10940
Prgm Dir: Maria E Masker, PT DPT
Tel: 914 341-4290   *Fax:* 914 341-4799
E-mail: mmasker@sunyorange.edu

New York University
Physical Therapist Assistant Prgm
School of Continuing and Prof Studies
594 Broadway, Rm 400
New York, NY 10012
Prgm Dir: Maureen Thornby, PhD PT
Tel: 212 992-8722   *Fax:* 212 995-4890
E-mail: mat2@nyu.edu

Touro College
Physical Therapist Assistant Prgm
27 W 23rd St
New York, NY 10010-4202
Prgm Dir: Christopher Kevin Wong, PT PhD OCS
Tel: 212 463-0400, Ext 606   *Fax:* 212 989-2054
E-mail: ckwong@touro.edu

Niagara County Community College
Physical Therapist Assistant Prgm
Div of Life Sciences
3111 Saunders Settlement Rd
Sanborn, NY 14132
Prgm Dir: Deborah K Matuch, MS PT
Tel: 716 614-6422   *Fax:* 716 614-6798
E-mail: matuch@niagaracc.suny.edu

Suffolk County Community College -
Ammerman Campus
Physical Therapist Assistant Prgm
Dept of Education, Health and Human Services
533 College Rd
Selden, NY 11784
Prgm Dir: Cheryl Gillespie, PT MA DPT
Tel: 516 451-4299, Ext 4017   *Fax:* 516 451-4697
E-mail: gillesc@sunysuffolk.edu

Onondaga Community College
Physical Therapist Assistant Prgm
4941 Onondaga Rd
Syracuse, NY 13215
Prgm Dir: Cynthia Warner, PT MEd
Tel: 315 498-2388   *Fax:* 315 498-2751
E-mail: warnerc@sunyocc.edu

North Carolina

Central Piedmont Community College
Physical Therapist Assistant Prgm
PO Box 35009
Charlotte, NC 28235
Prgm Dir: Ilene Weiner, MS PT
Tel: 704 330-6505   *Fax:* 704 330-6131
E-mail: ilene.weiner@cpcc.edu

Fayetteville Technical Community College
Physical Therapist Assistant Prgm
PO Box 35236
Fayetteville, NC 28303
Prgm Dir: Elaine M Eckel, MA PT
Tel: 910 678-8259   *Fax:* 910 678-8500
E-mail: eckele@faytechcc.edu

Caldwell Comm College & Tech Institute
Physical Therapist Assistant Prgm
2855 Hickory Blvd
Hudson, NC 28638
Prgm Dir: Martha Y Zimmerman, PT MA
Tel: 828 726-2605   *Fax:* 828 726-2489
E-mail: mzimmerman@cccti.edu

Guilford Technical Community College
Physical Therapist Assistant Prgm
601 High Point Rd, PO Box 309
Jamestown, NC 27282
Prgm Dir: Joey Jeffers, PT MA
Tel: 336 334-4822, Ext 2443   *Fax:* 336 454-2510
E-mail: jeffersj@gtcc.edu

Nash Community College
Physical Therapist Assistant Prgm
522 N Old Carriage Rd
PO Box 7488
Rocky Mount, NC 27804-0488
Prgm Dir: Tammie L Clark, PT MS
Tel: 252 443-4011, Ext 372   *Fax:* 252 443-0828
E-mail: tclark@nashcc.edu

Southwestern Community College
Physical Therapist Assistant Prgm
447 College Dr
Sylva, NC 28779
Prgm Dir: Debra M Klavohn, PT MA
Tel: 828 586-4091, Ext 331   *Fax:* 828 586-3129
E-mail: debm@southwesterncc.edu

Martin Commuity College
Physical Therapist Assistant Prgm
1161 Kehukee Park Rd
Williamston, NC 27892
Prgm Dir: Jean Lambert, PT PhD
Tel: 252 792-1521, Ext 237   *Fax:* 252 792-4425
E-mail: jlambert@martincc.edu

North Dakota

Williston State College
Physical Therapist Assistant Prgm
PO Box 1326, 1410 University Ave
Williston, ND 58802-1326
Prgm Dir: Robert Benson, MA PT LMT NCTMB
Tel: 701 774-4291   *Fax:* 701 774-4265
E-mail: robert.benson@wsc.nodak.edu

Ohio

Kent State University - Ashtabula Campus
Physical Therapist Assistant Prgm
3325 W 13th St
Ashtabula, OH 44004
Prgm Dir: Michael Blake, MS PT
Tel: 440 964-4333   *Fax:* 440 964-4269
E-mail: blake@ashtabula.kent.edu

Stark State College of Technology
Physical Therapist Assistant Prgm
Health Technologies Div
6200 Frank Ave NW
Canton, OH 44720
Prgm Dir: Wallace H Linville, PT MA
Tel: 330 966-5458, Ext 4619   *Fax:* 330 966-6586
E-mail: wlinville@starkstate.edu

University of Cincinnati
Physical Therapist Assistant Prgm
Department of Rehabilitation Sciences
College of Allied Health Sciences, French East Building
Cincinnati, OH 45267-0394
Prgm Dir: Tina Whalen, DPT MPA PT
Tel: 513 558-7485   *Fax:* 513 558-7474
E-mail: whalentf@uc.edu

Cuyahoga Community College
Physical Therapist Assistant Prgm
2900 Community College Ave, MHCS 126
Cleveland, OH 44115
Prgm Dir: Toby Sternheimer, MEd PT
Tel: 216 987-4502   *Fax:* 216 987-4386
E-mail: toby.sternheimer@tri-c.edu

Sinclair Community College
Physical Therapist Assistant Prgm
444 W Third St, Rm 3340
Dayton, OH 45402
Prgm Dir: Colleen Whittington, PT MHS
Tel: 937 512-5355   *Fax:* 937 512-2058
E-mail: colleen.whittington@sinclair.edu

Kent State University - East Liverpool Campus
Physical Therapist Assistant Prgm
400 E Fourth St
East Liverpool, OH 43920-3497
Prgm Dir: Thomas Rutledge, MS PT ATC
Tel: 330 382-7448   *Fax:* 330 382-7564
E-mail: trutledge@eliv.kent.edu

Lorain County Community College
Physical Therapist Assistant Prgm
1005 N Abbe Rd
Elyria, OH 44035
Prgm Dir: John T Myers, PTA MBA
Tel: 800 995-5222, Ext 7881   *Fax:* 216 366-4116
E-mail: jmyers@lorainccc.edu

Rhodes State College
Physical Therapist Assistant Prgm
4240 Campus Dr
Lima, OH 45804
Prgm Dir: Angela M Heaton, PT MSEd
Tel: 419 995-8813   *Fax:* 419 995-8818
E-mail: heaton.a@rhodesstate.edu

PROGRAMS

North Central State College
Physical Therapist Assistant Prgm
2441 Kenwood Circle, PO Box 698
Mansfield, OH 44901-0698
Prgm Dir: James L Hull, MBA PT
Tel: 419 755-4773   *Fax:* 419 755-4790
E-mail: jhull@ncstatecollege.edu

Washington State Community College
Physical Therapist Assistant Prgm
710 Colegate Dr
Marietta, OH 45750
Prgm Dir: Kimberly D Salyers, PTA MA Ed
Tel: 740 374-8716, Ext 1692   *Fax:* 740 373-7496
E-mail: ksalyers@wscc.edu

Marion Technical College
Physical Therapist Assistant Prgm
1467 Mt Vernon Ave
Marion, OH 43302-5694
Prgm Dir: Susan P Cotterman, PT MBA
Tel: 740 389-4636, Ext 356   *Fax:* 740 389-6136
E-mail: cottermans@mtc.edu

Hocking College
Physical Therapist Assistant Prgm
3301 Hocking Pkwy SEO 309
Nelsonville, OH 45764
Prgm Dir: Kathy Kropf, PT MEd
Tel: 740 753-3591, Ext 2867   *Fax:* 740 753-5105
E-mail: kropf_k@hocking.edu

Shawnee State University
Physical Therapist Assistant Prgm
940 2nd St
Portsmouth, OH 45662
Prgm Dir: Sam M Coppoletti, MPT ACCE CSCS
Tel: 740 351-3228   *Fax:* 740 351-3354
E-mail: scoppoletti@shawnee.edu

Clark State Community College
Physical Therapist Assistant Prgm
PO Box 570
Springfield, OH 45501-0570
Prgm Dir: Beth M Gustafson, PT MSEd
Tel: 937 328-8074   *Fax:* 937 328-6138
E-mail: gustafsonb@clarkstate.edu

Owens Community College
Physical Therapist Assistant Prgm
PO Box 10,000
30335 Oregon Rd
Toledo, OH 43699
Prgm Dir: Nancy Rupp, PT
Tel: 419 661-7084   *Fax:* 419 661-7251
E-mail: nrupp@owens.edu

Professional Skills Institute
Physical Therapist Assistant Prgm
20 Arco Dr
Toledo, OH 43607-1947
Prgm Dir: Colleen Macdonald-Mason, MS PT
Tel: 419 531-9610   *Fax:* 419 531-4732
E-mail: cm-mason@proskills.com

Zane State College
Physical Therapist Assistant Prgm
1555 Newark Rd
Zanesville, OH 43701
Prgm Dir: Barbara Shelby, PT MEd
Tel: 740 588-1315   *Fax:* 740 454-0035
E-mail: bshelby@zanestate.edu

Oklahoma

SW Oklahoma St Univ/Caddo Kiowa Tech Ctr
Physical Therapist Assistant Prgm
PO Box 190
Fort Cobb, OK 73038
Prgm Dir: LaMae Green, RPT
Tel: 405 643-3268   *Fax:* 405 643-2144
E-mail: lgreen@caddokiowa.com

Northeastern Oklahoma A&M College
Physical Therapist Assistant Prgm
Health Sciences Division
200 I Street NE
Miami, OK 74354
Prgm Dir: James D Compton, PT
Tel: 918 542-8441, Ext 6316   *Fax:* 918 540-6471
E-mail: jcompton@neoam.edu

Oklahoma City Community College
Physical Therapist Assistant Prgm
7777 S May Ave
Oklahoma City, OK 73159
Prgm Dir: Peggy DeCelle Newman, MHR PT
Tel: 405 682-1611, Ext 7305   *Fax:* 405 682-7826
E-mail: pnewman@okccc.edu

Carl Albert State College
Physical Therapist Assistant Prgm
1507 S McKenna
Poteau, OK 74953-5208
Prgm Dir: William L Carroll, MPT
Tel: 918 647-1358   *Fax:* 918 647-1327
E-mail: bcarroll@carlalbert.edu

Murray State College
Physical Therapist Assistant Prgm
One Murray Campus, NAH 116
Tishomingo, OK 73460
Prgm Dir: Gary Robinson, MS PT PCS
Tel: 580 371-2371, Ext 340   *Fax:* 580 371-9844
E-mail: grobinson@mscok.edu

Tulsa Community College
Physical Therapist Assistant Prgm
909 S Boston Ave
Tulsa, OK 74119
Prgm Dir: Suzanne Reese, MS PT
Tel: 918 595-7017   *Fax:* 918 595-7091
E-mail: sreese@tulsacc.edu

Oregon

Mt Hood Community College
Physical Therapist Assistant Prgm
26000 SE Stark St
Gresham, OR 97030
Prgm Dir: Jane Cedar, PT MS
Tel: 503 491-7464   *Fax:* 503 491-6047
E-mail: jane.cedar@mhcc.edu

Pennsylvania

Harcum College
Physical Therapist Assistant Prgm
750 Montgomery Ave
Bryn Mawr, PA 19010
Prgm Dir: Jacqueline Klaczak Kopack, MPT
Tel: 610 526-6059   *Fax:* 610 526-6031
E-mail: jkopack@harcum.edu

Butler County Community College
Physical Therapist Assistant Prgm
PO Box 1203
Butler, PA 16003-1203
Prgm Dir: Randall J Kruger, MPT
Tel: 724 287-8711, Ext 8372   *Fax:* 724 285-6047
E-mail: randy.kruger@bc3.edu

California University of Pennsylvania
Physical Therapist Assistant Prgm
Coll of Ed and Human Serv, Dept of Hlth Sci &
   Sport Studies
250 University Ave
California, PA 15419-1394
Prgm Dir: Jodi DeBlassio Dusi, MPT
Tel: 724 938-4562   *Fax:* 724 938-4542
E-mail: deblassio@cup.edu

Mount Aloysius College
Physical Therapist Assistant Prgm
7373 Admiral Peary Hwy
Cresson, PA 16630
Prgm Dir: Stacy A Sekely, PT DPT
Tel: 814 886-6428   *Fax:* 814 886-2978
E-mail: ssekely@mtaloy.edu

Penn State University - DuBois
Physical Therapist Assistant Prgm
College Place
DuBois, PA 15801
Prgm Dir: Barbara Reinard, PT MA
Tel: 814 375-4773
E-mail: ber125@psu.edu

Penn State University - Hazleton
Physical Therapist Assistant Prgm
76 University Dr
Hazleton, PA 18202
Prgm Dir: Rosemarie Petrilla
Tel: 717 450-3042   *Fax:* 717 450-3182
E-mail: rxp21@psu.edu

Comm College of Allegheny County
Physical Therapist Assistant Prgm
595 Beatty Rd
Monroeville, PA 15146
Prgm Dir: Norman L Johnson, PT DPT Ded
Tel: 724 325-6663   *Fax:* 724 325-6701
E-mail: njohnson@ccac.edu

Penn State University - Mont Alto Campus
Physical Therapist Assistant Prgm
Campus Dr
Mont Alto, PA 17237-9703
Prgm Dir: Thomas Glumac, PT
Tel: 717 749-6217   *Fax:* 717 749-6039
E-mail: txg3@psu.edu

Mercyhurst College
Physical Therapist Assistant Prgm
North East Campus
16 W Division St
North East, PA 16428
Prgm Dir: Janice Haas, PTA MS
Tel: 814 725-6305   *Fax:* 814 725-6339
E-mail: jhaas@mercyhurst.edu

Lehigh Carbon Community College
Physical Therapist Assistant Prgm
4525 Education Park Dr
Schnecksville, PA 18078-2598
Prgm Dir: Evelyn M Petrash, PT MS
Tel: 610 799-1515   *Fax:* 610 799-1527
E-mail: epetrash@lccc.edu

Penn State University - Shenango Campus
Physical Therapist Assistant Prgm
147 Shenango Ave
Sharon, PA 16146
Prgm Dir: Richard L Holzworth, MS PT
Tel: 724 983-2866   *Fax:* 724 983-2820
E-mail: rlh18@psu.edu

Central Pennsylvania College
Physical Therapist Assistant Prgm
Campus on College Hill and Valley Rds
Summerdale, PA 17093-0309
Prgm Dir: Krista M Wolfe, DPT ATC
Tel: 717 728-2276   *Fax:* 717 732-5254
E-mail: kristawolfe@centralpenn.edu

University of Pittsburgh - Titusville
Physical Therapist Assistant Prgm
504 E Main St
Titusville, PA 16354-2097
Prgm Dir: Malorie Kosht-Fedyshin, PT DPT
Tel: 814 827-4445   *Fax:* 814 827-5671
E-mail: mkosht@pitt.edu

Puerto Rico

University of Puerto Rico at Humacao
Physical Therapist Assistant Prgm
CUH Postal Station
100 CARR 908
Humacao, PR 00791-4300
Prgm Dir: Eneida Silva-Collazo, PT MPH
Tel: 787 850-9390   *Fax:* 787 850-9423
E-mail: e_silva@webmail.uprh.edu

Ponce Technological University College
Physical Therapist Assistant Prgm
Univ of Puerto Rico Regl Coll Admin
PO Box 7186
Ponce, PR 00732
Prgm Dir: Felix A Cuevas Guzman, MPT
Tel: 787 844-8181, Ext 2414   *Fax:* 787 844-8679
E-mail: fac401@yahoo.com

Rhode Island

Community College of Rhode Island
Physical Therapist Assistant Prgm
1 John H Chafee Blvd
Newport, RI 02840
Prgm Dir: Kimberly Crealey Rouillier, DPT MS
Tel: 401 851-1668   *Fax:* 401 851-1710
E-mail: krouillier@ccri.edu

South Carolina

Trident Technical College
Physical Therapist Assistant Prgm
PO Box 118067 AH-M
Charleston, SC 29423-8067
Prgm Dir: Lori Fischer, MS PT
Tel: 843 574-6480   *Fax:* 843 574-6585
E-mail: lori.fischer@tridenttech.edu

Midlands Technical College
Physical Therapist Assistant Prgm
PO Box 2408
Columbia, SC 29202
Prgm Dir: Lynn van Dijk, PT MBA
Tel: 803 822-3590   *Fax:* 803 822-3619
E-mail: vandijkl@midlandstech.edu

Greenville Technical College
Physical Therapist Assistant Prgm
PO Box 5616
Greenville, SC 29606-5616
Prgm Dir: Alicia Dittmar, MEd PT
Tel: 864 848-2036   *Fax:* 864 848-2038
E-mail: Alicia.Dittmar@gvltec.edu

South Dakota

Lake Area Technical Institute
Physical Therapist Assistant Prgm
230 11th St NE, PO Box 730
Watertown, SD 57201-0730
Prgm Dir: Christina Barrett, PT MEd
Tel: 605 886-5284, Ext 329   *Fax:* 605 882-6299
E-mail: barrettc@lakeareatech.edu

Tennessee

Chattanooga State Technical Comm College
Physical Therapist Assistant Prgm
4501 Amnicola Hwy
Chattanooga, TN 37406-1097
Prgm Dir: Laura P Warren, MS PT
Tel: 423 697-3171, Ext 4450   *Fax:* 423 634-3071
E-mail: laura.warren@chattanoogastate.edu

Volunteer State Community College
Physical Therapist Assistant Prgm
1480 Nashville Pike
Gallatin, TN 37066
Prgm Dir: Dennis Dipert, MS PT
Tel: 615 230-3336   *Fax:* 615 230-4816
E-mail: dennis.dipert@volstate.edu

Jackson State Community College
Physical Therapist Assistant Prgm
2046 N Parkway St
Jackson, TN 38301-3797
Prgm Dir: Jane David, PT DPT
Tel: 731 425-2612, Ext 214   *Fax:* 731 425-9551
E-mail: jdavid@jscc.edu

South College
Physical Therapist Assistant Prgm
3904 Lonas Dr
Knoxville, TN 37909
Prgm Dir: Kelly S Nash, MS PT
Tel: 865 251-1800, Ext 1839   *Fax:* 865 584-9816
E-mail: knash@southcollegetn.edu

Southwest Tennessee Community College
Physical Therapist Assistant Prgm
Union Ave Campus
737 Union Ave
Memphis, TN 38103-3322
Prgm Dir: Edward Zeno, MS PT
Tel: 901 333-5394   *Fax:* 901 333-5391
E-mail: ezeno@southwest.tn.edu

Walters State Community College
Physical Therapist Assistant Prgm
500 S Davy Crockett Pkwy
Morristown, TN 37813-6899
Prgm Dir: Ann Lowdermilk
Tel: 423 585-6986   *Fax:* 423 585-6955
E-mail: margaret.lowdermilk@ws.edu

Roane State Community College
Physical Therapist Assistant Prgm
701 Briarcliff Ave
Oak Ridge, TN 37830
Prgm Dir: Kurt Backstrom, MS PT
Tel: 865 481-2000, Ext 2117   *Fax:* 865 481-2019
E-mail: backstrom_ka@roanestate.edu

Texas

Amarillo College
Physical Therapist Assistant Prgm
PO Box 447
Amarillo, TX 79178
Prgm Dir: Kelly J Jones, MPT
Tel: 806 354-6043   *Fax:* 806 354-6076
E-mail: jones-kj@actx.edu

Austin Community College
Physical Therapist Assistant Prgm
Eastview Campus
3401 Webberville Rd
Austin, TX 78702
Prgm Dir: Jana Israel, PT MEd
Tel: 512 223-5938   *Fax:* 512 223-5897
E-mail: jisrael@austincc.edu

Blinn College
Physical Therapist Assistant Prgm
PO Box 6030
Bryan, TX 77805-6030
Prgm Dir: John K Hubbard, PhD PT
Tel: 979 209-7154   *Fax:* 979 209-7524
E-mail: John.Hubbard@Blinn.edu

Montgomery College
Physical Therapist Assistant Prgm
3200 College Park Dr
Conroe, TX 77384-4077
Prgm Dir: Renee Pruitt, MHA
Tel: 936 273-7470   *Fax:* 936 273-7050
E-mail: rpruitt@nhmccd.edu

Del Mar College
Physical Therapist Assistant Prgm
Div of Occupational Education and Tech
West Campus
Corpus Christi, TX 78404-3897
Prgm Dir: Russell Stowers, PTA MS
Tel: 361 698-1847   *Fax:* 361 698-1849
E-mail: rstowers@delmar.edu

El Paso Community College
Physical Therapist Assistant Prgm
Rio Grande Campus, PO Box 20500
El Paso, TX 79998
Prgm Dir: Debra L Tomacelli-Brock, MS PT
Tel: 915 831-4172   *Fax:* 915 831-4114
E-mail: DebraT@epcc.edu

Houston Community College
Physical Therapist Assistant Prgm
Coleman College of Health Science
1900 Pressler Dr
Houston, TX 77030-3799
Prgm Dir: Jan H Myers, PT MS
Tel: 713 718-7391   *Fax:* 713 718-6495
E-mail: jan.myers@hccs.edu

San Jacinto College South
Physical Therapist Assistant Prgm
13735 Beamer Rd
Houston, TX 77089-6099
Prgm Dir: Carolyn Hoffman, PT MS
Tel: 281 929-4697   *Fax:* 281 922-3487
E-mail: carolyn.hoffman@sjcd.edu

Tarrant County College - Northeast Campus
Physical Therapist Assistant Prgm
828 Harwood Rd
Hurst, TX 76054
Prgm Dir: Jill Pool, PTA MEd
Tel: 817 515-6555   *Fax:* 817 515-6700
E-mail: jill.pool@tccd.edu

Kilgore College
Physical Therapist Assistant Prgm
1100 Broadway
Kilgore, TX 75662
Prgm Dir: Carla Gleaton, MEd PT
Tel: 903 983-8148   *Fax:* 903 988-7596
E-mail: cgleaton@kilgore.edu

Laredo Community College
Physical Therapist Assistant Prgm
West End Washington St
Campus Box 153
Laredo, TX 78040
Prgm Dir: Consuelo Moreno, PT MS
Tel: 956 764-5724   *Fax:* 956 721-5431
E-mail: cmoreno@laredo.edu

South Texas College
Physical Therapist Assistant Prgm
PO Box 9701
McAllen, TX 78502-9701
Prgm Dir: Diana Salinas Hernandez, PT
Tel: 956 971-3725   *Fax:* 956 971-3723
E-mail: dianah@stcc.cc.tx.us

Odessa College
Physical Therapist Assistant Prgm
201 W University Blvd
Odessa, TX 79764
Prgm Dir: Lynn McKelvey, PT MS
Tel: 915 335-6842   *Fax:* 915 335-6846
E-mail: lmckelvey@odessa.edu

St Philip's College
Physical Therapist Assistant Prgm
1801 Martin Luther King Dr
San Antonio, TX 78203-2098
Prgm Dir: J Thomas Davis, PhD PT
Tel: 210 531-3440   *Fax:* 210 531-3459
E-mail: jdavis@accd.edu

McLennan Community College
Physical Therapist Assistant Prgm
1400 College Dr
Waco, TX 76708
Prgm Dir: Julie Pickle, PT MS
Tel: 254 299-8715   *Fax:* 254 299-8747
E-mail: jpickle@mclennan.edu

Wharton County Junior College
Physical Therapist Assistant Prgm
911 Boling Hwy
Wharton, TX 77488
Prgm Dir: Phil Carter, MEd PT
Tel: 979 532-6491, Ext 6373   *Fax:* 979 532-6489
E-mail: philc@wcjc.edu

Utah

Provo College
Physical Therapist Assistant Prgm
1450 W 820 N
Provo, UT 84601
Prgm Dir: Bradley Cordero, DPT MBA CSCS
Tel: 801 818-8910   *Fax:* 801 375-9728
E-mail: bradleycordero@provocollege.edu

Salt Lake Community College
Physical Therapist Assistant Prgm
PO Box 30808
4600 S Redwood Rd
Salt Lake City, UT 84130-0808
Prgm Dir: Diana N Ploeger, PT MEd
Tel: 801 957-4054   *Fax:* 801 957-5708
E-mail: diana.ploeger@slcc.edu

Virginia

Jefferson College of Health Sciences
Physical Therapist Assistant Prgm
Community Hospital of Roanoke Valley
PO Box 13186, 920 S Jefferson St
Roanoke, VA 24031-3186
Prgm Dir: Michael A Krackow, PhD PTA
Tel: 540 224-4478   *Fax:* 540 985-9722
E-mail: mkrackow@jchs.edu

Northern Virginia Community College
Physical Therapist Assistant Prgm
6699 Springfield Center Dr
Springfield, VA 22150
Prgm Dir: Patricia S Ottavio, MPH PT
Tel: 703 822-6570   *Fax:* 703 822-6619
E-mail: pottavio@nvcc.edu

Tidewater Community College
Physical Therapist Assistant Prgm
1700 College Crescent, Bldg E, Rm E101
Virginia Beach, VA 23453
Prgm Dir: Melanie C Basinger, PT MS
Tel: 757 822-7251   *Fax:* 757 427-1338
E-mail: mbasinger1@tcc.edu

Wytheville Community College
Physical Therapist Assistant Prgm
1000 E Main St
Wytheville, VA 24382
Prgm Dir: Geneva Overton, PTA MA
Tel: 276 223-4721   *Fax:* 276 223-4778
E-mail: wcoverg@wcc.vccs.edu

Washington

Green River Community College
Physical Therapist Assistant Prgm
Health Sciences Div, Mailstop OE-14
12401 SE 320th St
Auburn, WA 98002-3699
Prgm Dir: Barbara Brucker, PT DPT MEd
Tel: 253 833-9111, Ext 4343   *Fax:* 253 833-3498
E-mail: bbrucker@greenriver.edu

Whatcom Community College
Physical Therapist Assistant Prgm
237 W Kellogg Rd
Bellingham, WA 98226
Prgm Dir: Rebecca A Graves, PT MS
Tel: 360 676-2170, Ext 3311   *Fax:* 360 752-6767
E-mail: bgraves@whatcom.ctc.edu

Spokane Falls Community College
Physical Therapist Assistant Prgm
3410 W Fort George Wright Dr
MS3190
Spokane, WA 99224-5288
Prgm Dir: Mary Ann Sharkey, PT PhD
Tel: 509 533-4144   *Fax:* 509 533-4143
E-mail: maryannsh@spokanefalls.edu

West Virginia

Mountain State University
Physical Therapist Assistant Prgm
PO Box 9003
South Kanawha St
Beckley, WV 25801
Prgm Dir: Gina Brown, PTA MS ATC
Tel: 304 929-1458   *Fax:* 304 929-1600
E-mail: gbrown@mountainstate.edu

Fairmont State Univ
Cosponsor: Pierpont Comm & Tech College
Physical Therapist Assistant Prgm
Caperton Center
501 W Main St
Clarksburg, WV 26301
Prgm Dir: Beverly R Born, PT EdD
Tel: 304 367-4042   *Fax:* 304 367-4028
E-mail: bborn@fairmontstate.edu

Marshall Community & Technical College
Physical Therapist Assistant Prgm
2000 7th Ave
Cabell Hall #208
Huntington, WV 25755
Prgm Dir: Travis H Carlton, PTA MS
Tel: 304 696-3008   *Fax:* 304 696-2396
E-mail: carltont@marshall.edu

Wisconsin

Northeast Wisconsin Technical College
Physical Therapist Assistant Prgm
2740 W Mason St
Green Bay, WI 54307
Prgm Dir: Julie Siefert, PT MHS LAT ATC
Tel: 920 498-5566   *Fax:* 920 491-2660
E-mail: julie.siefert@nwtc.edu

Blackhawk Technical College
Physical Therapist Assistant Prgm
6004 Prairie Rd, County Trunk G
Janesville, WI 53547-5009
Prgm Dir: Ilene Larson, MS PT
Tel: 608 757-7698   *Fax:* 608 757-4407
E-mail: ilarson@blackhawk.edu

Gateway Technical College
Physical Therapist Assistant Prgm
3520 30th Ave
Kenosha, WI 53144
Prgm Dir: Jeffrey Kannel, PT MS
Tel: 262 564-2482   *Fax:* 262 564-2007
E-mail: kannelj@gtc.edu

Western Technical College
Physical Therapist Assistant Prgm
304 N Sixth St, PO Box C-908
La Crosse, WI 54602-0908
Prgm Dir: Mary Ann Herlitzke, MS PT
Tel: 608 785-9598   *Fax:* 608 785-9299
E-mail: herlitzkem@wwtc.edu

Milwaukee Area Technical College
Physical Therapist Assistant Prgm
Health Occupations Div
700 W State St
Milwaukee, WI 53233
Prgm Dir: Paul J Mansfield, MPT
Tel: 414 297-8078   *Fax:* 414 297-8651
E-mail: MansfieP@matc.edu

Includes:
- Doctor of Medicine (MD)
- Doctor of Osteopathic Medicine (DO)

Note: There are two types of physicians: MD—Doctor of Medicine—and DO—Doctor of Osteopathic Medicine. MDs also are known as allopathic physicians. Both MDs and DOs may use all accepted methods of treatment, including drugs and surgery, but DOs place special emphasis on the body's musculoskeletal system, preventive medicine, and holistic patient care, as well as practicing osteopathic manipulative treatment (OMT), the use of hands to diagnose illness and injury and to encourage the body's natural tendency toward good health. DOs are more likely than MDs to be primary care specialists, although they can practice in all specialties; approximately 65% of practicing osteopathic physicians specialize in primary care areas, such as pediatrics, family medicine, obstetrics and gynecology, and internal medicine.

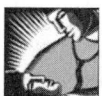

Career Description

Physicians, often referred to as doctors, serve a fundamental role in our society and have an effect upon all our lives. They diagnose illnesses and prescribe and administer treatment for people suffering from injury or disease. Physicians examine patients; obtain medical histories; and order, perform, and interpret diagnostic tests. They counsel patients on diet, hygiene, and preventive health care.

About one third of the nation's physicians are generalists—"primary care" doctors who provide lifelong medical services. These include internists, family physicians, and pediatricians. Generalists provide a wide range of services children and adults need. When patients' specific health needs require further treatment, generalist physicians send them to see a specialist physician.

Specialist physicians, such as neurologists, cardiologists, and ophthalmologists, differ from generalists in that they focus on treating a particular system or part of the body. They collaborate with generalist physicians to ensure that patients receive treatment for specific medical problems as well as complete and comprehensive care throughout life.

The most frequently entered areas of practice include the following:
- Emergency medicine
- Family medicine
- Internal medicine
- Obstetrics-gynecology
- Orthopedic surgery
- Pediatrics
- Psychiatry
- Surgery

Employment Characteristics

Many physicians—primarily general and family practitioners, general internists, pediatricians, ob/gyns, and psychiatrists—work in small private offices or clinics, often assisted by a small staff of nurses and other administrative or clinical personnel. Increasingly, physicians are practicing in groups or health care organizations, including hospitals, that provide backup coverage and allow for more time off. These physicians often work as part of a team coordinating care for a population of patients; they are less independent than solo practitioners of the past.

Other physicians work in research, academic settings, or with health maintenance organizations, pharmaceutical companies, medical device manufacturers, health insurance companies, or in corporations directing health and safety programs.

Many physicians work long, irregular hours. Over one third of full-time physicians worked 60 hours or more a week in 2004. Only 8 percent of all physicians worked part-time, compared with 16 percent for all occupations. Physicians must travel frequently between office and hospital to care for their patients. Those who are on call deal with many patients' concerns over the phone and may make emergency visits to hospitals or nursing homes at all hours of the day or night.

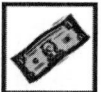

Salary

Data from the US Bureau of Labor Statistics show that, among the highest paying occupations, physicians moved from 12th place in 1997 to fourth place in 2005, behind airline pilots, economics teachers, and judges. Physicians had the largest upward change in the rankings (see www.bls.gov/opub/cwc/print/ cm20070824ar01p1.htm).

Employment Outlook

Employment of physicians is projected to grow faster than average for all occupations through the year 2014 due to continued expansion of health care industries. The growing and aging population will drive overall growth in the demand for physician services, as consumers continue to demand high levels of care using the latest technologies, diagnostic tests, and therapies. In addition to employment growth, job openings will result from the need to replace physicians who retire over the 2004-14 period.

Demand for physicians' services is highly sensitive to changes in consumer preferences, health care reimbursement policies, and legislation. For example, if changes to health coverage result in consumers facing higher out-of-pocket costs, they may demand fewer physician services. Demand for physician services may also be tempered by patients relying more on other health care providers—such as physician assistants, nurse practitioners, optometrists, and nurse anesthetists—for some health care services. In addition, new technologies will increase physician productivity. Telemedicine will allow physicians to treat patients or consult with other providers remotely. Increasing use of electronic medical records, test and prescription orders, billing, and scheduling may also improve physician productivity.

Opportunities for individuals interested in becoming physicians and surgeons are expected to be very good. Reports of shortages in some specialties or geographic areas should attract new entrants, encouraging schools to expand programs. Because physician training is so lengthy, however, employment change happens gradually. In the short term, to meet increased demand, experienced physicians may work longer hours, delay retirement, or take measures to increase productivity, such as using more support staff to provide services. Opportunities should be particularly good in rural and low-income areas, because some physicians find these areas unattractive due to less control over work hours, isolation from medical colleagues, or other reasons.

Unlike their predecessors, newly trained physicians face radically different choices of where and how to practice. New physicians are much less likely to enter solo practice and more likely to take salaried jobs in group medical practices, clinics, and health networks.

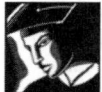

Educational Programs

Award, Length. After completing a bachelor's degree, allopathic physicians complete 4 years of medical school in the US, graduating with a doctor of medicine degree (MD); osteopathic physicians earn a doctor of osteopathic medicine degree (DO). (Some medical schools offer combined undergraduate and medical school programs that last 6 rather than the customary 8 years.) Next, allopathic physicians complete a residency program of 3 to 5 years in their chosen specialty (eg, neurology, surgery, internal medicine); some also complete an additional fellowship of 1 to 3 years in a subspecialty, such as cardiology, pain medicine, or neonatal-perinatal medicine.

Following graduation, osteopathic graduates complete an approved 12-month internship, which serves as the link between predoctoral and postdoctoral clinical training and provides a year of maturation and transition from application of predoctoral knowledge to clinical decision-making skills. The internship exposes graduates to core disciplines including internal medicine, family medicine, general surgery, obstetrics/gynecology, pediatrics and emergency medicine. Many graduates then choose to complete a residency program in a specialty area.

Prerequisites. Premedical students must complete undergraduate work in physics, biology, mathematics, English, and inorganic and organic chemistry. Students also take courses in the humanities and the social sciences. Some students volunteer at local hospitals or clinics to gain practical experience in the health professions. The minimum educational requirement for entry into a medical school is 3 years of college; most applicants, however, have at least a bachelor's degree, and many have advanced degrees. In addition, the Medical College Admission Test (MCAT) is required by most US medical schools.

The pathway is substantially similar for osteopathic physicians. Osteopathic medical school applicants typically have a bachelor's degree, with undergraduate studies that include 1 year each of English, biological sciences, physics, general chemistry, and organic chemistry. Other requirements may include genetics, mathematics, and psychology. Most prospective DO students major in sciences with an emphasis in biology or chemistry; however, applicants may major in any discipline as long as they meet the minimum course and grade requirements. Applicants must also take the MCAT.

Curriculum. Students spend most of the first 2 years of medical school in laboratories and classrooms, taking courses such as anatomy, biochemistry, physiology, pharmacology, psychology, microbiology, pathology, medical ethics, and laws governing medicine. They also learn to take medical histories, examine patients, and diagnose illnesses. During their last 2 years, students work with patients under the supervision of experienced physicians in hospitals and clinics, learning acute, chronic, preventive, and rehabilitative care. Through rotations in internal medicine, family medicine, obstetrics and gynecology, pediatrics, psychiatry, and surgery, they gain experience in diagnosing and treating illness.

Similarly, osteopathic medical students spend their first 2 years of school in lectures and laboratories, learning a core set of clinical examination skills and taking courses that cover the various systems of the body, including anatomy, physiology, microbiology,

histology, osteopathic principles and practices (including osteopathic manipulative medicine), pharmacology, clinical skills, and doctor/patient communication. Many osteopathic colleges have students assigned to work with physicians beginning early in the first year. This process continues throughout the second year in conjunction with the necessary science courses. In the third and fourth years, osteopathic medical students spend time learning about and exploring the major specialties in medicine through clinical clerkships in both in-patient and ambulatory care settings.

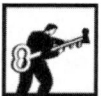

Licensure and Certification

Licensure, which is required of physicians in all US states and jurisdictions, ensures that practicing physicians have appropriate education and training and that they abide by recognized standards of professional conduct while serving their patients. Candidates for first licensure must complete a rigorous examination (for MDs, Steps 1, 2, and 3 of the United States Medical Licensing Examination; for DOs, Levels 1, 2 and 3 of the Comprehensive Osteopathic Medical Licensing Examination) designed to assess a physician's ability to apply knowledge, concepts, and principles that are important in health and disease and that constitute the basis of safe and effective patient care. All applicants must submit proof of medical education and training and provide details about their work history. Finally, applicants may have to reveal information regarding past medical history (including the use of habit-forming drugs and emotional or mental illness), arrests, and convictions.

The majority of physicians choose to become board certified, which is an optional, voluntary process, although it is required by many hospitals and managed care organizations. Certification involves testing and assessment of knowledge, skills, and experience to determine whether a physician is qualified to provide quality patient care in a given specialty/subspecialty. Certification in medical specialties and subspecialties is offered to MDs through the 24 boards of the American Board of Medical Specialties. In the past, physicians were required to recertify every 7 to 10 years, primarily by a written examination; this process is being replaced by Maintenance of Certification, an ongoing rather than periodic process that will require the assessment and improvement of practice performance.

For osteopathic physicians, the Board of Trustees of the American Osteopathic Association (AOA), through the Bureau of Osteopathic Specialists, is the certifying body in osteopathic medicine; there are 19 certifying boards.

Inquiries

MD Education, Careers, Resources
American Medical Association
515 N State Street
Chicago, IL 60610
www.ama-assn.org/go/becominganmd
E-mail: becominganmd@ama-assn.org

Association of American Medical Colleges
Careers in Medicine
2450 N Street NW
Washington, DC 20037-1126
www.aamc.org/students/considering/careers.htm
E-mail: careersinmedicine@aamc.org

DO Education, Careers, Resources
American Osteopathic Association
142 E Ontario Street
Chicago, IL 60611
800 621-1773 or 312 202-8000
www.osteopathic.org

American Association of Colleges of Osteopathic Medicine
5550 Friendship Blvd, Suite 310
Chevy Chase, MD 20815-7231
www.aacom.org

MD Program Accreditation
Liaison Committee on Medical Education
c/o American Medical Association
515 N State Street
Chicago, IL 60610
www.lcme.org

DO Program Accreditation
Commission on Osteopathic College Accreditation
American Osteopathic Association
142 E Ontario Street
Chicago, IL 60611
800 621-1773 or 312 202-8000
www.osteopathic.org

Note: Adapted in part from the Bureau of Labor Statistics, US Department of Labor, *Occupational Outlook Handbook*, 2006-07 Edition, Physicians and Surgeons, on the Internet at www.bls.gov/oco/ocos074.htm.

Physician (allopathic)

Alabama

University of Alabama School of Medicine
Allopathic Medicine Prgm
School of Medicine
Birmingham, AL 35294
www.ua.edu

University of South Alabama
Allopathic Medicine Prgm
College of Medicine
Mobile, AL 36688
www.southalabama.edu/com

Alberta, Canada

University of Calgary
Allopathic Medicine Prgm
Faculty of Medicine
Calgary, AB T2N 4N1
http://faculty.med.ucalgary.ca

University of Alberta
Allopathic Medicine Prgm
Faculty of Medicine and Dentistry
Edmonton, AB T6G 2R7
www.med.ualberta.ca

Arizona

University of Arizona
Allopathic Medicine Prgm
College of Medicine
Tucson, AZ 85721
www.medicine.arizona.edu

Arkansas

University of Arkansas at Little Rock
Allopathic Medicine Prgm
College of Medicine
Little Rock, AR 72204
www.uams.edu/COM/

British Columbia, Canada

University of British Columbia
Allopathic Medicine Prgm
Faculty of Medicine
Vancouver, BC V6T 1Z3
www.med.ubc.ca

California

University of California - Davis
Allopathic Medicine Prgm
School of Medicine
Davis, CA 95817
www.ucdmc.ucdavis.edu/medschool

University of CA - Irvine School of Medicine
Allopathic Medicine Prgm
Irvine, CA 92697
www.ucihs.uci.edu

Loma Linda University
Allopathic Medicine Prgm
School of Medicine
Loma Linda, CA 92350
www.llu.edu/llu/medicine

University of California - Los Angeles
Allopathic Medicine Prgm
David Geffen School of Medicine
Los Angeles, CA 90095
http://dgsom.healthsciences.ucla.edu

University of Southern California
Allopathic Medicine Prgm
Keck School of Medicine
Los Angeles, CA 90089
www.usc.edu/schools/medicine/ksom.html

Stanford University School of Medicine
Allopathic Medicine Prgm
Palo Alto, CA 94305
http://med.stanford.edu/

Univ of California San Diego Med Ctr
Allopathic Medicine Prgm
School of Medicine
San Diego, CA 92103
http://medicine.ucsd.edu/

University of California - San Francisco
Allopathic Medicine Prgm
School of Medicine
San Francisco, CA 94143
http://medschool.ucsf.edu/

Colorado

University of Colorado at Denver
Allopathic Medicine Prgm
Health Sciences Center
School of Medicine
Denver, CO 80217
www.uchsc.edu/som

Connecticut

University of Connecticut
Allopathic Medicine Prgm
School of Medicine
Farmington, CT 06269
http://medicine.uchc.edu

Yale University School of Medicine
Allopathic Medicine Prgm
New Haven, CT 06510
www.med.yale.edu/ysm

District of Columbia

George Washington University
Allopathic Medicine Prgm
School of Medicine and Health Sciences
Washington, DC 20007
www.gwumc.edu/Smhs

Georgetown University Medical Center
Allopathic Medicine Prgm
Washington, DC 20007
http://gumc.georgetown.edu

Howard University
Allopathic Medicine Prgm
College of Medicine
Washington, DC 20007
www.med.howard.edu

Florida

University of Florida
Allopathic Medicine Prgm
College of Medicine
Gainesville, FL 32611
www.med.ufl.edu

Leonard M Miller School of Medicine at the University of Miami
Allopathic Medicine Prgm
Miami, FL 33136
www.med.miami.edu

Florida State University
Allopathic Medicine Prgm
College of Medicine
Tallahassee, FL 32306
http://med.fsu.edu/

University of South Florida
Allopathic Medicine Prgm
College of Medicine
Tampa, FL 33620
http://health.usf.edu/medicine/home.html

Georgia

Emory University
Allopathic Medicine Prgm
School of Medicine
Atlanta, GA 30322
www.med.emory.edu

Morehouse School of Medicine
Allopathic Medicine Prgm
Atlanta, GA 30310
www.msm.edu

Medical College of Georgia
Allopathic Medicine Prgm
School of Medicine
Augusta, GA 30912
www.mcg.edu/som/index.asp

Mercer University
Allopathic Medicine Prgm
School of Medicine
Macon, GA 31207
http://medicine.mercer.edu/

Hawaii

University of Hawaii
Allopathic Medicine Prgm
John A Burns School of Medicine`
Honolulu, HI 96813
http://jabsom.hawaii.edu/jabsom

Illinois

Northwestern University
Allopathic Medicine Prgm
The Feinburg School of Medicine
Chicago, IL 60611
www.medschool.northwestern.edu

Rush University
Allopathic Medicine Prgm
Rush Medical College
Chicago, IL 60612
www.rushu.rush.edu/health/dept.html

University of Chicago Division of the Biological Sciences
Allopathic Medicine Prgm
The Pritzker School of Medicine
Chicago, IL 60637
pritzker.bsd.uchicago.edu

University of Illinois at Chicago
Allopathic Medicine Prgm
College of Medicine
Chicago, IL 60612
www.uic.edu/depts/mcam

Loyola University Medical Center
Allopathic Medicine Prgm
Stritch School of Medicine
Maywood, IL 60153
www.meddean.luc.edu

Rosalind Franklin Univ of Medicine & Science
Allopathic Medicine Prgm
The Chicago Medical School
North Chicago, IL 60064
www.rosalindfranklin.edu/cms

Southern Illinois University
Allopathic Medicine Prgm
School of Medicine
Springfield, IL 62794
www.siumed.edu

Indiana

Indiana University
Allopathic Medicine Prgm
School of Medicine
Indianapolis, IN 46202
www.medicine.iu.edu

Iowa

University of Iowa
Allopathic Medicine Prgm
Roy J and Lucille Carver College of Medicine
Iowa City, IA 52242
www.medicine.uiowa.edu

Kansas

University of Kansas Medical Center
Allopathic Medicine Prgm
School of Medicine
Kansas City, KS 66160
www.kumc.edu/som

Kentucky

University of Kentucky
Allopathic Medicine Prgm
College of Medicine
Lexington, KY 40506
www.mc.uky.edu/medicine

University of Louisville
Allopathic Medicine Prgm
School of Medicine
Louisville, KY 40292
http://louisville.edu/medschool/

Louisiana

Louisiana State Univ Health Sciences Center
Allopathic Medicine Prgm
School of Medicine
New Orleans, LA 70112
www.medschool.lsuhsc.edu

Tulane University
Allopathic Medicine Prgm
School of Medicine
New Orleans, LA 70118
www.som.tulane.edu

Louisiana State U Hlth Sci Ctr - Shreveport
Allopathic Medicine Prgm
School of Medicine
Shreveport, LA 71103
www.sh.lsuhsc.edu

Manitoba, Canada

University of Manitoba
Allopathic Medicine Prgm
Faculty of Medicine
Winnipeg, MB R3E 3P5
www.umanitoba.ca/faculties/medicine

Maryland

Johns Hopkins School of Medicine
Allopathic Medicine Prgm
Baltimore, MD 21205
www.hopkinsmedicine.org/som

University of Maryland
Allopathic Medicine Prgm
School of Medicine
Baltimore, MD 21201
http://medschool.umaryland.edu/

Uniformed Serv Univ of the Hlth Sci
Allopathic Medicine Prgm
F Edward Hebert School of Medicine
Bethesda, MD 20814
www.usuhs.mil/medschool/fehsom.html

Massachusetts

Boston University
Allopathic Medicine Prgm
School of Medicine
Boston, MA 02118
www.bumc.bu.edu

Harvard Medical School
Allopathic Medicine Prgm
Boston, MA 02118
http://hms.harvard.edu/hms/

Tufts University
Allopathic Medicine Prgm
School of Medicine
Boston, MA 02118
www.tufts.edu/med/

University of Massachusetts - Boston Medical School
Allopathic Medicine Prgm
Worcester, MA 01655
www.umassmed.edu

Michigan

University of Michigan Medical School
Allopathic Medicine Prgm
Ann Arbor, MI 48109
www.med.umich.edu/medschool

Wayne State University
Allopathic Medicine Prgm
School of Medicine
Detroit, MI 48202
www.med.wayne.edu

Michigan State University
Allopathic Medicine Prgm
College of Human Medicine
East lansing, MI 48824
http://humanmedicine.msu.edu/

Minnesota

University of Minnesota - Minneapolis Medical School
Allopathic Medicine Prgm
Minneapolis, MN 55455
www.med.umn.edu

Mayo School of Health Sciences
Allopathic Medicine Prgm
Rochester, MN 55905
www.mayo.edu/mshs

Mississippi

University of Mississippi
Allopathic Medicine Prgm
School of Medicine
Jackson, MS 38677
http://som.umc.edu/

Missouri

University of Missouri - Columbia
Allopathic Medicine Prgm
School of Medicine
Columbia, MO 65212
www.muhealth.org/~medicine

University of Missouri - Kansas City
Allopathic Medicine Prgm
School of Medicine
Kansas City, MO 64110
http://research.med.umkc.edu

Saint Louis University
Allopathic Medicine Prgm
School of Medicine
St Louis, MO 63104
http://medschool.slu.edu/

Washington University
Allopathic Medicine Prgm
St Louis School of Medicine
St Louis, MO 63110
http://medschool.wustl.edu/

Nebraska

Creighton University
Allopathic Medicine Prgm
School of Medicine
Omaha, NE 68178
www2.creighton.edu/medschool/

University of Nebraska - Omaha
Allopathic Medicine Prgm
College of Medicine
Omaha, NE 68182
www.unmc.edu/dept/com/

Nevada

University of Nevada - Reno
Allopathic Medicine Prgm
School of Medicine
Reno, NV 89557
www.unr.edu/med/

Newfoundland, Canada

Memorial University of Newfoundland
Allopathic Medicine Prgm
Faculty of Medicine
St John's, NF A1C 5S7
www.med.mun.ca

New Hampshire

Dartmouth Medical School
Allopathic Medicine Prgm
Hanover, NH 03755
http://dms.dartmouth.edu

New Jersey

Univ of Medicine & Dent of New Jersey Medical School
Allopathic Medicine Prgm
Newark, NJ 07107
www.umdnj.edu

UMDNJ - Robert Wood Johnson Medical School
Allopathic Medicine Prgm
Piscataway, NJ 08854
http://rwjms.umdnj.edu/

New Mexico

University of New Mexico School of Medicine
Allopathic Medicine Prgm
Albuquerque, NM 87131
http://hsc.unm.edu/som

New York

Albany Medical College
Allopathic Medicine Prgm
Albany, NY 12208
www.amc.edu

SUNY Downstate Medical Center
Allopathic Medicine Prgm
Downstate Medical Center College of Medicine
Brooklyn, NY 11203
www.hscbklyn.edu/college_of_medicine

University at Buffalo - SUNY
Allopathic Medicine Prgm
School of Medicine and Biomedical Sciences
Buffalo, NY 14260
www.smbs.buffalo.edu

Columbia University
Allopathic Medicine Prgm
College of Physicians and Surgeons
New York, NY 10032
www.cumc.columbia.edu/dept/ps

Cornell University
Allopathic Medicine Prgm
Weill Medical College
New York, NY 10021
www.med.cornell.edu

Mt Sinai School of Medicine
Allopathic Medicine Prgm
New York University
New York, NY 10029
www.mssm.edu

New York Medical College
Allopathic Medicine Prgm
New York, NY 10595
www.nymc.edu

New York University
Allopathic Medicine Prgm
School of Medicine
New York, NY 10016
www.med.nyu.edu

Yeshiva University
Allopathic Medicine Prgm
Albert Einstein College of Medicine
New York, NY 10033
www.yu.edu

University of Rochester
Allopathic Medicine Prgm
School of Medicine and Dentistry
Rochester, NY 14627
www.urmc.rochester.edu/smd

University at Stony Brook
Allopathic Medicine Prgm
Health Sciences Center School of Medicine
Stony Brook, NY 11794
www.stonybrookmedicalcenter.org/education/som.cfm

SUNY Upstate Medical University
Allopathic Medicine Prgm
Syracuse, NY 13210
www.upstate.edu

North Carolina

University of North Carolina Hospitals
Allopathic Medicine Prgm
School of Medicine
Chapel Hill, NC 27514
www.med.unc.edu

Duke University Medical Center
Allopathic Medicine Prgm
School of Medicine
Durham, NC 27710
http://medschool.duke.edu/

East Carolina University
Allopathic Medicine Prgm
The Brody School of Medicine
Greenville, NC 27834
www.ecu.edu/med

Wake Forest University School of Medicine
Allopathic Medicine Prgm
Winston-Salem, NC 27157
www1.wfubmc.edu/school

North Dakota

University of North Dakota
Allopathic Medicine Prgm
School of Medicine and Health Sciences
Grand Forks, ND 58202
www.med.und.nodak.edu

Nova Scotia, Canada

Dalhousie University
Allopathic Medicine Prgm
Faculty of Medicine
Halifax, NS B3H 4H7
www.medicine.dal.ca

Ohio

University of Cincinnati
Allopathic Medicine Prgm
College of Medicine
Cincinnati, OH 45267
www.med.uc.edu

Case Western Reserve University
Allopathic Medicine Prgm
School of Medicine
Cleveland, OH 44106
http://casemed.case.edu/

Ohio State University
Allopathic Medicine Prgm
College of Medicine and Public Health
Columbus, OH 43210
http://sph.osu.edu/

Wright State University
Allopathic Medicine Prgm
School of Medicine
Dayton, OH 45401
www.med.wright.edu

Northeastern Ohio Univ College of Medicine
Allopathic Medicine Prgm
Rootstown, OH 44272
www.neoucom.edu

University of Toledo
Allopathic Medicine Prgm
College of Medicine
Toledo, OH 43614
http://hsc.utoledo.edu/med

Oklahoma

University of Oklahoma
Allopathic Medicine Prgm
College of Medicine
Oklahoma City, OK 73190
www.medicine.ouhsc.edu

Ontario, Canada

McMaster University
Allopathic Medicine Prgm
School of Medicine
Hamilton, ON L8N 3Z5
www.mcmaster.ca/

Queen's University
Allopathic Medicine Prgm
Faculty of Health Sciences
Kingston, ON K7L 3N6
http://meds.queensu.ca/

University of Western Ontario
Allopathic Medicine Prgm
Schulich School of Medicine
London, ON N6A 5B8
www.schulich.uwo.ca/education/admissions/medicine/

University of Ottawa
Allopathic Medicine Prgm
Faculty of Medicine
Ottawa, ON K1H 8M5
www.medicine.uottawa.ca

Northern Ontario Medical School
Allopathic Medicine Prgm
Thunder Bay & Sudbury, ON P7B 5E1
www.normed.ca

University of Toronto
Allopathic Medicine Prgm
Faculty of Medicine
Toronto, ON M5S 1A6
www.facmed.utoronto.ca

Oregon

Oregon Health & Science University
Allopathic Medicine Prgm
School of Medicine
Portland, OR 97239
www.ohsuhealth.com

Pennsylvania

Penn State University
Allopathic Medicine Prgm
College of Medicine
Hershey, PA 17033
www.hmc.psu.edu/college

Drexel University
Allopathic Medicine Prgm
College of Medicine
Philadelphia, PA 19104
www.drexelmed.edu

Hospital of the Univ of Pennsylvania
Allopathic Medicine Prgm
School of Medicine
Philadelphia, PA 19106
www.med.upenn.edu

Temple University
Allopathic Medicine Prgm
School of Medicine
Philadelphia, PA 19140
www.temple.edu/medicine

Thomas Jefferson University
Allopathic Medicine Prgm
Jefferson Medical College
Philadelphia, PA 19107
www.jefferson.edu/jchp/home/

University of Pittsburgh
Allopathic Medicine Prgm
School of Medicine
Pittsburgh, PA 15260
www.medschool.pitt.edu

Puerto Rico

Universidad Central del Caribe
Allopathic Medicine Prgm
School of Medicine
Bayamon, PR 00960
www.uccaribe.edu

Ponce School of Medicine
Allopathic Medicine Prgm
Ponce, PR 00732
www.psm.edu

University of Puerto Rico
Allopathic Medicine Prgm
School of Medicine
San Juan, PR 00936
www.md.rcm.upr.edu

Quebec, Canada

McGill University
Allopathic Medicine Prgm
Faculty of Medicine
Montreal, QC H3G 1Y6
www.medicine.mcgill.ca

University de Montreal
Allopathic Medicine Prgm
Faculty of Medicine
Montreal, QC H3C 3J7
www.umontreal.ca

University Laval
Allopathic Medicine Prgm
Faculty of Medicine
Quebec City, QC G1K 7P4
http://w3.fmed.ulaval.ca/site_fac/

University of Sherbrooke
Allopathic Medicine Prgm
Faculty of Medicine
Sherbrooke, QC J1K 2R1
www.usherbrooke.ca/medecine

Rhode Island

Brown Medical School
Allopathic Medicine Prgm
Providence, RI 02912
http://bms.brown.edu

Saskatchewan, Canada

University of Saskatchewan
Allopathic Medicine Prgm
College of Medicine
Saskatoon, SK S7N 0W3

South Carolina

Medical University of South Carolina
Allopathic Medicine Prgm
College of Medicine
Charleston, SC 29425
www.musc.edu/com/COM1.shtml

University of South Carolina
Allopathic Medicine Prgm
School of Medicine
Columbia, SC 29203
www.med.sc.edu

South Dakota

University of South Dakota
Allopathic Medicine Prgm
School of Medicine
Vermillion, SD 57069
www.usd.edu/med

Tennessee

East Tennessee State University
Allopathic Medicine Prgm
James H Quillen College of Medicine
Johnson City, TN 37614
http://com.etsu.edu

University of Tennessee Health Science Ctr
Allopathic Medicine Prgm
College of Medicine
Memphis, TN 38163
www.utmem.edu/Medicine

Meharry Medical College
Allopathic Medicine Prgm
School of Medicine
Nashville, TN 37208
www.mmc.edu

Vanderbilt University
Allopathic Medicine Prgm
School of Medicine
Nashville, TN 37232
www.mc.vanderbilt.edu/medschool/

Texas

Texas A&M University
Allopathic Medicine Prgm
Health Science Center College of Medicine
College Station, TX 77845
http://medicine.tamhsc.edu/

Univ of Texas Southwestern Med Ctr
Allopathic Medicine Prgm
Southwestern Medical School
Dallas, TX 75390
www8.utsouthwestern.edu

University of Texas Medical Branch
Allopathic Medicine Prgm
Galveston, TX 77555
www.utmb.edu

Baylor College of Medicine
Allopathic Medicine Prgm
Houston, TX 77030
www.bcm.edu

Univ of Texas Medical School at Houston
Allopathic Medicine Prgm
Houston, TX 77225
http://med.uth.tmc.edu

Texas Tech Univ Health Sciences Center
Allopathic Medicine Prgm
School of Medicine
Lubbock, TX 79430
www.ttuhsc.edu/som

University of Texas Health Science Center
Allopathic Medicine Prgm
San Antonio, TX 78229
www.uthscsa.edu

Utah

University of Utah
Allopathic Medicine Prgm
School of Medicine
Salt Lake City, UT 84132
http://uuhsc.utah.edu/som/

Vermont

University of Vermont
Allopathic Medicine Prgm
College of Medicine
Burlington, VT 05405
www.med.uvm.edu

Virginia

University of Virginia
Allopathic Medicine Prgm
School of Medicine
Charlottesville, VA 22908
www.healthsystem.virginia.edu

Eastern Virginia Medical School
Allopathic Medicine Prgm
Medical College of Hampton Roads
Norfolk, VA 23507
www.evms.edu

Virginia Commonwealth University
Allopathic Medicine Prgm
School of Medicine
Richmond, VA 23298
www.medschool.vcu.edu

Washington

University of Washington
Allopathic Medicine Prgm
School of Medicine
Seattle, WA 98195
www.uwmedicine.org

West Virginia

Marshall University
Allopathic Medicine Prgm
Joan C Edwards School of Medicine
Huntington, WV 25701
http://musom.marshall.edu/

West Virginia University
Allopathic Medicine Prgm
School of Medicine
Morgantown, WV 26506
www.hsc.wvu.edu/som

Wisconsin

**University of Wisconsin - Madison Medical
School**
Allopathic Medicine Prgm
Madison, WI 53705
www.med.wisc.edu

Medical College of Wisconsin
Allopathic Medicine Prgm
Milwaukee, WI 53226
www.mcw.edu

Physician (osteopathic)

Arizona

Midwestern University - Glendale Campus
Osteopathic Medicine Prgm
Arizona College of Osteopathic Medicine
19555 N 59th Ave
Glendale, AZ 85308
Tel: 623 572-3300

AT Still University of Health Sciences
Osteopathic Medicine Prgm
College of Osteopathic Medicine-Mesa
5850 E Still Circle
Mesa, AZ 85206
Tel: 480 219-6000

California

Western Univ of Health Sciences
Osteopathic Medicine Prgm
College of Osteopathic Medicine of the Pacific
309 E 2nd St/College Plaza
Pomona, CA 91766-1889
Tel: 909 623-6116

Touro University Mare Island
Osteopathic Medicine Prgm
College of Osteopathic Medicine-CA
Vallejo, CA 94592
Tel: 707 638-5200

Colorado

Rocky Vista Univ Coll of Osteopathic Medicine
Osteopathic Medicine Prgm
3449 Chambers Rd, Ste B
Aurora, CO 80011
Tel: 303 373-2008

Florida

Lake Erie Coll of Osteopathic Medicine
Osteopathic Medicine Prgm
5000 Lakewood Ranch Blvd
Bradenton, FL 34211
Tel: 941 756-0690

Nova Southeastern University
Osteopathic Medicine Prgm
College of Osteopathic Medicine
3200 S University Dr
Fort Lauderdale, FL 33328
Tel: 800 356-0026   *Fax:* 954 262-2250

Georgia

Georgia Campus - PA Coll of Osteopathic Med
Osteopathic Medicine Prgm
625 Old Peachtree Rd
Suwanee, GA 30024
Tel: 678 225-7500

Illinois

Midwestern University
Osteopathic Medicine Prgm
Chicago College of Osteopathic Medicine
555 31st St
Downers Grove, IL 60515
Tel: 630 969-4400

Iowa

Des Moines University
Osteopathic Medicine Prgm
College of Osteopathic Medicine
3200 Grand Ave
Des Moines, IA 50312
Tel: 515 271-1450

Kentucky

Pikeville College
Osteopathic Medicine Prgm
School of Osteopathic Medicine
147 Sycamore St
Pikeville, KY 41501
Tel: 606 218-5400

Maine

University of New England
Osteopathic Medicine Prgm
College of Osteopathic Medicine
11 Hills Beach Rd
Biddeford, ME 04005
Tel: 800 477-4863

Michigan

Michigan State University
Osteopathic Medicine Prgm
College of Osteopathic Medicine
A-309 E Fee Hall
East Lansing, MI 48824
Tel: 517 353-7740

Missouri

Kansas City Univ of Medicine and Bioscience
Osteopathic Medicine Prgm
College of Osteopathic Medicine
1750 Independence Ave
Kansas City, MO 64106
Tel: 800 234-4847

Kirksville College of Osteopathic Medicine
Cosponsor: - AT Still University of Health Sciences
Osteopathic Medicine Prgm
800 W Jefferson
Kirksville, MO 63501
Tel: 660 626-2237

Nevada

Touro University - Nevada
Osteopathic Medicine Prgm
College of Osteopathic Medicine
874 American Pacific
Henderson, NV 89014
Tel: 702 777-8687

New Jersey

Univ of Medicine & Dent of New Jersey
Osteopathic Medicine Prgm
School of Osteopathic Medicine
Academic Center, One Medical Center Dr
Stratford, NJ 08084
Tel: 856 566-6000

New York

Touro College
Osteopathic Medicine Prgm
Touro College of Osteopathic Medicine
2090 Adam Clayton Powell Blvd, 6th Fl
New York, NY 10027
Tel: 212 851-1199, Ext 2004

New York Institute of Technology
Osteopathic Medicine Prgm
College of Osteopathic Medicine
PO Box 8000
Old Westbury, NY 11568
Tel: 516 626-6947

Ohio

Ohio University
Osteopathic Medicine Prgm
College of Osteopathic Medicine
Grosvenor, Irvine Halls
Athens, OH 45701
Tel: 800 345-1560

Oklahoma

Oklahoma State University
Osteopathic Medicine Prgm
College of Osteopathic Medicine
1111 W 17th St
Tulsa, OK 74107
Tel: 800 799-1972

Pennsylvania

Lake Erie Coll of Osteopathic Medicine - Erie
Osteopathic Medicine Prgm
1858 W Grandview Blvd
Erie, PA 16509
Tel: 814 866-6641

Robert Morris College/Allegheny Gen Hosp
Osteopathic Medicine Prgm
School of Osteopathic Medicine
6001 University Blvd
Moon Township, PA 15108-2574
Tel: 412 397-3947

Philadelphia College of Osteopathic Medicine
Osteopathic Medicine Prgm
4170 City Ave
Philadelphia, PA 19131
Tel: 215 871-6701

Tennessee

Lincoln Memorial University
Osteopathic Medicine Prgm
DeBusk College of Osteopathic Medicine
6965 Cumberland Gap Pkwy
Harrogate, TN 37752
Tel: 423 869-3611

Texas

Univ of North Texas Hlth Sci Ctr at Ft Worth
Osteopathic Medicine Prgm
Texas College of Osteopathic Medicine
3500 Camp Bowie Blvd
Fort Worth, TX 76107-2970
Tel: 817 735-2205

Virginia

Edward Via Virginia Coll of Opteopathic Med
Osteopathic Medicine Prgm
2265 Kraft Dr
Blacksburg, VA 24060
Tel: 540 231-4000

West Virginia

West Virginia of Osteopathic Medicine
Osteopathic Medicine Prgm
400 N Lee St
Lewisburg, WV 24901
Tel: 304 647-6373

Physician Assistant

History

The profession of physician assistant (PA) originated in the mid 1960s with leadership from Duke University, the University of Colorado, the University of Washington, and Wake Forest University. The early 1970s brought a rapid growth in the number of such educational programs, which were supported initially with $6.1 million appropriated under the authority of the Health Manpower Act of 1972. The funding also supported some of the initial organization and administration of the national program for the accreditation of educational programs in this field, specifically those designed to prepare individuals as assistants to primary care physicians. Since 1992, the number of accredited PA programs has more than doubled from 55 to 137. While the Accreditation Review Commission on Education for the Physician Assistant (ARC-PA) accredits the program to award the professional credential "PA," currently 80% of the institutions that sponsor PA programs also award an advanced academic degree.

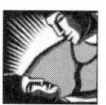

Career Description

The physician assistant is academically and clinically prepared to practice medicine with the direction and responsible supervision of a doctor of medicine or osteopathy. The physician-PA team relationship is fundamental to the PA profession and enhances the delivery of high-quality health care. Within the physician-PA relationship, PAs make clinical decisions and provide a broad range of diagnostic, therapeutic, preventive, and health maintenance services. The clinical role of PAs includes primary and specialty care in medical and surgical practice settings. PA practice is centered on patient care and may include educational, research, and administrative activities.

The role of the physician assistant demands intelligence, sound judgment, intellectual honesty, appropriate interpersonal skills, and the capacity to react to emergencies in a calm and reasoned manner. An attitude of respect for self and others, adherence to the concepts of privilege and confidentiality in communicating with patients, and a commitment to the patient's welfare are essential attributes of the graduate PA.

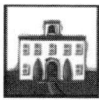

Employment Characteristics

The 2006 Physician Assistant Census, published by the American Academy of Physician Assistants, indicates that of the more than 63,600 practicing physician assistants, about 36% are practicing in primary care. Family practice is the most common specialty for physician assistants (27%), followed by surgery and surgical subspecialties, emergency medicine, subspecialties of internal medicine, general internal medicine, and dermatology.

The majority of physician assistants practice in ambulatory care settings. Solo and group practices employ 57% of all physician assistants. The number of physician assistants employed by hospitals is 22%, owing in part to the number of physician assistants working as house staff. The government employs almost 10% of the physician assistant workforce, primarily in the military and the Department of Veterans Affairs. The remaining members of the profession are practicing in community health centers, managed care organizations, freestanding urgent care centers, correctional facilities, and other settings.

Physician assistants work an average of 44.3 hours per week. The number of patient visits for physician assistants in outpatient settings averages 94.6 per week; in inpatient settings the average is 63.7 patient visits per week. Forty percent of physician assistants have on-call responsibilities that average 94 hours per month.

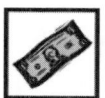

Salary

AAPA data indicated that the average PA salary in 2006 was $84,396. Salaries vary depending on the experience of the individual, the practice specialty, job responsibilities, and the regional cost of living. Refer to Section IV, Table 5 of this *Directory* for more information, or see www.ama-assn.org/ go/hpsalary.

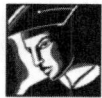

Educational Programs

Length. Although 25 to 27 months is most common, the length of programs varies, largely owing to a difference in student selection criteria and in the educational objectives of the individual program. Most PA programs award a master's degree upon completion.

Prerequisites. Although requirements differ widely, a majority of programs require 2 years of undergraduate study and some work experience in health care. A balance of study in the applied behavioral sciences and the biological sciences is advised for students who wish to qualify for admission to a physician assistant program. Students entering PA programs generally hold a bachelor's degree.

Curriculum. Accreditation standards require competency-based curricula. The professional curriculum for PA education includes basic medical, behavioral, and social sciences; clinical preparatory sciences, patient assessment, and supervised clinical practice; health policy; and professional practice issues. Four-year programs are designed to provide the student with a balance of traditional liberal arts courses and biological and applied behavioral science courses. These courses are prerequisites to clinical didactic and supervised clinical practice instruction common to both 2-year and 4-year programs. Supervised clinical practice rotations in pediatrics, family medicine, general internal medicine, prenatal care and women's health, geriatrics, emergency medicine, psychiatry/behavioral medicine, and general surgery offer advanced applied content and supervised clinical work experience in dealing with commonly encountered demands for the primary health care of individuals from infancy through childhood, adolescence, and the various phases of adulthood. These experiences are provided in outpatient, emergency, inpatient, and long-term care clinical settings.

Licensure

All 50 states, the District of Columbia, and the majority of US territories have enacted laws regulating the practice of physician assistants. In order to practice as a physician assistant, an individual must meet the state's licensing criteria and have a supervising physician. All 50 states and the District of Columbia allow physicians to delegate prescriptive authority to the PAs they supervise.

Inquiries

Careers
American Academy of Physician Assistants
950 N Washington Street
Alexandria, VA 22314
703 836-2272
703 684-1924 Fax
E-mail: aapa@aapa.org
www.aapa.org

Physician Assistant Education Association
300 North Washington Street, Suite 505
Alexandria, VA 22314-2544
703 548-5538
703 548-5539 Fax
E-mail: info@PAEAonline.org
www.paeaonline.org

National Certification
National Commission on Certification of Physician Assistants
12000 Findley Road, Suite 200
Duluth, GA 30097
678 417-8100
www.nccpa.net

Program Accreditation
Accreditation Review Commission on Education for the Physician Assistant (ARC-PA)
John McCarty, Executive Director
12000 Findley Road, Suite 240
Duluth, GA 30097
770 476-1224
770 476-1738 Fax
Email: arc-pa@arc-pa.org
www.arc-pa.org

Physician Assistant

Alabama

University of Alabama at Birmingham
Surgical Physician Assistant Prgm
Sch of Health Professions
1705 University Blvd, RMSB 481
Birmingham, AL 35294-1212
www.uab.edu
Prgm Dir: Herbert Ridings, MA PA-C
Tel: 205 996-2911   *Fax:* 205 934-3780
E-mail: hridings@uab.edu

University of South Alabama
Physician Assistant Prgm
Dept of Physician Asst Studies
1504 Springhill Ave, Ste 4410
Mobile, AL 36604-3273
www.southalabama.edu/alliedhealth/pa
Prgm Dir: Cheryl Vrettos, PA-C MHS
Tel: 251 434-3641   *Fax:* 251 434-3646
E-mail: pastudies@usouthal.edu

Arizona

Midwestern University - Glendale Campus
Physician Assistant Prgm
19555 N 59th Ave
Glendale, AZ 85308
www.midwestern.edu
Prgm Dir: Kevin Lohenry, MPAS PA-C
Tel: 623 572-3311   *Fax:* 623 572-3227
E-mail: klohen@midwestern.edu

AT Still University of Health Sciences
Physician Assistant Prgm
5850 E Still Circle
Mesa, AZ 85206
Prgm Dir: Albert F Simon, DHSc PA-C
Tel: 480 219-6040   *Fax:* 480 219-6100
E-mail: afsimon@atsu.edu

Arkansas

Harding University
Physician Assistant Prgm
915 E Market Ave
HU 12231
Searcy, AR 72149-2231
www.harding.edu/paprogram
Prgm Dir: Michael Murphy, MD
Tel: 501 279-5642   *Fax:* 501 268-2111
E-mail: paprogram@harding.edu

California

University of Southern California
Physician Assistant Prgm
1000 S Fremont Ave, Unit 7
Bldg A6, 4th Fl
Alhambra, CA 91803
Prgm Dir: Rosslynn Byous, PA-C DPA
Tel: 626 457-4262   *Fax:* 626 457-4262
E-mail: byous@usc.edu

Loma Linda University
Physician Assistant Prgm
Nichol Hall, Rm 2033
Loma Linda, CA 92350
Prgm Dir: Kenrick Bourne, DrPH PA-C
Tel: 909 558-1000, Ext 87289   *Fax:* 909 558-0495
E-mail: kbourne@llu.edu

Charles R Drew Univ of Med & Science
Physician Assistant Prgm
1731 E 120th St
Los Angeles, CA 90059
Prgm Dir: Sunil Singhania, DO
Tel: 323 563-5950   *Fax:* 323 563-4833
E-mail: singhania_sunil@hotmail.com

Riverside County Regional Medical Center
Cosponsor: Riverside Community College
Physician Assistant Prgm
Moreno Valley Campus
16130 Lasselle St
Moreno Valley, CA 92551-2045
Prgm Dir: Delores Middleton, MSEd PA-C
Tel: 951 571-6118   *Fax:* 951 571-6221
E-mail: delores.middleton@rcc.edu

Samuel Merritt College
Physician Assistant Prgm
450 30th St, 4th Fl, Rm 4708
Oakland, CA 94609
Prgm Dir: Lorraine Petti, MS PA-C
Tel: 510 869-6623   *Fax:* 510 869-6951
E-mail: Lpetti@samuelmerritt.edu

Stanford University School of Medicine
Physician Assistant Prgm
Primary Care Associate Prgm
1215 Welch Rd, Ste Modular G
Palo Alto, CA 94305
Prgm Dir: Sherry Stolberg, MGPGP PA-C
Tel: 650 725-5340   *Fax:* 650 723-9692
E-mail: stolberg@stanford.edu

Western Univ of Health Sciences
Physician Assistant Prgm
Primary Care PA Program
309 E Second St
Pomona, CA 91766-1854
www.westernu.edu
Prgm Dir: Roy Guizado, MS PA-C
Tel: 909 469-5378   *Fax:* 909 469-5407
E-mail: roygpac@westernu.edu

University of California - Davis
Physician Assistant Prgm
2516 Stockton Blvd, Ste 254
Sacramento, CA 95817-2297
www.ucdmc.ucdavis.edu/fnppa/
Prgm Dir: Shelly Stewart
Tel: 916 734-3551   *Fax:* 916 452-2112
E-mail: shelly.stewart@ucdmc.ucdavis.edu

Touro University Mare Island
Physician Assistant Prgm
1310 Johnson Ln
Vallejo, CA 94592
Prgm Dir: Lauren Padilla
Tel: 707 638-5978   *Fax:* 707 638-5955
E-mail: lpadilla@touro.edu

San Joaquin Valley College - Visalia
Physician Assistant Prgm
8400 W Mineral King
Visalia, CA 93291
Prgm Dir: Leslie W Howard, BS PA
Tel: 559 651-2500   *Fax:* 559 651-3161
E-mail: lesh@sjvc.edu

Colorado

U of Colorado (Denver) Health Sciences Center
Physician Assistant Prgm
Child Hlth Associate, PA Program
Mail Stop F543, PO Box 6508
Aurora, CO 80045
www.uchsc.edu/chapa
Prgm Dir: Anita Duhl Glicken, MSW
Tel: 303 724-1338   *Fax:* 303 724-1350
E-mail: anita.glicken@uchsc.edu

Red Rocks Community College
Physician Assistant Prgm
Campus Box 38
13300 W Sixth Ave
Lakewood, CO 80228
Prgm Dir: Jim Keller, MPH PA-C
Tel: 303 914-6287   *Fax:* 303 914-6806
E-mail: jim.keller@rrcc.edu

Connecticut

Quinnipiac University
Physician Assistant Prgm
275 Mt Carmel Ave
Hamden, CT 06518-1908
www.quinnipiac.edu/x1040.xml
Prgm Dir: Cynthia Booth-Lord, MHS PA-C
Tel: 203 582-5297 *Fax:* 203 582-5303
E-mail: Cynthia.Lord@quinnipiac.edu

Yale University School of Medicine
Physician Assistant Prgm
47 College St Ste 220
New Haven, CT 06510-3209
www.paprogram.yale.edu
Prgm Dir: Mary Warner, MMSc PA-C
Tel: 203 785-2860 *Fax:* 203 785-3601
E-mail: mary.warner@yale.edu

District of Columbia

George Washington University
Physician Assistant Prgm
900 23rd St NW, Ste 6148
Washington, DC 20037
Prgm Dir: James Cawley, MPH PA-C
Tel: 202 994-6670 *Fax:* 202 994-7647
E-mail: purljfc@aol.com

Howard University
Physician Assistant Prgm
6th and Bryant Sts NW
Washington, DC 20059
Prgm Dir: Shelly LS Powers, MA PA-C
Tel: 202 806-7536, Ext 5955 *Fax:* 202 806-4476
E-mail: spowers@howard.edu

Florida

Nova Southeastern University - Ft Lauderdale
Physician Assistant Prgm
3200 S University Dr
Fort Lauderdale, FL 33328
www.nova.edu/pa
Prgm Dir: William H Marquardt, MA PA-C
Tel: 954 262-1252 *Fax:* 954 262-2285
E-mail: marquard@nova.edu

University of Florida
Physician Assistant Prgm
College of Medicine
PO Box 100176
Gainesville, FL 32610-0176
www.med.ufl.edu/pap/apply
Prgm Dir: Wayne D Bottom, PA-C MPH
Tel: 352 265-7955 *Fax:* 352 265-7996
E-mail: wayne.bottom@medicine.ufl.edu

Miami Dade College
Physician Assistant Prgm
950 NW 20th St
Miami, FL 33127-4693
Prgm Dir: Pete A Gutierrez, MD MMS PA-C
Tel: 305 237-4261 *Fax:* 305 237-4278
E-mail: pgutier2@mdc.edu

Barry University
Physician Assistant Prgm
11300 NE 2nd Ave, Box SGMS-PA
Miami Shores, FL 33161-6695
www.barry.edu
Prgm Dir: Doreen C Parkhurst, MD
Tel: 305 899-4065, Ext 4065 *Fax:* 305 899-4083
E-mail: dparkhurst@mail.barry.edu

Nova Southeastern University - Naples
Physician Assistant Prgm
2655 Northbrooke Dr
Naples, FL 33328
Prgm Dir: Julie B Keena, MMSc PA-C
Tel: 239 591-4528, Ext 10 *Fax:* 239 495-5925
E-mail: jkeena@nsu.nova.edu

Nova Southeastern University - Orlando
Physician Assistant Prgm
4850 Millenia Blvd
Orlando, FL 32839
Prgm Dir: J Dyda, Jr, PA-C DHSc
Tel: 407 264-5151 *Fax:* 407 264-5140
E-mail: dyda@nsu.nova.edu

Georgia

Emory University
Physician Assistant Prgm
School of Medicine
1462 Clifton Rd, Ste 280
Atlanta, GA 30322
www.emorypa.org
Prgm Dir: Dana Sayre-Stanhope, PA-C
Tel: 404 727-7857 *Fax:* 404 727-7836
E-mail: dsayres@emory.edu

Mercer University
Physician Assistant Prgm
3001 Mercer University Dr
Atlanta, GA 30341
Prgm Dir: Bradford W Schwarz, MS PA-C
Tel: 678 547-6085 *Fax:* 678 547-6384
E-mail: Schwarz_BW@Mercer.edu

Medical College of Georgia
Physician Assistant Prgm
Health Sciences Building, Rm EC-3304
987 St Sebastian Way
Augusta, GA 30912
Prgm Dir: Bonnie A Dadig, EdD PA-C
Tel: 706 721-3246 *Fax:* 706 721-3990
E-mail: bdadig@mcg.edu

South University
Physician Assistant Prgm
709 Mall Blvd
Savannah, GA 31406
Prgm Dir: Robert J Philpot, PhD PA-C
Tel: 912 201-8024 *Fax:* 912 201-8070
E-mail: rphilpot@southuniversity.edu

Idaho

Idaho State University
Physician Assistant Prgm
921 S 8th Ave, Stop 8253
1021 S Red Hill Rd
Pocatello, ID 83209-8253
www.isu.edu/paprog
Prgm Dir: John Schroeder, PA-C JD
Tel: 208 282-4726 *Fax:* 208 282-4969
E-mail: schrjohn@isu.edu

Illinois

Southern Illinois University Carbondale
Physician Assistant Prgm
School of Allied Health and School of Medicine
Lindegren Hall Rm 129 MC 6516
Carbondale, IL 62901-6516
http://mccoy.lib.siu.edu/~paprogram/
Prgm Dir: Laurie Dunn-Ryznyk, MPAS PA-C
Tel: 618 453-8850 *Fax:* 618 453-7216
E-mail: ldunn@siumed.edu

Malcolm X College
Physician Assistant Prgm
1900 W Van Buren St, Rm 3241
Chicago, IL 60612-3197
Prgm Dir: Kathy Rayford
Tel: 312 850-3532 *Fax:* 312 850-3536
E-mail: krayford@ccc.edu

Midwestern University
Physician Assistant Prgm
555 31st St
Downers Grove, IL 60515-1235
www.midwestern.edu
Prgm Dir: Alyson Smith, MS PA-C
Tel: 630 515-6034 *Fax:* 630 971-6402
E-mail: asmith@midwestern.edu

Rosalind Franklin Univ of Medicine & Science
Physician Assistant Prgm
3333 Green Bay Rd
North Chicago, IL 60064-3095
Prgm Dir: Patrick Knott, PhD PA-C
Tel: 847 578-8689 *Fax:* 847 578-8690
E-mail: Patrick.Knott@RosalindFranklin.edu

Indiana

University of Saint Francis
Physician Assistant Prgm
Department of Physician Assistant Studies
2701 Spring St
Fort Wayne, IN 46808
Prgm Dir: Dawn LaBarbera, PhD PA-C
Tel: 260 399-8559 *Fax:* 260 434-7773
E-mail: dlabarbera@sf.edu

Butler University/Clarian Health
Physician Assistant Prgm
College of Pharm and Hlth Sci
4600 Sunset Ave
Indianapolis, IN 46208-3485
www.butler.edu/cophs/?pg=2077&parentID=2041
Prgm Dir: John A Lucich, MD
Tel: 317 940-6147 *Fax:* 317 940-6172
E-mail: jlucich@butler.edu

Iowa

Des Moines University
Physician Assistant Prgm
3200 Grand Ave
Des Moines, IA 50312-4198
www.dmu.edu
Prgm Dir: Jolene R Kelly, MPAS PA-C
Tel: 515 271-1685 *Fax:* 515 271-7176
E-mail: Jolene.Kelly@dmu.edu

University of Iowa
Physician Assistant Prgm
Roy J and Lucille A Carver College of Medicine
5167 Westlawn
Iowa City, IA 52242-1100
www.medicine.uiowa.edu/pa/
Prgm Dir: David P Asprey, PhD PA-C
Tel: 319 335-8920 *Fax:* 319 335-8923
E-mail: david-asprey@uiowa.edu

Kansas

Wichita State University
Physician Assistant Prgm
Campus Box 43
1845 N Fairmount
Wichita, KS 67260-0043
http://chp.wichita.edu/pa
Prgm Dir: Richard Muma, PhD MPH
Tel: 316 978-3011 *Fax:* 316 978-3025
E-mail: richard.muma@wichita.edu

Kentucky

University of Kentucky
Physician Assistant Prgm
Dept of Clinical Sciences
900 S Limestone St, Ste 205
Lexington, KY 40536-0200
Prgm Dir: Doris Rapp, PharmD PA-C
Tel: 859 323-1100, Ext 80514   *Fax:* 859 257-2454
E-mail: darapp1@email.uky.edu

Louisiana

Our Lady of the Lake College
Physician Assistant Prgm
7443 Picardy Ave
Baton Rouge, LA 70808
Prgm Dir: Elaine E Grant, PA-C MPH
Tel: 225 214-6988   *Fax:* 225 490-1650
E-mail: egrant@ololcollege.edu

Louisiana State U Hlth Sci Ctr - Shreveport
Physician Assistant Prgm
1501 Kings Hwy, PO Box 33932
Shreveport, LA 71130-3932
www.sh.lsuhsc.edu/ah/
Prgm Dir: Kim Meyer, MPAS PA-C
Tel: 318 675-7744   *Fax:* 318 675-6937
E-mail: kmeyer1@LSUHSC.edu

Maine

University of New England
Physician Assistant Prgm
716 Stevens Ave
Portland, ME 04103-2670
www.une.edu/chp/pa
Prgm Dir: Erich Fogg, PA-C MMSc
Tel: 207 221-4529   *Fax:* 207 221-4711
E-mail: EFogg@une.edu

Maryland

Anne Arundel Community College
Physician Assistant Prgm
101 College Pkwy
Arnold, MD 21012-1895
www.aacc.edu/physassist
Prgm Dir: Mary Jo Bondy, MHS PA-C
Tel: 410 777-7392   *Fax:* 410 777-7099
E-mail: mjbondy@aacc.edu

Towson University
Cosponsor: CCBC Essex
Physician Assistant Prgm
7201 Rossville Blvd
Baltimore, MD 21237-3855
Prgm Dir: Donna Sewell, MS PA-C
Tel: 410 780-6616   *Fax:* 410 780-6405
E-mail: dsewell@ccbcmd.edu

University of Maryland Eastern Shore
Physician Assistant Prgm
Modular 934-5 Backbone Rd
Princess Anne, MD 21853
Prgm Dir: Darlene Jackson-Bowen, MPAS PA-C
Tel: 410 651-8932   *Fax:* 410 651-7586
E-mail: dljackson-bowen@umes.edu

Massachusetts

Mass College of Pharmacy & Health Sciences
Physician Assistant Prgm
179 Longwood Ave
Boston, MA 02115
Prgm Dir: Gloria Stewart, EdD PA-C ATC
Tel: 617 735-1576   *Fax:* 617 732-1027
E-mail: gloria.stewart@mcphs.edu

Northeastern University
Physician Assistant Prgm
360 Huntington Ave, 202 Robinson
Boston, MA 02115-5000
www.bouve.neu.edu/Graduate/Health/pap.html
Prgm Dir: Rosann M Ippolito, PhD
Tel: 617 373-3195   *Fax:* 617 373-3338
E-mail: r.ippolito@neu.edu

Springfield College
Physician Assistant Prgm
263 Alden St
Springfield, MA 01109-3797
Prgm Dir: Jennifer Hixon, MS PA-C
Tel: 413 748-3554   *Fax:* 413 748-3595
E-mail: jhixon@spfldcol.edu

Michigan

University of Detroit Mercy
Physician Assistant Prgm
4001 West McNichols Rd
Detroit, MI 48221
http://healthprofessions.udmercy.edu/paprogram
Prgm Dir: Suzanne York, MPH PA-C
Tel: 313 993-1930   *Fax:* 313 993-1271
E-mail: warnimsk@udmercy.edu

Wayne State University
Physician Assistant Prgm
College of Pharmacy and Health Sciences
259 Mack Ave, Ste 2590
Detroit, MI 48201
Prgm Dir: Stephanie Joseph Gilkey, MS PA-C
Tel: 313 577-1368   *Fax:* 313 577-5467

Grand Valley State University
Physician Assistant Prgm
Center for Health Sciences
301 Michigan St NE, Ste 200
Grand Rapids, MI 49503
www.gvsu.edu/pa
Prgm Dir: Wallace Boeve, EdD PA-C
Tel: 616 331-5988   *Fax:* 616 331-5999
E-mail: boevew@gvsu.edu

Western Michigan University
Physician Assistant Prgm
1903 W Michigan Ave
Kalamazoo, MI 49008-5138
www.wmich.edu/hhs/pa
Prgm Dir: Eric Vangsnes, PhD PA-C
Tel: 269 387-5315   *Fax:* 269 387-3319
E-mail: eric.vangsnes@wmich.edu

Central Michigan University
Physician Assistant Prgm
HPB 1222
Mount Pleasant, MI 48859
Prgm Dir: Ahmad Hakemi, MD
Tel: 989 774-1273   *Fax:* 989 774-2433
E-mail: hakem1a@cmich.edu

Minnesota

Augsburg College
Physician Assistant Prgm
2211 Riverside Ave, CB 149
Minneapolis, MN 55454
Prgm Dir: Dawn B Ludwig, PhD PA-C
Tel: 612 330-1399   *Fax:* 612 330-1757
E-mail: ludwig@augsburg.edu

Missouri

Missouri State University
Physician Assistant Prgm
901 S National Ave
Springfield, MO 65897
Prgm Dir: Steve Dodge, MD
Tel: 417 836-6151   *Fax:* 417 836-6406
E-mail: stevedodge@missouristate.edu

Saint Louis University Doisy College of Health Sciences
Physician Assistant Prgm
3437 Caroline St
3025 Doisy College of Health Sciences
St Louis, MO 63104
www.slu.edu/x6078.xml
Prgm Dir: Anne C Hart Garazini, MEd PA-C
Tel: 314 977-8521   *Fax:* 314 977-8649
E-mail: paprog@slu.edu

Montana

Rocky Mountain College
Physician Assistant Prgm
1511 Poly Dr
Billings, MT 59102-1796
pa.rocky.edu
Prgm Dir: Joseph Tritchler, PA-C MS MT(ASCP)SBB
Tel: 406 657-1191   *Fax:* 406 657-1194
E-mail: tritchlj@rocky.edu

Nebraska

Union College
Physician Assistant Prgm
3800 S 48th St
Lincoln, NE 68506
Prgm Dir: Michael J Huckabee, MPAS PA-C
Tel: 402 486-2527   *Fax:* 402 486-2559
E-mail: mihuckab@ucollege.edu

University of Nebraska Medical Center
Physician Assistant Prgm
984300 Nebraska Medical Center
Omaha, NE 68198-4300
www.unmc.edu/alliedhealth/pa
Prgm Dir: James E Somers, PhD PA
Tel: 402 559-9495   *Fax:* 402 559-7996
E-mail: dklandon@unmc.edu

Nevada

Touro University - Nevada
Physician Assistant Prgm
874 American Pacific Dr
Henderson, NV 89014
Prgm Dir: Vicki Chan-Padgett, PA-C MPAS
Tel: 702 856-3262   *Fax:* 702 856-3346
E-mail: dculmone@touro.edu

New Hampshire

Mass College of Pharmacy & Health Sciences
Physician Assistant Prgm
1260 Elm St
Manchester, NH 03101
Prgm Dir: Scott L Massey, PhD PA-C
Tel: 603 314-1708   *Fax:* 603 314-0303
E-mail: scott.massey@mcphs.edu

New Jersey

Univ of Medicine & Dent of New Jersey
Physician Assistant Prgm
Robert Wood Johnson Med Sch
675 Hoes Ln
Piscataway, NJ 08854-5635
www.shrp.umdnj.edu/programs/paweb
Prgm Dir: Ruth Fixelle, EdM PA-C
Tel: 732 235-4445 *Fax:* 732 235-4820
E-mail: r.fixelle@umdnj.edu

Seton Hall University
Physician Assistant Prgm
400 S Orange Ave
South Orange, NJ 07079
Prgm Dir: Carol Biscardi, PA-C MS
Tel: 973 275-2027 *Fax:* 973 275-2370
E-mail: biscarca@shu.edu

New Mexico

University of New Mexico
Physician Assistant Prgm
School of Medicine
Dept of Family and Community Medicine MSC 09 5040
Albuquerque, NM 87131-0001
http://hsc.unm.edu/som/fcm/pap/
Prgm Dir: Nikki Katalanos, PhD PA-C
Tel: 505 272-9864 *Fax:* 505 272-9828
E-mail: nkatalanos@salud.unm.edu

University of St Francis
Physician Assistant Prgm
4401 Silver Ave SE, Ste B
Albuquerque, NM 87108
Prgm Dir: William Riesterer, PA-C MPAS
Tel: 505 266-5565 *Fax:* 505 266-5585
E-mail: wriesterer@stfrancis.edu

New York

Albany Medical College
Physician Assistant Prgm
Albany Medical College Mail Code 4
47 New Scotland Ave
Albany, NY 12208-3412
www.amc.edu/pa
Prgm Dir: David Irvine, DHSc RPA-C
Tel: 518 262-5251 *Fax:* 518 262-6698
E-mail: irvined@mail.amc.edu

Daemen College
Physician Assistant Prgm
4380 Main St
Amherst, NY 14226-3592
Prgm Dir: Gregg Shutts, MS RPA-C
Tel: 716 839-8563 *Fax:* 716 839-8252
E-mail: gshutts@daemen.edu

Touro College - Bay Shore
Physician Assistant Prgm
Bay Shore PA Prgm, Winthrop University
    Hospital Ext Ctr
1700 Union Blvd
Bay Shore, NY 11706
www.touro.edu
Prgm Dir: Joseph Tommasino, PhD RPAC
Tel: 631 665-1600, Ext 271 *Fax:* 631 665-6086
E-mail: jtpaphd@aol.com

Mercy College
Physician Assistant Prgm
Graduate Program in Physician Assistant Studies
1200 Waters Place
Bronx, NY 10461
Prgm Dir: Theresa Horvath, MPH PA-C
Tel: 914 674-7626 *Fax:* 718 678-8605
E-mail: thorvath@mercy.edu

Long Island University
Physician Assistant Prgm
Division of Physician Assistant Studies
Long Island University
Brooklyn, NY 11201
www.brooklyn.liu.edu/health/bsphyass.html
Prgm Dir: Elizabeth Salzer, RPA-C MA
Tel: 718 488-1505 *Fax:* 718 246-6364
E-mail: elizabeth.salzer@liu.edu

SUNY Downstate Medical Center
Physician Assistant Prgm
450 Clarkson Ave, PO Box 1222
Brooklyn, NY 11203
Prgm Dir: Rena Mitchell, MS CHES RPA-C
Tel: 718 270-2324 *Fax:* 718 270-7459
E-mail: rena.mitchell@downstate.edu

D'Youville College
Physician Assistant Prgm
320 Porter Ave
Buffalo, NY 14201-1084
www.dyc.edu
Prgm Dir: Maureen F Finney, RPA-C MS
Tel: 716 829-7713 *Fax:* 716 829-7732
E-mail: finneym@dyc.edu

St John's University
Physician Assistant Prgm
175-05 Horace Harding Expressway
Fresh Meadows, NY 11365
Prgm Dir: Niels Schmidt, PA-C
Tel: 718 990-8417 *Fax:* 718 357-4588
E-mail: schmidtn@stjohns.edu

Hofstra University
Physician Assistant Prgm
113 Monroe Lecture Center
Hempstead, NY 11549-1270
Prgm Dir: Anne M Bozzarelli, PA-C MHS
Tel: 516 463-4804 *Fax:* 516 463-5177
E-mail: Anne.M.Bozzarelli@hofstra.edu

CUNY York College
Physician Assistant Prgm
94-20 Guy R Brewer Blvd, Rm 1E12
Jamaica, NY 11451
Prgm Dir: Robert Brugna, MBA PA-C
Tel: 718 262-2823 *Fax:* 718 262-2504
E-mail: rabrugna@york.cuny.edu

City University of New York, The City College
Cosponsor: The Sophie Davis School of Biomedical
    Education
Physician Assistant Prgm
138th St and Convent Ave, Harris Hall, Ste 15
New York, NY 10031
Prgm Dir: Adrian Llewellyn, RPA-C MPAS
Tel: 212 650-7745, Ext 7745 *Fax:* 212 650-6697
E-mail: allewellyn@ccny.cuny.edu

Pace University - Lenox Hill Hospital
Physician Assistant Prgm
1 Pace Plaza, Rm Y-31
New York, NY 10038-1598
www.pace.edu/dyson/paprogram
Prgm Dir: Kathleen T Roche, RPA-C RN FNP MPA
Tel: 212 346-1241 *Fax:* 212 346-1503
E-mail: kroche@pace.edu

Touro College
Physician Assistant Prgm
Manhattan PA Program
27-33 W 23rd St
New York, NY 10010
www.touro.edu/shs/pany
Prgm Dir: Nadja Graff, PhD
Tel: 212 463-0400, Ext 788 *Fax:* 212 741-0195
E-mail: ngraff@touro.edu

Weill Med College/Cornell Univ Med Sch
Physician Assistant Prgm
575 Lexington Ave
New York, NY 10022
Prgm Dir: Gerard J Marciano, PA-C MS
Tel: 646 962-7277 *Fax:* 646 962-7290
E-mail: gjm2001@med.cornell.edu

New York Institute of Technology
Physician Assistant Prgm
NYCOM II, Rm 352
Northern Blvd , PO Box 8000
Old Westbury, NY 11568-8000
http://iris.nyit.edu/hpbls/pas
Prgm Dir: Salvatore Barese, EdD PA-C
Tel: 516 686-3881 *Fax:* 516 686-3795
E-mail: pa@nyit.edu

Rochester Institute of Technology
Physician Assistant Prgm
153 Lomb Memorial Dr
Bldg 75, CBET
Rochester, NY 14623
www.rit.edu/~676www/main_pa.html
Prgm Dir: Heidi B Miller, MPH PA-C
Tel: 585 475-5945 *Fax:* 585 475-5809
E-mail: hbmscl@rit.edu

Wagner College/Staten Island University
Physician Assistant Prgm
Concord Site
1034 Targee St, Spring Bldg
Staten Island, NY 10304
Prgm Dir: Nora Lowy, PA-C
Tel: 718 390-4610 *Fax:* 718 390-4662
E-mail: nlowy@siuh.edu

Stony Brook University
Physician Assistant Prgm
SHTM-HSC, L2-424
Stony Brook, NY 11794-8202
www.hsc.stonybrook.edu/shtm/
Prgm Dir: Paul Lombardo, MPS RPAC
Tel: 631 444-3190 *Fax:* 631 444-1404
E-mail: paul.lombardo@stonybrook.edu

Le Moyne College
Physician Assistant Prgm
1416 Salt Springs Rd
Syracuse, NY 13214-1399
Prgm Dir: Linda G Allison, MD MPH
Tel: 315 445-4745 *Fax:* 315 445-4602
E-mail: allisolg@lemoyne.edu

North Carolina

Duke University Medical Center
Physician Assistant Prgm
Department of Community and Family Medicine
DUMC 3848
Durham, NC 27710-0001
http://pa.mc.duke.edu
Prgm Dir: Patricia Dieter, MPA PA-C
Tel: 919 681-3259 *Fax:* 919 681-9666
E-mail: patricia.dieter@duke.edu

Methodist University
Physician Assistant Prgm
5105 B College Center Dr
5107 College Center Dr
Fayetteville, NC 28311-1498
www.methodist.edu/paprogram
Prgm Dir: E Ronald Foster, MA MPAS PAC
Tel: 910 630-7495 *Fax:* 910 630-7218
E-mail: fosterr@methodist.edu

East Carolina University
Physician Assistant Prgm
College of Allied Health Sciences
Dept of Physician Assistant Studies
Greenville, NC 27834-4353
www.ecu.edu/pa
Prgm Dir: Larry Dennis, MPAS PA-C
Tel: 252 744-1100   *Fax:* 252 744-1110
E-mail: dennisl@ecu.edu

Wake Forest University School of Medicine
Physician Assistant Prgm
Medical Center Blvd
Winston-Salem, NC 27157-1006
www.wfubmc.edu/paprogram
Prgm Dir: James Van Rhee, MS PA-C
Tel: 336 716-2905   *Fax:* 336 716-4432
E-mail: jvanrhee@wfubmc.edu

North Dakota

University of North Dakota
Physician Assistant Prgm
School of Medicine and Health Sciences, Rm 4128
Family & Community Medicine
Grand Forks, ND 58202-9037
www.med.und.nodak.edu/depts/pa/
Prgm Dir: Mary Ann Laxen, MAB PA-C
Tel: 701 777-2344   *Fax:* 701 777-2491
E-mail: mlaxen@medicine.nodak.edu

Ohio

University of Findlay
Physician Assistant Prgm
1000 N Main St
Findlay, OH 45840
Prgm Dir: Cynthia Pentz
Tel: 419 434-6983   *Fax:* 419 434-6557
E-mail: pentz@findlay.edu

Kettering College of Medical Arts
Physician Assistant Prgm
3737 Southern Blvd
Kettering, OH 45429
www.kcma.edu
Prgm Dir: Susan Wulff, MS PA-C
Tel: 937 298-3399, Ext 55625   *Fax:* 937 395-8095
E-mail: sue.wulff@kcma.edu

Marietta College
Physician Assistant Prgm
215 Fifth St
Marietta, OH 45750
Prgm Dir: Peter Hogan, PhD
Tel: 740 376-4950   *Fax:* 740 376-4951
E-mail: hoganp@marietta.edu

Cuyahoga Community College
Cosponsor: Cleveland State University
Physician Assistant Prgm
11000 Pleasant Valley Rd
Parma, OH 44130
www.tri-c.edu/pa
Prgm Dir: Sharon Luke, MSHS PA-C
Tel: 216 987-5123   *Fax:* 216 987-5066
E-mail: sharon.luke@tri-c.edu

University of Toledo
Physician Assistant Prgm
3015 Arlington Ave
Toledo, OH 43614
www.utoledo.edu
Prgm Dir: Patricia Hogue, MS PA-C
Tel: 419 383-5408   *Fax:* 419 383-5880
E-mail: patricia.hogue@utoledo.edu

Oklahoma

Univ of Oklahoma Health Sciences Center
Physician Assistant Prgm
PO Box 26901
Oklahoma City, OK 73190
Prgm Dir: Dan McNeill, PhD PA
Tel: 405 271-2058   *Fax:* 405 271-3621
E-mail: daniel-mcneill@ouhsc.edu

University of Oklahoma - Tulsa
Physician Assistant Prgm
4502 E 41st St
Tulsa, OK 74135-2512
Prgm Dir: Steven Meixel, MD

Oregon

Pacific University
Physician Assistant Prgm
222 SE 8th Ave, Ste 551
Hillsboro, OR 97123
www.pacificu.edu/pa/
Prgm Dir: Randy Randolph, PA-C MPAS
Tel: 503 352-7299   *Fax:* 503 352-7280
E-mail: randolph@pacificu.edu

Oregon Health & Science University
Physician Assistant Prgm
3181 SW Sam Jackson Park Rd, GH 219
Portland, OR 97239-3098
www.ohsu.edu/pa
Prgm Dir: Ted J Ruback, MS PA-C
Tel: 503 494-1484   *Fax:* 503 494-1409
E-mail: paprgm@ohsu.edu

Pennsylvania

DeSales University
Physician Assistant Prgm
2755 Station Ave
Center Valley, PA 18034-9568
Prgm Dir: Christine Bruce, MHSA PA-C
Tel: 610 282-1100, Ext 1415   *Fax:* 610 282-1893
E-mail: Christine.Bruce@desales.edu

Pennsylvania College of Optometry
Physician Assistant Prgm
8360 Old York Rd
Elkins Park, PA 19027
Prgm Dir: George S Bottomley, DVM PA-C
E-mail: gbottomley@pco.edu

Gannon University
Physician Assistant Prgm
109 University Square
Erie, PA 16541-0001
Prgm Dir: Michele Roth-Kauffman, JD MPAS PA-C
Tel: 814 871-5643   *Fax:* 814 871-5502
E-mail: roth-kauffman@gannon.edu

Arcadia University
Physician Assistant Prgm
450 S Easton Rd
Glenside, PA 19038
Prgm Dir: Michael Dryer, MPH PA-C
Tel: 215 572-2083   *Fax:* 215 881-8746
E-mail: dryer@arcadia.edu

Seton Hill University
Physician Assistant Prgm
Seton Hill Dr
Greensburg, PA 15601
Prgm Dir: Cathy Shallenberger, MS PA-C
Tel: 724 830-1097   *Fax:* 724 838-7846
E-mail: shallenberger@setonhill.edu

Lock Haven University
Physician Assistant Prgm
401 N Fairview St
104 Annex Building
Lock Haven, PA 17745
www.lhup.edu
Prgm Dir: Walter Eisenhauer, MEd MMSc PA-C
Tel: 570 484-2168   *Fax:* 570 484-2540
E-mail: weisenha@lhup.edu

St Francis University
Physician Assistant Prgm
Sullivan Hall Rm 104
PO Box 600
Loretto, PA 15940-0600
www.francis.edu/PhysAsst/PAHome.shtml
Prgm Dir: Donna Yeisley, MEd PA-C
Tel: 814 472-3130   *Fax:* 814 472-3137
E-mail: pa@francis.edu

Drexel University
Physician Assistant Prgm
245 N 15th St, MS 504
Philadelphia, PA 19102
Prgm Dir: Patrick C Auth, PhD MS PA-C
Tel: 215 762-1432   *Fax:* 215 762-1164
E-mail: pa27@drexel.edu

Philadelphia College of Osteopathic Medicine
Physician Assistant Prgm
4190 City Ave
Rowland Hall
Philadelphia, PA 19131
Prgm Dir: John Cavenagh, PhD PA-C
Tel: 215 871-6772   *Fax:* 215 871-6702
E-mail: johnca@pcom.edu

Philadelphia University
Physician Assistant Prgm
School of Science and Health
School House Ln and Henry Ave
Philadelphia, PA 19144-5497
Prgm Dir: Michael Rackover, PA-C MS
Tel: 215 951-2908   *Fax:* 215 951-2526
E-mail: rackoverm@philau.edu

Chatham University
Physician Assistant Prgm
Woodland Rd
Pittsburgh, PA 15232-2826
Prgm Dir: Luis A Ramos, MS PA-C
Tel: 412 365-1405   *Fax:* 412 365-1623
E-mail: lramos@chatham.edu

Duquesne University
Physician Assistant Prgm
Rangos Sch of Health Sciences
Health Sciences Bldg, Ste 405
Pittsburgh, PA 15282
Prgm Dir: Bridget Calhoun, MPH PA-C
Tel: 412 396-5914   *Fax:* 412 396-4118
E-mail: calhoun@duq.edu

Marywood University
Physician Assistant Prgm
2300 Adams Ave
Scranton, PA 18509
www.marywood.edu/departments/PA_Program/
   program.stm
Prgm Dir: Karen Arscott, DO MSc
Tel: 570 348-6211, Ext 2175   *Fax:* 570 348-6020
E-mail: arscott@marywood.edu

King's College
Physician Assistant Prgm
133 N River St
Wilkes-Barre, PA 18711-0851
www.kings.edu/paprog
Prgm Dir: Frances Feudale, DO FACEP
Tel: 570 208-5853, Ext 5768   *Fax:* 570 208-6018
E-mail: fafeudal@kings.edu

Pennsylvania College of Technology
Physician Assistant Prgm
One College Ave #123
Williamsport, PA 17701
Prgm Dir: Joseph Mileto, Jr, MHSc PA-C
Tel: 570 320-2400, Ext 2777   *Fax:* 570 321-5557
E-mail: jmileto@pct.edu

South Carolina

Medical University of South Carolina
Physician Assistant Prgm
PO Box 250962
151 B Rutledge Ave
Charleston, SC 29425
www.musc.edu/chp/pa
Prgm Dir: Reamer L Bushardt, PharmD RPh PA-C
Tel: 843 792-3789   *Fax:* 843 792-0506
E-mail: busharrl@musc.edu

South Dakota

University of South Dakota
Physician Assistant Prgm
414 E Clark St
Vermillion, SD 57069-2390
Prgm Dir: Wade Nilson, MPAS PA-C
Tel: 605 677-5128   *Fax:* 605 677-6569
E-mail: wnilson@usd.edu

Tennessee

South College
Physician Assistant Prgm
3904 Lonas Dr
Knoxville, TN 37909
Prgm Dir: Ken Harbert, PhD CHES PA-C

Trevecca Nazarene University
Physician Assistant Prgm
333 Murfreesboro Rd
Nashville, TN 37210-2877
Prgm Dir: G Michael Moredock, MD
Tel: 615 248-1225   *Fax:* 615 248-1622
E-mail: mmoredock@trevecca.edu

Texas

Univ of Texas Southwestern Med Ctr
Physician Assistant Prgm
5323 Harry Hines Blvd, V4.114
Dallas, TX 75390-9090
www.utsouthwestern.edu
Prgm Dir: Venetia Orcutt, PhD PA-C
Tel: 214 648-1701   *Fax:* 214 648-1003
E-mail: venetia.orcutt@utsouthwestern.edu

Univ of Texas - Pan American
Physician Assistant Prgm
1201 West University Dr
Edinburg, TX 78541
www.panam.edu/dept/pasp
Prgm Dir: Frank Ambriz, BS MPAS PA-C
Tel: 956 316-7049   *Fax:* 956 381-2438
E-mail: frankambriz@utpa.edu

Interservice
Interservice Physician Assistant Prgm
MCCS-HMP Physician Assistant Branch Rm 1202
3151 Scott Rd, Ste 1230
Fort Sam Houston, TX 78234-6138
Prgm Dir: Col William L Tozier
Tel: 210 221-8004   *Fax:* 210 221-8493

Univ of North Texas Hlth Sci Ctr at Ft Worth
Physician Assistant Prgm
3500 Camp Bowie Blvd
Fort Worth, TX 76107-2699
Prgm Dir: Henry Lemke, MMS PA-C
Tel: 817 735-2301   *Fax:* 817 735-2529
E-mail: hlemke@hsc.unt.edu

University of Texas Medical Branch
Physician Assistant Prgm
301 University Blvd
Galveston, TX 77555-1145
www.sahs.utmb.edu/pas
Prgm Dir: Richard R Rahr, EdD PA-C
Tel: 409 772-3047   *Fax:* 409 772-9710
E-mail: rrahr@utmb.edu

Baylor College of Medicine
Physician Assistant Prgm
One Baylor Plaza-Rm BTA 107C
Houston, TX 77030-3411
Prgm Dir: Carl E Fasser, PA
Tel: 713 798-5405   *Fax:* 713 798-6128
E-mail: cfasser@bcm.edu

Texas Tech Univ Health Sciences Center
Physician Assistant Prgm
3600 N Garfield
Midland, TX 79705
www.ttuhsc.edu/sah/mpa/
Prgm Dir: Elvin E Maxwell, Jr, MA MPAS PA-C
Tel: 432 620-9905, Ext 233   *Fax:* 432 620-8605
E-mail: ed.maxwell@ttuhsc.edu

Univ of Texas Hlth Sci Ctr at San Antonio
Physician Assistant Prgm
7703 Floyd Curl Dr MC6249
San Antonio, TX 78229-3900
www.uthscsa.edu
Prgm Dir: Judith Colver, MMS PA-C
Tel: 210 567-8810   *Fax:* 210 567-8846
E-mail: colver@uthscsa.edu

Utah

University of Utah Health Science Center
Cosponsor: Utah Medical Association
Physician Assistant Prgm
375 Chipeta Way Ste A
Salt Lake City, UT 84108
www.utah.edu/upap
Prgm Dir: Don M Pedersen, PhD PA-C
Tel: 801 585-7426   *Fax:* 801 581-5807
E-mail: dpedersen@upap.utah.edu

Virginia

James Madison University
Physician Assistant Prgm
Dept of Health Sciences
MSC 4301
Harrisonburg, VA 22807
www.jmu.edu/healthsci/paweb
Prgm Dir: James B Hammond, MA PA-C
Tel: 540 568-8171   *Fax:* 540 568-3336
E-mail: hammonjb@jmu.edu

Eastern Virginia Medical School
Physician Assistant Prgm
700 W Olney
Lewis Hall, Ste 1100
Norfolk, VA 23507
www.evms.edu
Prgm Dir: Thomas Parish, DHSc PA-C
Tel: 757 446-7158, Ext 7126   *Fax:* 757 446-7403
E-mail: parishtg@evms.edu

Jefferson College of Health Sciences
Physician Assistant Prgm
PO Box 13186
Roanoke, VA 24031-4016
www.jchs.edu
Prgm Dir: Wilton C Kennedy, MMSc PA-C
Tel: 540 985-4016   *Fax:* 540 224-4551
E-mail: wkennedy@jchs.edu

Shenandoah University
Physician Assistant Prgm
MOB II, Ste 430
190 Campus Blvd
Winchester, VA 22601
www.su.edu/pa
Prgm Dir: Anthony Miller, MEd PA-C
Tel: 540 545-7257   *Fax:* 540 542-6210
E-mail: amiller@su.edu

Washington

University of Washington
Physician Assistant Prgm
MEDEX Northwest
4311 11th Ave NE, Ste 200
Seattle, WA 98105-4608
www.medex.washington.edu
Prgm Dir: Ruth Ballweg, MPA PA-C
Tel: 206 616-4001, Ext 6343   *Fax:* 206 616-3889
E-mail: medex@u.washington.edu

West Virginia

Mountain State University
Physician Assistant Prgm
PO Box 9003
Beckley, WV 25802-2830
Prgm Dir: Debra Campbell, PA-C
Tel: 304 929-1451   *Fax:* 304 256-5571
E-mail: dcampbell@mountainstate.edu

Alderson-Broaddus College
Physician Assistant Prgm
500 College Hill Dr
PO Box 2036
Philippi, WV 26416
www.ab.edu
Prgm Dir: Michael W Holt, MS PA
Tel: 304 457-6290   *Fax:* 304 457-6308
E-mail: holtmw@mail.ab.edu

Wisconsin

University of Wisconsin - La Crosse
Cosponsor: Gundersen Lutheran & Mayo School of
Health Science
Physician Assistant Prgm
1725 State St, 4031 HSC
La Crosse, WI 54601-3767
www.uwlax.edu/pastudies
Prgm Dir: Edward Malone, MD
Tel: 608 785-8470   *Fax:* 608 785-6647
E-mail: malone.edwa@uwlax.edu

University of Wisconsin - Madison
Physician Assistant Prgm
1300 University Ave, 1135 MSC
Madison, WI 53706
Prgm Dir: Virginia Snyder, PhD PA-C
Tel: 608 263-5620   *Fax:* 608 263-6434
E-mail: aktyler@wisc.edu

Marquette University
Physician Assistant Prgm
PO Box 1881
Milwaukee, WI 53201-1881
Prgm Dir: Tim Gengembre, PA-C MS MBA PhD
Tel: 414 288-5688   *Fax:* 414 288-7951
E-mail: tim.gengembre@marquette.edu

Physician Assistant

Programs*	Class Capacity	Begins	Length (months)	Award	Res. Tuition	Non-res. Tuition	Stipend	1	2	3	4
Alabama											
University of Alabama at Birmingham	32	Aug	27	MSPAS	$9,400	$23,500				•	
University of South Alabama (Mobile)	36	May	27	MHS	$8,700	$17,400				•	
Arizona											
Midwestern University - Glendale Campus	86	Jun	27	MMS	$28,928	$28,928			•	•	
Arkansas											
Harding University (Searcy)	32	Jun	26	MS	$23,300	$23,300				•	
California											
University of California - Davis (Sacramento)	60	Jul	24	Cert	$10,469	$30,181		•		•	•
University of Southern California (Alhambra)	50	Aug	33	MPAP	$36,000	$36,000			•	•	
Western Univ of Health Sciences (Pomona)	98	Aug	24	MS	$26,700	$26,700				•	
Colorado											
U of Colorado (Denver) Health Sciences Center (Aurora)	40	May	36	Cert, MPAS	$10,466	$32,200				•	
Connecticut											
Quinnipiac University (Hamden)	54	May	27	MHS	$27,555	$27,555				•	
Yale University School of Medicine (New Haven)	32	Sep	27	MMSc	$26,500	$26,500				•	
District of Columbia											
George Washington University	55	Aug-MSHS Jul-PA/MPH	24, 36	Cert, MSHS, PA/MPH	$33,000	$33,000					
Florida											
Barry University (Miami Shores)	69	Aug	28	Cert, MCMSc	$23,625	$23,625			•	•	•
Miami Dade College	40	Aug	24	AS	$11,313	$15,786				•	
Nova Southeastern Univ - Ft Lauderdale	90	Jun	27	Dipl, MMS	$20,950	$21,640				•	
University of Florida (Gainesville)	60	Jun Jul	24	Cert, MPAS	$10,495	$35,703				•	
Georgia											
Emory University (Atlanta)	52	Aug	28	MMSC	$21,000	$21,000				•	•
Idaho											
Idaho State University (Pocatello)	50	Aug	24	Cert, MPAS	$23,370	$38,025				•	
Illinois											
Midwestern University (Downers Grove)	84	Jun	27	Cert, MMS	$22,864	$25,327				•	
Rosalind Franklin Univ of Medicine & Science (North Chicago)	60	May	24	MS	$20,714	$20,714				•	
Southern Illinois University Carbondale	24	Jun	26	MSPA	$20,000	$40,000				•	•
Indiana											
Butler University/Clarian Health (Indianapolis)	50	Aug	30	Dipl, MPAS	$28,140	$28,140				•	
University of Saint Francis (Fort Wayne)	25	May	27	Dipl, MS	$28,500	$28,500					
Iowa											
Des Moines University	44	Jun	25	MS	$23,190	$23,190				•	
University of Iowa (Iowa City)	26	May	25	Cert, MPAS	$9,417	$27,396				•	
Kansas											
Wichita State University	42	Jun	26	MPA	$8,500	$23,000				•	
Kentucky											
University of Kentucky (Lexington)	54	Jan	31	Dipl, MSPAS	$11,168	$21,260				•	
Louisiana											
Louisiana State U Hlth Sci Ctr - Shreveport	36	May	27	Dipl, BS	$6,000	$8,500				•	
Our Lady of the Lake College (Baton Rouge)	30	Jan	28	Masters	$500	$500 per credit hour				•	
Maine											
University of New England (Portland)	40	Jun	24	Cert, MS	$28,500	$28,500					•
Maryland											
Anne Arundel Community College (Arnold)	40	May	25	Cert	$9,910	$19,960				•	
Massachusetts											
Mass College of Pharmacy & Health Sciences (Boston)	40	Sep	30	MPAS	$26,000	$26,000				•	
Northeastern University (Boston)	34	Aug	24	MS	$23,460	$23,460				•	
Michigan											
Grand Valley State University (Grand Rapids)	30	Aug	32	MPAS	$15,745	$25,550				•	
University of Detroit Mercy	45	Sep	24, 36	MS	$30,060	$30,060		•		•	•
Wayne State University (Detroit)	50	May	24	MS	$13,360	$28,044				•	
Western Michigan University (Kalamazoo)	40	Aug	24	MS	$9,840	$19,390				•	
Minnesota											
Augsburg College (Minneapolis)	28	May	36	Cert, MS	$27,000	$27,000				•	
Missouri											
Saint Louis Univ Doisy Coll of Health Sciences (St Louis)	34	Aug	27	MMS	$30,232	$30,232				•	
Montana											
Rocky Mountain College (Billings)	28	Jul	26	MPAS	$27,000	$27,000				•	

*Data are shown only for programs that completed the 2007 AMA Survey of Health Professions Education Programs.
‡Key to Offers: 1: Evening or weekend classes; 2: Non-English instruction; 3: Cultural competence instruction; 4: Distance education component.

Physician Assistant

Programs*	Class Capacity	Begins	Length (months)	Award	Res. Tuition	Non-res. Tuition	Stipend	Offers:‡ 1	2	3	4
Nebraska											
University of Nebraska Medical Center (Omaha)	40	Aug	28	MPAS	$10,406	$28,032				•	
New Jersey											
Seton Hall University (South Orange)	90	Sep	36	MS	$28,000	$28,000				•	
Univ of Medicine & Dent of New Jersey (Piscataway)	50	Aug	36	MS	$14,112	$21,168			•	•	
New Mexico											
University of New Mexico (Albuquerque)	14	Jun	25	Dipl, Cert, BS	$7,515	$18,146				•	
New York											
Albany Medical College	40	Jan	28	MS	$18,000	$18,000				•	
D'Youville College (Buffalo)	40	Aug	54	BS/MS	$18,800	$18,800		•		•	•
Hofstra University (Hempstead)	40	Sep	27	Dipl, Cert, BS	$33,000	$33,000				•	
Long Island University (Brooklyn)	42	Aug	24	Cert, BS	$23,400	$23,400				•	
Mercy College (Bronx)	40	Jun	27	Dipl, BS, MS	$28,350	$28,350			•	•	
New York Institute of Technology (Old Westbury)	40	Sep	30	BS, MS	$25,000	$25,000				•	
Pace University - Lenox Hill Hospital (New York)	50	Jul	26	BS	$38,000	$38,000					
Rochester Institute of Technology	25	Sep	48	BS	$25,362	$25,362		•		•	
St John's University (Fresh Meadows)	150	Aug	22	Cert	$15,500	$16,500					
Stony Brook University	40	Jul	24	MS	$11,218	$17,031				•	
Touro College (New York)	30	Aug	28	BS	$14,700	$14,700		•		•	
Touro College - Bay Shore	55	Sep Jan	23	Dipl, Cert, BS	$15,800	$15,800					
North Carolina											
Duke University Medical Center (Durham)	56	Aug	24	Cert, MHS	$27,032	$27,032				•	
East Carolina University (Greenville)	40	Aug	27	Cert, MS	$16,446	$54,842				•	
Methodist University (Fayetteville)	30	Aug	28	MMS	$25,000	$25,000			•	•	
Wake Forest University School of Medicine (Winston-Salem)	48	Jun	24	MMS	$21,655	$21,655			•	•	
North Dakota											
University of North Dakota (Grand Forks)	60	Jun	24	MPAS	$30,000	$30,000				•	
Ohio											
Cuyahoga Community College (Parma)	52	May	27	Cert, MSHS	$35,000	$42,000					
Kettering College of Medical Arts	40	May	27	MPAS	$27,265	$27,265				•	
Marietta College	22	Jun	27	MS	$29,334	$29,334				•	
University of Toledo	30	Aug	27	MSBS	$9,280	$21,135				•	
Oklahoma											
Univ of Oklahoma Health Sciences Center (Oklahoma City)	50	Jul	30	MHS	$6,594	$15,592					
Oregon											
Oregon Health & Science University (Portland)	36	Jun	26	MPAS	$25,668	$25,668			•	•	
Pacific University (Hillsboro)	42	Jun 6	27	MS	$24,762	$24,762			•	•	
Pennsylvania											
Chatham University (Pittsburgh)	50	Aug	24	MPAS	$30,014	$30,014				•	
Gannon University (Erie)	40	Aug	60, 24	MPAS	$22,100	$22,100				•	
King's College (Wilkes-Barre)	44	Aug	24	MSPAS	$23,450	$23,450				•	
Lock Haven University	48	May	24	MHS	$13,925	$20,888				•	
Marywood University (Scranton)	30	May	27	MS	$26,000	$26,000				•	
Pennsylvania College of Technology (Williamsport)	30	Aug	24	BS	$16,688	$21,000				•	
Philadelphia College of Osteopathic Medicine	55	Jun	26	Cert, MS	$25,300	$25,300				•	
Philadelphia University	50	Aug	25	Cert, MS	$29,253	$29,253				•	
St Francis University (Loretto)	55	May	24	MPAS	$35,812	$35,812					
South Carolina											
Medical University of South Carolina (Charleston)	60	May	27	Dipl, MSPAS	$16,245	$34,191			•	•	•
South Dakota											
University of South Dakota (Vermillion)	20	Aug	28	MS	$5,583	$16,375				•	
Tennessee											
Trevecca Nazarene University (Nashville)	40	May	27	MS-MEd	$60,000	$60,000			•	•	•
Texas											
Texas Tech Univ Health Sciences Center (Midland)	48	Jun	27	MPAS	$11,500	$25,000			•	•	
Univ of North Texas Hlth Sci Ctr at Ft Worth (Fort Worth)	36	Jul	34	MPAS	$5,970	$19,582				•	
Univ of Texas - Pan American (Edinburg)	33	Jun	24	BS	$4,534	$15,390	$1,000			•	
Univ of Texas Hlth Sci Ctr at San Antonio	30	Aug	33	MPAS	$7,410	$13,828				•	•
Univ of Texas Southwestern Med Ctr (Dallas)	36	May	31	Dipl, MPAS	$4,970	$17,790			•	•	
University of Texas Medical Branch (Galveston)	70	Aug	26, 48	MPAS	$9,200	$25,000				•	
Utah											
University of Utah Health Science Center (Salt Lake City)	36	May	27	Cert, MS	$23,770	$35,392				•	
Virginia											
Eastern Virginia Medical School (Norfolk)	50	Jan	27	MPA	$20,967	$22,014			•	•	
James Madison University (Harrisonburg)	25	Aug	28	MPAS						•	

*Data are shown only for programs that completed the 2007 AMA Survey of Health Professions Education Programs.
‡Key to Offers: 1: Evening or weekend classes; 2: Non-English instruction; 3: Cultural competence instruction; 4: Distance education component.

Physician Assistant

Programs*	Class Capacity	Begins	Length (months)	Award	Res. Tuition	Non-res. Tuition	Stipend	Offers:‡ 1	2	3	4
Jefferson College of Health Sciences (Roanoke)	70	Aug	24	BS	$27,460	$27,460				•	
Shenandoah University (Winchester)	38	Aug	27	Masters	$26,560	$26,560				•	
Washington											
University of Washington (Seattle)	80	Jun	24	Cert, BCHS	$19,316	$19,316				•	
West Virginia											
Alderson-Broaddus College (Philippi)	45	Aug	32	MPAS	$19,830	$19,830			•		
Wisconsin											
University of Wisconsin - La Crosse	14	Jun	24	Cert, MS PAS	$9,500	$30,075					

*Data are shown only for programs that completed the 2007 AMA Survey of Health Professions Education Programs.
‡Key to Offers: 1: Evening or weekend classes; 2: Non-English instruction; 3: Cultural competence instruction; 4: Distance education component.

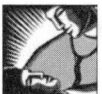

Career Description

The human foot is a complex structure. It contains 26 bones—plus muscles, nerves, ligaments, and blood vessels—and is designed for balance and mobility. The 52 bones in the feet make up about one fourth of all the bones in the human body. Podiatrists, also known as doctors of podiatric medicine (DPMs), diagnose and treat disorders, diseases, and injuries of the foot and lower leg.

Podiatrists treat corns, calluses, ingrown toenails, bunions, heel spurs, and arch problems; ankle and foot injuries, deformities, and infections; and foot complaints associated with diseases such as diabetes. To treat these problems, podiatrists prescribe drugs, order physical therapy, set fractures, and perform surgery. They also fit corrective inserts called orthotics, design plaster casts and strappings to correct deformities, and design custom-made shoes. Podiatrists may use a force plate or scanner to help design the orthotics: Patients walk across a plate connected to a computer that "reads" their feet, picking up pressure points and weight distribution. From the computer readout, podiatrists order the correct design or recommend another kind of treatment.

To diagnose a foot problem, podiatrists also order x rays and laboratory tests. The foot may be the first area to show signs of serious conditions such as arthritis, diabetes, and heart disease. For example, patients with diabetes are prone to foot ulcers and infections due to poor circulation. Podiatrists consult with and refer patients to other health practitioners when they detect symptoms of these disorders.

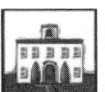

Employment Characteristics

Most podiatrists have a solo practice, although more are forming group practices with other podiatrists or health practitioners. Some specialize in surgery, orthopedics, primary care, or public health. Besides these board-certified specialties, podiatrists may practice other specialties, such as sports medicine, pediatrics, dermatology, radiology, geriatrics, or diabetic foot care.

Podiatrists who are in private practice are responsible for running a small business. They may hire employees, order supplies, and keep records, among other tasks. In addition, some educate the community on the benefits of foot care through speaking engagements and advertising.

In addition to working in their own offices, podiatrists also may spend time visiting patients in nursing homes or performing surgery at hospitals or ambulatory surgical centers. Those with private practices set their own hours, but may work evenings and weekends to accommodate their patients.

Opportunities are also available in academia and management: Podiatrists may advance to become professors at colleges of podiatric medicine, department chiefs in hospitals, or general health administrators. Podiatrists can also be commissioned officers in the Armed Forces and US Public Health Service or work in the Department of Veterans Affairs or in municipal health departments.

Salary

Podiatrists enjoy very high earnings. Median annual earnings of salaried podiatrists were $94,400 in 2004. Additionally, a survey by *Podiatry Management*

reported median net income of $113,000 in 2004. Podiatrists in partnerships tended to earn higher net incomes than those in solo practice. Self-employed podiatrists must provide for their own health insurance and retirement.

For more information, see www.ama-assn.org/go/hpsalary.

Employment Outlook

Employment of podiatrists is expected to grow about as fast as average for all occupations through 2014.

More people will turn to podiatrists for foot care because of the rising number of injuries sustained by a more active and increasingly older population. Additional job openings will result from podiatrists who retire from the occupation, particularly members of the baby-boom generation. However, relatively few job openings from this source are expected because the occupation is small and most podiatrists remain in it until they retire.

Medicare and most private health insurance programs cover acute medical and surgical foot services, as well as diagnostic x rays and leg braces. Details of such coverage vary among plans. However, routine foot care, including the removal of corns and calluses, ordinarily is not covered unless the patient has a systemic condition that has resulted in severe circulatory problems or areas of desensitization in the legs or feet. Like dental services, podiatric care is often discretionary and, therefore, more dependent on disposable income than some other medical services.

Employment of podiatrists would grow even faster were it not for continued emphasis on controlling the costs of specialty health care. Insurers balance the cost of sending patients to podiatrists against the cost and availability of other practitioners, such as physicians and physical therapists. Opportunities will be better for board-certified podiatrists, because many managed care organizations require board certification. Opportunities for newly trained podiatrists will be better in group medical practices, clinics, and health networks than in traditional solo practices. Establishing a practice will be most difficult in the areas surrounding colleges of podiatric medicine, where podiatrists are concentrated.

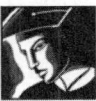

Educational Programs

Award, Length. Graduates receive the degree of Doctor of Podiatric Medicine (DPM) after completing the 4-year program.

Prerequisites. Admission to a college of podiatric medicine requires completion of at least 90 semester hours of undergraduate study, an acceptable grade point average, and suitable scores on the Medical College Admission Test (some colleges also may accept the Dental Admission Test or the Graduate Record Exam). All colleges require 8 semester hours each of biology, inorganic chemistry, organic chemistry, and physics, as well as 6 hours of English. The science courses should be those designed for premedical students. Potential podiatric medical students also are evaluated on the basis of extracurricular and community activities, personal interviews, and letters of recommendation. About 95 percent of podiatric students have at least a bachelor's degree. In general, those interested in the field should possess scientific aptitude, manual dexterity, interpersonal skills, and good business sense.

Curriculum. Colleges of podiatric medicine offer a core curriculum similar to that in other schools of medicine. During the first 2 years, students receive classroom instruction in basic sciences, including anatomy, chemistry, pathology, and pharmacology. Third- and fourth-year students have clinical rotations in private practices, hospitals, and clinics. During these rotations, they learn how to take general and podiatric histories, perform routine physical examinations, interpret tests and findings, make diagnoses, and perform therapeutic procedures.

Advanced Training. Most graduates complete a 2- to 4-year hospital-based residency program after receiving a DPM. Residents receive advanced training in podiatric medicine and surgery and serve clinical rotations in anesthesiology, internal medicine, pathology, radiology, emergency medicine, and orthopedic and general surgery.

Licensure and Certification

All states and the District of Columbia require a license for the practice of podiatric medicine. Each state defines its own licensing requirements, although many states grant reciprocity to podiatrists who are licensed in another state. Applicants for licensure must be graduates of an accredited college of podiatric medicine and must pass written and oral examinations. Some states permit applicants to substitute the examination of the National Board of Podiatric Medical Examiners, given in the second and fourth years of podiatric medical college, for part or all of the written state examination. Most states also require the completion of a postdoctoral residency program of at least 2 years and continuing education for license renewal.

Podiatrists can achieve certification in orthopedics, primary medicine, and surgery. Certification means that the DPM meets higher standards than those required for licensure. Each certification board requires advanced training, the completion of written and oral examinations, and experience as a practicing podiatrist. Most managed-care organizations prefer to contract with board-certified podiatrists.

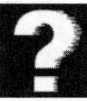

Inquiries

Education, Careers, Resources
American Podiatric Medical Association
9312 Old Georgetown Road
Bethesda, MD 20814-1621
www.apma.org/careers

American Association of Colleges of Podiatric Medicine
15850 Crabbs Branch Way, Suite 320
Rockville, MD 20855-2622
800 922-9266
www.aacpm.org

Licensure
National Board of Podiatric Medical Examiners
PO Box 510
Bellefonte, PA 16823
www.nbpme.info

Program Accreditation
American Podiatric Medical Association
Council on Podiatric Medical Education (CPME)
9312 Old Georgetown Road
Bethesda, MD 20814-1621
301 581-9200
301 571-4903 Fax
www.cpme.org

Note: Adapted in part from the Bureau of Labor Statistics, US Department of Labor, *Occupational Outlook Handbook*, 2006-07 Edition, Podiatrists, on the Internet at www.bls.gov/oco/ocos075.htm (visited August 27, 2007).

Podiatrist

Arizona

Midwestern University - Glendale Campus
Podiatric Medicine Prgm
Arizona Podiatric Medicine Program
19555 N 59th Ave
Glendale, AZ 85308
www.midwestern.edu/azpod

California

Samuel Merritt College
Podiatric Medicine Prgm
California School of Podiatric Medicine
370 Hawthorne Ave
Oakland, CA 94609
www.samuelmerritt.edu

Florida

Barry University
Podiatric Medicine Prgm
11300 NE Second Ave
Miami Shores, FL 33161
www.barry.edu/gms/podiatry

Illinois

Rosalind Franklin Univ of Medicine & Science
Podiatric Medicine Prgm
Dr William M Scholl College of Podiatric Medicine
3333 Green Bay Rd
North Chicago, IL 60064
www.rosalindfranklin.edu

Iowa

Des Moines University
Podiatric Medicine Prgm
College of Podiatric Medicine and Surgery
3200 Grand Ave
Des Moines, IA 50312
www.dmu.edu/cpms

New York

New York College of Podiatric Medicinie
Podiatric Medicine Prgm
1800 Park Ave
New York, NY 10035
www.nycpm.edu

Ohio

Ohio College of Podiatric Medicine
Podiatric Medicine Prgm
10515 Carnegie Ave
Cleveland, OH 44106
www.ocpm.edu

Pennsylvania

Temple University
Podiatric Medicine Prgm
School of Podiatric Medicine
Eighth at Race St
Philadelphia, PA 19107
http://podiatry.temple.edu

Polysomnographic technologists perform sleep tests and work with physicians to provide information needed for the diagnosis of sleep disorders. The technologist monitors brain waves, eye movements, muscle activity, multiple breathing variables, and blood oxygen levels during sleep using specialized recording equipment. The technologist interprets the recording as it happens and responds appropriately to emergencies. Technologists provide support services related to the treatment of sleep-related problems, including helping patients use devices for the treatment of breathing problems during sleep and helping individuals develop good sleep habits.

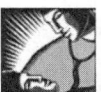

Career Description

The technologist gathers and analyzes patient information and physician orders to ensure that the appropriate test is performed. Technologists explain the sleep study procedures to the patient. Before a sleep study, technologists prepare and calibrate equipment required for testing and make adjustments if necessary. They apply electrodes and sensors according to accepted published standards; perform appropriate calibrations to ensure proper signals and make adjustments if necessary; and perform positive airway pressure (PAP) mask fitting. PAP consists of a machine (air pump) that is connected to a mask worn over the patient's nose by a hose; the machine gently pushes the air into the patient's nose and down the airway to prevent it from collapsing during sleep, as in the case of sleep apnea.

There are several types of tests, including the Multiple Sleep Latency Test (MSLT, measures daytime sleepiness), Maintenance of Wakefulness Test (MWT, measures ability to stay awake), parasomnia studies (eg, unusual behaviors during sleep), and oxygen and PAP titration (eg, adjusting the air pressure of the PAP machine to find the right pressure that will keep the airway from collapsing). The polysomnographic technologist follows these protocols to ensure appropriate data collection. Technologists follow "lights out" procedures to obtain baseline values. They then perform data collection while keeping track of study quality and making any necessary adjustments. The technologist keeps a log of observations, including sleep stages and clinical events, changes in procedure, and significant events. This helps in the interpretation of polysomnographic results.

During the sleep study the technologist must ensure patient safety, apply PAP at the correct pressure level when appropriate, and administer oxygen as directed. At the end of the study the technologist follows "lights on" procedures to ensure that data have been collected correctly. Polysomnographic technologists must be comfortable working with newborn, child, teenage, adult, and geriatric patients.

After the sleep study the technologist scores sleep/wake stages using professionally accepted guidelines; scores clinical events (such as respiratory events, cardiac events, limb movements, arousals, etc) according to center-specific protocols; and generates accurate reports by tabulating sleep/wake and clinical event data.

All polysomnographic technologists must comply with laws, regulations, guidelines, and standards regarding safety and infection control issues. They perform routine and complex equipment care and maintenance and evaluate sleep study-related equipment and inventory. Current CPR (cardiopulmonary resuscitation) or BCLS (basic cardiac life support) certification is required.

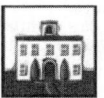

Employment Characteristics

Most polysomnographic technologists work in sleep disorders centers. Sleep disorders centers may be located within or affiliated with a hospital, or may be "freestanding" (in a physician's office or professional building). Some senior technologists may spend all or part of their time scoring sleep recordings, performing daytime tests, and managing a center, but most of the polysomnographic technologists' work is done at night. Typical shifts are three to four 10- to 12-hour shifts per week. The recommended workload is two patients per night. Salaries and benefits are competitive with other allied health professions.

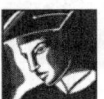

Educational Programs

Length. A 2-year program leading to an associate's degree is preferred. However, some programs provide a certificate after a year of training.

Curriculum. The curriculum of an accredited program focuses on correct performance of polysomnographic procedures and patient safety. Students learn principles of physiological monitoring and the pathophysiology of sleep disorders. Through lecture and observation they gain experience with study protocols.

Inquiries

Careers
Christopher Waring, Coordinator
Association of Polysomnographic Technologists
One Westbrook Corporate Center, Suite 920
Westchester, IL 60154
708 492-0796
708 273-9344 Fax
E-mail: cwaring@aptweb.org

Certification
Cathi Eifert, CAE, Executive Director
Board of Registered Polysomnographic Technologists (BRPT)
8201 Greensboro Drive, Suite 300
McLean, VA 22102
703 610-9020
703 610-9005 Fax
E-mail: brpt@amg-inc.com

Program Accreditation
Commission on Accreditation of Allied Health Education Programs (CAAHEP) in collaboration with:
Committee on Accreditation of Polysomnographic Technologist Education
Richard S Rosenberg, PhD, Coordinator
One Westbrook Corporate Center, Suite 920
Westchester, IL 60154
708 492-0930
708 492-0943 Fax
E-mail: rrosenberg@aasmnet.org

Polysomnographic Technologist

California

Orange Coast College
Polysomnographic Technology Prgm
2701 Fairview Rd
PO Box 5005
Costa Mesa, CA 92628-5005
http://occonline.occ.cccd.edu/online/wbanoczi
Prgm Dir: Walter Banoczi, REEG/EP T CNIM RPSGT
Tel: 714 432-5591   *Fax:* 714 432-5534
E-mail: wbanoczi@cccd.edu

Massachusetts

Northern Essex Community College
Polysomnographic Technology Prgm
45 Franklin St
Lawrence, MA 01841
Prgm Dir: Bonnie McGuire, RPSGT CRT
Tel: 978 738-7223, Ext 7223   *Fax:* 978 738-7450
E-mail: bmcguire@necc.mass.edu

Michigan

Baker College of Flint
Polysomnographic Technology Prgm
1050 W Bristol Rd
Flint, MI 48507
www.baker.edu
Prgm Dir: Christine Robinson, BA AAS RRT RPSGT
Tel: 810 766-4288, Ext 2037   *Fax:* 810 766-2055
E-mail: christine.robinson@baker.edu

Minnesota

Minneapolis Community & Technical Coll
Polysomnographic Technology Prgm
7501 Hennepin Ave
Minneapolis, MN 55403
Prgm Dir: Chad Whittlef
Tel: 612 659-6000
E-mail: chad.whittlef@minneapolis.edu

Ohio

Sleep Care Inc
Polysomnographic Technology Prgm
7634 Rivers Edge Dr
Columbus, OH 43235
Prgm Dir: Jennifer Brickner-York, MPH RPSGT CHES
Tel: 866 320-8989   *Fax:* 866 291-8990
E-mail: jennifer@sleepcareinc.com

Tennessee

Volunteer State Community College
Polysomnographic Technology Prgm
1420 Nashville Pike
Gallatin, TN 37066
Prgm Dir: Anthony Manasco, BS RPSGT
Tel: 615 230-3349
E-mail: anthony.manasco@volstate.edu

Roane State Community College
Polysomnographic Technology Prgm
132 Hayfield Rd
Knoxville, TN 37922
www.roanestate.edu
Prgm Dir: Donna Plumlee, RPSGT/REEGT
Tel: 865 539-6904   *Fax:* 865 539-6907
E-mail: plumleedw@roanestate.edu

Polysomnographic Technologist

Programs*	Class Capacity	Begins	Length (months)	Award	Res. Tuition	Non-res. Tuition	Stipend	Offers:‡ 1	2	3	4
California											
Orange Coast College (Costa Mesa)	24	Aug (odd yrs)	22	AS	$663	$3,876		•			
Massachusetts											
Northern Essex Community College (Lawrence)	25	Sep	9	Cert	$2,520	$8,304		•		•	
Michigan											
Baker College of Flint	25	Sep	22	AAS	$16,655	$16,655		•		•	
Ohio											
Sleep Care Inc (Columbus)	16	Varies	4	Cert	$10,000	$10,000				•	
Tennessee											
Roane State Community College (Knoxville)	20	Aug	12	Cert	$2,705	$8,121				•	

*Data are shown only for programs that completed the 2007 AMA Survey of Health Professions Education Programs.
‡Key to Offers: 1: Evening or weekend classes; 2: Non-English instruction; 3: Cultural competence instruction; 4: Distance education component.

Psychologist

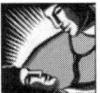

Career Description

Psychologists study the human mind and human behavior. Research psychologists investigate the physical, cognitive, emotional, or social aspects of human behavior. Psychologists in health service provider fields provide mental health care in hospitals, clinics, schools, or private settings. Psychologists employed in applied settings, such as business, industry, government, or nonprofits, provide training, conduct research, design systems, and act as advocates for psychology.

Like other social scientists, psychologists formulate hypotheses and collect data to test their validity. Research methods vary with the topic under study. Psychologists sometimes gather information through controlled laboratory experiments or by administering personality, performance, aptitude, or intelligence tests. Other methods include observation, interviews, questionnaires, clinical studies, and surveys.

Psychologists apply their knowledge to a wide range of endeavors, including health and human services, management, education, law, and sports. In addition to working in a variety of settings, psychologists usually specialize in one of a number of different areas.

Clinical psychologists—who constitute the largest specialty—work most often in counseling centers, independent or group practices, hospitals, or clinics. They help mentally and emotionally disturbed clients adjust to life and may assist medical and surgical patients in dealing with illnesses or injuries. Some clinical psychologists work in physical rehabilitation settings, treating patients with spinal cord injuries, chronic pain or illness, stroke, arthritis, and neurological conditions. Others help people deal with times of personal crisis, such as divorce or the death of a loved one.

Clinical psychologists often interview patients and give diagnostic tests. They may provide individual, family, or group psychotherapy and may design and implement behavior modification programs. Some clinical psychologists collaborate with physicians and other specialists to develop and implement treatment and intervention programs for patients. Other clinical psychologists work in universities and medical schools, where they train graduate students in the delivery of mental health and behavioral medicine services. Some administer community mental health programs.

Areas of specialization within clinical psychology include:

- *Health psychologists*, who promote good health through health maintenance counseling programs designed to help people achieve goals, such as stopping smoking or losing weight
- *Neuropsychologists*, who study the relation between the brain and behavior. They often work in stroke and head injury programs
- *Geropsychologists*, who deal with the special problems faced by the elderly.

Often, clinical psychologists will consult with other medical personnel regarding the best treatment for patients, especially treatment that includes medication. Clinical psychologists generally are not permitted to prescribe medication to treat patients; only psychiatrists and other medical doctors may prescribe certain medications. Louisiana and New Mexico, however, currently allow clinical psychologists to prescribe medication, with some limitations, and similar proposals have been made in other states.

In addition to clinical psychologists, other types of psychologists include:

- Counseling psychologists
- School psychologists
- Industrial-organizational psychologists
- Developmental psychologists
- Social psychologists
- Experimental or research psychologists

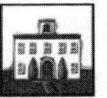

Employment Characteristics

A psychologist's working conditions are determined by type of practice and place of employment. Clinical psychologists in private practice have their own offices and set their own hours. They often offer evening and weekend hours to accommodate their clients. Those employed in hospitals, nursing homes, and other health care facilities may work shifts that include evenings and weekends, while those who work in schools and clinics generally work regular hours.

Increasingly, many psychologists are working as part of a team, consulting with other psychologists and professionals. Many experience pressures because of deadlines, tight schedules, and overtime. Their routine may be interrupted frequently. Travel may be required in order to attend conferences or conduct research.

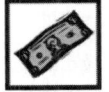

Salary

Median annual earnings of wage and salary clinical, counseling, and school psychologists in May 2004 were $54,950. The middle 50 percent earned between $41,850 and $71,880. The lowest 10 percent earned less than $32,280, and the highest 10 percent earned more than $92,250. Median annual earnings in the industries employing the largest numbers of clinical, counseling, and school psychologists in May 2004 were:

- Offices of other health practitioners — $64,460
- Elementary and secondary schools — $58,360
- Outpatient care centers — $46,850
- Individual and family services — $42,640

For more information, see www.ama-assn.org/go/hpsalary.

Employment Outlook

Employment of psychologists is expected to grow faster than average for all occupations through 2014, because of increased demand for psychological services in schools, hospitals, social service agencies, mental health centers, substance abuse treatment clinics, consulting firms, and private companies.

Clinical and counseling psychologists will be needed to help people deal with depression and other mental disorders, marriage and family problems, job stress, and addiction. The rise in health care costs associated with unhealthy lifestyles, such as smoking, alcoholism, and obesity, has made prevention and treatment more critical. An increase in the number of employee assistance programs, which help workers deal with personal problems, also should spur job growth in clinical and counseling specialties.

Demand should be particularly strong for persons holding doctorates from leading universities in applied specialties, such as counseling, health, and school psychology. Psychologists with extensive training in quantitative research methods and computer science may have a competitive edge over applicants without this experience.

Master's degree holders in fields other than industrial-organizational psychology will face keen competition for jobs, because of the limited number of positions that require only a master's degree. Master's degree holders may find jobs as psychological assistants or counselors, providing mental health services under the direct supervision of a licensed psychologist. Still others may find jobs involving research and data collection and analysis in universities, government, or private companies.

Opportunities directly related to psychology will be limited for bachelor's degree holders. Some may find jobs as assistants in rehabilitation centers or in other jobs involving data collection and analysis. Those who meet state certification requirements may become high school psychology teachers.

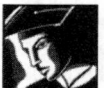

Educational Programs

Award, Length. A doctoral degree, either a PhD or a Doctor of Psychology (PsyD) degree, generally requires 5 to 7 years of graduate study.

Prerequisites. Competition for admission to graduate psychology programs is keen. Some universities require applicants to have an undergraduate major in psychology. Others prefer only coursework in basic psychology with courses in the biological, physical, and social sciences and in statistics and mathematics.

Aspiring psychologists who are interested in direct patient care must be emotionally stable, mature, and able to deal effectively with people. Sensitivity, compassion, good communication skills, and the ability to lead and inspire others are particularly important qualities for persons wishing to do clinical work and counseling. Research psychologists should be able to do detailed work both independently and as part of a team. Patience and perseverance are vital qualities, because achieving results in the psychological treatment of patients or in research may take a long time.

Curriculum. The PhD degree culminates in a dissertation based on original research. Courses in quantitative research methods, which include the use of computer-based analysis, are an integral part of graduate study and are necessary to complete the dissertation. The PsyD may be based on practical work and examinations rather than a dissertation. In clinical or counseling psychology, the requirements for the doctoral degree include at least a 1-year internship.

Licensure, Certification, Registration

Psychologists in independent practice or those who offer any type of patient care—including clinical, counseling, and school psychologists—must meet certification or licensing requirements in all states and the District of Columbia. Licensing laws vary by state and type of position and require licensed or certified psychologists to limit their practice to areas in which they have developed professional competence through training and experience. Clinical and counseling psychologists usually require a doctorate in psychology, the completion of an approved internship, and 1 to 2 years of professional experience. In addition, all states require that applicants pass an examination. Most state licensing boards administer a standardized test, and many supplement that with additional oral or essay questions. Some states require continuing education for licensure renewal.

The American Board of Professional Psychology (ABPP) recognizes professional achievement by awarding specialty certification, primarily in clinical psychology, clinical neuropsychology, and counseling, forensic, industrial-organizational, and school psychology. Requirements for ABPP certification include a doctorate in psychology, postdoctoral training in one's specialty, 5 years of experience, professional endorsements, and a passing grade on an examination.

Inquiries

Education, Careers, Resources

American Psychological Association, Research Office and Education Directorate
750 1st Street NE
Washington, DC 20002-4242
www.apa.org/students

Licensure, Certification

Association of State and Provincial Psychology Boards
PO Box 241245
Montgomery, AL 36124-1245
www.asppb.org

American Board of Professional Psychology
300 Drayton Street, 3rd Floor
Savannah, GA 31401
www.abpp.org

Psychologist

Alabama

Auburn University (PhD)
Psychology Prgm
Department of Psychology
Auburn, AL 36849

University of Alabama - Birmingham (PhD)
Psychology Prgm
Medical Psychology Program
Birmingham, AL 35294

University of Alabama - Tuscaloosa (PhD)
Psychology Prgm
Department of Psychology
Tuscaloosa, AL 35487

Arizona

Argosy University - Phoenix (PsyD)
Psychology Prgm
Phoenix, AZ 85021

Arizona State University (PhD)
Psychology Prgm
Department of Psychology
Tempe, AZ 85287

University of Arizona (PhD)
Psychology Prgm
Department of Psychology
Tucson, AZ 85721

Arkansas

University of Arkansas for Medical Sciences (PhD)
Psychology Prgm
Department of Psychology
Fayetteville, AR 72701

British Columbia, Canada

Simon Fraser University (PhD)
Psychology Prgm
Burnaby, BC V5A 1S6

University of British Columbia (PhD)
Psychology Prgm
Department of Psychology
Vancouver, BC V6T 1Z4

University of Victoria (PhD)
Psychology Prgm
Victoria, BC V8W 3P5

California

Alliant International University - Los Angeles (PhD)
Psychology Prgm
Alhambra, CA 91803

Azusa Pacific University (PsyD)
Psychology Prgm
Department of Graduate Psychology
Azusa, CA 91702

The Wright Insitute (PsyD)
Psychology Prgm
Berkeley, CA 94704

University of California - Berkeley (PhD)
Psychology Prgm
Department of Psychology
Berkeley, CA 94720

Alliant International University - Fresno (PhD)
Psychology Prgm
Fresno, CA 93727

Alliant International University - Fresno (PsyD)
Psychology Prgm
Fresno, CA 93727

Biola University (PhD)
Psychology Prgm
La Mirada, CA 90639

Biola University (PsyD)
Psychology Prgm
La Mirada, CA 90639

University of La Verne (PhD)
Psychology Prgm
Department of Psychology
La Verne, CA 91750

Loma Linda University (PsyD)
Psychology Prgm
Loma Linda, CA 92350

Loma Linda University (PsyD)
Psychology Prgm
Department of Psychology
Loma Linda, CA 92350

Alliant International University - Los Angeles (PsyD)
Psychology Prgm
Los Angeles, CA 91803

Pepperdine University (PhD)
Psychology Prgm
Department of Psychology
Los Angeles, CA 90045

University of California - Los Angeles (PhD)
Psychology Prgm
Department of Psychology
Los Angeles, CA 90095

University of Southern California (PhD)
Psychology Prgm
Department of Psychology
Los Angeles, CA 90089

Pacific Graduate School of Psychology
Cosponsor: Stanford Univ Med Sch Consortium (PsyD)
Psychology Prgm
Palo Alto, CA 94303

Pacific Graduate School of Psychology (PhD)
Psychology Prgm
Palo Alto, CA 94303

Fuller Theological Seminary (PhD)
Psychology Prgm
Pasadena, CA 91101

Fuller Theological Seminary (PsyD)
Psychology Prgm
Pasadena, CA 91101

John F Kennedy University (PsyD)
Psychology Prgm
Pleasant Hill, CA 94523

Biola University - San Francisco (PsyD)
Psychology Prgm
Point Richmond, CA 94804

Alliant International University - San Diego (PhD)
Psychology Prgm
San Diego, CA 92131

Alliant International University - San Diego (PsyD)
Psychology Prgm
San Diego, CA 92131

San Diego State University (PhD)
Psychology Prgm
Joint doctoral program in clinical psychology
San Diego, CA 92120

Alliant International University - San Francisco Bay (PsyD)
Psychology Prgm
San Francisco, CA 94133

California Institute of Integral Studies (PsyD)
Psychology Prgm
San Francisco, CA 94103

Fielding Graduate University (PhD)
Psychology Prgm
Santa Barbara, CA 93105

Colorado

University of Colorado at Boulder (PhD)
Psychology Prgm
Department of Psychology
Boulder, CO 80309

University of Colorado at Denver (PhD)
Psychology Prgm
Department of Psychology
Denver, CO 80208

University of Colorado at Denver (PsyD)
Psychology Prgm
Denver, CO 80208

Connecticut

University of Hartford (PsyD)
Psychology Prgm
Graduate Institute of Professional Psychology
Hartford, CT 06105

Yale University School of Medicine (PhD)
Psychology Prgm
Department of Psychology
New Haven, CT 06520

University of Connecticut (PhD)
Psychology Prgm
Department of Psychology
Storrs, CT 06269

Delaware

University of Delaware (PhD)
Psychology Prgm
Department of Psychology
Newark, DE 19716

District of Columbia

American University (PhD)
Psychology Prgm
Washington, DC 20016

Catholic University of America (PhD)
Psychology Prgm
Department of Psychology
Washington, DC 20064

Gallaudet University (PhD)
Psychology Prgm
Department of Psychology
Washington, DC 20002

George Washington University
Psychology Prgm
Department of Psychology
Washington, DC 20052

George Washington University (PsyD)
Psychology Prgm
Washington, DC 20037

Howard University (PhD)
Psychology Prgm
Department of Psychology
Washington, DC 20059

Florida

University of Miami (PhD)
Psychology Prgm
Department of Psychology
Coral Gables, FL 33124

Nova Southeastern University (PhD)
Psychology Prgm
Department of Psychology
Fort Lauderdale, FL 33314

Nova Southeastern University (PsyD)
Psychology Prgm
Fort Lauderdale, FL 33314

University of Florida (PhD)
Psychology Prgm
Department of Clinical and Health Psychology
Gainesville, FL 32610

Florida Institute of Technology (PsyD)
Psychology Prgm
Melbourne, FL 32901

Carlos Albizu University (PsyD)
Psychology Prgm
Miami, FL 33172

University of Central Florida (PhD)
Psychology Prgm
Department of Psychology
Orlando, FL 32816

Florida State University (PhD)
Psychology Prgm
Department of Psychology
Tallahassee, FL 32306

Argosy University - Tampa (PsyD)
Psychology Prgm
Tampa, FL 33614

University of South Florida (PhD)
Psychology Prgm
Department of Psychology
Tampa, FL 33620

Georgia

University of Georgia
Psychology Prgm
Department of Psychology
Athens, GA 30602

Argosy University - Atlanta Campus (PsyD)
Psychology Prgm
Atlanta, GA 30328

Emory University (PhD)
Psychology Prgm
Department of Psychology
Atlanta, GA 30322

Georgia State University (PhD)
Psychology Prgm
Department of Psychology
Atlanta, GA 30303

Hawaii

Argosy University - Hawaii Campus (PsyD)
Psychology Prgm
Honolulu, HI 96813

University of Hawaii (PhD)
Psychology Prgm
Department of Psychology
Honolulu, HI 96822

Idaho

Idaho State University (PhD)
Psychology Prgm
Department of Psychology
Pocatello, ID 83209

Illinois

Southern Illinois University Carbondale (PhD)
Psychology Prgm
Department of Psychology
Carbondale, IL 62901

Univ of Illinois at Urbana-Champaign (PhD)
Psychology Prgm
Department of Psychology
Champaign, IL 61820

Adler School of Professional Psychology (PsyD)
Psychology Prgm
Department of Psychology
Chicago, IL 60601

Argosy University - Chicago Campus (PsyD)
Psychology Prgm
Chicago, IL 60654

Chicago School of Professional Psychology (PsyD)
Psychology Prgm
Chicago, IL 60610

DePaul University (PhD)
Psychology Prgm
Chicago, IL 60614

Illinois Institute of Technology (PhD)
Psychology Prgm
Institute of Psychology
Chicago, IL 60616

Loyola University of Chicago (PhD)
Psychology Prgm
Department of Psychology
Chicago, IL 60626

Northwestern University Medical School - Chicago (PhD)
Psychology Prgm
Department of Psychiatry and Behavioral Sciences
Chicago, IL 60611

Roosevelt University (PsyD)
Psychology Prgm
School of Psychology
Chicago, IL 60605

University of Illinois at Chicago (PhD)
Psychology Prgm
Department of Psychology
Chicago, IL 60607

Northern Illinois University (PhD)
Psychology Prgm
Department of Psychology
DeKalb, IL 60115

Northwestern University - Evanston (PhD)
Psychology Prgm
Department of Psychology
Evanston, IL 60208

Rosalind Franklin Univ of Medicine & Science (PhD)
Psychology Prgm
Department of Psychology
North Chicago, IL 60064

Argosy University - Schaumburg (PsyD)
Psychology Prgm
Schaumburg, IL 60173

Wheaton College (PsyD)
Psychology Prgm
Wheaton, IL 60187

Indiana

Indiana University - Bloomington (PsyD)
Psychology Prgm
Department of Psychological and Brain Sciences
Bloomington, IN 47405

Indiana Univ-Purdue U-Indianapolis (PhD)
Psychology Prgm
Department of Psychology
Indianapolis, IN 46202

University of Indianapolis (PsyD)
Psychology Prgm
School of Psychological Sciences
Indianapolis, IN 46227

Indiana State University (PhD)
Psychology Prgm
Department of Psychology
Terre Haute, IN 47809

Purdue University (PhD)
Psychology Prgm
Department of Psychological Sciences
West Lafayette, IN 47907

Iowa

University of Iowa (PhD)
Psychology Prgm
Department of Psychology
Iowa City, IA 52242

Kansas

University of Kansas (PhD)
Psychology Prgm
Lawrence, KS 66045

University of Kansas (PhD)
Psychology Prgm
Department of Psychology
Lawrence, KS 66045

Wichita State University (PhD)
Psychology Prgm
Department of Psychology
Wichita, KS 67260

Kentucky

University of Kentucky (PhD)
Psychology Prgm
Department of Psychology
Lexington, KY 40506

Spalding University (PsyD)
Psychology Prgm
School of Professional Psychology
Louisville, KY 40203

University of Louisville (PhD)
Psychology Prgm
Department of Psychology and Brain Sciences
Louisville, KY 40292

Louisiana

Louisiana State University (PhD)
Psychology Prgm
Department of Psychology
Baton Rouge, LA 70803

Maine

University of Maine - Orono (PsyD)
Psychology Prgm
Department of Psychology
Orono, ME 04469

Manitoba, Canada

University of Manitoba (PhD)
Psychology Prgm
Department of Psychology
Winnipeg, MB R3T 2N2

Maryland

Loyola College of Maryland (PhD)
Psychology Prgm
Department of Psychology
Baltimore, MD 21210

University of Maryland Baltimore County (PhD)
Psychology Prgm
Department of Psychology
Baltimore, MD 21250

Uniformed Serv Univ of the Hlth Sci (PhD)
Psychology Prgm
Bethesda, MD 20814

Univ of Maryland at College Park (PsyD)
Psychology Prgm
Department of Psychology
College Park, MD 20742

Massachusetts

University of Massachusetts - Amherst (PhD)
Psychology Prgm
Department of Psychology
Amherst, MA 01003

Boston University - Boston (PhD)
Psychology Prgm
Department of Psychology
Boston, MA 02215

Massachusetts Sch of Prof Psychology Inc (PsyD)
Psychology Prgm
Boston, MA 02132

Suffolk University (PhD)
Psychology Prgm
Department of Psychology
Boston, MA 02114

University of Massachusetts - Boston (PsyD)
Psychology Prgm
Department of Psychology
Boston, MA 02125

Clark University (PhD)
Psychology Prgm
Department of Psychology
Worcester, MA 01610

Michigan

University of Michigan (PhD)
Psychology Prgm
Department of Psychology
Ann Arbor, MI 48109

University of Detroit Mercy (PhD)
Psychology Prgm
Department of Psychology
Detroit, MI 48221

Wayne State University (PhD)
Psychology Prgm
Department of Psychology
Detroit, MI 48202

Michigan State University (PhD)
Psychology Prgm
Department of Psychology
East Lansing, MI 48824

Western Michigan University (PhD)
Psychology Prgm
Department of Psychology
Kalamazoo, MI 49008

Central Michigan University (PhD)
Psychology Prgm
Department of Psychology
Mount Pleasant, MI 48859

Eastern Michigan University (PhD)
Psychology Prgm
Department of Psychology
Ypsilanti, MI 48197

Minnesota

Argosy University - Twin Cities (PsyD)
Psychology Prgm
Eagan, MN 55121

University of Minnesota - Minneapolis (PhD)
Psychology Prgm
Department of Psychology
Minneapolis, MN 55455

Mississippi

University of Southern Mississippi (PhD)
Psychology Prgm
Department of Psychology
Hattiesburg, MS 39406

Jackson State University (PsyD)
Psychology Prgm
Department of Psychology
Jackson, MS 39217

University of Mississippi (PhD)
Psychology Prgm
Department of Psychology
University, MS 38677

Missouri

University of Missouri - Columbia (PhD)
Psychology Prgm
Department of Psychological Sciences
Columbia, MO 65211

University of Missouri - Kansas City (PhD)
Psychology Prgm
Department of Psychology
Kansas City, MO 64110

Forest Institute of Professional Psychology (PsyD)
Psychology Prgm
Springfield, MO 65807

Saint Louis University (PhD)
Psychology Prgm
St Louis, MO 63103

University of Missouri - St Louis (PhD)
Psychology Prgm
Department of Psychology
St Louis, MO 63121

Washington University (PhD)
Psychology Prgm
Department of Psychology
St Louis, MO 63130

Montana

University of Montana (PhD)
Psychology Prgm
Department of Psychology
Missoula, MT 59812

Nebraska

University of Nebraska - Lincoln (PhD)
Psychology Prgm
Department of Psychology
Lincoln, NE 68588

Nevada

University of Nevada - Las Vegas (PhD)
Psychology Prgm
Department of Psychology
Las Vegas, NV 89154

University of Nevada - Reno (PhD)
Psychology Prgm
Department of Psychology
Reno, NV 89557

New Brunswick, Canada

University of New Brunswick (PhD)
Psychology Prgm
Fredericton, NB E3B 6E4

New Hampshire

Antioch University New England (PsyD)
Psychology Prgm
Department of Clinical Psychology
Keene, NH 03431

New Jersey

Rutgers University (PhD)
Psychology Prgm
Department of Psychology
Piscataway, NJ 08854

Rutgers University - SUNJ (PsyD)
Psychology Prgm
Piscataway, NJ 08854

Fairleigh Dickinson University (PhD)
Psychology Prgm
School of Psychology
Teaneck-Hackensack Campus
Teaneck, NJ 07666

New Mexico

University of New Mexico (PhD)
Psychology Prgm
Department of Psychology
Albuquerque, NM 87131

New York

SUNY at Albany (PhD)
Psychology Prgm
Department of Psychology
Albany, NY 12222

Binghamton University / SUNY (PhD)
Psychology Prgm
Binghamton, NY 13902

Fordham University (PhD)
Psychology Prgm
Bronx, NY 10458

Yeshiva University (PhD)
Psychology Prgm
Jack and Pearl Resnick Campus
Bronx, NY 10461

Yeshiva University (PsyD)
Psychology Prgm
Albert Einstein College of Medicine Campus
Bronx, NY 10461

Long Island University (PsyD)
Psychology Prgm
Department of Psychology
Brooklyn, NY 11201

Long Island University
Cosponsor: CW Post Campus (PsyD)
Psychology Prgm
Brookville, NY 11548

University at Buffalo - SUNY (PhD)
Psychology Prgm
Department of Psychology
Buffalo, NY 14260

Adelphi University (PhD)
Psychology Prgm
Demar Institute of Advanced Psychological Studies
Garden City, NY 11530

St John's University (PhD)
Psychology Prgm
Department of Psychology
Jamaica, NY 11439

City University of New York, The City College (PhD)
Psychology Prgm
Department of Psychology
New York, NY 10038

Columbia University Teachers College (PhD)
Psychology Prgm
Department of Clinical Psychology
New York, NY 10027

New York University (PhD)
Psychology Prgm
Department of Psychology
New York, NY 10003

The New School (PhD)
Psychology Prgm
New York, NY 10003

University of Rochester (PhD)
Psychology Prgm
Department of Clinical and Social Sciences in Psychology
Rochester, NY 14627

SUNY at Stony Brook (PhD)
Psychology Prgm
Stony Brook, NY 11794

Syracuse University (PhD)
Psychology Prgm
Department of Psychology
Syracuse, NY 13244

North Carolina

University of North Carolina - Chapel Hill (PhD)
Psychology Prgm
Department of Psychology
Chapel Hill, NC 27599

Duke University (PhD)
Psychology Prgm
Durham, NC 27708

University of North Carolina - Greensboro (PhD)
Psychology Prgm
Department of Psychology
Greensboro, NC 27402

North Dakota

University of North Dakota (PhD)
Psychology Prgm
Department of Psychology
Grand Forks, ND 58202

Ohio

Ohio University (PhD)
Psychology Prgm
Department of Psychology
Athens, OH 45701

Bowling Green State University (PhD)
Psychology Prgm
Department of Psychology
Bowling Green, OH 43403

University of Cincinnati (PhD)
Psychology Prgm
Department of Psychology
Cincinnati, OH 45221

Xavier University (PsyD)
Psychology Prgm
Department of Psychology
Cincinnati, OH 45207

Case Western Reserve University (PhD)
Psychology Prgm
Department of Psychology
Cleveland, OH 44106

Ohio State University (PhD)
Psychology Prgm
Department of Psychology
Columbus, OH 43210

Wright State University (PsyD)
Psychology Prgm
School of Professional Psychology
Dayton, OH 45435

Kent State University (PhD)
Psychology Prgm
Department of Psychology
Kent, OH 44242

Miami University (PhD)
Psychology Prgm
Department of Psychology
Oxford, OH 45056

University of Toledo (PhD)
Psychology Prgm
Department of Psychology
Toledo, OH 43606

Oklahoma

Oklahoma State University (PhD)
Psychology Prgm
Department of Psychology
Stillwater, OK 74078

University of Tulsa (PhD)
Psychology Prgm
Department of Psychology
Tulsa, OK 74104

Ontario, Canada

University of Ottawa (PhD)
Psychology Prgm
School of Psychology
Ottawa, ON K1N 6N5

York University (PhD)
Psychology Prgm
Programme in Clinical-Development Psychology
Toronto, ON M3J 1P3

York University (PhD)
Psychology Prgm
Clinical Program-Adult Emphasis
Toronto, ON M3J 1P3

University of Waterloo (PhD)
Psychology Prgm
Waterloo, ON N2L 3G1

Oregon

University of Oregon (PhD)
Psychology Prgm
Department of Psychology
Eugene, OR 97403

Pacific University (PsyD)
Psychology Prgm
School of Professional Psychology
Forest Grove, OR 97116

George Fox University (PsyD)
Psychology Prgm
Graduate Department of Clinical Psychology
Newberg, OR 97132

Pennsylvania

Widener University (PsyD)
Psychology Prgm
School of Human Service Professions
Chester, PA 19013

Immaculata University (PsyD)
Psychology Prgm
Graduate Division
Immaculata, PA 19345

Indiana University of Pennsylvania (PsyD)
Psychology Prgm
Department of Psychology
Indiana, PA 15705

Chestnut Hill College (PsyD)
Psychology Prgm
Philadelphia, PA 19118

Drexel University (PhD)
Psychology Prgm
Department of Psychology
Philadelphia, PA 19102

La Salle University (PhD)
Psychology Prgm
Department of Psychology
Philadelphia, PA 19141

Philadelphia College of Osteopathic Medicine (PhD)
Psychology Prgm
Department of Psychology
Philadelphia, PA 19131

Temple University (PhD)
Psychology Prgm
Department of Psychology
Philadelphia, PA 19122

University of Pennsylvania (PhD)
Psychology Prgm
Philadelphia, PA 19104

Duquesne University (PhD)
Psychology Prgm
Department of Psychology
Pittsburgh, PA 15282

University of Pittsburgh (PhD)
Psychology Prgm
Department of Psychology
Pittsburgh, PA 15260

Marywood University (PhD)
Psychology Prgm
Department of Psychology and Counseling
Scranton, PA 18509

Penn State University - University Park (PhD)
Psychology Prgm
Department of Psychology
University Park, PA 16802

Puerto Rico

Ponce School of Medicine (PsyD)
Psychology Prgm
Clinical Psychology Doctoral Program
Ponce, PR 00732

Carlos Albizu University (PhD)
Psychology Prgm
San Juan, PR 00902

Carlos Albizu University (PsyD)
Psychology Prgm
San Juan, PR 00902

Quebec, Canada

Concordia University (PhD)
Psychology Prgm
Department of Psychology
Montreal, QC H4B 1R6

McGill University (PhD)
Psychology Prgm
Montreal, QC H3A 1B1

Rhode Island

University of Rhode Island (PhD)
Psychology Prgm
Department of Psychology
Kingston, RI 02881

Saskatchewan, Canada

University of Saskatchewan (PhD)
Psychology Prgm
Department of Psychology
Saskatoon, SK S7N 5A5

South Carolina

University of South Carolina (PhD)
Psychology Prgm
Department of Psychology
Columbia, SC 29208

South Dakota

University of South Dakota (PhD)
Psychology Prgm
Department of Psychology
Vermillion, SD 57069

Tennessee

University of Tennessee - Knoxville - Knoxville (PhD)
Psychology Prgm
Department of Psychology
Knoxville, TN 37996

University of Memphis (PhD)
Psychology Prgm
Department of Psychology
Memphis, TN 38152

Vanderbilt University (PhD)
Psychology Prgm
Department of Psychology
Nashville, TN 37203

Texas

University of Texas at Austin (PhD)
Psychology Prgm
Department of Psychology
Austin, TX 78712

Texas A&M University (PhD)
Psychology Prgm
Department of Psychology
College Station, TX 77843

Univ of Texas Southwestern Med Ctr (PhD)
Psychology Prgm
Division of Psychology
Dallas, TX 75390

University of North Texas
Cosponsor: North Texas Health Sciences Center (Consortium) (PhD)
Psychology Prgm
Denton, TX 76203

University of North Texas (PhD)
Psychology Prgm
Department of Psychology
Denton, TX 76203

University of Houston (PsyD)
Psychology Prgm
Department of Psychology
Houston, TX 77204

Sam Houston State University (PhD)
Psychology Prgm
Department of Psychology and Philosophy
Huntsville, TX 77341

Texas Tech University (PhD)
Psychology Prgm
Department of Psychology
Lubbock, TX 79409

Baylor University - Waco (PsyD)
Psychology Prgm
Department of Psychology
Waco, TX 76798

Utah

Brigham Young University - Provo (PhD)
Psychology Prgm
Department of Psychology
Provo, UT 84602

University of Utah (PhD)
Psychology Prgm
Department of Psychology
Salt Lake City, UT 84112

Vermont

University of Vermont (PhD)
Psychology Prgm
Department of Psychology
Burlington, VT 05405

Virginia

Argosy University - Washington (PsyD)
Psychology Prgm
Arlington, VA 22209

Virginia Polytechnic Inst & State Univ (PhD)
Psychology Prgm
Department of Psychology
Blacksburg, VA 24061

University of Virginia (PhD)
Psychology Prgm
Dept of Human Services
Curry School of Education
Charlottesville, VA 22904

University of Virginia (PhD)
Psychology Prgm
Department of Psychology
Charlottesville, VA 22904

George Mason University (PhD)
Psychology Prgm
Department of Psychology
Fairfax, VA 22030

Regent University (PsyD)
Psychology Prgm
School of Psychology and Counseling
Virginia Beach, VA 23464

Virginia Consortium Program in Clinical Psych (PsyD)
Psychology Prgm
Virginia Beach, VA 23453

Washington

Washington State University (PhD)
Psychology Prgm
Department of Psychology
Pullman, WA 99164

Seattle Pacific University (PhD)
Psychology Prgm
Department of Graduate Psychology
Seattle, WA 98119

University of Washington (PhD)
Psychology Prgm
Department of Psychology
Seattle, WA 98195

West Virginia

Marshall University (PhD)
Psychology Prgm
Department of Psychology
Huntington, WV 25755

West Virginia University (PhD)
Psychology Prgm
Department of Psychology
Morgantown, WV 26506

Wisconsin

University of Wisconsin - Madison (PhD)
Psychology Prgm
Department of Psychology
Madison, WI 53706

Marquette University (PhD)
Psychology Prgm
Department of Psychology
Milwaukee, WI 53201

University of Wisconsin - Milwaukee (PhD)
Psychology Prgm
Department of Psychology
Milwaukee, WI 53201

Wyoming

University of Wyoming (PhD)
Psychology Prgm
Department of Psychology
Laramie, WY 82071

Includes:
- Magnetic resonance technologist
- Medical dosimetrist
- Radiation therapist
- Radiographer

Magnetic Resonance Technologist

Magnetic resonance technologists use radiowaves, magnetic fields, and computerized equipment to produce images of body tissues. MR technologists strive to provide quality patient care while producing patient images that permit accurate diagnoses. MR technologists use problem-solving and critical-thinking skills to adapt procedural requirements to the patient and specific area of study.

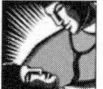
Career Description
Magnetic resonance technologists apply knowledge of anatomy, physiology, positioning, and MR protocols in the performance of their responsibilities. They must be able to communicate effectively with patients, other health professionals, and the public. The MR technologist must show competence and compassion in meeting the special needs of the patient.

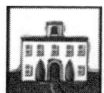
Employment Characteristics
Magnetic resonance technologists are employed in health care facilities—including hospitals, specialized imaging centers, urgent care clinics, and physician offices—and as educators or imaging department administrators.

Salary
Salary and benefits are generally competitive with other health professions and vary according to experience and employment location. Refer to Section IV, Table 5 of this *Directory* for more information, or see www.ama-assn.org/go/hpsalary.

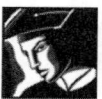
Educational Programs
Length. Program length varies, depending on program design, objectives, and the degree or certificate awarded.

Curriculum. Many, though not all, programs require certification as a radiographer as a prerequisite. The curriculum of an accredited program includes an extensive component of technical and professional courses, including an emphasis on structured competency-based clinical education. Contact a particular program for information on specific courses and prerequisites.

Medical Dosimetrist

Medical dosimetrists, in collaboration with radiation oncologists and medical physicists, generate radiation dose distributions and dose calculations to design radiation treatment plans that will deliver a prescribed dose of radiation to a defined anatomic area.

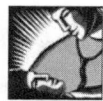
Career Description
Medical dosimetrists apply knowledge of anatomy and physiology, oncologic pathology, radiation biology, radiation oncology techniques, treatment planning and dosimetry procedures, and computer computation in the performance of their duties. The medical dosimetrist accepts responsibility for designing a radiation oncologist (physician)-prescribed course of radiation therapy, considering dose-limiting structures and the need for special casts and immobilization devices. They must be able to communicate effectively with other health care professionals.

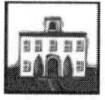
Employment Characteristics
Medical dosimetrists are employed in health care facilities, including hospitals and cancer centers.

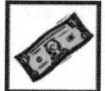
Salary
Salary and benefits vary with experience and employment location but are competitive with other health specialties. See Section IV, Table 5 of this *Directory* for more information, or www.ama-assn.org/go/hpsalary.

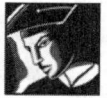
Educational Programs
Length. Program length varies, depending on program design, objectives, and the degree or certificate awarded.

Curriculum. Most programs require prerequisite work in radiation therapy or radiation physics. The curriculum of an accredited program includes an extensive component of technical and professional courses, including an emphasis on structured, competency-based clinical education. Interested individuals should contact a particular program for information on specific courses and prerequisites.

Radiation Therapist

Radiation therapists deliver prescribed doses of radiation to patients for therapeutic purposes. In fulfilling this primary responsibility, radiation therapists provide appropriate patient care; apply problem-solving and critical thinking skills in the administration of treatment protocols, tumor localization, and dosimetry; and maintain appropriate patient records. Radiation therapists are particularly concerned with the principles of radiation protection for patients, themselves, and others.

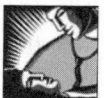
Career Description
Radiation therapists apply knowledge of anatomy and physiology, oncologic pathology, radiation biology, radiation oncology techniques, treatment planning procedures, and dosimetry in the performance of their duties. They must also communicate effectively with patients, health professionals, and the public.

The radiation therapist accepts responsibility for administering a radiation oncologist (physician)-prescribed course of radiation therapy, providing patient care during treatment, and maintaining treatment records. Radiation therapists also evaluate and assess treatment delivery components, evaluate and assess the daily physiologic and psychologic responsiveness of patients, and ensure quality care for patients undergoing radiation therapy. Additional duties may include tumor localization, dosimetry, patient follow-up, and patient education. Radiation therapists must display competence and compassion in meeting the special needs of the oncology patient.

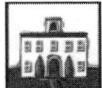

Employment Characteristics

Radiation therapists are employed in health care facilities, including hospitals, cancer centers and private offices; they are also employed in settings where their responsibilities focus on education, management, research, and sales.

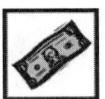

Salary

In 2004, radiation therapist salary averaged $72,300. Salaries and benefits vary with experience and employment location. Some states require licensure as a condition of practice. Refer to Section IV, Table 5 of this Directory for more information, or see www.ama-assn.org/go/hpsalary.

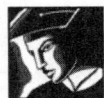

Educational Programs

Length. Programs may be 1, 2, or 4 years, depending on program design, objectives, and the degree or certificate awarded.

Curriculum. The curriculum of an accredited program includes an extensive component of technical and professional courses, including an emphasis on structured, competency-based clinical education. Interested individuals should contact a particular program for information on specific courses and prerequisites.

Radiographer

Radiographers use radiation equipment to produce images of the tissues, organs, bones, and vessels of the body, as prescribed by physicians, to assist in the diagnosis of disease or injury. Radiographers continually strive to provide quality patient care and are particularly concerned with limiting radiation exposure to patients, themselves, and others. Radiographers use problem-solving and critical-thinking skills to perform medical imaging procedures by adapting variable technical parameters of the procedure to the condition of the patient.

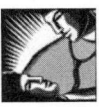

Career Description

Radiographers apply knowledge of anatomy, physiology, positioning, radiographic technique, and radiation biology and protection in the performance of their responsibilities. They must be able to communicate effectively with patients, other health professionals, and the public. Additional duties may include evaluating radiologic equipment, conducting a radiographic quality assurance program, providing patient education, and managing a medical imaging department. The radiographer must display competence and compassion in meeting the special needs of the patient.

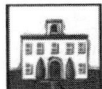

Employment Characteristics

Radiographers are employed in health care facilities—including hospitals, specialized imaging centers, urgent care clinics, and private physician offices—and as educators or imaging department administrators. Thirty-five states require licensure as a condition of practice.

Salary

In 2004, radiographer salary averaged $59,735. Salaries and benefits vary according to experience and employment location. Refer to Section IV, Table 5 of this Directory for more information, or see www.ama-assn.org/go/hpsalary.

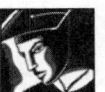

Educational Programs

Length. Programs are generally 2 to 4 years, depending on program design, objectives, and the degree or certificate awarded.

Curriculum. The curriculum of an accredited program includes an extensive component of technical and professional courses, including an emphasis on structured competency-based clinical education. Contact a particular program for information on specific courses and prerequisites.

Post Primary Specialties in Radiologic Technology

Practitioners of the following post primary specialties in radiologic technology are eligible for certification by the American Registry of Radiologic Technologists. Candidates for certification must be certified in radiography, radiation therapy, or nuclear medicine and document specific clinical competencies to be eligible for the certification examination.

- Bone Densitometry
- Breast Sonography
- Cardiac-Interventional Radiography
- Computed Tomography
- Magnetic Resonance Imaging
- Mammography
- Quality Management
- Vascular Sonography
- Vascular-interventional Radiography

Inquiries

Careers/Curriculum
American Society of Radiologic Technologists
15000 Central Avenue SE
Albuquerque, NM 87123
505 298-4500
www.asrt.org

American Association of Medical Dosimetrists
c/o Credentialing Services
One Physics Ellipse
College Park, MD 20740
301 209-3320   301 209-3343 Fax
E-mail: aamd@aapm.org
www.medicaldosimetry.org

Certification/Registration
American Registry of Radiologic Technologists
1255 Northland Drive
Mendota Heights, MN 55120
651 687-0048

Program Accreditation
Joint Review Committee on Education in Radiologic Technology
20 N Wacker Drive, Suite 2850
Chicago, IL 60606-3182
312 704-5300   312 704-5304 Fax
E-mail: mail@jrcert.org
www.jrcert.org

Magnetic Resonance Technologist

Georgia

Ogeechee Technical College
Magnetic Resonance Prgm
One Joe Kennedy Blvd
Statesboro, GA 30458
Prgm Dir: Lynda A Tinker, MA RT(R)(M)(CT)(QM)
Tel: 912 871-1642
E-mail: ltinker@ogeecheetech.edu

Pennsylvania

Thomas Jefferson University
Magnetic Resonance Prgm
130 S 9th St, Ste 1005
Philadelphia, PA 19107
Prgm Dir: Richard H Weening, PhD RT(R)(CT)(MR)
Tel: 215 503-0059
E-mail: richard.weening@jefferson.edu

Medical Dosimetrist

Illinois

Southern Illinois University Carbondale
Medical Dosimetry Prgm
MC 6615
Carbondale, IL 62901
Prgm Dir: Kevin S Collins, MS Ed RT(R)(T) CMD
Tel: 618 453-8800
E-mail: kscollin@siu.edu

North Carolina

University of North Carolina Hospitals
Medical Dosimetry Prgm
101 Manning Dr
Chapel Hill, NC 27514-7512
Prgm Dir: Robert D Adams, EdD RT(R)(T) CMD
Tel: 919 966-1101, Ext 247
E-mail: robert_adams@med.unc.edu

Texas

Univ of Texas M D Anderson Cancer Ctr
Medical Dosimetry Prgm
1515 Holcombe Blvd, Unit 190
Houston, TX 77030
Prgm Dir: Melissa Jane Chapman, MEd CMD
Tel: 713 792-3455
E-mail: mchapman@mdanderson.org

Wisconsin

University of Wisconsin - La Crosse
Medical Dosimetry Prgm
1725 State St 4033 HSC
LaCrosse, WI 54601
Prgm Dir: Nishele D Lenards, BS RT(R)(T)
Tel: 608 785-5071
E-mail: lenards.nish@uwlax.edu

Radiation Therapist

Alabama

University of Alabama at Birmingham
Radiation Therapy Prgm
1705 University Blvd
RMSB 437
Birmingham, AL 35294-1212
www.uab.edu/rtt
Prgm Dir: Pamela C Cartright, MA Ed RT(R)(T)
Tel: 205 934-3443   *Fax:* 205 975-7302
E-mail: pamcartr@uab.edu

Arkansas

Central Arkansas Radiation Therapy Inst
Radiation Therapy Prgm
PO Box 55050
Little Rock, AR 72215
www.carti.com
Prgm Dir: Debra G Tomlinson, MA RT(R)(T)
Tel: 501 603-8866   *Fax:* 501 603-9573
E-mail: dtomlinson@carti.com

Arkansas State University
Radiation Therapy Prgm
PO Box 910
State University, AR 72467
Prgm Dir: Tracy B White, MS RT(R)(T)
Tel: 870 972-2976   *Fax:* 870 972-2004
E-mail: twhite@astate.edu

California

City of Hope
Radiation Therapy Prgm
1500 E Duarte Rd
Duarte, CA 91010-0269
www.cityofhope.org
Prgm Dir: Christine Forell, BS RT(R)(T)
Tel: 626 301-8247   *Fax:* 626 930-5334
E-mail: cforell@coh.org

Loma Linda University
Radiation Therapy Prgm
Nichol Hall Rm A829
Loma Linda, CA 92350
Prgm Dir: Carol A L Davis, RT(T)
Tel: 909 558-7368   *Fax:* 909 558-0264
E-mail: cadavis@ahs.llumc.edu

California State University - Long Beach
Radiation Therapy Prgm
1250 Bellflower Blvd
Long Beach, CA 90840-4902
Prgm Dir: Stephanie Eatmon, EdD RT(R)(T) FASRT
Tel: 562 985-7507   *Fax:* 562 985-2384
E-mail: seatmon@csulb.edu

Kaiser Permanente Sch of Allied Hlth Sciences
Radiation Therapy Prgm
938 Marina Way S
Richmond, CA 94804
Prgm Dir: Roma-Dakini Alexander, BS RT(R)(T) CRT
Tel: 510 231-5062   *Fax:* 510 231-5001
E-mail: Roma.D.Alexander@kp.org

City College of San Francisco
Radiation Therapy Prgm
50 Phelan Ave, Box S91
San Francisco, CA 94112
Prgm Dir: Les K Yim, BS RT(T)(R)
Tel: 415 239-3458   *Fax:* 415 239-3930
E-mail: lyim@ccsf.edu

Connecticut

Hartford Hospital
Radiation Therapy Prgm
80 Seymour St
Hartford, CT 06115-5037
http://harthosp.org
Prgm Dir: Nora Uricchio, MEd RT(R)(T)
Tel: 860 545-3956   *Fax:* 860 545-6461
E-mail: nuricch@harthosp.org

Gateway Community College
Radiation Therapy Prgm
88 Bassett Rd
North Haven, CT 06473
www.gwcc.commnet.edu
Prgm Dir: Gina M Finn, RT(T)
Tel: 203 285-2392   *Fax:* 203 285-2400
E-mail: gfinn@gwcc.commnet.edu

District of Columbia

Howard University
Radiation Therapy Prgm
515½ W Street NW
Washington, DC 20059
Prgm Dir: Adrienne D Harrison, MS RT(T)
Tel: 202 806-5920   *Fax:* 202 806-4476
E-mail: aharrison@howard.edu

Florida

21st Cent Oncology Inc Sch-Rad Therapy Tech
Radiation Therapy Prgm
Cape Coral Office
1419 SE 8th Terrace
Cape Coral, FL 33990
Prgm Dir: Claire Marie Skowronski, MS RT(R)(T) CMD
Tel: 239 573-5972
E-mail: cskowronski@rtsx.com

Halifax Medical Center
Radiation Therapy Prgm
303 N Clyde Morris Blvd, PO Box 2830
Daytona Beach, FL 32120-2830
https://halifax-cancer.org
Prgm Dir: Belinda H Phillips, BS RT(R)(T)
Tel: 386 254-4075, Ext 3510   *Fax:* 386 254-4231
E-mail: belinda.phillips@halifax.org

Miami Dade College
Radiation Therapy Prgm
Medical Center Campus
950 NW 20th St
Miami, FL 33127
www.mdc.edu
Prgm Dir: Deborah Hughes, MBA
Tel: 305 237-4034   *Fax:* 305 237-4278
E-mail: dhughes@mdc.edu

Hillsborough Community College
Radiation Therapy Prgm
PO Box 30030
Tampa, FL 33614
Prgm Dir: Karen M Nelson, MS RT(R)(T)
Tel: 813 253-7372   *Fax:* 813 253-7491
E-mail: knelson@hccfl.edu

Georgia

Grady Health System
Radiation Therapy Prgm
80 Jesse Hill Jr Dr SE, PO Box 26095
Atlanta, GA 30303-3050
www.gradyhealthsystem.org
Prgm Dir: Kevin Kindle, BS RT(T)
Tel: 404 616-5024   *Fax:* 404 616-3512
E-mail: kkindle@gmh.edu

Medical College of Georgia
Radiation Therapy Prgm
Ga Radiation Therapy Center
821 St Sebastian Way, Bldg HK
Augusta, GA 30912
www.mcg.edu
Prgm Dir: Anne Marie Vann, MEd CMD RT(R)(T)
Tel: 706 721-2971   *Fax:* 706 721-7248
E-mail: amvann@mcg.edu

Coosa Valley Technical College
Radiation Therapy Prgm
One Maurice Culberson Dr
Rome, GA 30161
Prgm Dir: Susan Y Lanham, MEd(L) BS RT(T)
Tel: 706 295-6962
E-mail: slanham@coosavalleytech.edu

Armstrong Atlantic State University
Radiation Therapy Prgm
11935 Abercorn St
Savannah, GA 31419-1997
Prgm Dir: Lee Braswell, Jr, MPH RT(T)
Tel: 912 927-5360, Ext 7429   *Fax:* 912 921-5838
E-mail: braswele@mail.armstrong.edu

Illinois

Northwestern Memorial Hospital
Radiation Therapy Prgm
251 E Huron St
Galter Pavilion LC-178
Chicago, IL 60611
www.nmh.org
Prgm Dir: Sandy L Piehl, MPA RT(R)(T)
Tel: 312 926-2733   *Fax:* 312 926-6374
E-mail: spiehl@nmh.org

Swedish American Hospital
Radiation Therapy Prgm
1401 E State St
Rockford, IL 61104
Prgm Dir: Leia Levy, MAdEd RT(T)
Tel: 815 961-2038   *Fax:* 815 966-3966
E-mail: llevy@swedishamerican.org

Indiana

Indiana University Northwest
Radiation Therapy Prgm
3400 Broadway St
Gary, IN 46408-1197
Prgm Dir: Dorothy B Rytczak, BS RT(R)(T)
Tel: 219 981-4204   *Fax:* 219 980-6649
E-mail: drytczak@iun.edu

Indiana University
Radiation Therapy Prgm
School of Medicine, Dept of Radiation Oncology
535 Barnhill Dr, RT 041
Indianapolis, IN 46202
Prgm Dir: Donna Kay Dunn, MS RT(T)
Tel: 317 274-1302   *Fax:* 317 274-4723
E-mail: dodunn@iupui.edu

Iowa

University of Iowa Hospitals & Clinics
Radiation Therapy Prgm
200 Hawkins Dr, LL West Addition PFP
Iowa City, IA 52242-1009
Prgm Dir: Mindi J TenNapel, MBA RT(R)(T)
Tel: 319 356-8286   *Fax:* 319 356-1530
E-mail: mindi-tennapel@uiowa.edu

Kentucky

Univ of Kentucky Hospital
Radiation Therapy Prgm
800 Rose St, Rm C-15
Lexington, KY 40536-0293
www.mc.uky.edu/radiationmedicine/
Prgm Dir: David Lockhart, BS RT(R)(T)
Tel: 859 323-6486   *Fax:* 859 257-4931
E-mail: dklock2@uky.edu
Notes: Currently inactive

James Graham Brown Cancer Center
Radiation Therapy Prgm
University of Louisville Hospital
529 S Jackson St
Louisville, KY 40202
Prgm Dir: Mellonie F Brown, BS RT(T)
Tel: 502 562-4656   *Fax:* 502 562-3209
E-mail: mellonbr@ulh.org

Louisiana

Delgado Community College
Radiation Therapy Prgm
615 City Park Ave
New Orleans, LA 70119
www.dcc.edu
Prgm Dir: Sylvia P Sandberg, BS RT(R)(T)
Tel: 504 671-6230   *Fax:* 504 483-4609
E-mail: ssandb@dcc.edu

Maine

Southern Maine Community College
Radiation Therapy Prgm
Two Fort Rd
South Portland, ME 04106
www.smccME.edu
Prgm Dir: Dennis T Leaver, MS RT(R)(T)
Tel: 207 741-5593   *Fax:* 207 741-5593
E-mail: dleaver@smccME.edu

Maryland

Community College of Baltimore County - Essex Campus
Radiation Therapy Prgm
7201 Rossville Blvd
Baltimore, MD 21237-9987
Prgm Dir: Dionne M Johnson, MEd RT(T)
Tel: 410 780-6709   *Fax:* 410 780-6946
E-mail: djohnson3@ccbcmd.edu

Massachusetts

Caritas Labour, College
Radiation Therapy Prgm
2120 Dorchester Ave
Boston, MA 02124-5698
www.laboure.edu
Prgm Dir: Pauline E Clancy, MS RT(T)
Tel: 617 296-8300, Ext 4044   *Fax:* 617 296-7947
E-mail: pauline_clancy@laboure.edu

Mass College of Pharmacy & Health Sciences
Radiation Therapy Prgm
179 Longwood Ave
Boston, MA 02115-5896
www.mcphs.edu
Prgm Dir: Susan B Belinsky, EdD RT(R)(T)
Tel: 617 732-2261   *Fax:* 617 732-2075
E-mail: sbelinsky@mcphs.edu

Suffolk University
Radiation Therapy Prgm
Physics Department
41 Temple St
Boston, MA 02114
Prgm Dir: Gina C Passmore, MS RT(T)
Tel: 617 573-1995   *Fax:* 617 367-5063
E-mail: gpassmore@suffolk.edu

UMass Memorial Medical Center
Radiation Therapy Prgm
Radiation Oncology Department
55 Lake Ave N
Worcester, MA 01655
Prgm Dir: Patricia E Webster, MS RT(T)
Tel: 508 856-5551   *Fax:* 508 856-5006
E-mail: WebsterP@ummhc.org

Michigan

Wayne State University
Radiation Therapy Prgm
Eugene Applebaum College of Pharmacy and
   Health Sciences
259 Mack Ave
Detroit, MI 48201
www.wayne.edu
Prgm Dir: Adam F Kempa, MEd RT(T)
Tel: 313 577-1137   *Fax:* 313 577-0908
E-mail: aa1156@wayne.edu

University of Michigan - Flint
Radiation Therapy Prgm
H2108 William S White Bldg
303 E Kearsley St
Flint, MI 48502-1950
Prgm Dir: Kelly A Brown, BS RT(T)
Tel: 810 237-6502   *Fax:* 810 762-3003
E-mail: brownkel@umflint.edu

Grand Valley State University
Radiation Therapy Prgm
301 Michigan St NE, Ste 200
Grand Rapids, MI 49503
Prgm Dir: Bonita Pawloski, BS RT(R)(T)
Tel: 616 331-5949
E-mail: pawloskb@gvsu.edu

Baker College of Jackson
Radiation Therapy Prgm
2800 Springport Rd
Jackson, MI 49202
Prgm Dir: Terilynn K Fedchenko, BS RT(R)(T)
Tel: 517 780-4562   *Fax:* 517 789-7331
E-mail: teri.fedchenko@baker.edu

William Beaumont Hospital
Radiation Therapy Prgm
3601 W 13 Mile Rd
Royal Oak, MI 48073-6769
www.beaumonthospitals.com
Prgm Dir: Laura L Ochs, MEd RT(T)
Tel: 248 551-7156   *Fax:* 248 551-7166
E-mail: lochs@beaumont.edu

Minnesota

Argosy University - Twin Cities
Radiation Therapy Prgm
1515 Cental Parkway
Eagan, MN 55121
Prgm Dir: Laura J Peterson, MEd RT(R)(T)
Tel: 651 846-3404   *Fax:* 651 994-0895
E-mail: lpeterson@argosy.edu

Fairview University
Radiation Therapy Prgm
420 Delaware St SE
MMC Box 494
Minneapolis, MN 55455
Prgm Dir: Patricia M Fountinelle, MS RT(R)(T) CMD
Tel: 612 273-5107   *Fax:* 612 273-6411
E-mail: pfounti1@fairview.org

Mayo School of Health Sciences
Radiation Therapy Prgm
Sch of Hlth Sciences
200 First St SW
Rochester, MN 55905
www.mayo.edu/mshs
Prgm Dir: Leila A Bussman-Yeakel, BS RT(R)(T)
Tel: 507 284-4148   *Fax:* 507 284-0079
E-mail: bussmanyeakel.leila@mayo.edu

Missouri

CoxHealth
Radiation Therapy Prgm
3850 S National Ave, Ste 100
Springfield, MO 65807
www.coxhealth.com
Prgm Dir: Benjamin J Morris, BS RT(R)(T)(CT)
Tel: 417 269-5363   *Fax:* 417 269-6979
E-mail: benjamin.morris@coxhealth.com

Lester E Cox Medical Center South
Radiation Therapy Prgm
3850 S National Ave, Ste 100
Springfield, MO 65807
Prgm Dir: Sarah J Friend, BS RT(R)(T)
Tel: 417 269-5363
E-mail: sarah.friend@coxhealth.com

**Saint Louis University Doisy College of
   Health Sciences**
Radiation Therapy Prgm
3437 Caroline St
St Louis, MO 63104
Prgm Dir: Kathleen O Kienstra, MAT RT(R)(T)
Tel: 314 977-8630   *Fax:* 314 454-5239
E-mail: kkienst1@slu.edu

Nebraska

University of Nebraska Medical Center
Radiation Therapy Prgm
984545 Nebraska Medical Center
Omaha, NE 68198-4545
www.unmc.edu/alliedhealth/rste
Prgm Dir: Lisa Bartenhagen, MS RT(R)(T)
Tel: 402 559-4236   *Fax:* 402 559-2181
E-mail: labarten@unmc.edu

New Hampshire

New Hampshire Technical Institute
Radiation Therapy Prgm
31 College Dr
Concord, NH 03301
Prgm Dir: Amy C VonKadich, MEd RT(T)
Tel: 603 271-0700
E-mail: avonkadich@nhctc.edu

New Jersey

Cooper University Hospital
Radiation Therapy Prgm
One Cooper Plaza
Camden, NJ 08103
Prgm Dir: Karen D Ljunggren, BS RT(R)(T)(CT)
Tel: 856 342-2734   *Fax:* 609 365-8504
E-mail: Ljunggren-Karen@cooperhealth.edu

St Barnabas Medical Center
Radiation Therapy Prgm
94 Old Short Hills Rd
Livingston, NJ 07039
www.sbhcs.com
Prgm Dir: Jennie S Lichtenberger, MAS RT(T)(R)(M)
Tel: 973 322-5628   *Fax:* 973 322-5648
E-mail: jlichtenberger@sbhcs.com

Muhlenberg Regional Medical Center
Radiation Therapy Prgm
Park Ave and Randolph Rd
Plainfield, NJ 07061
Prgm Dir: Beverly S Nias, MS RT(R)(T) ARRT
Tel: 908 668-2637   *Fax:* 908 226-4568
E-mail: bnias@solarishs.org

New York

New York Methodist Hospital
Radiation Therapy Prgm
506 Sixth St, Box 159008
Brooklyn, NY 11215-9008
Prgm Dir: Mary Reynolds, BA RT(T)
Tel: 718 645-3500, Ext 121   *Fax:* 718 780-3637
E-mail: marybreynolds@aol.com

Erie Community College
Radiation Therapy Prgm
121 Ellicott St
Buffalo, NY 14203
Prgm Dir: Patricia A Bennewitz, MSEd RT(T)
Tel: 716 851-1048, Ext 1048   *Fax:* 716 851-1129
E-mail: bennewitz@ecc.edu

Nassau Community College
Radiation Therapy Prgm
One Education Dr
Garden City, NY 11530
Prgm Dir: Catherine Smyth, MA RT(T)
Tel: 516 572-7491   *Fax:* 516 572-9750
E-mail: cquane@aol.com

Memorial Sloan-Kettering Cancer Ctr
Radiation Therapy Prgm
School of Radiation Therapy
1275 York Ave / Box 22
New York, NY 10065
www.mskcc.org/schoolofradiationtherapy
Prgm Dir: Wilson H Apollo, BA RT(T)
Tel: 212 639-6835   *Fax:* 212 717-3090
E-mail: apollow@mskcc.org

SUNY Upstate Medical University
Radiation Therapy Prgm
750 E Adams St
Syracuse, NY 13210
www.upstate.edu
Prgm Dir: Joan E O'Brien, MSEd RT(T)
Tel: 315 464-8448   *Fax:* 315 464-6940
E-mail: obrienj@upstate.edu

North Carolina

Pitt Community College
Radiation Therapy Prgm
PO Drawer 7007
Greenville, NC 27835-7007
http://www.health.pittcc.edu/rad/radiation.htm
Prgm Dir: Elaine Spencer, BS RT(T)
Tel: 252 493-7452   *Fax:* 252 321-4451
E-mail: espencer@email.pittcc.edu

Forsyth Technical Community College
Radiation Therapy Prgm
2100 Silas Creek Pkwy
Winston-Salem, NC 27104
www.forsythtech.edu
Prgm Dir: Christina R Gibson, MPH RT(R)(T)
Tel: 336 734-7184   *Fax:* 336 734-7444
E-mail: cgibson@forsythtech.edu

Ohio

Aultman Hospital
Radiation Therapy Prgm
2600 Sixth St SW
Canton, OH 44710
Prgm Dir: Victoria Migge, MS RT(R)(T)
Tel: 330 363-4853   *Fax:* 330 588-2601
E-mail: vmigge@aultman.com

University of Cincinnati
Cosponsor: Raymond Walters College
Radiation Therapy Prgm
234 Goodman Ave, ML 757
Cincinnati, OH 45219
Prgm Dir: Carolyn Hollan, MS RT(R)(T)
Tel: 513 584-9099   *Fax:* 513 584-4007
E-mail: carolyn.hollan@uc.edu

Cleveland Clinic Foundation
Radiation Therapy Prgm
9500 Euclid Ave, T28
Cleveland, OH 44195
Prgm Dir: Patricia A Barrett, MS RT(R)(T) CMD
Tel: 216 444-5484   *Fax:* 216 445-1217
E-mail: barretp1@ccf.org

A G James Cancer Hosp & Research Inst
Radiation Therapy Prgm
300 W Tenth Ave
Columbus, OH 43210
Prgm Dir: Ruth M Hackworth, BS RT(R)(T)
Tel: 614 293-6203   *Fax:* 614 293-4044
E-mail: ruth.hackworth@osumc.edu

Oklahoma

Univ of Oklahoma Health Sciences Center
Radiation Therapy Prgm
PO Box 26901 Rm 451
Oklahoma City, OK 73190
www.ah.ouhsc.edu/main/
Prgm Dir: Stacy L Anderson, MS RT(T) CMD
Tel: 405 271-6477, Ext 41169   *Fax:* 405 271-1424
E-mail: stacy-anderson@ouhsc.edu

Oregon

Oregon Health & Science University
Radiation Therapy Prgm
3181 SW Sam Jackson Park Rd, GH 124
Portland, OR 97239-3098
http://euston.ohsu.edu/radiation_therapy
Prgm Dir: Anne M Maddeford, MS MAcOM RT(T) LAc
Tel: 503 494-6708   *Fax:* 503 494-2730
E-mail: maddefoa@ohsu.edu

Pennsylvania

Gwynedd-Mercy College
Radiation Therapy Prgm
1325 Sumneytown Pike
PO Box 901
Gwynedd Valley, PA 19437-0901
www.gmc.edu
Prgm Dir: Patricia J Giordano, MS RT(R)(T)
Tel: 215 542-4658   *Fax:* 215 641-5559
E-mail: giordano.p@gmc.edu

Thomas Jefferson University
Radiation Therapy Prgm
130 S Ninth St, Ste 1013
Philadelphia, PA 19107
Prgm Dir: Donna M Powell, BS RT(T) CMD
Tel: 215 503-1434
E-mail: donna.powell@jefferson.edu

Comm College of Allegheny County
Radiation Therapy Prgm
808 Ridge Ave, M607
Pittsburgh, PA 15212-6097
www.ccac.edu
Prgm Dir: Elizabeth Anne Harkay, BS RT(T)
Tel: 412 237-2752   *Fax:* 412 237-6579
E-mail: eharkay@ccac.edu

South Carolina

Spartanburg Community College
Radiation Therapy Prgm
PO Box 4386
Spartanburg, SC 29305-4386
Prgm Dir: M Lynne Eggert, BS RT(R)(T)
Tel: 864 591-9417   *Fax:* 864 591-3881
E-mail: eggertl@sccsc.edu

Tennessee

Chattanooga State Technical Comm College
Radiation Therapy Prgm
4501 Amnicola Hwy
Chattanooga, TN 37406
Prgm Dir: Lisa Legg, MA RT(R)(T)
Tel: 423 697-3336   *Fax:* 423 697-3324
E-mail: lisa.legg@chattanoogastate.edu

Baptist College of Health Sciences
Radiation Therapy Prgm
1003 Monroe Ave
Memphis, TN 38104
www.bchs.edu
Prgm Dir: Beverly K Coker, MA RT(R)(T)
Tel: 901 572-2645   *Fax:* 901 572-2750
E-mail: beverly.coker@bchs.edu

Vanderbilt University Medical Center
Radiation Therapy Prgm
Center for Radiation Oncology
The Vanderbilt Clinic B 902
Nashville, TN 37232-5671
Prgm Dir: April D Tingler, BS RT(R)(T)
Tel: 615 343-4304   *Fax:* 615 343-0161
E-mail: april.d.tingler@vanderbilt.edu

Texas

Amarillo College
Radiation Therapy Prgm
PO Box 447
Amarillo, TX 79105-9973
www.actx.edu
Prgm Dir: Tony Tackitt, MEd RT(T)
Tel: 806 354-6063   *Fax:* 806 354-6076
E-mail: tackitt-tm@actx.edu

Galveston College
Radiation Therapy Prgm
4015 Ave Q
Galveston, TX 77550-2782
Prgm Dir: Hubert Callahan, MSRS RT(R)(T)
Tel: 409 944-1492   *Fax:* 409 772-3014
E-mail: hcallaha@gc.edu

Univ of Texas M D Anderson Cancer Ctr
Radiation Therapy Prgm
1515 Holcombe Blvd, PO Unit 190
Houston, TX 77030-4009
Prgm Dir: Shaun T Caldwell, MS RT(R)(T)
Tel: 713 792-3455   *Fax:* 713 792-0956
E-mail: scaldwell@mdanderson.org

Texas State University - San Marcos
Radiation Therapy Prgm
601 University Dr
San Marcos, TX 78666
Prgm Dir: Ronnie G Lozano, MSRS RT(T)(ARRT)
Tel: 512 245-9081   *Fax:* 512 245-1477
E-mail: rl10@txstate.edu

Virginia

University of Virginia Health System
Cosponsor: University of Virginia Medical Center
Radiation Therapy Prgm
PO Box 800383
Charlottesville, VA 22908-0383
www.healthsystem.virginia.edu/radonc
Prgm Dir: Frances R Taylor, BA RT(R)(T)
Tel: 434 243-2760   *Fax:* 434 982-3262
E-mail: frt@virginia.edu

Virginia Commonwealth University
Radiation Therapy Prgm
701 W Grace St, Ste 2100
Box 843057
Richmond, VA 23298-3057
Prgm Dir: Melanie Dempsey, RTT CMD
Tel: 804 828-9104   *Fax:* 804 828-5778
E-mail: mcdempsey@vcu.edu

Virginia Western Community College
Radiation Therapy Prgm
PO Box 14007
Roanoke, VA 24038
Prgm Dir: Carole S Graham, MS RT(R)(T)
Tel: 540 981-7731   *Fax:* 540 981-7528
E-mail: cgraham@vw.vccs.edu

Washington

Bellevue Community College
Radiation Therapy Prgm
3000 Landerholm Circle SE, Rm B243
Bellevue, WA 98007-6484
www.bellevuecollege.edu
Prgm Dir: Julius B Armstrong, MBA RT(T)
Tel: 425 564-5079   *Fax:* 425 564-4193
E-mail: jarmstro@bcc.ctc.edu

West Virginia

West Virginia University Hospitals
Radiation Therapy Prgm
PO Box 8150/Medical Ctr Dr
Morgantown, WV 26506-8150
www.wvuhradtech.com
Prgm Dir: Christina M Paugh, MA RT(R)(T)
Tel: 304 598-4715   *Fax:* 304 598-4717
E-mail: paughc@wvuh.com

Wisconsin

Moraine Park Technical College
Radiation Therapy Prgm
235 N National Ave
Fond du Lac, WI 54936
Prgm Dir: Kerry J Stehlik, MS RT(R)(T)
Tel: 920 924-6395
E-mail: kstehlik@excel.net

University of Wisconsin - La Crosse
Radiation Therapy Prgm
1725 State St, 4094 HSC
La Crosse, WI 54601
Prgm Dir: Nishele D Lenards, BS RT(R)(T)
Tel: 608 785-5017   *Fax:* 608 785-8460
E-mail: lenards.nish@uwlax.edu

Radiation Therapist

Programs*	Class Capacity	Begins	Length (months)	Award	Res. Tuition	Non-res. Tuition	Stipend	Offers:‡ 1	2	3	4
Alabama											
University of Alabama at Birmingham	50	Aug Jan	18	Dipl, Cert, BS	$10,002	$20,004				•	•
Arkansas											
Central Arkansas Radiation Therapy Inst (Little Rock)	15	Aug	12	Cert	$3,000	$3,000				•	
California											
City of Hope (Duarte)	14	Oct	12	Cert	$3,000	$3,000				•	
Connecticut											
Gateway Community College (North Haven)	28	Jun	22	AS	$4,029	$9,940		•			
Hartford Hospital	16	Sep	24, 16	Cert	$3,000	$3,000				•	
Florida											
Halifax Medical Center (Daytona Beach)	8	Rotating	15	Cert	$2,800	$2,800				•	
Miami Dade College	58	Aug	24, 12	AS	$2,654	$8,807				•	
Georgia											
Armstrong Atlantic State University (Savannah)	15	Jun	24	BS	$4,575	$15,987				•	•
Coosa Valley Technical College (Rome)	34	Fall quarter	12, 21	Dipl, Cert, AAS	$1,480	$0					
Grady Health System (Atlanta)	16	Sep	12	Cert	$8,000	$8,000				•	
Medical College of Georgia (Augusta)	14	Aug	21	Cert, BS	$5,691	$20,127					
Illinois											
Northwestern Memorial Hospital (Chicago)	8	Aug	12	Cert, BS	$5,000	$5,000				•	
Swedish American Hospital (Rockford)	10	Aug	17, 22	Cert	$3,000	$3,000				•	
Indiana											
Indiana University (Indianapolis)	14	Jun	48	BS	$9,654	$23,769				•	
Indiana University Northwest (Gary)	10	Jul	22	BS	$5,000	$14,750					
Kentucky											
Univ of Kentucky Hospital (Lexington)	6	Sep	12	Cert	$1,500	$1,500				•	
Louisiana											
Delgado Community College (New Orleans)	8	Each 16 Months	16	Cert	$1,800	$7,400				•	
Maine											
Southern Maine Community College (South Portland)	11	Sep	15, 24	AS	$3,192	$5,620		•			
Massachusetts											
Caritas Labour, College (Boston)	19	Sep	24	AS	$16,625	$0		•			
Mass College of Pharmacy & Health Sciences (Boston)	60	Sep	33, 21	BS	$22,000	$22,000				•	
UMass Memorial Medical Center (Worcester)	7	Sep	15	Cert	$4,500	$4,500				•	
Michigan											
Wayne State University (Detroit)	28	Sep	48	BS (RT)	$9,978	$21,178				•	
William Beaumont Hospital (Royal Oak)	6	Sep	24	Cert	$4,256	$4,256				•	
Minnesota											
Mayo School of Health Sciences (Rochester)	8	Sep	12	Cert	$9,000	$9,000				•	
Missouri											
CoxHealth (Springfield)	4	Late Sep	14	Cert	$3,500	$3,500				•	
Nebraska											
University of Nebraska Medical Center (Omaha)	19	Aug	12	Dipl, BS	$7,290	$21,650				•	•
New Jersey											
St Barnabas Medical Center (Livingston)	12	Sep	12	Cert	$7,000	$7,000				•	
New York											
Erie Community College (Buffalo)	17	Sep	24	AAS	$2,500	$5,000					
Memorial Sloan-Kettering Cancer Ctr (New York)	20	Sep	24	Cert	$3,000	$3,000				‡	
SUNY Upstate Medical University (Syracuse)	15	Aug	20	BS	$5,798	$14,146				•	
North Carolina											
Forsyth Technical Community College (Winston-Salem)	22	Aug	24, 12	AAS	$2,000	$10,000					
Pitt Community College (Greenville)	30	Aug	12	Dipl	$1,500	$7,800					
Ohio											
A G James Cancer Hosp & Research Inst (Columbus)	10	Sep	15	Cert	$3,000	$3,000					
Cleveland Clinic Foundation	9	Jul	12	Cert	$3,500	$3,500				•	

*Data are shown only for programs that completed the 2007 AMA Survey of Health Professions Education Programs.
‡Key to Offers: 1: Evening or weekend classes; 2: Non-English instruction; 3: Cultural competence instruction; 4: Distance education component.

Radiation Therapist

Programs*	Class Capacity	Begins	Length (months)	Award	Res. Tuition	Non-res. Tuition	Stipend	Offers:‡ 1	2	3	4
Oklahoma											
Univ of Oklahoma Health Sciences Center (Oklahoma City)	12	Aug	48	BS	$3,522	$7,400				•	
Oregon											
Oregon Health & Science University (Portland)	8	Aug	24	BS	$11,731	$20,864				•	
Pennsylvania											
Comm College of Allegheny County (Pittsburgh)	30	Aug	24, 12	Cert, AS	$3,500	$10,500				•	
Gwynedd-Mercy College (Gwynedd Valley)	13	Sep	20, 40	Cert, BS	$22,000	$22,000				•	
Tennessee											
Baptist College of Health Sciences (Memphis)	8	Fall	48	BS	$7,900	$0		•			
Chattanooga State Technical Comm College	54	Aug	12	Cert	$3,475	$14,330					•
Texas											
Amarillo College	15	Jun	24	AAS	$2,066	$4,600				•	
Virginia											
University of Virginia Health System (Charlottesville)	12	Aug	16	Cert	$4,000	$4,000				•	
Virginia Western Community College (Roanoke)	20		15	Cert	$4,087	$0					
Washington											
Bellevue Community College	25	Sep	24	AA	$4,000	$4,000				•	
West Virginia											
West Virginia University Hospitals (Morgantown)	4	Jul	12	Cert	$2,000	$2,000				•	
Wisconsin											
University of Wisconsin - La Crosse	23	Sep	23	BS	$6,500	$19,000				•	

*Data are shown only for programs that completed the 2007 AMA Survey of Health Professions Education Programs.
‡Key to Offers: 1: Evening or weekend classes; 2: Non-English instruction; 3: Cultural competence instruction; 4: Distance education component.

Radiographer

Alabama

Carraway Methodist Medical Center
Radiography Prgm
1600 Carraway Blvd
Birmingham, AL 35242
Prgm Dir: Robert N Odom, JD RT(R)
Tel: 205 502-6920   *Fax:* 205 502-5365
E-mail: odomb@carraway.com

Jefferson State Community College
Radiography Prgm
2601 Carson Rd
GLB Rm 251
Birmingham, AL 35215
www.jeffstateonline.com
Prgm Dir: Christie W Bolton, MEd RT(R)
Tel: 205 856-6017   *Fax:* 205 856-7725
E-mail: cbolton@jeffstateonline.com

University of Alabama at Birmingham
Radiography Prgm
1705 University Blvd
RMSB 447
Birmingham, AL 35294-1212
http://main.uab.edu/shrp/
Prgm Dir: Audrey Harris, MA Ed RT(R)(CT)(M)(QM)
Tel: 205 934-7539   *Fax:* 205 975-7302
E-mail: radprof@uab.edu

George C Wallace Community College
Radiography Prgm
1141 Wallace Dr
Dothan, AL 36303
Prgm Dir: G Bates Gilmore, BS RT(R)
Tel: 334 556-2299   *Fax:* 334 983-3600
E-mail: bgilmore@wallace.edu

Gadsden State Community College
Radiography Prgm
PO Box 227
Gadsden, AL 35902-0227
http://gadsdenstate.edu
Prgm Dir: Deborah Gay Utz, MEd RT(R)
Tel: 256 549-8468   *Fax:* 256 549-8458
E-mail: gutz@gadsdenstate.edu

Wallace State Community College
Radiography Prgm
PO Box 2000
Hanceville, AL 35077-2000
Prgm Dir: Terrie Gammon, PhD RT(R)(M)
Tel: 256 352-8309   *Fax:* 256 352-8320
E-mail: terrie.gammon@wallacestate.edu

Crestwood Medical Center
Radiography Prgm
One Hospital Dr SE
Huntsville, AL 35801
Prgm Dir: Ronald A Murphree, BS RT(R)
Tel: 256 880-4587
E-mail: ronald.murphree@triadhospitals.com

Huntsville Hospital
Radiography Prgm
101 Sivley Rd
Huntsville, AL 35801
http://huntsvillehospital.org
Prgm Dir: Cheryl Dutton, BS RT(R)
Tel: 256 265-8928   *Fax:* 256 265-9417
E-mail: cdutton@hhsys.org

University of South Alabama
Radiography Prgm
1504 Springhill Ave, Ste 2515
Mobile, AL 36604-3273
Prgm Dir: Charles W Newell, EdD RT(R)(MR)(CV)(CT)
Tel: 251 434-3456   *Fax:* 251 434-3458
E-mail: cnewell@jaguar1.usouthal.edu

Baptist Medical Center South
Radiography Prgm
2169 Normandie Dr
Montgomery, AL 36111
www.baptistfirst.org
Prgm Dir: Paul H Littlefield, EdS RT(R)
Tel: 334 281-3061   *Fax:* 334 281-3671
E-mail: plittlefield@baptistfirst.org

Southern Union State Community College
Radiography Prgm
1701 Lafayette Pkwy
Opelika, AL 36801
http://suscc.edu
Prgm Dir: Carol Southern, EdD RT(R)(CT)
Tel: 334 745-6437, Ext 5517   *Fax:* 334 745-6342
E-mail: jcs@suscc.edu

DCH Regional Medical Center
Radiography Prgm
809 University Blvd E
Tuscaloosa, AL 35401
www.dchsystem.com
Prgm Dir: Dena F Ennis, MA Ed RT(R)
Tel: 205 759-6009   *Fax:* 205 345-8521
E-mail: dennis@dchsystem.com

Arizona

Pima Medical Institute - Mesa
Radiography Prgm
957 S Dobson Rd
Mesa, AZ 85202
Prgm Dir: Nancy M Daugherty, BS RT(R)
Tel: 480 644-0267, Ext 120   *Fax:* 480 649-5249
E-mail: ndaugherty@pmi.edu

Apollo College
Radiography Prgm
2701 W Bethany Home Rd
Phoenix, AZ 85017
Prgm Dir: Joanne S Greathouse, EdS RT(R) FAERS FASRT
Tel: 602 433-1333, Ext 21112   *Fax:* 602 433-1414
E-mail: jgreathouse@apollocollege.edu

GateWay Community College
Radiography Prgm
108 N 40th St
Phoenix, AZ 85034
www.gatewaycc.edu
Prgm Dir: Mary Carrillo, MBA RT(R)(M)(CDT)
Tel: 602 286-8542   *Fax:* 602 286-8480
E-mail: carrillo@gwmail.maricopa.edu

Pima Community College
Radiography Prgm
2202 W Anklam Rd, HRP 220
Tucson, AZ 85709-0080
Prgm Dir: Randall D Dings, BS RT(R)
Tel: 520 206-6916   *Fax:* 520 206-3027
E-mail: rdings@pima.edu

Pima Medical Institute - Tucson
Radiography Prgm
3350 E Grant Rd
Tucson, AZ 85716
Prgm Dir: Michael T Hawkes, BSRS RT(R)
Tel: 520 881-1284
E-mail: mhawkes@pmi.edu

Arizona Western College
Radiography Prgm
PO Box 929
Yuma, AZ 85366-0929
Prgm Dir: Victoria Holas, MEd RT(R)
Tel: 928 314-9574
E-mail: victoria.holas@azwestern.edu

Arkansas

South Arkansas Community College
Radiography Prgm
300 S West Ave
PO Box 7010
El Dorado, AR 71731-7010
www.southark.edu
Prgm Dir: Deborah M Edney, MBA RT(R)
Tel: 870 862-8131, Ext 226   *Fax:* 870 864-7104
E-mail: dedney@southark.edu

University of Arkansas for Medical Sciences
Radiography Prgm
AHEC-Northwest
2907 E Joyce St
Fayetteville, AR 72703
Prgm Dir: Stanley R Olejniczak, MS RT(R)
Tel: 479 521-7615   *Fax:* 479 684-6501
E-mail: solejniczak@ahecnw.uams.edu

University of Arkansas - Fort Smith
Radiography Prgm
5201 Grand Ave
PO Box 3649
Fort Smith, AR 72913-3649
Prgm Dir: Nancy G Hawking, EdD RT(R)
Tel: 501 788-7852   *Fax:* 501 788-7869
E-mail: nhawking@uafortsmith.edu

North Arkansas College
Radiography Prgm
1515 Pioneer Dr
Harrison, AR 72601
www.northark.edu
Prgm Dir: Sondra L Richards, MS RT(R)(M)
Tel: 870 391-3318   *Fax:* 870 391-3250
E-mail: srichard@northark.edu

National Park Community College
Radiography Prgm
101 College Dr
Hot Springs, AR 71913-9174
Prgm Dir: Timothy J Skaife, MA RT(R)
Tel: 501 760-4282   *Fax:* 501 760-4141
E-mail: tskaife@npcc.edu

Baptist Health Schools Little Rock
Radiography Prgm
School of Radiography
11900 Colonel Glenn Rd, Ste 1000
Little Rock, AR 72210-2820
http://baptist-health.com
Prgm Dir: Brenda A Simmons, BS RT(R)
Tel: 501 202-7942   *Fax:* 501 202-7712
E-mail: bsimmons@baptist-health.org

Saint Vincent Health System
Radiography Prgm
Two St Vincent Circle
Little Rock, AR 72205-5499
www.stvincenthealth.com/radtech
Prgm Dir: Frank Porter, RT(R) (QM)
Tel: 501 552-2971   *Fax:* 501 552-4236
E-mail: fporter@stvincenthealth.com

University of Arkansas for Medical Sciences
Radiography Prgm
4301 W Markham St, Slot 563
Little Rock, AR 72205
www.uams.edu/chrp/rad-tech
Prgm Dir: Joseph R Bittengle, MEd RT(R)
Tel: 501 686-6510   *Fax:* 501 686-6513
E-mail: bittenglejosephr@uams.edu

Southeast Arkansas College
Radiography Prgm
1900 Hazel St
Pine Bluff, AR 71603
Prgm Dir: Tina M Pierce, BS RT(R)(M)
Tel: 870 543-5941   *Fax:* 870 543-5912
E-mail: tpierce@seark.edu

Arkansas State University - Jonesboro
Radiography Prgm
PO Box 910
State University, AR 72467
www.clt.astate.edu/RadSci/
Prgm Dir: Raymond F Winters, MS RT(R)
Tel: 870 972-3073, Ext 3329   *Fax:* 870 972-2004
E-mail: rwinters@astate.edu

University of Arkansas for Medical Sciences
Radiography Prgm
300 E Sixth St
Texarkana, AR 71854
www.uams.edu/chrp/rad-tech
Prgm Dir: William M Pedigo, MPA RT(R)
Tel: 870 779-6029   *Fax:* 870 779-6045
E-mail: pedigowilliamm@uams.edu

California

Cabrillo College
Radiography Prgm
6500 Soquel Dr
Aptos, CA 95003
www.cabrillo.edu
Prgm Dir: Ann S Smeltzer, BS RT(R)(M)
Tel: 831 479-5056   *Fax:* 831 479-5748
E-mail: ansmeltz@cabrillo.edu

Bakersfield College
Radiography Prgm
Radiologic Technology Program
1801 Panorama Dr
Bakersfield, CA 93305
www.bakersfieldcollege.edu
Prgm Dir: Nancy J Perkins, MA RT(R)(M)
Tel: 661 395-4284   *Fax:* 661 395-4295
E-mail: nperkins@bakersfieldcollege.edu

Mills-Peninsula Health Services
Radiography Prgm
1501 Trousdale Dr
Burlingame, CA 94010
www.mills-peninsula.org
Prgm Dir: Patricia Sperry, MS ARRT(R)(CT)
Tel: 650 696-5519   *Fax:* 650 696-5995
E-mail: sperryp@sutterhealth.org

Pima Medical Institute
Radiography Prgm
780 Bay Blvd, Ste 101
Chula Vista, CA 91910
Prgm Dir: Lisa F Schmidt, PhD RT(R)(M)
Tel: 619 425-3200, Ext 121   *Fax:* 619 425-0182
E-mail: lschmidt@pmi.edu

Arrowhead Regional Medical Center
Radiography Prgm
400 N Pepper Ave
Colton, CA 92324-1819
Prgm Dir: Morris Hunter, MA RT(R)
Tel: 909 580-3540   *Fax:* 909 580-1561
E-mail: hunterm@armc.sbcounty.gov

Orange Coast College
Radiography Prgm
2701 Fairview Rd, PO Box 5005
Costa Mesa, CA 92628-5005
Prgm Dir: Loren A Sachs, MA RT(R)(CV)(CT)(MR)
Tel: 714 432-5540   *Fax:* 714 432-5534
E-mail: laschs@occ.cccd.edu

Cypress College
Radiography Prgm
9200 Valley View St
Cypress, CA 90630-5897
http://CypressCollege.edu
Prgm Dir: Robert J Parelli, MA RT(R)
Tel: 714 484-7000, Ext 47286   *Fax:* 714 527-2175
E-mail: rparelli@cypresscollege.edu

Fresno City College
Radiography Prgm
1101 E University Ave
Fresno, CA 93741
Prgm Dir: Joseph J Shultz, MEd RT(R)
Tel: 559 244-2618   *Fax:* 559 244-2626
E-mail: Joseph.Shultz@FresnoCityCollege.edu

Loma Linda University
Radiography Prgm
School of Allied Health Professions
Loma Linda, CA 92350
www.llu.edu/llu/sahp
Prgm Dir: Mark J Clements, MA RT(R)
Tel: 909 558-4931, Ext 47272   *Fax:* 909 558-7965
E-mail: mclements@llu.edu

Foothill Community College
Radiography Prgm
12345 El Monte Rd
Los Altos Hills, CA 94022-4599
www.foothill.edu
Prgm Dir: Bonnie M Wheeler, MA RT(R)(M)
Tel: 650 949-7563   *Fax:* 650 949-7686
E-mail: WheelerBonny@foothill.edu

Charles R Drew Univ of Med & Science
Radiography Prgm
1731 E 120th St
Los Angeles, CA 90059
Prgm Dir: Eugene Hasson, MS RT(R)
Tel: 323 563-5835, Ext 5885   *Fax:* 323 357-3419
E-mail: euhasson@cdrewu.edu

East Los Angeles Education and Career Center
Radiography Prgm
2100 Marengo St
Los Angeles, CA 90033
Prgm Dir: Alicia Ortiz, MEd RT(R)(M)
Tel: 323 223-1283, Ext 161   *Fax:* 323 223-6365
E-mail: aokp2@sbcglobal.net

Los Angeles City College
Radiography Prgm
855 N Vermont Ave
Los Angeles, CA 90029
www.lacitycollege.edu
Prgm Dir: John G Radtke, MA RT(R)(N)
Tel: 323 953-4000, Ext 2943   *Fax:* 323 953-4013
E-mail: JGR5150@Yahoo.com

Yuba Community College
Radiography Prgm
2088 N Beale Rd
Marysville, CA 95901
www.yccd.edu/radtech
Prgm Dir: Angela Willson, PhD MPA RT(R)(M)(QM)
Tel: 530 741-6960   *Fax:* 530 741-3541
E-mail: awillson@yccd.edu

Merced College
Radiography Prgm
3600 M St
Merced, CA 95348-2898
www.mccd.edu/alliedhealth/radtechhp.htm
Prgm Dir: K Judy Rose, MA RT(R)
Tel: 209 384-6132   *Fax:* 209 384-6167
E-mail: rose.j@mccd.edu

Moorpark College
Radiography Prgm
7075 Campus Rd
Moorpark, CA 93021
www.moorparkcollege.net
Prgm Dir: Guadalupe Aldana, MS RT(R)
Tel: 805 378-1400, Ext 1632   *Fax:* 805 378-1548
E-mail: laldana@vcccd.net

Maric College
Radiography Prgm
6180 Laurel Canyon Blvd, Ste 101
North Hollywood, CA 91606
Prgm Dir: Maria A Kelly, BFA RT(R)(CT)
Tel: 818 763-2563, Ext 247
E-mail: mkelly@mariccollege.edu

California State University - Northridge
Radiography Prgm
18111 Nordhoff St
Northridge, CA 91330-8285
www.csun.edu/~vchsc02t/
Prgm Dir: Anita M Slechta, MS RT(R)(M)
Tel: 818 677-2475   *Fax:* 818 677-2045
E-mail: anita.slechta@csun.edu

Merritt College
Radiography Prgm
12500 Campus Dr
Oakland, CA 94619
http://merritt.peralta.edu
Prgm Dir: Jennifer L Yates, MS RT(R)(M)(BD)
Tel: 510 436-2427   *Fax:* 510 434-3870
E-mail: jyates@peralta.edu

Pasadena City College
Radiography Prgm
1570 E Colorado Blvd
Pasadena, CA 91106-2003
Prgm Dir: Leavon Spires, MA BS RT(R)(T) CRT
Tel: 626 585-7469   *Fax:* 626 585-7977
E-mail: lxspires@pasadena.edu

Chaffey College
Radiography Prgm
5885 Haven Ave
Rancho Cucamonga, CA 91737
Prgm Dir: Andrea Guillen Dutton, MEd RT(R)(M)
Tel: 909 477-8978   *Fax:* 909 477-8984
E-mail: andrea.dutton@chaffey.edu

Canada College
Radiography Prgm
4200 Farm Hill Blvd
Redwood City, CA 94061
Prgm Dir: Rafael A Rivera, RT(R)
Tel: 650 306-3283   *Fax:* 650 306-3281
E-mail: riverar@smccd.net

Kaiser Permanente Sch of Allied Hlth Sciences
Cosponsor: Richmond Medical Center
Radiography Prgm
938 Marina Way S
Richmond, CA 94804
www.kpsahs.org
Prgm Dir: Gregory J Wheeler, BA CRT
Tel: 510 231-5032   *Fax:* 510 231-5129
E-mail: Gregory.Wheeler@kp.org

Naval School of Health Sciences, San Diego
Radiography Prgm
34101 Farenholt Ave
San Diego, CA 92134
Prgm Dir: John F Somersall, BS RT(R)
Tel: 619 532-9522   *Fax:* 619 532-8189
E-mail: john.somersall@med.navy.mil

San Diego Mesa College
Radiography Prgm
7250 Mesa College Dr
San Diego, CA 92111
Prgm Dir: Catherine M Bertsch, BS RT(R)(M)(MR)
Tel: 916 388-2666   *Fax:* 916 388-2929
E-mail: cbertsch@sdccd.edu

City College of San Francisco
Radiography Prgm
50 Phelan Ave, Box S69
San Francisco, CA 94112
www.ccsf.edu/dmi
Prgm Dir: Kyle R Thornton, MA Ed CRT RT
Tel: 415 239-3694   *Fax:* 415 239-3930
E-mail: kthornto@ccsf.edu

Central California School of Continuing Edu
Radiography Prgm
3195 McMillan #F
San Luis Obispo, CA 93401
www.ccsce.org
Prgm Dir: Robert Desch, MS BA RT(R)
Tel: 805 543-9123   *Fax:* 805 543-6330
E-mail: ccsce@ccsce.org

Santa Barbara City College
Radiography Prgm
721 Cliff Dr
Santa Barbara, CA 93109-2394
Prgm Dir: Debra S McMahan, MSHS RT(R)
Tel: 805 965-0581, Ext 2504   *Fax:* 805 963-7222
E-mail: mcmahan@sbcc.edu

Santa Rosa Junior College
Radiography Prgm
1501 Mendocino Ave
Santa Rosa, CA 95401-4395
Prgm Dir: Xuan M Ho, PhD RT(R)
Tel: 707 527-4346   *Fax:* 707 527-4426
E-mail: xho@santarosa.edu

San Joaquin General Hospital
Radiography Prgm
PO Box 1020
Stockton, CA 95201
Prgm Dir: John S Job, MA RT(R)
Tel: 209 468-6233   *Fax:* 209 468-6038
E-mail: jjob@sjgh.org

El Camino College
Radiography Prgm
16007 S Crenshaw Blvd
Torrance, CA 90506
Prgm Dir: Dawn N Guzman, MEd RT(R)(M)
Tel: 310 660-3247   *Fax:* 310 660-3806
E-mail: dguzman@elcamino.edu

LA County Harbor UCLA Medical Center
Radiography Prgm
1000 W Carson St, Box 27
PO Box 2910
Torrance, CA 90509-2910
Prgm Dir: Tuyen T Bui, MSHS RT(R)
Tel: 310 222-2825   *Fax:* 310 618-9500
E-mail: tubui@ladhs.org

Mt San Antonio College
Radiography Prgm
1100 N Grand Ave
Walnut, CA 91789-1399
Prgm Dir: David L McLaughlin, BS RT(R)
Tel: 909 594-5611, Ext 4527   *Fax:* 909 468-3938
E-mail: dmclaugh@mtsac.edu

Colorado

Red Rocks Community College
Radiography Prgm
5420 Miller St
Arvada, CO 80002
www.rrcc.edu/medicalimaging
Prgm Dir: John F Trombly, BSRS
Tel: 303 914-6034   *Fax:* 303 420-9572
E-mail: john.trombly@rrcc.edu

Concorde Career College - Aurora
Radiography Prgm
111 N Havana St
Aurora, CO 80010
www.concorde.edu
Prgm Dir: Richard M Crabb, MPA RT(R)(MR)
Tel: 720 207-0499   *Fax:* 303 839-5478
E-mail: rcrabb@concorde.edu

Memorial Hospital
Radiography Prgm
1400 E Boulder
175 S Union, Ste 240
Colorado Springs, CO 80909
http://memorialhealthsystem.com
Prgm Dir: Elaine R Ivan, MA RT(R)(M)
Tel: 719 365-8291   *Fax:* 719 365-5374
E-mail: elaine.ivan@memorialhealthsystem.com

Centura Health-St Anthony Hospitals
Radiography Prgm
1601 Lowell Blvd
Denver, CO 80204-1597
Prgm Dir: Wayne J Stellick, MA Ed RT(R)
Tel: 303 899-5265   *Fax:* 303 899-5134
E-mail: waynestellick@centura.org

Community College of Denver - Lowry Campus
Radiography Prgm
1070 Alton Way, Bldg 849
Denver, CO 80230
Prgm Dir: Donna R Kimrey, RT(R)
Tel: 303 365-8379   *Fax:* 303 365-8396
E-mail: donna.kimrey@ccd.edu

Pima Medical Institute - Denver
Radiography Prgm
7475 Dakin St, Ste 100
Denver, CO 80221
Prgm Dir: Ryan Z Minic, MPH RT(R)
Tel: 303 426-1800   *Fax:* 303 450-4048
E-mail: rminic@pmi.edu

Mesa State College
Radiography Prgm
1100 North Ave
Grand Junction, CO 81501
www.mesastate.edu
Prgm Dir: Bette Schans, PhD RT(R)
Tel: 970 248-1651   *Fax:* 970 248-1133
E-mail: bschans@mesastate.edu

Connecticut

St Vincent's College
Radiography Prgm
2800 Main St
Bridgeport, CT 06606
www.stvincentscollege.edu
Prgm Dir: Terry K Hine, MAT RT(R)(M)
Tel: 203 576-5072   *Fax:* 203 581-6533
E-mail: thine@stvincentscollege.edu

Danbury Hospital
Radiography Prgm
24 Hospital Ave
Danbury, CT 06810
www.danburyhospital.org
Prgm Dir: Ruthanna T Shanley, RT(R) RDMS
Tel: 203 739-7182   *Fax:* 203 739-8944
E-mail: ruth.shanley@danhosp.org

Quinnipiac University
Radiography Prgm
Mt Carmel Ave
Hamden, CT 06518-0008
http://qcinet.quinnipiac.edu/q.html
Prgm Dir: William F Hennessy, MHS RT(R)(M)(QM)
Tel: 203 582-5214   *Fax:* 203 582-8706
E-mail: Bill.Hennessy@quinnipiac.edu

Capital Community College
Radiography Prgm
950 Main St
Hartford, CT 06103-1207
Prgm Dir: Paul Creech, Esq, MPH JD RT(R)
Tel: 860 906-5155   *Fax:* 860 906-5148
E-mail: pcreech@ccc.commnet.edu

Hartford Hospital
Radiography Prgm
560 Hudson St
Hartford, CT 06106
www.harthosp.org/alliedhealth/radiography
Prgm Dir: Pamela M Cooke, MEd RT(R)(M)
Tel: 860 545-3955   *Fax:* 860 545-6461
E-mail: pcooke@harthosp.org

Middlesex Community College
Radiography Prgm
100 Training Hill Rd
Middletown, CT 06457
Prgm Dir: Elaine Lisitano, BA RT(R)(M)
Tel: 860 344-6505   *Fax:* 860 358-8887
E-mail: elaine_lisitano@midhosp.org

Gateway Community College
Radiography Prgm
88 Bassett Rd
North Haven, CT 06473
Prgm Dir: Julie A Austin, BS RT(R)(M)
Tel: 203 285-2382   *Fax:* 203 285-2400
E-mail: jaustin@gwcc.commnet.edu

Stamford Hospital
Radiography Prgm
Shelburne Rd W Broad St/Box 9317
Stamford, CT 06904-9317
www.stamhealth.org
Prgm Dir: Dorothy A Saia, MA RT(R)(M)
Tel: 203 276-7877   *Fax:* 203 276-7352
E-mail: dsaia@stamhealth.org

Naugatuck Valley Community College
Radiography Prgm
750 Chase Pkwy
Waterbury, CT 06708
www.nvcc.commnet.edu
Prgm Dir: James P Pronovost, MS RT(R)
Tel: 203 575-8266   *Fax:* 203 575-8146
E-mail: jpronovost@nvcc.commnet.edu

University of Hartford
Radiography Prgm
200 Bloomfield Ave
DANA HALL RM 433
West Hartford, CT 06117
www.hartford.edu
Prgm Dir: Azmi A Bani-Baker, MHP RT(R)(MR)
Tel: 860 768-5499   *Fax:* 860 768-5706
E-mail: banibaker@hartford.edu

Windham Community Memorial Hospital
Radiography Prgm
112 Mansfield Ave
Willimantic, CT 06226
Prgm Dir: Mark K Patros, BS RT(R)
Tel: 860 456-6713   *Fax:* 860 456-6838
E-mail: mpatros@wcmh.org

Delaware

Delaware Technical & Community College - Owens Campus
Radiography Prgm
PO Box 610, Seashore Hwy
Georgetown, DE 19947
Prgm Dir: Christy A Moriarty, MEd RT(R)
Tel: 302 855-5934   *Fax:* 302 858-5460
E-mail: cmoriart@dtcc.edu

Delaware Technical & Community College - Wilmington
Radiography Prgm
333 Shipley St
Wilmington, DE 19802
Prgm Dir: Theresa A Foy, MEd RT(R)
Tel: 302 765-4594   *Fax:* 302 765-4599
E-mail: tfoy@christianacare.org

District of Columbia

University of the District of Columbia
Radiography Prgm
4200 Connecticut Ave NW
Washington, DC 20008
Prgm Dir: McDonald G Kpadeh, MEd RT(R)
Tel: 202 274-5882   *Fax:* 202 274-5952
E-mail: kpadeh@udc.edu

Washington Hospital Center
Radiography Prgm
110 Irving St NW
Washington, DC 20010
Prgm Dir: Mitchell Bieber, BA RT(R)
Tel: 202 877-6434   *Fax:* 202 877-8625
E-mail: Mitchell.Bieber@medstar.net

Florida

West Boca Medical Center
Radiography Prgm
21644 State Rd 7
Boca Raton, FL 33428
Prgm Dir: Raymond Mata, BS RT(R)
Tel: 561 488-8173   *Fax:* 561 488-8379
E-mail: Ray.Mata@tenethealth.com

Bethesda Memorial Hospital
Radiography Prgm
2815 S Seacrest Blvd
Boynton Beach, FL 33435
Prgm Dir: Charles E Lockett, Jr, BS RT(R)(CV)
Tel: 561 737-7733, Ext 4792   *Fax:* 561 734-2545
E-mail: Eddie.Lockett@BethesdaHealthcare.com

Manatee Community College
Radiography Prgm
5840 26th St W
Bradenton, FL 32406-1849
www.mccfl.edu/radiography
Prgm Dir: Patrick W Patterson, MS RT(R)(N) CNMT
Tel: 941 752-5245   *Fax:* 941 727-6443
E-mail: patterp@mccfl.edu

Brevard Community College
Radiography Prgm
1519 Clearlake Rd
Cocoa, FL 32922
www.brevardcc.edu
Prgm Dir: Susan A Sheehan, MS RT(R)(M) (QM)
Tel: 321 433-7591   *Fax:* 321 433-7599
E-mail: sheehans@brevardcc.edu

Halifax Medical Center
Radiography Prgm
303 N Clyde Morris Blvd
Daytona Beach, FL 32114
Prgm Dir: Darcie J Nethery, PhD RT(R)
Tel: 386 254-4075, Ext 3509   *Fax:* 386 254-4231
E-mail: darcie.nethery@halifax.org

Keiser University - Daytona Beach
Radiography Prgm
1800 Business Park Blvd
Daytona Beach, FL 32114
Prgm Dir: Gloria E Wyatt, BS RT(R)
Tel: 386 274-5060, Ext 108   *Fax:* 386 274-2725
E-mail: gwyatt@keisercollege.edu

Keiser University
Radiography Prgm
1500 NW 49th St
Fort Lauderdale, FL 33309
www.keisercollege.edu
Prgm Dir: Theresa S Reid-Paul, MBA/HCM RT(R)
Tel: 954 776-4456, Ext 410   *Fax:* 954 776-5157
E-mail: terryr@keiseruniversity.edu

MedVance Institute - Ft Lauderdale Campus/KI
Radiography Prgm
Ft Lauderdale/KIMC Investments, Inc
4850 W Oakland Park Blvd, Ste 200
Fort Lauderdale, FL 33313
www.medvance.edu
Prgm Dir: Marie C Hamilton, MEd RT(R)(M)
Tel: 954 587-7100, Ext 206   *Fax:* 954 587-7704
E-mail: marie.hamilton@medvance.edu

Edison College
Radiography Prgm
PO Box 60210
8099 College Pkwy SW
Fort Myers, FL 33906-6210
Prgm Dir: James E Mayhew, MS RT(R)(QM)
Tel: 239 489-9110   *Fax:* 239 985-8352
E-mail: jmayhew@edison.edu

Indian River Community College
Radiography Prgm
3209 Virginia Ave
Fort Pierce, FL 34982
Prgm Dir: Gary Shaver, EdD RT(R)
Tel: 772 462-4368   *Fax:* 772 462-7816
E-mail: gshaver@ircc.edu

Santa Fe Community College
Radiography Prgm
3000 NW 83rd St
Gainesville, FL 32602-6200
http://inst.sfcc.edu/~health/xray/
Prgm Dir: Barbara A Konter, BSRS RT(R)
Tel: 352 395-5702   *Fax:* 352 395-5711
E-mail: bobbie.konter@sfcc.edu

Mayo Clinic Jacksonville
Radiography Prgm
4500 San Pablo Rd
Jacksonville, FL 32224
www.mayo.edu/mshs
Prgm Dir: Myke Kudlas, MEd RT(R)(QM)
Tel: 904 953-8663   *Fax:* 904 953-2894
E-mail: kudlas.myke@mayo.edu

Shands Jacksonville
Radiography Prgm
School of Radiologic Technology
655 W Eighth St
Jacksonville, FL 32209
www.shandsjacksonville.org/schools/radtech
Prgm Dir: Thomas A Graham, BS RT(R)
Tel: 904 244-3274   *Fax:* 904 244-6070
E-mail: thomas.graham@jax.ufl.edu

St Vincent's Medical Center
Radiography Prgm
PO Box 2982
Jacksonville, FL 32204
Prgm Dir: Kevin F Nevins, MSHA RT(R)(QM)
Tel: 904 308-8552   *Fax:* 904 308-5109
E-mail: knevins@jaxhealth.com

Lakeland Regional Medical Center
Radiography Prgm
1324 Lakeland Hills Blvd, PO Box 95448
Lakeland, FL 33805
http://lrmc.com
Prgm Dir: Lynn C Sadler, MSRS RT(R)(QM)
Tel: 863 687-1100, Ext 3769   *Fax:* 863 687-1471
E-mail: lynn.sadler@lrmc.com

Keiser University - Melbourne Campus
Radiography Prgm
900 S Babcock St
Melbourne, FL 32901
www.keiseruniversity.edu
Prgm Dir: Theresa D Roberts, MHS RT(R)(MR)
Tel: 321 409-4800, Ext 136   *Fax:* 321 725-3766
E-mail: troberts@keiseruniversity.edu

Jackson Mem Medical Center
Cosponsor: Univ of Miami
Radiography Prgm
1611 NW 12th Ave
Miami, FL 33136-1094
https://www.um-jmh.org or https://www.jhsmiami.org
Prgm Dir: Courtney P Glenn, MSM RT(R)
Tel: 305 585-6811   *Fax:* 305 585-6579
E-mail: cglenn@um-jmh.org, cglenn@jhsmiami.org

MedVance Institute
Radiography Prgm
Miami/KIMC Investments, Inc
9035 Sunset Dr, Ste 200
Miami, FL 33173
Prgm Dir: Judith Wilhite, BA RT(R)(M)
Tel: 305 596-5553
E-mail: jwilhite@medvance.edu

Miami Dade College
Radiography Prgm
Medical Center Campus
950 NW 20th St
Miami, FL 33127
Prgm Dir: Merlinn R Zolfaghari, MS RT(R)
Tel: 305 237-4292   *Fax:* 305 237-4116
E-mail: Merlin.Zolfaghari@mdc.edu

Marion County School of Radiologic Tech
Radiography Prgm
1014 SW Seventh Rd
Ocala, FL 34474
www.mcctae.com
Prgm Dir: Timothy Richardson, BS RT(R)
Tel: 352 671-7222   *Fax:* 352 671-7216
E-mail: Timothy.Richardson@marion.k12.fl.us

Florida Hospital College of Health Sciences
Radiography Prgm
671 Winyah Dr
Orlando, FL 32803
Prgm Dir: Genese M Gibson, MA RT(R)(M)(QM)
Tel: 407 895-7747, Ext 1077   *Fax:* 407 303-7820
E-mail: genese_gibson@fhchs.edu

University of Central Florida
Radiography Prgm
HPA2, Room 210K
4000 Central Florida Blvd
Orlando, FL 32816-2220
www.ucf.edu
Prgm Dir: Thomas J Edwards III, EdD RT(R)(QM)
Tel: 407 823-2174   *Fax:* 407 823-6138
E-mail: tedwards@mail.ucf.edu

Valencia Community College
Radiography Prgm
PO Box 3028
Orlando, FL 32802
http://valenciacc.edu/asdegrees/as.asp
Prgm Dir: Julie McCaughtry, BS RT(R)(CT)
Tel: 407 582-1192   *Fax:* 407 582-1278
E-mail: jmccaughtry@valenciacc.edu

Palm Beach Community College
Radiography Prgm
3160 PGA Blvd
Palm Beach Gardens, FL 33418-2893
www.pbcc.edu/x1284.xml
Prgm Dir: Vicki E Shaver, EdD RT(R)
Tel: 561 207-5067   *Fax:* 561 207-5011
E-mail: shaverv@pbcc.edu

MedVance Institute - West Palm Beach Campus
Radiography Prgm
1630 S Congress Ave
Palm Springs, FL 33461
www.medvance.org
Prgm Dir: Julie M Slusser, BS RT(R)(M)
Tel: 561 304-3466, Ext 128   *Fax:* 561 423-9251
E-mail: julie.slusser@medvance.edu

Gulf Coast Community College
Radiography Prgm
School of Radiography
5230 W US Hwy 98
Panama City, FL 32401-1041
Prgm Dir: Dee Ann VanDerSchaaf, RT(R)
Tel: 850 913-3318   *Fax:* 850 747-3246
E-mail: dvanderschaaf@gulfcoast.edu

Pensacola Junior College
Radiography Prgm
Warrington Campus
5555 W Hwy 98
Pensacola, FL 32507-1097
http://pjc.edu
Prgm Dir: Marilyn K Coseo, EdD
Tel: 850 484-2305   *Fax:* 850 484-2390
E-mail: mcoseo@pjc.edu

Keiser University - Sarasota
Radiography Prgm
6151 Lake Osprey Dr
Sarasota, FL 34240
www.keiseruniversity.edu
Prgm Dir: Kathleen M Drotar, MA Ed RT(R)(N)(T)
Tel: 941 907-3900   *Fax:* 941 907-2889
E-mail: kdrotar@keiseruniversity.edu

Hillsborough Community College
Radiography Prgm
PO Box 30030
Tampa, FL 33630-3030
www.hccfl.edu
Prgm Dir: Beth E Wyckoff, MA Ed RT(R)
Tel: 813 253-7371   *Fax:* 813 253-7226
E-mail: bwyckoff@hccfl.edu

Polk Community College
Radiography Prgm
999 Avenue H NE
Winter Haven, FL 33881-4299
Prgm Dir: Barbara A Koontz, MA RT(R)(M)
Tel: 863 297-1010, Ext 5722   *Fax:* 863 297-1036
E-mail: bkoontz@polk.edu

Georgia

North Metro Technical College
Radiography Prgm
5198 Ross Rd
Acworth, GA 30102
Prgm Dir: Deanne D Collins, BS RT(R)
Tel: 770 975-4055   *Fax:* 770 956-6601
E-mail: dcollins@northmetrotech.edu

Albany Technical College
Radiography Prgm
1704 S Slappey Blvd
Albany, GA 31701
Prgm Dir: Kelley R Castro, MEd RT(R)
Tel: 229 430-3619   *Fax:* 229 430-3601
E-mail: kcastro@albanytech.edu

Athens Technical College
Radiography Prgm
800 US Hwy 29 N
Athens, GA 30601-1500
www.athenstech.edu
Prgm Dir: Douglas A Baker, MS RT(R)
Tel: 706 355-5070   *Fax:* 706 369-5753
E-mail: dbaker@athenstech.edu

Emory University
Radiography Prgm
Medical Imaging Program
PO Box 25901
Atlanta, GA 30322
www.radiology.emory.edu/medimag
Prgm Dir: Dawn Couch Moore, MMSc RT(R)
Tel: 404 727-3200   *Fax:* 404 712-7256
E-mail: dawn.moore@emoryhealthcare.org

Grady Health System
Radiography Prgm
80 Jesse Hill Jr Dr SE
PO Box 26095
Atlanta, GA 30303-3050
www.gradyhealthsystem.org
Prgm Dir: Cheryl T Pressly, BMSc RT(R)
Tel: 404 616-3611   *Fax:* 404 616-3512
E-mail: cpressly@gmh.edu

University Hospital
Radiography Prgm
1350 Walton Way
Augusta, GA 30901-3599
Prgm Dir: Patricia S Graham, MBA RT(R)
Tel: 706 774-8646   *Fax:* 706 774-5079
E-mail: pgraham@uh.org

Coastal Georgia Community College
Radiography Prgm
3700 Altama Ave
Brunswick, GA 31520-3644
www.cgcc.peachnet.edu
Prgm Dir: Dianne T Castor, BSEd RT(R)
Tel: 912 264-7381   *Fax:* 912 262-3283
E-mail: dcastor@cgcc.edu

Columbus Technical College
Radiography Prgm
928 Manchester Expwy
Columbus, GA 31904-6572
www.columbustech.edu
Prgm Dir: Patricia A Mansell, MS RT(R)(M)
Tel: 706 641-5277   *Fax:* 706 641-5284
E-mail: pmansell@Columbustech.edu

Dalton State College
Radiography Prgm
650 College Dr
Dalton, GA 30720
Prgm Dir: Susan West, MEd RT(R)
Tel: 706 272-2605 *Fax:* 706 272-2699
E-mail: swest@daltonstate.edu

DeKalb Medical Center
Radiography Prgm
2701 N Decatur Rd
Decatur, GA 30033
www.dekalbmedicalcenter.org
Prgm Dir: Lashaun D Taylor, MS RT(R)
Tel: 404 501-5306 *Fax:* 404 501-1883
E-mail: Shaun_Taylor@dkmc.org

West Central Technical College
Radiography Prgm
4600 Timber Ridge Dr
Douglasville, GA 30135
www.westcentraltech.edu
Prgm Dir: S Paige Saylors, MSHA RT(R)(M)(QM)
Tel: 770 947-7222 *Fax:* 770 947-3818
E-mail: psaylors@westcentraltech.edu

Heart of Georgia Technical College
Radiography Prgm
560 Pinehill Rd
Dublin, GA 31021
Prgm Dir: Roslyn Johnson, BAS RT(R)
Tel: 478 274-7882 *Fax:* 478 275-6642
E-mail: rjohnson@hgtc.org

Griffin Technical College
Radiography Prgm
501 Varsity Rd
Griffin, GA 30223-2042
www.griffintech.edu
Prgm Dir: Deborah R Dawson, BMSc RT(R)
Tel: 770 229-3225 *Fax:* 770 229-3294
E-mail: ddawson@griffintech.edu

West Georgia Technical College
Radiography Prgm
303 Fort Dr
LaGrange, GA 30240
www.westgatech.edu
Prgm Dir: Wanda W Barbee, MEd RT(R)
Tel: 706 756-4552, Ext 4552 *Fax:* 706 845-4339
E-mail: wbarbee@westgatech.edu

Gwinnett Technical College
Radiography Prgm
5150 Sugarloaf Pkwy
Lawrenceville, GA 30043
http://gwinnetttech.edu
Prgm Dir: James A Sass, MEd RT(R)(M)(QM)
Tel: 678 226-6326 *Fax:* 770 685-1338
E-mail: jsass@gwinnetttech.edu

Moultrie Technical College
Radiography Prgm
800 Veterans Pkwy N
Moultrie, GA 31788
Prgm Dir: Alfred L Jones, BS RT(R)
Tel: 229 891-7000 *Fax:* 229 891-7010
E-mail: ajones@moultrietech.edu

Lanier Technical College
Radiography Prgm
2990 Landrum Education Dr
Oakwood, GA 30566
www.laniertech.edu
Prgm Dir: Robert R Wells, BS RT(R)(CT)
Tel: 770 535-5928
E-mail: rwells@laniertech.edu

Coosa Valley Technical College
Radiography Prgm
1 Maurice Culberson Dr
Rome, GA 30161
Prgm Dir: Mark H Layne, MEd RT(R)(CT)(MR)
Tel: 706 295-6955 *Fax:* 706 295-6984
E-mail: mlayne@coosavalleytech.edu

Armstrong Atlantic State University
Cosponsor: Armstrong Atlantic State University
Radiography Prgm
11935 Abercorn St
Savannah, GA 31419
www.armstrong.edu
Prgm Dir: Sharyn D Gibson, EdD RT(R)
Tel: 912 927-5360 *Fax:* 912 921-5838
E-mail: sharyn.gibson@mail.armstrong.edu

Ogeechee Technical College
Radiography Prgm
One Joe Kennedy Blvd
Statesboro, GA 30458
www.ogeecheetech.edu
Prgm Dir: Lynda Tinker, MA RT(R)(M)(CT)(QM)
Tel: 912 681-5500, Ext 1642 *Fax:* 912 871-1162
E-mail: ltinker@ogeechee.org

Valdosta Technical College
Radiography Prgm
4089 Val Tech Rd
Valdosta, GA 31603
Prgm Dir: Linda L Booth, BS RT(R)
Tel: 229 245-2461 *Fax:* 229 259-5567
E-mail: lbooth@valdostatech.edu

Southeastern Technical College
Radiography Prgm
3001 E First St
Vidalia, GA 30474
Prgm Dir: Tara Weldon Carter, BS RT(R)(M)(CT)
RDMS
Tel: 912 538-3152 *Fax:* 912 538-3106
E-mail: tcarter@southeasterntech.edu

Middle Georgia Technical College
Radiography Prgm
80 Cohen Walker Dr
Warner Robins, GA 31088
www.middlegatech.edu
Prgm Dir: Patricia Melnick, MEd RT(R)(M)
Tel: 478 988-6800, Ext 4047 *Fax:* 478 988-6875
E-mail: pmelnick@middlegatech.edu

Okefenokee Technical College
Radiography Prgm
1701 Carswell Ave
Waycross, GA 31503
Prgm Dir: Donna L Yeomans, RT(R)
Tel: 912 287-5837 *Fax:* 912 287-4865
E-mail: dyeomans@okefenokeetech.edu

Hawaii

Kapi'olani Community College
Radiography Prgm
4303 Diamond Head Rd
Honolulu, HI 96816
http://programs.kcc.hawaii.edu
Prgm Dir: Harry K Nakayama, BS RT(R)
Tel: 808 734-9251 *Fax:* 808 734-9126
E-mail: hnakayam@hawaii.edu

Idaho

Boise State University
Radiography Prgm
College of Health Sciences
1910 University Dr
Boise, ID 83725
http://radsci.boisestate.edu
Prgm Dir: Darlene K Travis, BS RT(R)(T)(CV)
Tel: 208 426-3290 *Fax:* 208 426-4459
E-mail: dtravis@boisestate.edu

College of Southern Idaho
Radiography Prgm
315 Falls Ave
Twin Falls, ID 83303-1238
www.csi.edu/radiologic_technology/
Prgm Dir: O Gary Lauer, PhD RT(R)
Tel: 208 732-6719 *Fax:* 208 736-4743
E-mail: glauer@csi.edu

Illinois

Southwestern Illinois College
Radiography Prgm
2500 Carlyle Rd
Belleville, IL 62221-9989
Prgm Dir: Rhonda K Kern, MBA RT(R)
Tel: 618 235-2700, Ext 5303 *Fax:* 618 235-2052
E-mail: rhonda.kern@swic.edu

Kaskaskia College
Radiography Prgm
27210 College Rd
Centralia, IL 62801
www.kc.cc.il.us
Prgm Dir: Mimi L Polczynski, MS ED RT(R)(M)(CT)
Tel: 618 545-3000, Ext 3363 *Fax:* 618 545-3028
E-mail: mpolczynski@kc.cc.il.us

Parkland College
Radiography Prgm
2400 W Bradley Ave
Champaign, IL 61821-1899
Prgm Dir: Kimberly A Mills, BS RT(R)(CT)
Tel: 217 351-2436 *Fax:* 217 373-3830
E-mail: kmills@parkland.edu

Advocate Illinois Masonic Medical Center
Radiography Prgm
836 W Wellington Ave
Chicago, IL 60657
www.advocatehealth.com
Prgm Dir: Philis George, BS RT(R)(M)
Tel: 773 296-8951 *Fax:* 773 296-8960
E-mail: philis.george@advocatehealth.com

Advocate Trinity Hospital
Radiography Prgm
2320 E 93rd St
Chicago, IL 60617
Prgm Dir: Joann Kern, BS RT(R)
Tel: 773 967-5292 *Fax:* 773 967-3954
E-mail: joann.kern@advocatehealth.com

Malcolm X College
Radiography Prgm
1900 W Van Buren St
Chicago, IL 60612
www.ccc.edu/malcolmx
Prgm Dir: Geraldine Williams, MEd RT(R)
Tel: 312 850-7373 *Fax:* 312 850-7372
E-mail: glwilliams@ccc.edu

Wright College
Radiography Prgm
4300 N Narragansett Ave
Chicago, IL 60634
http://wright.ccc.edu
Prgm Dir: Dennis M King, MHS RT(R)
Tel: 773 481-8880 *Fax:* 773 481-8892
E-mail: dking@ccc.edu

Danville Area Community College
Radiography Prgm
2000 E Main St
Danville, IL 61832
www.dacc.edu
Prgm Dir: Alberto Bello, Jr, MEd RT(R)(CV)
Tel: 217 443-8552   *Fax:* 217 443-8595
E-mail: abello@dacc.edu

Sauk Valley Community College
Radiography Prgm
173 Illinois Rte 2
Dixon, IL 61021-9112
www.svcc.edu
Prgm Dir: Stan Shippert, MEd RT(R)(MR)(CT)
Tel: 815 288-5511, Ext 342   *Fax:* 815 288-5651
E-mail: shippes@svcc.edu

St Francis Hospital
Cosponsor: Resurrection Health Care
Radiography Prgm
355 Ridge Ave
Evanston, IL 60202
Prgm Dir: Mary Ellen Newton, MS RT(R)(M)
Tel: 847 316-5810   *Fax:* 847 316-5811
E-mail: mnewton@reshealthcare.org

College of DuPage
Radiography Prgm
425 Fawell Blvd
Glen Ellyn, IL 60137-6599
http://cod.edu
Prgm Dir: Gina M Carrier, MBA MS RT(R)
Tel: 630 942-2434   *Fax:* 630 858-5409
E-mail: carrier@cod.edu

College of Lake County
Radiography Prgm
19351 W Washington St
Grayslake, IL 60030-1198
Prgm Dir: Lynn Platz Wiechert, MS RT(R)(CT)
Tel: 847 543-2880   *Fax:* 847 543-3880
E-mail: lwiechert@clcillinois.edu

McDonough District Hospital
Radiography Prgm
525 E Grant St
Macomb, IL 61455
Prgm Dir: Vincent E Staub, BS RT(R)
Tel: 309 833-4101, Ext 12461   *Fax:* 309 836-1551
E-mail: vestaub@mdh.org

Kishwaukee College
Radiography Prgm
21193 Malta Rd
Malta, IL 60150-9699
www.kishwaukeecollege.edu
Prgm Dir: Carol Guschl, BS RT(R)(QM)
Tel: 815 825-2086, Ext 257   *Fax:* 815 825-2072
E-mail: guschl@kishwaukeecollege.edu

Bloomington-Normal School of Radiography
Radiography Prgm
900 Franklin Ave
Normal, IL 61761
Prgm Dir: Lisa R Aberle, BS RT(R)(CV)
Tel: 309 452-2834   *Fax:* 309 392-2835
E-mail: laberle@bromenn.org

Olney Central College
Radiography Prgm
305 N West St
Olney, IL 62450
Prgm Dir: Carol Kocher, BA RT(R)(M)
Tel: 618 395-7777, Ext 2239   *Fax:* 618 392-3293
E-mail: kocherc@iecc.edu

Moraine Valley Community College
Radiography Prgm
9000 W College Parkway
Palos Hills, IL 60465
www.morainevalley.edu
Prgm Dir: Michael A Gatto, BS RT(R)
Tel: 708 974-5316   *Fax:* 708 974-0185
E-mail: gatto@morainevalley.edu

Illinois Central College
Radiography Prgm
Thomas K Thomas Bldg
201 SW Adams St
Peoria, IL 61635-0001
www.icc.edu
Prgm Dir: Diane L Schulz, MEd RT(R) FASRT
Tel: 309 999-4659   *Fax:* 309 673-9626
E-mail: dschulz@icc.edu

OSF St Francis Medical Center
Radiography Prgm
530 NE Glen Oak Ave
Peoria, IL 61637
www.osfsaintfrancis.org
Prgm Dir: Suzanne M Yezek, MS RT(R)(M)
Tel: 309 655-2782   *Fax:* 309 655-2172
E-mail: Suzanne.M.Yezek@osfhealthcare.org

Blessing Hospital
Radiography Prgm
Box 7005, Broadway at 11th St
Quincy, IL 62305-7005
Prgm Dir: Rhonda L Brinks, BS RT(R)
Tel: 217 223-8400, Ext 6160   *Fax:* 217 223-6898
E-mail: rbrinks@blessinghospital.com

Triton College
Radiography Prgm
2000 N Fifth Ave
River Grove, IL 60171
www.triton.edu
Prgm Dir: Catherine T Lekostaj, MA RT(R)
Tel: 708 456-0300, Ext 3370   *Fax:* 708 583-3336
E-mail: clekosta@triton.edu

Trinity College of Nursing & Health Sciences
Radiography Prgm
2122 25th Ave
Rock Island, IL 61201-5317
www.trinityqc.com/homepage_col.cfm?id=1835
Prgm Dir: Diana Werderman, MS Ed RT(R)
Tel: 309 779-7776   *Fax:* 309 779-7796
E-mail: werdermand@ihs.org

Rockford Memorial Hospital
Radiography Prgm
2400 N Rockton Ave
Rockford, IL 61103
www.rhsnet.org
Prgm Dir: Patricia Griesman, MS RT(R)
Tel: 815 971-5480   *Fax:* 815 968-3407
E-mail: pgriesman@rhsnet.org

Swedish American Hospital
Radiography Prgm
1250 E State St
Rockford, IL 61104-2315
www.swedishamerican.org
Prgm Dir: Amy C Meagher, BS RT(R)
Tel: 815 489-4959   *Fax:* 815 489-4975
E-mail: ameagher@swedishamerican.org

South Suburban College
Radiography Prgm
15800 S State St
South Holland, IL 60473
http://wwww.southsuburbancollege.edu
Prgm Dir: Shari J McGovern, BSRS RT(R)
Tel: 708 296-2000, Ext 2634   *Fax:* 708 210-5792
E-mail: smcgovern@southsuburbancollege.edu

Lincoln Land Community College
Radiography Prgm
5250 Shepherd Rd
PO Box 19256
Springfield, IL 62794-9256
www.llcc.edu
Prgm Dir: William J Callaway, BA RT(R)
Tel: 217 786-2408, Ext 217   *Fax:* 217 786-2824
E-mail: bill.callaway@llcc.edu

Indiana

Columbus Regional Hospital
Radiography Prgm
2400 E 17th St
Columbus, IN 47201
www.crh.org
Prgm Dir: Karen A Frazier, MS RT(R)
Tel: 812 376-5354   *Fax:* 812 376-5988
E-mail: kfrazier@crh.org

University of Southern Indiana
Radiography Prgm
8600 University Blvd
Evansville, IN 47712
Prgm Dir: Martin A Reed, PhD RT(R)
Tel: 812 464-1894   *Fax:* 812 465-7092
E-mail: mreed@usi.edu

Fort Wayne School of Radiography
Radiography Prgm
700 Broadway
Fort Wayne, IN 46802
Prgm Dir: Elizabeth Ann Lewis, BS RT(R)
Tel: 260 425-3990   *Fax:* 260 425-3887
E-mail: fwsr@fwi.com

University of Saint Francis
Radiography Prgm
2701 Spring St
Fort Wayne, IN 46808
Prgm Dir: Donna J Lyke, MS RT(R)(M)(QM)
Tel: 260 434-7671   *Fax:* 260 434-7697
E-mail: dlyke@sf.edu

Indiana University Northwest
Radiography Prgm
3400 Broadway St
Gary, IN 46408-1197
Prgm Dir: Arlene Adler, MEd RT(R) FAERS
Tel: 219 980-6540   *Fax:* 219 980-6649
E-mail: aadler@iun.edu

Hancock Regional Hospital
Radiography Prgm
801 N State St
Greenfield, IN 46140
www.hancockregional.org
Prgm Dir: Vaughn Sutton, BS RT(R)
Tel: 317 468-4468   *Fax:* 317 468-4549
E-mail: vsutton@hancockregional.org

Ball State University
Radiography Prgm
1701 N Senate Blvd
Wile Hall 643
Indianapolis, IN 46202
www.bsu.edu/physiology-health/radiography/
Prgm Dir: Donna L Long, MSM RT(R)(M)(QM)
Tel: 317 962-3284   *Fax:* 317 962-2102
E-mail: dlong2@clarian.org

Community Health Network
Radiography Prgm
1500 N Ritter Ave
Indianapolis, IN 46219
www.ecommunity.com/radiologyschool/
Prgm Dir: Meryem Cole, BS RT(R)
Tel: 317 355-5867   *Fax:* 317 351-7733
E-mail: mcole@ecommunity.com

Indiana University
Radiography Prgm
541 Clinical Dr 120
Indianapolis, IN 46202-5111
http://ww2.indyrad.iupui.edu/RadWeb/
Prgm Dir: Bruce W Long, MS RT(R)(CV) FASRT
Tel: 317 274-5254   *Fax:* 317 274-4074
E-mail: blong@iupui.edu

Ivy Tech Community College
Radiography Prgm
9301 E 59th St
Indianapolis, IN 46216
Prgm Dir: Ann Sisel, MS RT(R)(M)
Tel: 317 921-4438   *Fax:* 317 546-3808
E-mail: asisel@ivytech.edu

St Vincent Health/St Joseph Hospital
Radiography Prgm
2001 W 86th St
Indianapolis, IN 46260
www.stvincent.org/education/radiography
Prgm Dir: Mark E Adkins, MS Ed RT(R)(QM)
Tel: 317 338-3879
E-mail: meadkins@stvincent.org

Indiana University - Kokomo
Radiography Prgm
2300 S Washington St
Kokomo, IN 46902
www.iuk.edu/~koalhe/
Prgm Dir: John O Hughey, MS RT(R)
Tel: 765 455-9329   *Fax:* 765 455-9310
E-mail: johughey@iuk.edu

King's Daughters' Hospital & Health Services
Radiography Prgm
One King's Daughter's Dr
PO Box 447
Madison, IN 47250
www.kdhhs.org
Prgm Dir: Deborah A Bazinet, MHSA RT(R)(M)
Tel: 812 265-5211, Ext 50633   *Fax:* 812 265-0184
E-mail: bazinetd@kdhhs.org

Ivy Tech Community College - Marion
Radiography Prgm
1015 E 3rd St
Marion, IN 46952
Prgm Dir: Debra Dillman, MSRS RT(R)
Tel: 765 651-3111, Ext 413
E-mail: ddillman@ivytech.edu

Ball Memorial Hospital
Radiography Prgm
2401 University Ave
Muncie, IN 47303-3499
Prgm Dir: Susan J Hinds, RT(R)
Tel: 765 747-4372   *Fax:* 765 747-4415
E-mail: shinds@chsmail.org

Reid Hospital & Health Care Services
Radiography Prgm
1401 Chester Blvd
Richmond, IN 47374
www.reidhosp.com
Prgm Dir: Roger A Preston, MSRS RT(R)
Tel: 765 983-3167   *Fax:* 765 983-3260
E-mail: prestoro@reidhosp.com

Indiana University South Bend
Radiography Prgm
1700 Mishawaka Ave, PO Box 7111
South Bend, IN 46634
www.iusb.edu
Prgm Dir: James H Howard, MSEd RT(R)
Tel: 574 520-5569   *Fax:* 574 520-5576
E-mail: jhhoward@iusb.edu

Ivy Tech Community College - Terre Haute
Radiography Prgm
8000 S Education Dr
Terre Haute, IN 47802
www.goivytech.net
Prgm Dir: Lou Ann Wisbey, BS RT(R)(T)
Tel: 812 298-2242   *Fax:* 812 299-2441
E-mail: lwisbey@ivytech.edu

Good Samaritan Hospital
Radiography Prgm
520 S Seventh St
Vincennes, IN 47591
Prgm Dir: Roger D Sterling, BS RT(R)
Tel: 812 885-8011   *Fax:* 812 885-3445
E-mail: rsterling@gshvin.org

Iowa

Scott Community College
Radiography Prgm
500 Belmont Rd
Bettendorf, IA 52722-5649
Prgm Dir: Jan M Jacobs, MA RT(R)
Tel: 563 441-4265   *Fax:* 563 441-4204
E-mail: jjacobs@eicc.edu

St Luke's Hospital
Cosponsor: Mercy Medical Center
Radiography Prgm
PO Box 3026
1026 A Ave NE
Cedar Rapids, IA 52406-3026
www.isrt.org/mstl.htm
Prgm Dir: Dana D Schmitz, MEd RT(R)
Tel: 319 369-7077   *Fax:* 319 368-5721
E-mail: schmitdd@crstlukes.com

Jennie Edmundson Memorial Hospital
Radiography Prgm
933 E Pierce St
Council Bluffs, IA 51503
www.bestcare.org
Prgm Dir: Kristin E Schnitker, BA RT(R)
Tel: 712 396-6746   *Fax:* 712 396-6227
E-mail: kris.schnitker@nmhs.org

Iowa Methodist Med Ctr/Iowa Hlth - Des Moines
Radiography Prgm
1200 Pleasant St
Des Moines, IA 50309-1453
www.iowahealth.org
Prgm Dir: Suzanne E Crandall, EdD RT(R)
Tel: 515 241-6883   *Fax:* 515 241-8015
E-mail: crandase@ihs.org

Mercy College of Health Sciences
Radiography Prgm
928 Sixth Ave
Des Moines, IA 50309
Prgm Dir: Angela Sapp, BS RT(R)
Tel: 515 643-6616   *Fax:* 515 643-6698
E-mail: asapp@mercydesmoines.org

Iowa Central Community College
Radiography Prgm
330 Ave M
Fort Dodge, IA 50501
www.iowacentral.com
Prgm Dir: Chantel Gruver, BS RT(R) RDMS RVT
Tel: 515 574-1302   *Fax:* 515 576-5656
E-mail: Gruver_c@iowacentral.com

University of Iowa Hospitals & Clinics
Radiography Prgm
Radiology, C-723 GH
200 Hawkins Dr
Iowa City, IA 52242-1077
www.radiology.uiowa.edu/radtech
Prgm Dir: Kathy Martensen, MA RT(R)
Tel: 319 356-4332   *Fax:* 319 384-9574
E-mail: kathy-martensen@uiowa.edu

Mercy Medical Center - North Iowa
Radiography Prgm
1000 Fourth St SW
Mason City, IA 50401
Prgm Dir: Janet L Moore, BS RT(R)(M)(QM)
Tel: 641 422-6079   *Fax:* 641 422-5301
E-mail: moorejl@mercyhealth.com

Indian Hills Community College
Radiography Prgm
525 Grandview
Ottumwa, IA 52501
www.ihcc.cc.ia.us
Prgm Dir: Jeanette DeWitt, BS RT(R)(M)(CT)
Tel: 515 683-5164, Ext 5316   *Fax:* 515 683-5184
E-mail: jdewitt@ihcc.cc.ia.us

Northeast Iowa Community College
Radiography Prgm
Peosta Campus
10250 Sundown Rd
Peosta, IA 52068
Prgm Dir: Angela K Kronlage, MA RT(R)
Tel: 563 556-5110, Ext 311   *Fax:* 563 556-5058
E-mail: kronlagea@portal.nicc.edu

St Luke's College
Radiography Prgm
2720 Stone Park Blvd
Sioux City, IA 51104
www.stlukescollege.edu
Prgm Dir: Deanna Butcher, MA RT(R)
Tel: 712 279-3734   *Fax:* 712 233-8017
E-mail: butchedl@stlukes.org

Allen College
Radiography Prgm
1825 Logan Ave
Waterloo, IA 50703
www.allencollege.edu
Prgm Dir: Peggy S Fortsch, EdD RT(R)
Tel: 319 226-2031   *Fax:* 319 226-2051
E-mail: fortscps@ihs.org

Covenant Medical Center
Radiography Prgm
3421 W 9th St
Waterloo, IA 50702
Prgm Dir: Kenneth K Helfrick, BA RT(R)(QM)
Tel: 319 272-7296   *Fax:* 319 272-7105
E-mail: Helfrick.Ken@wfhc.org

Kansas

Fort Hays State University
Radiography Prgm
600 Park St
Hays, KS 67601-4099
Prgm Dir: Michael E Madden, PhD RT(R)(CT)(MR)
Tel: 785 628-5678   *Fax:* 785 628-4076
E-mail: mmadden@fhsu.edu

Hutchinson Community College
Radiography Prgm
815 N Walnut
Hutchinson, KS 67501
www.hutchcc.edu
Prgm Dir: Renee Kautzer, MS RT(R)
Tel: 620 665-4954   *Fax:* 620 665-4988
E-mail: kautzerr@hutchcc.edu

Labette Community College
Radiography Prgm
200 S 14th St
Parsons, KS 67357
www.labette.edu
Prgm Dir: V June Downing, EdS RT(R)
Tel: 620 820-1158   *Fax:* 620 421-1539
E-mail: juned@labette.edu

Washburn University
Radiography Prgm
1700 SW College Ave
Topeka, KS 66621
www.washburn.edu
Prgm Dir: Jera J Roberts, EdS RT(R)(M)
Tel: 785 670-2173   *Fax:* 785 670-1027
E-mail: jera.roberts@washburn.edu

Newman University
Radiography Prgm
3100 McCormick Ave
Wichita, KS 67213
http://newmanu.edu
Prgm Dir: Ronald Shipley, MS RT(R)
Tel: 316 942-4291, Ext 2351   *Fax:* 316 942-4483
E-mail: shipleyr@newmanu.edu

Kentucky

King's Daughters' Medical Center
Radiography Prgm
2201 Lexington Ave
Ashland, KY 41101
Prgm Dir: Krista M Lambert, BS RT(R)(MR)
Tel: 606 327-4637   *Fax:* 606 327-7425
E-mail: krista.lambert@kdmc.net

Bowling Green Technical College
Radiography Prgm
1845 Loop Dr
Bowling Green, KY 42101
www.bowlinggreen.kctcs.edu
Prgm Dir: Diane Button, MA RT(R)(M)
Tel: 270 901-1077   *Fax:* 270 901-1139
E-mail: diane.button@kctcs.edu

Elizabethtown Community & Technical College
Radiography Prgm
620 College Street Rd
Elizabethtown, KY 42701
www.elizabethtown.kctcs.edu
Prgm Dir: Penelope Logsdon, MA RT(R)
Tel: 270 706-8649   *Fax:* 270 766-5131
E-mail: penelope.logsdon@kctcs.edu

Hazard Community & Technical College
Cosponsor: Southeast Community College
Radiography Prgm
One Community College Dr
Hazard, KY 41701
www.hazard.kctcs.edu
Prgm Dir: Homer Terry, MS RT(R)(M)(QM)
Tel: 606 436-5721, Ext 73389   *Fax:* 606 439-1600
E-mail: homer.terry@kctcs.edu

Northern Kentucky University
Radiography Prgm
227 Albright Health Ctr
Highland Heights, KY 41099-2104
Prgm Dir: Trina L Koscielicki, MEd RT(R)
Tel: 859 572-5477   *Fax:* 859 572-1314
E-mail: koscielicki@nku.edu

Bluegrass Community and Technical College
Radiography Prgm
470 Cooper Dr
Lexington, KY 40502-0235
Prgm Dir: Sarajane Doty, MS Ed RT(R)
Tel: 859 246-6238   *Fax:* 859 246-4671
E-mail: sarajane.doty@kctcs.edu

St Joseph Healthcare
Radiography Prgm
One St Joseph Dr
Lexington, KY 40504
www.saintjosephhealthcare.org/radiology
Prgm Dir: Robyn A Bradley, BS RT(R)(M)
Tel: 859 313-2282   *Fax:* 859 313-3104
E-mail: bradleyr@sjhlex.org

Jefferson Community and Technical College
Radiography Prgm
109 E Broadway St
Louisville, KY 40202
Prgm Dir: Kimberly A Hayse, BS RT(R)(CI)
Tel: 502 629-5180   *Fax:* 502 629-2088
E-mail: kimberly.hayse@kctcs.edu

Spencerian College
Radiography Prgm
4627 Dixie Hwy
Louisville, KY 40216
www.spencerian.edu
Prgm Dir: Mary Kaye Griffin, BSH
Tel: 502 447-1000, Ext 7846   *Fax:* 502 447-4574
E-mail: mgriffin@spencerian.edu

Madisonville Community College
Radiography Prgm
750 N Laffoon St
Health Campus
Madisonville, KY 42431
Prgm Dir: Tonia R Gibson, BS RT(R)
Tel: 270 824-7552, Ext 182   *Fax:* 270 824-7069
E-mail: tonia.gibson@kctcs.edu

Morehead State University
Radiography Prgm
150 University Blvd
Reed Hall 408
Morehead, KY 40351
Prgm Dir: Barbara L Dehner, MSRS RT(R)(M)(CT)
FAERS
Tel: 606 783-2651   *Fax:* 606 783-5051
E-mail: b.dehner@moreheadstate.edu

Owensboro Community & Technical College
Radiography Prgm
4800 New Hartford Rd
Owensboro, KY 42303
Prgm Dir: Nadine Joy Menser, MS RT(R)(T)
Tel: 270 686-4633   *Fax:* 270 686-4662
E-mail: joy.menser@kctcs.edu

West Kentucky Community & Technical College
Radiography Prgm
4810 Alben Barkley Dr, PO Box 7380
PO Box 7380
Paducah, KY 42002-7408
www.westkentucky.kctcs.edu
Prgm Dir: Deborah Smith, BS RT(R)(M)
Tel: 270 534-3479   *Fax:* 270 534-3498
E-mail: deborah.smith@kctcs.edu

Southeast Kentucky Comm & Tech College
Radiography Prgm
3300 US Highway 25E S
Pineville, KY 40977
www.secc.kctcs.edu/AcademicAffairs/AlliedHealth/RadiographyP/
Prgm Dir: Joseph Paul Hutson, MS RT(R)
Tel: 606 248-2118   *Fax:* 606 248-2166
E-mail: paul.hutson@kctcs.edu

Somerset Community College
Radiography Prgm
808 Monticello St
Somerset, KY 42501
Prgm Dir: Shanda L Catron, RT(R)
Tel: 606 451-6755
E-mail: shanda.catron@kctcs.edu

St Catharine College
Radiography Prgm
2735 Bardstown Rd
St Catharine, KY 40061
www.sccky.edu
Prgm Dir: Donna J Crum, MS RT(R)(CT)
Tel: 859 336-5082, Ext 1333   *Fax:* 859 336-9383
E-mail: dcrum@sccky.edu

Louisiana

Baton Rouge General Medical Center
Radiography Prgm
3600 Florida Blvd, PO Box 2511
Baton Rouge, LA 70806
www.brgeneral.org
Prgm Dir: Catherine W Lennier, RT(R)
Tel: 225 387-7157   *Fax:* 225 381-6168
E-mail: cathy.lennier@brgeneral.org

MedVance Institute
Radiography Prgm
Baton Rouge, KIMC Investments, Inc
9255 Interline Ave
Baton Rouge, LA 70809
Prgm Dir: Kacey A Roberts, BS RT(R)
Tel: 225 248-1015, Ext 217   *Fax:* 225 248-9517
E-mail: kroberts@medvance.org

Our Lady of the Lake College
Radiography Prgm
7434 Perkins Rd
Baton Rouge, LA 70808
www.ololcollege.edu
Prgm Dir: Debbie Gallerson, MEd RT(R)
Tel: 225 768-1737   *Fax:* 225 768-0819
E-mail: dgallers@ololcollege.edu

Louisiana State University - Eunice
Radiography Prgm
PO Box 1129
Eunice, LA 70535
www.lsue.edu/radtech/
Prgm Dir: Robert L McLaughlin, Jr, MA RT(R)
Tel: 337 550-1340   *Fax:* 337 550-1289
E-mail: rmclaugh@lsue.edu

North Oaks Medical Center
Radiography Prgm
School of Radiologic Technology
PO Box 2668
Hammond, LA 70404
www.northoaks.org
Prgm Dir: Marsha J Talbert, BA RT(R)
Tel: 985 345-9805   *Fax:* 985 345-9894
E-mail: talbertm@northoaks.org

Lafayette General Medical Center
Radiography Prgm
1214 Coolidge Ave
PO Box 52009 OCS
Lafayette, LA 70505
www.lgmc.com
Prgm Dir: Charlotte S Powell, MS RS LRT
Tel: 337 289-8457   *Fax:* 337 289-8458
E-mail: cpowell@lgmc.com

McNeese State University
Radiography Prgm
Box 92000
Lake Charles, LA 70609
www.faculty.mcneese.edu/gbradley/
Prgm Dir: Gregory L Bradley, MEd RT(R)
Tel: 337 475-5657   *Fax:* 337 475-5664
E-mail: bradleyg1@aol.com

Career Technical College
Radiography Prgm
2319 Louisville Ave
Monroe, LA 71201
Prgm Dir: Tonya L Krone, MA RT(R)(M)
Tel: 318 998-5638
E-mail: tkrone@careertc.com

University of Louisiana at Monroe
Radiography Prgm
700 University Ave
Monroe, LA 71209-0450
Prgm Dir: Brett H Bennett, MEd RT(R)
Tel: 318 342-1629   *Fax:* 318 342-1635
E-mail: bbennett@ulm.edu

Delgado Community College
Radiography Prgm
615 City Park Ave
New Orleans, LA 70119-4399
Prgm Dir: Carleen Boudreaux, MS RT(R)(M)
Tel: 504 483-4429   *Fax:* 504 483-4609
E-mail: cboudr@dcc.edu

Our Lady of Holy Cross College
Cosponsor: Ochsner Clinic Foundation
Radiography Prgm
1516 Jefferson Hwy
New Orleans, LA 70121
Prgm Dir: Carl J Tholen, MEd RT(R)(CT)
Tel: 504 842-3705   *Fax:* 504 842-2459
E-mail: ctholen@ochsner.org

Northwestern State University
Radiography Prgm
College of Nursing
1800 Line Ave
Shreveport, LA 71101-4653
www.nsula.edu
Prgm Dir: Laura S Aaron, PhD RT(R)(M)(QM)
Tel: 318 677-3100   *Fax:* 318 677-3127
E-mail: carwilel@nsula.edu

Southern Univ at Shreveport
Radiography Prgm
610 Texas St, #331
Shreveport, LA 71101
Prgm Dir: Shelia S Swift, BS RT(R)
Tel: 318 674-3339
E-mail: sswift@susla.edu

Maine

Eastern Maine Community College
Radiography Prgm
354 Hogan Rd
Bangor, ME 04401
www.emcc.edu
Prgm Dir: Susan Roeder, MEd RT(R)(N)
Tel: 207 974-4659   *Fax:* 207 974-4608
E-mail: sroeder@emcc.edu

Kennebec Valley Community College
Radiography Prgm
92 Western Ave
Fairfield, ME 04937
Prgm Dir: Michelle Luciano, MC RT(R)
Tel: 207 453-5043
E-mail: mluciano@kvcc.me.edu

Central Maine Medical Center
Radiography Prgm
300 Main St
Lewiston, ME 04240-0305
www.cmmc.org
Prgm Dir: Judith Ripley, BS RT(R)
Tel: 207 795-5974   *Fax:* 207 795-2476
E-mail: ripleyj@cmhc.org
Notes: Hospital-based program affiliated with Central
   Maine Community College in Auburn, ME for an
   associate degree.

Mercy Hospital
Radiography Prgm
144 State St
Portland, ME 04101
Prgm Dir: Brenda M Rice, BS RT(R)
Tel: 207 879-3501   *Fax:* 207 879-2452
E-mail: riceb@mercyme.com

Southern Maine Community College
Radiography Prgm
Two Fort Rd
South Portland, ME 04106
www.smccme.edu
Prgm Dir: Sally A Doe, MS RT(R)
Tel: 207 741-5596   *Fax:* 207 741-5590
E-mail: sdoe@smccme.edu

Maryland

Anne Arundel Community College
Radiography Prgm
101 College Pkwy
Arnold, MD 21012-1895
Prgm Dir: Thomas A Luby, Jr, MBA RT(R)(QM)
Tel: 410 777-7025   *Fax:* 410 777-7099
E-mail: taluby@aacc.edu

Greater Baltimore Medical Center
Radiography Prgm
6701 N Charles St
Baltimore, MD 21204
http://GBMC.ORG/education/radiology
Prgm Dir: Brenda Schuette, BA RT(R)(M)(QM)
Tel: 443 849-2463   *Fax:* 443 849-2866
E-mail: bschuette@gbmc.org

Johns Hopkins Hospital
Radiography Prgm
Schools of Medical Imaging
600 N Wolfe St
Baltimore, MD 21287
www.radiologycareers.rad.jhmi.edu
Prgm Dir: Sandra Moore, MA RT(R)(M)
Tel: 410 528-8210   *Fax:* 410 528-8308
E-mail: semoore@jhmi.edu

**Community College of Baltimore County -
   Essex Campus**
Radiography Prgm
7201 Rossville Blvd
Baltimore County, MD 21237-9987
Prgm Dir: Erin V Cordray, BA RT(R)
Tel: 410 780-6666   *Fax:* 410 780-6405
E-mail: ecordray@ccbcmd.edu

Allegany College of Maryland
Radiography Prgm
12401 Willowbrook Rd SE
Cumberland, MD 21502-2596
www.allegany.edu
Prgm Dir: Cathy A Kline, BA RT(R)
Tel: 301 784-5560   *Fax:* 301 784-5015
E-mail: ckline@allegany.edu

Hagerstown Community College
Radiography Prgm
11400 Robinwood Dr
Hagerstown, MD 21742-6590
Prgm Dir: Brenda J Hassinger, MS RT(R)(M)
Tel: 301 790-2800, Ext 205   *Fax:* 301 739-0737
E-mail: hassingerb@hagerstowncc.edu

Prince George's Community College
Radiography Prgm
301 Largo Rd
Largo, MD 20774-2199
http://academic.pgcc.edu/alliedhealth
Prgm Dir: Angela Dopkowski Anderson, MA
   RT(R)(CT)(QM)
Tel: 301 322-0569   *Fax:* 301 386-7528
E-mail: aanderson@pgcc.edu

Wor-Wic Community College
Radiography Prgm
32000 Campus Dr
Salisbury, MD 21804
Prgm Dir: Karie A Solembrino, BS RT(R)(CT)
Tel: 410 572-8741   *Fax:* 410 572-8730
E-mail: ksolembrino@worwic.edu

Holy Cross Hospital
Radiography Prgm
1500 Forest Glen Rd
Silver Spring, MD 20910
Prgm Dir: Staci M Maier, MHA RT (R)
Tel: 301 754-7889   *Fax:* 301 754-7371
E-mail: maiers@holycrosshealth.org

Montgomery College
Radiography Prgm
7600 Takoma Ave
Takoma Park, MD 20912
Prgm Dir: Rose M Aehle, MS RT(R)(M)
Tel: 240 567-5564   *Fax:* 240 567-5561
E-mail: rose.aehle@montgomerycollege.edu

Washington Adventist Hospital
Radiography Prgm
7600 Carroll Ave
Takoma Park, MD 20912
Prgm Dir: Lyndsay M Bower, RT(R)
Tel: 301 891-6236   *Fax:* 301 891-6558
E-mail: lbower@ahm.com

Chesapeake College
Radiography Prgm
PO Box 8
Wye Mills, MD 21679
www.chesapeake.edu
Prgm Dir: Linda Burchett Blythe, BSRS RT(R)
Tel: 410 822-5400, Ext 5927   *Fax:* 410 770-3764
E-mail: lblythe@chesapeake.edu

Massachusetts

Middlesex Community College - Bedford
Radiography Prgm
Springs Rd
Bedford, MA 01730
Prgm Dir: William Darmody, MEd RT(R)(MR)
Tel: 781 280-3942   *Fax:* 781 275-4911
E-mail: darmodyw@middlesex.mass.edu

Bunker Hill Community College
Radiography Prgm
Medical Imaging Program
250 New Rutherford Ave
Boston, MA 02129-2925
Prgm Dir: Donna Misrati, MBA RT(R)(CT)
Tel: 617 228-2197   *Fax:* 617 228-2052
E-mail: dmisrati@bhcc.mass.edu

Mass College of Pharmacy & Health Sciences
Radiography Prgm
179 Longwood Ave
Boston, MA 02115
Prgm Dir: Lisa S Fanning, MEd RT(R)(CT)
Tel: 617 879-5033   *Fax:* 617 732-2075
E-mail: lisa.fanning@mcphs.edu

MGH Institute of Health Professions
Radiography Prgm
Charlestown Navy Yard
36 1st Ave
Boston, MA 02129-4557
www.mghihp.edu
Prgm Dir: Richard Terrass, MEd RT(R)
Tel: 617 726-0781   *Fax:* 617 726-8022
E-mail: rterrass@mghihp.edu

Roxbury Community College
Radiography Prgm
1234 Columbus Ave
Boston, MA 02120
www.rcc.mass.edu/nursing
Prgm Dir: Georgeann Jenkins, RT(R)(M)
Tel: 617 427-0060, Ext 5408
E-mail: GJenkins@rcc.mass.edu

Massasoit Community College
Radiography Prgm
One Massasoit Blvd
Brockton, MA 02302
www.massasoit.mass.edu
Prgm Dir: Nancy J Sutcliffe, MEd RT(R)(QM)
Tel: 508 588-9100, Ext 1784   *Fax:* 508 427-1262
E-mail: NSutcliffe@Massasoit.Mass.edu

North Shore Community College
Radiography Prgm
One Ferncroft Rd, PO Box 3340
Danvers, MA 01923-0840
www.northshore.edu
Prgm Dir: Christine E Wiley, MEd RT(R)(M)
Tel: 978 762-4163   *Fax:* 978 762-4022
E-mail: cwiley@northshore.edu

Massachusetts Bay Community College
Radiography Prgm
19 Flagg Dr
Framingham, MA 01702
Prgm Dir: Micheal Glisson, PhD RT(R)
Tel: 508 270-4031   *Fax:* 508 270-4131
E-mail: mglisson@massbay.edu

Holyoke Community College
Radiography Prgm
303 Homestead Ave
Holyoke, MA 01040
Prgm Dir: Holly S Martin, BSRS RT(R)(CT)
Tel: 413 552-2460
E-mail: hmartin@hcc.mass.edu

Northern Essex Community College
Radiography Prgm
45 Franklin St
Lawrence, MA 01841-4911
www.necc.mass.edu
Prgm Dir: Nancy Garcia, MEd RT(R)
Tel: 978 738-7493   *Fax:* 978 738-7146
E-mail: ngarcia@necc.mass.edu

Regis College
Cosponsor: Lawrence Memorial
Radiography Prgm
170 Governors Ave
Medford, MA 02155
www.lmregis.org
Prgm Dir: James V Lampka, MS RT(R)
Tel: 781 306-6658   *Fax:* 781 306-6710
E-mail: jlampka@lmh.edu

Springfield Technical Community College
Radiography Prgm
One Armory Sq, PO Box 9000
Springfield, MA 01102-9000
www.stcc.edu
Prgm Dir: Anthony J Kapadoukakis, PhD RT(R)
Tel: 413 755-4850   *Fax:* 413 733-0688
E-mail: akapadoukakis@stcc.edu

Quinsigamond Community College
Radiography Prgm
670 W Boylston St
Worcester, MA 01606-2092
www.qcc.mass.edu/radiography
Prgm Dir: Linda LeFave, MEd RT(R)(M)(QM)
Tel: 508 854-4289   *Fax:* 508 852-6943
E-mail: lindal@qcc.mass.edu

Michigan

Washtenaw Community College
Radiography Prgm
4800 E Huron River Dr
Ann Arbor, MI 48106-0978
www.wccnet.edu
Prgm Dir: Connie Foster, MA RT(R) RDMS
Tel: 734 973-3418   *Fax:* 734 677-5078
E-mail: cfoster@wccnet.edu

Kellogg Community College
Radiography Prgm
450 North Ave
Battle Creek, MI 49017-3397
www.kellogg.edu
Prgm Dir: Janis M Karazim, MA RT(R)(M)
Tel: 269 965-3931, Ext 2315   *Fax:* 269 565-2059
E-mail: karazimj@kellogg.edu

Lake Michigan College
Radiography Prgm
2755 E Napier Ave
Benton Harbor, MI 49022-1899
Prgm Dir: Kerry T Mohney, RT(R)(M) BS MA
Tel: 269 927-8100, Ext 5093   *Fax:* 269 927-8186
E-mail: mohney@lakemichigancollege.edu

Ferris State University
Radiography Prgm
901 S State St
Big Rapids, MI 49307-9989
Prgm Dir: Lisa L Wall, MEd RT(R)
Tel: 231 591-2326   *Fax:* 231 591-3788
E-mail: walll@ferris.edu

Baker College of Clinton Township
Radiography Prgm
34950 Little Mack Ave
Clinton Township, MI 48035-4701
Prgm Dir: Christopher P Woodward, BS RT(R)
Tel: 586 790-9401
E-mail: christopher.woodward@baker.edu

Henry Ford Community College
Radiography Prgm
Health Careers Division
5101 Evergreen Rd
Dearborn, MI 48128
Prgm Dir: Sharon W Wu, BS RT(R)
Tel: 313 317-6595   *Fax:* 313 317-6569
E-mail: swu@hfcc.edu

Sinai-Grace Hospital
Radiography Prgm
6071 W Outer Dr
Detroit, MI 48235
www.sinaigrace.org
Prgm Dir: Mary Elizabeth Beam, BS RT(R)
Tel: 313 966-6866   *Fax:* 313 966-1272
E-mail: mbeam@dmc.org

St John Health
Cosponsor: St John Hospital and Medical Center
Radiography Prgm
22101 Moross Rd
Detroit, MI 48236-2172
www.stjohn.org
Prgm Dir: Denise R Allen, MBA RT(R)(M)(QM)
Tel: 313 343-4544   *Fax:* 313 343-3359
E-mail: denise.allen@stjohn.org

Wayne State University
Radiography Prgm
Detroit, MI 48202
www.cphs.wayne.edu
Prgm Dir: Kathleen Kath, MS RT(R)
Tel: 313 916-1348   *Fax:* 313 916-3049
E-mail: kathy@rad.hfh.edu

Hurley Medical Center
Radiography Prgm
One Hurley Plaza
Flint, MI 48503-5993
www.hurleymc.com
Prgm Dir: Dawn Sturk, MS RT(R)
Tel: 810 257-9835   *Fax:* 810 257-9009
E-mail: dsturk1@hurleymc.com

Grand Rapids Community College
Radiography Prgm
143 Bostwick St NE
Grand Rapids, MI 49503
Prgm Dir: Deborah C Nordman, MS RT(R)(M)
Tel: 616 234-3735   *Fax:* 616 234-4317
E-mail: dnordman@grcc.edu

Mid Michigan Community College
Radiography Prgm
1375 S Clare Ave
Harrison, MI 48625-9447
Prgm Dir: John Skinner, MEd MSA RT(R)
Tel: 989 386-6646   *Fax:* 989 386-9088
E-mail: jskinner@midmich.edu

Lansing Community College
Radiography Prgm
Dept 3100 Health and Human Service Careers
PO Box 40010
Lansing, MI 48901-7210
www.lcc.edu
Prgm Dir: Brian W Pickford, MS RT(R)
Tel: 517 483-5379   *Fax:* 517 483-1508
E-mail: pickforb@lcc.edu

Marquette General Health System
Radiography Prgm
420 W Magnetic Ave
Marquette, MI 49855
www.mgh.org
Prgm Dir: JoAnna Perucco, MS RT(R)(M)
Tel: 906 225-4916   *Fax:* 906 225-4943
E-mail: jlperucco@mgh.org

Baker College of Muskegon
Radiography Prgm
1903 Marquette Ave
Muskegon, MI 49442-1490
Prgm Dir: Cameron J Vander Stel, MBA RT(R)
Tel: 231 777-5224
E-mail: cameron.vanderstel@baker.edu

Baker College of Owosso
Radiography Prgm
1020 S Washington St
Owosso, MI 48867-4400
Prgm Dir: Kathleen M Wallen, BS RT(R)
Tel: 989 729-3416   *Fax:* 989 729-3411
E-mail: kathleen.wallen@baker.edu

Port Huron Hospital
Radiography Prgm
1221 Pine Grove, PO Box 5011
Port Huron, MI 48061-5011
www.porthuronhospital.org
Prgm Dir: Monica S Rowling, MS RT(R)(M)
Tel: 810 989-3163   *Fax:* 810 989-3197
E-mail: mrowling@porthuronhosp.org

William Beaumont Hospital
Radiography Prgm
3601 W 13 Mile Rd
Royal Oak, MI 48073
www.beaumont.edu
Prgm Dir: Terese A Trost, MA RT(R)
Tel: 248 898-6048   *Fax:* 248 898-5015
E-mail: ttrost@beaumont.edu

Oakland Community College - Southfield
Radiography Prgm
22322 Rutland Dr
Southfield, MI 48075-4793
Prgm Dir: Carolyn Nacy, BS RT(R) RDMS
Tel: 248 233-2918   *Fax:* 248 233-2891
E-mail: ceoneill@oaklandcc.edu

Providence Hospital
Radiography Prgm
16001 W Nine Mile Rd, PO Box 2043
Southfield, MI 48037
www.realmedicine.org/Providence
Prgm Dir: Mary A Kleven, MAOM RT(R)(M)
Tel: 248 849-3293   *Fax:* 248 424-5397
E-mail: Mary.Kleven@stjohn.org

Delta College
Radiography Prgm
1961 Delta Rd
University Center, MI 48710
Prgm Dir: Brett Cone, MBA RT(R)
Tel: 989 686-9533   *Fax:* 989 667-2230
E-mail: bret_cone_2000@yahoo.com

Minnesota

Riverland Community College
Radiography Prgm
1600 8th Ave NW
Austin, MN 55912
Prgm Dir: Eugene D Frank, MA RT(R) FASRT
Tel: 507 433-0645   *Fax:* 507 433-0515
E-mail: gfrank@river.cc.mn.us

Lake Superior College
Radiography Prgm
2101 Trinity Rd
Duluth, MN 55811-2741
www.lsc.edu
Prgm Dir: Nancy A Fredrickson, RT(R)
Tel: 218 725-7714   *Fax:* 218 733-7615
E-mail: n.fredrickson@lsc.edu

Argosy University - Twin Cities
Radiography Prgm
1515 Central Parkway
Eagan, MN 55121
www.argosyu.edu
Prgm Dir: Stacy L Nelson, RT(R)
Tel: 651 846-3535
E-mail: snelson@argosy.edu

Northland Community & Technical College
Radiography Prgm
2022 Central Ave NE
East Grand Forks, MN 56721-2702
www.northlandcollege.edu
Prgm Dir: Debra King, BS RT(R)
Tel: 218 773-3441, Ext 567   *Fax:* 218 773-4502
E-mail: deb.king@northlandcollege.edu

Fairview University
Radiography Prgm
School of Radiologic Technology
6545 France Ave, Ste 450
Edina, MN 55435
Prgm Dir: Linda A Dehrer-Wendt, BS RT(R)
Tel: 952 836-3544   *Fax:* 952 836-3925
E-mail: ldehrer1@fairview.org

College of St Catherine - Minneapolis
Radiography Prgm
601 25th Ave S
Minneapolis, MN 55454
www.stkate.edu
Prgm Dir: Alan Bode, MA RT(R)(QM)
Tel: 651 690-7887   *Fax:* 651 690-7849
E-mail: ajbode@stkate.edu

Veterans Affairs Medical Center
Radiography Prgm
One Veterans Dr
Minneapolis, MN 55417
Prgm Dir: Michael C Stori, MS RT(R)(CT)
Tel: 612 467-2546   *Fax:* 612 727-5635
E-mail: michael.stori@med.va.gov

North Memorial Medical Center
Radiography Prgm
3300 N Oakdale
Robbinsdale, MN 55422
www.northmemorial.com
Prgm Dir: Joni E Gosch, MS RT(R)
Tel: 763 520-5337   *Fax:* 763 520-8770
E-mail: joni.gosch@northmemorial.com

Mayo School of Health Sciences
Radiography Prgm
Siebens Rm 1119
200 First St SW
Rochester, MN 55905
www.mayo.edu/mshs
Prgm Dir: Beverly J Tupper, MS RT(R)(CV)
Tel: 507 284-3169   *Fax:* 507 284-0656
E-mail: tupper.beverly@mayo.edu

St Cloud Hospital
Radiography Prgm
1406 Sixth Ave N
St Cloud, MN 56303
www.centracare.com
Prgm Dir: John Falconer, BA RT(R)
Tel: 320 255-5719, Ext 53001   *Fax:* 320 255-5730
E-mail: falconerj@centracare.com

Methodist Hospital
Radiography Prgm
6500 Excelsior Blvd
St Louis Park, MN 55426
Prgm Dir: Linda C Olson, RT(R)
Tel: 952 993-5410   *Fax:* 952 993-6531
E-mail: olsonli@parknicollet.com

Century College
Radiography Prgm
3300 Century Ave N
White Bear Lake, MN 55110
www.century.edu
Prgm Dir: Diane J Fleury-Evans, MA RT(R)
Tel: 651 779-3334   *Fax:* 651 779-5779
E-mail: diane.fleury@century.edu

Rice Memorial Hospital
Radiography Prgm
301 Becker Ave SW
Willmar, MN 56201-3302
Prgm Dir: Luther Linn, RT(R)
Tel: 320 231-4553   *Fax:* 320 231-4865
E-mail: llinn@rice.willmar.mn.us

Mississippi

Northeast Mississippi Community College
Radiography Prgm
Cunningham Blvd
Booneville, MS 38829
www.nemcc.edu
Prgm Dir: Jennifer C Davis, MA RT(R)(T)
Tel: 662 720-7364   *Fax:* 662 720-1165
E-mail: jcdavis@nemcc.edu

Jones County Junior College
Radiography Prgm
900 S Court St
Ellisville, MS 39437
www.jcjc.edu
Prgm Dir: Timothy S Cochran, MS RT(R)
Tel: 601 477-4159   *Fax:* 601 477-4152
E-mail: sandy.cochran@jcjc.edu

Itawamba Community College
Radiography Prgm
602 W Hill St
Fulton, MS 38843-0999
Prgm Dir: Deborah G Shell, MEd RT(R)
Tel: 662 862-8345   *Fax:* 662 862-8350
E-mail: dgshell@iccms.edu

Mississippi Gulf Coast Community College
Radiography Prgm
PO Box 100
Gautier, MS 39553
www.mgccc.edu
Prgm Dir: Judy S Lewis, MEd
    RT(R)(M)(CT)(QM)(ARRT)
Tel: 228 497-9602, Ext 7710   *Fax:* 228 497-7676
E-mail: judy.lewis@mgccc.edu

Pearl River Community College
Radiography Prgm
5448 US Hwy 49 S
Hattiesburg, MS 39401
Prgm Dir: C David Armstrong, MEd RT(R)
Tel: 601 554-5484   *Fax:* 601 554-5553
E-mail: darmstrong@prcc.edu

University of Mississippi Medical Center
Radiography Prgm
2500 N State St
Jackson, MS 39216-4505
Prgm Dir: Mark R Gray, BA RT(R)
Tel: 601 984-2605   *Fax:* 601 984-4986
E-mail: mgray@radiology.umsmed.edu

Meridian Community College
Radiography Prgm
910 Hwy 19 N
Meridian, MS 39307
Prgm Dir: Seena Shazowee Edgerton, MBA RT(R)(M)
Tel: 601 484-8609, Ext 609   *Fax:* 601 484-8704
E-mail: sedgerton@meridiancc.edu

Mississippi Delta Community College
Radiography Prgm
PO Box 668
Moorhead, MS 38761
Prgm Dir: Alice K Pyles, MS RS RT(R)
Tel: 601 246-6504   *Fax:* 601 246-6507
E-mail: apyles@msdelta.edu

Hinds Community College
Radiography Prgm
PMB 10458
Raymond, MS 39154-9799
www.hindscc.edu
Prgm Dir: Stephen C Compton, BS RT(R)
Tel: 601 376-4826   *Fax:* 601 376-4962
E-mail: sccompton@hindscc.edu

Copiah-Lincoln Community College
Radiography Prgm
PO Box 649
Wesson, MS 39191
www.colin.edu/careertech/Radiology
Prgm Dir: Billie Faye Sartin, BS RT(R)
Tel: 601 643-8496   *Fax:* 601 643-8214
E-mail: bfsartin@colin.edu

Missouri

Southeast Missouri Hospital College of Nursing and Health Sciences
Radiography Prgm
2001 William St, 2nd Fl
Cape Girardeau, MO 63703
www.sehcollege.org
Prgm Dir: Peter J Barger, MSEd RT(R)(CT)
Tel: 573 334-6825, Ext 30   *Fax:* 573 339-4628
E-mail: pbarger@sehosp.org

University of Missouri - Columbia
Radiography Prgm
School of Health Professions
605 Lewis Hall
Columbia, MO 65211
www.umshp.org/rs/
Prgm Dir: Patricia A Tew, MS RT(R)(CT)
Tel: 573 884-2623   *Fax:* 573 884-1490
E-mail: tewp@health.missouri.edu

Mineral Area Regional Medical Center
Cosponsor: Farmington Missouri Hospital Company, LLC
Radiography Prgm
1212 Weber Rd
Farmington, MO 63640-3398
www.marmc.net
Prgm Dir: Brandi N Grindel, BS RT(R)
Tel: 573 701-7387   *Fax:* 573 756-6109
E-mail: Brandi_Grindel@chs.net

Sanford-Brown College
Radiography Prgm
Fenton Campus
1345 Smizer Mill Rd
Fenton, MO 63026
Prgm Dir: Angela Jean Bland, BS RT(R)
Tel: 636 651-1677   *Fax:* 636 651-1733
E-mail: abland@sbc-fenton.com

Nichols Career Center
Radiography Prgm
605 Union St
Jefferson City, MO 65101
www.jcps.k12.mo.us/education/school
Prgm Dir: Ronda Wahl, PhD RT(R)
Tel: 573 659-3238   *Fax:* 573 659-3154
E-mail: ronda.wahl@jcps.k12.mo.us

Missouri Southern State University
Radiography Prgm
3950 E Newman Rd
Joplin, MO 64801-1595
Prgm Dir: Alan D Schiska, MS RT(R) RDMS
Tel: 417 625-3118
E-mail: schiska-A@mssu.edu

Avila University
Radiography Prgm
11901 Wornall Rd
Kansas City, MO 64145-9990
Prgm Dir: Carole A Hillestad, MSEd RT(R)
Tel: 816 501-3624   *Fax:* 816 501-2457
E-mail: hillestadca@mail.avila.edu

Colorado Technical University
Radiography Prgm
520 E 19th Ave
Kansas City, MO 64116
Prgm Dir: Jessica L Langley, MS RT(R)(CT)
Tel: 816 303-7864   *Fax:* 816 472-0688
E-mail: jlangley@kc.coloradotech.edu

Metropolitan Community College - Penn Valley
Radiography Prgm
3201 SW Trafficway
Kansas City, MO 64111
www.mcckc.edu
Prgm Dir: Judith E Taylor, MEd RT(R)(M)
Tel: 816 759-4243   *Fax:* 816 759-4553
E-mail: Judy.Taylor@mcckc.edu

Research Medical Center
Radiography Prgm
2316 E Meyer Blvd
Kansas City, MO 64132-1199
http://researchmedicalcenter.com
Prgm Dir: Cheryl S Johnson, MS RT(R)
Tel: 816 276-3390   *Fax:* 816 276-3138
E-mail: cheryl.johnson2@hcamidwest.com

Saint Luke's Hospital
Radiography Prgm
4401 Wornall Rd
Kansas City, MO 64111
www.saint-lukes.org
Prgm Dir: Mary D Wooldrige, BS RT(R)
Tel: 816 932-8292   *Fax:* 816 932-2322
E-mail: mwooldridge@saint-lukes.org

Rolla Technical Center
Radiography Prgm
500 Forum Dr
Rolla, MO 65401-3699
Prgm Dir: Waneta M Odgen, MEd RT(R)(M)
Tel: 573 458-0160, Ext 16190   *Fax:* 573 458-0164
E-mail: mogden@rolla.k12.mo.us

State Fair Community College
Radiography Prgm
3201 W 16th St
Sedalia, MO 65301
Prgm Dir: Ruth Ann Pfremmer, MBA RT(R)
Tel: 660 596-7405   *Fax:* 660 530-5820
E-mail: rpfremmer@sfccmo.edu

CoxHealth
Radiography Prgm
1423 N Jefferson Ave
Springfield, MO 65802
Prgm Dir: David Frazier, MEd RT(R)(QM)
Tel: 417 269-4074   *Fax:* 417 269-4250
E-mail: david.frazier@coxhealth.com

St John's Regional Health Center
Radiography Prgm
1235 E Cherokee St
Springfield, MO 65804-2263
www.stjohns.com
Prgm Dir: Joan Hedrick, MEd RT(R)(M)
Tel: 417 820-2982   *Fax:* 417 820-3427
E-mail: jfhedrick@sprg.mercy.net

Hillyard Technical Center
Radiography Prgm
3434 Faraon St
St Joseph, MO 64506
Prgm Dir: Shirley A Erickson, MBA RT(R)(N)
Tel: 816 671-4170
E-mail: shirley.erickson@sjsd.k12.mo.us

St John's Mercy Medical Center
Radiography Prgm
615 S New Ballas Rd
St Louis, MO 63141-8277
Prgm Dir: James E Ibaviosa, BA RT(R)(CV)
Tel: 314 569-6933, Ext 3326   *Fax:* 314 569-6343
E-mail: ibavje@stlo.mercy.net

St Louis Community College - Forest Park
Radiography Prgm
5600 Oakland Ave
St Louis, MO 63110
Prgm Dir: Vincent E Featherson, MA Ed RT(R)(M)
Tel: 314 644-9613   *Fax:* 314 951-9412
E-mail: vfeatherson@stlcc.edu

Montana

Benefis Healthcare
Radiography Prgm
500 15th Ave S
Great Falls, MT 59405
www.benefis.org
Prgm Dir: Thomas M Liston, RT(R)
Tel: 406 455-2164   *Fax:* 406 455-2162
E-mail: listthom@benefis.org
Notes: Currently inactive

Nebraska

Mary Lanning Memorial Hospital
Radiography Prgm
715 N St Joseph Ave
Hastings, NE 68901
https://www.mlmh.org
Prgm Dir: Jean M Korth, MS Ed ARRT(R)
Tel: 402 461-5087   *Fax:* 402 461-5059
E-mail: jkorth@mlmh.org

Southeast Community College
Radiography Prgm
8800 O St
Lincoln, NE 68520
www.southeast.edu
Prgm Dir: Bev Harvey, MEd RT(R)
Tel: 402 437-2759   *Fax:* 402 437-2404
E-mail: bharvey@southeast.edu

Alegent Health
Radiography Prgm
7500 Mercy Rd
Omaha, NE 68124
www.alegent.com
Prgm Dir: Luann Baylor, BGS RT(R)
Tel: 402 398-5527   *Fax:* 402 398-6650
E-mail: lbaylor@alegent.org

Clarkson College
Radiography Prgm
101 S 42nd St
Omaha, NE 68131-2739
Prgm Dir: Ellen L Collins, MS RT(R)(M)
Tel: 402 552-6140   *Fax:* 402 552-6019
E-mail: collins@clarksoncollege.edu

University of Nebraska Medical Center
Radiography Prgm
984545 Nebraska Medical Center
Omaha, NE 68198-4545
www.unmc.edu/alliedhealth/rste
Prgm Dir: Connie L Mitchell, MA RT(R)(CT)
Tel: 402 559-6945   *Fax:* 402 559-4667
E-mail: clmitche@unmc.edu

Regional West Medical Center
Radiography Prgm
School of Radiologic Technology
4021 Ave B
Scottsbluff, NE 69361
www.rwhs.org
Prgm Dir: Daniel R Gilbert, MSEd RT(R)(CV)(MR)(CT)(QM)
Tel: 308 630-1155   *Fax:* 308 630-1983
E-mail: gilberd@rwmc.net

Nevada

Pima Medical Institute
Radiography Prgm
3333 E Flamingo Rd
Las Vegas, NV 89121
Prgm Dir: Jennifer L Beirdneau, BS RT(R)(MR)
Tel: 702 458-9650, Ext 235
E-mail: jbeirdneau@pmi.edu

University of Nevada - Las Vegas
Radiography Prgm
4505 Maryland Pkwy
Las Vegas, NV 89154-3017
www.unlv.edu
Prgm Dir: George Pales, PhD RT(R)(MR)(T)
Tel: 702 895-3296   *Fax:* 702 895-1312
E-mail: GPales@ccmail.nevada.edu

Truckee Meadows Community College
Radiography Prgm
7000 Dandini Blvd, RDMT 417
Reno, NV 89512-3999
www.tmcc.edu/x-ray
Prgm Dir: Deborah K Baker, BS RT(R)
Tel: 775 673-7121   *Fax:* 775 673-7034
E-mail: dbaker@tmcc.edu

New Hampshire

New Hampshire Technical Institute
Radiography Prgm
31 College Dr
Concord, NH 03301-7412
www.nhti.edu
Prgm Dir: Kevin P Barry, MEd RT(R) RDMS RDCS
Tel: 603 271-7154   *Fax:* 603 271-7148
E-mail: kbarry@nhctc.edu

Lebanon College
Radiography Prgm
15 Hanover St
Lebanon, NH 03766
Prgm Dir: Karen Amadon Burgess, MEd RT(R)(M)
Tel: 603 448-2445, Ext 125
E-mail: kburgess@lebanoncollege.edu

New Jersey

Cooper University Hospital
Radiography Prgm
One Cooper Plaza
Camden, NJ 08103
www.cooperhealth.org
Prgm Dir: Francis Williams, BS RT(R)
Tel: 856 342-2397   *Fax:* 856 968-8532
E-mail: williams-frank@cooperhealth.edu

Middlesex County College
Radiography Prgm
2600 Woodbridge Ave, PO Box 3050
Edison, NJ 08818-3050
www.middlesexcc.edu
Prgm Dir: Albert M Snopek, BS RT(R)(M)(CV)(QM)
Tel: 732 906-2583   *Fax:* 732 906-7784
E-mail: asnopek@middlesexcc.edu

Englewood Hospital & Medical Center
Radiography Prgm
350 Engle St
Englewood, NJ 07631
www.englewoodhospital.com
Prgm Dir: Pamela Woodward, MS
   RT(R)(M)(MR)(QM)(CT)
Tel: 201 894-3481   *Fax:* 201 816-0168
E-mail: pamela.woodward@ehmc.com

Christ Hospital
Radiography Prgm
Hudson Area School of Radiologic Technology
176 Palisade Ave
Jersey City, NJ 07306
www.christhospital.org
Prgm Dir: Kenneth Lee, DHS RT(R)(M)
Tel: 201 795-8520   *Fax:* 201 795-5818
E-mail: klee@christhospital.org

Brookdale Community College
Radiography Prgm
765 Newman Springs Rd
Lincroft, NJ 07738
www.brookdalecc.edu/fac/radtech
Prgm Dir: Terry M Konn, PhD RT(R)
Tel: 732 224-2696   *Fax:* 732 224-2998
E-mail: tkonn@brookdalecc.edu

Essex County College
Radiography Prgm
303 University Ave
Newark, NJ 07102
Prgm Dir: Ronald M Kopec, MAEd RT(R)
Tel: 973 877-3437   *Fax:* 973 877-1930
E-mail: kopec@essex.edu

Bergen Community College
Radiography Prgm
400 Paramus Rd
Paramus, NJ 07652
www.bergen.edu
Prgm Dir: William L Leonard, MA RT(R)
Tel: 201 447-7944   *Fax:* 201 612-3876
E-mail: wleonard@bergen.edu

Passaic County Community College
Radiography Prgm
One College Blvd
Paterson, NJ 07505-1179
http://pccc.edu
Prgm Dir: Eileen Maloney, MEd RT(R)(M)FASRT
Tel: 973 684-5280   *Fax:* 973 684-5843
E-mail: emaloney@pccc.edu

Burlington County College
Radiography Prgm
601 Pemberton Browns Mills Rd
Pemberton, NJ 08068
www.bcc.edu
Prgm Dir: Elizabeth Price, MS RT(R)(M)(CT)
Tel: 609 894-9311, Ext 1407   *Fax:* 609 726-0628
E-mail: eprice@bcc.edu

Muhlenberg Regional Medical Center
Radiography Prgm
Park Ave and Randolph Rd
Plainfield, NJ 07061
http://muhlenbergschools.org
Prgm Dir: Valerie L Carlisle, MEd RT(R)
Tel: 908 668-2966   *Fax:* 908 226-4568
E-mail: VCarlisle@solarishs.org

County College of Morris
Radiography Prgm
214 Center Grove Rd
Randolph, NJ 07869
Prgm Dir: Denise M Vill'Neuve, MA RT(R)(M)(CT)
Tel: 973 328-5354   *Fax:* 973 328-5379
E-mail: dvillneuve@ccm.edu

The Valley Hospital
Radiography Prgm
223 N Van Dien Ave
Ridgewood, NJ 07450
Prgm Dir: Maureen K Wolf, BS RT(R)(N)
Tel: 201 447-8221   *Fax:* 201 251-3280
E-mail: mwolf@valleyhealth.com

Shore Memorial Hospital
Radiography Prgm
1 E New York Ave
Somers Point, NJ 08244-2387
www.shorememorial.org
Prgm Dir: Richard L Fries, BS RT(R)
Tel: 609 653-3924   *Fax:* 609 653-3566
E-mail: rfries@shorememorial.org

Mercer County Community College
Radiography Prgm
1200 Old Trenton Rd, PO Box B
Trenton, NJ 08690
www.mccc.edu
Prgm Dir: Sandra L Kerr, MA RT(R)(M)
Tel: 609 586-4800, Ext 3337   *Fax:* 609 570-3831
E-mail: kerr@mccc.edu

St Francis Medical Center
Radiography Prgm
601 Hamilton Ave
Trenton, NJ 08629-1986
www.stfrancismedical.com
Prgm Dir: Theresa M Levitsky, MA RT(R)(CV)(M)(QM)
Tel: 609 599-5234   *Fax:* 609 599-5529
E-mail: tlevitsky@che-east.org

Cumberland County College
Radiography Prgm
College Dr, PO Box 1500
Vineland, NJ 08362-1500
Prgm Dir: Robert P Champa, MA RT(R)
Tel: 609 691-8600, Ext 264   *Fax:* 609 691-9489
E-mail: rchampa@cccnj.net

Pascack Valley Hospital
Radiography Prgm
Old Hook Rd
Westwood, NJ 07675-3181
Prgm Dir: Colleen Smorra, MS RT(R)(M)(MR)
Tel: 201 358-3219   *Fax:* 201 358-3216
E-mail: csmorra@pvhospital.org

New Mexico

Pima Medical Institute - Albuquerque
Radiography Prgm
2201 San Pedro NE, Bldg 3, Ste 100
Albuquerque, NM 87110
Prgm Dir: James G Murrell, MSRS RT(R)(M)(CT)(QM)
Tel: 505 881-1234   *Fax:* 505 884-8371
E-mail: jmurrell@pmi.edu

Clovis Community College
Radiography Prgm
417 Schepps Blvd
Clovis, NM 88101
www.clovis.edu
Prgm Dir: Jeannie Kilgore, MEd RT(R)
Tel: 505 769-4996   *Fax:* 505 769-4190
E-mail: jeannie.kilgore@clovis.edu

Northern New Mexico College
Radiography Prgm
921 Paseo de Onate
Espanola, NM 87532
Prgm Dir: Michael P Frain, MA RT(R)
Tel: 505 747-2218   *Fax:* 505 747-5415
E-mail: frainm@nnmc.edu

Dona Ana Community College
Radiography Prgm
MSC 3DA PO Box 30001
3400 S Espina St
Las Cruces, NM 88003-8001
http://dacc.nmsu.edu
Prgm Dir: Annja M Cox, MA RT(R)(M)
Tel: 505 527-7581   *Fax:* 505 527-7765
E-mail: acox@nmsu.edu

New York

Broome Community College
Radiography Prgm
Upper Front St, PO Box 1017
Binghamton, NY 13902
www.sunybroome.edu
Prgm Dir: Nancy E Button, MS RT(R)
Tel: 607 778-5070   *Fax:* 607 778-5467
E-mail: button_n@sunybroome.edu

Bronx Community College
Cosponsor: City University of New York
Radiography Prgm
University Ave and W 181st St
CP Hall Rm 222
Bronx, NY 10453
www.bcc.cuny.edu
Prgm Dir: Virginia M Mishkin, MS RT(R)(M)(QM)
Tel: 718 289-5396   *Fax:* 718 289-6373
E-mail: virginia.mishkin@bcc.cuny.edu

Hostos Community College of CUNY
Radiography Prgm
475 Grand Concourse
Bronx, NY 10451
Prgm Dir: Allen Solomon, MSEd RT(R)
Tel: 718 518-4123   *Fax:* 718 518-4194
E-mail: asolomon@hostos.cuny.edu

Long Island College Hospital
Radiography Prgm
339 Hicks St
Brooklyn, NY 11201
Prgm Dir: Sergeo Guilbaud, BS RT(R)
Tel: 718 780-1681   *Fax:* 718 780-1592
E-mail: sguilbau@chpnet.org

New York City College of Technology
Radiography Prgm
300 Jay St
Brooklyn, NY 11201-2983
Prgm Dir: Mary Alice Browne, MS RT(R)(CV)(CT)(MR)
Tel: 718 260-5360, Ext 5360   *Fax:* 718 260-5540
E-mail: mabrowne@citytech.cuny.edu

New York Methodist Hospital
Radiography Prgm
Bartone Center of Allied Health Education
1401 Kings Hwy, 2nd Fl
Brooklyn, NY 11229
www.nym.org/education/bartone
Prgm Dir: Joanne M Durney, BS RT(R)(M)
Tel: 718 645-3500, Ext 107   *Fax:* 718 780-3494
E-mail: jdurney@nymahe.org

Long Island University - C W Post Campus
Radiography Prgm
720 Northern Blvd
Brookville, NY 11548-1300
Prgm Dir: James F Joyce, MS RT(R)(M)(QM)
Tel: 516 299-3075   *Fax:* 516 299-3081
E-mail: jjoyce@liu.edu

Trocaire College
Radiography Prgm
360 Choate Ave
Buffalo, NY 14220
Prgm Dir: Nancy L Augustyn, MSEd RT(R)
Tel: 716 826-1200, Ext 1243   *Fax:* 716 828-6107
E-mail: augustynn@trocaire.edu

Arnot Ogden Medical Center
Radiography Prgm
600 Roe Ave
Elmira, NY 14905-1676
www.arnothealth.org
Prgm Dir: Ellen R Richards, MPS RT(R)
Tel: 607 737-4289   *Fax:* 607 737-4116
E-mail: erichards@aomc.org

Nassau Community College
Radiography Prgm
One Education Dr
Garden City, NY 11530
Prgm Dir: Jeffrey T Miller, BS RT(R)
Tel: 516 572-7539   *Fax:* 516 572-7565
E-mail: millerjt@ncc.edu

Glens Falls Hospital
Radiography Prgm
School of Radiologic Technology
126 South St
Glens Falls, NY 12801
Prgm Dir: Roger F Weeden, Jr, BA RT(R)
Tel: 518 926-7025   *Fax:* 518 926-3747
E-mail: rweeden@glensfallshosp.org

St James Mercy Health
Radiography Prgm
St James Mercy Hospital
411 Canisteo St
Hornell, NY 14843
www.stjamesmercy.org
Prgm Dir: Lynne M Freeland, MS RT(R)
Tel: 607 324-8265   *Fax:* 607 324-8214
E-mail: lfreelan@sjmh.org

Woman's Christian Association Hospital
Radiography Prgm
207 Foote Ave
Jamestown, NY 14701-0840
Prgm Dir: Christina Slojkowski, BS RT(R)
Tel: 716 664-8366   *Fax:* 716 664-8312
E-mail: Christina.Slojkowski@wcahospital.org

Orange County Community College
Radiography Prgm
115 South St
Middletown, NY 10940
Prgm Dir: Robert M Misiak, RT(R)
Tel: 845 341-4275   *Fax:* 845 341-4511
E-mail: rmmisiak@sunyorange.edu

Winthrop University Hospital
Radiography Prgm
259 First St
Ste 127
Mineola, NY 11501
www.winthrop-radiology.com
Prgm Dir: Mary Jo Perry, MS RT(R)(M)
Tel: 516 663-2536, Ext 2819   *Fax:* 516 663-2587
E-mail: mperry@winthrop.org

Bellevue Hospital Center
Radiography Prgm
First Ave and 27th St, C&D Bldg, Rm D510
New York, NY 10016
Prgm Dir: Andrew C Richter, BS RT(R)
Tel: 212 562-4895   *Fax:* 212 562-8260
E-mail: richtera@bellevue.nychhc.org

Harlem Hospital Center
Radiography Prgm
506 Lenox Ave
Kountz Pavilion Rm 415
New York, NY 10037
Prgm Dir: William Hall, MPH RT(R) (MR)
Tel: 212 939-3480   *Fax:* 212 939-3479
E-mail: wah47@columbia.edu

Robt J Hochstim Sch Rad/S Nassau Comm Hosp
Radiography Prgm
One Healthy Way
Oceanside, NY 11572
http://snch.org
Prgm Dir: Gina Collins, MPA RT(R)(M)
Tel: 516 632-4678   *Fax:* 516 336-2983
E-mail: gcollins@snch.org

Champlain Valley Phys Hospital Med Ctr
Radiography Prgm
75 Beekman St
Plattsburgh, NY 12901
www.cvph.org
Prgm Dir: Fayrene M Ashline, BS RT(R)(M)(N)
Tel: 518 562-7510   *Fax:* 518 562-7486
E-mail: fashline@cvph.org

St John's University
Radiography Prgm
8000 Utopia Pkwy
Queens, NY 11439
Prgm Dir: Caroline Burns, MS RT(R)(M)
Tel: 718 990-8403
E-mail: burnsc@stjohns.edu

Peconic Bay Medical Center
Radiography Prgm
1300 Roanoke Ave
Riverhead, NY 11901
Prgm Dir: William L DeCamp, BS RT(R)(CT)
Tel: 631 548-6173   *Fax:* 631 548-6751
E-mail: xrayschool@centralsuffolkhospital.org

Monroe Community College
Radiography Prgm
1000 E Henrietta Rd
Rochester, NY 14623-5780
www.monroecc.edu
Prgm Dir: Eileen M Doyle, MPA RT(R)
Tel: 585 292-2379   *Fax:* 585 292-3834
E-mail: edoyle@monroecc.edu

Mercy Medical Center
Radiography Prgm
PO Box 9024
1000 N Village Ave
Rockville Centre, NY 11571-9024
Prgm Dir: Barbara Geiger, MA RT(R)(M)
Tel: 516 705-2272   *Fax:* 516 705-1079
E-mail: barbara.geiger@chsli.org

Niagara County Community College
Radiography Prgm
3111 Saunders Settlement Rd
Sanborn, NY 14132
Prgm Dir: Carolyn Cianciosa, MS RT(R)
Tel: 716 614-6416   *Fax:* 716 614-6879
E-mail: sciera@niagaracc.suny.edu

North Country Community College
Radiography Prgm
23 Santanoni Ave, PO Box 89
Saranac Lake, NY 12983-0089
Prgm Dir: Bonnie S Clinebell, BS RT(R)(M)
Tel: 518 891-2915, Ext 255   *Fax:* 518 891-2915
E-mail: bclinebell@nccc.edu

SUNY Upstate Medical University
Radiography Prgm
Medical Imaging Sciences Program
750 E Adams St
Syracuse, NY 13210
Prgm Dir: David A Clemente, MSEd RT(R)(MR)
Tel: 315 464-6929   *Fax:* 315 464-4561
E-mail: clementd@upstate.edu

Faxton - St Luke's Healthcare
Radiography Prgm
Champlain Ave, PO Box 479
Utica, NY 13503-0479
Prgm Dir: Rosemary Morin, MS RT(R)
Tel: 315 798-6136   *Fax:* 315 798-6295
E-mail: xrayed@dreamscape.com

St Elizabeth Medical Center
Radiography Prgm
2209 Genesee St
Utica, NY 13501
www.stemc.org
Prgm Dir: Janice M Lutz, MPS RT(R)(M)
Tel: 315 798-8258   *Fax:* 315 734-3084
E-mail: jlutz@stemc.org

Westchester Community College
Radiography Prgm
75 Grasslands Rd
Valhalla, NY 10595-1698
Prgm Dir: Barbara Chakmakjian, MS RT(R)(M)
Tel: 914 606-6682   *Fax:* 914 606-7832
E-mail: barbara.chakmakjian@sunywcc.edu

St Joseph's Medical Center
Radiography Prgm
127 S Broadway
Yonkers, NY 10701
Prgm Dir: Rose P LaBate, BS RT(R)(M)
Tel: 914 934-3000
E-mail: labate99@yahoo.com

North Carolina

Asheville-Buncombe Technical Comm College
Radiography Prgm
340 Victoria Rd
Asheville, NC 28801
www.abtech.edu
Prgm Dir: Debra J Reese, MPH RT(R)
Tel: 828 254-1921, Ext 282   *Fax:* 828 281-9846
E-mail: dreese@abtech.edu

University of North Carolina - Chapel Hill
Radiography Prgm
Medical School
CB 7130 E Wing
Chapel Hill, NC 27599-7130
Prgm Dir: Joy J Renner, MA RT(R)
Tel: 919 966-5147   *Fax:* 919 966-6951
E-mail: jrenner@med.unc.edu

Carolinas College of Health Sciences
Radiography Prgm
PO Box 32861
1200 Blythe Blvd
Charlotte, NC 28232-2861
www.CarolinasCollege.edu
Prgm Dir: Roy M Smither II, MA RT(R)
Tel: 704 355-2446   *Fax:* 704 355-5967
E-mail: roy.smither@carolinashealthcare.org

Presbyterian Healthcare
Radiography Prgm
200 Hawthorne Ln/PO Box 33549
Charlotte, NC 28204
www.presbyterian.org
Prgm Dir: Elizabeth S Shields, BS RT(R)
Tel: 704 384-5104   *Fax:* 704 384-5684
E-mail: esshields@novanthealth.org

Fayetteville Technical Community College
Radiography Prgm
PO Box 35236
Fayetteville, NC 28303-0236
Prgm Dir: Anita L McKnight, BHS RT(R)
Tel: 910 678-8303   *Fax:* 910 678-8500
E-mail: mcknigha@faytechcc.edu

Moses Cone Health System
Radiography Prgm
1200 N Elm St
Greensboro, NC 27401-1020
www.mosescone.com/radtech
Prgm Dir: Rene Parrish, BS RT(R)
Tel: 336 832-7487   *Fax:* 336 832-7465
E-mail: rene.parrish@mosescone.com

Pitt Community College
Radiography Prgm
PO Drawer 7007, Hwy 11 S
Greenville, NC 27835-7007
www.pittcc.edu
Prgm Dir: Louise R Cox, BA RT(R)(CV)(M)
Tel: 252 493-7464   *Fax:* 252 321-4451
E-mail: lcox@email.pittcc.edu

Vance-Granville Community College
Radiography Prgm
PO Box 917
Henderson, NC 27536
Prgm Dir: Angela M Thomas, BA RT(R)
Tel: 919 258-4737, Ext 3517   *Fax:* 252 738-3319
E-mail: thomasa@vgcc.edu

Caldwell Comm College & Tech Institute
Radiography Prgm
2855 Hickory Blvd
Hudson, NC 28638
Prgm Dir: Rosanne Y Annas, BS RT(R)
Tel: 704 726-2358   *Fax:* 704 726-2489
E-mail: rannas@cccti.edu

Lenoir Community College
Radiography Prgm
PO Box 188
Kinston, NC 28502-0188
Prgm Dir: Bobby G Austin, MSRS
    RT(R)(CV)(M)(CT)(MR)
Tel: 252 527-6223, Ext 814   *Fax:* 252 233-6893
E-mail: baustin@lenoircc.edu

Carteret Community College
Radiography Prgm
3505 Arendell St
Morehead City, NC 28557-2989
Prgm Dir: Elaine M Fuge, MEd RT(R)
Tel: 252 222-6165   *Fax:* 252 222-6074
E-mail: fugee@carteret.edu

Wilkes Regional Medical Center
Radiography Prgm
1508 West D St, PO Box 609
North Wilkesboro, NC 28659
www.wilkesregional.com
Prgm Dir: Linda G Vickery, BS RT(R)(CT)
Tel: 336 661-0214   *Fax:* 336 667-0740
E-mail: lvickery@wilkesregional.com

Sandhills Community College
Radiography Prgm
3395 Airport Rd
Pinehurst, NC 28374
www.sandhills.edu
Prgm Dir: Kay B Nardo, BA RT(R)(CV)
Tel: 910 695-3916   *Fax:* 910 693-2060
E-mail: nardok@sandhills.edu

Wake Technical Community College
Radiography Prgm
9101 Fayetteville Rd
Raleigh, NC 27603-5696
Prgm Dir: Deborah J Wood, MEd RT(R)(M)
Tel: 919 250-4290   *Fax:* 919 250-4329
E-mail: djwood@waketech.edu

Edgecombe Community College
Radiography Prgm
225 Tarboro St
Rocky Mount, NC 27801
Prgm Dir: Deborah L Rossi, MS LRT
Tel: 252 446-0346, Ext 386   *Fax:* 252 985-2212
E-mail: rossid@edgecombe.edu

Rowan-Cabarrus Community College
Radiography Prgm
PO Box 1595
Salisbury, NC 28145-1595
www.rowancabarrus.edu
Prgm Dir: Frankie Lyons, MHA RT(R)(M)
Tel: 704 216-3719   *Fax:* 704 642-0750
E-mail: lyonsf@rowancabarrus.edu

Cleveland Community College
Radiography Prgm
137 S Post Rd
Shelby, NC 28152
www.clevelandcommunitycollege.edu
Prgm Dir: Alease Rousseau, BS RT(R)
Tel: 704 484-4091, Ext 4091   *Fax:* 704 484-5304
E-mail: rousseau@cleveland.cc.nc.us

Johnston Community College
Radiography Prgm
PO Box 2350
Smithfield, NC 27577-2350
www.johnstoncc.edu
Prgm Dir: Ann P Jackson, BS RT(R)
Tel: 919 209-2156   *Fax:* 919 209-2153
E-mail: jacksona@johnstoncc.edu

Southwestern Community College
Radiography Prgm
447 College Dr
Sylva, NC 28779
Prgm Dir: Meg Rollins, MS RT(R)(N)
Tel: 828 586-4091, Ext 320   *Fax:* 828 586-3129
E-mail: mrollins@southwesterncc.edu

Cape Fear Community College
Radiography Prgm
411 N Front St
Wilmington, NC 28401
Prgm Dir: Donna M Collentine, MA RT(R)
Tel: 910 362-7298   *Fax:* 910 362-7087
E-mail: dcollentine@cfcc.edu

Forsyth Technical Community College
Radiography Prgm
2100 Silas Creek Pkwy
Winston-Salem, NC 27103
Prgm Dir: Linda W Yurko, MA RT(R)(M)
Tel: 336 734-7180   *Fax:* 336 734-7444
E-mail: lyurko@forsythtech.edu

North Dakota

Medcenter One
Radiography Prgm
300 N 7th St
Bismarck, ND 58506-5525
www.medcenterone.com
Prgm Dir: Cindy Hanson, MS RT(R)
Tel: 701 323-5470   *Fax:* 701 323-5479
E-mail: chanson@mohs.org

MeritCare Medical Center
Radiography Prgm
801 N Broadway
Fargo, ND 58122
Prgm Dir: Mary Jo Bergman, MEd MS RN RT(R)
Tel: 701 364-1728
E-mail: mary.jo.bergman@meritcare.com

Trinity Health
Radiography Prgm
407 3rd St NE
Minot, ND 58701
www.trinityhealth.org
Prgm Dir: Debbie Hornbacher Brandt, MS RT(R)
Tel: 701 857-5000, Ext 5620   *Fax:* 701 857-5620
E-mail: deb.hornbacher@trinityhealth.org

Ohio

Children's Hospital Medical Ctr of Akron
Radiography Prgm
One Perkins Square
Akron, OH 44308
www.akronchildrens.org
Prgm Dir: David L Whipple, MEd RT(R)
Tel: 330 543-8849, Ext 3   *Fax:* 330 543-8282
E-mail: dwhipple@chmca.org

University of Cincinnati
Cosponsor: Raymond Walters College
Radiography Prgm
9555 Plainfield Rd
Blue Ash, OH 45236
Prgm Dir: Angie Arnold, MEd RT(R)
Tel: 513 745-5659   *Fax:* 513 936-7113
E-mail: angie.arnold@uc.edu

Aultman Hospital
Radiography Prgm
2600 Sixth St SW
Canton, OH 44710
Prgm Dir: Robin R Williams, BA RT(R)
Tel: 330 363-5352
E-mail: rwilliams@aultman.com

Mercy Medical Center
Radiography Prgm
1320 Mercy Dr NW
Canton, OH 44708
Prgm Dir: Gary F Greathouse, MS RT(R)
Tel: 330 489-1273, Ext 1273   *Fax:* 330 430-2772
E-mail: gary.greathouse@csauh.com

Collins Career Center
Radiography Prgm
11627 St Rte 243
Chesapeake, OH 45619
Prgm Dir: Teresa Lynn Williamson, BA
   RT(R)(M)(CT)(BD)
Tel: 740 867-6641, Ext 362
E-mail: williamsontl@collins-cc.k12.oh.us

Xavier University
Radiography Prgm
3800 Victory Pkwy
Cincinnati, OH 45207-4331
www.xavier.edu
Prgm Dir: Donna J Endicott, MEd RT(R)
Tel: 513 745-3358   *Fax:* 513 745-1079
E-mail: endicott@xavier.edu

Columbus State Community College
Radiography Prgm
550 E Spring St
GR389
Columbus, OH 43216
www.cscc.edu/radiography
Prgm Dir: James J Byrne, MEd RT(R)
Tel: 800 621-6407, Ext 5215   *Fax:* 614 287-6059
E-mail: jbyrne@cscc.edu

Sinclair Community College
Radiography Prgm
444 W Third St
Dayton, OH 45402-1460
Prgm Dir: Debra Schwartz, BS RT(R)(M)
Tel: 937 512-2159   *Fax:* 937 512-2058
E-mail: debra.schwartz@sinclair.edu

Lorain County Community College
Radiography Prgm
1005 N Abbe Rd, HS223
Elyria, OH 44035
www.lorainccc.edu
Prgm Dir: Jeffrey J Walmsley, MEd RT(R)(QM)
Tel: 440 366-7197   *Fax:* 440 366-4116
E-mail: jwalmsle@lorainccc.edu

Cleveland Clinic
Radiography Prgm
18901 Lakeshore Blvd
Euclid, OH 44119
www.cchseast.org/schools
Prgm Dir: Gloria A Albrecht, BS RT(R)
Tel: 216 692-7512   *Fax:* 216 692-7806
E-mail: galbrech@cchseast.org

Kettering College of Medical Arts
Radiography Prgm
3737 Southern Blvd
Kettering, OH 45429
http://kcma.edu
Prgm Dir: Lawrence Beneke, MSEd RT(R)(CT)
Tel: 937 298-3399, Ext 55696   *Fax:* 937 395-8484
E-mail: larry.beneke@kcma.org

Lakeland Community College
Radiography Prgm
7700 Clocktower Dr
Kirtland, OH 44094-5198
Prgm Dir: Jack A Thomas, MS RT(R)(QM)
Tel: 440 525-7074   *Fax:* 440 525-7433
E-mail: jthomas@lakelandcc.edu

Rhodes State College
Radiography Prgm
4240 Campus Dr
Lima, OH 45804-3597
Prgm Dir: Dennis F Spragg, MSEd RT(R)(CT)(QM)
Tel: 419 995-8257   *Fax:* 419 995-8818
E-mail: Spragg.D@rhodesstate.edu

North Central State College
Radiography Prgm
2441 Kenwood Circle, PO Box 698
Mansfield, OH 44901-0698
www.ncstatecollege.edu
Prgm Dir: Ellen M Johnson, BS RT(R)
Tel: 419 755-4809   *Fax:* 419 755-5630
E-mail: ejohnson@ncstatecollege.edu

Marietta Memorial Hospital
Radiography Prgm
401 Matthew St
Marietta, OH 45750
Prgm Dir: Paul E Richards, Jr, MA RT(R)
Tel: 740 374-8716, Ext 1720   *Fax:* 740 373-7496
E-mail: prichards@wscc.edu

Marion Technical College
Radiography Prgm
1467 Mt Vernon Ave
Marion, OH 43302-5694
www.mtc.edu
Prgm Dir: Linda Rizzo, BS RT(R)
Tel: 740 389-4636, Ext 246   *Fax:* 740 725-4018
E-mail: rizzol@mtc.edu

Central Ohio Technical College
Radiography Prgm
1179 University Dr
Newark, OH 43055-1767
www.cotc.edu
Prgm Dir: Linnea A Hopewell, MEd RT(R)(M)(QM)
Tel: 740 366-9387   *Fax:* 740 366-5047
E-mail: hopewell@cotc.edu

Cuyahoga Community College
Radiography Prgm
Western Campus
11000 Pleasant Valley Rd
Parma, OH 44130-5199
www.tri-c.edu
Prgm Dir: Marilyn A Rep, BA RT(R)
Tel: 216 987-5264   *Fax:* 216 987-5066
E-mail: marilyn.rep@tri-c.edu

Shawnee State University
Radiography Prgm
940 Second St
Portsmouth, OH 45662-4344
www.shawnee.edu
Prgm Dir: William W Sykes, MBA
   RT(R)(M)(CT)(MR)(QM)
Tel: 740 351-3253   *Fax:* 740 351-3354
E-mail: bsykes@shawnee.edu

Kent State University - Salem Campus
Radiography Prgm
2491 State Route 45 S
Salem, OH 44460-9412
www.salem.kent.edu
Prgm Dir: Janice J Gibson, MEd RT(R)
Tel: 330 337-4223   *Fax:* 330 337-4122
E-mail: jjgibso1@kent.edu

Jefferson Community College
Radiography Prgm
4000 Sunset Blvd
Steubenville, OH 43952-3598
www.jcc.edu
Prgm Dir: Shelly Gaumer, MS Ed RT(R)
Tel: 740 264-5591, Ext 168   *Fax:* 740 264-1338
E-mail: sgaumer@jcc.edu

Mercy College of Northwest Ohio
Radiography Prgm
2221 Madison Ave
Toledo, OH 43624-1132
Prgm Dir: Linda S Wheatley, PhD RT(R)(MR)
Tel: 419 251-8958   *Fax:* 419 251-1730
E-mail: linda.wheatley@mercycollege.edu

Owens Community College
Radiography Prgm
PO Box 10,000
Toledo, OH 43699-1947
Prgm Dir: Catherine A Ford, BS RT(R)
Tel: 567 661-7261   *Fax:* 567 661-7251
E-mail: catherine_ford@owens.edu

Zane State College
Radiography Prgm
1555 Newark Rd
Zanesville, OH 43701
Prgm Dir: Tricia D Leggett, MSEd RT(R)(QM)
Tel: 740 588-1271   *Fax:* 740 454-0035
E-mail: tleggett@zanestate.edu

Oklahoma

Western Oklahoma State College
Radiography Prgm
2801 N Main
Altus, OK 73521-1397
www.wosc.edu
Prgm Dir: Nancy J Estes, MSRS RT(R)(M)
Tel: 580 477-7823   *Fax:* 580 477-7865
E-mail: nancy.estes@wosc.edu

Autry Technology Center
Radiography Prgm
1201 W Willow
Enid, OK 73703
www.autrytech.com
Prgm Dir: Sharon Johnson, MS RT(R)(T)
Tel: 580 242-2750, Ext 134   *Fax:* 580 233-8262
E-mail: sjohnson@autrytech.com

Great Plains Technology Center
Radiography Prgm
4500 W Lee Blvd
Lawton, OK 73505
www.gptech.org
Prgm Dir: Carrie L Baxter, MEd RT(R)(M)(CT)
Tel: 580 355-6371, Ext 5577   *Fax:* 580 250-5583
E-mail: cbaxter@gptech.org

Rose State College
Radiography Prgm
6420 SE 15th St
Midwest City, OK 73110-2799
Prgm Dir: Jonnye Griffin, MA RT(R)(QM)(M)
Tel: 405 733-7568   *Fax:* 405 736-0338
E-mail: jgriffin@rose.edu

Bacone College
Radiography Prgm
2299 Old Bacone Rd
Muskogee, OK 74403-1568
Prgm Dir: Stephanie A Stephens, BSRS RT(R)(M)
Tel: 918 781-7326   *Fax:* 918 781-7214
E-mail: stephens@bacone.edu

Indian Capital Technology Center
Radiography Prgm
2403 N 41st St E
Muskogee, OK 74403-1799
Prgm Dir: Ernest A Briggs, MS RT(R)
Tel: 918 687-6383, Ext 243   *Fax:* 866 877-9987
E-mail: ernieb@ictctech.com

Metro Technology Centers
Radiography Prgm
1720 Springlake Dr
Oklahoma City, OK 73111
www.metrotech.org
Prgm Dir: Barbara J Harper, MEd RT(R)
Tel: 405 605-4634   *Fax:* 405 424-9403
E-mail: barbara.harper@metrotech.org

Univ of Oklahoma Health Sciences Center
Radiography Prgm
801 NE 13th St, CHB-451
PO Box 26901
Oklahoma City, OK 73126
Prgm Dir: Jeffrey L Berry, MS RT(R)(CT)
Tel: 405 271-6477, Ext 41165   *Fax:* 405 271-1424
E-mail: jeff-berry@ouhsc.edu

Carl Albert State College
Radiography Prgm
1507 S McKenna
Poteau, OK 74953
www.carlalbert.edu
Prgm Dir: Linda Pearson, PhD RT(R)(M)(QM)
Tel: 918 635-3312   *Fax:* 918 635-3524
E-mail: lpearson@carlalbert.edu

Southwestern Oklahoma State University
Radiography Prgm
409 E Mississippi
Sayre, OK 73662-1236
www.swosu.edu/sayre
Prgm Dir: Chris Stufflebean, MBA RT(R)
Tel: 580 928-5533, Ext 155   *Fax:* 580 928-5533
E-mail: chris.stufflebean@swosu.edu

Meridian Technology Center
Radiography Prgm
1312 S Sangre Rd
Stillwater, OK 74074-1841
Prgm Dir: Tanya Lynn Vasso, RT(R)(M)
Tel: 405 377-3333, Ext 336   *Fax:* 405 377-9604
E-mail: tanyav@meridian-technology.com

Tulsa Community College
Radiography Prgm
909 S Boston Ave
Tulsa, OK 74119-7263
www.tulsacc.edu
Prgm Dir: Benedict J Middleton, MS RT(R)
Tel: 918 595-7012   *Fax:* 918 595-7091
E-mail: rmiddlet@tulsacc.edu

Tulsa Technology Center
Radiography Prgm
801 E 91st St
Tulsa, OK 74132
www.tulsatech.org
Prgm Dir: Kathleen M Davis, MS RT(R)
Tel: 918 828-4230   *Fax:* 918 828-4219
E-mail: kathy.davis@tulsatech.org

Oregon

Portland Community College
Radiography Prgm
12000 SW 49th Ave, PO Box 19000
Portland, OR 97280-0990
Prgm Dir: Virginia Vanderford, MEd RT(R)(M)
Tel: 503 977-4907   *Fax:* 503 977-8240
E-mail: vvanderf@pcc.edu

Pennsylvania

Northampton Community College
Radiography Prgm
3835 Green Pond Rd
Bethlehem, PA 18020
www.northampton.edu
Prgm Dir: Zoland Z Zile III, MS RT(R)(QM)
Tel: 610 861-5387   *Fax:* 610 861-4581
E-mail: zzile@northampton.edu

Bradford Regional Medical Center
Cosponsor: University of Pittsburgh at Bradford
Radiography Prgm
116 Interstate Pkwy
Bradford, PA 16701
http://BRMC.com
Prgm Dir: Scott Gregoire, BS RT(R)
Tel: 814 362-8292   *Fax:* 814 362-8643
E-mail: sgregoire@mail.bfdmed.org

Harcum College
Radiography Prgm
130 S Bryn Mawr Ave
Bryn Mawr, PA 19010-3158
Prgm Dir: Julie A Taddeo, BS RT(R)
Tel: 610 526-6127   *Fax:* 610 526-6141
E-mail: jtaddeo@harcum.edu

Holy Spirit Hospital
Radiography Prgm
503 N 21st St
Camp Hill, PA 17011-2288
www.hsh.org/home.htm
Prgm Dir: Kevin L Otto, MS RT(R)
Tel: 717 763-2123   *Fax:* 717 763-2963
E-mail: kotto@hsh.org

Clearfield Hospital
Radiography Prgm
809 Turnpike Ave, PO Box 992
Clearfield, PA 16830
Prgm Dir: Sandra L Alsop, RT(R)(M)(CT)
Tel: 814 768-2230   *Fax:* 814 768-2258
E-mail: salsop@clearfieldhosp.org

Misericordia Unversity
Radiography Prgm
Medical Imaging
301 Lake St
Dallas, PA 18612-1098
www.misericordia.edu/mi
Prgm Dir: Elaine Halesey, EdD RT(R)(QM)
Tel: 570 674-6480   *Fax:* 570 674-3052
E-mail: ehalesey@misericordia.edu

Geisinger Medical Center
Radiography Prgm
100 N Academy Ave
Danville, PA 17822-2007
Prgm Dir: Kenneth A Roszel, MS RT(R)
Tel: 570 271-6301   *Fax:* 570 271-5976
E-mail: kroszel@geisinger.edu

Gannon University
Radiography Prgm
109 University Square
Erie, PA 16541-0001
www.gannon.edu
Prgm Dir: Cynthia L Liotta, MS RT(R)(CT)
Tel: 814 871-5644   *Fax:* 814 871-5662
E-mail: liotta@gannon.edu

Conemaugh Memorial Medical Center
Radiography Prgm
1086 Franklin St
Johnstown, PA 15905-4398
Prgm Dir: Gloria J Mongelluzzo, MEd RT(R)(M)
Tel: 814 534-9582   *Fax:* 814 534-9945
E-mail: gmongell@conemaugh.org

Armstrong County Memorial Hospital
Radiography Prgm
Armstrong Center for Medicine and Health
One Nolte Dr
Kittanning, PA 16201
www.acmh.org
Prgm Dir: Paula Keister, BS RT(R)(M)
Tel: 724 543-8206   *Fax:* 724 543-8652
E-mail: keisterp@acmh.org

Lancaster Gen Coll of Nursing & Hlth Sciences
Radiography Prgm
410 N Lime St
Lancaster, PA 17602
www.LancasterGeneral.org
Prgm Dir: Robin L Harclerode, MEd RT(R)
Tel: 717 544-4865   *Fax:* 717 544-5970
E-mail: rlharcle@lancastergeneral.org

Mansfield University
Radiography Prgm
Elliott Hall
Mansfield, PA 16933
www.mansfield.edu
Prgm Dir: Jo Ann Hanlon, BS RT(R)(M)
Tel: 570 882-4007, Ext 4007   *Fax:* 570 882-6509
E-mail: hanlon_joann@guthrie.org

Ohio Valley General Hospital
Radiography Prgm
25 Heckel Rd
McKees Rocks, PA 15136
Prgm Dir: Lori A Fazio, BA RT(R)
Tel: 412 777-6200   *Fax:* 412 777-6866
E-mail: lfazio@ohiovalleyhospital.org

Comm College of Allegheny County
Radiography Prgm
595 Beatty Rd
Monroeville, PA 15146-1395
www.ccac.edu
Prgm Dir: August B Kellermann III, PhD RT(R)
Tel: 724 325-6754   *Fax:* 724 325-6701
E-mail: akellermann@ccac.edu

Jameson Hospital
Radiography Prgm
1000 S Mercer St
New Castle, PA 16101
Prgm Dir: David W Hyser, BS RT(R)
Tel: 724 656-6134   *Fax:* 724 656-6148
E-mail: dhyser@jamesonhealthsystem.com

Penn State University - New Kensington
Radiography Prgm
3550 Seventh St, RR 780
New Kensington, PA 15068
Prgm Dir: Debra A Majetic, MAHE RT(R)
Tel: 724 334-6738   *Fax:* 724 334-6111
E-mail: dak25@psu.edu

Bucks County Community College
Radiography Prgm
275 Swamp Rd, Tyler Hall 302A
Newtown, PA 18940
Prgm Dir: Maria Elena A Leodore, BS RT(R)
Tel: 215 504-8475   *Fax:* 215 504-8504
E-mail: leodorem@bucks.edu

Albert Einstein Medical Center
Radiography Prgm
5501 Old York Rd
Philadelphia, PA 19141
http://einsteinxray.org
Prgm Dir: Bonnie L Benson, RT(R)
Tel: 215 456-6234   *Fax:* 215 456-3232
E-mail: bensonb@einstein.edu

Community College of Philadelphia
Radiography Prgm
1700 Spring Garden St
Philadelphia, PA 19130-3991
www.ccp.edu
Prgm Dir: Sally M Rensch, MPP RT(R)
Tel: 215 751-8424   *Fax:* 215 751-8937
E-mail: srensch@ccp.edu

Drexel University
Radiography Prgm
245 N 15th St, MS 206
Philadelphia, PA 19102-1192
www.drexel.edu
Prgm Dir: La Vetta N Reliford, MSRS RT(R)
Tel: 215 762-3990 *Fax:* 215 762-3990
E-mail: lnr25@drexel.edu

Holy Family University
Radiography Prgm
Grant and Frankford Aves
9701 Frankford Ave
Philadelphia, PA 19114
www.holyfamily.edu
Prgm Dir: Kermit Cy Whaley, EdD MPH RT(R)
Tel: 267 341-3566, Ext 3275
E-mail: cwhaley@holyfamily.edu

St Christopher Hospital School of Rad Tech
Radiography Prgm
Erie Ave at Front
Philadelphia, PA 19134
Prgm Dir: Celestine Coleman, BS RT(R)
Tel: 215 427-6751 *Fax:* 215 427-6845
E-mail: Celestine.Coleman@tenethealth.com

Thomas Jefferson University
Radiography Prgm
130 S Ninth St, Ste 1010
Philadelphia, PA 19107-5233
www.tju.edu/chp
Prgm Dir: Frances H Gilman, MS RT(R)(CT)(MR)(CV)
Tel: 215 503-1865 *Fax:* 215 503-1031
E-mail: frances.gilman@jefferson.edu

Univ of Penn MC/Hosp of the Univ of Penn
Radiography Prgm
3400 Spruce St Basement Donner Building
Philadelphia, PA 19104
www.uphs.upenn.edu/radiology/educ/RTed/
Prgm Dir: Joanne M Niewood, MEd RT(R)(CT)
Tel: 215 662-7511 *Fax:* 215 614-0330
E-mail: joanne.niewood@uphs.upenn.edu

UPMC Health System
Radiography Prgm
UPMC Presbyterian School of Medical Imaging
Murdock Bldg, Ste 206
Pittsburgh, PA 15213-2582
http://schoolofmedicalimaging.upmc.com
Prgm Dir: Denise Csonka Lake, MEd RT(R)(M)
Tel: 412 647-3528 *Fax:* 412 647-3713
E-mail: laked@upmc.edu

Western School of Health & Business -
** Pittsburgh**
Radiography Prgm
421 7th Ave
Pittsburgh, PA 15219
Prgm Dir: Kimberly A Doss, MS RT(R)
Tel: 412 281-2600, Ext 144 *Fax:* 412 281-0819
E-mail: kdoss@western-school.com

Montgomery County Community College
Radiography Prgm
101 College Dr
Pottstown, PA 19464
www.mc3.edu/aa/career/programs/rt.htm
Prgm Dir: Debra J Poelhuis, MS RT(R)(M)
Tel: 610 718-1813 *Fax:* 610 718-1983
E-mail: dpoelhui@mc3.edu

Reading Hospital & Medical Center
Radiography Prgm
School of Health Sciences
PO Box 16052
Reading, PA 19612-6052
www.readinghospital.org
Prgm Dir: Kathleen R Jackson, BS RT(R)
Tel: 610 988-8993 *Fax:* 610 988-8400
E-mail: jacksonk@readinghospital.org

St Joseph Medical Center
Radiography Prgm
2500 Bernville Rd
Reading, PA 19605
Prgm Dir: Cynthia L Keane, RT(R)
Tel: 610 378-2237 *Fax:* 610 898-5767
E-mail: cynthiakeane@catholichealth.net

Penn State University - Schuylkill Haven
Radiography Prgm
200 University Dr
Schuylkill Haven, PA 17972-0308
Prgm Dir: David K Rill, MEd RT(R)
Tel: 570 385-6108 *Fax:* 570 385-6105
E-mail: dkr7@psu.edu

Johnson College
Radiography Prgm
3427 N Main Ave
Scranton, PA 18508-1495
www.johnson.edu
Prgm Dir: Jane Maas, BS RT(R)
Tel: 570 342-6404, Ext 176
E-mail: jmaas@johnson.edu

UPMC Northwest
Radiography Prgm
100 Fairfield Dr
Seneca, PA 16346
Prgm Dir: Walter G Jones, Sr, BS RT(R)
Tel: 814 677-1433 *Fax:* 814 677-1440
E-mail: joneswg@upmc.edu

Sewickley Vlly Hosp/Heritage Valley Hlth Sys
Radiography Prgm
720 Blackburn Rd
Sewickley, PA 15143
Prgm Dir: Joyce E Cirelli, MS RT(R)
Tel: 724 773-4761, Ext 4761 *Fax:* 412 749-4241
E-mail: jcirelli@hvhs.org

Sharon Regional Health System
Radiography Prgm
740 E State St
Sharon, PA 16146-3395
Prgm Dir: Robert Piccirillo, RT(R) MBA
Tel: 724 983-5603 *Fax:* 724 983-5614
E-mail: rpiccirillo@srhs-pa.org

Crozer-Keystone Medical Center
Radiography Prgm
One Medical Center Blvd
Upland, PA 19013
Prgm Dir: Eileen Ottaviano, MEd RT(R)
Tel: 610 447-2578 *Fax:* 610 447-6137
E-mail: eileen.ottaviano@crozer.org

Washington Hospital
Radiography Prgm
155 Wilson Ave
Washington, PA 15301
http://washingtonhospital.org
Prgm Dir: Karen C Williams, MA RT(R)(QM)
Tel: 724 223-3326 *Fax:* 724 250-4417
E-mail: kwilliams@washingtonhospital.org

Wilkes-Barre General Hospital
Radiography Prgm
575 N River St
Wilkes-Barre, PA 18764
www.wvhcs.org
Prgm Dir: Kathleen A Smith, BA RT(R)
Tel: 570 552-1760 *Fax:* 570 552-2476
E-mail: ksmith@wvhcs.org

Pennsylvania College of Technology
Radiography Prgm
One College Ave
Williamsport, PA 17701-5799
www.pct.edu
Prgm Dir: Robert J Slothus, MS RT(R)
Tel: 570 320-2400, Ext 7409 *Fax:* 570 321-5556
E-mail: rslothus@pct.edu

Abington Memorial Hospital
Radiography Prgm
2500 Maryland Rd
Willow Grove, PA 19090-1284
www.amh.org
Prgm Dir: Gail J Hoffman, MA Ed RT(R)
Tel: 215 481-5516 *Fax:* 215 481-5490
E-mail: ghoffman@amh.org

York Hospital/WellSpan Health
Radiography Prgm
37 Monument Rd, Ste 101
York, PA 17403
www.wellspan.org/body.cfm?id=306
Prgm Dir: Tracy L Szczypinski, BS RT(R)(CV)
Tel: 717 851-4438 *Fax:* 717 812-3809
E-mail: tszczypinski@wellspan.org

Puerto Rico

Universidad Central del Caribe
Radiography Prgm
PO Box 60327
Bayamon, PR 00960-6032
www.uccaribe.edu
Prgm Dir: Jose Rafael Moscoso-Alvarez, EdD LT
Tel: 787 798-3001, Ext 2330 *Fax:* 787 785-3425
E-mail: jose.moscoso@uccaribe.edu

Universidad del Este
Radiography Prgm
PO Box 2010
Carolina, PR 00984-2010
Prgm Dir: Denise Nazario Pagan, MPH LT
Tel: 787 257-7373, Ext 2106
E-mail: dnazario@suagm.edu

Inter American University of Puerto Rico
Radiography Prgm
PO Box 5100
San German, PR 00683-9801
Prgm Dir: Sara L Torres, MBA RT(R)
Tel: 787 264-1912, Ext 7438 *Fax:* 787 892-6350
E-mail: sara@sg.inter.edu

University of Puerto Rico
Radiography Prgm
GPO Box 5067
San Juan, PR 00936-5067
Prgm Dir: Juan Melendez-Sostre, MEd MPH RT(R)
Tel: 787 751-4434, Ext 4609 *Fax:* 787 751-4434
E-mail: juanmelendez@cprs.rcm.upr.edu

Rhode Island

Community College of Rhode Island
Radiography Prgm
Flanagan Campus
1762 Louisquisset Pike
Lincoln, RI 02865-4585
www.ccri.edu
Prgm Dir: Sharon E Perkins, MEd RT(R)(M)
Tel: 401 333-7144 *Fax:* 401 333-7441
E-mail: sperkins@ccri.edu

Rhode Island Hospital
Radiography Prgm
3 Davol Square
Bldg A, 4th Flr
Providence, RI 02903
www.lifespan.org/diagimag
Prgm Dir: Ellen E Alexandre, BS RT(R)
Tel: 401 528-8531, Ext 223 *Fax:* 401 457-0219
E-mail: ealexandre@lifespan.org

South Carolina

Aiken Technical College
Radiography Prgm
PO Drawer 696
Aiken, SC 29802-0696
Prgm Dir: James A Pitzer, MS RT(R)
Tel: 803 593-9231, Ext 1635   *Fax:* 803 593-3106
E-mail: pitzerj@atc.edu

AnMed Health Medical Center
Radiography Prgm
800 N Fant St
Anderson, SC 29621
Prgm Dir: Gaye Nichols, RT(R)
Tel: 864 260-3705   *Fax:* 864 261-1319
E-mail: gnichols@anmed.com

Technical College of the Lowcountry
Radiography Prgm
PO Box 1288
Beaufort, SC 29901
www.tcl.edu
Prgm Dir: John W Eichinger, MS RS RT(R)(CT)
Tel: 843 470-8397   *Fax:* 843 525-8268
E-mail: jeichinger@tcl.edu

Trident Technical College
Radiography Prgm
7000 Rivers Ave
PO Box 118067
Charleston, SC 29423-8067
http://tridenttech.edu
Prgm Dir: Krista R Gentry, MA RT(R)
Tel: 843 574-6077   *Fax:* 843 574-6585
E-mail: krista.gentry@tridenttech.edu

Midlands Technical College
Radiography Prgm
PO Box 2408
Columbia, SC 29202
www.midlandstech.edu
Prgm Dir: C William Mulkey, EdD RT(R)
Tel: 803 822-3482   *Fax:* 803 822-3417
E-mail: mulkeyb@midlandstech.edu

Horry - Georgetown Technical College
Radiography Prgm
Hwy 501 E, PO Box 261966
Conway, SC 29528-6066
Prgm Dir: Beckey Miller, MS RT(R)
Tel: 843 349-5384   *Fax:* 843 349-7880
E-mail: beckey.miller@hgtc.edu

Florence-Darlington Technical College
Radiography Prgm
PO Box 100548
Florence, SC 29501-0548
www.fdtc.edu
Prgm Dir: E Yancy Wells, BS RT(R)
Tel: 843 676-8529   *Fax:* 843 292-0851
E-mail: Yancy.Wells@fdtc.edu

Greenville Technical College
Radiography Prgm
PO Box 5616
Greenville, SC 29606
www.gvltec.edu
Prgm Dir: Janet K Hirt, BS RT(R)(MR)
Tel: 864 250-8316   *Fax:* 864 250-8462
E-mail: jan.hirt@gvltec.edu

Piedmont Technical College
Radiography Prgm
PO Box 1467, Emerald Rd
Greenwood, SC 29648-1467
Prgm Dir: William Lee Balentine Sr, MSM RT(R)
Tel: 864 941-8523   *Fax:* 864 941-8684
E-mail: balentine.l@ptc.edu

Orangeburg Calhoun Technical College
Radiography Prgm
3250 St Matthews Rd
Orangeburg, SC 29118-8299
Prgm Dir: Frances W Andrews, BHS RT(R)
Tel: 803 535-1356   *Fax:* 803 535-1350
E-mail: andrewsf@octech.edu

York Technical College
Radiography Prgm
452 S Anderson Rd
Rock Hill, SC 29730
Prgm Dir: Michele Rutan Wells, BS RT(R)(M)RDMS
Tel: 803 981-7036   *Fax:* 803 327-8059
E-mail: mwells@yorktech.com

Spartanburg Community College
Radiography Prgm
PO Drawer 4386
Spartanburg, SC 29305-4386
Prgm Dir: Deborah B Jennings, MS RT(R)(M)(QM)
Tel: 864 592-4722   *Fax:* 864 591-3881
E-mail: jenningsd@sccsc.edu

South Dakota

Presentation College
Radiography Prgm
1500 N Main St
Aberdeen, SD 57401
Prgm Dir: Nancy J Vander Hoek, MSRS RT(R)(M)
Tel: 605 229-8545   *Fax:* 605 229-8518
E-mail: nancy.vanderhoek@presentation.edu

Mitchell Technical Institute
Radiography Prgm
821 N Capital
Mitchell, SD 57301
Prgm Dir: Eric A Schaffer, BS RT(R)(CT)
Tel: 605 995-3068
E-mail: eric.schaffer@mitchelltech.edu

Rapid City Regional Hospital
Radiography Prgm
353 Fairmont Blvd, PO Box 6000
Rapid City, SD 57709-6000
www.rcrh.org
Prgm Dir: Jerilyn Jo Powell, BS RT(R) RDMS RVT
Tel: 605 719-8433   *Fax:* 605 719-1436
E-mail: jpowell2@rcrh.org

Avera McKennan Hospital
Radiography Prgm
800 E 21st St, PO Box 5045
Sioux Falls, SD 57117-5045
Prgm Dir: Stephen Cooper, MBA RT(R)
Tel: 605 322-1720   *Fax:* 605 322-1701
E-mail: stephen.cooper@mckennan.org

Sanford Medical Center
Radiography Prgm
1305 W 18th St, PO Box 5039
Sioux Falls, SD 57117-5039
Prgm Dir: Kenneth G Lee, BS RT(R)
Tel: 605 333-6466   *Fax:* 605 333-1554
E-mail: leek@sanfordhealth.org

Avera Sacred Heart Hospital
Radiography Prgm
501 Summit St
Yankton, SD 57078-9967
www.averasacredheart.com
Prgm Dir: Anessa M Van Osdel, BS RT(R)(M)
Tel: 605 668-8158   *Fax:* 605 668-8153
E-mail: avanosdel@shhservices.com

Tennessee

Chattanooga State Technical Comm College
Radiography Prgm
4501 Amnicola Hwy
Chattanooga, TN 37406-1097
www.chattanoogastate.edu/allied_health/rad_tech/
  rad_tech_main.asp
Prgm Dir: Margery Sanders, MBA RT(R)(M)(QM)
Tel: 423 697-4450, Ext 4211   *Fax:* 423 634-3071
E-mail: margery.sanders@chattanoogastate.edu

Columbia State Community College
Radiography Prgm
PO Box 1315
1665 Hampshire Pike
Columbia, TN 38402-1315
Prgm Dir: Brenda M Coleman, MSRS RT(R)
Tel: 931 540-2745, Ext 2745   *Fax:* 931 540-2798
E-mail: bcoleman@columbiastate.edu

MedVance Institute
Radiography Prgm
Cookeville/KIMC Investments, Inc
1025 Highway 111
Cookeville, TN 38501
Prgm Dir: William H May, MEd RT(R) FASRT
Tel: 931 526-3660, Ext 233   *Fax:* 931 372-2603
E-mail: bill.may@medvance.edu

East Tennessee State University
Radiography Prgm
Nave Center, 1000 Jason Witten Way
Elizabethton, TN 37643
Prgm Dir: Shirley J Cherry, MBA RT(R)
Tel: 423 547-4912   *Fax:* 423 547-4921
E-mail: cherrys@etsu.edu

Volunteer State Community College
Radiography Prgm
1480 Nashville Pike
Gallatin, TN 37066-3188
www.volstate.edu
Prgm Dir: Monica M (White) Korpady, MS RT(R)(M)
Tel: 615 230-3651   *Fax:* 615 230-3224
E-mail: mkorpady@volstate.edu

Jackson State Community College
Radiography Prgm
2046 N Parkway St
Jackson, TN 38301-3797
www.jscc.edu/academics/8uallied/rad.htm
Prgm Dir: Gerald L Graddy, MS RT(R)
Tel: 731 424-3520, Ext 299   *Fax:* 731 425-9551
E-mail: ggraddy@jscc.edu

South College
Radiography Prgm
3904 Lonas Dr
Knoxville, TN 37909
www.southcollegetn.edu
Prgm Dir: Donna Shehane, EdD RT(R)
Tel: 865 251-1885   *Fax:* 865 584-9816
E-mail: dshehane@southcollegetn.edu

Univ of Tennessee Medical Ctr at Knoxville
Radiography Prgm
Radiology Dept
1924 Alcoa Hwy
Knoxville, TN 37920-6999
www.utmedicalcenter.org/
Prgm Dir: Clyde R Hembree, MBA RT(R)
Tel: 865 544-9005   *Fax:* 865 544-8581
E-mail: chembree@mc.utmck.edu

Baptist College of Health Sciences
Radiography Prgm
1003 Monroe Ave
Memphis, TN 38104
www.bchs.edu
Prgm Dir: Wanda Lillie, MS RT(R)
Tel: 901 572-2646   *Fax:* 901 572-2750
E-mail: wanda.lillie@bchs.edu

Methodist University Hospital
Radiography Prgm
1265 Union Ave
Memphis, TN 38104
www.methodisthealth.org
Prgm Dir: Peggy D Franklin, BS RT(R)
Tel: 901 726-8099   *Fax:* 901 726-2870
E-mail: franklip@methodisthealth.org

Southwest Tennessee Community College
Radiography Prgm
PO Box 780
Memphis, TN 38101-0780
www.southwest.tn.edu
Prgm Dir: Thomas H Wolfe, MSRS RT(R)
Tel: 901 333-5417   *Fax:* 901 333-5102
E-mail: thwolfe@southwest.tn.edu

MedVance Institute
Radiography Prgm
Nashville/KIMC Investments Inc
2400 Parman Pl, Ste 3
Nashville, TN 37203
Prgm Dir: Craig T Shephard, MS RT(R)
Tel: 615 320-5917
E-mail: craig.shephard@medvance.edu

Nashville General Hospital
Radiography Prgm
1818 Albion St
Nashville, TN 37208
Prgm Dir: Kenneth W Jones, MEd RT(R)
Tel: 615 341-4440   *Fax:* 615 341-4906
E-mail: ken.w.jones@nashville.gov

Roane State Community College
Radiography Prgm
701 Briarcliff Ave
Oak Ridge, TN 37830
Prgm Dir: Jean Reif Robinson, BA RT(R)
Tel: 865 481-2015   *Fax:* 865 481-2019
E-mail: robinsonjr@roanestate.edu

Texas

Hendrick Medical Center
Radiography Prgm
1900 Pine
Abilene, TX 79601-2316
https://www.ehendrick.org/radiography
Prgm Dir: Richard K Bower, MEd RT(R)
Tel: 325 670-2427   *Fax:* 325 670-2990
E-mail: rbower@ehendrick.org

Amarillo College
Radiography Prgm
PO Box 447
Amarillo, TX 79178
www.actx.edu/radiography
Prgm Dir: Bill Crawford, BAAS RT(R)
Tel: 806 354-6070   *Fax:* 806 354-6076
E-mail: crawford-be@actx.edu

Austin Community College
Radiography Prgm
3401 Webberville Rd
Austin, TX 78702
Prgm Dir: Rudy L Garza, MS RT(R)
Tel: 512 223-5817   *Fax:* 512 223-5901
E-mail: rudygarz@austincc.edu

Lamar Institute of Technology
Radiography Prgm
PO Box 10061
Beaumont, TX 77710
www.lit.edu
Prgm Dir: Brenda A Barrow, MEd RT(R)(CT)
Tel: 409 880-8845, Ext 8848   *Fax:* 409 880-8955
E-mail: brenda.barrow@lit.edu

Memorial Hermann Baptist Hospital Beaumont
Radiography Prgm
PO Drawer 1591
Beaumont, TX 77704
www.mhbh.org
Prgm Dir: Carolyn M Nicholas, MEd RT(R)(M)
Tel: 409 212-5726   *Fax:* 409 212-5743
E-mail: carolyn.nicholas@mhbh.org

Univ Tx at Brownsville/Tx Southmost Coll
Radiography Prgm
80 Ft Brown
Brownsville, TX 78520
Prgm Dir: Manuel Gavito, BS RT(R)
Tel: 956 554-5010   *Fax:* 956 554-8910
E-mail: otivag@utb.edu

Blinn College
Radiography Prgm
PO Box 6030
Bryan, TX 77805-6030
Prgm Dir: M Elia Flores, MEd RT(R)
Tel: 979 209-7566   *Fax:* 979 209-7289
E-mail: sflores@blinn.edu

Montgomery College
Radiography Prgm
3200 College Park Dr
Conroe, TX 77384
Prgm Dir: Francis Ozor, EdD RT(R)
Tel: 936 273-7360   *Fax:* 936 273-7054
E-mail: francis.c.ozor@nhmccd.edu

Del Mar College
Radiography Prgm
101 Baldwin and Ayers Sts
Corpus Christi, TX 78404
Prgm Dir: Ismael Garcia, BAAS RT(R)
Tel: 361 698-2858, Ext 2826   *Fax:* 361 698-2811
E-mail: igarcia@delmar.edu

Cy-Fair College
Radiography Prgm
9191 Barker Cypress Rd
Cypress, TX 77433
www.cy-faircollege.com
Prgm Dir: Cynthia B Robertson, MEd RT(R)
Tel: 281 290-3966   *Fax:* 281 290-5282
E-mail: cynthia.b.robertson@nhmccd.edu

Baylor University Med Center
Radiography Prgm
3616 Worth St
Dallas, TX 75246
Prgm Dir: Terri Wyly, MS RT(R)(T)
Tel: 214 820-3780   *Fax:* 214 820-7773
E-mail: terriwy@baylorhealth.edu

El Centro College
Radiography Prgm
Main and Lamar Sts
Dallas, TX 75202-3604
Prgm Dir: Debra Kendall, BS RT(R)(CV)(QA)(CT)
Tel: 214 860-2303   *Fax:* 214 860-2268
E-mail: dkendall@dcccd.edu

El Paso Community College
Radiography Prgm
PO Box 20500
El Paso, TX 79998
www.epcc.edu
Prgm Dir: Christl E Thompson, MA RT(R)
Tel: 915 831-4098   *Fax:* 915 831-4234
E-mail: christlt@epcc.edu

US Army Medical Dept Center & School
Radiography Prgm
3151 Scott Rd
Ste 1316, MCCS-HCR
Fort Sam Houston, TX 78234-6137
Prgm Dir: Brunhilde S Green, MA RT(R)
Tel: 210 221-8958   *Fax:* 210 221-7611
E-mail: brunhilde.green@amedd.army.mil

Career Centers of Texas - Ft Worth Campus
Radiography Prgm
2001 Beach St, Ste 201
Fort Worth, TX 76103
Prgm Dir: Carolyn A Johnson, BS RT(R)
Tel: 817 413-2000
E-mail: cjohnson@cct-fw.com

Galveston College
Radiography Prgm
4015 Ave Q
Galveston, TX 77550-2782
Prgm Dir: Deborah M Scroggins, MS
   RT(R)(CV)(M)(CT)
Tel: 409 772-9463   *Fax:* 409 772-3014
E-mail: dscroggi@gc.edu

Harris County Hosp Dist/Ben Taub Gen Hosp
Radiography Prgm
c/o Lyndon B Johnson General Hospital
5656 Kelley St
Houston, TX 77026
Prgm Dir: Hazel E Bourne, MS RT(R)
Tel: 713 873-2276   *Fax:* 713 873-2416
E-mail: hazel_bourne@hchd.tmc.edu

Houston Community College
Radiography Prgm
Coleman College for Health Sciences
1900 Pressler Dr, MC 1637-512
Houston, TX 77030
www.hccs.edu
Prgm Dir: Lynne Y Davis, EdD RT(R)
Tel: 713 718-7367   *Fax:* 713 718-7608
E-mail: lynne.davis@hccs.edu

MedVance Institute
Radiography Prgm
Houston/KIMC Investments Inc
6220 Westpark, Ste 180
Houston, TX 77057
Prgm Dir: Imran Ayub, MA RT(R)
Tel: 713 266-6594, Ext 224
E-mail: iayub@medvance.edu

Memorial Hermann Healthcare System
Radiography Prgm
Technical Education Center
921 Gessner
Houston, TX 77024
Prgm Dir: Rita J Robinson, BS RT(R)
Tel: 713 932-4861   *Fax:* 713 932-3701
E-mail: rita_robinson@mhhs.org

Tarrant County College - Northeast Campus
Radiography Prgm
828 W Harwood Rd
Hurst, TX 76054-3219
www.tccd.edu
Prgm Dir: Mark Holt, MS RT(R)
Tel: 817 515-6569   *Fax:* 817 515-6700
E-mail: mark.holt@tccd.edu

Laredo Community College
Radiography Prgm
West End Washington St
Laredo, TX 78040-4395
www.laredo.edu
Prgm Dir: Oscar Gomez, BAAS RT(R)
Tel: 956 721-5386   *Fax:* 956 721-5431
E-mail: ogomez@laredo.edu

Covenant Medical Center
Radiography Prgm
2002 W Loop 289, Ste 120
Lubbock, TX 79407
Prgm Dir: Lori Oswalt, MS RT(R)(MR)
Tel: 806 725-0456   *Fax:* 806 797-4350
E-mail: ljordan@covhs.org

South Plains College
Radiography Prgm
Reese Center
819 Gilbert Dr
Lubbock, TX 79416
www.southplainscollege.edu
Prgm Dir: Denny Barnes, BS RT(R)
Tel: 806 885-3048, Ext 4629   *Fax:* 806 885-5608
E-mail: dbarnes@southplainscollege.edu

Angelina College
Radiography Prgm
PO Box 1768
3500 S First
Lufkin, TX 75902
Prgm Dir: Angie L Wilcox, MEd RT(R)(CT)
Tel: 936 633-5413, Ext 5413   *Fax:* 936 633-3207
E-mail: awilcox@angelina.edu

Midland College
Radiography Prgm
3600 N Garfield
Midland, TX 79705-6399
www.midland.edu
Prgm Dir: Quinn B Carroll, MEd RT(R)
Tel: 915 685-4600, Ext 4592   *Fax:* 915 685-4762
E-mail: eskimo@midland.edu

Odessa College
Radiography Prgm
201 W University Blvd
Odessa, TX 79764
www.odessa.edu/dept/radiology
Prgm Dir: Carolyn Leach, BS RT(R)
Tel: 432 335-6449   *Fax:* 432 335-6846
E-mail: sleach@odessa.edu

San Jacinto College Central
Radiography Prgm
8060 Spencer Hwy, PO Box 2007
Pasadena, TX 77501-2007
Prgm Dir: Tunde B Breaker, MBA RT(R)
Tel: 281 476-1871   *Fax:* 281 478-2754
E-mail: tunde.breaker@sjcd.edu

Baptist Health System
Radiography Prgm
8400 Datapoint Dt
Ste 226
San Antonio, TX 78229
Prgm Dir: Anna Y Flores, BS RT(R)(M)
Tel: 210 297-9160   *Fax:* 210 297-0941
E-mail: aflores@baptisthealthsystem.com

St Philip's College
Radiography Prgm
1801 Martin Luther King Dr
San Antonio, TX 78203-2098
Prgm Dir: Donna Laird, BS RT(R)(M)
Tel: 210 531-3422   *Fax:* 210 531-3503
E-mail: dlaird@accd.edu

USAF School of Health Care Sciences
Radiography Prgm
939 Missile Rd, 382 TRS/XYAF
Sheppard AFB, TX 76311-2246
Prgm Dir: MSgt Timothy L Owens, BS RT(R)
Tel: 940 676-3808   *Fax:* 940 676-2210
E-mail: timothy.owens@sheppard.af.mil

Tyler Junior College
Radiography Prgm
PO Box 9020
Tyler, TX 75711
www.tjc.edu
Prgm Dir: Nathan D Stallings, BS RT(R)
Tel: 903 510-2596   *Fax:* 903 510-2880
E-mail: nsta@tjc.edu

Citizens Medical Center
Radiography Prgm
2701 Hospital Dr
Victoria, TX 77901
http://citizensmedicalcenter.org
Prgm Dir: Mary Jane Reynolds, BS RT(R)(T)
Tel: 361 572-5062   *Fax:* 361 572-5091
E-mail: mjreynolds@cmcvtx.org

McLennan Community College
Radiography Prgm
1400 College Dr
Waco, TX 76708
Prgm Dir: Heather Zanek, MSRS RT(R) CT
Tel: 254 299-8342   *Fax:* 254 299-8397
E-mail: hzanek@mclennan.edu

Wharton County Junior College
Radiography Prgm
911 Boling Hwy, Ste J230
Wharton, TX 77488
www.wcjc.edu
Prgm Dir: Sharla S Walker, MS RT(R)(M)(QM)
Tel: 979 532-6379   *Fax:* 979 532-6489
E-mail: sharlaw@wcjc.cc.tx.us

Midwestern State University
Radiography Prgm
3410 Taft Blvd
Wichita Falls, TX 76308-2099
Prgm Dir: Nadia Bugg, PhD RT(R) FAERS
Tel: 940 397-4571   *Fax:* 940 397-4845
E-mail: nadia.bugg@mwsu.edu

Utah

Dixie State College of Utah
Radiography Prgm
225 South 700 East
St George, UT 84770
Prgm Dir: Sherry M Floerchinger, MA RT(R)(N)(QM)
Tel: 435 652-7857
E-mail: floerchinge@dixie.edu

Salt Lake Community College
Radiography Prgm
Jordan Campus
3491 W Wights Fort Rd
West Jordan, UT 84088
Prgm Dir: David L Neil, MAOM RT(R)
Tel: 801 957-3112   *Fax:* 801 957-3300
E-mail: david.neil@slcc.edu

Vermont

Champlain College
Radiography Prgm
163 S Willard St, PO Box 670
Burlington, VT 05402-0670
www.champlain.edu
Prgm Dir: Susyn Dees, MS RT(R)(CT)
Tel: 802 865-6469   *Fax:* 802 860-2750
E-mail: dees@champlain.edu

Virginia

University of Virginia Health System
Cosponsor: University of Virginia Medical Center
Radiography Prgm
Jefferson Park Ave, Radiology Box 800377
Charlottesville, VA 22908
www.med.virginia.edu
Prgm Dir: Jody Crane, BS RTR-BD
Tel: 434 924-9344   *Fax:* 434 982-0626
E-mail: jdc5s@virginia.edu

Danville Regional Medical Center
Radiography Prgm
142 South Main St
Danville, VA 24541
Prgm Dir: Kevin L Murray, MSEd RT(R)(QM)
Tel: 434 799-2271
E-mail: murrayk@drhsi.org

Mary Washington Hospital
Cosponsor: MediCorp Health System
Radiography Prgm
2300 Fall Hill Ave, Ste 260
Fredericksburg, VA 22401
Prgm Dir: Donna Carroll Van Norman, MEd RT(R)(M)
Tel: 540 741-1802   *Fax:* 540 741-3507
E-mail: Donna.CarrollVanNorman@medicorp.org

Rockingham Memorial Hospital
Radiography Prgm
235 Cantrell Ave
Harrisonburg, VA 22801-3293
Prgm Dir: Russell Crank, BA RT(R)
Tel: 540 433-4532   *Fax:* 540 433-4423
E-mail: rcrank@rhcc.com

Central Virginia Community College
Radiography Prgm
3506 Wards Rd
Lynchburg, VA 24502-2498
www.cvcc.vccs.edu
Prgm Dir: Eddie W Haynes, MEd RT(R)
Tel: 434 832-7683   *Fax:* 434 832-7835
E-mail: haynese@cvcc.vccs.edu

ACT College
Radiography Prgm
8870 Rixlew Ln Ste 201
Manassas, VA 20109
Prgm Dir: Therese A Henry, BBA RT(R)(M)
Tel: 703 365-9286, Ext 472   *Fax:* 703 365-9288
E-mail: thenry@actcollege.edu

Medical Careers Institute
Radiography Prgm
1001 Omni Blvd, Ste 200
Newport News, VA 23606
www.medical.edu
Prgm Dir: Charles W Phaneuf, MS RT(R)
Tel: 757 873-2423   *Fax:* 757 873-2472
E-mail: cphaneuf@medical.edu

Riverside School of Health Careers
Cosponsor: Newport News Public Schools
Radiography Prgm
School of Radiologic Technology
316 Main St
Newport News, VA 23601
www.riversideonline.com/rshc
Prgm Dir: Pamela Gebhart-Cline, MSFE RT(R)(M)
Tel: 757 240-2206   *Fax:* 757 240-2201
E-mail: pam.cline@rivhs.com

Southside Regional Medical Center
Radiography Prgm
801 S Adams St
Petersburg, VA 23803
Prgm Dir: Pamela J G Shelton, MBA RT(R)
Tel: 804 862-5883   *Fax:* 804 862-5171
E-mail: pshelton@chs.net

Naval School of Health Sciences
Radiography Prgm
1001 Holcomb Rd
Portsmouth, VA 23708-5200
Prgm Dir: Tony L Ellison, BS RT(R)
Tel: 757 953-6420   *Fax:* 757 953-5033
E-mail: tlellison@hsp.med.navy.mil

Southwest Virginia Community College
Radiography Prgm
PO Box SVCC
Richlands, VA 24641-1510
www.sw.vccs.edu
Prgm Dir: Donald B Lowe, MEd RT(R)
Tel: 540 964-7306   *Fax:* 540 964-7715
E-mail: don.lowe@sw.edu

Bon Secours St Mary's Hospital
Radiography Prgm
8550 Magellan Pkwy Ste 700
Richmond, VA 23227
Prgm Dir: Kimberly Likens-Perry, MSEd RT(R)
Tel: 804 627-5307   *Fax:* 804 627-5304
E-mail: kim_likens@bshsi.com

Virginia Commonwealth University
Radiography Prgm
701 W Grace St, Ste 2100
Box 843057
Richmond, VA 23284-3057
www.sahp.vcu.edu/radsci
Prgm Dir: Terri L Fauber, EdD RT(R)(M)
Tel: 804 828-9104   *Fax:* 804 828-5778
E-mail: tfauber@vcu.edu

Virginia Western Community College
Radiography Prgm
3095 Colonial Ave SW
PO Box 14007
Roanoke, VA 24038
Prgm Dir: Shirl Duke Lamanca, MSEd RT(R)
Tel: 540 857-6285   *Fax:* 540 857-6224
E-mail: slamanca@vw.vccs.edu

Tidewater Community College
Radiography Prgm
1700 College Crescent
Virginia Beach, VA 23453
Prgm Dir: Kim B Utley, MS RT(R)
Tel: 757 822-7253   *Fax:* 757 822-7466
E-mail: kutley@tcc.edu

Winchester Medical Center Inc
Radiography Prgm
1840 Amherst St
PO Box 3340
Winchester, VA 22601
Prgm Dir: John D Orndoff, BS RT(R)
Tel: 540 536-8136   *Fax:* 540 536-8827
E-mail: jorndorf@valleyhealthlink.com

Washington

Pima Medical Institute - Seattle
Radiography Prgm
9709 Third Ave NE, #400
Seattle, WA 98115
http://pmi.edu
Prgm Dir: Jacqueline Kralik, BAS RT(R)(CT)(MR)
Tel: 206 322-6100, Ext 114   *Fax:* 206 324-1985
E-mail: jkralik@pmi.edu

Apollo College
Radiography Prgm
10102 E Knox Ste 200
Spokane, WA 99206
Prgm Dir: Susan Johnson
Tel: 509 532-8888   *Fax:* 509 533-5983
E-mail: sjohnson@apollocollege.edu

Spokane Community College
Radiography Prgm
1810 N Greene St, MS 1090
Spokane, WA 99217
Prgm Dir: Deborah K Miller, MEd RT(R)(CV)(M)
Tel: 509 624-5012   *Fax:* 509 624-3546
E-mail: Millerdk2@shmc.org

Tacoma Community College
Radiography Prgm
6501 S 19th St, Building 19
Tacoma, WA 98466
www.tacomacc.edu
Prgm Dir: Michael Mixdorf, MEd RT(R)(CT)
Tel: 253 566-5168   *Fax:* 253 566-5273
E-mail: mmixdorf@tcc.ctc.edu

West Virginia

Mountain State University
Radiography Prgm
Box 9003
Beckley, WV 25802-9003
Prgm Dir: Jason M Wilcox, BS RT(R)
Tel: 800 766-6067, Ext 1465   *Fax:* 304 929-1617
E-mail: jwilcox@mountainstate.edu

Bluefield State College
Radiography Prgm
219 Rock St
Bluefield, WV 24701
www.bluefieldstate.edu
Prgm Dir: Melissa Oxley Haye, MS RT(R)
Tel: 304 327-4145   *Fax:* 304 327-4219
E-mail: mhaye@bluefieldstate.edu

University of Charleston
Radiography Prgm
2300 MacCorkle Ave SE
Charleston, WV 25304
Prgm Dir: Joan L Clark, MS RT(R)(M)
Tel: 304 357-4839   *Fax:* 304 357-4769
E-mail: joanclark@ucwv.edu

United Hospital Center
Radiography Prgm
3 Hospital Plaza/PO Box 1680
Clarksburg, WV 26302-1680
www.uhcwv.org
Prgm Dir: Rosemary Trupo, MBA RT(R)
Tel: 304 624-2895, Ext 1   *Fax:* 304 624-2856
E-mail: trupor@uhcwv.org

St Mary's Medical Center
Cosponsor: Marshall Community and Technical College
Radiography Prgm
School for Medical Imaging
2900 First Ave
Huntington, WV 25702
www.st-marys.org
Prgm Dir: Rita Fisher-Carroll, PhD RT(R)(CV)(CT)
Tel: 304 526-1259   *Fax:* 304 526-1487
E-mail: rfisher@st-marys.org

West Virginia University Hospitals
Radiography Prgm
Medical Center Dr
Box 8062
Morgantown, WV 26506
www.wvuhradtech.com
Prgm Dir: Jay S Morris, MA RT(R)(CV)
Tel: 304 598-4251   *Fax:* 304 598-4702
E-mail: morrisj@wvuh.com

Southern West Virginia Comm & Tech College
Radiography Prgm
PO Box 2900
Mount Gay, WV 25637
www.southern.wvnet.edu
Prgm Dir: Eva M Hallis, MS RT(R)
Tel: 304 792-7098, Ext 267   *Fax:* 304 792-7028
E-mail: evah@southern.wvnet.edu

Ohio Valley Medical Center
Radiography Prgm
2000 Eoff St
Wheeling, WV 26003
Prgm Dir: Catherine M Ball, MS RT(R)(M)
Tel: 304 234-8781   *Fax:* 304 234-8410
E-mail: cball@ovrh.org

Wheeling Hospital
Radiography Prgm
One Medical Park
Wheeling, WV 26003-0668
www.wheelinghospital.com
Prgm Dir: Misty D Kahl, MS RT(R)
Tel: 304 243-3173   *Fax:* 304 243-3130
E-mail: mkahl@wheelinghospital.com

Wisconsin

Lakeshore Technical College
Radiography Prgm
1290 North Ave
Cleveland, WI 53015-1414
Prgm Dir: James R Odau, MS RT(R)
Tel: 920 693-1840   *Fax:* 920 693-8955
E-mail: james.odau@gotoltc.edu

Chippewa Valley Technical College
Radiography Prgm
620 W Clairemont Ave
Eau Claire, WI 54701-6162
Prgm Dir: Shelly Y Olson, MS RT(R)
Tel: 715 833-6675   *Fax:* 715 833-6470
E-mail: solson@cvtc.edu

Wisconsin Indianhead Technical College
Radiography Prgm
235 N National Ave
Fond du Lac, WI 54936
Prgm Dir: Dyan Hannam, MS Ed R(R)
Tel: 920 924-3243
E-mail: dhannam@morainepark.edu

Bellin Health Hosp/Bellin Health Systems Inc
Radiography Prgm
744 S Webster, PO Box 23400
Green Bay, WI 54305-3400
www.bellin.org/careers
Prgm Dir: Randy Griswold, MPA RT(R)
Tel: 920 433-3497   *Fax:* 920 433-5811
E-mail: rcgris@bellin.org

Blackhawk Technical College
Radiography Prgm
6004 Prairie Rd, PO Box 5009
Janesville, WI 53547
www.blackhawk.edu
Prgm Dir: Joseph W Ipsen, MEd RT(R)
Tel: 608 757-7703   *Fax:* 608 743-4578
E-mail: jipsen@blackhawk.edu

Western Technical College
Radiography Prgm
304 N Sixth St, PO Box C-908
La Crosse, WI 54602-0908
Prgm Dir: Bob Raasch, MEPD RT R
Tel: 608 789-4738   *Fax:* 608 785-9299
E-mail: raaschb@westerntc.edu

Madison Area Technical College
Radiography Prgm
3550 Anderson St
Madison, WI 53704-2599
Prgm Dir: Kay Parish, MA RT(R) RDMS
Tel: 608 258-2478   *Fax:* 608 258-2480
E-mail: kparish@matcmadison.edu

University of Wisconsin Hospital and Clinics
Radiography Prgm
600 Highland Ave
E3/311 Radiology
Madison, WI 53792-3252
www.uwhealth.org/radtechschool
Prgm Dir: Karen L Tvedten, MEd RT(R)
Tel: 608 263-9029   *Fax:* 608 263-9208
E-mail: KTvedten@uwhealth.org

St Joseph's Hospital
Radiography Prgm
611 St Joseph Ave
Marshfield, WI 54449
Prgm Dir: Susan M Duncan, MBA RT(R)
Tel: 715 387-7184   *Fax:* 715 389-5431
E-mail: duncans@stjosephs-marshfield.org

Aurora St Luke's Medical Center
Radiography Prgm
180 W Grange Ave
Milwaukee, WI 53207
www.aurora.org/radtech
Prgm Dir: Debra J Biggins, BA RT(R)(CV)(M)(QM)
Tel: 414 747-4335   *Fax:* 414 747-4366
E-mail: debra.biggins@aurora.org

Columbia St Mary's Hospitals
Radiography Prgm
Columbia St Mary's School of Radiologic Technology
2025 E Newport Ave
Milwaukee, WI 53211
www.ccon.edu/SORT.htm
Prgm Dir: Jayne L Wisniewski, BS RT(R)
Tel: 414 961-8158   *Fax:* 414 961-4121
E-mail: jwisnie1@columbia-stmarys.org

Froedtert Memorial Lutheran Hospital
Radiography Prgm
9200 W Wisconsin Ave
Milwaukee, WI 53226
www.froedtert.com
Prgm Dir: Susan Lura Sanson, MEd RT(R)(QM)
Tel: 414 805-4999   *Fax:* 414 805-4990
E-mail: ssanson@fmlh.edu

Milwaukee Area Technical College
Radiography Prgm
700 W State St
Milwaukee, WI 53233-1443
www.matc.edu
Prgm Dir: Bradley J Rothe, BS RT(R)(CT)
Tel: 414 297-6645   *Fax:* 414 297-6851
E-mail: RotheB@matc.edu

Wheaton Franciscan Healthcare - St Joseph
Radiography Prgm
Glendale Campus, 2400 West Villard Ave
Milwaukee, WI 53209
Prgm Dir: Diane E Wingenter, MS RT(R)
Tel: 414 527-5149   *Fax:* 414 527-5156
E-mail: Diane.Wingenter@wfhc.org

Theda Clark Regional Medical Center
Radiography Prgm
130 Second St
PO Box 2021
Neenah, WI 54957
www.thedacare.org
Prgm Dir: Troy Albrecht, MS RT(R)(CT)
Tel: 920 729-3146   *Fax:* 920 729-2118
E-mail: troy.albrecht@thedacare.org

Mercy Medical Center/Affinity Health System
Radiography Prgm
500 S Oakwood Rd
Oshkosh, WI 54904
Prgm Dir: James R Werner, BS RT(R)
Tel: 920 223-0135   *Fax:* 920 223-1727
E-mail: jwerner@affinityhealth.org

Wheaton Franciscan Healthcare - All Saints
Radiography Prgm
3801 Spring St
Racine, WI 53405
Prgm Dir: Linda Szolwinski, BS RT(R)(M)
Tel: 262 687-8962
E-mail: Linda.Szolwinski@wfhc.org

Northcentral Technical College
Radiography Prgm
1000 Campus Dr
Wausau, WI 54401-1899
Prgm Dir: Steven J Hommerding, PhD ABDRT(R)
Tel: 715 675-3331, Ext 1326   *Fax:* 715 675-5621
E-mail: hommerdi@ntc.edu

Wyoming

Casper College
Radiography Prgm
125 College Dr
Casper, WY 82601
http://caspercollege.edu
Prgm Dir: Laurie Weaver, MS RT(R)
Tel: 307 268-2587   *Fax:* 307 268-3034
E-mail: lweaver@caspercollege.edu

Laramie County Community College
Radiography Prgm
1400 E College Dr
Cheyenne, WY 82007
www.lccc.wy.edu/radiography
Prgm Dir: Starla L Mason, MS RT(R)(QM)
Tel: 307 778-1391   *Fax:* 307 778-4386
E-mail: smason@lccc.wy.edu

Radiographer

Programs*	Class Capacity	Begins	Length (months)	Award	Res. Tuition	Non-res. Tuition	Stipend	Offers:‡ 1	2	3	4
Alabama											
Baptist Medical Center South (Montgomery)	16	Oct	22	Cert	$3,000	$3,000				•	
Crestwood Medical Center (Huntsville)	16	Jan	24	Cert	$2,000	$2,000					
DCH Regional Medical Center (Tuscaloosa)	20	Oct	24	Cert	$2,200	$2,200				•	
Gadsden State Community College	25	Aug	21	AAS	$3,420	$6,118				•	
Huntsville Hospital	15	Jul	24	Cert	$2,000	$2,000					
Jefferson State Community College (Birmingham)	37	Aug	22	AAS	$1,914	$3,514					•
Southern Union State Community College (Opelika)	32	Aug	21	AAS	$3,600	$7,200			•	•	•
University of Alabama at Birmingham	30	Aug	28	BS	$6,000	$12,424				•	
University of South Alabama (Mobile)	45	Aug	24	Cert, BS	$4,254	$8,509					
Arizona											
Apollo College (Phoenix)	25	Every 4 mos	24	AOS	$17,000	$17,000				•	
GateWay Community College (Phoenix)	64	Aug	22	Dipl, AAS	$2,600	$11,100		•		•	
Arkansas											
Arkansas State University - Jonesboro	40	Jun	24	AAS, BS	$5,200	$11,400					
Baptist Health Schools Little Rock	15	Jul	24	Cert	$4,000	$4,400				•	
North Arkansas College (Harrison)	21	Aug	22	AAS	$3,049	$6,039					
Saint Vincent Health System (Little Rock)	15	Jul	24	Cert	$8,000	$8,000				•	
South Arkansas Community College (El Dorado)	13	Aug	24	AAS	$2,494	$5,040				•	
University of Arkansas for Medical Sciences (Little Rock)	22	Aug	24, 36	AS, BS	$5,100	$11,730		•		•	•
University of Arkansas for Medical Sciences (Texarkana)	48	Aug	36, 48	AS, BS	$5,100	$11,890		•			
California											
Arrowhead Regional Medical Center (Colton)	10	Aug	24	Cert						•	
Bakersfield College	25	Jun	24	AS	$800	$6,000				•	
Cabrillo College (Aptos)	22	Aug	22	AS	$730	$4,994				•	
California State University - Northridge	30	Aug	55	BS	$3,042	$10,692		•		•	
Central California School of Continuing Edu (San Luis Obispo)	38	Year-round	24	Cert	$10,500	$10,500		•			
City College of San Francisco	20	Aug Jan	30	AS	$672	$5,434				•	
Cypress College	38	Aug	30	Cert, AS	$780	$4,680	$3,600	•		•	

*Data are shown only for programs that completed the 2007 AMA Survey of Health Professions Education Programs.
‡Key to Offers: 1: Evening or weekend classes; 2: Non-English instruction; 3: Cultural competence instruction; 4: Distance education component.

Radiographer

Programs*	Class Capacity	Begins	Length (months)	Award	Res. Tuition	Non-res. Tuition	Stipend	Offers:‡ 1	2	3	4
East Los Angeles Education and Career Center	15	Jan	11	Cert	$220	$220				•	•
Foothill Community College (Los Altos Hills)	35	Aug	22	AS	$1,500	$3,984				•	
Fresno City College	76	Aug	24	AS	$400	$3,660					
Kaiser Permanente Sch of Allied Hlth Sciences (Richmond)	55	Jul Oct	24, 27	Cert	$4,000	$4,000		•		•	
LA County Harbor UCLA Medical Center (Torrance)	14	Jul	24	Cert						•	
Loma Linda University	32	Sep	21	AS, BS	$11,517	$11,517				•	
Los Angeles City College	26	Sep	27	Cert, AS	$400	$3,915	$7,200	•		•	
Merced College	20	Aug	29	Cert, AS	$806	$4,988	$6,000			•	
Merritt College (Oakland)	32	Aug	24	Cert, AS	$1,350	$7,380				•	
Mills-Peninsula Health Services (Burlingame)	9	Jul	24	Cert	$0	$0	$1,200			•	
Moorpark College	26	Jun	24	AS	$750	$5,130				•	
Naval School of Health Sciences, San Diego	35	Feb Aug	12	Cert						•	
Santa Rosa Junior College	20	Aug	23	Cert, AS	$1,755	$11,872			•	•	
Yuba Community College (Marysville)	100	Aug	24	Cert, AS	$350	$2,500				•	
Colorado											
Concorde Career College - Aurora	24	Every 20 wks	22	AAS	$18,848	$18,848				•	
Memorial Hospital (Colorado Springs)	18	Aug	24	AAS	$4,000	$4,000				•	
Mesa State College (Grand Junction)	18	Aug	21	AAS	$4,000	$12,000				•	
Red Rocks Community College (Arvada)	20	Aug	21	AAS	$3,300	$7,500				•	
Connecticut											
Capital Community College (Hartford)	20	Sep	22	AS	$2,900	$8,400		•		•	
Danbury Hospital	12	Sep	24	Cert	$3,500	$3,500				•	
Hartford Hospital	28	Sep	24	Dipl, Cert	$3,000	$3,000				•	
Middlesex Community College (Middletown)	19	Jun	27	Dipl, Cert, AS	$3,800	$8,500				•	
Naugatuck Valley Community College (Waterbury)	24	Sep	22	AS	$3,458	$8,326		•		•	
Quinnipiac University (Hamden)	70	Sep	35	Cert, BS	$26,280	$26,280		•		•	
St Vincent's College (Bridgeport)	20	Sep	21	AS	$12,420	$12,420				•	
Stamford Hospital	14	Jul	24	Cert	$2,800	$2,800				•	
University of Hartford (West Hartford)	21	Sep	50	Cert, BS	$23,406	$23,406				•	
Delaware											
Delaware Tech & Comm Coll - Owens Campus (Georgetown)	26	Aug	22	AAS	$1,800	$3,600				•	
Delaware Technical & Community College - Wilmington	30	May Aug	24	AAS	$2,934	$7,335				•	
District of Columbia											
Washington Hospital Center	32	Sep	22	Cert	$2,500	$2,500				•	
Florida											
Bethesda Memorial Hospital (Boynton Beach)	9	Jul	24	Cert	$1,100	$0				•	
Brevard Community College (Cocoa)	32	Jun	23	AS	$2,400	$7,600					
Halifax Medical Center (Daytona Beach)	10	Jan	30	Cert	$2,800	$2,800				•	
Hillsborough Community College (Tampa)	25	Aug	22	AS	$2,519	$9,196					
Jackson Mem Medical Center (Miami)	21	Jun	24	Dipl	$2,500	$3,000				•	
Keiser University (Fort Lauderdale)	24	Jan May Sep	24	AS	$17,748	$17,748				•	
Keiser University - Melbourne Campus	120	Jan May Sep	24	AS	$17,748	$0					
Keiser University - Sarasota	96	Jan May Aug	24	AS	$17,748	$17,748				•	
Lakeland Regional Medical Center	14	Jul	24	Cert	$500	$500				•	
Manatee Community College (Bradenton)	30	May	23	AS/AAS	$3,090	$8,427				•	
Marion County School of Radiologic Tech (Ocala)	30	Aug	24	Cert	$3,400	$6,800				•	
Mayo Clinic Jacksonville	10	Aug	24	Cert, AAS	$1,500	$0				•	
MedVance Institute - Ft Lauderdale Campus/KI	62	Oct	24	AS	$10,631	$0				•	
MedVance Institute - West Palm Beach Campus (Palm Springs)	35	Jul	24	AS	$15,800	$0				•	
Palm Beach Community College (Palm Beach Gardens)	40	Jan	24	AS	$2,425	$6,352					
Pensacola Junior College	35	Jun	23	AAS	$2,541	$9,006		•		•	
Santa Fe Community College (Gainesville)	35	Aug	22	AS	$5,156	$16,055				•	
Shands Jacksonville	15	Jul	24	Cert	$750	$750					
University of Central Florida (Orlando)	16	Aug	24	BS	$5,224	$26,052		•		•	•
Valencia Community College (Orlando)	22	Aug	24	AS	$2,683	$10,085				•	
Georgia											
Albany Technical College	42	Jul	24	Dipl, Assoc	$1,812	$0		•		•	
Armstrong Atlantic State University (Savannah)	24	Jun	48	BS	$3,903	$13,860				•	
Athens Technical College	17	Sep	21	AAS	$1,528	$3,056					
Coastal Georgia Community College (Brunswick)	15	Aug	24	AS	$2,700	$9,843					
Columbus Technical College	15	Jan	24	AS	$1,900	$0					
Coosa Valley Technical College (Rome)	32	Jul	24	Dipl, AAS	$1,400	$2,800					
DeKalb Medical Center (Decatur)	42	Sep	24	Cert	$1,600	$1,600					
Emory University (Atlanta)	20	Fall semester	33	BMSc	$13,900	$13,900			•	•	
Grady Health System (Atlanta)	35	Sep	24	Cert	$4,300	$4,300					

*Data are shown only for programs that completed the 2007 AMA Survey of Health Professions Education Programs.
‡Key to Offers: 1: Evening or weekend classes; 2: Non-English instruction; 3: Cultural competence instruction; 4: Distance education component.

PROGRAMS

Programs*	Class Capacity	Begins	Length (months)	Award	Res. Tuition	Non-res. Tuition	Stipend	Offers:‡ 1	2	3	4
Griffin Technical College	22	Jul	24	AAT	$1,764	$3,528				•	
Gwinnett Technical College (Lawrenceville)	68	Sep	21	AS	$1,900	$3,380				•	
Lanier Technical College (Oakwood)	17	Oct	24	AAS	$2,537	$2,537					
Middle Georgia Technical College (Warner Robins)	16	Oct	24	Dipl, AAS	$1,860	$3,720				•	
Ogeechee Technical College (Statesboro)	15	Oct	21	Dipl	$2,124	$4,248				•	
Okefenokee Technical College (Waycross)	20	Jul	24	Dipl	$1,812	$0					
Southeastern Technical College (Vidalia)	24	Fall quarter	21	Dipl	$2,985	$0					
West Central Technical College (Douglasville)	18	Summer	24	AAS	$2,000	$0				•	
West Georgia Technical College (LaGrange)	20	Oct	21	AAS	$1,812	$3,300				•	
Hawaii											
Kapi'olani Community College (Honolulu)	25	Aug	23	AS	$1,410	$7,260					
Idaho											
Boise State University	26	Aug	29, 48	AS, BS	$5,990	$13,765		•		•	
College of Southern Idaho (Twin Falls)	34	Fall	22	AAS	$1,000	$2,800					
Illinois											
Advocate Illinois Masonic Medical Center (Chicago)	25	Sep	24	Cert	$3,000	$3,000				•	
Advocate Trinity Hospital (Chicago)	17	Aug	24	Dipl	$3,000	$3,000				•	
Blessing Hospital (Quincy)	16	Jul	24	Cert	$2,000	$2,000				•	
College of DuPage (Glen Ellyn)	72	Jun	24	AAS	$4,500	$13,500				•	
Danville Area Community College	15	Aug	24	AAS	$4,000	$7,000				•	
Illinois Central College (Peoria)	20	Aug	23	AAS	$2,700	$5,940				•	
Kaskaskia College (Centralia)	45	Aug	18, 21	AAS	$2,784	$4,712					
Kishwaukee College (Malta)	22	Aug	22	AAS	$3,500	$8,650					
Lincoln Land Community College (Springfield)	16	Jun	24	AAS	$3,494	$0		•		•	
Malcolm X College (Chicago)	35	Jun	24	AAS	$2,952	$5,237				•	
McDonough District Hospital (Macomb)	5	Aug	24	Cert	$500	$500					
Moraine Valley Community College (Palos Hills)	51	Jun	26	AAS	$1,320	$5,070		•		•	
OSF St Francis Medical Center (Peoria)	11	Jan	24	Cert	$1,500	$1,500					
Rockford Memorial Hospital	10	Jun	24	Cert	$1,600	$2,400					
Sauk Valley Community College (Dixon)	34	Aug	22	AAS	$3,000	$10,535					
South Suburban College (South Holland)	42	Aug	21	AAS	$2,340	$8,250					
St Francis Hospital (Evanston)	25	Aug	24	Dipl, Cert	$2,500	$0					
Swedish American Hospital (Rockford)	10	May	24	Cert	$1,500	$0					•
Trinity College of Nursing & Health Sciences (Rock Island)	16	Jun	23	AAS	$8,500	$8,500				•	•
Triton College (River Grove)	45	Aug	24	AAS	$1,980	$6,500					
Wright College (Chicago)	45	Aug	24	AAS	$3,720	$12,468					
Indiana											
Ball State University (Indianapolis)	20	May	14	AS	$667	$17,740				•	
Columbus Regional Hospital	6	Jul	24	Cert	$2,500	$2,500					
Community Health Network (Indianapolis)	14	Jun	24	Cert	$3,000	$3,000					
Fort Wayne School of Radiography	28	Jun	24	Cert	$3,300	$3,300				•	
Good Samaritan Hospital (Vincennes)	10	Jun	24	Cert	$2,000	$2,000					
Hancock Regional Hospital (Greenfield)	15	Jul	23	Cert	$3,500	$3,500				•	
Indiana University (Indianapolis)	37	Jun	22	AS	$6,428	$18,274				•	
Indiana University - Kokomo	24	Aug	21, 9	AS, BS	$4,600	$0				•	
Indiana University Northwest (Gary)	45	Jul	24	AS	$5,966	$14,761				•	
Indiana University South Bend	19	Jul	22	AS	$4,348	$11,419		•		•	
Ivy Tech Community College - Terre Haute	36	Aug	21	AS	$7,020	$14,280				•	•
King's Daughters' Hospital & Health Services (Madison)	6	Jul 1	24	Cert	$2,500	$2,500					
Reid Hospital & Health Care Services (Richmond)	11	Sep	24	Cert	$2,000	$2,000					
St Vincent Health/St Joseph Hospital (Indianapolis)	17	Aug	22	Cert	$5,000	$5,000					
University of Saint Francis (Fort Wayne)	24	Aug	22	AS				•	•	•	•
University of Southern Indiana (Evansville)	18	Jan	24	AS	$2,880	$7,029					
Iowa											
Allen College (Waterloo)	17	Jun	24	AS	$14,737	$14,737					
Indian Hills Community College (Ottumwa)	40	Aug	24	AAS	$4,515	$6,794		•	•		
Iowa Central Community College (Fort Dodge)	30	Sep	22	AAS	$4,020	$5,890				•	•
Iowa Methodist Med Ctr/Iowa Hlth - Des Moines	14	Jul	24	Cert	$3,000	$3,000				•	
Jennie Edmundson Memorial Hospital (Council Bluffs)	8	Aug	24	Cert	$2,000	$2,000				•	
Mercy College of Health Sciences (Des Moines)	38	Jun	24	AS	$18,900	$18,900				•	
Mercy Medical Center - North Iowa (Mason City)	12	Mid-Aug	24	Cert	$1,250	$1,250				•	
St Luke's College (Sioux City)	18	Aug	24	ASR	$12,920	$12,920				•	
St Luke's Hospital (Cedar Rapids)	23	Jun	24	Cert	$2,500	$2,500				•	
University of Iowa Hospitals & Clinics (Iowa City)	25	Jul	24	Cert	$5,500	$5,500				•	
Kansas											
Fort Hays State University	75	Jun	24	AS	$8,053	$111,164		•		•	
Hutchinson Community College	21	Aug	24	AASRT	$2,277	$3,450					

*Data are shown only for programs that completed the 2007 AMA Survey of Health Professions Education Programs.
‡Key to Offers: 1: Evening or weekend classes; 2: Non-English instruction; 3: Cultural competence instruction; 4: Distance education component.

Radiographer

Programs*	Class Capacity	Begins	Length (months)	Award	Res. Tuition	Non-res. Tuition	Stipend	Offers:‡ 1	2	3	4
Labette Community College (Parsons)	29	Jun	23	AAS	$2,070	$2,700					
Newman University (Wichita)	80	Aug	24	AS	$20,410	$20,410				•	
Washburn University (Topeka)	28	Aug	22	AS	$3,977	$9,030					
Kentucky											
Bluegrass Community and Technical College (Lexington)	40	Aug	24	AAS	$2,616	$7,848					•
Bowling Green Technical College	21	Aug	22	AAS	$3,565	$10,695					
Elizabethtown Community & Technical College	16	Aug	20	AAS	$2,548	$4,000				•	
Hazard Community & Technical College	22	Aug	22	AAS	$3,234	$8,820					•
Jefferson Community and Technical College (Louisville)	59	Aug	21	AAS	$109	$140				•	
Southeast Kentucky Comm & Tech College (Pineville)	25	Aug	22	Dipl, AAS	$3,450	$10,350				•	•
Spencerian College (Louisville)	15	Quarterly	27	AD	$40,410	$0				•	
St Catharine College	30	Aug	22	AS	$14,000	$0					
St Joseph Healthcare (Lexington)	12	Jun	24	Cert	$2,000	$2,000				•	
West Kentucky Community & Technical College (Paducah)	23	Aug	24	Dipl, AAS	$2,760	$8,280				•	
Louisiana											
Baton Rouge General Medical Center	16	Jul	24	Cert	$1,500	$1,500					
Lafayette General Medical Center	6	Sep	24	Cert	$7,000	$7,000					
Louisiana State University - Eunice	20	Jun	24	AS	$2,772	$6,522				•	
McNeese State University (Lake Charles)	21	Aug	21	BS	$4,239	$7,835					
North Oaks Medical Center (Hammond)	20	Jul	24	Cert	$4,000	$0				•	
Northwestern State University (Shreveport)	40	Jan	21	BS	$3,500	$9,400				•	•
Our Lady of Holy Cross College (New Orleans)	12	Aug	21	Dipl, BS-HS, AS-RS	$12,800	$12,800				•	
Our Lady of the Lake College (Baton Rouge)	28	Aug	18	AS	$8,475	$8,475				•	
University of Louisiana at Monroe	36	Aug	21	BSRT	$3,076	$9,028		•		•	
Maine											
Central Maine Medical Center (Lewiston)	13	Aug	24	Cert	$3,200	$3,200				•	
Eastern Maine Community College (Bangor)	20	Aug 27	23	AS	$3,315	$6,757					
Mercy Hospital (Portland)	11	Jul	24	Cert	$3,025	$3,025				•	
Southern Maine Community College (South Portland)	23	Sep	23	AS	$4,000	$0				•	
Maryland											
Allegany College of Maryland (Cumberland)	23	Jul	22	AAS	$3,400	$7,300					
Chesapeake College (Wye Mills)	13	Jun	24	AAS	$3,990	$9,415				•	
Greater Baltimore Medical Center	12	Aug	23	Cert	$2,500	$2,500					
Hagerstown Community College	35	May	24	AAS	$3,255	$6,825					
Holy Cross Hospital (Silver Spring)	11	Aug	22	Dipl, Cert	$1,000	$1,000					
Johns Hopkins Hospital (Baltimore)	22	Jun	18	Cert	$5,200	$5,200				•	
Montgomery College (Takoma Park)	30	Sep	24	AAS	$3,204	$8,820				•	
Prince George's Community College (Largo)	42	Aug	19	Dipl, AAS	$2,491	$4,372				•	
Wor-Wic Community College (Salisbury)	20	Jul	23	AAS	$2,660	$7,828		•		•	
Massachusetts											
Bunker Hill Community College (Boston)	129	Sep	22, 35	AS	$4,100	$10,700		•		•	•
Holyoke Community College	26	Sep	21	AS	$3,855	$10,623				•	
Mass College of Pharmacy & Health Sciences (Boston)	32	Sep	33	Cert, BS	$21,200	$21,200				•	
Massasoit Community College (Brockton)	35	Sep	21	AS	$888	$8,510				•	
MGH Institute of Health Professions (Boston)	42	Sep	17	Cert	$34,240	$34,240				•	•
North Shore Community College (Danvers)	20	Sep	21	AS	$4,002	$12,006				•	
Northern Essex Community College (Lawrence)	25	Sep	21	AS	$4,095	$13,260				•	
Quinsigamond Community College (Worcester)	26	Sep	22	AS	$5,200	$10,000				•	
Regis College (Medford)	32	Aug	22	AS	$18,000	$0			•	•	
Roxbury Community College (Boston)	26	Sep	16	AS	$3,500	$3,500				•	
Springfield Technical Community College	20	Sep	23	AS	$3,415	$9,590					
Michigan											
Hurley Medical Center (Flint)	7	Sep	24	Cert	$1,500	$0				•	
Kellogg Community College (Battle Creek)	22	May	24	AAS	$2,756	$4,307					
Lansing Community College	72	Aug	21	AAS	$3,250	$5,250				•	•
Marquette General Health System	10	Aug	24	Cert, Assoc	$2,450	$2,450				•	
Port Huron Hospital	7	Jul	24	Dipl	$2,000	$2,000					
Providence Hospital (Southfield)	12	Sep Oct	24	Cert	$1,500	$0				•	
Sinai-Grace Hospital (Detroit)	14	Jul	24	Cert	$500	$500					
St John Health (Detroit)	20	Sep	24	Cert	$750	$750				•	
Washtenaw Community College (Ann Arbor)	37	May 30	24	AAS	$6,800	$8,000				•	
Wayne State University (Detroit)	20	May	24	Cert, BS	$266	$612					
William Beaumont Hospital (Royal Oak)	12	Jan Jul	24	Cert	$500	$500				•	
Minnesota											
Argosy University - Twin Cities (Eagan)	21	Sep Jan May	24, 36	Dipl, AAS	$13,500	$0					•
Century College (White Bear Lake)	50	Aug	24	AAS	$146	$0				•	•
College of St Catherine - Minneapolis	18	Sep Feb	23	AAS	$460	$460				•	

*Data are shown only for programs that completed the 2007 AMA Survey of Health Professions Education Programs.
‡Key to Offers: 1: Evening or weekend classes; 2: Non-English instruction; 3: Cultural competence instruction; 4: Distance education component.

Radiographer

Programs*	Class Capacity	Begins	Length (months)	Award	Res. Tuition	Non-res. Tuition	Stipend	Offers:‡ 1	2	3	4
Fairview University (Edina)	20	Sep	24	Cert, AAS	$5,414	$5,414		•		•	
Lake Superior College (Duluth)	30	Aug	24, 18	AAS	$4,904	$9,808			•	•	
Mayo School of Health Sciences (Rochester)	40	Aug	24	Cert, AS	$6,500	$8,000				•	
Methodist Hospital (St Louis Park)	5	Jan Sep	24	Dipl	$1,000	$1,000					
North Memorial Medical Center (Robbinsdale)	6	Mar Sep	24	Cert	$1,500	$1,500					
Northland Community & Technical College (East Grand Forks)	16	Aug	24	AAS	$10,746	$21,493		•		•	
Rice Memorial Hospital (Willmar)	8	Aug	24	Cert	$3,000	$3,000					
St Cloud Hospital	9	Sep	24	Cert	$4,597	$4,597				•	
Veterans Affairs Medical Center (Minneapolis)	15	Sep	24	Cert						•	
Mississippi											
Copiah-Lincoln Community College (Wesson)	24	Aug	24	AAS	$1,800	$3,700					
Hinds Community College (Raymond)	51	Jun	24	AS	$2,100	$3,606					
Itawamba Community College (Fulton)	22	Aug	22	Dipl, AAS	$3,000	$5,480				•	
Jones County Junior College (Ellisville)	14	May	24	Dipl, AAS	$2,005	$4,616				•	
Mississippi Gulf Coast Community College (Gautier)	37	May	24	AAS	$2,235	$5,004				•	
Northeast Mississippi Community College (Booneville)	15	Jul	23	AAS	$1,830	$3,660				•	
Pearl River Community College (Hattiesburg)	20	Jun	24	AAS	$4,500	$9,000				•	
Missouri											
Colorado Technical University (Kansas City)	30	Jan Jul	24	AAS	$30,040	$0				•	
Metropolitan Community College - Penn Valley (Kansas City)	68	Jun	24	AAS	$3,000	$7,200		•			•
Mineral Area Regional Medical Center (Farmington)	24	Aug 13	22	Cert	$3,188	$3,188			•		
Nichols Career Center (Jefferson City)	14	Aug	24	Cert	$6,800	$6,800					
Research Medical Center (Kansas City)	15	Jul	24	Cert	$2,400	$2,400				•	
Saint Luke's Hospital (Kansas City)	20	Jul 10	24	Cert	$2,290	$2,290				•	
Sanford-Brown College (Fenton)	30	Every 20 wks	18	AAS						•	
SE Missouri Hosp Coll of Nursing and Health Sciences (Cape Girardeau)	17	Jul 25	22	Dipl, Assoc	$10,200	$0				•	
St John's Regional Health Center (Springfield)	24	Jul	23	Cert	$2,500	$2,500					
St Louis Community College - Forest Park	53	Aug	23	AAS	$3,240	$5,920				•	
State Fair Community College (Sedalia)	18	Aug	21	AAS	$3,542	$4,460				•	
University of Missouri - Columbia	12	Jun	24	BHS	$8,225	$20,650				•	•
Montana											
Benefis Healthcare (Great Falls)	6	Jul	24	Cert						•	
Nebraska											
Alegent Health (Omaha)	34	Aug	23	Dipl, Assoc	$2,525	$2,525				•	
Clarkson College (Omaha)	28	Aug	24	AS	$12,000	$12,000				•	
Mary Lanning Memorial Hospital (Hastings)	20	Aug	24	Dipl	$2,527	$2,527				•	
Regional West Medical Center (Scottsbluff)	14	Aug	24	Cert	$2,000	$2,000				•	
Southeast Community College (Lincoln)	70	Jul Jan	24	AAS	$6,262	$7,296					•
University of Nebraska Medical Center (Omaha)	20	Aug	21	BS	$9,440	$28,025		•		•	•
Nevada											
Truckee Meadows Community College (Reno)	16	Aug	24	AAS	$1,772	$7,157				•	
University of Nevada - Las Vegas	45	Aug	24	Cert	$2,370	$10,155				•	
New Hampshire											
New Hampshire Technical Institute (Concord)	35	Jun	24	Dipl, AS	$8,985	$17,116					
New Jersey											
Bergen Community College (Paramus)	42	Sep	24	AAS	$2,908	$5,816					
Brookdale Community College (Lincroft)	30	Sep	24	AAS	$3,800	$7,200				•	
Burlington County College (Pemberton)	14	May	24	AAS	$4,600	$0				•	
Christ Hospital (Jersey City)	25	Sep	12, 24	Cert	$9,250	$9,250				•	
Cooper University Hospital (Camden)	53	Sep	24	Cert	$3,000	$3,000					
County College of Morris (Randolph)	46	Sep	24	AAS	$6,000	$0					
Englewood Hospital & Medical Center	11	Jul	24	Cert	$5,000	$5,000				•	
Mercer County Community College (Trenton)	77	Aug	23	AAS	$3,876	$5,187		•		•	
Middlesex County College (Edison)	36	Sep	24	AAS	$4,240	$8,479				•	
Muhlenberg Regional Medical Center (Plainfield)	42	Sep	36	Dipl, AS	$2,886	$5,772				•	
Passaic County Community College (Paterson)	28	Sep	24	AAS	$3,022	$6,044				•	
Shore Memorial Hospital (Somers Point)	25	Aug	24	Cert	$4,000	$4,000				•	
St Francis Medical Center (Trenton)	8	Jul	24	Cert	$3,497	$3,497				•	
The Valley Hospital (Ridgewood)	13	Sep	24	Cert, AS	$14,610	$14,610				•	
New Mexico											
Clovis Community College	18	Aug	24	AAS	$785	$1,386					
Dona Ana Community College (Las Cruces)	23	Aug	21	AS	$1,216	$3,154					
New York											
Arnot Ogden Medical Center (Elmira)	7	Aug	24	Cert	$3,500	$3,500					
Bellevue Hospital Center (New York)	20	Oct	24	Cert	$4,500	$4,500				•	

*Data are shown only for programs that completed the 2007 AMA Survey of Health Professions Education Programs.
‡Key to Offers: 1: Evening or weekend classes; 2: Non-English instruction; 3: Cultural competence instruction; 4: Distance education component.

Radiographer

Programs*	Class Capacity	Begins	Length (months)	Award	Res. Tuition	Non-res. Tuition	Stipend	Offers:‡ 1	2	3	4
Bronx Community College	40	Aug	24	AAS	$2,800	$3,000				•	
Broome Community College (Binghamton)	30	Aug	21	AAS	$2,388	$4,776				•	•
Champlain Valley Phys Hospital Med Ctr (Plattsburgh)	14	Jul	24	Cert, AS	$6,000	$8,160					
Hostos Community College of CUNY (Bronx)	60	Sep	24	AAS	$4,200	$8,000					
Mercy Medical Center (Rockville Centre)	17	Sep	24	Cert	$4,250	$0					
Monroe Community College (Rochester)	46	Sep	21	AAS	$3,152	$6,304				•	
New York Methodist Hospital (Brooklyn)	14	Sep	24	Cert	$8,000	$8,000				•	
Peconic Bay Medical Center (Riverhead)	12	Sep	24	Cert	$4,000	$4,000					
Robt J Hochstim Sch Rad/S Nassau Comm Hosp (Oceanside)	10	Sep	24	Cert	$4,500	$4,500				•	
St Elizabeth Medical Center (Utica)	30	Sep	23	Cert	$3,750	$3,750				•	
St James Mercy Health (Hornell)	16	Aug	24	Cert	$4,600	$4,600				•	
Westchester Community College (Valhalla)	45	Sep	24	AAS	$3,350	$8,376					
Winthrop University Hospital (Mineola)	11	Sep	24	Cert	$4,500	$4,500				•	
North Carolina											
Asheville-Buncombe Technical Comm College	24	Aug	21	AAS	$1,680	$9,332				•	
Caldwell Comm College & Tech Institute (Hudson)	18	Aug	21	AAS	$1,824	$10,128					
Cape Fear Community College (Wilmington)	24	Fall semester	21	AAS	$1,189	$10,536				•	
Carolinas College of Health Sciences (Charlotte)	40	Aug	21	AAS	$5,250	$5,250					
Cleveland Community College (Shelby)	21	Aug	19	AAS	$1,106	$3,376				•	
Edgecombe Community College (Rocky Mount)	32	Aug	21	AAS	$1,435	$7,851				•	
Forsyth Technical Community College (Winston-Salem)	25	Aug Jan	21	AAS	$1,850	$8,395				•	
Johnston Community College (Smithfield)	36	Aug	21	AAS	$840	$4,552					
Lenoir Community College (Kinston)	24		21	AAS	$1,625	$1,625					
Moses Cone Health System (Greensboro)	20	Jul	24	Cert	$500	$500	$840			•	
Pitt Community College (Greenville)	35	Aug	21	AAS	$1,422	$7,902					
Presbyterian Healthcare (Charlotte)	10	Aug	23	Cert	$550	$550				•	
Rowan-Cabarrus Community College (Salisbury)	30	Aug	21	AAS	$1,704	$9,456				•	•
Sandhills Community College (Pinehurst)	18	Aug	21	AAS	$1,512	$8,398					
Vance-Granville Community College (Henderson)	31	Aug	21	AAS	$1,500	$8,200				•	•
Wilkes Regional Medical Center (North Wilkesboro)	21	Jun	24	Cert	$1,250	$1,250				•	
North Dakota											
Medcenter One (Bismarck)	6	Aug	24	Cert						•	
MeritCare Medical Center (Fargo)	8	Aug	24	Cert						•	
Trinity Health (Minot)	12	Jul	24	Cert	$2,500	$3,000				•	
Ohio											
Central Ohio Technical College (Newark)	35	Sep	21	AAS	$4,300	$8,925				•	
Children's Hospital Medical Ctr of Akron	34	Jul	24	Cert, AAS	$20,202	$20,202					
Cleveland Clinic (Euclid)	28	Aug	24	Cert	$3,375	$3,375				•	
Columbus State Community College	32	Summer Quarter	21	AAS	$4,345	$8,690		•			
Cuyahoga Community College (Parma)	24	Aug Jan	24	AAS	$2,960	$3,723		•		•	
Jefferson Community College (Steubenville)	16	Aug	24	AAS	$2,144	$5,270					
Kent State University - Salem Campus	38	Jun	24	AAS	$6,289	$16,364				•	
Kettering College of Medical Arts	27	Aug	22	AS	$11,680	$11,680		•			
Lorain County Community College (Elyria)	36	Aug	21	AAS	$3,300	$3,831				•	
Marietta Memorial Hospital	42	Sep	24	Cert, AAS	$4,104	$8,208				•	
Marion Technical College	16	Jun	23	AAS	$5,983	$0		•		•	
Mercy Medical Center (Canton)	30	Jul	24	Dipl	$4,500	$0					
North Central State College (Mansfield)	21	Jun	24	AAS	$5,681	$10,686				•	
Rhodes State College (Lima)	35	Sep	21	AAS	$5,077	$10,154				•	
Shawnee State University (Portsmouth)	23	May	24	AAS	$6,404	$10,380					
Xavier University (Cincinnati)	20	Aug	23	AS	$7,300	$7,300				•	
Oklahoma											
Autry Technology Center (Enid)	9	Aug	24	Cert	$2,670	$7,510				•	
Carl Albert State College (Poteau)	12	Fall	21	AAS	$2,083	$5,080				•	
Great Plains Technology Center (Lawton)	22	Jul	24	Cert, AAS	$1,875	$2,875				•	•
Indian Capital Technology Center (Muskogee)	30	Jul	23	Dipl	$1,500	$3,000				•	
Metro Technology Centers (Oklahoma City)	15	Aug	22	Cert	$3,350	$0		•			
Rose State College (Midwest City)	20	Aug	24	AAS	$2,581	$3,602				•	
Southwestern Oklahoma State University (Sayre)	17	Aug	24	AAS	$2,100	$5,040				•	
Tulsa Community College	40	Jun	24	Dipl, AAS	$2,821	$7,480					
Tulsa Technology Center	20	Aug	22	Cert	$3,320	$3,320				•	
Univ of Oklahoma Health Sciences Center (Oklahoma City)	30	Aug	48	BS	$5,960	$8,900				•	•
Western Oklahoma State College (Altus)	29	Fall	22	Dipl, AAS	$3,100	$0					
Pennsylvania											
Abington Memorial Hospital (Willow Grove)	30	Sep	24	Cert	$4,500	$4,500					
Albert Einstein Medical Center (Philadelphia)	20	Sep	24	Cert	$3,000	$3,000		•			
Armstrong County Memorial Hospital (Kittanning)	8	Jul	24	Cert	$3,000	$3,000					

*Data are shown only for programs that completed the 2007 AMA Survey of Health Professions Education Programs.
‡Key to Offers: 1: Evening or weekend classes; 2: Non-English instruction; 3: Cultural competence instruction; 4: Distance education component.

Radiographer

Programs*	Class Capacity	Begins	Length (months)	Award	Res. Tuition	Non-res. Tuition	Stipend	1	2	3	4
Bradford Regional Medical Center	10	Sep	24	Dipl	$5,000	$5,000				•	
Clearfield Hospital	6	Sep	24	Cert	$2,075	$2,075				•	
Comm College of Allegheny County (Monroeville)	75	Aug	24	AS	$1,092	$2,020		•			
Community College of Philadelphia	30	Jul	24	AAS	$2,863	$8,112				•	
Conemaugh Memorial Medical Center (Johnstown)	17	Sep	24	Cert	$4,075	$4,075					
Crozer-Keystone Medical Center (Upland)	24	Jul Jan	24	Cert	$4,500	$4,500					
Drexel University (Philadelphia)	30	Sep	21	Assoc	$14,300	$0					
Gannon University (Erie)	18	Aug	24	AS	$22,100	$22,100				•	
Holy Family University (Philadelphia)	30	Aug	20	AS, BSRT	$19,700	$19,700					
Holy Spirit Hospital (Camp Hill)	8	Jan	24	Cert	$1,800	$1,800				•	
Johnson College (Scranton)	60	Aug	21	AS	$12,858	$12,858					
Lancaster Gen Coll of Nursing & Hlth Sciences	21	Aug	21	AS	$13,370	$13,370				•	
Mansfield University	15	Aug	24	AAS	$6,508	$16,273				•	•
Misericordia Unversity (Dallas)	30	Aug	42	BS	$19,800	$19,800				•	
Montgomery County Community College (Pottstown)	26	Aug	24	AAS	$3,200	$10,000				•	
Northampton Community College (Bethlehem)	34	Aug	21	AAS	$3,450	$10,350				•	
Pennsylvania College of Technology (Williamsport)	30	Aug	24	AAS	$13,452	$0				•	
Reading Hospital & Medical Center	20	Aug	24	Cert	$3,300	$4,200				•	
Sharon Regional Health System	5	Aug	24	Cert	$2,500	$2,500				•	
St Christopher Hospital School of Rad Tech (Philadelphia)	65	Jul	24	Cert	$6,500	$6,500		•			
St Joseph Medical Center (Reading)	10	Jul	24	Cert	$1,000	$0					
Thomas Jefferson University (Philadelphia)	25	Sep	12	BS, MS	$23,685	$23,685				•	
Univ of Penn MC/Hosp of the Univ of Penn (Philadelphia)	52	Sep	24	Cert	$5,000	$5,000				•	
UPMC Health System (Pittsburgh)	49	Jul Jan	24	Cert	$5,000	$5,000		•			
UPMC Northwest (Seneca)	7	Jul	24	Cert	$5,000	$5,000					
Washington Hospital	15	Sep	24	Dipl	$7,500	$7,500					
Wilkes-Barre General Hospital	12	Sep	24	Cert	$5,000	$5,000				•	
York Hospital/WellSpan Health	26	Sep	24	Cert	$1,850	$1,850					
Puerto Rico											
Universidad Central del Caribe (Bayamon)	35	Aug	22	AS	$4,200	$0			•	•	
Rhode Island											
Community College of Rhode Island (Lincoln)	90	Jun	24	AAS	$3,056	$9,196				•	
Rhode Island Hospital (Providence)	20	Jun	24, 30	Cert	$3,750	$3,750		•		•	
South Carolina											
Aiken Technical College	20	Fall semester	24	Dipl, AS	$3,036	$0					
Florence-Darlington Technical College	42	Aug	21	AS	$1,595	$1,726					
Greenville Technical College	36	Aug	28	AS	$4,680	$9,792		•		•	•
Horry - Georgetown Technical College (Conway)	27	Aug	18	AHS	$4,380	$7,080					
Midlands Technical College (Columbia)	20/	Jun	24	AS	$4,500	$13,500				•	
Technical College of the Lowcountry (Beaufort)	32	Fall semester	24	Assoc	$4,500	$10,188					
Trident Technical College (Charleston)	59	May	24	AHS	$4,671	$8,847				•	•
York Technical College (Rock Hill)	20	May	24	AHS	$4,482	$10,296				•	
South Dakota											
Avera McKennan Hospital (Sioux Falls)	12	Sep	24	Cert	$1,250	$1,250					
Avera Sacred Heart Hospital (Yankton)	8	Sep	24	Cert	$900	$900					
Presentation College (Aberdeen)	20	Jun	36	BS	$12,300	$12,300				•	
Rapid City Regional Hospital	10	Jun	24	Cert	$1,250	$1,250				•	
Sanford Medical Center (Sioux Falls)	14	Jul	24	Cert	$1,000	$1,000					
Tennessee											
Baptist College of Health Sciences (Memphis)	20	Aug	20	BS	$7,900	$7,900					
Chattanooga State Technical Comm College	62	Aug	24	AAS	$3,163	$11,573				•	
East Tennessee State University (Elizabethton)	45	Aug	20	BS	$2,892	$9,396				•	
Jackson State Community College	31	Aug	24	AAS	$3,329	$12,317				•	
MedVance Institute (Cookeville)	32	Jan	24	AS	$14,500	$14,500				•	
Methodist University Hospital (Memphis)	22	Jul	24	Cert	$2,500	$2,500					
Nashville General Hospital	28	Oct	24	Cert	$4,500	$4,500				•	
South College (Knoxville)	106	Jan	18, 30	AS, BS	$16,800	$16,800		•		•	
Southwest Tennessee Community College (Memphis)	35	Jul	24	AAS	$2,400	$4,400					
Univ of Tennessee Medical Ctr at Knoxville	14	Jul	24	Cert	$2,500	$2,500				•	
Volunteer State Community College (Gallatin)	35	Jul	24	Dipl, AAS	$2,441	$8,781					
Texas											
Amarillo College	30	Aug	24	AAS	$1,800	$3,200					
Blinn College (Bryan)	18	Sep	24	AAS	$7,500	$0					
Career Centers of Texas - Ft Worth Campus (Fort Worth)	36	Jul	24	Dipl	$13,500	$0					
Citizens Medical Center (Victoria)	6	Jul	24	Cert	$1,000	$1,000				•	
Cy-Fair College (Cypress)	40	Aug	24	AAS	$1,596	$3,654				•	

*Data are shown only for programs that completed the 2007 AMA Survey of Health Professions Education Programs.

‡Key to Offers: 1: Evening or weekend classes; 2: Non-English instruction; 3: Cultural competence instruction; 4: Distance education component.

Radiographer

Programs*	Class Capacity	Begins	Length (months)	Award	Res. Tuition	Non-res. Tuition	Stipend	Offers:‡ 1	2	3	4
Del Mar College (Corpus Christi)	32	Jul	24	AAS	$1,224	$7,840					
El Centro College (Dallas)	54	Aug	23	AAS	$1,080	$1,800			•	•	
El Paso Community College	16	Jun	24	AAS	$2,180	$2,995				•	
Harris County Hosp Dist/Ben Taub Gen Hosp (Houston)	44	Jul	24	Cert	$1,650	$1,800				•	
Hendrick Medical Center (Abilene)	15	Jan Jul	24	Cert	$2,800	$2,800					
Houston Community College	125	Jun	24	AAS	$3,703	$7,321				•	
Lamar Institute of Technology (Beaumont)	38	Jun	48	AAS	$2,500	$8,000					
Laredo Community College	14	Sep	24	Dipl, AAS	$700	$0					
McLennan Community College (Waco)	42	Aug	24	AAS	$1,224	$3,384			•	•	
Memorial Hermann Baptist Hospital Beaumont	64	Jun	24	Cert	$4,800	$0					
Midland College	12	Aug	23	AAS	$1,988	$3,525					
Midwestern State University (Wichita Falls)	120	Sep	24	AAS	$7,550	$8,928					
Montgomery College (Conroe)	48	Jan	24	AAS	$5,300	$9,600				•	
Odessa College	17	Jul	24	AAS	$1,908	$2,448				•	
South Plains College (Lubbock)	32	Sep	24	AAS	$1,846	$3,408					
St Philip's College (San Antonio)	68	Jun	24	AAS	$1,300	$4,000				•	
Tarrant County College - Northeast Campus (Hurst)	40	Jul	22	AAS	$1,775	$2,237				•	•
Tyler Junior College	43	Aug	24	AAS	$1,801	$3,881				•	
Wharton County Junior College	18	Aug	24	AAS	$32	$64				•	
Utah											
Salt Lake Community College (West Jordan)	35	Aug	21	AAS	$3,167	$9,820		•		•	
Vermont											
Champlain College (Burlington)	23	Sep	21, 45	Dipl, AS, BS	$21,000	$0	$900			•	
Virginia											
Central Virginia Community College (Lynchburg)	20	Aug	24	AAS	$82	$257				•	
Mary Washington Hospital (Fredericksburg)	24	Aug	23	Cert	$3,500	$3,500				•	
Medical Careers Institute (Newport News)	15	Every 31 wks	18	AAS	$15,000	$15,000				•	
Riverside School of Health Careers (Newport News)	64	Sep	22	Cert	$8,000	$8,000				•	
Southwest Virginia Community College (Richlands)	36	Jul	24	AAS	$2,650	$8,250		•			
Tidewater Community College (Virginia Beach)	45	May	24	AAS	$3,258	$9,563				•	
University of Virginia Health System (Charlottesville)	20	Jul	24	Cert	$2,000	$2,000				•	
Virginia Commonwealth University (Richmond)	48	Aug	33	BS	$7,500	$23,000				•	
Washington											
Pima Medical Institute - Seattle	30	Apr Aug Dec	24	AS	$14,350	$14,350		•		•	•
Tacoma Community College	24	Sep	24	Dipl, CertAAS	$3,451	$5,009				•	
West Virginia											
Bluefield State College	34	May	24	AS	$4,715	$10,023		•			
Ohio Valley Medical Center (Wheeling)	10	Jul	24	Cert	$1,500	$1,500				•	
Southern West Virginia Comm & Tech College (Mount Gay)	40	Aug	21	Dipl, AAS	$2,300	$6,800		•		•	•
St Mary's Medical Center (Huntington)	40	Jul	24	Dipl, Cert, AAS	$6,000	$6,000				•	
United Hospital Center (Clarksburg)	15	Jun	24	Cert, AAS	$3,000	$3,000				•	
West Virginia University Hospitals (Morgantown)	18	Jul	24	Cert	$2,000	$2,000				•	
Wheeling Hospital	10	Jul	24	Cert	$1,500	$1,500				•	
Wisconsin											
Aurora St Luke's Medical Center (Milwaukee)	18	Sep	24	Cert	$2,000	$2,000				•	
Bellin Health Hosp/Bellin Health Systems Inc (Green Bay)	16	Aug	24	Dipl	$3,900	$3,900				•	
Blackhawk Technical College (Janesville)	18	Jun	24	AS	$92	$478					
Columbia St Mary's Hospitals (Milwaukee)	20	Sep	24	Cert	$5,000	$5,000				•	
Froedtert Memorial Lutheran Hospital (Milwaukee)	45	Sep	24	Cert	$5,000	$5,000				•	
Lakeshore Technical College (Cleveland)	16	Jan	22	AAS	$3,196	$16,496				•	•
Madison Area Technical College	22	Aug	24	AAS	$3,500	$0					
Mercy Medical Center/Affinity Health System (Oshkosh)	14	Sep	24	Cert	$10,000	$10,000					
Milwaukee Area Technical College	24	Aug	24	AAS	$3,981	$0				•	
Theda Clark Regional Medical Center (Neenah)	16	Sep	24	Cert	$3,250	$3,250				•	
University of Wisconsin Hospital and Clinics (Madison)	16	Sep	24	Dipl	$2,000	$2,000				•	
Western Technical College (La Crosse)	32	Aug	23	AAS	$3,354	$16,068					
Wheaton Franciscan Healthcare - St Joseph (Milwaukee)	10	Sep	24	Cert	$3,000	$3,000					
Wyoming											
Casper College	20	May	24	AS	$1,668	$4,644		•		•	
Laramie County Community College (Cheyenne)	18	Aug	24	AAS	$2,784	$6,752				•	

*Data are shown only for programs that completed the 2007 AMA Survey of Health Professions Education Programs.
‡Key to Offers: 1: Evening or weekend classes; 2: Non-English instruction; 3: Cultural competence instruction; 4: Distance education component.

PROGRAMS

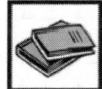

History

Initially, rehabilitation professionals were recruited from a variety of human service disciplines, including public health nursing, social work, and school counseling. Although educational programs began to appear in the 1940s, it was not until the availability of federal funding for rehabilitation counseling programs in 1954 that the profession began to grow and establish its own identity.

Historically, rehabilitation counselors primarily served working-age adults with disabilities. Today, the need for rehabilitation counseling services extends to persons of all age groups who have disabilities. Rehabilitation counselors also may provide general and specialized counseling to people with disabilities in public human service programs and private practice settings.

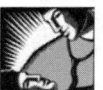

Career Description

Working directly with an individual with a disability or their advocates, a rehabilitation counselor is a special type of professional counselor who helps evaluate and coordinate needed services to assist people with disabilities in coping with limitations caused by such factors as cognitive and learning difficulties, environmental and societal discrimination and barriers, psychological conflict/distress, or loss of physical/functional ability.

Rehabilitation counselors assist people with physical, mental, or emotional disabilities to become or remain self-sufficient, productive citizens. Disabilities may result from:

- Congenital disability
- Illness and disease
- Work-related injuries
- Automobile accidents
- The stresses of war, work, and daily life
- The aging process

Rehabilitation counselors help individuals with disabilities deal with societal and personal problems, plan careers, and find and keep satisfying jobs. They also may work with individuals, professional organizations, and advocacy groups to address the environmental and social barriers that create obstacles for people with disabilities. The rehabilitation counselor builds bridges between the often isolated world of people with disabilities and their families, communities, and work environments. Major goals are to empower individuals to make informed choices, help individuals achieve positive mental health, and maximize opportunities for economic independence (obtain employment, if possible).

Other responsibilities for the rehabilitation counselor include:

- Evaluating an individual's potential for independent living and employment and arranging for medical and psychological services and vocational assessment, training, and job placement
- Evaluating medical and psychological reports and conferring with physicians and psychologists about the types of work individuals can perform
- Working with employers to identify and/or modify job responsibilities to accommodate individuals with disabilities

The rehabilitation counselor draws on knowledge from several fields, including psychology, medicine, psychiatry, sociology, social work, education, and law. Their specialized knowledge of disabilities and environmental factors that interact with disabilities, as well as specific knowledge and skills, differentiate rehabilitation counselors from other types of counselors.

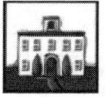

Employment Characteristics

Many rehabilitation counselors work in state or federal rehabilitation agencies or community rehabilitation programs. Others seek opportunities in the private or for-profit sector of rehabilitation. Because all state rehabilitation agencies follow the same general procedures, a rehabilitation counselor has geographical mobility and can find employment throughout the United States and its territories. Other potential employers include

- Comprehensive rehabilitation centers
- Universities and academic settings
- Insurance companies
- Substance abuse rehabilitation centers
- Correctional facilities
- Halfway houses
- Independent living centers

Reflecting this wide range of job opportunities, rehabilitation counselors are often employed in positions with different job titles, such as counselor, job placement specialist, substance abuse counselor, rehabilitation consultant, independent living specialist, or case manager. According to survey data from the Human Resources Development Committee of CSAVR, 2006, the average starting salary for rehabilitation counselors in the public sector is more than $34,300 and can range between $27,500 and $51,700. Average salaries in states that require the master's degree may be considerably higher. The salary ranges in the private sector are significantly higher. The average overall salary in the private sector is estimated at between $55,000 to $75,000-plus.

Refer to Section IV, Table 5 of this *Directory* for more information, or see www.ama-assn.org/go/hpsalary.

Employment Outlook

Rehabilitation counselors serve a large portion of the US population. An estimated 48 million Americans have physical, mental, or psychological disabilities that restrict their activities and prevent them from obtaining or maintaining jobs.

Consequently, the employment outlook for the profession is excellent. Based on national employment outlook studies and regional and state surveys, hundreds of rehabilitation counselor positions are expected to be available in the coming years for qualified master's-level professionals. Recent studies show that rehabilitation counselor education programs are not graduating sufficient numbers of qualified students to meet current and anticipated marketplace needs.

The roles and responsibilities of rehabilitation counselors have expanded greatly over the last 10 years, further increasing the attractiveness of a career in the profession. Rehabilitation counselors, for example, have begun to determine, coordinate, and arrange for rehabilitation and transition services for children within school systems. In addition, rehabilitation counselors are providing geriatric rehabilitation services to older persons with health problems, and workers injured on the job are increasingly receiving rehabilitation services through private rehabilitation counseling companies and employers' disability management and employee assistance programs. They may also become life-care planners assisting individuals who will experience major long-term disability. Many former teachers, attorneys, nurses, physical therapists, occupational therapists, clergy, and business people have found second careers as professional rehabilitation counselors.

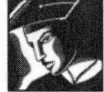

Educational Programs

Length. Rehabilitation counselor education programs typically provide between 18 and 24 months of academic and field-based clinical training. Clinical training consists of a practicum and a minimum of 600 hours of supervised internship experience. Clinical field experiences are available in a variety of community, state, federal, and private rehabilitation-related programs.

Prerequisites. Although no formal requirements exist, most rehabilitation counseling graduate students have undergraduate degrees in rehabilitation services, psychology, sociology, or other human services-related fields.

Curriculum. Rehabilitation counselors are trained in:
- Counseling theory, skills, and techniques
- Individual and group counseling
- Environmental assessment
- Psychosocial and medical aspects of disability, including human growth and development
- Social and cultural diversity
- Principles of psychiatric rehabilitation
- Case management and rehabilitation planning
- Issues and ethics in rehabilitation service delivery
- Technological adaptation
- Vocational evaluation and work adjustment
- Career counseling
- Research and program evaluation
- Job development and placement

In addition, students may enroll in courses such as marriage and family counseling, substance abuse rehabilitation, juvenile and adult offender rehabilitation, mental retardation, communication disorders, sign language, stress management, psychological testing, conflict management, crisis counseling, and rehabilitation administration.

Licensure, Certification, and Registration

Certification and licensure of rehabilitation counselors help protect the public and provide a means of identifying those individuals who possess the minimum training and meet supervised work experience standards established by professional groups and governmental agencies.

Certification. The Commission on Rehabilitation Counselor Certification (CRCC), an independent credentialing body incorpo-

rated in 1974, certifies rehabilitation counselors throughout the United States and in Canada who meet educational and work experience requirements, pass an examination, and maintain certification by completing 100 hours of acceptable continuing education credit every 5 years.

Licensure. A counseling license is a credential authorized by a state legislature that regulates the title and/or practice of professional counselors. Rehabilitation counselors are eligible for licensure as professional counselors in nearly all states that regulate counselors; licensure requirements include passing an examination, acquiring needed supervised counseling experience, and, in some states, completing specified coursework.

Registration. A number of state workers' compensation laws or regulations specify education, training, and/or credentials requirements for people providing rehabilitation counseling services to workers with disabilities. In these states, rehabilitation counselors pay a fee and provide proof of education and/or certification to register with the state workers' compensation agency. Many states also require the certified rehabilitation counselor (CRC) credential, although the permitted scope of services may vary from one state to the next.

Inquiries

National Council on Rehabilitation Education
Sharon Benshoff, Administrative Secretary
2012 West Norwood Drive
Carbondale, IL 62901
618 549-3267
E-mail: sbenshoff@ncre-admin.org
www.rehabeducators.org

Certification
Commission on Rehabilitation Counselor Certification
Cindy Chapman, Executive Director
300 North Martingale Road, Suite 460
Schaumburg, IL 60173
847 944-1325
www.crccertification.com

Program Accreditation
Council on Rehabilitation Education
300 North Martingale Road, Suite 460
Schaumburg, IL 60173
847 944-1345
847 944-1324 Fax
www.core-rehab.org

Rehabilitation Counselor

Alabama

Auburn University
Rehabilitation Counseling Prgm
Rehabilitation and Special Education
1228 Haley Center
Auburn University, AL 36849
Prgm Dir: E Davis Martin, Jr, EdD CRC NCC
Tel: 334 844-2083   *Fax:* 334 844-2080
E-mail: martiev@auburn.edu

University of Alabama at Birmingham
Rehabilitation Counseling Prgm
School of Education, Rm 157
901 S 13th St
Birmingham, AL 35294-1250
Prgm Dir: Patricia M Sheets
Tel: 205 934-8334   *Fax:* 205 934-3702
E-mail: psheets@uab.edu

Alabama A&M University
Rehabilitation Counseling Prgm
PO Box 580
Normal, AL 35762
www.aamu.edu
Prgm Dir: William Fennesee, RhD CRC
Tel: 256 372-4039   *Fax:* 256 372-5255
E-mail: william.fennesee@email.aamu.edu

Troy University
Rehabilitation Counseling Prgm
College of Education
228 General Academic Bldg
Troy, AL 36082
Prgm Dir: Mary Anne Templeton, PhD CRC
Tel: 334 670-3350   *Fax:* 334 670-3291
E-mail: mtempleton@troy.edu

University of Alabama
Rehabilitation Counseling Prgm
318 Graves Hall, PO Box 870231
Tuscaloosa, AL 35487-0231
Prgm Dir: Jamie Satcher, PhD
Tel: 205 348-1178   *Fax:* 205 348-7884
E-mail: Jsatcher@bamaed.ua.edu

Arizona

University of Arizona
Rehabilitation Counseling Prgm
Dept of Spec Educ and Rehab
College of Education
Tucson, AZ 85721
www.arizona.edu
Prgm Dir: Amos Sales, EdD CRC NCC
Tel: 520 621-0941   *Fax:* 520 621-3821
E-mail: sales@u.arizona.edu

Arkansas

University of Arkansas
Rehabilitation Counseling Prgm
Rehabilitation Education and Research Program
100 Graduate Education Bldg
Fayetteville, AR 72701
www.uark.edu/depts/coehp/RHAB.htm
Prgm Dir: Lynn Koch, PhD CRC
Tel: 479 575-8696   *Fax:* 479 575-3319
E-mail: lckoch@uark.edu

University of Arkansas at Little Rock
Rehabilitation Counseling Prgm
2801 S University Ave
Little Rock, AR 72204
www.ualr.edu/rc
Prgm Dir: Larry R Dickerson, PhD
Tel: 501 569-3428   *Fax:* 501 569-3547
E-mail: lrdickerson@ualr.edu

Arkansas State University
Rehabilitation Counseling Prgm
Dept of Psychology and Counseling
PO Box 1560
State University, AR 72467
Prgm Dir: Loretta McGregor, PhD CRC
Tel: 870 972-3064   *Fax:* 870 972-3962
E-mail: lmcgregor@astate.edu

California

California State University - Fresno
Rehabilitation Counseling Prgm
5005 N Maple Ave/MS ED 3
Fresno, CA 93740
http://education.csufresno.edu/cser/
Prgm Dir: Charles Arokiasamy, RhD CRC NCC CCM
Tel: 559 278-0325   *Fax:* 559 278-0045
E-mail: charlesa@csufresno.edu

California State University - Los Angeles
Rehabilitation Counseling Prgm
5151 State University Dr, King Hall C1064
Los Angeles, CA 90032
Prgm Dir: Martin Brodwin, PhD CRC
Tel: 323 343-4440   *Fax:* 323 343-5605
E-mail: mbrodwi@calstatela.edu

California State University - Sacramento
Rehabilitation Counseling Prgm
College of Education
6000 J St
Sacramento, CA 95819-6079
Prgm Dir: Guy Deaner, PhD
Tel: 916 278-6663   *Fax:* 916 278-3948
E-mail: deanerg@csus.edu

California State University - San Bernardino
Rehabilitation Counseling Prgm
School of Education
5500 University Pkwy
San Bernardino, CA 92407
Prgm Dir: Joseph Turpin, PhD CRC
Tel: 909 880-5662   *Fax:* 909 880-5992
E-mail: jturpin@csusb.edu

San Diego State University
Rehabilitation Counseling Prgm
Dept of Adm Rehab and Postsecondary Ed
3590 Camino del Rio N
San Diego, CA 92108-1716
Prgm Dir: Caren Sax, EdD CRC
Tel: 619 594-7183   *Fax:* 619 594-4208
E-mail: csax@mail.sdsu.edu

San Francisco State University
Rehabilitation Counseling Prgm
Dept of Counseling
1600 Holloway Ave
San Francisco, CA 94132
Prgm Dir: Leslie Zwillinger, PhD CRC
Tel: 415 338-1718   *Fax:* 415 338-0594
E-mail: lzwill@sfsu.edu

Colorado

University of Northern Colorado
Rehabilitation Counseling Prgm
School of Human Sciences
Gunter 1250, Box 132
Greeley, CO 80639
www.unco.edu/HHS/hs/hs.htm
Prgm Dir: Joseph Ososkie, PhD
Tel: 970 351-1579   *Fax:* 970 351-1255
E-mail: joe.ososkie@unco.edu

Connecticut

Central Connecticut State University
Rehabilitation Counseling Prgm
165 Stanley St
New Britain, CT 06050
Prgm Dir: Judith Rosenberg
E-mail: rosenbergj@ccsu.edu

District of Columbia

George Washington University
Rehabilitation Counseling Prgm
Dept of Counseling, Human/Org Studies
2134 G St NW, 3rd Fl
Washington, DC 20052
Prgm Dir: Jorge Garcia, RhD CRC LPC
Tel: 202 994-7126   *Fax:* 202 994-3436
E-mail: garcia@gwu.edu

Florida

Florida Atlantic University
Rehabilitation Counseling Prgm
777 Glades Rd
Boca Raton, FL 33431
Prgm Dir: Michael Frain, PhD CRC
Tel: 561 297-3626
E-mail: mfrain@fau.edu

University of Florida
Rehabilitation Counseling Prgm
Dept of Rehabilitation Counseling
PO Box 100175
Gainesville, FL 32610-0175
Prgm Dir: Linda Shaw, PhD CRC
Tel: 352 273-6745   *Fax:* 352 273-6048
E-mail: lshaw@phhp.ufl.edu

University of North Florida
Rehabilitation Counseling Prgm
Department of Public Health
1 University Dr
Jacksonville, FL 32224
www.unf.edu/brooks/cohrehab.htm
Prgm Dir: Jeanne Patterson, EdD CRC
Tel: 904 620-1428   *Fax:* 904 620-1035
E-mail: jpatters@unf.edu

Florida State University
Rehabilitation Counseling Prgm
205 Stone Bldg
Tallahassee, FL 32306
www.coe.fsu.edu/cerds/programs/RehabCounsel.html
Prgm Dir: Deborah Ebener, PhD CRC NCC
Tel: 850 644-1789   *Fax:* 850 644-8715
E-mail: debener@fsu.edu

University of South Florida
Rehabilitation Counseling Prgm
Dept of Rehabilitation and Mental Health Counseling
4202 E Fowler Ave, SOC 107
Tampa, FL 33620-8100
Prgm Dir: Charlotte Dixon, RhD CRC NCC
Tel: 813 974-0973   *Fax:* 813 974-8080
E-mail: dixon@cas.usf.edu

Georgia

Georgia State University
Rehabilitation Counseling Prgm
Counseling and Psych Services Dept
PO Box 3980
Atlanta, GA 30302-3980
http://education.gsu.edu/aae/ms/rehl
Prgm Dir: Roger Weed, PhD CRC CDMS CLCP LPC CCM
  FNRCA FIALCP
Tel: 404 413-8172   *Fax:* 404 413-8013
E-mail: rweed@gsu.edu

Fort Valley State University
Rehabilitation Counseling Prgm
1005 State College Dr
PO Box 31030-4313
Fort Valley, GA 31030-4313
Prgm Dir: Dothel Edwards, Jr, RhD CRC CLCP
Tel: 478 825-6237, Ext 6526 *Fax:* 478 827-3097
E-mail: edwardsd@fvsu.edu

Thomas University
Rehabilitation Counseling Prgm
Division of Counseling
1501 Millpond Rd
Thomasville, GA 31792
www.thomasu.edu
Prgm Dir: Theresa C Reese, PhD CRC
Tel: 229 226-1621, Ext 255 *Fax:* 229 226-1653
E-mail: treese@thomasu.edu

Hawaii

University of Hawaii
Rehabilitation Counseling Prgm
Dept of Counselor Education
1776 University Ave, WA2-221
Honolulu, HI 96822
Prgm Dir: Brenda Cartwright, PhD CRC
Tel: 808 956-4386 *Fax:* 808 956-3814
E-mail: bcartwri@hawaii.edu

Idaho

University of Idaho
Rehabilitation Counseling Prgm
Counseling, School Psychology, Special Education, and
   Education
College of Education Rm 206
Moscow, ID 83844-3083
Prgm Dir: Jerry Fischer, RhD CRC LPC
Tel: 208 885-5947 *Fax:* 208 885-6869
E-mail: jfischer@uidaho.edu

Illinois

Southern Illinois University Carbondale
Rehabilitation Counseling Prgm
Rehabilitation Institute
Ste 308
Carbondale, IL 62901-4609
Prgm Dir: Thomas Upton, PhD CRC
Tel: 618 453-8287 *Fax:* 618 453-8271
E-mail: tupton@siu.edu

Univ of Illinois at Urbana-Champaign
Rehabilitation Counseling Prgm
1206 S 4th, 121 Hoff
Champaign, IL 61820
Prgm Dir: David Strauser, PhD CRC
Tel: 217 333-2307 *Fax:* 217 333-2766
E-mail: strauser@uiuc.edu

Illinois Institute of Technology
Rehabilitation Counseling Prgm
Inst of Psych/Rm 252 Life Science Bldg
3105 S Dearborn St
Chicago, IL 60616
www.iit.edu/colleges/psych/
Prgm Dir: Chow Lam, PhD
Tel: 312 567-3515 *Fax:* 312 567-3493
E-mail: Lam@iit.edu

Northeastern Illinois University
Rehabilitation Counseling Prgm
5500 N St Louis Ave
Chicago, IL 60625
Prgm Dir: Kenneth F Currier, PhD CRC
Tel: 773 442-5550, Ext 5576 *Fax:* 773 442-5559
E-mail: k-currier@neiu.edu

Northern Illinois University
Rehabilitation Counseling Prgm
Dept of Communicative Disorders
Northern Illinois University
DeKalb, IL 60115
Prgm Dir: Deborah Gough, EdD
Tel: 815 753-6519 *Fax:* 815 753-9123
E-mail: dgough@niu.edu

Indiana

Ball State University
Rehabilitation Counseling Prgm
Dept of Counseling Psychology and Guidance Services
TC 622
Muncie, IN 47306-0585
Prgm Dir: Molly Tschopp, PhD CRC
Tel: 765 285-8569 *Fax:* 765 285-2067
E-mail: mktschopp@bsu.edu

Iowa

Drake University
Rehabilitation Counseling Prgm
Counseling, Leadership, and Adult Development
3206 University
Des Moines, IA 50311
Prgm Dir: Robert Stensrud, EdD CRC
Tel: 515 271-3061 *Fax:* 515 271-4140
E-mail: robert.stensrud@drake.edu

University of Iowa
Rehabilitation Counseling Prgm
N362 Lindquist Center
Iowa City, IA 52242-1529
www.coe164.education.uiowa.edu:8180/crsd/rehab
Prgm Dir: John Wadsworth, PhD CRC
Tel: 319 335-5246 *Fax:* 319 335-5291
E-mail: john-s-wadsworth@uiowa.edu

Kansas

Emporia State University
Rehabilitation Counseling Prgm
Campus Box 4036/1200 Commerical
Emporia, KS 66801
www.emporia.edu/counre/
Prgm Dir: Jim Costello, PhD
Tel: 620 341-5791 *Fax:* 620 341-6200
E-mail: jcostell@emporia.edu

Kentucky

University of Kentucky
Rehabilitation Counseling Prgm
224 Taylor Education Bldg
Lexington, KY 40506
www.uky.edu/Education/EDS/RC.html
Prgm Dir: Malachy Bishop, PhD CRC
Tel: 859 257-3834 *Fax:* 859 257-3835
E-mail: mbishop@uky.edu

Louisiana

Southern Univ and A&M College
Rehabilitation Counseling Prgm
229 Blanks Hall
Baton Rouge, LA 70813
Prgm Dir: Madan M Kundu, PhD CRC NCC LRC FNRCA
Tel: 225 771-2819 *Fax:* 225 771-2293
E-mail: kundusubr@aol.com

Louisiana State Univ Health Sciences Center
Rehabilitation Counseling Prgm
School of Allied Health Professions
1900 Gravier St, Ste 8A1
New Orleans, LA 70112-2262
Prgm Dir: John Dolan, RhD CRC
Tel: 504 568-4244 *Fax:* 504 568-4324
E-mail: jdolan@lsuhsc.edu

Maine

University of Southern Maine
Rehabilitation Counseling Prgm
400 Bailey Hall
Gorham, ME 04038
Prgm Dir: Stephen T Murphy, PhD CRC
Tel: 207 780-5319 *Fax:* 207 780-5043
E-mail: smurphy@usm.maine.edu

Maryland

Coppin State University
Rehabilitation Counseling Prgm
2500 W North Ave
Baltimore, MD 21216
Prgm Dir: Janet D Spry, EdD
Tel: 410 951-3514 *Fax:* 410 951-3511
E-mail: jspry@coppin.edu

University of Maryland
Rehabilitation Counseling Prgm
Counseling and Personnel Services Dept
Coll of Education, Benjamin Bldg Rm 3214
College Park, MD 20742
Prgm Dir: Ellen Fabian, PhD
Tel: 301 405-2872 *Fax:* 301 405-9995
E-mail: efabian@umd.edu

University of Maryland Eastern Shore
Rehabilitation Counseling Prgm
Ste 1062, Hazel Hall
Princess Anne, MD 21853
Prgm Dir: Maryam Rahimi, PhD CRC LCPC
Tel: 410 651-6514 *Fax:* 410 651-6736
E-mail: mrahimi@umes.edu

Massachusetts

Boston University
Rehabilitation Counseling Prgm
Sargent Coll of Hlth and Rehab Sciences
635 Commonwealth Ave
Boston, MA 02215
Prgm Dir: Arthur E Dell Orto, PhD CRC
Tel: 617 353-7486 *Fax:* 617 353-8914
E-mail: ado@bu.edu

University of Massachusetts - Boston
Rehabilitation Counseling Prgm
Counseling and School Psychology
Graduate College of Education
Boston, MA 02125-3393
Prgm Dir: Gonzalo Bacigalupe, EdD MPH
Tel: 617 287-7631 *Fax:* 617 287-7664
E-mail: gonzalo.bacigalupe@umb.edu

Springfield College
Rehabilitation Counseling Prgm
Rehabilitation and Disability Studies Dept
263 Alden St
Springfield, MA 01109-3797
www.spfldcol.edu
Prgm Dir: Thomas J Ruscio, EdD
Tel: 413 748-3566 *Fax:* 413 748-3787
E-mail: truscio@spfldcol.edu

Assumption College
Rehabilitation Counseling Prgm
Inst for Social and Rehab Services
500 Salisbury St
Worcester, MA 01609-1296
Prgm Dir: Lee Pearson, CRC
Tel: 508 767-7063   *Fax:* 508 798-2872
E-mail: lpearson@assumption.edu

Michigan

Wayne State University
Rehabilitation Counseling Prgm
Theoretical and Behavioral Foundation
323 College of Education, 5425 Gullen Mall
Detroit, MI 48202
Prgm Dir: George Parris, PhD LPC CCRC NCP ABDA
Tel: 313 577-1619   *Fax:* 313 577-5235
E-mail: gparris@wayne.edu

Michigan State University
Rehabilitation Counseling Prgm
Counseling, Educ Psych and Spec Educ
237 Erickson Hall
East Lansing, MI 48824-1034
Prgm Dir: John F Kosciulek, PhD CRC
Tel: 517 355-1838   *Fax:* 517 353-6393
E-mail: jkosciul@msu.edu

Western Michigan University
Rehabilitation Counseling Prgm
The Graduate College
3404 Sangren Hall, Mail Stop 5218
Kalamazoo, MI 49008
Prgm Dir: Jennipher Wiebold, PhD CRC
Tel: 616 387-3459   *Fax:* 616 387-3567
E-mail: Jennipher.wiebold@wmich.edu

Minnesota

Minnesota State University - Mankato
Rehabilitation Counseling Prgm
Dept of Speech, Hearing, and Rehabilitation Svcs
College of Allied Health and Nursing
Mankato, MN 56001
http://ahn.mnsu.edu/rehabilitation
Prgm Dir: Gerald Schneck, PhD CRC-MAC FVE NCC
Tel: 507 389-5438   *Fax:* 507 389-2821
E-mail: gerald.schneck@mnsu.edu

St Cloud State University
Rehabilitation Counseling Prgm
Dept of Counselor Education and Ed Psych
720 4th Ave S
St Cloud, MN 56301-4498
www.stcloudstate.edu/ceep/rehab
Prgm Dir: Brad W Kuhlman, PhD CRC
Tel: 320 308-1685   *Fax:* 320 308-4082
E-mail: bkuhlman@stcloudstate.edu

Mississippi

Jackson State University
Rehabilitation Counseling Prgm
PO Box 18829
Jackson, MS 39217
Prgm Dir: Dion Porter, CRC
Tel: 601 979-3364   *Fax:* 601 968-2213
E-mail: dion.porter@jsums.edu

Mississippi State University
Rehabilitation Counseling Prgm
Counseling, Ed Psych and Special Education
Mail Stop 9727
Mississippi State, MS 39762
www.msstate.edu/dept/rehab/Graduate/rehab.html
Prgm Dir: Charles Palmer, PhD
Tel: 662 325-7917   *Fax:* 662 325-3263
E-mail: cpalmer@colled.msstate.edu

Missouri

University of Missouri - Columbia
Rehabilitation Counseling Prgm
Dept of Educational, School, and Counseling Psychology
98 Corporate Lake Dr
Columbia, MO 65211
Prgm Dir: C David Roberts, PhD
Tel: 573 882-3807   *Fax:* 573 882-1728
E-mail: RobertsC@missouri.edu

Maryville University
Rehabilitation Counseling Prgm
650 Maryville University Dr
St Louis, MO 63141
Prgm Dir: Michael Kiener, PhD CRC
Tel: 314 529-9443   *Fax:* 314 529-9139
E-mail: mkiener@maryville.edu

Montana

Montana State University - Billings
Rehabilitation Counseling Prgm
Dept of Rehabilitation and Human Services
1500 N 30th St
Billings, MT 59101-0298
Prgm Dir: Kyle Colling
Tel: 406 657-2056   *Fax:* 406 657-2255
E-mail: kcolling@msubillings.edu

New Jersey

Univ of Medicine & Dent of New Jersey
Rehabilitation Counseling Prgm
Dept of Psychiatric Rehabilitation
1776 Raritan Rd
Scotch Plains, NJ 07076
http://shrp.umdnj.edu/programs/graduate.html
Prgm Dir: Janice Oursler, PhD CRC
Tel: 908 889-2462   *Fax:* 908 889-2432
E-mail: ourslejd@umdnj.edu

New York

SUNY at Albany
Rehabilitation Counseling Prgm
School of Education, Rm 220
1400 Washington Ave
Albany, NY 12222
Prgm Dir: Puspa M Das, PhD
Tel: 518 442-5042   *Fax:* 518 442-4953
E-mail: pdas@albany.edu

University at Buffalo - SUNY
Rehabilitation Counseling Prgm
Dept of Counseling, School, and Educ Psych
409 Baldy Hall
Buffalo, NY 14260-1000
Prgm Dir: Timothy Janikowski
Tel: 716 645-2484, Ext 1067   *Fax:* 716 645-6166
E-mail: tjanikow@buffalo.edu

Hofstra University
Rehabilitation Counseling Prgm
119 Hofstra University, 160 Hagedorn
Hempstead, NY 11549-1190
Prgm Dir: Jamie S Mitus, PhD
Tel: 516 463-7453   *Fax:* 516 463-6184
E-mail: Jamie.S.Mitus@hofstra.edu

CUNY Hunter College
Rehabilitation Counseling Prgm
Dept of Educ Found and Counseling Prgms
695 Park Ave
New York, NY 10021
Prgm Dir: John O'Neill, PhD CRC
Tel: 212 772-5188   *Fax:* 212 650-3198

Syracuse University
Rehabilitation Counseling Prgm
259 Huntington Hall
Syracuse, NY 13244
Prgm Dir: Dennis Gilbride, PhD CRC
Tel: 315 443-5264   *Fax:* 315 443-5732
E-mail: ddgilbri@syr.edu

North Carolina

University of North Carolina - Chapel Hill
Rehabilitation Counseling Prgm
CB 7205, 2088 Bondurant Hall
Chapel Hill, NC 27599
Prgm Dir: Charles Bernacchio, EdD CRC
Tel: 919 966-8788   *Fax:* 919 966-9007
E-mail: cbernacc@med.unc.edu

North Carolina A&T State University
Rehabilitation Counseling Prgm
1601 E Market St
Greensboro, NC 27411
Prgm Dir: Tyra Turner Whittaker, RhD CRC
E-mail: tnwhitta@ncat.edu

East Carolina University
Rehabilitation Counseling Prgm
Dept of Rehabilitation Studies
School of Allied Health Sciences
Greenville, NC 27858-4353
www.ecu.edu/rehb
Prgm Dir: Mark Stebnicki, PhD CRC LPC
Tel: 252 744-6300   *Fax:* 252 744-6302
E-mail: stebnickim@ecu.edu

Winston-Salem State University
Rehabilitation Counseling Prgm
Anderson Center
601 Martin Luther King Jr Dr
Winston-Salem, NC 27110
Prgm Dir: Yolanda Edwards
Tel: 336 750-2258   *Fax:* 336 750-2914
E-mail: edwardsyo@wssu.edu

Ohio

Ohio University
Rehabilitation Counseling Prgm
201 McCracken Hall
Athens, OH 45701
Prgm Dir: Jerry A Olsheski, PhD CRC LPC
Tel: 740 593-0032   *Fax:* 740 593-0799
E-mail: olsheski@ohio.edu

Bowling Green State University
Rehabilitation Counseling Prgm
School of Intervention Services
Bowling Green, OH 43403-0255
Prgm Dir: Jay R Stewart, PhD
Tel: 419 372-7301   *Fax:* 419 372-8265
E-mail: jstewar@bgnet.bgsu.edu

Ohio State University
Rehabilitation Counseling Prgm
356 Arps Hall, 1945 N High St
Columbus, OH 43210-1172
Prgm Dir: Michael Klein, PhD CRC
Tel: 614 292-8183   *Fax:* 614 292-4255
E-mail: klein.3@osu.edu

Wright State University
Rehabilitation Counseling Prgm
M052 Creative Arts Center
Dayton, OH 45435-0001
Prgm Dir: Jan La Forge, PhD CRC PC NCC
Tel: 937 775-2075   *Fax:* 937 775-2042
E-mail: jan.laforge@wright.edu

Kent State University
Rehabilitation Counseling Prgm
405 White Hall
Kent, OH 44242
Prgm Dir: Philip D Rumrill Jr, PhD CRC
Tel: 330 672-0600   *Fax:* 330 672-2512
E-mail: prumrill@kent.edu

Oklahoma

East Central University
Rehabilitation Counseling Prgm
Box C-1
Ada, OK 74820
www.ecok.edu
Prgm Dir: Randal Elston, EdD CRC NCC CVE
Tel: 580 559-5463   *Fax:* 580 559-5492
E-mail: relston@ecok.edu

Langston University
Rehabilitation Counseling Prgm
4205 N Lincoln Blvd
Oklahoma City, OK 73105
Prgm Dir: Corey L Moore, RhD CRC
Tel: 405 962-1671   *Fax:* 405 962-1628
E-mail: clmoore@lunet.edu

Oregon

Western Oregon University
Rehabilitation Counseling Prgm
Education Bldg 220
Monmouth, OR 97361
www.wou.edu/rehab
Prgm Dir: Julia Smith, PhD CRC LPC
Tel: 503 838-8444, Ext 88744   *Fax:* 503 838-8228
E-mail: smithj@wou.edu

Portland State University
Rehabilitation Counseling Prgm
PO Box 751
Portland, OR 97207-0751
www.webmail.pdx.edu
Prgm Dir: Hanoch Livneh, PhD CRC
Tel: 503 725-4719   *Fax:* 503 725-5599
E-mail: livnehh@pdx.edu

Pennsylvania

Edinboro University of Pennsylvania
Rehabilitation Counseling Prgm
322 Butterfield Hall
Edinboro, PA 16444
www.edinboro.edu/cwis/education/counseling/
  rehab_counseling.html
Prgm Dir: Susan H Packard, PhD CRC LPC NCC CAC
Tel: 814 732-2430   *Fax:* 814 732-2233
E-mail: spackard@edinboro.edu

University of Pittsburgh
Rehabilitation Counseling Prgm
5044 Forbes Tower
3600 Forbes at Atwood St
Pittsburgh, PA 15260
Prgm Dir: Michael McCue, PhD CRC
Tel: 412 383-6589   *Fax:* 412 383-6597
E-mail: mmccue@pitt.edu

University of Scranton
Rehabilitation Counseling Prgm
Dept of Counseling and Human Services
Scranton, PA 18510-4523
Prgm Dir: Lori A Bruch, EdD CRC CVE
Tel: 717 941-4308   *Fax:* 717 941-5882
E-mail: BruchL1@scranton.edu

Penn State University
Rehabilitation Counseling Prgm
327 Cedar Bldg
University Park, PA 16802-3110
www.ed.psu.edu/cecprs
Prgm Dir: Elias Mpofu, PhD CRC
Tel: 814 863-2411   *Fax:* 814 863-7750
E-mail: exm31@psu.edu

Puerto Rico

University of Puerto Rico
Rehabilitation Counseling Prgm
College of Social Science
PO Box 23345
San Juan, PR 00931-3345
Prgm Dir: Marilyn Mendoza Lugo
Tel: 787 764-0000, Ext 4206   *Fax:* 787 763-4199
E-mail: core@rrpac.upr.clu.edu

Rhode Island

Salve Regina University
Rehabilitation Counseling Prgm
100 Ochre Point Ave
Newport, RI 02840
Prgm Dir: Dimity Peter, PhD CRC
Tel: 401 341-3189   *Fax:* 401 341-2973
E-mail: dimity.peter@salve.edu

South Carolina

University of South Carolina
Rehabilitation Counseling Prgm
School of Medicine
3555 Harden St Ext, Ste B20
Columbia, SC 29208
Prgm Dir: Linda L Leech, PhD
Tel: 803 434-6170   *Fax:* 803 434-4301
E-mail: lleech@gw.mp.sc.edu

South Carolina State University
Rehabilitation Counseling Prgm
300 College St NE
Orangeburg, SC 29117-0001
Prgm Dir: C Brannon Underwood, PhD CRC NCC
Tel: 803 536-8908   *Fax:* 803 533-3636
E-mail: underwood@scsu.edu

Tennessee

University of Tennessee - Knoxville
Rehabilitation Counseling Prgm
A522 Claxton Complex
Knoxville, TN 37996-3452
Prgm Dir: Patrick L Dunn, PhD CRC
Tel: 865 974-8090   *Fax:* 865 974-0135
E-mail: pdunn4@utk.edu

University of Memphis
Rehabilitation Counseling Prgm
Dept of Counseling, Educ Psych and Research
119D Patterson Hall
Memphis, TN 38152
www.memphis.edu
Prgm Dir: Steve Zanskas, PhD CRC
Tel: 901 678-4021   *Fax:* 901 678-3215
E-mail: szanskas@memphis.edu

Texas

University of Texas at Austin
Rehabilitation Counseling Prgm
Special Education
1 University Station, D5300
Austin, TX 78712
Prgm Dir: Randall Parker, PhD
Tel: 512 232-5687   *Fax:* 512 232-5686
E-mail: r.parker@mail.utexas.edu

Univ of Texas Southwestern Med Ctr
Rehabilitation Counseling Prgm
5323 Harry Hines Blvd
Dallas, TX 75390-9088
Prgm Dir: Gerald William Casenave, PhD
Tel: 214 648-1740   *Fax:* 214 648-1771
E-mail: bobbie.vash@utsouthwestern.edu

University of North Texas
Rehabilitation Counseling Prgm
Dept of Rehab Social Work and Addiction
PO Box 311456
Denton, TX 76203
Prgm Dir: Rodney Isom, PhD CRC CDMS
Tel: 940 565-2234   *Fax:* 940 565-3960
E-mail: isom@unt.edu

Univ of Texas - Pan American
Rehabilitation Counseling Prgm
1201 W University Dr
Edinburg, TX 78539-2999
Prgm Dir: Irmo Marini, PhD CRC
Tel: 956 316-7036   *Fax:* 956 380-6499
E-mail: imarini@utpa.edu

Texas Tech University
Rehabilitation Counseling Prgm
Rehabilitation Sciences
3601 Fourth St, M/S 6225, Ste 2C-200
Lubbock, TX 79430-6225
Prgm Dir: Evans Spears, PhD CRC
Tel: 806 743-4208   *Fax:* 806 743-3518
E-mail: evans.spears@ttuhsc.edu

Stephen F Austin State University
Rehabilitation Counseling Prgm
Dept of Human Services
PO Box 13019/SFA Station
Nacogdoches, TX 75962-3019
www.sfasu.edu/hs
Prgm Dir: Robert O Choate, EdD NCC CRC LPC
Tel: 409 468-1147   *Fax:* 409 468-1342
E-mail: rchoate@sfasu.edu

Utah

Utah State University
Rehabilitation Counseling Prgm
Dept of Special Educ and Rehab
2865 Old Main Hill
Logan, UT 84322-2865
Prgm Dir: Julie Smart, PhD CRC LPC NCC ABDA CCFC
Tel: 435 797-3269   *Fax:* 435 797-3572
E-mail: jsmart@cc.usu.edu

Virginia

Virginia Commonwealth University
Rehabilitation Counseling Prgm
Dept of Rehab Counseling
1112 E Clay St, Box 980330
Richmond, VA 23298-0330
Prgm Dir: Amy J Armstrong, PhD
Tel: 804 827-0913   *Fax:* 804 828-1321
E-mail: rehabcnsling@vcu.edu

Washington

Western Washington University
Rehabilitation Counseling Prgm
6912 220th St SW
Ste 105
Mountlake Terrace, WA 98043
Prgm Dir: Elizabeth Swett, PhD CRC
Tel: 425 771-7435   *Fax:* 425 774-9303
E-mail: elizabeth.swett@wwu.edu

West Virginia

West Virginia University
Rehabilitation Counseling Prgm
502 Allen Hall, PO Box 6122
Morgantown, WV 26506-6122
Prgm Dir: Margaret K Glenn, EdD CRC
Tel: 304 293-2276   *Fax:* 304 293-4082
E-mail: mkglenn@mail.wvu.edu

Wisconsin

University of Wisconsin - Madison
Rehabilitation Counseling Prgm
Rehab Psych and Special Educ
432 N Murray St
Madison, WI 53706
Prgm Dir: Norman L Berven, PhD
Tel: 608 262-7917   *Fax:* 608 262-8108
E-mail: berven@education.wisc.edu

University of Wisconsin - Stout
Rehabilitation Counseling Prgm
Dept of Rehabilitation and Counseling
250F Vocational Rehabilitation
Menomonie, WI 54751
Prgm Dir: Michelle Hamilton, PhD CVE CRC
Tel: 715 232-1895   *Fax:* 715 232-2356
E-mail: hamiltonmi@uwstout.edu

Rehabilitation Counselor

Programs*	Class Capacity	Begins	Length (months)	Award	Res. Tuition	Non-res. Tuition	Stipend	Offers:‡ 1	2	3	4
Alabama											
Alabama A&M University (Normal)	30	Fall semester	24	MA	$6,870	$12,756		•		•	
Arizona											
University of Arizona (Tucson)	25	Aug	24	BA, MA	$2,678	$16,780	$3,500	•			
Arkansas											
University of Arkansas (Fayetteville)	40	Aug Jan Jun Jul	24	MS, PhD	$0	$0	$12,000			•	
University of Arkansas at Little Rock	25	Sep Jan Jun	18, 24	Cert, MA	$291	$291		•		•	•
California											
California State University - Fresno	40	Jan Aug	24	MS	$3,190	$15,000	$5,670	•		•	
Colorado											
University of Northern Colorado (Greeley)	25	Aug	24, 48	BS, MA	$2,708	$11,268		•		•	•
Florida											
Florida State University (Tallahassee)	70	Aug	27, 22	BS, MS/PhD	$248	$879		•		•	
University of North Florida (Jacksonville)	40	Fall	18	MS	$9,029	$30,318		•		•	
Georgia											
Georgia State University (Atlanta)	25	Aug	48	MS	$4,368	$17,464	$800	•		•	
Thomas University (Thomasville)	30	Rolling admission	24	MS	$9,000	$9,000		•		•	•
Idaho											
University of Idaho (Moscow)	12	Aug	24	MEd, MS	$6,000	$10,000	$9,000	•		•	
Illinois											
Illinois Institute of Technology (Chicago)	32	Aug	24, 36	Cert, MS	$22,410	$22,410	$6,000	•		•	•
Iowa											
University of Iowa (Iowa City)	22	Jun Sep	23, 48	MA, PhD	$5,689	$15,723		•		•	
Kansas											
Emporia State University	40	Aug Jan Jun	24	MS	$4,554	$12,126		•		•	•
Kentucky											
University of Kentucky (Lexington)	100	Aug	16	MRC	$7	$16,158	$4,800	•		•	•
Louisiana											
Louisiana State Univ Health Sciences Center (New Orleans)	30	Aug	12, 20	BS, MHS	$4,661	$8,404	$6,000	•			
Maryland											
Coppin State University (Baltimore)	12	Sep	30	MEd	$0	$2,196				•	
Massachusetts											
Springfield College	50	Sep Jan May	24, 18	Dipl, Cert, BS, MS/MEd	$21,570	$21,570	$12,250	•		•	•
Michigan											
Wayne State University (Detroit)	25	Sep	24, 48	MA, PhD	$8,422	$17,186	$6,000	•		•	
Minnesota											
Minnesota State University - Mankato	25	Late Aug	16, 20	MS	$7,673	$10,464				•	•
St Cloud State University	15	Sep	21	MS	$5,600	$8,800		•			
Mississippi											
Mississippi State University	15	Aug	24	MS	$3,874	$8,780		•		•	
Missouri											
University of Missouri - Columbia	15	Late Aug	24	MEd, MA	$8,000	$16,000	$5,000	•		•	
New Jersey											
Univ of Medicine & Dent of New Jersey (Scotch Plains)				Cert, MS				•		•	
North Carolina											
East Carolina University (Greenville)	65	Aug	24	Dipl, Cert, BS, MS/Ph	$4,500	$17,000		•		•	
Oklahoma											
East Central University (Ada)	15	Aug	20	MS	$3,800	$0		•			

*Data are shown only for programs that completed the 2007 AMA Survey of Health Professions Education Programs.
‡Key to Offers: 1: Evening or weekend classes; 2: Non-English instruction; 3: Cultural competence instruction; 4: Distance education component.

Rehabilitation Counselor

Programs*	Class Capacity	Begins	Length (months)	Award	Res. Tuition	Non-res. Tuition	Stipend	Offers:‡ 1	2	3	4
Oregon											
Portland State University	15	Sep	24	MS	$9,000	$14,000		•			
Western Oregon University (Monmouth)	15	Sep	22	MS	$14,000	$24,000	$8,000				
Pennsylvania											
Edinboro University of Pennsylvania	25	Aug Jan	30	MA	$6,048	$9,678		•		•	
Penn State University (University Park)	10	Late Aug	24	BS, MEd	$10,048	$19,724		•		•	
Tennessee											
University of Memphis	25	Aug Jan	18, 22	MS	$7,101	$15,837	$3,600	•		•	
Texas											
Stephen F Austin State University (Nacogdoches)	20	Jun Aug Jan	30	BSR, MA	$4,304	$10,928	$15,000	•			•

*Data are shown only for programs that completed the 2007 AMA Survey of Health Professions Education Programs.
‡Key to Offers: 1: Evening or weekend classes; 2: Non-English instruction; 3: Cultural competence instruction; 4: Distance education component.

Includes:
- Respiratory therapist (advanced)
- Respiratory therapist (entry-level)

Respiratory Therapist (Advanced)

Respiratory therapists work in a wide variety of settings to evaluate, treat, and manage patients of all ages with respiratory illnesses and other cardiopulmonary disorders. The advanced respiratory therapist participates in clinical decision-making and patient education, develops and implements respiratory care plans, applies patient-driven protocols, utilizes evidence-based clinical practice guidelines, and participates in health promotion, disease prevention, and disease management. The advanced level respiratory therapist may be required to exercise considerable independent judgment, under the supervision of a physician, in the respiratory care of patients.

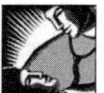

Career Description

In fulfillment of the advanced therapist role, the respiratory therapist may perform the following procedures:
- Acquiring and evaluating clinical data
- Assessing the cardiopulmonary status of patients
- Performing and assisting in the performance of prescribed diagnostic studies, such as obtaining blood samples, blood gas analysis, pulmonary function testing, and polysomnography
- Evaluating data to assess the appropriateness of prescribed respiratory care
- Establishing therapeutic goals for patients with cardiopulmonary disease
- Participating in the development and modification of respiratory care plans
- Performing case management of patients with cardiopulmonary and related diseases
- Initiating prescribed respiratory care treatments, evaluating and monitoring patient responses to such therapy, and modifying the prescribed therapy to achieve the desired therapeutic objectives
- Initiating and conducting prescribed pulmonary rehabilitation
- Providing patient, family, and community education
- Promoting cardiopulmonary wellness, disease prevention, and disease management
- Participating in life support activities as required and promoting evidence-based medicine, research, and clinical practice guidelines

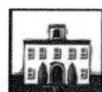

Employment Characteristics

Respiratory therapists are employed in a variety of settings that include acute care, chronic care, subacute care, extended care, and rehabilitation facilities; educational institutions; clinics; physician's offices; home care; sleep labs; diagnostic and research labs; and pharmaceutical companies.

Salary

The Human Resources Study from the American Association for Respiratory Care (AARC) indicated that advanced level respiratory therapists with an RRT (Registered Respiratory Therapist) credential earned an average salary of $57,803 in 2005. Refer to Section IV, Table 5 of this *Directory* for more information, or see www.ama-assn.org/go/hpsalary.

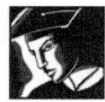

Educational Programs

Length. Advanced level respiratory therapists complete 2 or more years of formal training and education leading to an associate, baccalaureate, or graduate degree.

Prerequisite. Varies depending on degree awarded.

Curriculum. The knowledge and skills for performing these functions are achieved through formal college- or university-based programs of classroom, laboratory, and clinical preparation. Biological and physical sciences required include anatomy, physiology, chemistry, physics, microbiology, computer science, pharmacology, and pathophysiology. Coursework may also be required in mathematics, communications, psychology, medical ethics, and the social sciences. Professional coursework may include:
- Patient assessment, monitoring, and evaluation
- Diagnostic and therapeutic procedures
- Airway management and mechanical ventilatory support
- Infection control
- Basic and advanced life support
- Patient and caregiver education
- Rehabilitation and disease management
- Health promotion/disease prevention

Clinical training in all aspects of respiratory care applicable to pediatric, adult, and geriatric patients is also provided.

Respiratory Therapist (Entry-level)

The entry-level respiratory therapist performs general respiratory care procedures. Entry-level therapists may assume clinical responsibility for specified respiratory care modalities involving the application of therapeutic techniques under the supervision of an advanced-level therapist and/or a physician.

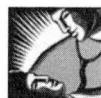

Career Description

In fulfillment of the entry-level role, the respiratory therapist may perform the following procedures:
- Review existing data in the patient records, including patient history and physical, blood gas results, pulmonary function results, imaging studies, and monitoring data
- Collect and evaluate additional pertinent clinical data and recommend procedures to obtain additional data
- Select, assemble, use, and troubleshoot equipment used in the delivery of respiratory care, ensure infection control, and perform quality control procedures

PROGRAMS

- Maintain records and communicate information regarding patient's clinical status to appropriate members of the health care team
- Maintain a patient's airway, including care of artificial airways
- Remove bronchial secretions, assure provision of adequate respiratory support, and evaluate and monitor patient's objective and subjective responses to respiratory care
- Modify therapeutic procedures and recommend modifications in the respiratory care plan based on patient's response
- Initiate, conduct, or modify respiratory care techniques in an emergency setting
- Act as an assistant to the physician performing special procedures
- Initiate and conduct pulmonary rehabilitation and home care within the prescription

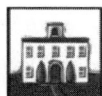

Employment Characteristics

Entry-level respiratory therapists are employed in hospitals, nursing care facilities, clinics, physicians' offices, home care companies, pulmonary function laboratories, and sleep labs.

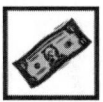

Salary

The Human Resources Study from the American Association for Respiratory Care (AARC) indicated that the average salary for respiratory therapists with a CRT (Certified Respiratory Therapist) credential was $56,035 in the year 2005. This same study indicated that the mean salary of all respiratory therapists at entry-level was $41,537 in year 2005. Refer to Section IV, Table 5 of this *Directory* for more information, or see www.ama-assn.org/go/hpsalary.

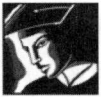

Educational Programs

Length. Educational programs for entry-level therapists are usually 2 years in length, leading to an associate degree.

Prerequisites. High school degree or equivalent.

Curriculum. The knowledge and skills of an entry-level therapist are acquired through formal programs of didactic, laboratory, and clinical preparation. Courses include biological and physical sciences basic to understanding the function of the cardiopulmonary system. Included are chemistry, biology, anatomy and physiology, physics, microbiology, mathematics, computer science, and psychology, as well as courses in basic equipment, therapeutic modalities, clinical medicine, and pathophysiology. Clinical training in routine and special procedures applicable to pediatric, adult, and geriatric patients is also provided.

Inquiries

Careers
American Association for Respiratory Care
11030 Ables Lane
Dallas, TX 75229
972 243-2272
www.aarc.org

Licensure/Certification/Registration
National Board for Respiratory Care
8310 Nieman Road
Lenexa, KS 66214
www.nbrc.org

Program Accreditation
Commission on Accreditation of Allied Health Education Programs (CAAHEP) in collaboration with:
Committee on Accreditation for Respiratory Care (CoARC)
1248 Harwood Road
Bedford, TX 76021
817 283-2835
817 354-8519 Fax
E-mail: bill@heasc.org

Respiratory Therapist (Advanced)

Alabama

University of Alabama at Birmingham
Respiratory Therapist (Advanced) Prgm
RMSB 486
1705 University Blvd
Birmingham, AL 35294-1212
Prgm Dir: Wesley M Granger, PhD RRT
Tel: 205 934-3783   *Fax:* 205 975-7302
E-mail: grangerw@uab.edu

George C Wallace Community College
Respiratory Therapist (Advanced) Prgm
1141 Wallace Dr
Dothan, AL 36303
Prgm Dir: Drayton Odom, BS RRT
Tel: 334 556-2291   *Fax:* 334 556-2422
E-mail: dodom@wallace.edu

Wallace State Community College
Respiratory Therapist (Advanced) Prgm
PO Box 2000
Hanceville, AL 35077-2000
www.wallacestate.edu
Prgm Dir: Paul D Taylor, DHSc RRT
Tel: 205 352-8310   *Fax:* 205 352-8320
E-mail: paul.taylor@wallacestate.edu

University of South Alabama
Respiratory Therapist (Advanced) Prgm
1504 Springhill Ave, Ste 2545
Mobile, AL 36604
www.usouthal.edu
Prgm Dir: William V Wojciechowski, MS RRT
Tel: 251 434-3405   *Fax:* 251 434-3941
E-mail: wwojciec@usouthal.edu

Shelton State Community College
Respiratory Therapist (Advanced) Prgm
3401 M L King Jr Blvd
Tuscaloosa, AL 35401
Prgm Dir: Bruce E Spruell, AS RRT
Tel: 205 391-2641   *Fax:* 205 391-2658
E-mail: bspruell@sheltonstate.edu

Arizona

Pima Medical Institute - Mesa
Respiratory Therapist (Advanced) Prgm
957 S Dobson Rd
Mesa, AZ 85202
www.pmi.edu
Prgm Dir: Cynthia Smathers, MEd RRT
Tel: 480 898-9898   *Fax:* 480 649-5249
E-mail: csmathers@pmi.edu

GateWay Community College
Respiratory Therapist (Advanced) Prgm
108 N 40th St
Phoenix, AZ 85034
Prgm Dir: Edward Hoskins, MEd RRT
Tel: 602 286-8503   *Fax:* 602 286-8478
E-mail: hoskins@gatewaycc.edu

Kaplan College
Respiratory Therapist (Advanced) Prgm
13610 N Black Canyon Hwy, Ste 104
Phoenix, AZ 85029
www.KC-Phoenix.com
Prgm Dir: Robert Brown, BS RRT AE-C
Tel: 602 548-1955   *Fax:* 602 926-1456
E-mail: brbrown@kaplan.edu

Pima Community College
Respiratory Therapist (Advanced) Prgm
2202 W Anklam Rd/HRP 242
Tucson, AZ 85709-0080
www.pima.edu
Prgm Dir: Jody Kosanke, MEd RRT-NPS
Tel: 520 206-3107   *Fax:* 520 206-3027
E-mail: Jody.Kosanke@pima.edu

Pima Medical Institute - Tucson
Respiratory Therapist (Advanced) Prgm
3350 E Grant Rd
Tucson, AZ 85716
Prgm Dir: Tammy Redasky, BS RRT
Tel: 520 881-1483   *Fax:* 520 881-1483
E-mail: leanna@qwest.net

Arkansas

NorthWest Arkansas Community College
Respiratory Therapist (Advanced) Prgm
One College Dr
Bentonville, AR 72712
www.nwacc.edu
Prgm Dir: Alan Clark, BA RRT
Tel: 479 619-4250   *Fax:* 479 619-4254
E-mail: aclark@nwacc.edu

University of Arkansas for Medical Sciences
Cosponsor: Central Arkansas Veterans Healthcare
   Services
Respiratory Therapist (Advanced) Prgm
CHRP
4301 W Markham St, Slot 704 (14B/NLR)
Little Rock, AR 72205
www.uams.edu/chrp/resp.htm
Prgm Dir: Erna L Boone, MEd RRT
Tel: 501 257-2348   *Fax:* 501 257-2349
E-mail: booneernal@uams.edu

Southeast Arkansas College
Respiratory Therapist (Advanced) Prgm
1900 Hazel St
Pine Bluff, AR 71603
www.seark.edu
Prgm Dir: Kathleen M Boyle, MEd MS RRT-NPS
Tel: 870 543-5924   *Fax:* 870 543-5912
E-mail: kboyle@seark.edu

University of Arkansas for Medical Sciences
Respiratory Therapist (Advanced) Prgm
UAMS AHEC-Southwest
300 E 6th St
Texarkana, AR 71854
www.uams.edu
Prgm Dir: Patrick Evans, RRT RN MEd
Tel: 870 779-6033   *Fax:* 870 779-6045
E-mail: evansdennisp@uams.edu

California

San Joaquin Valley College - Bakersfield
Respiratory Therapist (Advanced) Prgm
201 New Stine Rd
Bakersfield, CA 93309
Prgm Dir: Albert Ayotte, MBA RRT RCP
Tel: 661 834-0126, Ext 140   *Fax:* 661 834-1021
E-mail: albert.ayotte@sjvc.edu

Pima Medical Institute - Chula Vista
Respiratory Therapist (Advanced) Prgm
780 Bay Blvd
Chula Vista, CA 91910
Prgm Dir: Debra Volpe, Bs RCP RRT
Tel: 619 425-3200
E-mail: dvolpe@pmi.edu

Orange Coast College
Respiratory Therapist (Advanced) Prgm
2701 Fairview Rd, PO Box 5005
Costa Mesa, CA 92626
www.orangecoastcollege.edu
Prgm Dir: Daniel S Adelmann, MS RRT
Tel: 714 432-5541   *Fax:* 714 432-5534
E-mail: dadelman@occ.cccd.edu

Grossmont College
Respiratory Therapist (Advanced) Prgm
8800 Grossmont College Dr
El Cajon, CA 92020-1799
www.grossmont.edu/healthprofessions
Prgm Dir: Lorenda Seibold-Phalan, MA RRT-NPS RCP
Tel: 619 644-7448   *Fax:* 619 644-7961
E-mail: lorenda.seibold-phalan@gcccd.edu

Ohlone College
Respiratory Therapist (Advanced) Prgm
43600 Mission Blvd, PO Box 3909
Fremont, CA 94539
Prgm Dir: Carol McNamee-Cole, MA RRT
Tel: 510 659-6029   *Fax:* 510 659-6070
E-mail: hstory@ohlone.edu

Fresno City College
Respiratory Therapist (Advanced) Prgm
1101 E University Ave
Fresno, CA 93741
Prgm Dir: Steven L Boyd, MBA RRT
Tel: 559 244-2631   *Fax:* 559 244-2626
E-mail: steven.boyd@fresnocitycollege.edu

Loma Linda University
Respiratory Therapist (Advanced) Prgm
Nichol Hall, Rm 1926
Loma Linda, CA 92350
Prgm Dir: David Stanton, MS RPFT RCP RRT-NPS
Tel: 909 558-4932   *Fax:* 909 558-4701
E-mail: dstanton@llu.edu

Foothill Community College
Respiratory Therapist (Advanced) Prgm
12345 El Monte Rd
Los Altos Hills, CA 94022
Prgm Dir: Virginia Becchine, MA RRT
Tel: 650 949-7466   *Fax:* 650 949-7686
E-mail: becchinevirginia@foothill.edu

Modesto Junior College
Respiratory Therapist (Advanced) Prgm
435 College Ave
Modesto, CA 95350
Prgm Dir: David Nordin, BA RCP RRT
Tel: 209 575-6381   *Fax:* 209 575-6593
E-mail: nordind@yosemite.cc.ca.us

East Los Angeles College
Respiratory Therapist (Advanced) Prgm
1301 Avenida Cesar Chavez
Monterey Park, CA 91754
Prgm Dir: Michael R Carr, BA RRT
Tel: 323 265-8612, Ext 8612   *Fax:* 323 265-8684
E-mail: michael_carr@sbcglobal.net

Napa Valley College
Respiratory Therapist (Advanced) Prgm
2277 Napa Vallejo Hwy
Napa, CA 94558
Prgm Dir: Kate Benscoter, MEd RRT
Tel: 707 253-3145   *Fax:* 707 259-8933
E-mail: kbenscoter@napavalley.edu

Butte College
Respiratory Therapist (Advanced) Prgm
3536 Butte Campus Dr
Oroville, CA 95965
Prgm Dir: Donna Davis, BS RRT
Tel: 530 895-2827   *Fax:* 530 895-2472
E-mail: davisdo@butte.edu

San Joaquin Valley College
Respiratory Therapist (Advanced) Prgm
10641 Church St
Rancho Cucamonga, CA 91730
Prgm Dir: Ricardo Guzman, BA CRT RRT
Tel: 909 948-7582, Ext 243
E-mail: ricardo.guzman@sjvc.edu

American River College
Respiratory Therapist (Advanced) Prgm
4700 College Oak Dr
Sacramento, CA 95841
Prgm Dir: James L Warman, PhD RRT
Tel: 916 484-8876   *Fax:* 916 484-8030
E-mail: warmanj@arc.losrios.edu

Maric College - Salida
Respiratory Therapist (Advanced) Prgm
5172 Kiernan Ct
Salida, CA 95368
Prgm Dir: Thomas Ankeney, BA RRT CPFT
Tel: 209 543-7000
E-mail: tankeney@mariccollege.edu

Concorde Career College - San Bernardino
Respiratory Therapist (Advanced) Prgm
201 E Airport Dr, Ste A
San Bernardino, CA 92408
Prgm Dir: Robert Wandel, BS RRT
Tel: 909 884-8891
E-mail: rwandek@concorde.edu

Skyline College
Respiratory Therapist (Advanced) Prgm
3300 College Dr
San Bruno, CA 94066
Prgm Dir: Raymond Hernandez
Tel: 650 738-4457   *Fax:* 650 738-4299
E-mail: hernandezr@smccd.net

California College San Diego
Respiratory Therapist (Advanced) Prgm
2820 Camino Del Rio S
San Diego, CA 92108
Prgm Dir: Miguel Moreno, MD BSRT RRT RCP
Tel: 619 295-5785, Ext 1531   *Fax:* 619 295-5762
E-mail: miguel.moreno@cc-sd.edu

Los Angeles Valley College
Respiratory Therapist (Advanced) Prgm
5800 Fulton Ave
Valley Glen, CA 91401-4096
Prgm Dir: Frank Sinsheimer, EdD RRT RCP
Tel: 818 947-2562   *Fax:* 818 947-2850
E-mail: sinshefa@lavc.edu

Victor Valley Community College District
Respiratory Therapist (Advanced) Prgm
18422 Bear Valley Rd
Victorville, CA 92392-5849
Prgm Dir: Larry Boutcher, PhD RRT
Tel: 760 245-4271, Ext 2222   *Fax:* 760 951-5861
E-mail: boutcherl@vvc.edu

San Joaquin Valley College - Visalia
Respiratory Therapist (Advanced) Prgm
8400 W Mineral King
Visalia, CA 93291
www.sjvc.edu
Prgm Dir: Gaylene Mooney, MEd RRT-NPS
Tel: 559 622-1943   *Fax:* 559 651-3645
E-mail: Gaylene.Mooney@sjvc.edu

Mt San Antonio College
Respiratory Therapist (Advanced) Prgm
1100 N Grand Ave
Walnut, CA 91789
Prgm Dir: Terrance M Krider, BS RRT RCP
Tel: 909 594-5611, Ext 3930   *Fax:* 909 468-3938
E-mail: thood@mtsac.edu

Crafton Hills College
Respiratory Therapist (Advanced) Prgm
11711 Sand Canyon Rd
Yucaipa, CA 92399
Prgm Dir: Kenneth R Bryson, MEd BVE RCP RRT
Tel: 909 389-3284   *Fax:* 909 389-3229
E-mail: kbryson@crafton.sbccd.cc.ca.us

Colorado

T H Pickens Technical Center
Respiratory Therapist (Advanced) Prgm
500 Airport Blvd
Aurora, CO 80011-9307
Prgm Dir: Leigh Otto, BS RRT
Tel: 303 344-4910, Ext 27781   *Fax:* 303 326-1277
E-mail: leigho@pickens.aps.k12.co.us

Pima Medical Institute - Denver
Respiratory Therapist (Advanced) Prgm
7475 Dakin St
Denver, CO 80221
Prgm Dir: Amy Brown, BS RRT
Tel: 303 426-1800   *Fax:* 303 430-4048
E-mail: abrown@pmi.edu

Pueblo Community College
Respiratory Therapist (Advanced) Prgm
900 W Orman Ave
Pueblo, CO 81004
www.pueblocc.edu
Prgm Dir: Delia Lechtenberg, MA RRT
Tel: 719 549-3266   *Fax:* 719 549-3381
E-mail: delia.lechtenberg@pueblocc.edu

Connecticut

Quinnipiac University
Respiratory Therapist (Advanced) Prgm
Mt Carmel Ave
Hamden, CT 06518
Prgm Dir: Ronald G Beckett, RRT PhD
Tel: 203 582-8682   *Fax:* 203 582-8706
E-mail: ronald.beckett@quinnipiac.edu

Manchester Community College
Respiratory Therapist (Advanced) Prgm
Great Path, PO Box 1046
Manchester, CT 06045-1046
Prgm Dir: Nancy LaRoche-Shovak, MS RRT
Tel: 860 512-2714   *Fax:* 860 512-2714
E-mail: nlaroche-shovak@mcc.commnet.edu

Norwalk Hospital/Norwalk Community College
Respiratory Therapist (Advanced) Prgm
24 Maple St
Norwalk, CT 06856
www.norwalkhealth.org
Prgm Dir: Geraldine Bernacki, RRT
Tel: 203 852-2479   *Fax:* 203 852-2738
E-mail: geraldine.bernacki@norwalkhealth.org

Naugatuck Valley Community College
Respiratory Therapist (Advanced) Prgm
750 Chase Pkwy
Waterbury, CT 06708
www.nvcc.commnet.edu
Prgm Dir: Margaret Guerrera, BS RRT
Tel: 203 596-8662   *Fax:* 203 575-8146
E-mail: mguerrera@nvcc.commnet.edu

University of Hartford
Respiratory Therapist (Advanced) Prgm
200 Bloomfield Ave
West Hartford, CT 06117-1559
Prgm Dir: Peter W Kennedy, PhD RRT
Tel: 860 768-4823   *Fax:* 860 768-5706
E-mail: pkennedy@hartford.edu

Delaware

Delaware Technical & Community College - Owens Campus
Respiratory Therapist (Advanced) Prgm
PO Box 610
Georgetown, DE 19947
www.dtcc.edu/owens/rescare/
Prgm Dir: James G Little, MEd RRT
Tel: 302 855-5535   *Fax:* 302 858-5460
E-mail: jlittle@dtcc.edu

Delaware Technical & Community College - Wilmington
Cosponsor: Christiana Care Health Services
Respiratory Therapist (Advanced) Prgm
Ste 101, Medical Arts Complex
700 W Lea Blvd
Wilmington, DE 19802
Prgm Dir: Joseph Ciarlo, BS RRT
Tel: 302 765-4598   *Fax:* 302 765-4599
E-mail: jciarlo@christianacare.org

District of Columbia

University of the District of Columbia
Respiratory Therapist (Advanced) Prgm
4200 Connecticut Ave NW
Washington, DC 20008
Prgm Dir: Susan D Lockwood, MA RN RRT
Tel: 202 274-5925   *Fax:* 202 274-5952
E-mail: slockwood@udc.edu

Florida

Broward Community College
Respiratory Therapist (Advanced) Prgm
1000 Coconut Creek Blvd
Coconut Creek, FL 33066
Prgm Dir: John Prince, RRT
Tel: 954 969-2082   *Fax:* 954 973-2348
E-mail: jprince@broward.edu

Daytona Beach Community College
Respiratory Therapist (Advanced) Prgm
PO Box 2811
1200 W Internatonal Speedway Blvd
Daytona Beach, FL 32114
www.dbcc.edu
Prgm Dir: Michael R McCumber, EdD RRT
Tel: 386 506-3759   *Fax:* 386 506-3300
E-mail: mccumbm@dbcc.edu

Edison College
Respiratory Therapist (Advanced) Prgm
8099 College Pkwy SW
PO Box 60210
Fort Myers, FL 33906-6210
Prgm Dir: Jeffrey B Elsberry, PhD RRT
Tel: 239 489-9251   *Fax:* 239 985-8352
E-mail: jelsberry@edison.edu

Indian River Community College
Respiratory Therapist (Advanced) Prgm
3209 Virginia Ave
Fort Pierce, FL 34981
Prgm Dir: Georgette Rosenfeld, PhD RRT RN
Tel: 772 462-7542   *Fax:* 561 462-4900
E-mail: grosenfe@ircc.edu

Florida Community College - Jacksonville
Respiratory Therapist (Advanced) Prgm
North Campus, 4501 Capper Rd
Jacksonville, FL 32218
Prgm Dir: James R Woods, MS RRT RPFT
Tel: 904 766-6513   *Fax:* 904 766-5573
E-mail: jwoods@fccj.edu

ATI Health Education Centers
Respiratory Therapist (Advanced) Prgm
1395 NW 167th St, Ste 200
Miami, FL 33169
Prgm Dir: David Robbins, BS RRT
Tel: 305 628-1000, Ext 220   *Fax:* 305 628-1461
E-mail: rrobbins@atienterprises.edu

Miami Dade College
Respiratory Therapist (Advanced) Prgm
Medical Center Campus
950 NW 20th St
Miami, FL 33127
Prgm Dir: Randy De Kler, MS RRT
Tel: 305 237-4423   *Fax:* 305 237-4278
E-mail: rdekler@mdc.edu

University of Central Florida
Respiratory Therapist (Advanced) Prgm
Dept of Health Professions
HPA II-206, PO Box 162205
Orlando, FL 32816-2205
Prgm Dir: Jeffery Ludy, EdD RRT
Tel: 407 823-3888   *Fax:* 407 823-6138
E-mail: jludy@mail.ucf.edu

Valencia Community College
Respiratory Therapist (Advanced) Prgm
PO Box 3028
Orlando, FL 32802-9961
http://valenciacc.edu
Prgm Dir: Lynn W Capraun, MS RRT
Tel: 407 582-1550   *Fax:* 407 582-1278
E-mail: lcapraun@valenciacc.edu

Palm Beach Community College
Respiratory Therapist (Advanced) Prgm
3160 PGA Blvd
Palm Beach Gardens, FL 33410-2893
Prgm Dir: Thomas J Reid, BSRT RRT
Tel: 561 207-5068   *Fax:* 561 207-5011
E-mail: reidt@pbcc.edu

Gulf Coast Community College
Respiratory Therapist (Advanced) Prgm
5230 W US Hwy 98
Panama City, FL 32401
Prgm Dir: Bradley E Killion, BS RRT
Tel: 904 872-3837   *Fax:* 904 747-3246
E-mail: Bkillion@gulfcoast.edu

St Petersburg College
Respiratory Therapist (Advanced) Prgm
7200 66th St N
Pinellas Park, FL 33781
Prgm Dir: Stephen P Mikles, EdS RRT
Tel: 727 341-3627   *Fax:* 727 341-3744
E-mail: mikless@spjc.edu

Seminole Community College
Respiratory Therapist (Advanced) Prgm
100 Weldon Blvd
Sanford, FL 32773
www.scc-fl.edu/respiratory/
Prgm Dir: Steve Shideler, MS RRT
Tel: 407 708-2293   *Fax:* 407 708-2319
E-mail: shideles@scc-fl.edu

Florida A&M University
Respiratory Therapist (Advanced) Prgm
Ware-Rhaney Extension
Ste 328
Tallahassee, FL 32307
Prgm Dir: Alphonso Baldwin, PhD RRT RPFT
Tel: 850 561-2186   *Fax:* 850 561-2457
E-mail: alphonso.baldwin@famu.edu

Tallahassee Community College
Respiratory Therapist (Advanced) Prgm
444 Appleyard Dr
Tallahassee, FL 32304
Prgm Dir: Dewey Streetman, RRT
Tel: 850 201-8327   *Fax:* 850 201-8329
E-mail: streetmd@tcc.fl.edu

Hillsborough Community College
Respiratory Therapist (Advanced) Prgm
PO Box 30030
4001 Tampa Bay Blvd
Tampa, FL 33630-3030
Prgm Dir: Richard Palma
Tel: 813 253-7318   *Fax:* 813 253-7491
E-mail: rpalma@hccfl.edu

Georgia

Darton College
Respiratory Therapist (Advanced) Prgm
2400 Gillionville Rd
Albany, GA 31707
www.darton.edu
Prgm Dir: William F Thomas, MS RRT
Tel: 229 317-6896   *Fax:* 229 317-6682
E-mail: william.thomas@darton.edu

Athens Technical College
Respiratory Therapist (Advanced) Prgm
800 US Hwy 29 N
Athens, GA 30601-1500
Prgm Dir: Bruce A Ott, EdD RRT
Tel: 706 355-5104   *Fax:* 706 425-3104
E-mail: bott@athenstech.edu

Georgia State University
Respiratory Therapist (Advanced) Prgm
PO Box 4019
Atlanta, GA 30302-4019
http://chhs.gsu.edu/rt/
Prgm Dir: Lynda T Goodfellow, EdD RRT
Tel: 404 651-3091   *Fax:* 404 651-1584
E-mail: ltgoodfellow@gsu.edu

Augusta Technical College
Respiratory Therapist (Advanced) Prgm
3200 Augusta Tech Dr
Augusta, GA 30906
Prgm Dir: Rita Waller, MSN RRT RPSGT
Tel: 706 771-4194   *Fax:* 706 771-4181
E-mail: rwaller@augustatech.edu

Medical College of Georgia
Respiratory Therapist (Advanced) Prgm
815 St Sebastian Way, Rm HM-143
Augusta, GA 30912-0850
Prgm Dir: Arthur A Taft, PhD RRT
Tel: 706 721-3553   *Fax:* 706 721-0495
E-mail: ataft@mail.mcg.edu

Heart of Georgia Technical College
Respiratory Therapist (Advanced) Prgm
560 Pinehill Rd
Dublin, GA 31021
Prgm Dir: Natalie A Smith, BS RRT RPFT
Tel: 478 274-7881   *Fax:* 478 275-6642
E-mail: natalies@hgtc.org

Griffin Technical College
Respiratory Therapist (Advanced) Prgm
501 Varsity Rd
Griffin, GA 30223
www.griffintech.edu
Prgm Dir: Duane Reed, MA RRT
Tel: 770 233-6169   *Fax:* 770 229-3294
E-mail: dreed@griffintech.edu

Gwinnett Technical College
Respiratory Therapist (Advanced) Prgm
5150 Sugarloaf Pkwy
Lawrenceville, GA 30043-5702
www.gwinnetttech.edu
Prgm Dir: Robert P DeLorme, EdS RRT-NPS
Tel: 678 226-6658
E-mail: bdelorme@gwinnetttech.edu

Macon State College
Respiratory Therapist (Advanced) Prgm
100 College Station Dr
Macon, GA 31297
Prgm Dir: Charles R Matson, MEd RRT
Tel: 478 471-2789   *Fax:* 478 471-2787
E-mail: cmatson@maconstate.edu

Coosa Valley Technical College
Respiratory Therapist (Advanced) Prgm
One Maurice Culberson Dr
Rome, GA 30161
Prgm Dir: Zenia Bratton, BBA RRT
Tel: 706 295-6910   *Fax:* 706 295-6894
E-mail: zbratton@coosavalleytech.edu

Armstrong Atlantic State University
Respiratory Therapist (Advanced) Prgm
11935 Abercorn St
Savannah, GA 31419
www.armstrong.edu
Prgm Dir: Ross L Bowers III, MHS RRT
Tel: 912 921-7446   *Fax:* 912 921-5585
E-mail: bowersro@mail.armstrong.edu

Southwest Georgia Technical College
Respiratory Therapist (Advanced) Prgm
15689 US Hwy 19 N
Thomasville, GA 31792
http://southwestgatech.edu
Prgm Dir: Tammy A Miller, MEd CPFT RRT
Tel: 912 225-5094   *Fax:* 912 225-5289
E-mail: tmiller@southwestgatech.edu

Hawaii

Kapi'olani Community College
Respiratory Therapist (Advanced) Prgm
4303 Diamond Head Rd
Honolulu, HI 96816
Prgm Dir: Stephen F Wehrman, RRT RPFT AE-C
Tel: 808 734-9243   *Fax:* 808 734-9126
E-mail: wehrman@hawaii.edu

Idaho

Boise State University
Respiratory Therapist (Advanced) Prgm
College of Health Sciences
1910 University Dr, Rm HSR 116
Boise, ID 83725
http://respther.boisestate.edu
Prgm Dir: Lonny Ashworth
Tel: 208 426-3383   *Fax:* 208 426-4093
E-mail: lashwor@boisestate.edu

Illinois

Southwestern Illinois College
Respiratory Therapist (Advanced) Prgm
St Elizabeth's Hospital
211 S Third St
Belleville, IL 62222
www.swic.edu
Prgm Dir: Margaret J McMillin, MEd RRT
Tel: 618 234-8911, Ext 1989   *Fax:* 618 222-4658
E-mail: mmcmilli@sebh.org

Southern Illinois University Carbondale
Respiratory Therapist (Advanced) Prgm
School of Allied Health, 1365 Douglas Dr
College of Applied Sciences & Arts, MC6615
Carbondale, IL 62901
Prgm Dir: Stanley M Pearson, II, MSEd RRT
Tel: 618 453-7221   *Fax:* 618 453-7020
E-mail: stanman@siu.edu
Notes: Currently inactive

Kaskaskia College
Respiratory Therapist (Advanced) Prgm
27210 College Rd
Centralia, IL 62801
www.kaskaskia.edu
Prgm Dir: Sharon (Beth) Urban, RRT
Tel: 618 545-3352   *Fax:* 618 545-3389
E-mail: burban@kaskaskia.edu

Parkland College
Respiratory Therapist (Advanced) Prgm
2400 W Bradley Ave
Champaign, IL 61821
Prgm Dir: Terry Des Jardins, MEd RRT
Tel: 217 351-2224   *Fax:* 217 351-2581
E-mail: TDesJardins@parkland.edu

Malcolm X College
Respiratory Therapist (Advanced) Prgm
1900 W Van Buren St
Chicago, IL 60612-3197
Prgm Dir: George A West, MS RRT
Tel: 312 850-7382   *Fax:* 312 850-7453
E-mail: gwest@ccc.edu

Olive Harvey College
Respiratory Therapist (Advanced) Prgm
10001 W Woodlawn Ave, Rm 3317
Chicago, IL 60628
Prgm Dir: Sandra Barnes, MSHSA RRT NPS
Tel: 773 291-6568   *Fax:* 773 291-6304
E-mail: sbarnes@ccc.edu

Kankakee Community College
Respiratory Therapist (Advanced) Prgm
100 College Dr
Kankakee, IL 60901-6505
Prgm Dir: Nancy Stephens, BA MBA RRT
Tel: 815 802-8842   *Fax:* 815 802-8101
E-mail: nstephens@kcc.edu

Moraine Valley Community College
Respiratory Therapist (Advanced) Prgm
9000 W College Dr, Rm B-150
Palos Hills, IL 60465
www.morainevalley.edu
Prgm Dir: Laurie McKeown, MAEd RRT NPS
Tel: 708 608-4124   *Fax:* 708 608-4624
E-mail: McKeownL2@morainevalley.edu

Illinois Central College
Respiratory Therapist (Advanced) Prgm
201 SW Adams St
Peoria, IL 61635-0001
Prgm Dir: Carole (Kelly) Crawford-Jones, MS RRT
Tel: 309 999-4663   *Fax:* 309 673-9626
E-mail: kcrawfordjones@icc.edu

Triton College
Respiratory Therapist (Advanced) Prgm
2000 N Fifth Ave
River Grove, IL 60171
Prgm Dir: Kristine Anderson, MEd RRT-NPS CPFT
Tel: 708 456-0300, Ext 3429   *Fax:* 708 583-3121
E-mail: kanderso@triton.edu

Rock Valley College
Respiratory Therapist (Advanced) Prgm
4151 Samuelson Rd
Rockford, IL 61109-3272
www.rockvalleycollege.edu
Prgm Dir: John M Pace, BS CRT RRT
Tel: 815 921-3220   *Fax:* 815 921-3249
E-mail: j.pace@rockvalleycollege.edu

St John's Hospital
Cosponsor: Lincoln Land Community College
Respiratory Therapist (Advanced) Prgm
School of Respiratory Care
800 E Carpenter St
Springfield, IL 62769
Prgm Dir: Jan Szoke, RRT
Tel: 217 544-6464, Ext 44254   *Fax:* 217 535-3881
E-mail: jan.szoke@st-johns.org

Indiana

University of Southern Indiana
Respiratory Therapist (Advanced) Prgm
8600 University Blvd
Evansville, IN 47712
Prgm Dir: Robert Hooper, MA RRT
Tel: 812 464-1708   *Fax:* 812 465-7092
E-mail: rhooper@usi.edu

Ivy Tech Community College - Ft Wayne
Respiratory Therapist (Advanced) Prgm
3800 N Anthony Blvd
Fort Wayne, IN 46805
Prgm Dir: Jennifer Brink, BS RRT RPFT
Tel: 260 482-9171, Ext 4270   *Fax:* 260 480-4149
E-mail: jbrink@ivytech.edu

Indiana University Northwest
Respiratory Therapist (Advanced) Prgm
3400 Broadway NW Campus
Hawthorne Hall
Gary, IN 46408
Prgm Dir: Susan T Pearson, MPA RRT
Tel: 219 980-6548   *Fax:* 219 980-6649
E-mail: spearson@iun.edu

Clarian Health Partners Inc
Respiratory Therapist (Advanced) Prgm
I-65 at 21st St
PO Box 1367
Indianapolis, IN 46206-1367
www.clarian.org
Prgm Dir: Linda Van Scoder, EdD RRT
Tel: 317 962-8475   *Fax:* 317 962-2102
E-mail: lvanscoder@clarian.org

Indiana University
Respiratory Therapist (Advanced) Prgm
1140 W Michigan St, CF 224
Indianapolis, IN 46202
Prgm Dir: Deborah L Cullen, EdD RRT
Tel: 317 274-7381   *Fax:* 317 278-7383
E-mail: dcullen@iupui.edu

Ivy Tech Community College
Respiratory Therapist (Advanced) Prgm
Central Indiana Region
One W 26th St, PO Box 1763
Indianapolis, IN 46208-1763
Prgm Dir: Marcus D Stowe, MS RRT
Tel: 317 921-4410   *Fax:* 317 921-4753
E-mail: mstowe@ivytech.edu

Ivy Tech Community College - Lafayette
Respiratory Therapist (Advanced) Prgm
3101 S Creasy Ln
Lafayette, IN 47903
Prgm Dir: Peggy James, MBA RRT CPFT
Tel: 765 269-5207   *Fax:* 765 269-5248
E-mail: pjames@ivytech.edu

Ivy Tech Community College - Michigan City
Respiratory Therapist (Advanced) Prgm
3714 Franklin St
Michigan City, IN 46360
Prgm Dir: Susan Layhew, MA RRT
Tel: 219 879-9137   *Fax:* 219 879-9157
E-mail: slayhew@ivytech.edu

Ivy Tech Community College - Sellersburg
Respiratory Therapist (Advanced) Prgm
8204 Hwy 311
Sellersburg, IN 47172
Prgm Dir: Mark Kinkle, RRT CPFT
Tel: 812 246-3301
E-mail: mkinkle@ivytech.edu

Ivy Tech Community College - Terre Haute
Respiratory Therapist (Advanced) Prgm
8000 South Education Dr
Terre Haute, IN 47802
Prgm Dir: Jennifer Purdue, MA RRT RN
Tel: 812 298-2330
E-mail: jreece@ivytech.edu

Iowa

Des Moines Area Community College
Respiratory Therapist (Advanced) Prgm
2006 Ankeny Blvd
Ankeny, IA 50023
www.dmacc.edu
Prgm Dir: Kerry E George, MEd RRT FAARC
Tel: 515 964-6298   *Fax:* 515 964-6327
E-mail: kegeorge@dmacc.edu

Kirkwood Community College
Respiratory Therapist (Advanced) Prgm
6301 Kirkwood Blvd SW, PO Box 2068
Cedar Rapids, IA 52406-9973
Prgm Dir: H Kenneth Bronkhorst, MBA RRT
Tel: 319 398-4987   *Fax:* 319 398-1293
E-mail: ken.bronkhorst@kirkwood.edu

Northeast Iowa Community College
Respiratory Therapist (Advanced) Prgm
10250 Sundown Rd
Peosta, IA 52068
Prgm Dir: Amy Rausch, AAS RRT BS
Tel: 563 556-5110, Ext 274   *Fax:* 563 556-5058
E-mail: rauscha@nicc.edu

St Luke's College
Respiratory Therapist (Advanced) Prgm
2720 Stone Park Blvd
Sioux City, IA 51104
Prgm Dir: Allen W Barbaro, MS RRT
Tel: 712 279-7964   *Fax:* 712 233-8017
E-mail: barbaraw@stlukes.org

Hawkeye Community College
Respiratory Therapist (Advanced) Prgm
1501 E Orange Rd
PO Box 8015
Waterloo, IA 50704-8015
www.hawkeye.cc.ia.us
Prgm Dir: Jamie Bute, AAS RRT
Tel: 319 296-2320, Ext 1919   *Fax:* 319 296-4400
E-mail: jbute@hawkeyecollege.edu

Southeastern Community College
Respiratory Therapist (Advanced) Prgm
1500 W Agency Rd, PO Box 180
West Burlington, IA 52655-0180
www.scciowa.edu
Prgm Dir: Stacy Sells, BHS RRT-NPS CPFT
Tel: 319 208-5204   *Fax:* 319 752-4957
E-mail: ssells@scciowa.edu

Kansas

Bethany Med Ctr/Kansas City Kansas Comm Coll
Respiratory Therapist (Advanced) Prgm
7250 State Ave
Kansas City, KS 66112
Prgm Dir: C Michael Parrett, MBA RPFT RRT-NPS
Tel: 913 288-7245   *Fax:* 913 288-7649
E-mail: mparrett@kckcc.edu

University of Kansas Medical Center
Respiratory Therapist (Advanced) Prgm
3901 Rainbow Blvd, 4006 Delp, Mail Stop 1013
Kansas City, KS 66160
Prgm Dir: Barbara A Ludwig, MA RRT
Tel: 913 588-4634   *Fax:* 913 588-4631
E-mail: bludwig@kumc.edu

Seward County Community College
Respiratory Therapist (Advanced) Prgm
PO Box 1137
Liberal, KS 67901-1137
http://sccc.edu
Prgm Dir: Edward B Anderson, MS RRT
Tel: 316 626-3080   *Fax:* 316 626-3040
E-mail: eanderso@sccc.net

Johnson County Community College
Respiratory Therapist (Advanced) Prgm
12345 College Blvd
Overland Park, KS 66210
www.jccc.net/home/depts/001256
Prgm Dir: Clarissa M Craig, PhD RRT
Tel: 913 469-2583   *Fax:* 913 469-2315
E-mail: ccraig@jccc.edu

Labette Community College
Respiratory Therapist (Advanced) Prgm
200 S 14th St
Parsons, KS 67357
www.labette.edu
Prgm Dir: Connie S Crooks, BS RRT
Tel: 620 820-1160   *Fax:* 620 421-1539
E-mail: conniec@labette.edu

Washburn University
Respiratory Therapist (Advanced) Prgm
1700 College Ave SW
Topeka, KS 66621
www.washburn.edu/respiratory
Prgm Dir: Pat Munzer, DHSc RRT
Tel: 785 670-1404   *Fax:* 785 670-1027
E-mail: pat.munzer@washburn.edu

Newman University
Respiratory Therapist (Advanced) Prgm
3100 McCormick Ave
Wichita, KS 67213-2097
www.newmanu.edu
Prgm Dir: Meg Trumpp, MEd RRT AE-C
Tel: 316 942-4291, Ext 2344   *Fax:* 316 942-4483
E-mail: trumppm@newmanu.edu

Kentucky

Bowling Green Technical College
Respiratory Therapist (Advanced) Prgm
1845 Loop Dr
Bowling Green, KY 42101
Prgm Dir: M Marcia Fuller, BS RRT
Tel: 270 901-1078, Ext 2182   *Fax:* 270 901-1139
E-mail: mary.fuller@kctcs.edu

Northern Kentucky University
Respiratory Therapist (Advanced) Prgm
Nunn Dr/AHC-225
Highland Heights, KY 41099-8002
Prgm Dir: Debra Kasel, MEd RRT CPFT AE-C
Tel: 859 572-5608   *Fax:* 859 572-1314
E-mail: kaseld@nku.edu

Bluegrass Community and Technical College
Cosponsor: University of Kentucky
Respiratory Therapist (Advanced) Prgm
Rm 330 Oswald Bldg, Cooper Dr
Lexington, KY 40506-0235
Prgm Dir: James K Matchuny, BS RRT
Tel: 859 257-4872, Ext 4106   *Fax:* 859 257-9580
E-mail: jkmatc1@uky.edu

Jefferson Community and Technical College
Respiratory Therapist (Advanced) Prgm
109 E Broadway St
Louisville, KY 40202
www.jefferson.kctcs.edu
Prgm Dir: Joan Kruse, MEd RRT
Tel: 502 213-2197   *Fax:* 502 213-2343
E-mail: joan.kruse@kctcs.edu

Madisonville Community College
Respiratory Therapist (Advanced) Prgm
Health Campus
750 N Laffoon St
Madisonville, KY 42431
Prgm Dir: David F Pennaman, MS RRT
Tel: 270 824-7552
E-mail: david.pennaman@kctcs.edu

West Kentucky Community & Technical College
Respiratory Therapist (Advanced) Prgm
PO Box 7408
5200 Blandville Rd
Paducah, KY 42002-7408
Prgm Dir: Ruth Thompson, MS RRT
Tel: 270 534-3486   *Fax:* 270 554-6227
E-mail: Ruth.Thompson@kctcs.edu

Big Sandy Community & Technical College
Respiratory Therapist (Advanced) Prgm
Mayo Campus
513 Third St
Paintsville, KY 41240
www.bigsandy.kctcs.edu
Prgm Dir: Melissa Skeens, RRT NPS RPFT
Tel: 888 641-4132, Ext 82822   *Fax:* 606 789-9753
E-mail: melissa.skeens@kctcs.edu

Southeast Kentucky Comm & Tech College
Respiratory Therapist (Advanced) Prgm
3300 US Highway 25E S
Pineville, KY 40977
Prgm Dir: Michael Good, MS RRT-NPS RPFT
Tel: 606 248-2122   *Fax:* 606 248-2166
E-mail: mike.good@kctcs.edu

Louisiana

Bossier Parish Community College
Respiratory Therapist (Advanced) Prgm
6220 E Texas St
Bossier City, LA 71111
Prgm Dir: Dennis Wissing, PhD RRT
Tel: 318 675-6814   *Fax:* 318 675-6937
E-mail: dwissi@lsuhsc.edu

Nicholls State University
Respiratory Therapist (Advanced) Prgm
Dept of Allied Health Sciences
235 Civic Center Blvd
Houma, LA 70360
www.nicholls.edu
Prgm Dir: Errol Champagne, MEd RRT-NPS
Tel: 985 876-8848   *Fax:* 985 876-8856
E-mail: errol.champagne@nicholls.edu

Delgado Community College
Respiratory Therapist (Advanced) Prgm
615 City Park Ave
New Orleans, LA 70119
Prgm Dir: Diane M Olsen-Rawls, MHS RRT
Tel: 504 483-4114, Ext 4007   *Fax:* 504 483-4609
E-mail: dolsen@dcc.edu

Louisiana State Univ Health Sciences Center
Respiratory Therapist (Advanced) Prgm
1900 Gravier St
New Orleans, LA 70112
www.lsuhsc.edu/no/
Prgm Dir: John Zamjahn, PhD RRT
Tel: 504 568-4228   *Fax:* 504 599-0410
E-mail: jzamja@lsuhsc.edu

Our Lady of Holy Cross College
Cosponsor: Alton Ochsner School of Allied Health Sciences
Respiratory Therapist (Advanced) Prgm
4123 Woodland Dr
New Orleans, LA 70131
www.ochsner.org
Prgm Dir: Mary LaBiche, MEd RRT
Tel: 504 842-3736   *Fax:* 504 842-4372
E-mail: mlabiche@ochsner.org

Louisiana State U Hlth Sci Ctr - Shreveport
Respiratory Therapist (Advanced) Prgm
1501 Kings Hwy
Shreveport, LA 71130
Prgm Dir: Dennis R Payne, MD
Tel: 318 675-6814
E-mail: kpayne@lsuhsc.edu

Southern Univ at Shreveport
Respiratory Therapist (Advanced) Prgm
3050 Martin Luther King Jr Dr
Shreveport, LA 71107
Prgm Dir: JoAnn Warren, BA RRT
Tel: 318 674-3452   *Fax:* 318 676-5307
E-mail: jwarren@susla.edu

Maine

Kennebec Valley Community College
Respiratory Therapist (Advanced) Prgm
92 Western Ave
Fairfield, ME 04937-1367
www.kvcc.me.edu
Prgm Dir: Barbara A Larsson, MEd RRT
Tel: 207 453-5161   *Fax:* 207 453-5197
E-mail: blarsson@kvcc.me.edu

Southern Maine Community College
Respiratory Therapist (Advanced) Prgm
Two Fort Rd
South Portland, ME 04106
www.smccme.edu
Prgm Dir: Walter C Chop, MS RRT
Tel: 207 741-5592   *Fax:* 207 741-4560
E-mail: wchop@smccme.edu

Maryland

Baltimore City Community College
Respiratory Therapist (Advanced) Prgm
2901 Liberty Heights Ave
Baltimore, MD 21215
www.bccc.edu
Prgm Dir: William Cooper, RRT
Tel: 410 462-7776   *Fax:* 410 462-7401
E-mail: wcooper@bccc.edu

Community College of Baltimore County - Essex Campus
Respiratory Therapist (Advanced) Prgm
7201 Rossville Blvd
Baltimore, MD 21237
Prgm Dir: Barbara Schenk, BA RRT
Tel: 410 780-6760   *Fax:* 410 682-8044
E-mail: bschenk@ccbcmd.edu

Allegany College of Maryland
Respiratory Therapist (Advanced) Prgm
12401 Willowbrook Rd SE
Cumberland, MD 21502-2596
Prgm Dir: William R Rocks, EdD RRT
Tel: 301 784-5522   *Fax:* 301 784-5015
E-mail: brocks@allegany.edu

Frederick Community College
Respiratory Therapist (Advanced) Prgm
7932 Opossumtown Pike
Frederick, MD 21702
Prgm Dir: Mark L Paugh, PhD RRT
Tel: 301 846-2528   *Fax:* 301 846-2498
E-mail: mpaugh@frederick.edu

Prince George's Community College
Respiratory Therapist (Advanced) Prgm
301 Largo Rd
Largo, MD 20774
www.pgcc.edu
Prgm Dir: James Courtwright, RRT MSHP
Tel: 301 322-0860   *Fax:* 301 386-7528
E-mail: jcourtwright@pgcc.edu

Salisbury University
Respiratory Therapist (Advanced) Prgm
1101 Camden Ave
Salisbury, MD 21801
www.salisbury.edu
Prgm Dir: Robert Joyner, PhD RRT
Tel: 410 543-6365   *Fax:* 410 548-9185
E-mail: rljoyner@salisbury.edu

Columbia Union College
Respiratory Therapist (Advanced) Prgm
7600 Flower Ave
Takoma Park, MD 20912
Prgm Dir: Vicki Rosette, RRT RPFT
Tel: 301 891-4187   *Fax:* 301 891-4181
E-mail: vrosette@cuc.edu

Massachusetts

Northeastern University
Respiratory Therapist (Advanced) Prgm
249 Ryder Hall
360 Huntington Ave
Boston, MA 02115
www.spcs.neu.edu/ms_respther/
Prgm Dir: Scott Stanley, EdD RRT FAARC
Tel: 617 373-5382
E-mail: s.stanley@neu.edu

Massasoit Community College
Respiratory Therapist (Advanced) Prgm
One Massasoit Blvd
Brockton, MA 02301
www.massasoit.mass.edu
Prgm Dir: Martha DeSilva, MEd RRT
Tel: 508 588-9100, Ext 1787   *Fax:* 508 427-1262
E-mail: mdesilva@massasoit.mass.edu

North Shore Community College
Respiratory Therapist (Advanced) Prgm
One Ferncroft Rd, PO Box 3340
Danvers, MA 01923-0840
Prgm Dir: Geraldine Twomey, MEd RRT RN
Tel: 978 762-4166   *Fax:* 978 762-4022
E-mail: gtwomey@northshore.edu

Northern Essex Community College
Respiratory Therapist (Advanced) Prgm
45 Franklin St
Lawrence, MA 01841
Prgm Dir: Saleh Daher, BS RRT CPFT NPS
Tel: 978 738-7217, Ext 7217   *Fax:* 978 738-7450
E-mail: sdaher@necc.mass.edu

Berkshire Community College
Respiratory Therapist (Advanced) Prgm
1350 West St
Pittsfield, MA 01201
http://Berkshirecc.edu
Prgm Dir: Thomas P Carey, Jr, RRT MPH
Tel: 413 236-4526   *Fax:* 413 448-2700
E-mail: tcarey@berkshirecc.edu

Springfield Technical Community College
Respiratory Therapist (Advanced) Prgm
One Armory Sq
Springfield, MA 01105
Prgm Dir: Lee J Robinson, MEd RRT
Tel: 413 755-4829   *Fax:* 413 755-4764
E-mail: robinson@stcc.edu

Quinsigamond Community College
Respiratory Therapist (Advanced) Prgm
670 W Boylston St
Worcester, MA 01606-2092
www.qcc.mass.edu
Prgm Dir: Lynda A Nesbitt, MA RRT
Tel: 508 854-4398   *Fax:* 508 852-6943
E-mail: lyndan@qcc.mass.edu

Michigan

Ferris State University
Respiratory Therapist (Advanced) Prgm
200 Ferris Dr/VFS 210A
Big Rapids, MI 49307-2740
www.ferris.edu
Prgm Dir: Gary Jeromin, MA RRT LRT
Tel: 231 591-2318
E-mail: jeromig@ferris.edu

Macomb Community College
Respiratory Therapist (Advanced) Prgm
44575 Garfield Rd, E Bldg, Rm 219
Clinton Township, MI 48038-1139
www.macomb.edu
Prgm Dir: Mary E Alstead, BS RRT NPS
Tel: 586 286-2150   *Fax:* 586 286-2098
E-mail: alsteadm@macomb.edu

Henry Ford Community College
Respiratory Therapist (Advanced) Prgm
Health Careers Education Center
5101 Evergreen Rd
Dearborn, MI 48128-1495
Prgm Dir: Debra Szymanski, MA RRT
Tel: 313 317-6580   *Fax:* 313 317-6569
E-mail: dszyman@hfcc.edu

Mott Community College
Respiratory Therapist (Advanced) Prgm
1401 E Court St
Flint, MI 48503
Prgm Dir: David L Panzlau, MA RRT
Tel: 810 232-6563   *Fax:* 810 762-5619
E-mail: dpanzlau@mcc.edu

Kalamazoo Valley Community College
Respiratory Therapist (Advanced) Prgm
Texas Township Campus
6767 West O Ave, PO Box 4070
Kalamazoo, MI 49003-4070
Prgm Dir: Albert W Moss, MA RRT
Tel: 269 488-4288   *Fax:* 269 488-4458
E-mail: amoss@kvcc.edu

Monroe County Community College
Respiratory Therapist (Advanced) Prgm
1555 S Raisinville Rd
Monroe, MI 48161
Prgm Dir: Bonnie Boggs, RRT
Tel: 734 384-4268   *Fax:* 734 384-4187
E-mail: bboggs@monroecc.edu

Muskegon Community College
Respiratory Therapist (Advanced) Prgm
221 S Quarterline Rd
Muskegon, MI 49442
http://muskegon.cc.mi.us/~devriesd/resp-home.htm
Prgm Dir: Daniel Knue, MM RRT-NPS
Tel: 231 777-0370   *Fax:* 231 777-0490
E-mail: Dan.Knue@muskegoncc.edu

Oakland Community College - Southfield
Respiratory Therapist (Advanced) Prgm
22322 Rutland Dr
Southfield, MI 48075
Prgm Dir: Sue J Work, MSA RRT-NPS
Tel: 248 233-2919   *Fax:* 248 233-2891
E-mail: sjwork@oaklandcc.edu

Delta College
Respiratory Therapist (Advanced) Prgm
1961 Delta Rd
University Center, MI 48710
Prgm Dir: Earl B Gregory, MS RRT
Tel: 989 686-9489   *Fax:* 989 667-2211
E-mail: ebgregor@alpha.delta.edu

Minnesota

Lake Superior College
Respiratory Therapist (Advanced) Prgm
2101 Trinity Rd
Duluth, MN 55811
Prgm Dir: Cynthia Annable, RRT NPS RPFT
Tel: 218 733-5925   *Fax:* 218 723-4921
E-mail: c.annable@lsc.edu

Northland Community & Technical College
Respiratory Therapist (Advanced) Prgm
2022 Central Ave NE
East Grand Forks, MN 56721
www.northlandcollege.edu
Prgm Dir: Anthony Sorum, BA RRT
Tel: 218 773-4791, Ext 4791   *Fax:* 218 773-4502
E-mail: tony.sorum@northlandcollege.edu

College of St Catherine - Minneapolis
Respiratory Therapist (Advanced) Prgm
601 25th Ave S
Minneapolis, MN 55454
www.stkate.edu/RC
Prgm Dir: John E Boatright, MA RRT
Tel: 651 690-7819   *Fax:* 651 690-7849
E-mail: jeboatright@stkate.edu

Mayo School of Health Sciences
Respiratory Therapist (Advanced) Prgm
200 First St SW
1009 Siebens
Rochester, MN 55905
Prgm Dir: Vanessa King, MED RRT
Tel: 507 284-0174   *Fax:* 507 284-2818
E-mail: king.vanessa@mayo.edu

Saint Paul College
Respiratory Therapist (Advanced) Prgm
235 Marshall Ave
St Paul, MN 55102
Prgm Dir: Joseph Buhain, RRT RCP EMT-B
Tel: 651 846-1501   *Fax:* 651 221-1416
E-mail: joseph.buhain@saintpaul.edu

Mississippi

Northeast Mississippi Community College
Respiratory Therapist (Advanced) Prgm
Cunningham Blvd
Booneville, MS 38829
www.nemcc.edu
Prgm Dir: Beverly Prince, RRT BS
Tel: 662 720-7387   *Fax:* 662 728-1165
E-mail: biprince@nemcc.edu

Itawamba Community College
Respiratory Therapist (Advanced) Prgm
602 W Hill St
Fulton, MS 38843
http://iccms.edu
Prgm Dir: James Harold Plunkett, MS RRT
Tel: 601 862-8149, Ext 8149   *Fax:* 601 862-8350
E-mail: hjplunkett@iccms.edu

Mississippi Gulf Coast Community College
Respiratory Therapist (Advanced) Prgm
PO Box 100
Gautier, MS 39553
Prgm Dir: Donald Hayes, AS RRT
Tel: 228 497-7711, Ext 290   *Fax:* 228 497-7676
E-mail: donald.hayes@mgccc.edu

Pearl River Community College
Respiratory Therapist (Advanced) Prgm
Forrest County Voc-Tech Ctr
5448 US Hwy 49 S
Hattiesburg, MS 39401
Prgm Dir: Lori Anderson
Tel: 601 554-5521   *Fax:* 601 554-5487
E-mail: landerson@prcc.edu

Hinds Community College
Respiratory Therapist (Advanced) Prgm
1750 Chadwick Dr
Jackson, MS 39204
Prgm Dir: Shirley Miller, RRT BSEd
Tel: 601 371-3517   *Fax:* 601 376-4541
E-mail: slmiller@hindscc.edu

Meridian Community College
Respiratory Therapist (Advanced) Prgm
910 Hwy 19 N
Meridian, MS 39307
www.meridiancc.edu
Prgm Dir: Steve W Arinder, RRT BS MPH
Tel: 601 484-8752   *Fax:* 601 482-3936
E-mail: sarinder@meridiancc.edu

Copiah-Lincoln Community College
Respiratory Therapist (Advanced) Prgm
Natchez Campus Career and Technical Sch
30 Campus Dr
Natchez, MS 39120-5398
www.colin.edu
Prgm Dir: Walton B Wilson, BS RRT
Tel: 601 446-1161   *Fax:* 601 446-1298
E-mail: walt.wilson@colin.edu

Northwest Mississippi Community College
Respiratory Therapist (Advanced) Prgm
5197 WE Ross Pkwy
Southaven, MS 38671
Prgm Dir: Regina K Clark, MEd RRT
Tel: 601 280-6151   *Fax:* 601 280-6161
E-mail: r_clark@northwestms.edu

Missouri

Cape Girardeau Career & Technology Center
Respiratory Therapist (Advanced) Prgm
1080 S Silver Springs Rd
Cape Girardeau, MO 63703
Prgm Dir: Kenneth L Pfau, BS RRT
Tel: 573 334-0449, Ext 320   *Fax:* 573 334-5930
E-mail: pfauk@cape.k12.mo.us

University of Missouri - Columbia
Respiratory Therapist (Advanced) Prgm
605 Lewis Hall
Columbia, MO 65211
Prgm Dir: Rosemary G Hogan, RRT MEd
Tel: 573 882-8034   *Fax:* 573 884-1490
E-mail: hoganr@health.missouri.edu

Hannibal Career & Technical Center
Cosponsor: Hannibal LaGrange College
Respiratory Therapist (Advanced) Prgm
School of Respiratory Care
4550 McMasters Ave
Hannibal, MO 63401
www.hannibal.k12.mo.us
Prgm Dir: Linda E Smith, BS RRT RCP
Tel: 573 221-4430, Ext 164   *Fax:* 573 221-1385
E-mail: LSmith@hannibal.k12.mo.us

Missouri Southern State University
Respiratory Therapist (Advanced) Prgm
3950 E Newman Rd
Joplin, MO 64801-1595
Prgm Dir: Glenda Pippin, BS RRT CPFT
Tel: 417 659-4405   *Fax:* 417 659-4408
E-mail: pippin-g@mssu.edu

Concorde Career College - Kansas City
Respiratory Therapist (Advanced) Prgm
3239 Broadway Blvd
Kansas City, MO 64111
Prgm Dir: Lana C Conrad, BS RRT
Tel: 816 531-5223, Ext 403   *Fax:* 816 756-3231
E-mail: lconrad@concorde.edu

Rolla Technical Center
Respiratory Therapist (Advanced) Prgm
500 Forum Dr
Rolla, MO 65401
Prgm Dir: Diane R Oldfather
Tel: 573 458-0160
E-mail: doldfather@rolla.k12.mo.us

Ozarks Technical Community College
Respiratory Therapist (Advanced) Prgm
1001 E Chestnut Expressway
Springfield, MO 65802
www.otc.edu
Prgm Dir: Doug Pursley, MEd RRT
Tel: 417 447-8823   *Fax:* 417 447-8841
E-mail: pursleyd@otc.edu

St Louis Community College - Forest Park
Respiratory Therapist (Advanced) Prgm
5600 Oakland Ave
St Louis, MO 63110
Prgm Dir: James R Brennan, MEd RRT
Tel: 314 644-9079   *Fax:* 314 951-9412
E-mail: jbrennan@stlcc.edu

Montana

Montana State Univ - Great Falls Coll of Tech
Respiratory Therapist (Advanced) Prgm
2100 16th Ave S
Great Falls, MT 59405
www.msugf.edu
Prgm Dir: Leonard Bates, MEd RRT
Tel: 406 771-4360   *Fax:* 406 771-4313
E-mail: lbates@msugf.edu

University of Montana
Respiratory Therapist (Advanced) Prgm
909 S Avenue W
Missoula, MT 59801
Prgm Dir: Robert Wafstet, MS RRT
Tel: 406 243-7821   *Fax:* 406 243-7899
E-mail: Robert.Wafstet@umontana.edu

Nebraska

Southeast Community College
Respiratory Therapist (Advanced) Prgm
8800 O St
Lincoln, NE 68520-1299
Prgm Dir: Charlotte Pasco, BA RRT
Tel: 402 437-2781   *Fax:* 402 437-2404
E-mail: cpasco@southeast.edu

Alegent Health
Cosponsor: Midland Lutheran College/UNK
Respiratory Therapist (Advanced) Prgm
6901 N 72nd St
Omaha, NE 68122
http://Alegent.com
Prgm Dir: Todd Klopfenstein, BS RRT
Tel: 402 572-2312   *Fax:* 402 572-3157
E-mail: tklopfen@alegent.org

Metropolitan Community College
Respiratory Therapist (Advanced) Prgm
PO Box 3777
Omaha, NE 68103
Prgm Dir: Jerald A Moss, RRT MPA
Tel: 402 738-4653   *Fax:* 402 738-4005
E-mail: jmoss@metropo.mccneb.edu

NE Methodist Coll Nursing & Allied Hlth
Respiratory Therapist (Advanced) Prgm
720 N 87th St
Omaha, NE 68114
www.methodistcollege.edu
Prgm Dir: Christine Hamilton, MA RRT AE-C
Tel: 402 354-7065   *Fax:* 402 354-7130
E-mail: Chris.Hamilton@methodistcollege.edu

Nevada

College of Southern Nevada
Respiratory Therapist (Advanced) Prgm
Cardiorespiratory Sciences
6375 W Charleston Blvd, W1B
Las Vegas, NV 89146-1124
Prgm Dir: Tracy Sherman, MEd RRT-NPS
Tel: 702 651-5849   *Fax:* 702 651-7926
E-mail: tracy.sherman@csn.edu

Pima Medical Institute
Respiratory Therapist (Advanced) Prgm
3333 E Flamingo Rd
Las Vegas, NV 89121
Prgm Dir: Bill Pifer, BS RRT
Tel: 702 458-9650
E-mail: bpifer@pmi.edu

New Hampshire

New Hampshire Comm Tech Coll - Claremont
Respiratory Therapist (Advanced) Prgm
One College Dr
Claremont, NH 03743
Prgm Dir: John Marcley, MEd RRT
Tel: 603 542-7744, Ext 2530   *Fax:* 603 543-1844
E-mail: jmarcley@nhctc.edu

New Jersey

Northwest NJ Consortium Resp Care Educ
Respiratory Therapist (Advanced) Prgm
Saint Clares Hospital
400 Blackwell St
Dover, NJ 07801
Prgm Dir: Dianne Adams, MA RRT
Tel: 973 537-3906   *Fax:* 973 537-3996
E-mail: dadams@saintclares.org

Brookdale Community College
Respiratory Therapist (Advanced) Prgm
765 Newman Springs Rd
Lincroft, NJ 07738
www.brookdalecc.edu
Prgm Dir: Carol Schedel, MA RRT
Tel: 732 224-2692   *Fax:* 732 224-2998
E-mail: cschedel@brookdalecc.edu

Univ of Medicine & Dent of New Jersey
Respiratory Therapist (Advanced) Prgm
School of Health Related Professions
65 Bergen St
Newark, NJ 07101
Prgm Dir: Albert J Heuer, PhD RRT
Tel: 973 972-2418   *Fax:* 973 972-5258
E-mail: heueraj@umdnj.edu

Bergen Community College
Respiratory Therapist (Advanced) Prgm
400 Paramus Rd
Paramus, NJ 07652
www.bergen.edu/academics/respiratory_therapy/
Prgm Dir: Robert A Muller, MA RRT
Tel: 201 612-5337   *Fax:* 201 612-3876
E-mail: rmuller@bergen.edu

Univ of Medicine & Dent of New Jersey
Respiratory Therapist (Advanced) Prgm
Sch of Hlth Related Professions
UEC 40 E Laurel Rd
Stratford, NJ 08084
Prgm Dir: Alan Realey, BS RRT
Tel: 856 566-2891   *Fax:* 856 566-2894
E-mail: realeyam@umdnj.edu

New Mexico

Central New Mexico Community College
Respiratory Therapist (Advanced) Prgm
525 Buena Vista SE
Albuquerque, NM 87106
Prgm Dir: John Blewett, RRT
Tel: 505 224-4138   *Fax:* 505 224-4120
E-mail: jblewett@cnm.edu

Dona Ana Community College
Respiratory Therapist (Advanced) Prgm
Box 30001, Dept 3DA
3400 S Espina St
Las Cruces, NM 88003-0001
Prgm Dir: Virginia Durant, MA RRT
Tel: 505 527-7607   *Fax:* 505 527-7765
E-mail: vdurant@nmsu.edu

Eastern New Mexico University - Roswell Campus
Respiratory Therapist (Advanced) Prgm
PO Box 6000
52 University Blvd
Roswell, NM 88202-6000
www.roswell.enmu.edu
Prgm Dir: Gina Buldra, BS RRT RCP
Tel: 505 624-7217   *Fax:* 505 624-7100
E-mail: gina.buldra@roswell.enmu.edu

New York

Genesee Community College
Respiratory Therapist (Advanced) Prgm
1 College Rd
Batavia, NY 14020-1519
Prgm Dir: Ronald M Jacobs, MBA RRT-NPS
Tel: 585 343-0055, Ext 6633   *Fax:* 585 343-0433
E-mail: rmjacobs@genesee.edu

Long Island University - Brooklyn Campus
Respiratory Therapist (Advanced) Prgm
University Plaza
Brooklyn, NY 11201
Prgm Dir: Thomas J Johnson, RRT
Tel: 718 488-1492   *Fax:* 718 488-1432
E-mail: tjohnson@liu.edu

Nassau Community College
Respiratory Therapist (Advanced) Prgm
One Education Dr
Garden City, NY 11530
http://ncc.edu
Prgm Dir: Mary B Smith, RRT NPS
Tel: 516 572-7911   *Fax:* 516 572-7565
E-mail: smithmb@ncc.edu

CUNY Borough of Manhattan Community Coll
Respiratory Therapist (Advanced) Prgm
199 Chambers St
New York, NY 10007
Prgm Dir: Everett W Flannery, MPS RRT
Tel: 212 346-8731   *Fax:* 212 346-8738
E-mail: eflannery@bmcc.cuny.edu

Molloy College
Respiratory Therapist (Advanced) Prgm
1000 Hempstead Ave
PO Box 5002
Rockville Centre, NY 11571-5002
www.molloy.edu
Prgm Dir: Robert Tralongo, MBA RT RRT-NPS CPFT
Tel: 516 678-5000, Ext 6337 *Fax:* 516 256-2252
E-mail: rtralongo@molloy.edu

Stony Brook University
Respiratory Therapist (Advanced) Prgm
Sch of Health Tech and Management
Stony Brook, NY 11794-8203
Prgm Dir: James A Ganetis, MS RRT
Tel: 631 444-3180 *Fax:* 631 444-7621
E-mail: kaxton@epo.hsc.sunysb.edu

Onondaga Community College
Respiratory Therapist (Advanced) Prgm
Rte 173
Syracuse, NY 13215
www.sunyocc.edu
Prgm Dir: Daniel Cleveland, RRT BS
Tel: 315 498-2458 *Fax:* 315 498-2751
E-mail: clevelad@sunyocc.edu

SUNY Upstate Medical University
Respiratory Therapist (Advanced) Prgm
750 E Adams St
Syracuse, NY 13210
www.upstate.edu/chp/csrc/
Prgm Dir: Joseph G Sorbello, MSEd RRT RT
Tel: 315 464-5580 *Fax:* 315 464-6876
E-mail: sorbellj@upstate.edu

Hudson Valley Community College
Respiratory Therapist (Advanced) Prgm
80 Vandenburgh Ave
Troy, NY 12180
Prgm Dir: Patricia G Hyland, MEd RRT
Tel: 518 629-7454 *Fax:* 518 629-7594
E-mail: hylanpat@hvcc.edu

Mohawk Valley Community College
Respiratory Therapist (Advanced) Prgm
1101 Sherman Dr
Utica, NY 13501
Prgm Dir: Lorie Phillips, MS RRT
Tel: 315 792-5664 *Fax:* 315 731-5855
E-mail: lphillips@mvcc.edu

Westchester Community College
Respiratory Therapist (Advanced) Prgm
75 Grasslands Rd
Valhalla, NY 10595
www.sunywcc.edu
Prgm Dir: Jose Quinones, MS RRT-NPS RPFT
Tel: 914 606-6883 *Fax:* 914 606-7832
E-mail: jose.quinones@sunywcc.edu

Erie Community College - North Campus
Respiratory Therapist (Advanced) Prgm
6205 Main St
Williamsville, NY 14221
Prgm Dir: James J Bierl, MS RRT NPS
Tel: 716 851-1531 *Fax:* 716 851-1429
E-mail: bierl@ecc.edu

North Carolina

Stanly Community College
Respiratory Therapist (Advanced) Prgm
141 College Dr
Albemarle, NC 28001
Prgm Dir: Tammy P Crump, PhD RRT
Tel: 704 991-0267, Ext 267 *Fax:* 704 991-0110
E-mail: tcrump5648@stanly.edu

Central Piedmont Community College
Respiratory Therapist (Advanced) Prgm
PO Box 35009
Charlotte, NC 28235
www.cpcc.edu
Prgm Dir: Brian Stearns, RRT
Tel: 704 330-6274 *Fax:* 704 330-6131
E-mail: brian.stearns@cpcc.edu

Durham Technical Community College
Respiratory Therapist (Advanced) Prgm
1637 Lawson St, Drawer 11307
Durham, NC 27703
www.durhamtech.edu
Prgm Dir: Richard D Miller, PhD RRT RCP
Tel: 919 686-3643 *Fax:* 919 686-3693
E-mail: millerr@durhamtech.edu

Fayetteville Technical Community College
Respiratory Therapist (Advanced) Prgm
2201 Hull Rd
Fayetteville, NC 28303
Prgm Dir: Ruth A Baldwin, MA RRT
Tel: 910 678-8316 *Fax:* 910 678-8500
E-mail: baldwinr@faytechcc.edu

Pitt Community College
Respiratory Therapist (Advanced) Prgm
PO Drawer 7007
Greenville, NC 27834
www.pittcc.edu
Prgm Dir: Donna V Neal, PhD RRT RCP
Tel: 252 493-7378 *Fax:* 252 321-4451
E-mail: dneal@email.pittcc.edu

Catawba Valley Community College
Respiratory Therapist (Advanced) Prgm
2550 Hwy 70 SE
Hickory, NC 28602
www.cvcc.edu
Prgm Dir: Catherine A Bitsche, MA RRT
Tel: 828 327-7000, Ext 4391 *Fax:* 828 327-7276
E-mail: cbitsche@cvcc.edu

Robeson Community College
Respiratory Therapist (Advanced) Prgm
PO Box 1420
Lumberton, NC 28359
Prgm Dir: Kelli Heustess, RCP RRT CPFT
Tel: 910 272-3400 *Fax:* 910 272-3416
E-mail: kheustes@robeson.cc.nc.us

Carteret Community College
Respiratory Therapist (Advanced) Prgm
3505 Arendell St
Morehead City, NC 28557
www.carteret.edu
Prgm Dir: Trisha J Miller, BS RRT CPFT RCP
Tel: 252 222-6169 *Fax:* 252 222-6074
E-mail: tjm@carteret.edu

Sandhills Community College
Respiratory Therapist (Advanced) Prgm
3395 Airport Rd
Pinehurst, NC 28374
www.sandhills.edu
Prgm Dir: William L Croft, MS RRT-NPS RCP
Tel: 910 695-3836 *Fax:* 910 692-6918
E-mail: croftb@sandhills.edu

Edgecombe Community College
Respiratory Therapist (Advanced) Prgm
225 Tarboro St
Rocky Mount, NC 27801
www.edgecombe.edu
Prgm Dir: Ralph D Webb, BAS RRT RCP
Tel: 252 446-0436, Ext 330 *Fax:* 252 985-2212
E-mail: webbrd@edgecombe.edu

Southwestern Community College
Respiratory Therapist (Advanced) Prgm
447 College Dr
Sylva, NC 28779-9578
Prgm Dir: Mitchell Fischer, JD RRT RCP
Tel: 828 586-4091, Ext 472 *Fax:* 828 586-3381
E-mail: mfischer@southwesterncc.edu

Rockingham Community College
Respiratory Therapist (Advanced) Prgm
PO Box 38
Wentworth, NC 27375-0038
Prgm Dir: Thomas W Harding, MS RRT RPFTRCP
Tel: 336 342-4261, Ext 2339 *Fax:* 336 634-1253
E-mail: hardingt@rockinghamcc.edu

Forsyth Technical Community College
Respiratory Therapist (Advanced) Prgm
2100 Silas Creek Pkwy
302A Bob Greene Hall
Winston-Salem, NC 27103-5197
www.forsythtech.edu
Prgm Dir: Perry W Sheppard, MEd RRT-NPS RPFT RCP
Tel: 336 734-7427 *Fax:* 336 734-7444
E-mail: psheppard@forsythtech.edu

North Dakota

University of Mary/St Alexius Medical Ctr
Cosponsor: University of Mary and St Alexius Medical
Center
Respiratory Therapist (Advanced) Prgm
900 E Broadway, PO Box 5510
Bismarck, ND 58502
http://st.alexius.org/about_stas/allied_schools/
Prgm Dir: Wilmer D Beachey, PhD RRT
Tel: 701 530-7757 *Fax:* 701 530-7701
E-mail: wbeachey@primecare.org

NDSU/MeritCare Hospital Consortium
Respiratory Therapist (Advanced) Prgm
MeritCare Hospital
PO Box MC
Fargo, ND 58122-0207
www.ndsu.edu/rc/
Prgm Dir: Gary Brown, BA RRT
Tel: 701 234-6147 *Fax:* 701 234-6942
E-mail: gary.brown@meritcare.com

Ohio

University of Akron
Respiratory Therapist (Advanced) Prgm
302 E Buchtel Mall
Akron, OH 44325-3702
Prgm Dir: LaVerne Yousey, MS RRT
Tel: 330 972-7906 *Fax:* 330 972-2016
E-mail: laverne@uakron.edu

Stark State College of Technology
Respiratory Therapist (Advanced) Prgm
6200 Frank Ave NW
Canton, OH 44720-7299
www.starkstate.edu
Prgm Dir: Peter R Castillo, MEd RRT
Tel: 330 966-5458, Ext 4311 *Fax:* 330 966-6586
E-mail: pcastillo@starkstate.edu

Collins Career Center
Cosponsor: Marshall Community and Technical College
Respiratory Therapist (Advanced) Prgm
11627 State Route 243
Chesapeake, OH 45619
www.collins-cc.k12.oh.us
Prgm Dir: Keith Terry, MS RRT RN
Tel: 740 867-6641, Ext 411 *Fax:* 740 867-9626
E-mail: KATerry@collins-cc.k12.oh.us

Cincinnati State Tech & Comm College
Respiratory Therapist (Advanced) Prgm
3520 Central Pkwy
Cincinnati, OH 45223
Prgm Dir: Debra Lierl, MEd RRT
Tel: 513 569-1690   *Fax:* 513 569-1559
E-mail: debra.lierl@cincinnatistate.edu

Columbus State Community College
Respiratory Therapist (Advanced) Prgm
550 E Spring St
Columbus, OH 43215
www.cscc.edu/Respiratory/
Prgm Dir: Susan L Donohue, MEd RCP RRT
Tel: 614 287-2633   *Fax:* 614 287-6080
E-mail: sdonohue@cscc.edu

Ohio State University
Respiratory Therapist (Advanced) Prgm
431 Atwell Hall
453 W Tenth Ave
Columbus, OH 43210
Prgm Dir: F Herbert Douce, MS RRT-NPS RPFT
Tel: 614 292-8445   *Fax:* 614 292-0210
E-mail: douce.2@osu.edu

Sinclair Community College
Respiratory Therapist (Advanced) Prgm
444 W Third St
Dayton, OH 45402
Prgm Dir: Cynthia Beckett, PhD RRT RPFT
Tel: 937 512-2849   *Fax:* 937 512-2058
E-mail: cynthia.beckett@sinclair.edu

Bowling Green State University
Respiratory Therapist (Advanced) Prgm
One University Dr
Huron, OH 44839-9791
www.firelands.bgsu.edu/programs/rt
Prgm Dir: Rod C Roark, MS RRT
Tel: 419 433-5560, Ext 20865   *Fax:* 419 433-9696
E-mail: rroark@bgnet.bgsu.edu

Kettering College of Medical Arts
Respiratory Therapist (Advanced) Prgm
3737 Southern Blvd
Kettering, OH 45429
www.kcma.edu
Prgm Dir: Nancy E Colletti, MS RRT CPFT RCIS
Tel: 937 298-3399, Ext 55644   *Fax:* 937 395-8635
E-mail: nancy.colletti@kcma.edu

Lakeland Community College
Respiratory Therapist (Advanced) Prgm
7700 Clocktower Dr
Kirtland, OH 44094-5198
www.lakelandcc.edu
Prgm Dir: Catherine J Kenny, MEd RRT
Tel: 440 525-7343   *Fax:* 440 525-7433
E-mail: ckenny@lakelandcc.edu

Rhodes State College
Respiratory Therapist (Advanced) Prgm
4240 Campus Dr
Lima, OH 45804
Prgm Dir: Letitia A Hatfield, MS RRT CPFT
Tel: 419 995-8366   *Fax:* 419 995-8818
E-mail: hatfield.t@rhodesstate.edu

North Central State College
Respiratory Therapist (Advanced) Prgm
2441 Kenwood Circle, PO Box 698
Mansfield, OH 44901
www.ncstatecollege.edu
Prgm Dir: Robert A Slabodnick, MEd BS RRT/NPS
Tel: 419 755-4891, Ext 4891   *Fax:* 419 755-5630
E-mail: rslabod@ncstatecollege.edu

Washington State Community College
Respiratory Therapist (Advanced) Prgm
710 Colegate Dr
Marietta, OH 45750
www.wscc.edu
Prgm Dir: James R Kinker, PhD RRT
Tel: 614 374-8716, Ext 1605   *Fax:* 614 373-7496
E-mail: rkinker@wscc.edu

Cuyahoga Community College
Respiratory Therapist (Advanced) Prgm
11000 Pleasant Valley Rd
Parma, OH 44130
Prgm Dir: David A Lucas, MS RRT
Tel: 216 987-5267   *Fax:* 216 987-5066
E-mail: david.lucas@tri-c.edu

Shawnee State University
Respiratory Therapist (Advanced) Prgm
940 Second St
Portsmouth, OH 45662
Prgm Dir: Donald L Thomas, MS RRT
Tel: 740 351-3235   *Fax:* 740 351-3354
E-mail: dthomas@shawnee.edu

Jefferson Community College
Respiratory Therapist (Advanced) Prgm
4000 Sunset Blvd
Steubenville, OH 43952
www.jcc.edu
Prgm Dir: Cynthia Carducci, MEd RRT
Tel: 740 264-5591, Ext 171   *Fax:* 740 264-9504
E-mail: ccarducci@jcc.edu

University of Toledo
Respiratory Therapist (Advanced) Prgm
College of Health Science and Human Service
2801 W Bancroft St
Toledo, OH 43606
www.utoledo.edu
Prgm Dir: Suzanne Spacek, MEd RRT-NPS CPFT
Tel: 419 530-4556   *Fax:* 419 530-4780
E-mail: suzanne.spacek@utoledo.edu

Youngstown State University
Respiratory Therapist (Advanced) Prgm
One University Plaza
Youngstown, OH 44555
www.ysu.edu
Prgm Dir: Louis N Harris, EdD RRT
Tel: 330 941-1764   *Fax:* 330 941-2921
E-mail: lnharris01@ysu.edu

Oklahoma

Rose State College
Respiratory Therapist (Advanced) Prgm
6420 SE 15th St
Midwest City, OK 73110
www.rose.edu/cstudent/hsdiv/res_prog/
Prgm Dir: Kathe Rowe, BSEd RRT-NPS
Tel: 405 733-7571   *Fax:* 405 736-0338
E-mail: krowe@rose.edu

Francis Tuttle Technology Center
Cosponsor: Oklahoma City Community College
Respiratory Therapist (Advanced) Prgm
12777 N Rockwell Ave
Oklahoma City, OK 73142-2789
Prgm Dir: Lezli Heyland, BS RRT
Tel: 405 717-4269   *Fax:* 405 717-4789
E-mail: lheyland@francistuttle.com

Tulsa Community College
Respiratory Therapist (Advanced) Prgm
909 S Boston Ave
Tulsa, OK 74119
Prgm Dir: Gary Persing, BS RRT
Tel: 918 595-7015   *Fax:* 918 595-7091
E-mail: gpersing@tulsacc.edu

Oregon

Lane Community College
Respiratory Therapist (Advanced) Prgm
4000 E 30th Ave
Eugene, OR 97405-0640
www.lanecc.edu
Prgm Dir: Roger H Hecht, AS RRT
Tel: 541 463-5624   *Fax:* 541 463-4151
E-mail: hechtr@lanecc.edu

Mt Hood Community College
Respiratory Therapist (Advanced) Prgm
26000 SE Stark St
Gresham, OR 97030
Prgm Dir: George Hicks, MS RRT
Tel: 503 491-7172   *Fax:* 503 491-6047
E-mail: hicksg@mhcc.edu

Oregon Institute of Technology
Respiratory Therapist (Advanced) Prgm
202 S Riverside
Medford, OR 97501
Prgm Dir: James L Hulse, MPH RRT-NPS RPFT
Tel: 541 245-7516   *Fax:* 541 774-4203
E-mail: james.hulse@oit.edu

Pennsylvania

West Chester University
Cosponsor: Bryn Mawr Hospital
Respiratory Therapist (Advanced) Prgm
130 S Bryn Mawr Ave
Bryn Mawr, PA 19010
http://health-sciences.wcupa.edu/health/
Prgm Dir: Brian Kellar, MS RRT-NPS RPFT AE-C
Tel: 610 526-3347   *Fax:* 610 526-3821
E-mail: kellarb@mlhs.org

Gannon University
Respiratory Therapist (Advanced) Prgm
109 University Square
Erie, PA 16541
www.gannon.edu/programs/under/respcare.asp
Prgm Dir: Charles Cornfield, MS RRT
Tel: 814 871-5637   *Fax:* 814 871-5662
E-mail: cornfield@gannon.edu

Gwynedd-Mercy College
Respiratory Therapist (Advanced) Prgm
1325 Sumneytown Pike
PO Box 901
Gwynedd Valley, PA 19437
Prgm Dir: William F Galvin, MSEd RRT CPFT AE-C
Tel: 215 641-5536   *Fax:* 215 641-5559
E-mail: Galvin.w@gmc.edu

Harrisburg Area Community College
Respiratory Therapist (Advanced) Prgm
One HACC Dr
Harrisburg, PA 17110
Prgm Dir: Bradley A Leidich, MSEd RRT
Tel: 717 780-2315   *Fax:* 717 780-2551
E-mail: baleidic@hacc.edu

University of Pittsburgh - Johnstown
Respiratory Therapist (Advanced) Prgm
227 Krebs Hall
450 Schoolhouse Rd
Johnstown, PA 15904
Prgm Dir: Bruce J Colbert, MS RRT
Tel: 814 269-2960   *Fax:* 814 269-2044
E-mail: bcolbert@pitt.edu

Millersville University of Pennsylvania
Cosponsor: Lancaster Regional Medical Center
Respiratory Therapist (Advanced) Prgm
PO Box 1002
Millersville, PA 17551-0302
www.muweb.millersville.edu/~rtp
Prgm Dir: John M Hughes, RRT MEd AE-C
Tel: 717 735-3167   *Fax:* 717 544-5970
E-mail: muprt@comcast.net

Western School of Health & Business - Monroeville
Respiratory Therapist (Advanced) Prgm
One Monroeville Center, Ste 125
Monroeville, PA 15246
Prgm Dir: Michael Mehall, BS RRT
Tel: 412 373-9038   *Fax:* 412 281-0319
E-mail: mmehall@western-school.com

Luzerne County Community College
Respiratory Therapist (Advanced) Prgm
1333 S Prospect St
Nanticoke, PA 18634
www.luzerne.edu
Prgm Dir: Christopher Tino, BS RRT
Tel: 570 740-0467   *Fax:* 570 740-0526
E-mail: ctino@luzerne.edu

Community College of Philadelphia
Respiratory Therapist (Advanced) Prgm
1700 Spring Garden St
Philadelphia, PA 19130
www.ccp.edu
Prgm Dir: Frank M Alsis, EdD RRT
Tel: 215 751-8423   *Fax:* 215 751-8937
E-mail: falsis@ccp.edu

Comm College of Allegheny County
Respiratory Therapist (Advanced) Prgm
808 Ridge Ave
Pittsburgh, PA 15212
www.ccac.edu
Prgm Dir: Thomas A Roop, RRT
Tel: 412 237-2607   *Fax:* 412 237-6579
E-mail: troop@ccac.edu

Indiana University of Pennsylvania
Respiratory Therapist (Advanced) Prgm
4800 Friendship Ave
Pittsburgh, PA 15224
Prgm Dir: William J Malley, MS RRT
Tel: 412 578-7000   *Fax:* 412 578-4651
E-mail: gmeyers@wpahs.org

Reading Area Community College
Respiratory Therapist (Advanced) Prgm
Ten S Second St, PO Box 1706
Reading, PA 19603
www.racc.edu
Prgm Dir: James H Cicman, BHS RRT
Tel: 610 372-4721, Ext 5435   *Fax:* 610 372-4264
E-mail: jcicman@racc.edu

Mansfield University
Cosponsor: Robert Packer Hospital
Respiratory Therapist (Advanced) Prgm
One Guthrie Square
Sayre, PA 18840
www.guthrie.org/RespRx
Prgm Dir: Larry Vosburgh, BS RRT
Tel: 570 882-4513   *Fax:* 570 882-6509
E-mail: vosburgh_larry@guthrie.org

Crozer-Keystone Medical Center
Cosponsor: Delaware County Community College
Respiratory Therapist (Advanced) Prgm
One Medical Center Blvd
Upland, PA 19013
Prgm Dir: Patti L Curran, MEd RRT RPFT
Tel: 610 447-2440   *Fax:* 610 447-6353
E-mail: Patti.Curran@Crozer.org

York College of Pennsylvania
Cosponsor: York Hospital
Respiratory Therapist (Advanced) Prgm
1001 S George St
York, PA 17405
www.wellspan.org
Prgm Dir: Mark Simmons, MSEd RPFT RRT-NPS
Tel: 717 851-2464   *Fax:* 717 851-2934
E-mail: msimmons@wellspan.org

Rhode Island

Community College of Rhode Island
Respiratory Therapist (Advanced) Prgm
1762 Louisquisset Pike
Lincoln, RI 02865-4585
www.ccri.edu/alliedhealth
Prgm Dir: Joanne Jacobs, MA RRT AE-C
Tel: 401 333-7024   *Fax:* 401 333-7441
E-mail: jjacobs@ccri.edu

South Carolina

Trident Technical College
Respiratory Therapist (Advanced) Prgm
PO Box 118067
7000 Rivers Ave
Charleston, SC 29423
www.tridenttech.edu
Prgm Dir: Ann R Moore, MS RRT CPFT
Tel: 843 574-6101   *Fax:* 843 574-6585
E-mail: ann.moore@tridenttech.edu

Midlands Technical College
Respiratory Therapist (Advanced) Prgm
PO Box 2408
Columbia, SC 29202
Prgm Dir: Linda H Ackerman, MA RRT
Tel: 803 822-3433   *Fax:* 803 822-3079
E-mail: ackermanl@midlandstech.edu

Florence-Darlington Technical College
Respiratory Therapist (Advanced) Prgm
PO Box 100548
Florence, SC 29501-0548
www.fdtc.edu
Prgm Dir: John A Evans, BS RRT
Tel: 843 661-8148   *Fax:* 843 661-8306
E-mail: john.evans@fdtc.edu

Greenville Technical College
Respiratory Therapist (Advanced) Prgm
PO Box 5616
Greenville, SC 29606
www.gvltec.edu
Prgm Dir: Jim Woody, MinED RRT
Tel: 864 228-5073   *Fax:* 864 228-5079
E-mail: Jim.Woody@gvltec.edu

Piedmont Technical College
Respiratory Therapist (Advanced) Prgm
PO Box 1467, Emerald Rd
Greenwood, SC 29647
Prgm Dir: Jane C Walker, BSN RN
Tel: 864 941-8526   *Fax:* 864 941-8684
E-mail: walker.j@ptc.edu

Tri-County Technical College
Respiratory Therapist (Advanced) Prgm
PO Box 587
Pendleton, SC 29670
Prgm Dir: Tom Baxter, MHRD RRT
Tel: 864 646-1354   *Fax:* 864 646-1892
E-mail: tbaxter@tctc.edu

Spartanburg Community College
Respiratory Therapist (Advanced) Prgm
PO Drawer 4386
Spartanburg, SC 29305-4386
Prgm Dir: Randall W Anderson, RRT
Tel: 864 592-4938   *Fax:* 864 592-4881
E-mail: andersonr@stcsc.edu

South Dakota

Dakota State University
Respiratory Therapist (Advanced) Prgm
Science Center
Madison, SD 57042-1799
www.dsu.edu
Prgm Dir: Bruce Feistner, MSS RRT
Tel: 605 322-8613   *Fax:* 605 322-6666
E-mail: bruce.feistner@dsu.edu

Tennessee

Chattanooga State Technical Comm College
Respiratory Therapist (Advanced) Prgm
4501 Amnicola Hwy
Chattanooga, TN 37406
Prgm Dir: Sharon Hall
Tel: 423 697-4772   *Fax:* 423 634-3071
E-mail: sharon.hall@chattanoogastate.edu

Columbia State Community College
Respiratory Therapist (Advanced) Prgm
1665 Hampshire Pike
Columbia, TN 38402
www.columbiastate.edu/respiratory
Prgm Dir: R David Johnson
Tel: 931 540-2663   *Fax:* 931 540-2795
E-mail: david.johnson@columbiastate.edu

East Tennessee State University
Respiratory Therapist (Advanced) Prgm
1000 West E St, ETSU Nave Center
Elizabethton, TN 37643
Prgm Dir: Douglas E Masini, EdD RPFT RRT FAARC
Tel: 423 547-4916   *Fax:* 423 547-4921
E-mail: masini@etsu.edu

Volunteer State Community College
Respiratory Therapist (Advanced) Prgm
1480 Nashville Pike
Gallatin, TN 37066-3188
www.volstate.edu
Prgm Dir: Cory E Martin, BS RRT
Tel: 888 335-8722, Ext 3349   *Fax:* 615 230-3224
E-mail: Cory.Martin@volstate.edu

Roane State Community College
Respiratory Therapist (Advanced) Prgm
276 Patton Ln
Harriman, TN 37748
www.roanestate.edu
Prgm Dir: Lesha Hill, BS RRT
Tel: 865 539-6904   *Fax:* 865 539-6907
E-mail: hillla@roanestate.edu

Jackson State Community College
Respiratory Therapist (Advanced) Prgm
2046 N Parkway St
Jackson, TN 38301-3797
www.jscc.edu
Prgm Dir: Cathy K Garner, MS RRT-NPS
Tel: 731 424-3520, Ext 235   *Fax:* 731 425-9551
E-mail: cgarner@jscc.edu

Baptist College of Health Sciences
Respiratory Therapist (Advanced) Prgm
1003 Monroe Ave
Memphis, TN 38104
www.bchs.edu
Prgm Dir: Brian J Parker, MPH RRT-NPS RPFT AE-C
Tel: 901 572-2568   *Fax:* 901 572-2750
E-mail: brian.parker@bchs.edu

Concorde Career College - Memphis
Respiratory Therapist (Advanced) Prgm
5100 Poplar Ave, Ste 132
Memphis, TN 38137
Prgm Dir: Michael Camp, BS RRT
Tel: 901 761-9494   *Fax:* 901 843-9442
E-mail: mcamp@concorde.edu

Tennessee State University
Respiratory Therapist (Advanced) Prgm
3500 John A Merritt Blvd
Nashville, TN 37209
Prgm Dir: Thomas John, PhD RRT
Tel: 615 963-7420   *Fax:* 615 963-7422
E-mail: tjohn@tnstate.edu

Texas

Alvin Community College
Respiratory Therapist (Advanced) Prgm
3110 Mustang Rd
Alvin, TX 77511
www.alvincollege.edu
Prgm Dir: Diane Flatland, MS RRT-NPS CPFT LP
Tel: 281 756-3658   *Fax:* 281 756-3860
E-mail: dflatland@alvincollege.edu

Amarillo College
Respiratory Therapist (Advanced) Prgm
PO Box 447
Amarillo, TX 79178
www.actx.edu/respiratory
Prgm Dir: William A Young, MS RRT
Tel: 806 354-6058   *Fax:* 806 354-6076
E-mail: young-wa@actx.edu

Lamar Institute of Technology
Respiratory Therapist (Advanced) Prgm
PO Box 10061
Beaumont, TX 77710
Prgm Dir: Gwen Walden, BS RRT NPS CPFT RCP
Tel: 409 880-8852   *Fax:* 409 880-8955
E-mail: gwen.walden@lit.edu

Univ Tx at Brownsville/Tx Southmost Coll
Respiratory Therapist (Advanced) Prgm
83 Ft Brown
Brownsville, TX 78520
Prgm Dir: John L McCabe, PhD RRT
Tel: 956 554-5010   *Fax:* 956 554-5012
E-mail: john.mccabe@utb.edu

Del Mar College
Respiratory Therapist (Advanced) Prgm
101 Baldwin Blvd
Corpus Christi, TX 78404
Prgm Dir: Jeffrey T Watson, BA RRT-NPS
Tel: 361 698-2835   *Fax:* 361 698-2811
E-mail: jwatson@delmar.edu

ATI-Career Training
Respiratory Therapist (Advanced) Prgm
10003 Technology Blvd West
Dallas, TX 75220
Prgm Dir: Rudy Schatke, MS RRT RCP
Tel: 214 902-8191, Ext 201   *Fax:* 214 366-0881
E-mail: rschatke@atienterprises.edu

El Centro College
Respiratory Therapist (Advanced) Prgm
Main and Lamar Sts
Dallas, TX 75202
Prgm Dir: Gary L Peschka, MEd RRT RCP
Tel: 214 860-2279   *Fax:* 214 860-2268
E-mail: glp5547@dcccd.edu

University of Texas Medical Branch
Respiratory Therapist (Advanced) Prgm
School of Allied Health Sciences
301 University Blvd
Galveston, TX 77555-1146
www.sahs.utmb.edu/programs/rc/
Prgm Dir: Jon O Nilsestuen, PhD RRT FAARC
Tel: 409 772-5693   *Fax:* 409 772-3014
E-mail: jnilsest@utmb.edu

Houston Community College
Respiratory Therapist (Advanced) Prgm
1900 Galen Dr
Houston, TX 77030
Prgm Dir: Romar S Reyes, MEd RRT
Tel: 713 718-7384   *Fax:* 713 718-7136
E-mail: romar.reyes@hccs.edu

Texas Southern University
Respiratory Therapist (Advanced) Prgm
3100 Cleburne Ave
Houston, TX 77004
Prgm Dir: Reginald G Allen
Tel: 713 313-7265, Ext 7377   *Fax:* 713 313-1094
E-mail: allen_rg@tsu.edu

Tarrant County College - Northeast Campus
Respiratory Therapist (Advanced) Prgm
828 Harwood Rd
Hurst, TX 76054
Prgm Dir: John D Hiser, MEd RRT FAARC
Tel: 817 515-6574   *Fax:* 817 515-6700
E-mail: john.hiser@tccd.edu

Kingwood College - NHMCCD
Respiratory Therapist (Advanced) Prgm
20,000 Kingwood Dr
Kingwood, TX 77339
www.nhmccd.edu
Prgm Dir: Kenny P McCowen, RRT
Tel: 281 312-1608   *Fax:* 281 312-1490
E-mail: kmccowen@nhmccd.edu

South Plains College
Respiratory Therapist (Advanced) Prgm
Reese Center
819 Gilbert Dr
Lubbock, TX 79416
www.southplainscollege.edu
Prgm Dir: Khris Segrist, BS RRT
Tel: 806 885-3048, Ext 4625   *Fax:* 806 885-5608
E-mail: ksegrist@southplainscollege.edu

Angelina College
Respiratory Therapist (Advanced) Prgm
PO Box 1768
Lufkin, TX 75902-1768
Prgm Dir: Michael Parks, MEd RRT
Tel: 936 633-5419
E-mail: mparks@angelina.edu

Collin County Community College
Respiratory Therapist (Advanced) Prgm
2200 W University Dr
McKinney, TX 75071
www.ccccd.edu/rcp
Prgm Dir: Abe Johnson, ThM RRT RCP
Tel: 972 548-6870   *Fax:* 972 548-6722
E-mail: ajohnson@ccccd.edu

Midland College
Respiratory Therapist (Advanced) Prgm
3600 N Garfield
Midland, TX 79705
www.midland.edu
Prgm Dir: Robert Weidmann, BS RPFT RRT-NPS RCP
Tel: 432 685-5549   *Fax:* 432 685-5575
E-mail: rweidmann@midland.edu

San Jacinto College Central
Respiratory Therapist (Advanced) Prgm
8060 Spencer Hwy, PO Box 2007
Pasadena, TX 77505-2007
http://sjcd.edu
Prgm Dir: Larry P Vandiver, MPH RRT
Tel: 281 476-1864   *Fax:* 281 478-2754
E-mail: larry.vandiver@sjcd.edu

Univ of Texas Hlth Sci Ctr at San Antonio
Respiratory Therapist (Advanced) Prgm
7703 Floyd Curl Dr MC6248
San Antonio, TX 78229-3900
Prgm Dir: David Vines
Tel: 210 567-8850   *Fax:* 210 567-8852
E-mail: vines@uthscsa.edu

Texas State University - San Marcos
Respiratory Therapist (Advanced) Prgm
601 University Dr
Health Professions Bldg, Rm 350A
San Marcos, TX 78666-4616
www.health.txstate.edu/RC
Prgm Dir: S Gregory Marshall, PhD RRT RPSGT
Tel: 512 245-8243   *Fax:* 512 245-7978
E-mail: sm10@txstate.edu

Temple College
Respiratory Therapist (Advanced) Prgm
2600 S First St
Temple, TX 76504
www.templejc.edu
Prgm Dir: William M Cornelius III, MHSM RRT-NPS
Tel: 254 298-8928   *Fax:* 254 298-8676
E-mail: bill.cornel@templejc.edu

Tyler Junior College
Respiratory Therapist (Advanced) Prgm
PO Box 9020
Tyler, TX 75711
Prgm Dir: Marty Partida, MHA RRT-NPS
Tel: 903 510-2481   *Fax:* 903 510-2592
E-mail: mpar@tjc.edu

Victoria College
Respiratory Therapist (Advanced) Prgm
2200 E Red River
Victoria, TX 77901
Prgm Dir: Chris E Kallus, MEd RRT RCP
Tel: 361 572-6491   *Fax:* 361 582-2542
E-mail: chris.kallus@victoriacollege.edu

Weatherford College
Respiratory Therapist (Advanced) Prgm
225 College Park Dr
Weatherford, TX 76086
Prgm Dir: Tonya Edwards, BS RRT RPFT RCP
Tel: 817 594-5471, Ext 452   *Fax:* 817 598-6455
E-mail: edwardst@wc.edu

Midwestern State University
Respiratory Therapist (Advanced) Prgm
3410 Taft Blvd
Wichita Falls, TX 76308
Prgm Dir: Ann Medford, MA RRT
Tel: 940 397-4653   *Fax:* 940 397-4513
E-mail: ann.medford@mwsu.edu

Utah

Stevens-Henager College
Respiratory Therapist (Advanced) Prgm
383 W Vine St
5831 S Royalton Dr
Murray, UT 84107
http://stevenshenager.edu
Prgm Dir: Max Eskelson, RRT BSBA
Tel: 801 281-7600, Ext 3042
E-mail: max.eskelson@intermountainmail.com

Weber State University
Respiratory Therapist (Advanced) Prgm
3904 University Circle
Ogden, UT 84408-3904
http://weber.edu/dchp.xml
Prgm Dir: Paul Eberle, PhD RRT
Tel: 801 626-6840   *Fax:* 801 626-7075
E-mail: peberle@weber.edu

Vermont

Vermont Technical College
Respiratory Therapist (Advanced) Prgm
201 Lawrence Place, Box 1A
Williston, VT 05495
www.vtc.edu
Prgm Dir: Faye Bacon, MEd RRT
Tel: 802 879-5972   *Fax:* 802 879-5645
E-mail: fbacon@vtc.edu

Virginia

Mountain Empire Community College
Respiratory Therapist (Advanced) Prgm
3441 Mountain Empire Rd
Big Stone Gap, VA 24219
www.me.vccs.edu/programs/aas-degrees/respiratory.pdf
Prgm Dir: Michael W Cook, MA RRT
Tel: 540 523-2400, Ext 277   *Fax:* 540 523-5458
E-mail: mcook@me.vccs.edu

Central Virginia Community College
Respiratory Therapist (Advanced) Prgm
3506 Wards Rd
Lynchburg, VA 24502
www.cvcc.vccs.edu
Prgm Dir: Martha N Crawley, MEd RRT
Tel: 804 832-7685   *Fax:* 804 832-7835
E-mail: crawleym@cvcc.vccs.edu

Southwest Virginia Community College
Respiratory Therapist (Advanced) Prgm
Box SVCC
Richlands, VA 24641-1101
www.sw.edu/sarc
Prgm Dir: Joseph S DiPietro, PhD RRT
Tel: 276 964-7306   *Fax:* 276 964-7715
E-mail: Joe.DiPietro@sw.edu

J Sargeant Reynolds Community College
Respiratory Therapist (Advanced) Prgm
PO Box 85622
Richmond, VA 23285-5622
www.reynolds.edu
Prgm Dir: Nakia Austin, RRT
Tel: 804 523-5009   *Fax:* 804 786-5298
E-mail: naustin@reynolds.edu

Jefferson College of Health Sciences
Respiratory Therapist (Advanced) Prgm
920 S Jefferson St, PO Box 13186
Roanoke, VA 24031
Prgm Dir: Sharon Hatfield, RRT
Tel: 540 985-8263   *Fax:* 540 985-9773
E-mail: shatfield@jchs.edu

Northern Virginia Community College
Respiratory Therapist (Advanced) Prgm
6699 Springfield Center Dr
Springfield, VA 22150
www.nvcc.edu/medical/health/respiratory/
Prgm Dir: Kathy Grilliot, MS Ed RRT-NPS
Tel: 703 822-6563   *Fax:* 703 822-6619
E-mail: kgrilliot@nvcc.edu

Tidewater Community College
Respiratory Therapist (Advanced) Prgm
1700 College Crescent
Virginia Beach, VA 23456
Prgm Dir: Gary Cross, BS RRT
Tel: 757 822-7263   *Fax:* 757 427-1338
E-mail: gcross@tcc.edu

Shenandoah University
Respiratory Therapist (Advanced) Prgm
1775 N Sector Ct
Winchester, VA 22601-5195
Prgm Dir: William A O'Neill, MA RRT
Tel: 540 665-5516   *Fax:* 540 665-5519
E-mail: woneill@su.edu

Washington

Highline Community College
Respiratory Therapist (Advanced) Prgm
2400 S 240th St
Des Moines, WA 98198-9800
Prgm Dir: Robert W Hirnle
Tel: 206 878-3710, Ext 3471   *Fax:* 206 870-3780
E-mail: bhirnle@highline.edu

Seattle Central Community College
Respiratory Therapist (Advanced) Prgm
1701 Broadway, 2BE3210
Seattle, WA 98122
Prgm Dir: Robert I C McCallum, BS RRT
Tel: 206 587-4056   *Fax:* 206 587-6337
E-mail: rmccallum@sccd.ctc.edu

Spokane Community College
Respiratory Therapist (Advanced) Prgm
N 1810 Greene St
Spokane, WA 99217
www.scc.spokane.edu/?resp
Prgm Dir: Gary White, MEd RRT RPFT
Tel: 509 533-7310   *Fax:* 509 533-8621
E-mail: gwhite@scc.spokane.edu

Tacoma Community College
Respiratory Therapist (Advanced) Prgm
6501 S 19th St
Tacoma, WA 98466
Prgm Dir: Ken Lizzi, MPH RRT
Tel: 253 566-5231   *Fax:* 253 566-5273
E-mail: klizzi@tacomacc.edu

West Virginia

Carver Career Center
Respiratory Therapist (Advanced) Prgm
4799 Midland Dr
Charleston, WV 25306
Prgm Dir: Donna Peters, BA RRT
Tel: 304 348-1965, Ext 115   *Fax:* 304 348-1938
E-mail: peters_946@hotmail.com

West Virginia Northern Community College
Respiratory Therapist (Advanced) Prgm
1704 Market St
Wheeling, WV 26003
Prgm Dir: Ralph C Lucki, MEd RRT
Tel: 304 233-5900, Ext 5511   *Fax:* 304 232-8185
E-mail: rlucki@northern.wvnet.edu

Wheeling Jesuit University
Respiratory Therapist (Advanced) Prgm
316 Washington Ave
Wheeling, WV 26003
www.wju.edu
Prgm Dir: Marybeth Emmerth, MS RRT CPFT
Tel: 304 243-2208   *Fax:* 304 243-6246
E-mail: memmerth@wju.edu

Wisconsin

Chippewa Valley Technical College
Respiratory Therapist (Advanced) Prgm
620 W Clairemont Ave
Eau Claire, WI 54701
Prgm Dir: Terry L Gonderzik
Tel: 715 833-6200
E-mail: tgonderzik@cvtc.edu

Northeast Wisconsin Technical College
Respiratory Therapist (Advanced) Prgm
2740 W Mason St, PO Box 19042
Green Bay, WI 54307
Prgm Dir: Katherine A Schlitz
Tel: 920 498-5533   *Fax:* 920 498-5673
E-mail: katherine.schlitz@nwtc.edu

Western Technical College
Respiratory Therapist (Advanced) Prgm
304 N Sixth St, PO Box C-908
La Crosse, WI 54602-0908
Prgm Dir: Robert A Milisch, MEd RRT
Tel: 608 785-9244   *Fax:* 608 785-9087
E-mail: milischr@wwtc.edu

Madison Area Technical College
Respiratory Therapist (Advanced) Prgm
3550 Anderson St
Madison, WI 53704
www.matcmadison.edu
Prgm Dir: Gail Walker, MS RRT
Tel: 608 246-6698   *Fax:* 608 246-6013
E-mail: gwalker@matcmadison.edu

Mid-State Technical College
Respiratory Therapist (Advanced) Prgm
2600 W Fifth St
Marshfield, WI 54449
www.mstc.edu
Prgm Dir: Barbara Hughes, RRT MS
Tel: 715 389-7053   *Fax:* 715 389-2864
E-mail: barbara.hughes@mstc.edu

Milwaukee Area Technical College
Respiratory Therapist (Advanced) Prgm
700 W State St
Milwaukee, WI 53233
Prgm Dir: Mark J Hoffman, MS RRT
Tel: 414 297-7130   *Fax:* 414 297-7990
E-mail: HoffmanM@matc.edu

Respiratory Therapist (Advanced)

Programs*	Class Capacity	Begins	Length (months)	Award	Res. Tuition	Non-res. Tuition	Stipend	Offers:‡ 1	2	3	4
Alabama											
Shelton State Community College (Tuscaloosa)	35	Aug	17, 24	AAS	$2,573	$4,445					
University of South Alabama (Mobile)	30	Aug	24	BS	$4,422	$8,844					
Wallace State Community College (Hanceville)	35	Aug	21	AAS	$2,160	$4,320					
Arizona											
GateWay Community College (Phoenix)	30	Aug Jan	24	AAS	$2,400	$10,320					
Kaplan College (Phoenix)	20	13x/yr	18, 24	AOS	$15,030	$15,030		•			
Pima Community College (Tucson)	28	Aug 22	22	AAS	$1,750	$6,752				•	
Pima Medical Institute - Mesa	30	Feb Jun Oct	24	Dipl, AS	$24,575	$0				•	
Arkansas											
NorthWest Arkansas Community College (Bentonville)	14	Aug	21	AAS	$5,250	$7,900			•	•	
Southeast Arkansas College (Pine Bluff)	16	Aug	16	AAS	$2,300	$4,600					
University of Arkansas for Medical Sciences (Little Rock)	24	Aug	21, 36	BS	$6,086	$13,974					•
University of Arkansas for Medical Sciences (Texarkana)	12	Aug	21, 33	BS	$5,783	$14,457					•
California											
Butte College (Oroville)	24	Aug	22	Cert, AS	$772	$6,272				•	
California College San Diego	60	Apr Sep	18, 24	AS, BS	$18,000	$0					
Crafton Hills College (Yucaipa)	30	Aug	12, 24	Cert, AS	$650	$6,337					
Grossmont College (El Cajon)	45	Aug	18	AS	$663	$3,850				•	
Loma Linda University	20	Sep	21	Cert, BS	$22,440	$22,440				•	
Orange Coast College (Costa Mesa)	28	Aug	22	AS	$754	$4,466					
San Joaquin Valley College (Rancho Cucamonga)	30	Aug	17	AS	$25,200	$25,200					
San Joaquin Valley College - Bakersfield	24	Varies	18	AS	$11,685	$0					
San Joaquin Valley College - Visalia	24	Varies	18	AS	$11,445	$0					
Colorado											
Pima Medical Institute - Denver	24	Apr Aug Dec	22	AOS	$24,340	$24,340				•	
Pueblo Community College	35	Aug	20	AAS	$2,118	$8,586					•
Connecticut											
Naugatuck Valley Community College (Waterbury)	37	Sep	24	AS	$2,828	$8,444			•	•	
Norwalk Hospital/Norwalk Community College	15	Sep	24	AS	$2,232	$6,696				•	
University of Hartford (West Hartford)	15	Sep	48	Cert, BS	$25,800	$0		•		•	
Delaware											
Delaware Tech & Comm Coll - Owens Campus (Georgetown)	20	Jun	24	AAS	$3,258	$8,145					
Delaware Technical & Community College - Wilmington	15	Aug	24	AAS	$2,376	$5,940				•	
Florida											
Daytona Beach Community College	28	Aug	21	AAS	$2,650	$10,010				•	
Gulf Coast Community College (Panama City)	16	Aug	21	AAS	$1,627	$6,243					
Indian River Community College (Fort Pierce)	17	Aug	21	AS	$2,400	$8,850					
Seminole Community College (Sanford)	24	Aug	20	AS	$3,000	$8,000		•			
University of Central Florida (Orlando)	20	Aug	20	BS	$3,432	$13,254				•	•
Valencia Community College (Orlando)	24	Jan	20	AS	$5,297	$19,912		•			
Georgia											
Armstrong Atlantic State University (Savannah)	20	Aug	21	BS	$3,804	$15,216		•			
Coosa Valley Technical College (Rome)	22	Apr	24	AAS	$1,500	$3,000				•	
Darton College (Albany)	20	Aug	21	AAS	$4,000	$0				•	
Georgia State University (Atlanta)	50	Aug	22	BS, MS	$163	$649				•	•
Griffin Technical College	20	Jul	14	AS	$1,528	$3,056					
Gwinnett Technical College (Lawrenceville)	20	Mar	15	AAS	$1,900	$3,388					
Southwest Georgia Technical College (Thomasville)	20	Jul	24	AAS	$1,208	$2,416		•			•
Idaho											
Boise State University	24	Aug	33	AS, BS	$5,100	$13,000				•	•
Illinois											
Kankakee Community College	16	Jan	24	Dipl, Cert, AAS	$3,600	$6,195				•	•
Kaskaskia College (Centralia)	24	Aug	21	AAS	$2,318	$4,446					
Moraine Valley Community College (Palos Hills)	32	Aug	21	AAS	$2,664	$7,659				•	
Rock Valley College (Rockford)	15	Aug	22	AAS	$2,450	$8,600		•			
Southern Illinois University Carbondale	25	Aug	16, 28	Cert, AAS	$7,205	$18,273				•	
Southwestern Illinois College (Belleville)	30	Aug	22	Dipl, AAS	$4,828	$19,925				•	
Indiana											
Clarian Health Partners Inc (Indianapolis)	30	Aug	48	BS	$182	$362				•	
Ivy Tech Community College - Ft Wayne	28	Aug	21	AS	$3,171	$6,412		•			
Ivy Tech Community College - Lafayette	60	Aug	21	AS	$3,600	$6,413		•			•
Ivy Tech Community College - Michigan City	20	Aug	20	AS	$6,405	$13,030				•	
Ivy Tech Community College - Terre Haute	14	Aug	34	AS	$91	$185					
University of Southern Indiana (Evansville)	14	Aug	24	AS	$5,835	$13,903					

*Data are shown only for programs that completed the 2007 AMA Survey of Health Professions Education Programs.
‡Key to Offers: 1: Evening or weekend classes; 2: Non-English instruction; 3: Cultural competence instruction; 4: Distance education component.

Respiratory Therapist (Advanced)

Programs*	Class Capacity	Begins	Length (months)	Award	Res. Tuition	Non-res. Tuition	Stipend	1	2	3	4
Iowa											
Des Moines Area Community College (Ankeny)	24	Aug	23	AAS	$4,055	$8,110				•	
Hawkeye Community College (Waterloo)	20	Aug	22	AAS	$8,058	$16,117					
Southeastern Community College (West Burlington)	20	Aug	22	AAS	$6,000	$7,000				•	
St Luke's College (Sioux City)	14	Aug	22	AS	$14,400	$0					
Kansas											
Johnson County Community College (Overland Park)	20	Jun	24	AAS	$2,400	$5,400		•		•	
Labette Community College (Parsons)	25	Aug	22	Dipl, AAS	$2,800	$3,400				•	
Newman University (Wichita)	20	Aug	28	ASHS	$17,008	$17,008				•	
Seward County Community College (Liberal)	18	Aug	24	AAS	$4,650	$6,375					•
Washburn University (Topeka)	18	Aug	22	AS	$7,122	$15,669					•
Kentucky											
Big Sandy Community & Technical College (Paintsville)	25	Aug	24	AAS	$115	$345		•		•	•
Jefferson Community and Technical College (Louisville)	20	Aug	19	AAS	$3,510	$5,235	$60			•	
Northern Kentucky University (Highland Heights)	16	Aug	21	AAS	$5,950	$11,400					
Southeast Kentucky Comm & Tech College (Pineville)	24	Aug	22	AAS	$3,335	$7,000		•			•
Louisiana											
Louisiana State Univ Health Sciences Center (New Orleans)	15	May	24	BS, MHS	$5,035	$8,160				•	
Nicholls State University (Houma)	15	Aug	10	Cert, AS, BS	$3,555	$9,003					
Our Lady of Holy Cross College (New Orleans)	8	Aug	14	BS	$6,720	$6,720				•	
Maine											
Kennebec Valley Community College (Fairfield)	14	Sep	18	AS	$3,034	$6,355		•		•	
Southern Maine Community College (South Portland)	20	Sep	21	AS	$2,900	$5,800					
Maryland											
Allegany College of Maryland (Cumberland)	24	Aug Sep	17	AAS	$3,690	$8,282					
Baltimore City Community College	25	Aug	20	AAS	$1,673	$3,923					
Prince George's Community College (Largo)	24	Aug	21	AAS	$2,967	$7,349				•	
Salisbury University	30	Sep	24	BS	$4,974	$10,908					
Massachusetts											
Berkshire Community College (Pittsfield)	20	Sep Jan	17	Dipl, AS	$3,900	$8,350		•			
Massasoit Community College (Brockton)	28	Sep	18	Cert, AS	$4,180	$12,046				•	
Northeastern University (Boston)	20	Sep	16	MS	$19,071	$19,071		•			
Quinsigamond Community College (Worcester)	20	Sep	18	AS	$120	$326		•		•	
Michigan											
Ferris State University (Big Rapids)	24	Aug	24	AAS	$7,200	$14,640		•		•	•
Macomb Community College (Clinton Township)	40	Aug	21	AAS	$2,448	$3,744				•	
Muskegon Community College	30	Sep	28	AAS	$5,500	$7,000		•			•
Minnesota											
College of St Catherine - Minneapolis	16	Sep	48	BA/BS	$18,000	$18,000				•	
Mayo School of Health Sciences (Rochester)	20	Sep	24	Dipl, BAS	$9,000	$9,000				•	•
Northland Community & Technical College (East Grand Forks)	25	Aug	27	AAS	$4,913	$9,826		•		•	
Mississippi											
Copiah-Lincoln Community College (Natchez)	15	Aug	12, 21	AS	$1,800	$3,600					
Itawamba Community College (Fulton)	16	Aug	17	AAS	$600	$1,475					
Meridian Community College	15	Aug	21	AAS	$1,750	$2,640					
Northeast Mississippi Community College (Booneville)	15	Aug	22	AAS	$915	$1,830					
Missouri											
Concorde Career College - Kansas City	10	Fall Spring	6	Cert	$6,516	$6,516					
Hannibal Career & Technical Center	20	Aug	24	AAS	$240	$240				•	
Ozarks Technical Community College (Springfield)	20	Aug	21	AAS	$2,964	$4,864				•	
Montana											
Montana State Univ - Great Falls Coll of Tech	15	Sep	20	AAS	$3,486	$10,096					
University of Montana (Missoula)	16	Aug	24	AAS	$3,298	$8,959				•	
Nebraska											
Alegent Health (Omaha)	15	Aug	11	Cert, BS	$20,000	$20,000				•	
Metropolitan Community College (Omaha)	21	Sep	21	AAS	$3,500	$5,000					
NE Methodist Coll Nursing & Allied Hlth (Omaha)	14	Aug Jan Jun	24, 48	AS, BS	$11,940	$11,940			•	•	•
Southeast Community College (Lincoln)	30	Jul Mar	18	AAS	$6,463	$6,888				•	•
Nevada											
College of Southern Nevada (Las Vegas)	35	Sep	22	AAS	$1,450	$4,100		•		•	•
New Hampshire											
New Hampshire Comm Tech Coll - Claremont	15	Sep	21	AS	$12,768	$27,396					•
New Jersey											
Bergen Community College (Paramus)	30	Sep	22	Cert, AAS	$3,869	$7,263					
Brookdale Community College (Lincroft)	25	Sep	18	AAS	$3,090	$6,750				•	

*Data are shown only for programs that completed the 2007 AMA Survey of Health Professions Education Programs.

‡Key to Offers: 1: Evening or weekend classes; 2: Non-English instruction; 3: Cultural competence instruction; 4: Distance education component.

Respiratory Therapist (Advanced)

Programs*	Class Capacity	Begins	Length (months)	Award	Res. Tuition	Non-res. Tuition	Stipend	Offers:‡ 1	2	3	4
Univ of Medicine & Dent of New Jersey (Newark)	32	May	12, 15	AS, BS	$7,500	$15,000				•	
New Mexico											
Eastern New Mexico University - Roswell Campus	20	Aug	18	AS	$684	$1,944				•	•
New York											
Molloy College (Rockville Centre)	28	Sep	24	AAS	$17,640	$17,640					
Nassau Community College (Garden City)	24	Sep	24	AAS	$3,310	$6,620		•		•	
Onondaga Community College (Syracuse)	25	Jan	24	AAS	$3,742	$7,485		•		•	•
SUNY Upstate Medical University (Syracuse)	20	Aug	21	BS	$4,350	$10,610		•		•	•
Westchester Community College (Valhalla)	36	Sep	24	AAS	$3,350	$8,376		•			
North Carolina											
Carteret Community College (Morehead City)	25	Aug	22	AAS	$1,895	$10,121				•	•
Catawba Valley Community College (Hickory)	15	Aug	21	AAS	$1,722	$9,561		•			
Central Piedmont Community College (Charlotte)	25	Aug	21	AAS	$1,422	$7,110					
Durham Technical Community College	25	Aug	21	AAS	$1,896	$11,199				•	
Edgecombe Community College (Rocky Mount)	15	Aug	21	AAS	$2,016	$11,198					
Forsyth Technical Community College (Winston-Salem)	25	Aug	21	AAS	$1,580	$8,780				•	
Pitt Community College (Greenville)	18	Aug	21	AAS	$39	$219				•	
Sandhills Community College (Pinehurst)	18	Aug	21	AAS	$1,216	$6,752					
Southwestern Community College (Sylva)	17	Aug	21	AAS	$1,302	$6,336				•	
Stanly Community College (Albemarle)	24	Aug	21	AAS	$1,600	$8,000		•			
North Dakota											
NDSU/MeritCare Hospital Consortium (Fargo)	12	May	13	Cert, BS	$4,774	$12,747					
University of Mary/St Alexius Medical Ctr (Bismarck)	10	Aug	20	Cert, BS	$14,000	$14,000				•	
Ohio											
Bowling Green State University (Huron)	30	Aug	28	AAS	$5,448	$14,850		•		•	•
Collins Career Center (Chesapeake)	24	Aug	22	Dipl, AAS	$5,550	$5,550				•	
Columbus State Community College	35	Sep	21	AAS	$4,385	$9,625				•	
Jefferson Community College (Steubenville)	21	Aug	21	AAS	$3,060	$4,182				•	
Kettering College of Medical Arts	24	Aug	22	AS	$0	$14,858				•	•
Lakeland Community College (Kirtland)	20	Aug	21	AAS	$3,685	$9,657		•			
North Central State College (Mansfield)	24	Sep	21	AAS	$4,194	$8,388		•			
Rhodes State College (Lima)	26	Jul	24	AAS	$6,091	$12,183				•	
Sinclair Community College (Dayton)	50	Sep	21	AAS	$2,271	$3,710					
Stark State College of Technology (Canton)	20	Aug	21	AAS	$127	$187		•			
University of Toledo	25	May	24	BS	$6,816	$15,627		•			•
Washington State Community College (Marietta)	24	Sep	21	AAS	$4,290	$8,580		•	•		
Youngstown State University	20	Aug	46	Cert, BSRC	$7,509	$12,717		•	•		
Oklahoma											
Rose State College (Midwest City)	24	Aug	12	AAS	$3,765	$7,470				•	•
Oregon											
Lane Community College (Eugene)	20	Sep	21	AAS	$3,540	$12,174	$1,485	•		•	
Mt Hood Community College (Gresham)	30	Sep	18	Cert, AAS	$3,013	$9,821					
Pennsylvania											
Comm College of Allegheny County (Pittsburgh)	35	Aug	22	AS	$3,400	$6,500					
Community College of Philadelphia	36	Sep	22	Cert, AAS	$5,000	$10,000		•		•	
Crozer-Keystone Medical Center (Upland)	16	Sep	22	AAS	$4,998	$12,117		•			
Gannon University (Erie)	16	Aug	24, 48	Cert, AS, BS	$22,110	$22,110					
Luzerne County Community College (Nanticoke)	24	Jun	24	AAS	$3,200	$6,400					
Mansfield University (Sayre)	20	Aug	21	AAS	$5,038	$12,598		•		•	
Millersville University of Pennsylvania	10	Aug	16	Cert, BS	$5,190	$12,974				•	
Reading Area Community College	20	Jun Sep Jan Mar	12, 24	Cert, AAS	$2,448	$4,896					
University of Pittsburgh - Johnstown	30	Sep	20	Dipl, Cert, AS	$10,888	$21,136				•	
West Chester University (Bryn Mawr)	25	Aug	48	BS	$4,906	$12,266					•
York College of Pennsylvania	12	Sep	36, 48	AS, BS	$12,000	$12,000					
Rhode Island											
Community College of Rhode Island (Lincoln)	24	Jun	24	AAS	$2,390	$7,000				•	
South Carolina											
Florence-Darlington Technical College	20	Aug	24	AS	$5,178	$7,929					
Greenville Technical College	25	Aug	24	AS	$4,785	$5,187				•	
Trident Technical College (Charleston)	24	May	24	AS	$4,671	$5,187					
South Dakota											
Dakota State University (Madison)	32	Sep Jun	21, 44	AS, BS	$3,635	$5,450				•	
Tennessee											
Baptist College of Health Sciences (Memphis)	10	Aug	22	BHS	$6,900	$6,900		•		•	•
Columbia State Community College	24	Aug	21	AAS	$2,100	$8,500					
Jackson State Community College	20	Aug	21	AAS	$2,617	$9,693				•	

*Data are shown only for programs that completed the 2007 AMA Survey of Health Professions Education Programs.
‡Key to Offers: 1: Evening or weekend classes; 2: Non-English instruction; 3: Cultural competence instruction; 4: Distance education component.

Respiratory Therapist (Advanced)

Programs*	Class Capacity	Begins	Length (months)	Award	Res. Tuition	Non-res. Tuition	Stipend	Offers:‡ 1	2	3	4
Roane State Community College (Harriman)	20	Aug	21	AAS	$1,115	$3,338					
Volunteer State Community College (Gallatin)	14	Aug	4, 8	Cert	$100	$378					•
Texas											
Alvin Community College	22	Aug	21	AAS	$2,733	$5,466				•	
Amarillo College	21	Aug	23	AAS	$1,773	$3,573					
Angelina College (Lufkin)	20	Aug	21	AAS	$546	$1,096					
Collin County Community College (McKinney)	25	Aug	22	Cert, AAS	$1,406	$4,028					
Del Mar College (Corpus Christi)	18	Sep	21	AAS	$2,500	$5,000					
Kingwood College - NHMCCD	24	Jan Sep	24	AAS	$2,976	$5,616		•		•	
Midland College	20	Aug	20, 23	AAS	$1,759	$2,155					
San Jacinto College Central (Pasadena)	30	Aug	24	AAS	$1,790	$2,865				•	
South Plains College (Lubbock)	30	Aug	22	AAS	$2,500	$2,800				•	
Tarrant County College - Northeast Campus (Hurst)	30	Aug	21	AAS	$2,050	$2,583					
Temple College	25	Aug	24	Cert, AAS	$2,634	$6,170				•	
Texas State University - San Marcos	40	Sep	48	Cert, BSRC	$5,866	$13,882				•	•
Tyler Junior College	30	Aug	16	AAS	$3,200	$5,800		•		•	
University of Texas Medical Branch (Galveston)	25	Aug	24	BSRC	$2,200	$14,432				•	•
Victoria College	18	Aug	21	AAS	$1,614	$2,514				•	•
Utah											
Stevens-Henager College (Murray)	25	Every 9 mos	22, 30	Dipl, AS, BSRT	$38,500	$0		•		•	•
Weber State University (Ogden)	20	Aug	33	AS, BS	$3,500	$10,500				•	
Vermont											
Vermont Technical College (Williston)	27	Aug	18	AS	$8,760	$16,704				•	
Virginia											
Central Virginia Community College (Lynchburg)	20	Aug	21	AAS	$1,506	$6,486				•	
J Sargeant Reynolds Community College (Richmond)	36	Jan	7	Cert	$2,323	$7,052		•			
Mountain Empire Community College (Big Stone Gap)	30	Jun	18	AAS	$5,987	$12,668					
Northern Virginia Community College (Springfield)	45	Aug	22, 23	AAS	$3,800	$14,450				•	
Southwest Virginia Community College (Richlands)	24	Aug	22	AAS	$2,616	$8,719		•		•	
Washington											
Spokane Community College	24	Sep	22	AAS	$3,000	$8,034				•	
Tacoma Community College	24	Jun	24	AAS	$3,272	$9,185				•	
West Virginia											
Carver Career Center (Charleston)	25	Jul	22	Dipl, AS	$4,150	$4,150		•		•	
West Virginia Northern Community College (Wheeling)	40	Aug	21	AAS	$1,824	$5,808		•		•	
Wheeling Jesuit University	12	Sep	48	BS	$21,000	$21,000				•	
Wisconsin											
Madison Area Technical College	26	Aug	22	AAS	$5,003	$15,121					•
Mid-State Technical College (Marshfield)	24	Aug	22	AS	$3,125	$15,932		•		•	

*Data are shown only for programs that completed the 2007 AMA Survey of Health Professions Education Programs.
‡Key to Offers: 1: Evening or weekend classes; 2: Non-English instruction; 3: Cultural competence instruction; 4: Distance education component.

PROGRAMS

Respiratory Therapist (Entry-Level)

Arkansas

Univ of Arkansas Comm Coll - Hope
Respiratory Therapist (Entry-Level) Prgm
Hwy 29 S, PO Box 140
Hope, AR 71801
www.uacch.edu
Prgm Dir: Ken LeJeune, MS RRT
Tel: 870 722-8275   *Fax:* 870 777-5957
E-mail: klejeune@uacch.edu

Black River Technical College
Respiratory Therapist (Entry-Level) Prgm
PO Box 468
Hwy 304 East
Pocahontas, AR 72455
Prgm Dir: Eric G Johnson, BS RRT
Tel: 870 248-4000, Ext 4153   *Fax:* 870 248-4100
E-mail: eric.johnson@blackrivertech.edu

California

Hacienda LaPuente Adult Education
Respiratory Therapist (Entry-Level) Prgm
Excelsior College
Willow Adult Campus
La Puente, CA 91746
Prgm Dir: Kevin Booth, AB RRT RCP
Tel: 626 934-2800, Ext 2995   *Fax:* 626 855-3169
E-mail: kmbooth@hlpusd.k12.ca.us

Concorde Career College - North Hollywood
Respiratory Therapist (Entry-Level) Prgm
12412 Victory Blvd
North Hollywood, CA 91606
Prgm Dir: Marlyn H Haberwood, RRT BSHS
Tel: 818 766-8151, Ext 253   *Fax:* 818 766-1587
E-mail: mhaberwood@concorde.edu

California College San Diego
Respiratory Therapist (Entry-Level) Prgm
2820 Camino Del Rio S
San Diego, CA 92108
Prgm Dir: Edward Moser, MBA RRT
Tel: 619 295-5785   *Fax:* 619 477-4360
E-mail: emoser@cc-sd.edu

Simi Valley Adult School
Respiratory Therapist (Entry-Level) Prgm
3192 Los Angeles Ave
Simi Valley, CA 93065
Prgm Dir: Christine R Kingston, BS RRT
Tel: 805 579-6262   *Fax:* 805 522-8902
E-mail: ronk@simi.tec.ca.us

El Camino College
Respiratory Therapist (Entry-Level) Prgm
16007 S Crenshaw Blvd
Torrance, CA 90506
www.elcamino.edu/respiratorycare
Prgm Dir: Louis M Sinopoli, EdD RRT FAARC AE-C
Tel: 310 660-3248   *Fax:* 310 660-3378
E-mail: sinopoli@elcamino.edu

Crafton Hills College
Respiratory Therapist (Entry-Level) Prgm
11711 Sand Canyon Rd
Yucaipa, CA 92399
Prgm Dir: Kenneth R Bryson, MEd BE RCP RRT
Tel: 909 389-3284   *Fax:* 909 389-3229
E-mail: kbryson@crafton.sbccd.cc.ca.us

Colorado

T H Pickens Technical Center
Respiratory Therapist (Entry-Level) Prgm
500 Airport Blvd
Aurora, CO 80011
Prgm Dir: Leigh Otto, BS RRT
Tel: 303 344-4910, Ext 27781   *Fax:* 303 326-1277
E-mail: leigho@pickens.aps.k12.co.us

Illinois

St Augustine College
Respiratory Therapist (Entry-Level) Prgm
1333 W Argyle
Chicago, IL 60640
Prgm Dir: Shirley Thomason, AS RRT
Tel: 773 878-7182   *Fax:* 773 878-0937
E-mail: sthomason@staugustine.edu

Kansas

Bethany Med Ctr/Kansas City Kansas Comm Coll
Respiratory Therapist (Entry-Level) Prgm
7250 State Ave
Kansas City, KS 66112
Prgm Dir: C Michael Parrett, MBA RPFT RRT-NPS
Tel: 913 288-7245   *Fax:* 913 288-7649
E-mail: mparrett@kckcc.edu

Kentucky

Maysville Comm & Tech College
Respiratory Therapist (Entry-Level) Prgm
609 Viking Dr
Morehead, KY 40351
Prgm Dir: Marlene Vice, RRT
Tel: 606 783-1538, Ext 442   *Fax:* 606 784-9876
E-mail: marlene.vice@kctcs.edu

Laurel Technical College - Rockcastle
Respiratory Therapist (Entry-Level) Prgm
PO Box 275
Mount Vernon, KY 40456
Prgm Dir: Carl Baker, RRT
Tel: 606 256-4346   *Fax:* 606 256-4337
E-mail: carl.baker@kctcs.edu

West Kentucky Community & Technical College
Respiratory Therapist (Entry-Level) Prgm
5200 Blandville Rd
PO Box 7408
Paducah, KY 42002-7408
Prgm Dir: Ruth Thompson, MS RRT
Tel: 270 534-3486   *Fax:* 270 538-3498
E-mail: ruth.thompson@kctcs.edu

Southeast Kentucky Comm & Tech College
Respiratory Therapist (Entry-Level) Prgm
3300 US Highway 25E S
Pineville, KY 40977
Prgm Dir: Michael S Good, MS RRT RPFT
Tel: 606 248-2122   *Fax:* 606 248-2166
E-mail: mike.good@kctcs.edu

Louisiana

Our Lady of the Lake College
Cosponsor: LSU Health Sciences Center
Respiratory Therapist (Entry-Level) Prgm
7434 Perkins Rd
Baton Rouge, LA 70808
www.ololcollege.edu
Prgm Dir: Jackie Bush, BS RRT
Tel: 225 768-1786   *Fax:* 225 768-0819
E-mail: jbush@ololcollege.edu

Bossier Parish Community College
Respiratory Therapist (Entry-Level) Prgm
6220 E Texas St
Bossier City, LA 71111
Prgm Dir: Dennis Wissing, PhD RRT
Tel: 318 675-6814   *Fax:* 318 675-6937
E-mail: dwissi@lsuhsc.edu

Louisiana State University - Eunice
Respiratory Therapist (Entry-Level) Prgm
PO Box 1129
Eunice, LA 70535
www.lsue.edu
Prgm Dir: Kathleen B Warner, BS RRT-NPS
Tel: 337 457-7311, Ext 341   *Fax:* 337 550-1289
E-mail: kreynold@lsue.edu

Louisiana Tech College
Respiratory Therapist (Entry-Level) Prgm
West Jefferson Campus
475 Manhattan Blvd
Harvey, LA 70058
www.dcc.edu
Prgm Dir: Toy B Smoot, RRT MEd
Tel: 504 671-6713   *Fax:* 504 736-7120
E-mail: tsmoot@dcc.edu

Nicholls State University
Respiratory Therapist (Entry-Level) Prgm
235 Civic Center Blvd
Houma, LA 70360
Prgm Dir: Errol Champagne, MEd RRT-NPS
Tel: 985 876-8848   *Fax:* 985 876-8856
E-mail: errol.champagne@nicholls.edu

Michigan

Monroe County Community College
Respiratory Therapist (Entry-Level) Prgm
1555 S Raisinville Rd
Monroe, MI 48161
Prgm Dir: Bonnie Boggs, BS RRT
Tel: 734 384-4268   *Fax:* 734 384-4187
E-mail: bboggs@monroeccc.edu

Minnesota

Northland Community & Technical College
Respiratory Therapist (Entry-Level) Prgm
2022 Central Ave NE
East Grand Forks, MN 56721
www.northlandcollege.edu
Prgm Dir: Anthony Sorum, BA RRT
Tel: 218 773-4791, Ext 4791   *Fax:* 218 773-4502
E-mail: tony.sorum@northlandcollege.edu
Notes: Currently inactive

Missouri

Cape Girardeau Career & Technology Center
Cosponsor: Mineral Area College
Respiratory Therapist (Entry-Level) Prgm
1080 S Silver Spring Rd
Cape Girardeau, MO 63703
Prgm Dir: Kenneth L Pfau, BS RRT
Tel: 573 334-0449, Ext 320   *Fax:* 573 334-5930
E-mail: pfauk@cape.k12.mo.us

Sanford-Brown College
Respiratory Therapist (Entry-Level) Prgm
1203 Smizer Mill Rd
Fenton, MO 63026
Prgm Dir: Monica Engh, BHS RRT
Tel: 636 349-4900, Ext 125   *Fax:* 636 349-9170
E-mail: mengh@sbcstlouis.sanfordbrown.com

Missouri Southern State University
Respiratory Therapist (Entry-Level) Prgm
3950 E Newman Rd
Joplin, MO 64801
Prgm Dir: Glenda Pippin
Tel: 417 659-4405   *Fax:* 417 659-4408
E-mail: pippin-g@mssu.edu

Concorde Career College - Kansas City
Respiratory Therapist (Entry-Level) Prgm
3239 Broadway Blvd
Kansas City, MO 64111
www.concordecareercolleges.com
Prgm Dir: Lana Conrad, BS RRT
Tel: 816 531-5223, Ext 403   *Fax:* 816 756-3231
E-mail: lconrad@concorde.edu

Ohio

University of Toledo
Respiratory Therapist (Entry-Level) Prgm
2801 W Bancroft St
Toledo, OH 43606
Prgm Dir: Suzanne Spacek, MEd RRT-NPS CPFT
Tel: 419 530-4556   *Fax:* 419 530-4780
E-mail: suzanne.spacek@utoledo.edu

Oklahoma

Great Plains Technology Center
Respiratory Therapist (Entry-Level) Prgm
4500 W Lee Blvd
Lawton, OK 73505
www.gptech.org/rsp
Prgm Dir: Jack Powers, RRT
Tel: 580 250-5572   *Fax:* 580 250-5583
E-mail: jpowers@gptech.org

Pennsylvania

Gwynedd-Mercy College
Respiratory Therapist (Entry-Level) Prgm
1325 Sumneytown Pike
PO Box 901
Gwynedd Valley, PA 19437
Prgm Dir: William F Galvin, MSEd RRT CPFT AE-C
Tel: 215 641-5536   *Fax:* 215 641-5559
E-mail: galvin.w@gmc.edu

Harrisburg Area Community College
Respiratory Therapist (Entry-Level) Prgm
One HACC Dr
Harrisburg, PA 17110
Prgm Dir: Bradley A Leidich, RRT MSEd
Tel: 717 780-2315   *Fax:* 717 780-2551
E-mail: baleidic@hacc.edu

Reading Area Community College
Respiratory Therapist (Entry-Level) Prgm
Ten S Second St, PO Box 1706
Reading, PA 19603
www.racc.edu
Prgm Dir: James H Cicman, BHS RRT
Tel: 610 372-4721, Ext 5435   *Fax:* 610 607-6254
E-mail: jcicman@racc.edu
Notes: Currently inactive

York College of Pennsylvania
Cosponsor: York Hospital
Respiratory Therapist (Entry-Level) Prgm
1001 S George St
York, PA 17405
www.wellspan.org
Prgm Dir: Mark Simmons, MSEd RPFT RRT-NPS
Tel: 717 851-2464   *Fax:* 717 851-2934
E-mail: msimmons@wellspan.org

Tennessee

Volunteer State Community College
Respiratory Therapist (Entry-Level) Prgm
1480 Nashville Pike
Gallatin, TN 37066-3188
Prgm Dir: Cory E Martin, BS RRT
Tel: 615 452-8600, Ext 3349   *Fax:* 615 230-3224
E-mail: Cory.Martin@volstate.edu

Walters State Community College
Respiratory Therapist (Entry-Level) Prgm
500 S Davy Crockett Pkwy
Morristown, TN 37813
www.ws.edu
Prgm Dir: Robert G McGee, RRT MS
Tel: 423 798-7941   *Fax:* 423 798-7944
E-mail: robert.mcgee@ws.edu

Texas

SWT/HMC Respiratory Care School Consortium
Respiratory Therapist (Entry-Level) Prgm
1900 Pine St
Abilene, TX 79601
Prgm Dir: Jeff Lawrence, MS RRT
Tel: 915 670-2368   *Fax:* 915 670-2114
E-mail: jlawrenc@hendrickhealth.org

Univ Tx at Brownsville/Tx Southmost Coll
Respiratory Therapist (Entry-Level) Prgm
80 Ft Brown
Brownsville, TX 78520
Prgm Dir: John L McCabe, PhD RRT
Tel: 956 554-5010   *Fax:* 956 554-5012
E-mail: john.mccabe@utb.edu

US Army Medical Dept Center & School
Respiratory Therapist (Entry-Level) Prgm
Department of Medical Science
Physician's Extender Branch Bldg 1151,
  2651 McIdoe Rd
Fort Sam Houston, TX 78234
www.cs.amedd.army.mil/dms/91v
Prgm Dir: Jon P O'Hora, RRT MSHP
Tel: 210 295-4411   *Fax:* 210 295-4317
E-mail: jon.ohora@cen.amedd.army.mil

USAF School of Health Care Sciences
Respiratory Therapist (Entry-Level) Prgm
USAF Cardiopulmonary Lab Technologist Program
383 TRS/XUFC, 939 Missile Rd
Sheppard AFB, TX 76311
Prgm Dir: MSgt Shane A Pearson, MAED RRT RPFT CCT
Tel: 940 676-3812   *Fax:* 940 676-2210
E-mail: shane.pearson@sheppard.af.mil

Utah

Weber State University
Respiratory Therapist (Entry-Level) Prgm
3904 University Circle
Ogden, UT 84408-3904
Prgm Dir: Georgine L Bills, MBA RRT
Tel: 801 626-7071   *Fax:* 801 626-7075
E-mail: gbills@weber.edu

Virginia

J Sargeant Reynolds Community College
Respiratory Therapist (Entry-Level) Prgm
PO Box 85622
Richmond, VA 23285-5622
www.reynolds.edu
Prgm Dir: Nakia Austin, RRT
Tel: 804 523-5009   *Fax:* 804 786-5298
E-mail: naustin@reynolds.edu

Respiratory Therapist (Entry-Level)

Programs*	Class Capacity	Begins	Length (months)	Award	Res. Tuition	Non-res. Tuition	Stipend	Offers:‡ 1	2	3	4
Arkansas											
Univ of Arkansas Comm Coll - Hope	21	Jul	29	AAS	$2,123	$4,306					
California											
Crafton Hills College (Yucaipa)	35	Aug	24	Cert, AS	$620	$6,045					
El Camino College (Torrance)	15	Jan Feb	28	Cert, AS	$200	$1,000		•		•	
Kentucky											
Southeast Kentucky Comm & Tech College (Pineville)	24	Aug	12, 18	AAS	$3,335	$7,000		•			
Louisiana											
Louisiana State University - Eunice	20	Aug	24	AS	$2,945	$6,946					•
Louisiana Tech College (Harvey)	15	Spring	12, 24	AAS	$1,037	$2,074				•	•
Nicholls State University (Houma)	15	Aug	24	Cert, AS	$4,697	$11,734					
Our Lady of the Lake College (Baton Rouge)	20	Jan	24	Dipl, AS	$3,280	$3,280				•	

*Data are shown only for programs that completed the 2007 AMA Survey of Health Professions Education Programs.
‡Key to Offers: 1: Evening or weekend classes; 2: Non-English instruction; 3: Cultural competence instruction; 4: Distance education component.

Respiratory Therapist (Entry-Level)

Programs*	Class Capacity	Begins	Length (months)	Award	Res. Tuition	Non-res. Tuition	Stipend	Offers:‡ 1	2	3	4
Minnesota											
Northland Community & Technical College (East Grand Forks)	25	Aug	24	AAS	$4,913	$9,826				•	
Missouri											
Concorde Career College - Kansas City	30	Every 10-12 wks	15	AS	$19,936	$19,936					
Oklahoma											
Great Plains Technology Center (Lawton)	12	Jan	12, 16	AAS	$1,925	$2,640					
Pennsylvania											
Reading Area Community College	20	Jun	24	Cert, AAS	$2,448	$4,896					
York College of Pennsylvania	12	Sep	24	AS	$12,000	$12,000					
Tennessee											
Walters State Community College (Morristown)	22	Jun	24	AAS	$3,000	$0					
Texas											
US Army Medical Dept Center & School (Fort Sam Houston)	70	Feb May Sep	9	Dipl						•	
USAF School of Health Care Sciences (Sheppard AFB)	14	Varies	11	Cert, AS							
Virginia											
J Sargeant Reynolds Community College (Richmond)	60	Aug	16	AAS	$5,335	$16,194		•			

*Data are shown only for programs that completed the 2007 AMA Survey of Health Professions Education Programs.
‡Key to Offers: 1: Evening or weekend classes; 2: Non-English instruction; 3: Cultural competence instruction; 4: Distance education component.

Speech-Language Pathologist

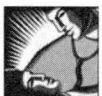

Career Description

Speech-language pathologists are professionals educated in the study of human communication, its development, and its disorders. Speech-language pathologists work with people who cannot make speech sounds or cannot make them clearly; those with speech rhythm and fluency problems, such as stuttering; people with voice quality problems, such as inappropriate pitch or harsh voice; those with problems understanding and producing language; those who wish to improve their communication skills by modifying an accent; those with cognitive communication impairments, such as attention, memory, and problem-solving disorders; and those with hearing loss who use hearing aids or cochlear implants, in order to develop auditory skills and improve communication. They also work with people who have swallowing difficulties.

Speech and language difficulties can result from a variety of causes, including stroke, brain injury or deterioration, developmental delays, cerebral palsy, cleft palate, voice pathology, mental retardation, hearing impairment, or emotional problems. Speech-language pathologists use written and oral tests, as well as special instruments, to diagnose the nature and extent of impairment and to record and analyze speech, language, and swallowing irregularities. For individuals with little or no speech capability, speech-language pathologists may select augmentative or alternative communication methods, including automated devices and sign language, and teach their use. They help patients develop, or recover, reliable communication skills so patients can fulfill their educational, vocational, and social roles.

Speech-language pathologists often work with education and other health care professionals, such as teachers, physicians, social workers, and psychologists, to evaluate and treat clients. They counsel individuals and their families concerning communication disorders and how to cope with the stress and misunderstanding that often accompany them. They also work with family members to recognize and change behavior patterns that impede communication and treatment and show them communication-enhancing techniques to use at home.

A graduate degree is required to work in most settings as a speech-language pathologist. A doctoral degree (PhD) is preferred in some career paths, such as college teaching, research, and private practice.

Working with an understanding of the full range of human communication and its disorders, speech-language pathologists:

- Evaluate and diagnose speech, language, and swallowing disorders in individuals of all ages, from infants to the elderly
- Treat speech, language, and swallowing disorders

In addition, speech-language pathologists may:

- Prepare future professionals in colleges and universities
- Engage in research to enhance knowledge about human communication processes and investigate behavioral patterns associated with communication disorders

Employment Characteristics

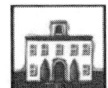

Speech-language pathologists may work in a wide range of settings, including schools, universities, hospitals, rehabilitation centers, skilled nursing facilities, community clinics, geriatric facilities, home health care services, and public health departments, or in private practice.

Salary

Salaries of speech-language pathologists depend on educational background, specialty, and experience, along with the geographical location and type of setting in which they work. According to the ASHA 2006 Schools Survey Salary Report, the median salary for ASHA-certified speech-language pathologists was $52,131 for those employed on an academic year (ie, 9-10 month) basis and $57,000 for those on a calendar year (ie, 11-12 month). The 2006 median starting salary for certified speech-language pathologists in school settings with 1 to 3 years' experience was $40,041 for an academic year appointment. The median calendar year salary for management positions was $80,000. According to the ASHA 2005 Health Care Survey Salary Report, the median salary for ASHA-certified speech-language pathologists was $60,000. The 2005 median starting salary for certified speech-language pathologists in health care settings with 1 to 3 years' experience was $52,694. The median calendar year salary for management positions was $72,985. Good benefits packages, such as insurance programs and leave, are usually available to speech-language pathologists.

Refer to Section IV, Table 5 of this Directory for more information, or see www.ama-assn.org/go/hpsalary.

Employment Outlook

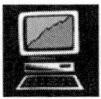

Employment of speech-language pathologists is expected to grow about as fast as the average for all occupations through the year 2014 (www.bls.gov/oco/ocos099.htm#outlook). More frequent recognition of problems in preschool and school-age children by teachers and parents, combined with the increased numbers of older citizens, and medical advances, has created a growing need for speech and language services. Additionally, opportunities for employment in research and higher education are expected to increase as baby boomers currently in these positions retire. Clinical opportunities will be especially strong for those with bilingual and multicultural expertise. There are shortages of qualified personnel in some areas of the country, especially in inner city, rural, and less populated areas. Job opportunities in medically related areas are expected to grow at an above average rate. Although competition for positions in some areas is keen, the potential for private practice and contract work is increasing rapidly. Many states now require that all newborns be screened for hearing loss and receive appropriate early intervention services. Greater awareness of the importance of early identification and diagnosis of speech, language, swallowing, and hearing disorders will also increase employment opportunities.

Educational Programs

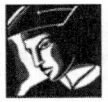

Approximately 245 universities in the United States offer graduate education programs in speech-language pathology that prepare students for entry into practice.

Length. Full-time study usually takes at least 2 years, including summers, to complete a master's degree program in speech-language pathology. In addition, most agencies require a 9- to 12-month postgraduate clinical experience to fulfill credentialing requirements.

Prerequisites. Course work in the biological sciences, physical sciences, mathematics, and behavioral or social sciences are required for graduate study. Undergraduate programs in communication sciences and disorders will provide a background in linguistics, phonetics, psychology, normal speech, and language development, and introductory course work in speech-language pathology. Excellent oral and written communication skills are expected.

Curriculum. Graduate programs should offer a curriculum to allow a student to meet the knowledge and skills necessary to enter practice in speech-language pathology. A typical graduate program of study includes course content in normal and abnormal communication development; diagnostic and treatment procedures, articulation, expressive and receptive language, voice disorders, fluency, swallowing, and ethics. Opportunities to work in a variety of different clinical settings and with a diverse range of clients should be provided during the graduate program of study.

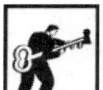

Licensure and Certification

In most states, speech-language pathologists must comply with state regulatory (licensure) standards and/or have state teacher certification to practice in specific settings. A graduate degree, completion of a 9- to

12-month clinical experience, and passage of a national examination are typically required to achieve the credentials. Individuals should contact the appropriate state licensure board or teacher certification agency for more information about requirements. ASHA offers the Certificate of Clinical Competence in Speech-Language Pathology (CCC-SLP), a nationally recognized credential that offers certificate holders ease in qualifying for state credentials because those requirements are similar or identical to ASHA's CCC requirements, recognition as a "highest qualified provider" of speech-language services for reimbursement, and increased opportunities for employment or promotion, as certain positions in hospitals, educational programs, or private practices may require ASHA certification.

Inquiries

For information about a specific program, write to the director of the speech-language pathology program in care of the institution listed.

For additional information about the professions or academic program accreditation, contact:

American Speech-Language-Hearing Association (ASHA)
2200 Research Boulevard
Rockville, MD 20850
800 498-2071
www.asha.org

Speech-Language Pathologist

Alabama

Auburn University
Speech-Language Pathology Prgm
Dept of Communication
1199 Haley Center
Auburn University, AL 36849-5232
Prgm Dir: Lawrence F Molt, PhD
Tel: 334 844-9600   *Fax:* 334 844-4585
E-mail: moltlaw@auburn.edu

University of South Alabama
Speech-Language Pathology Prgm
Dept of Speech Pathology and Audiology
2000 University Commons
Mobile, AL 36688-0002
Prgm Dir: Paul Dagenais, PhD CCC-SLP
Tel: 334 380-2600, Ext 4-2608   *Fax:* 334 380-2699
E-mail: pdagenais@usouthal.edu

University of Montevallo
Speech-Language Pathology Prgm
Comm Science and Disorders
Station 6720
Montevallo, AL 35115-6720
Prgm Dir: Mary Beth Armstrong, PhD CCC-SLP
Tel: 205 665-6720   *Fax:* 205 665-6721
E-mail: armstrom@montevallo.edu

Alabama A&M University
Speech-Language Pathology Prgm
Dept of Special Education
PO Box 580
Normal, AL 35762
Prgm Dir: Terry D Douglas, PhD CCC-SLP
Tel: 256 851-5533   *Fax:* 256 851-5538
E-mail: tdouglas@aamu.edu

University of Alabama
Speech-Language Pathology Prgm
Dept of Comm Disorders
PO Box 870242
Tuscaloosa, AL 35487-0242
www.as.ua.edu/comdis/
Prgm Dir: Karen Steckol, PhD CCC-SLP
Tel: 205 348-7131   *Fax:* 205 348-1845
E-mail: ksteckol@bama.ua.edu

Arizona

Northern Arizona University
Speech-Language Pathology Prgm
Communication Sciences and Disorders
NAU Box 15045
Flagstaff, AZ 86011-5045
Prgm Dir: Katherine Mahosky, MS
Tel: 928 523-2969, Ext 7444   *Fax:* 928 523-0034
E-mail: katherine.mahosky@nau.edu

Arizona State University
Speech-Language Pathology Prgm
Speech and Hearing Science
PO Box 870102
Tempe, AZ 85287-0102
www.asu.edu/clas/shs
Prgm Dir: William Yost, PhD
Tel: 602 965-2905   *Fax:* 602 965-8516
E-mail: william.yost@asu.edu

University of Arizona
Speech-Language Pathology Prgm
Dept of Speech and Hearing
PO Box 210071
Tucson, AZ 85721-0071
Prgm Dir: Elena Plante, PhD
Tel: 520 621-1644   *Fax:* 520 621-9901
E-mail: eplante@email.arizona.edu

Arkansas

University of Central Arkansas
Speech-Language Pathology Prgm
Box 4985
Conway, AR 72035-0001
www.uca.edu/chas
Prgm Dir: John Lowe III, PhD CCC-SLP
Tel: 501 450-3176   *Fax:* 501 450-5474
E-mail: jlowe@uca.edu

University of Arkansas
Speech-Language Pathology Prgm
Program in Communication Disorders
410 Arkansas Ave
Fayetteville, AR 72701
Prgm Dir: Barbara Shadden, PhD CCC-SLP BND
Tel: 501 575-4509   *Fax:* 501 575-4507
E-mail: bshadde@uark.edu

University of Arkansas for Medical Sciences
Cosponsor: University of Arkansas at Little Rock
Speech-Language Pathology Prgm
Dept of Audiology and Speech Pathology
2801 S University Ave
Little Rock, AR 72204-1099
www.uams.edu/chrp/
Prgm Dir: Thomas Guyette, PhD
Tel: 501 569-3155   *Fax:* 501 569-3157
E-mail: guyettethomasw@uams.edu

Arkansas State University
Speech-Language Pathology Prgm
PO Box 910
State University, AR 72467-0904
Prgm Dir: Richard A Neeley, PhD
Tel: 870 972-3106   *Fax:* 870 972-2040
E-mail: meeley@astate.edu

California

California State University - Chico
Speech-Language Pathology Prgm
Dept of Communication
1st & Normal Sts
Chico, CA 95929-0350
Prgm Dir: Suzanne Miller, PhD
Tel: 530 898-4379   *Fax:* 530 898-6612
E-mail: sbmiller@csuchico.edu

California State University - Fresno
Speech-Language Pathology Prgm
Dept of Communicative Sci and Disorder
5048 N Jackson
Fresno, CA 93740-8022
Prgm Dir: Donald Freed
Tel: 209 278-2423   *Fax:* 209 278-5187
E-mail: donfr@csufresno.edu

California State University - Fullerton
Speech-Language Pathology Prgm
Dept of Human Communication Studies
800 N State College Blvd
Fullerton, CA 92834
www.fullerton.edu
Prgm Dir: Edith Li, PhD
Tel: 714 278-3260   *Fax:* 714 278-3377
E-mail: edithli@fullerton.edu

California State University - East Bay
Speech-Language Pathology Prgm
Communicative Sciences and Disorders
25800 Carlos Bee Blvd
Hayward, CA 94542-3065
Prgm Dir: Janet Patterson, PhD CCC-SLP
Tel: 510 885-7557   *Fax:* 510 885-2186
E-mail: janet.patterson@csueastbay.edu

Loma Linda University
Speech-Language Pathology Prgm
Nichol Hall, Rm A804
Loma Linda, CA 92350
http://llu.edu
Prgm Dir: Paige Shaughnessy, PhD
Tel: 909 558-4998, Ext 47397   *Fax:* 909 558-4305
E-mail: pshaughnessy@llu.edu

California State University - Long Beach
Speech-Language Pathology Prgm
Communicative Disorders
1250 Bellflower Blvd
Long Beach, CA 90840-2501
Prgm Dir: Carolyn Conway Madding, PhD
Tel: 562 985-5283   *Fax:* 562 985-4584
E-mail: madding@csulb.edu

California State University - Los Angeles
Speech-Language Pathology Prgm
Communication Disorders
5151 State University Dr
Los Angeles, CA 90032
www.calstatela.edu
Prgm Dir: Miles Peterson, PhD
Tel: 323 343-4690   *Fax:* 323 343-4698
E-mail: mpeters@calstatela.edu

California State University - Northridge
Speech-Language Pathology Prgm
Dept of Communicative Disorders
18111 Nordhoff St
Northridge, CA 91330-8279
Prgm Dir: J Stephen Sinclair, PhD
Tel: 818 667-2852   *Fax:* 818 677-2632
E-mail: steve.sinclair@csun.edu

University of Redlands
Speech-Language Pathology Prgm
University of Redlands, Truesdail Center for
   Communication Disorders
PO Box 3080, 1200 E Colton Ave
Redlands, CA 92373-0999
www.redlands.edu
Prgm Dir: Christopher Walker, PhD
Tel: 909 748-8061   *Fax:* 909 335-5192
E-mail: christopher_walker@redlands.edu

California State University - Sacramento
Speech-Language Pathology Prgm
Dept of Speech Pathology and Audiology
6000 J St
Sacramento, CA 95819-6071
www.csus.edu
Prgm Dir: Laureen O'Hanlon, PhD
Tel: 916 278-4661   *Fax:* 916 278-7730
E-mail: ohanlon@csus.edu

San Diego State University
Speech-Language Pathology Prgm
School of Speech, Language and Hearing Sciences
5500 Campanile Dr
San Diego, CA 92182-1518
http://chhs.sdsu.edu/SLHS/
Prgm Dir: Beverly Wulfeck, PhD
Tel: 619 594-7746   *Fax:* 619 594-7109
E-mail: bwulfeck@mail.sdsu.edu

San Francisco State University
Speech-Language Pathology Prgm
1600 Holloway Ave
Burk Hall Rm 104
San Francisco, CA 94132-4158
Prgm Dir: Marcia Raggio, PhD
Tel: 415 338-1001   *Fax:* 415 338-0916
E-mail: mraggio@sfsu.edu

San Jose State University
Speech-Language Pathology Prgm
Speech and Hearing Ctr
One Washington Square
San Jose, CA 95192-0079
Prgm Dir: Gloria Weddington, PhD
Tel: 408 924-3688   *Fax:* 408 924-3641
E-mail: novakjm@sjsu.edu

University of the Pacific
Speech-Language Pathology Prgm
Dept of Speech-Language Pathology
3601 Pacific Ave
Stockton, CA 95211
Prgm Dir: Robert E Hanak, AuD CCC-A
Tel: 209 946-2381   *Fax:* 209 946-2647
E-mail: rhanyak@pacific.edu

Colorado

University of Colorado at Boulder
Speech-Language Pathology Prgm
2501 Kittredge Loop Rd
Campus Box 409
Boulder, CO 80309-0409
Prgm Dir: Susan M Moore, JD MA-CCC-SLP
Tel: 303 492-5284   *Fax:* 303 492-3274
E-mail: susan.moore@colorado.edu

University of Northern Colorado
Speech-Language Pathology Prgm
Audiology and Speech-Language Sciences
Gunter 1400, Box 140
Greeley, CO 80639-0030
Prgm Dir: Ellen Meyer Gregg, PhD CCC-SLP
Tel: 970 351-1597   *Fax:* 970 351-2974
E-mail: ellen.gregg@unco.edu

Connecticut

Southern Connecticut State University
Speech-Language Pathology Prgm
Communication Disorders
501 Crescent St
New Haven, CT 06515
www.southernct.edu/dept
Prgm Dir: Deborah Weiss, PhD
Tel: 203 392-6615   *Fax:* 203 392-5968
E-mail: weissd1@southernct.edu

University of Connecticut
Speech-Language Pathology Prgm
Communication Sciences
850 Bolton Rd, Unit 1085
Storrs, CT 06269-1085
Prgm Dir: Carl Coelho, PhD CCC-SLP
Tel: 860 486-2817   *Fax:* 860 486-4948
E-mail: coelho@uconn.edu

District of Columbia

Gallaudet University
Speech-Language Pathology Prgm
Audiology and Speech-Lang Path
800 Florida Ave NE
Washington, DC 20002-3695
Prgm Dir: James J Mahshie, PhD
Tel: 202 651-5329   *Fax:* 202 651-5324
E-mail: james.mahshie@gallaudet.edu

George Washington University
Speech-Language Pathology Prgm
Dept of Speech and Hearing Science
1922 F Street NW
Washington, DC 20052
www.gwu.edu/sphr
Prgm Dir: Geralyn M Schulz, PhD CCC-SLP
Tel: 202 994-7362   *Fax:* 202 994-2589
E-mail: schulz@gwu.edu

Howard University
Speech-Language Pathology Prgm
Communication Sciences and Disorders
525 Bryant St NW
Washington, DC 20059
Prgm Dir: Ovetta Harris
Tel: 202 806-6990   *Fax:* 202 806-4046
E-mail: oharris@howard.edu

University of the District of Columbia
Speech-Language Pathology Prgm
Communication Sciences
4200 Connecticut Ave NW
Washington, DC 20008
Prgm Dir: April Massey
Tel: 202 274-5546   *Fax:* 202 274-5230
E-mail: amassey@udc.edu

Florida

Florida Atlantic University
Speech-Language Pathology Prgm
Communication Sciences and Disorders
777 Glades Rd, PO Box 3091
Boca Raton, FL 33431-0991
Prgm Dir: Deena Louise Wener, PhD CCC-SLP
Tel: 561 297-6074   *Fax:* 561 297-2268
E-mail: wener@fau.edu

University of Florida
Speech-Language Pathology Prgm
Communication Processes and Disorders
335 Dauer Hall, PO Box 117420
Gainesville, FL 32611-7420
Prgm Dir: Kenneth J Logan, PhD
Tel: 352 392-2113   *Fax:* 352 846-0243
E-mail: logan@csd.ufl.edu

Florida International University
Speech-Language Pathology Prgm
HLS 143, University Park
Miami, FL 33199
Prgm Dir: Elaine Ramos, PhD
Tel: 305 348-2710   *Fax:* 305 348-2740
E-mail: csd@fiu.edu

Nova Southeastern University
Speech-Language Pathology Prgm
Comm Sciences and Disorders
1750 NE 167th st
North Miami, FL 33162-3017
Prgm Dir: Wren Newman
Tel: 954 262-7756   *Fax:* 954 272-3606
E-mail: newmanw@nova.edu

University of Central Florida
Speech-Language Pathology Prgm
Communicative Disorders
PO Box 162215
Orlando, FL 32826-2215
Prgm Dir: R Jane Lieberman
Tel: 407 823-2215   *Fax:* 407 823-4816
E-mail: jlieberm@mail.ucf.edu

Florida State University
Speech-Language Pathology Prgm
Communication Disorders
107 RRC (R-89)
Tallahassee, FL 32306-1200
www.fsu.edu/~commdis
Prgm Dir: Howard Goldstein, PhD
Tel: 850 644-2253   *Fax:* 850 644-8994
E-mail: howard.goldstein@comm.fsu.edu

University of South Florida
Speech-Language Pathology Prgm
Comm Sciences and Disorders
4202 E Fowler Ave PCD 1017
Tampa, FL 33620-8150
www.usf.edu
Prgm Dir: Theresa Chisolm, PhD
Tel: 813 974-2006   *Fax:* 813 974-0822
E-mail: chisolm@cas.usf.edu

Georgia

University of Georgia
Speech-Language Pathology Prgm
Comm Sciences and Disorders
516 Aderhold Hall
Athens, GA 30602
Prgm Dir: Albert R DeChicchis, PhD
Tel: 706 542-4561   *Fax:* 706 542-5348
E-mail: alde@uga.edu

Georgia State University
Speech-Language Pathology Prgm
Communication Disorders
33 Gilmer St SE
Atlanta, GA 30303-3086
Prgm Dir: Collen M O'Rourke, PhD
Tel: 404 651-2310   *Fax:* 404 651-4901
E-mail: corourke@gsu.edu

Armstrong Atlantic State University
Speech-Language Pathology Prgm
11935 Abercorn St
Savannah, GA 31419-1997
www.armstrong.edu
Prgm Dir: Donna R Brooks, PhD
Tel: 912 921-7319
E-mail: Donna.Brooks@armstrong.edu

Valdosta State University
Speech-Language Pathology Prgm
Dept of Special Education
1500 N Patterson St
Valdosta, GA 31698-0102
Prgm Dir: Corine Myers-Jennings
Tel: 912 333-5932
E-mail: cmjennin@valdosta.edu

Hawaii

University of Hawaii
Speech-Language Pathology Prgm
Dept of Speech Pathology and Audiology
1410 Lower Campus Dr
Honolulu, HI 96822
Prgm Dir: James T Yates, PhD
Tel: 808 956-8279   *Fax:* 808 956-5482
E-mail: jyates@hawaii.edu

Idaho

Idaho State University
Speech-Language Pathology Prgm
Communication Sciences & Disorders and Education of
   the Deaf
650 Memorial Dr, Bldg 68, Box 8116
Pocatello, ID 83209-8116
www.isu.edu/departments/spchpath
Prgm Dir: Toni Seikel
Tel: 208 282-4196   *Fax:* 208 282-4571
E-mail: seikel@isu.edu

Illinois

Southern Illinois University Carbondale
Speech-Language Pathology Prgm
Comm Disorders and Sciences
1025 Lincoln Dr, Rehn Hall #308
Carbondale, IL 62901-4609
Prgm Dir: Kenneth O Simpson, PhD
Tel: 618 536-8262   *Fax:* 618 453-8271
E-mail: ksimpson@siu.edu

Univ of Illinois at Urbana-Champaign
Speech-Language Pathology Prgm
220 Speech and Hearing Sci Bldg
901 S 6th St
Champaign, IL 61820
www.shs.uiuc.edu
Prgm Dir: Nicoline G Ambrose, PhD
Tel: 217 333-2230   *Fax:* 217 244-2235
E-mail: rdc@uiuc.edu

Eastern Illinois University
Speech-Language Pathology Prgm
Comm Disorders and Sciences
600 Lincoln Ave
Charleston, IL 61920-3099
www.eiu.edu/~commdis/
Prgm Dir: Gail J Richard, PhD
Tel: 217 581-2712   *Fax:* 217 581-7105
E-mail: gjrichard@eiu.edu

Rush University Medical Center
Speech-Language Pathology Prgm
Communication Disorders and Sciences
1653 W Congress Pkwy
Chicago, IL 60612
Prgm Dir: Richard K Peach, PhD
Tel: 312 942-3289   *Fax:* 312 942-7211
E-mail: richard_k_peach@rush.edu

Saint Xavier University
Speech-Language Pathology Prgm
Comm Disorders and Sciences
3700 W 103rd St
Chicago, IL 60655
www.sxu.edu
Prgm Dir: Michael Flahive, PhD
Tel: 773 298-3566   *Fax:* 773 298-3007
E-mail: flahive@sxu.edu

Northern Illinois University
Speech-Language Pathology Prgm
Communicative Disorders
DeKalb, IL 60115-2899
Prgm Dir: Pamela Jackson, PhD
Tel: 815 753-6510   *Fax:* 815 753-9123
E-mail: plj@niu.edu

Southern Illinois University
Speech-Language Pathology Prgm
Founders Hall, Rm 1300
Campus Box 1147
Edwardsville, IL 62026-1147
Prgm Dir: Jean M Harrison, EdD
Tel: 618 650-3668   *Fax:* 618 650-3307
E-mail: jeharri@siue.edu

Northwestern University
Speech-Language Pathology Prgm
Comm Sciences and Disorders
2240 Campus Dr
Evanston, IL 60208
www.communication.northwestern.edu/csd/
Prgm Dir: Charles Larson, PhD
Tel: 847 491-2468   *Fax:* 847 467-7141
E-mail: clarson@northwestern.edu

Western Illinois University
Speech-Language Pathology Prgm
Dept of Communication
121 Memorial Hall
Macomb, IL 61455-1390
Prgm Dir: Maureen Marx, PhD
Tel: 309 298-1955, Ext 244   *Fax:* 309 298-2049
E-mail: m-marx@wiu.edu

Illinois State University
Speech-Language Pathology Prgm
Speech Pathology and Audiology
Fairchild Hall #204
Normal, IL 61790-4720
www.ilstu.edu
Prgm Dir: Joe Smaldino, PhD
Tel: 309 438-8643   *Fax:* 309 438-5221
E-mail: wsmoski@ilstu.edu

Governors State University
Speech-Language Pathology Prgm
Communication Disorders
University Park, IL 60466
Prgm Dir: Jay Lubinsky
Tel: 708 534-4598   *Fax:* 708 235-2195
E-mail: j-lubinsky@govst.edu

Indiana

Indiana University - Bloomington
Speech-Language Pathology Prgm
Speech and Hearing Sciences
200 S Jordan Ave
Bloomington, IN 47405-7002
Prgm Dir: Phil Connell, PhD
Tel: 812 855-4156   *Fax:* 812 855-5531
E-mail: pconnell@indiana.edu

Ball State University
Speech-Language Pathology Prgm
Speech Pathology and Audiology
2000 University Ave
Muncie, IN 47306
Prgm Dir: Mary Jo Germani
Tel: 765 285-8160   *Fax:* 765 285-5623
E-mail: mgermani@bsu.edu

Indiana State University
Speech-Language Pathology Prgm
Department of Communication Disorders
8th & Sycamore St
Terre Haute, IN 47809
Prgm Dir: James L Campbell, PhD
Tel: 812 237-4389   *Fax:* 812 237-8137
E-mail: jcampbell2@isugw.indstate.edu

Purdue University
Speech-Language Pathology Prgm
Audiology and Speech Sciences
500 Oval Dr
West Lafayette, IN 47907-2038
Prgm Dir: Robert Novak
Tel: 765 494-3789   *Fax:* 765 494-9771
E-mail: novakr@purdue.edu

Iowa

University of Northern Iowa
Speech-Language Pathology Prgm
Communicative Disorders
Cedar Falls, IA 50614-0356
Prgm Dir: Clifford Highnam, PhD
Tel: 319 273-2496   *Fax:* 319 273-6384
E-mail: Clifford.Highnam@uni.edu

University of Iowa
Speech-Language Pathology Prgm
Speech Pathology and Audiology
Iowa City, IA 52242
Prgm Dir: Paul Abbas, PhD
Tel: 319 335-8718   *Fax:* 319 335-8851
E-mail: paul-abbas@uiowa.edu

Kansas

Fort Hays State University
Speech-Language Pathology Prgm
Communication Disorders
600 Park St
Hays, KS 67601
www.fhsu.edu/commdis/
Prgm Dir: Amy Finch, PhD
Tel: 785 628-5366, Ext 4496   *Fax:* 785 628-5271
E-mail: afinch@fhsu.edu

University of Kansas
Speech-Language Pathology Prgm
Intercampus Program in Communicative Disorders
3001 Dole Center
Lawrence, KS 66045
www.ku.edu/~splh/ipcd
Prgm Dir: Hugh Catts
Tel: 785 864-0630   *Fax:* 785 864-3974
E-mail: catts@ku.edu

Kansas State University
Speech-Language Pathology Prgm
Comm Sciences and Disorders
Justin Hall 303
Manhattan, KS 66506-1403
Prgm Dir: Robert Garcia
Tel: 785 532-6879   *Fax:* 785 532-5505
E-mail: rgarcia@humec.ksu.edu

Wichita State University
Speech-Language Pathology Prgm
Communication Sciences and Disorders
1845 N Fairmount
Wichita, KS 67260-0075
Prgm Dir: Kathy Coufal, PhD
Tel: 316 978-3171   *Fax:* 316 978-3291
E-mail: kathy.coufal@wichita.edu

Kentucky

Western Kentucky University
Speech-Language Pathology Prgm
1 Big Red Way
TPH, Rm 113
Bowling Green, KY 42101-3576
Prgm Dir: Joseph Etienne, PhD
Tel: 502 745-4302   *Fax:* 502 745-6474
E-mail: joseph.etienne@wku.edu

University of Kentucky
Speech-Language Pathology Prgm
Communication Disorders
900 S Limestone St, Ste 124G
Lexington, KY 40504-0200
Prgm Dir: Judith L Page, PhD
Tel: 859 323-1100, Ext 80571   *Fax:* 859 323-8957
E-mail: jpage01@uky.edu

University of Louisville
Speech-Language Pathology Prgm
Surgery/Graduate Program in Communicative Disorders
Health Sciences Center, Myers Hall
Louisville, KY 40292
Prgm Dir: Barbara M Baker, PhD
Tel: 502 852-5274   *Fax:* 502 852-0865
E-mail: barbara.baker@louisville.edu

Murray State University
Speech-Language Pathology Prgm
Communication Disorders
125 Alexander Hall
Murray, KY 42071-3340
Prgm Dir: Pearl Gordon Payne, PhD
Tel: 502 762-2446   *Fax:* 502 762-3963
E-mail: pearl.payne@murraystate.edu

Eastern Kentucky University
Speech-Language Pathology Prgm
Communication Disorders
245 Wallace Bldg
Richmond, KY 40475-3102
www.specialed.eku.edu/CD
Prgm Dir: Charlotte Hubbard, PhD, CCC-SLP
Tel: 859 622-4442   *Fax:* 859 622-4443
E-mail: charlotte.hubbard@eku.edu

Louisiana

Louisiana State Univ and A&M College
Speech-Language Pathology Prgm
Communication Disorders
Music/Dramatic Arts Bldg #163
Baton Rouge, LA 70803-2606
Prgm Dir: Paul R Hoffman
Tel: 225 578-2545   *Fax:* 225 578-2528
E-mail: cdhoff@lsu.edu

Southern Univ and A&M College
Speech-Language Pathology Prgm
Speech Pathology and Audiology
PO Box 11295
Baton Rouge, LA 70813
Prgm Dir: Regina Enwefa, PhD
Tel: 225 771-3950   *Fax:* 225 771-5652
E-mail: carolynp@subr.edu

Southeastern Louisiana University
Speech-Language Pathology Prgm
Department of Communication Sciences and Disorders
PO Box 10879 - SLU
Hammond, LA 70402
www.selu.edu/csd
Prgm Dir: Paula S Currie, PhD CCC-S
Tel: 504 549-2214   *Fax:* 504 549-5030
E-mail: pcurrie@selu.edu

University of Louisiana at Lafayette
Speech-Language Pathology Prgm
Department of Communicative Disorders
PO Box 43170
Lafayette, LA 70504
http://speechandlanguage.louisiana.edu
Prgm Dir: Martin Ball, PhD
Tel: 337 482-6721   *Fax:* 337 482-6195
E-mail: mjball@louisiana.edu

University of Louisiana at Monroe
Speech-Language Pathology Prgm
Department of Communicative Disorders
College of Health Sciences
Monroe, LA 71209-1032
www.ulm.edu/codi
Prgm Dir: Judy Fellows, PhD
Tel: 318 342-1392   *Fax:* 318 342-3199
E-mail: fellows@ulm.edu

Louisiana State Univ Health Sciences Center
Speech-Language Pathology Prgm
Communication Disorders
1900 Gravier St
New Orleans, LA 70112
www.alliedhealth.lsuhsc.edu
Prgm Dir: Sylvia M Davis, PhD
Tel: 504 568-4348   *Fax:* 504 568-4352
E-mail: sdavis2@lsuhsc.edu

Louisiana Tech University
Speech-Language Pathology Prgm
Dept of Speech
PO Box 3165
Ruston, LA 71272
www.latech.edu
Prgm Dir: Sheryl Shoemaker, AuD
Tel: 318 257-4764   *Fax:* 318 257-4492
E-mail: sshoemaker@latech.edu

Louisiana State U Hlth Sci Ctr - Shreveport
Speech-Language Pathology Prgm
Mollie E Webb Speech and Hearing Center
3735 Blair Dr
Shreveport, LA 71106
Prgm Dir: Thomas W Powell, PhD
Tel: 318 632-2015   *Fax:* 318 632-2003
E-mail: tpowel@lsuhsc.edu

Maine

University of Maine - Orono
Speech-Language Pathology Prgm
Communication Sciences and Disorders
5724 Dunn Hall
Orono, ME 04469-5724
www.umaine.edu/comscidis/
Prgm Dir: Nancy E Hall, PhD
Tel: 207 581-2006   *Fax:* 207 581-2060
E-mail: nhall@maine.edu

Maryland

Loyola College of Maryland
Speech-Language Pathology Prgm
Speech-Language Pathology and Audiology
4501 N Charles St
Baltimore, MD 21210
Prgm Dir: Marie R Kerins, EdD CCC-SLP
Tel: 410 617-2632, Ext 2632   *Fax:* 410 617-7634
E-mail: mkerins@loyola.edu

Univ of Maryland at College Park
Speech-Language Pathology Prgm
Hearing and Speech Science
Lefrak Hall
College Park, MD 20742
www.bsos.umd.edu/hesp/
Prgm Dir: Nan Ratner, EdD CCC
Tel: 301 405-4214   *Fax:* 301 314-2023
E-mail: nratner@hesp.umd.edu

Towson University
Speech-Language Pathology Prgm
Audiology, Speech Language Pathology and Deaf Studies
8000 York Rd
Towson, MD 21252-0001
Prgm Dir: Sharon Glennen, PhD
Tel: 410 704-4153   *Fax:* 410 704-4131
E-mail: sglennen@towson.edu

Massachusetts

University of Massachusetts - Amherst
Speech-Language Pathology Prgm
Communication Disorders
715 N Pleasant St
Amherst, MA 01003-9304
Prgm Dir: Jane Baran, PhD
Tel: 413 545-0131   *Fax:* 413 545-0803
E-mail: baran@comdis.umass.edu

Boston University
Speech-Language Pathology Prgm
Sargent Coll of Hlth and Rehab Sciences
635 Commonwealth Ave
Boston, MA 02215
www.bu.edu/sargent
Prgm Dir: Kristine Strand, EdD
Tel: 617 353-3188   *Fax:* 617 353-5074
E-mail: ksushi@bu.edu

Emerson College
Speech-Language Pathology Prgm
Communication Disorders
120 Beacon St
Boston, MA 02116-4624
Prgm Dir: Cynthia L Bartlett, PhD
Tel: 617 824-8730   *Fax:* 617 824-8735
E-mail: Cynthia_Bartlett@emerson.edu

MGH Institute of Health Professions
Speech-Language Pathology Prgm
Comm Sciences and Disorders
36 1st Ave
Boston, MA 02129-4557
www.mghihp.edu
Prgm Dir: Gregory Lof, Acting Dir, PhD CCC-SLP
Tel: 617 724-6313   *Fax:* 617 726-8022
E-mail: glof@mghihp.edu

Northeastern University
Speech-Language Pathology Prgm
Speech-Language Pathology and Audiology
106 Forsyth Bldg, 360 Huntington Ave
Boston, MA 02115
Prgm Dir: Linda J Ferrier, PhD
Tel: 617 373-3698   *Fax:* 617 373-2239
E-mail: l.ferrier@neu.edu

Worcester State College
Speech-Language Pathology Prgm
Communication Disorders
486 Chandler St
Worcester, MA 01602-2597
Prgm Dir: Linda Larrivee, PhD
Tel: 508 929-8055   *Fax:* 508 929-8175
E-mail: llarrivee@worcester.edu

Michigan

Wayne State University
Speech-Language Pathology Prgm
Communication Sciences and Disorders
207 Rackham Building
Detroit, MI 48202
www.clas.wayne.edu/CSD
Prgm Dir: Alex Johnson, PhD
Tel: 313 577-3339   *Fax:* 313 577-8885
E-mail: ajohnson@wayne.edu

Michigan State University
Speech-Language Pathology Prgm
101 Oyer Bldg
East Lansing, MI 48824-1220
Prgm Dir: Michael W Casby, PhD
Tel: 517 353-8780   *Fax:* 517 353-3176
E-mail: casby@msu.edu

Western Michigan University
Speech-Language Pathology Prgm
Speech Pathology and Audiology
Kalamazoo, MI 49008-5355
Prgm Dir: John M Hanley, PhD
Tel: 616 387-8045   *Fax:* 616 381-8044
E-mail: john.hanley@wmich.edu

Central Michigan University
Speech-Language Pathology Prgm
Communication Disorders
HPB 2187
Mount Pleasant, MI 48859
Prgm Dir: Mary Jane Lack
Tel: 989 774-1323   *Fax:* 989 774-2799
E-mail: Lack1mj@cmich.edu

Eastern Michigan University
Speech-Language Pathology Prgm
110 Porter Bldg
Ypsilanti, MI 48197
Prgm Dir: Bill P Cupples
Tel: 734 487-7120, Ext 2674   *Fax:* 734 487-2473
E-mail: willie.cupples@emich.edu

Minnesota

University of Minnesota - Duluth
Speech-Language Pathology Prgm
Communicative Disorders
1207 Ordean Court, 221 Bohannon Hall
Duluth, MN 55812
www.d.umn.edu/csd
Prgm Dir: Mark Mizuko, PhD
Tel: 218 726-7974   *Fax:* 218 726-8693
E-mail: cd@d.umn.edu

Minnesota State University - Mankato
Speech-Language Pathology Prgm
Communication Disorders
103 Armstrong Hall
Mankato, MN 56001
http://ahn.mnsu.edu/cd/
Prgm Dir: Bruce Poburka, PhD
Tel: 507 389-1414   *Fax:* 507 389-2821
E-mail: bruce.poburka@mnsu.edu

University of Minnesota - Minneapolis
Speech-Language Pathology Prgm
115 Shevlin Hall
164 Pillsbury Dr SE
Minneapolis, MN 55455
Prgm Dir: Jennifer Windsor, PhD
Tel: 612 624-3322   *Fax:* 612 624-7586
E-mail: slhs@umn.edu

Minnesota State University - Moorhead
Speech-Language Pathology Prgm
Speech-Language-Hearing Sciences
1104 7th Ave S
Moorhead, MN 56563
Prgm Dir: Bruce R Hanson, MS
Tel: 218 477-2286   *Fax:* 218 477-4392
E-mail: hansonbr@mnstate.edu

St Cloud State University
Speech-Language Pathology Prgm
A216 Education Bldg
720 4th Ave S
St Cloud, MN 56301
www.stcloudstate.edu/csd
Prgm Dir: Monica Devers, PhD
Tel: 320 308-2092   *Fax:* 320 308-6441
E-mail: mcdevers@stcloudstate.edu

Mississippi

Mississippi University for Women
Speech-Language Pathology Prgm
PO Box W-1340
Columbus, MS 39701
Prgm Dir: Robert F Oyler, PhD
Tel: 601 329-7270   *Fax:* 601 329-7460
E-mail: royler@muw.edu

University of Southern Mississippi
Speech-Language Pathology Prgm
Dept of Speech and Hearing Sciences
PO Box 5092
Hattiesburg, MS 39406-5092
www.usm.edu/shs
Prgm Dir: Brett Kemker, PhD
Tel: 601 266-5216   *Fax:* 601 266-5224
E-mail: brett.kemker@usm.edu

Jackson State University
Speech-Language Pathology Prgm
Dept of Communication Disorders
University Center, 3825 Ridgewood Rd, Box 23
Jackson, MS 39211-6453
Prgm Dir: Zenobia Bagli, PhD
Tel: 601 432-6713   *Fax:* 601 432-6844
E-mail: zbagli@jsums.edu

University of Mississippi
Speech-Language Pathology Prgm
Communicative Disorders
PO Box 1848
University, MS 38677
Prgm Dir: Carolyn Wiles Higdon, PhD
Tel: 662 915-7652   *Fax:* 662 915-5717
E-mail: chigdon@olemiss.edu

Missouri

Southeast Missouri State University
Speech-Language Pathology Prgm
Dept of Communication Disorders
One University Plaza
Cape Girardeau, MO 63701-4799
Prgm Dir: Sakina S Drummond, PhD
Tel: 573 651-2155   *Fax:* 573 651-2155
E-mail: ssdrummond@semovm.semo.edu

University of Missouri - Columbia
Speech-Language Pathology Prgm
Communication Science and Disorders
303 Lewis Hall
Columbia, MO 65211
www.umshp.org/csd/
Prgm Dir: Barbara McLay, MA CCC-A
Tel: 573 882-3873   *Fax:* 573 884-8686
E-mail: mclayb@health.missouri.edu

Rockhurst University
Speech-Language Pathology Prgm
Communication Sciences and Disorders
1100 Rockhurst Rd
Kansas City, MO 64110
Prgm Dir: Dennis Ingrisano, PhD
Tel: 816 501-4742   *Fax:* 816 501-4169
E-mail: dennis.ingrisano@rockhurst.edu

Truman State University
Speech-Language Pathology Prgm
Communication Disorders
Barnett Hall 222
Kirksville, MO 63501
http://comdis.truman.edu
Prgm Dir: Janet L Gooch, PhD
Tel: 660 785-4669   *Fax:* 660 785-7424
E-mail: jquinzer@truman.edu

Missouri State University
Speech-Language Pathology Prgm
Communication Disorders
901 S National Ave
Springfield, MO 65804-0095
Prgm Dir: Neil J DiSarno, PhD
Tel: 417 836-5368, Ext 66511   *Fax:* 417 836-4242
E-mail: neildisarno@missouristate.edu

Fontbonne University
Speech-Language Pathology Prgm
Communication Disorders and Deaf Education
6800 Wydown Blvd
St Louis, MO 63105
Prgm Dir: Lynne Shields, PhD CCC-SLP
Tel: 314 889-1407   *Fax:* 314 719-8016
E-mail: lshields@fontbonne.edu

Saint Louis University
Speech-Language Pathology Prgm
Communication Sciences & Disorders
3570 Lindell Blvd
St Louis, MO 63108
www.slu.edu/x10651.xml
Prgm Dir: Travis Threats, PhD CCC-SLP
Tel: 314 977-2940   *Fax:* 314 977-3360
E-mail: threatst@slu.edu

University of Central Missouri
Speech-Language Pathology Prgm
Speech Pathology and Audiology
Martin Bldg 41
Warrensburg, MO 64093
Prgm Dir: Carl Harlan
Tel: 660 543-4918   *Fax:* 660 543-8234
E-mail: harlan@ucmo.edu

Nebraska

University of Nebraska - Kearney
Speech-Language Pathology Prgm
Communication Disorders Department
College of Education
Kearney, NE 68849-4597
www.unk.edu/departments/cdis
Prgm Dir: Laurence M Hilton, PhD CCC-SLP
Tel: 308 865-8300   *Fax:* 308 865-8397
E-mail: hiltonlm@unk.edu

University of Nebraska - Lincoln
Speech-Language Pathology Prgm
Dept of Special Education and
    Communication Disorders
301 Barkley Center
Lincoln, NE 68583-0738
www.unl.edu/barkley/
Prgm Dir: John Bernthal, PhD
Tel: 402 472-5496   *Fax:* 402 472-7697
E-mail: jbernthal1@unl.edu

University of Nebraska - Omaha
Speech-Language Pathology Prgm
Special Education and Communication Disorders
6001 Dodge St
Omaha, NE 68182-0054
Prgm Dir: Mary J Friehe, PhD
Tel: 402 554-2211   *Fax:* 402 554-3572
E-mail: mfriehe@mail.unomaha.edu

Nevada

University of Nevada - Reno
Speech-Language Pathology Prgm
Dept of Speech Pathology and Audiology
Redfield Bldg/152
Reno, NV 89557-0046
www.unr.edu/spa
Prgm Dir: Thomas Watterson, PhD
Tel: 775 784-4887   *Fax:* 775 784-4095
E-mail: twatterson@medicine.nevada.edu

New Hampshire

University of New Hampshire
Speech-Language Pathology Prgm
Dept of Communication Sciences and Disorders
4 Library Way, Hewitt Hall
Durham, NH 03824
Prgm Dir: Stephen Calculator, PhD CCC-SLP
Tel: 603 862-3836   *Fax:* 603 862-4511
E-mail: stephen.calculator@unh.edu

New Jersey

College of New Jersey
Speech-Language Pathology Prgm
Special Education, Language and Literacy, Speech
    Pathology
2000 Pennington Rd
Ewing, NJ 08628-0718
Prgm Dir: Jasper B Phelps, PhD
Tel: 609 771-2308   *Fax:* 609 637-5172
E-mail: phelps@tcnj.edu

Seton Hall University
Speech-Language Pathology Prgm
400 S Orange Ave
South Orange, NJ 07079-2689
www.shu.edu
Prgm Dir: Robert Orlikoff, PhD CCC-SLP
Tel: 973 313-6185   *Fax:* 973 275-2171
E-mail: orlikoro@shu.edu

Kean University
Speech-Language Pathology Prgm
Dept of Communication Disorders and Deafness
1000 Morris Ave
Union, NJ 07083
Prgm Dir: Barbara Glazewski, EdD
Tel: 908 737-5407   *Fax:* 908 527-3232
E-mail: bglazews@kean.edu

Montclair State University
Speech-Language Pathology Prgm
Dept of Communication Sciences and Disorders
Speech Bldg
Upper Montclair, NJ 07043
Prgm Dir: Sarita Eisenberg
Tel: 973 655-7363   *Fax:* 973 655-7072
E-mail: speechclinic@mail.montclair.edu

William Paterson Univ of New Jersey
Speech-Language Pathology Prgm
Communication Disorders
300 Pompton Rd
Wayne, NJ 07470
Prgm Dir: Carole E Gelfer
Tel: 973 720-2208   *Fax:* 973 720-3357
E-mail: gelferc@wpunj.edu

New Mexico

University of New Mexico
Speech-Language Pathology Prgm
Dept of Speech and Hearing Sciences
MSC01 1195, 1 University of New Mexico,
    1700 Lomas Blvd NE
Albuquerque, NM 87131-0001
www.unm.edu/~sphrsci/
Prgm Dir: Philip Dale, PhD
Tel: 505 277-4453   *Fax:* 505 277-0968
E-mail: dalep@unm.edu

New Mexico State University
Speech-Language Pathology Prgm
Dept of Special Education/Communication Disorders
PO Box 30001/MSC 3SPE
Las Cruces, NM 88003
http://web.nmsu.edu/~nmsucd
Prgm Dir: Connie Stout, PhD
Tel: 505 646-2402   *Fax:* 505 646-7712
E-mail: cestout@nmsu.edu

Eastern New Mexico University
Speech-Language Pathology Prgm
Dept of Communicative Disorders
Station 3
Portales, NM 88130
Prgm Dir: Linda J Weems, PhD
Tel: 505 562-2156   *Fax:* 505 562-2380
E-mail: linda.weems@enmu.edu

New York

College of St Rose
Speech-Language Pathology Prgm
Communication Disorders Dept
432 Western Ave, Box 100
Albany, NY 12203-1490
Prgm Dir: David DeBonis, PhD
Tel: 518 458-5461   *Fax:* 518 458-5446
E-mail: coopermd@rosnet.strose.edu

CUNY Herbert H Lehman College
Speech-Language Pathology Prgm
Dept of Speech-Language-Hearing Sciences
250 Bedford Park Blvd W
Bronx, NY 10468-1589
Prgm Dir: Joyce West, PhD
Tel: 718 960-8134   *Fax:* 718 960-7376
E-mail: speech@lehman.cuny.edu

CUNY Brooklyn College
Speech-Language Pathology Prgm
Speech-Language Pathology and Audiology
2900 Bedford Ave
Brooklyn, NY 11210
http://http//www.brooklyn.cuny.edu
Prgm Dir: Gail B Gurland, PhD
Tel: 718 951-5186   *Fax:* 718 951-4363
E-mail: ggurland@brooklyn.cuny.edu

Long Island University - Brooklyn Campus
Speech-Language Pathology Prgm
Dept of Communication Sciences and Disorders
One University Plaza
Brooklyn, NY 11201-8423
Prgm Dir: Elaine Geller, PhD
Tel: 718 780-4122   *Fax:* 718 780-4007
E-mail: elaine.geller@liu.edu

Touro College
Speech-Language Pathology Prgm
1610 E 19th St
Brooklyn, NY 11229
Prgm Dir: Hindy Lubinsky
Tel: 718 787-1602   *Fax:* 718 787-1137
E-mail: Hlubintouro@yahoo.com

Long Island University - C W Post Campus
Speech-Language Pathology Prgm
Communication Sciences and Disorders
720 Northern Blvd
Brookville, NY 11548-1300
Prgm Dir: Dianne Slavin, PhD
Tel: 516 299-2436   *Fax:* 516 299-3151
E-mail: dslavin@liu.edu

Buffalo State, SUNY
Speech-Language Pathology Prgm
208 Ketchum Hall
1300 Elmwood Ave
Buffalo, NY 14222
Prgm Dir: Constance Dean Qualls, PhD
Tel: 716 878-5502   *Fax:* 716 878-5711
E-mail: westlenl@buffalostate.edu

University at Buffalo - SUNY
Speech-Language Pathology Prgm
Dept of Communicative Disorders and Sciences
122 Cary Hall
Buffalo, NY 14214-3005
www.wings.buffalo.edu/cds
Prgm Dir: Elaine Stathopoulos, PhD
Tel: 716 829-2797, Ext 625   *Fax:* 716 829-3979
E-mail: stathop@buffalo.edu

Mercy College
Speech-Language Pathology Prgm
555 Broadway, Main Hall, Rm G15
Dobbs Ferry, NY 10522
Prgm Dir: Helen Buhler, PhD
Tel: 914 674-7743   *Fax:* 914 674-7597
E-mail: hbuhler@mercy.edu

SUNY Fredonia
Speech-Language Pathology Prgm
Dept of Speech Pathology and Audiology
W123 Thompson Hall
Fredonia, NY 14063
Prgm Dir: Kim L Tillery, PhD
Tel: 716 673-3202   *Fax:* 716 673-3235
E-mail: tillery@fredonia.edu

Adelphi University
Speech-Language Pathology Prgm
Hy Weinberg Center
158 Cambridge Ave
Garden City, NY 11530
Prgm Dir: Susan Lederer, PhD
Tel: 516 877-4770   *Fax:* 516 877-4783
E-mail: lederer@adelphi.edu

SUNY College of Geneseo
Speech-Language Pathology Prgm
Dept of Communicative Disorders and Sciences
1 College Circle, 218 Sturgis
Geneseo, NY 14454
Prgm Dir: Linda I House, PhD
Tel: 716 245-5328   *Fax:* 716 345-5434
E-mail: house@geneseo.edu

Hofstra University
Speech-Language Pathology Prgm
Dept of Speech-Language-Hearing Sciences
110 Hofstra University
Hempstead, NY 11550
www.hofstra.edu
Prgm Dir: Carole Ferrand, PhD
Tel: 516 463-5508   *Fax:* 516 463-5260
E-mail: sphctf@hofstra.edu

Ithaca College
Speech-Language Pathology Prgm
Speech Pathology and Audiology
953 Danby Rd
Ithaca, NY 14850-7185
http://departments.ithaca.edu/slpa/
Prgm Dir: E W Testut, PhD
Tel: 607 274-3248   *Fax:* 607 274-1137
E-mail: testut@ithaca.edu

SUNY at New Paltz
Speech-Language Pathology Prgm
Dept of Communication Disorders
600 Hawk Dr
New Paltz, NY 12561-2499
Prgm Dir: Elizabeth Hester, PhD
Tel: 845 257-3600   *Fax:* 845 257-3605
E-mail: hestere@newpaltz.edu

Columbia University Teachers College
Speech-Language Pathology Prgm
Speech and Language Pathology and Audiology
525 W 120th St, Box 206
New York, NY 10027
Prgm Dir: John H Saxman, PhD
Tel: 212 678-3895   *Fax:* 212 678-8233
E-mail: saxman@tc.columbia.edu

CUNY Hunter College
Speech-Language Pathology Prgm
Communication Sciences Program
425 E 25th St
New York, NY 10010-2590
Prgm Dir: Dava E Waltzman, PhD
Tel: 212 481-4467   *Fax:* 212 481-4458
E-mail: dwaltzma@hunter.cuny.edu

New York University
Speech-Language Pathology Prgm
Dept of Speech-Language Pathology and Audiology
719 Broadway, Ste 200
New York, NY 10003
www.nyu.edu/education/speech/
Prgm Dir: Celia Stewart, PhD
Tel: 212 998-5230   *Fax:* 212 995-4356
E-mail: cs8@nyu.edu

SUNY College at Plattsburgh
Speech-Language Pathology Prgm
Dept of Communication Disorders and Sciences
224 Sibley Hall, 101 Broad St
Plattsburgh, NY 12901
Prgm Dir: Patrick Coppens, PhD
Tel: 518 564-2170   *Fax:* 518 564-5110
E-mail: patrick.coppens@Plattsburgh.edu

St John's University
Speech-Language Pathology Prgm
Speech and Hearing Ctr
8000 Utopia Pkwy
Queens, NY 11439
Prgm Dir: Donna Geffner, CCC-SLP CCC-A
Tel: 718 990-6480   *Fax:* 718 990-1917

Nazareth College of Rochester
Speech-Language Pathology Prgm
Dept of Comm Sci and Disorder Speech-Lang Pathology
4245 East Ave
Rochester, NY 14618-3790
Prgm Dir: Lisa Durant-Jones, MS
Tel: 585 389-2775   *Fax:* 585 389-2791
E-mail: ldurant4@naz.edu

Syracuse University
Speech-Language Pathology Prgm
Dept of Communication Sciences and Disorders
805 S Crouse Ave
Syracuse, NY 13244-2280
Prgm Dir: Raymond H Colton, PhD
Tel: 315 443-9637   *Fax:* 315 443-1113
E-mail: rhcolton@syr.edu

New York Medical College
Speech-Language Pathology Prgm
School of Public Health
Valhalla, NY 10595
www.nymc.edu/slp
Prgm Dir: Ben C Watson, PhD CCC-SLP
Tel: 914 594-4239   *Fax:* 914 594-4853
E-mail: slp_sph@nymc.edu

North Carolina

Appalachian State University
Speech-Language Pathology Prgm
Dept of Language, Reading and Exceptionalities
124 Edwin Duncan Hall, Box 32085
Boone, NC 28608-2085
Prgm Dir: Donna M Brown
Tel: 828 262-2182   *Fax:* 828 262-6767
E-mail: browndm@appstate.edu

University of North Carolina - Chapel Hill
Speech-Language Pathology Prgm
Division of Speech and Hearing Sciences
CB 7190 Wing D Medical School
Chapel Hill, NC 27599-7190
Prgm Dir: Jackson Roush, PhD
Tel: 919 966-1006   *Fax:* 919 966-0100
E-mail: jroush@med.unc.edu

Western Carolina University
Speech-Language Pathology Prgm
Human Services, Communication Sciences and
   Disorders
Killian 204, G30 McKee Bldg
Cullowhee, NC 28723-9043
Prgm Dir: Billy T Ogletree, PhD
Tel: 828 227-7310   *Fax:* 828 227-7021
E-mail: fischer@email.wcu.edu

North Carolina Central University
Speech-Language Pathology Prgm
Department of Communication Disorders
712 Cecil St
Durham, NC 27707
http://web.nccu.edu/soe/
Prgm Dir: Diane M Scott, PhD
Tel: 919 530-7473   *Fax:* 919 530-7975
E-mail: discott@nccu.edu

University of North Carolina - Greensboro
Speech-Language Pathology Prgm
Communication Sciences and Disorders
300 Ferguson Bldg/UNCG, Box 26170
Greensboro, NC 27402-6170
www.uncg.edu/csd
Prgm Dir: Celia R Hooper, PhD
Tel: 336 334-4657   *Fax:* 336 334-4475
E-mail: crhooper@uncg.edu

East Carolina University
Speech-Language Pathology Prgm
Dept of Communication Sciences and Disorders
College of Allied Health Science
Greenville, NC 27858-4353
www.ecu.edu/csd
Prgm Dir: Gregg D Givens
Tel: 252 744-6102   *Fax:* 252 744-6081
E-mail: givensg@ecu.edu

North Dakota

University of North Dakota
Speech-Language Pathology Prgm
Dept of Communication Sciences and Disorders
PO Box 8040
Grand Forks, ND 58202-8040
Prgm Dir: Wayne Swisher, PhD
Tel: 701 777-3232   *Fax:* 701 777-3650
E-mail: wayne_swisher@und.nodak.edu

Minot State University
Speech-Language Pathology Prgm
Dept of Communication Disorders
500 University Ave W
Minot, ND 58707
www.minotstateu.edu
Prgm Dir: Thomas A Linares, PhD
Tel: 701 858-3031   *Fax:* 701 858-3845
E-mail: thomas.linares@minotstateu.edu

Ohio

University of Akron
Speech-Language Pathology Prgm
School of Speech-Language and Audiology
Polsky Building, Rm 188K
Akron, OH 44325-3001
www.uakron.edu/sslpa
Prgm Dir: Roberta DePompei, PhD
Tel: 330 972-6114   *Fax:* 330 972-7884
E-mail: rdepom1@uakron.edu

Ohio University
Speech-Language Pathology Prgm
School of Hearing, Speech and Language Sciences
Grover Center W218
Athens, OH 45701-2979
Prgm Dir: Brooke Hallowell, PhD
Tel: 740 593-0903   *Fax:* 740 593-0287
E-mail: hsls@ohio.edu

Bowling Green State University
Speech-Language Pathology Prgm
Dept of Communication Disorders
200 Health Center
Bowling Green, OH 43403-0149
Prgm Dir: Larry Small, PhD
Tel: 419 372-6031   *Fax:* 419 372-8089
E-mail: lsmall@bgsu.edu

University of Cincinnati
Speech-Language Pathology Prgm
Communication Sciences and Disorders
Mail Station 379
Cincinnati, OH 45221-0379
Prgm Dir: Nancy Creaghead, PhD
Tel: 513 558-8501   *Fax:* 513 558-8500
E-mail: nancy.creaghead@uc.edu

Case Western Reserve University
Speech-Language Pathology Prgm
Dept of Communication Sciences
11206 Euclid Ave
Cleveland, OH 44106-7154
Prgm Dir: Angela Ciccia, PhD
Tel: 216 368-2470   *Fax:* 216 368-6078
E-mail: cosigrad@case.edu

Cleveland State University
Speech-Language Pathology Prgm
Dept of Speech and Hearing
2121 Euclid Ave, MC 430
Cleveland, OH 44115
Prgm Dir: Ben Wallace, PhD
Tel: 216 687-3717   *Fax:* 216 687-6983
E-mail: b.wallace@csuohio.edu

Ohio State University
Speech-Language Pathology Prgm
Dept of Speech and Hearing Sciences
110 Pressey Hall, 1070 Carmack Rd
Columbus, OH 43210-1002
Prgm Dir: Robert Allen Fox, PhD
Tel: 614 292-8207   *Fax:* 614 292-7504
E-mail: fox.2@osu.edu

Kent State University
Speech-Language Pathology Prgm
School of Speech Pathology and Audiology
A104 Music & Speech Bldg
Kent, OH 44242
http://dept.kent.edu/spa
Prgm Dir: Lynn E Rowan, PhD
Tel: 330 672-2672   *Fax:* 330 672-2643
E-mail: lrowan@kent.edu

Miami University
Speech-Language Pathology Prgm
Dept of Speech Pathology and Audiology
2 Bachelor Hall
Oxford, OH 45056-3414
Prgm Dir: Kathleen M Hutchinson
Tel: 513 529-2500   *Fax:* 513 529-2502
E-mail: hutchik@muohio.edu

University of Toledo
Speech-Language Pathology Prgm
Public Health and Rehabilitative Services
2801 W Bancroft St
Toledo, OH 43606
Prgm Dir: Lee W Ellis, PhD
Tel: 419 530-4065   *Fax:* 419 530-8774
E-mail: lee.ellis@utoledo.edu

Oklahoma

University of Central Oklahoma
Speech-Language Pathology Prgm
Special Services, Speech-Language Pathology
100 N University Dr
Edmond, OK 73034
Prgm Dir: Scott F McLaughlin, PhD
Tel: 405 974-5705   *Fax:* 405 974-3822
E-mail: SMcLaughlin@ucok.edu

Univ of Oklahoma Health Sciences Center
Speech-Language Pathology Prgm
Communication Disorders
825 NE 14th, PO Box 26901
Oklahoma City, OK 73190
Prgm Dir: Stephen Painton, PhD
Tel: 405 271-4214, Ext 46054   *Fax:* 405 271-3360
E-mail: stephen-painton@ouhsc.edu

Oklahoma State University
Speech-Language Pathology Prgm
Dept of Communication Sciences and Disorders
110 Hanner Bldg
Stillwater, OK 74078-5062
www.cas.okstate.edu/cdis
Prgm Dir: Randolph Deal, PhD
Tel: 405 744-6021   *Fax:* 405 744-8070
E-mail: randolph.deal@okstate.edu

Northeastern State University
Speech-Language Pathology Prgm
600 N Vinita, Special Services Bldg
Tahlequah, OK 74464-7051
Prgm Dir: Karen Patterson, PhD
Tel: 918 456-5511, Ext 3769   *Fax:* 918 458-9605
E-mail: pattersk@nsuok.edu

University of Tulsa
Speech-Language Pathology Prgm
Department of Communication Disorders
600 S College Ave
Tulsa, OK 74104-3189
Prgm Dir: Paula Cadogan, EdD
Tel: 918 631-2504   *Fax:* 918 631-3668
E-mail: paula-cadogan@utulsa.edu

Oregon

University of Oregon
Speech-Language Pathology Prgm
Communication Disorders and Sciences
5284 University of Oregon
Eugene, OR 97403-5284
Prgm Dir: Kathleen Roberts, PhD CCC-A
Tel: 541 346-2480   *Fax:* 541 346-2564
E-mail: robertsk@uoregon.edu

Portland State University
Speech-Language Pathology Prgm
Speech and Hearing Sciences
PO Box 751
Portland, OR 97207-0751
Prgm Dir: Thomas Dolan, PhD
Tel: 503 725-3533   *Fax:* 503 725-9171
E-mail: dolant@pdx.edu

Pennsylvania

Bloomsburg University
Speech-Language Pathology Prgm
Dept of Audiology and Speech Pathology
400 E 2nd St, Centennial Hall
Bloomsburg, PA 17815-1301
Prgm Dir: Dianne Angelo, PhD
Tel: 570 389-4436   *Fax:* 570 389-5022
E-mail: dangelo@bloomu.edu

California University of Pennsylvania
Speech-Language Pathology Prgm
Dept of Communication Disorders
250 University Ave
California, PA 15419
Prgm Dir: Barbara H Bonfanti, PhD
Tel: 724 938-4175   *Fax:* 724 938-1526
E-mail: bonfanti@cup.edu

Clarion University of Pennsylvania
Speech-Language Pathology Prgm
Dept of Communication Sciences and Disorders
840 Wood St, 118 Keeling Health Center
Clarion, PA 16214-1232
Prgm Dir: Colleen A McAleer, PhD
Tel: 814 393-2581   *Fax:* 814 393-2206
E-mail: cmcaleer@clarion.edu

East Stroudsburg University
Speech-Language Pathology Prgm
Speech Pathology and Audiology
LaRue Hall
East Stroudsburg, PA 18301-2999
Prgm Dir: Jane Page, PhD
Tel: 570 422-3247   *Fax:* 570 422-3850
E-mail: jpage@po-box.esu.edu

Edinboro University of Pennsylvania
Speech-Language Pathology Prgm
Speech, Language and Hearing Department
115A Compton Hall
Edinboro, PA 16444
www.edinboro.edu
Prgm Dir: Charlotte Molrine, PhD
Tel: 814 732-2432   *Fax:* 814 732-2612
E-mail: cmolrine@edinboro.edu

Indiana University of Pennsylvania
Speech-Language Pathology Prgm
Special Education and Clinical Svcs
203 Davis Hall, 570 S 11th St
Indiana, PA 15705
www.iup.edu
Prgm Dir: David W Stein, PhD CCC-SLP
Tel: 724 357-2450   *Fax:* 724 357-7716
E-mail: dwstein@iup.edu

La Salle University
Speech-Language Pathology Prgm
1900 W Olney Ave
Philadelphia, PA 19141
www.lasalle.edu/speech
Prgm Dir: Barbara Amster, PhD CCC-SLP
Tel: 215 951-1986   *Fax:* 215 951-5171
E-mail: amster@lasalle.edu

Temple University
Speech-Language Pathology Prgm
Communication Sciences
1701 N 13th St, 109 Weiss Hall
Philadelphia, PA 19122
Prgm Dir: Brian Goldstein, PhD
Tel: 215 204-7543   *Fax:* 215 204-5954
E-mail: CHP@temple.edu

Duquesne University
Speech-Language Pathology Prgm
600 Forbes Ave
Pittsburgh, PA 15282
www.slp.duq.edu
Prgm Dir: Mikael Kimelman, PhD
Tel: 412 396-4225   *Fax:* 412 396-4196
E-mail: speech-lang@duq.edu

University of Pittsburgh
Speech-Language Pathology Prgm
Communication Science and Disorders
4033 Fobes Tower, Atwood St
Pittsburgh, PA 15260
www.shrs.pitt.edu/csd/
Prgm Dir: Malcolm McNeil, PhD
Tel: 412 383-6540   *Fax:* 412 383-6555
E-mail: mcneil@pitt.edu

Marywood University
Speech-Language Pathology Prgm
Dept of Communication Sciences and Disorders
McGowan Center, 2300 Adams Ave
Scranton, PA 18509-1598
www.marywood.edu
Prgm Dir: Mona Griffer, EdD CCC-SLP
Tel: 570 348-6211, Ext 2363   *Fax:* 570 961-4708
E-mail: griffer@marywood.edu

Penn State University
Speech-Language Pathology Prgm
Dept of Communication Sciences and Disorders
110 Moore Bldg
University Park, PA 16802-3100
Prgm Dir: Gordon Blood, PhD
Tel: 814 865-3177 *Fax:* 814 863-3759
E-mail: F2X@psu.edu

West Chester University
Speech-Language Pathology Prgm
Dept of Communicative Disorders
201 Carter Dr
West Chester, PA 19383
Prgm Dir: Michael S Weiss, PhD
Tel: 610 436-3401 *Fax:* 610 436-3388
E-mail: mweiss@wcupa.edu

Rhode Island

University of Rhode Island
Speech-Language Pathology Prgm
Dept of Communicative Disorders
Independence Sq, Ste 1
Kingston, RI 02881-0821
Prgm Dir: Jay Singer, PhD
Tel: 401 874-5969 *Fax:* 401 874-4404
E-mail: DrJay@uri.edu

South Carolina

Medical University of South Carolina
Speech-Language Pathology Prgm
Communication Sciences and Disorders Program
77 President St, Ste 117
Charleston, SC 29425
Prgm Dir: Jennifer Horner, PhD
Tel: 843 792-0365 *Fax:* 843 792-0710
E-mail: hornerj@musc.edu

University of South Carolina
Speech-Language Pathology Prgm
Dept of Communication Sciences and Disorders
Columbia, SC 29208
Prgm Dir: Elaine M Frank, PhD
Tel: 803 777-5052 *Fax:* 803 777-3081
E-mail: efrank@sc.edu

South Carolina State University
Speech-Language Pathology Prgm
Speech Pathology and Audiology
300 College St NE, PO Box 7427
Orangeburg, SC 29117
Prgm Dir: Gwendolyn Wilson, EdD
Tel: 803 536-8074 *Fax:* 803 536-8593
E-mail: gdwilson@scsu.edu

South Dakota

University of South Dakota
Speech-Language Pathology Prgm
Dept of Communication Disorders
414 E Clark St
Vermillion, SD 57069-2390
www.usd.edu/dcom
Prgm Dir: Teri J Bellis, PhD
Tel: 605 677-5474 *Fax:* 605 677-5767
E-mail: tbellis@usd.edu

Tennessee

East Tennessee State University
Speech-Language Pathology Prgm
Dept of Communicative Disorders
PO Box 70643
Johnson City, TN 37614-0643
Prgm Dir: Nancy J Scherer, PhD
Tel: 423 439-4272 *Fax:* 423 439-4607
E-mail: scherern@etsu.edu

University of Tennessee - Knoxville
Speech-Language Pathology Prgm
Dept of Audiology and Speech
578 S Stadium Hall
Knoxville, TN 37996-0740
Prgm Dir: Patricia M Visser
Tel: 865 974-5019 *Fax:* 865 974-1539
E-mail: pvisser@utk.edu

University of Memphis
Speech-Language Pathology Prgm
School of Audiology and Speech-Language Pathology
807 Jefferson Ave
Memphis, TN 38105
www.ausp.memphis.edu
Prgm Dir: Maurice Mendel, PhD
Tel: 901 678-5800 *Fax:* 901 525-1282
E-mail: mmendel@memphis.edu

Tennessee State University
Speech-Language Pathology Prgm
330 10th Ave N, Ste A
PO Box 131
Nashville, TN 37203-3401
Prgm Dir: Harold R Mitchell, PhD
Tel: 615 963-7081 *Fax:* 615 963-7119
E-mail: hmitchell@tnstate.edu

Vanderbilt University Medical Center
Speech-Language Pathology Prgm
Hearing and Speech Sciences
1114 19th Ave S
Nashville, TN 37212
Prgm Dir: Fred H Bess, PhD
Tel: 615 936-5000 *Fax:* 615 936-5014
E-mail: fred.h.bess@vanderbilt.edu

Texas

Abilene Christian University
Speech-Language Pathology Prgm
ACU Box 28058
Abilene, TX 79699-8058
www.acu.edu/academics/cehs/programs/
  comm_disorders/
Prgm Dir: Brenda Bender, PhD CCC-SLP
Tel: 325 674-2074 *Fax:* 325 674-2552
E-mail: brenda.bender@acu.edu

University of Texas at Austin
Speech-Language Pathology Prgm
Communication Sciences and Disorders
1 University Station A1100
Austin, TX 78712-1089
http://csd.utexas.edu/graduate.html
Prgm Dir: Craig Champlin, PhD
Tel: 512 471-4119 *Fax:* 512 471-2957
E-mail: champlin@mail.utexas.edu

Lamar University
Speech-Language Pathology Prgm
Dept of Speech and Hearing Sciences
Box 10076, Lamar Station
Beaumont, TX 77710
Prgm Dir: William Harn, PhD
Tel: 409 880-8179 *Fax:* 409 880-2265
E-mail: harnwe@hal.lamar.edu

West Texas A&M University
Speech-Language Pathology Prgm
PO Box 60757
Canyon, TX 79016-0001
www.wtamu.edu
Prgm Dir: Howard Wilson, PhD
Tel: 806 651-5102 *Fax:* 806 651-5105
E-mail: hwilson@mail.wtamu.edu

University of Texas at Dallas
Speech-Language Pathology Prgm
Program in Communication Disorders
1966 Inwood Rd
Dallas, TX 75235-7298
Prgm Dir: Robert D Stillman, PhD
Tel: 214 905-3060 *Fax:* 214 905-3006
E-mail: stillman@utdallas.edu

Texas Woman's University
Speech-Language Pathology Prgm
Comm Sciences and Disorders
Box 425737, TWU Station
Denton, TX 76204-5737
Prgm Dir: Kathleen K Millary, PhD
Tel: 940 898-2025 *Fax:* 940 898-2070
E-mail: F_Millay@twu.edu

University of North Texas
Speech-Language Pathology Prgm
Dept of Speech and Hearing Sciences
PO Box 305010
Denton, TX 76203-5010
Prgm Dir: Jeffrey Cokely
Tel: 940 565-2481 *Fax:* 940 565-4058
E-mail: cokely@unt.edu

Univ of Texas - Pan American
Speech-Language Pathology Prgm
Health Science and Human Services West 1.264
1201 W University Dr
Edinburg, TX 78541
www.panam.edu/dept/commdisorder
Prgm Dir: Teri Mata-Pistokache, PhD
Tel: 956 316-7040 *Fax:* 956 318-5238
E-mail: tmpistok@utpa.edu

University of Texas at El Paso
Speech-Language Pathology Prgm
1101 N Campbell St
El Paso, TX 79902
Prgm Dir: Anthony P Salvatore, PhD
Tel: 915 747-7250 *Fax:* 915 747-7207
E-mail: asalvatore@utep.edu

Texas Christian University
Speech-Language Pathology Prgm
Dept of Communication Sciences and Disorders
TCU Box 297450
Fort Worth, TX 76129
Prgm Dir: William Ryan, PhD
Tel: 817 257-7621 *Fax:* 817 257-5692
E-mail: w.ryan@tcu.edu

University of Houston
Speech-Language Pathology Prgm
Communication Disorders
100 Clinical Research Services
Houston, TX 77204-6018
Prgm Dir: Lynn S Bliss
Tel: 713 743-2897 *Fax:* 713 743-2926
E-mail: lbliss@uh.edu

Texas A&M University - Kingsville
Speech-Language Pathology Prgm
Communication Sciences and Disorders
MSC 177A, 700 University Blvd
Kingsville, TX 78363
Prgm Dir: Shari Schlehuser Beams, PhD
Tel: 361 593-3401 *Fax:* 361 593-3404
E-mail: kfsls01@tamuk.edu

Texas Tech Univ Health Sciences Center
Speech-Language Pathology Prgm
Dept of Speech, Language, and Hearing Sciences
STOP 6073 - 3601 4th St
Lubbock, TX 79430
www.ttuhsc.edu/SAH
Prgm Dir: Sherry Sancibrian
Tel: 806 743-5660, Ext 232 *Fax:* 806 743-5670
E-mail: sherry.sancibrian@ttuhsc.edu

Stephen F Austin State University
Speech-Language Pathology Prgm
Communication Sciences and Disorders Program
PO Box 13019 SFA
Nacogdoches, TX 75962
Prgm Dir: Michael McKaig, PhD
Tel: 936 468-1252   *Fax:* 936 468-7096
E-mail: mmckaig@sfasu.edu

Our Lady of the Lake University
Speech-Language Pathology Prgm
Comm and Learning Disorders
411 S 24th St
San Antonio, TX 78207
www.ollusa.edu
Prgm Dir: Mary Ann Acevedo, PhD
Tel: 210 431-3938   *Fax:* 210 434-9360
E-mail: acevm@lake.ollusa.edu

Texas State University - San Marcos
Speech-Language Pathology Prgm
Department of Communication Disorders
Health Professions Bldg, 601 University Dr
San Marcos, TX 78666-4616
www.health.txstate.edu/cdis/cdis.html
Prgm Dir: Maria Diana Gonzales, PhD CCC-SLP
Tel: 512 245-2330, Ext 2035   *Fax:* 512 245-2029
E-mail: mg29@txstate.edu

Baylor University
Speech-Language Pathology Prgm
Dept of Communication Sciences and Disorders
One Bear Place # 97332
Waco, TX 76798
Prgm Dir: J David Garrett, PhD
Tel: 254 710-2567   *Fax:* 254 710-2590
E-mail: David_Garrett@baylor.edu

Utah

Utah State University
Speech-Language Pathology Prgm
Comm Disorders and Deaf Educ
1000 Old Main Mill
Logan, UT 84322-1000
www.usu.edu
Prgm Dir: Beth E Foley, PhD
Tel: 435 797-1388   *Fax:* 435 797-0221
E-mail: bethf@cc.usu.edu

Brigham Young University
Speech-Language Pathology Prgm
Communication Disorders
136 John Taylor Bldg
Provo, UT 84602-8641
www.byu.edu/mse/
Prgm Dir: David McPherson, PhD
Tel: 801 422-5117   *Fax:* 801 422-0197
E-mail: david_mcpherson@byu.edu

University of Utah Health Science Center
Speech-Language Pathology Prgm
Communication Sciences and Disorders
1201 Behavioral Science Bldg
Salt Lake City, UT 84112
www.health.utah.edu/cmdis/
Prgm Dir: Bruce Smith, PhD
Tel: 801 581-6725   *Fax:* 801 571-7955
E-mail: bruce.smith@hsc.utah.edu

Vermont

University of Vermont
Speech-Language Pathology Prgm
Communication Sciences
Pomeroy Hall, 489 Main St
Burlington, VT 05405
http://http:/www.uvm.edu/~cmsi/
Prgm Dir: Patricia Prelock, PhD
Tel: 802 656-2529   *Fax:* 802 656-2528
E-mail: Patricia.Prelock@uvm.edu

Virginia

University of Virginia
Speech-Language Pathology Prgm
Communication Disorders
2205 Fontaine Ave, Ste 202
Charlottesville, VA 22908-0781
Prgm Dir: Randall R Robey, PhD
Tel: 434 924-6354   *Fax:* 434 924-4612
E-mail: rrr7w@virginia.edu

Hampton University
Speech-Language Pathology Prgm
Dept of Communicative Sciences and Disorders
Hampton, VA 23668
Prgm Dir: Robert Martin Screen, PhD
Tel: 757 727-5435   *Fax:* 757 727-5765
E-mail: robert.screen@hamptonu.edu

James Madison University
Speech-Language Pathology Prgm
Communication Sciences and Disorders
Harrisonburg, VA 22807
Prgm Dir: Vicki Reed, EdD
Tel: 540 568-6440   *Fax:* 540 568-8077
E-mail: reedva@jmu.edu

Old Dominion University
Speech-Language Pathology Prgm
Speech Pathology and Audiology
Child Study Ctr
Norfolk, VA 23529-0136
Prgm Dir: Nicholas G Bountress, PhD
Tel: 757 683-4117   *Fax:* 757 683-5593
E-mail: nboontre@odu.edu

Radford University
Speech-Language Pathology Prgm
Dept of Communication Sciences and Disorders
PO Box 6961
Radford, VA 24142
Prgm Dir: Calaire M Waldron, PhD CCC-SLP
Tel: 540 831-7666   *Fax:* 540 831-7669
E-mail: cwaldron@radford.edu

Washington

Western Washington University
Speech-Language Pathology Prgm
Dept of Communication Sciences and Disorders
Parks Hall 17, MS 9078
Bellingham, WA 98225-9078
www.wwu.edu/~csd
Prgm Dir: Barbara Mathers-Schmidt, PhD
Tel: 360 650-3172   *Fax:* 360 650-2843
E-mail: barbara.mathers-schmidt@wwu.edu

Washington State University
Speech-Language Pathology Prgm
Dept of Speech and Hearing Sciences
201 Daggy Hall, Box 642420
Pullman, WA 99164-2420
Prgm Dir: Gail Chermak
Tel: 509 335-4525   *Fax:* 509 335-8357
E-mail: chermak@wsu.edu

University of Washington
Speech-Language Pathology Prgm
Speech and Hearing Sciences
Seattle, WA 98195-6246
Prgm Dir: Pamela E Souza, PhD
Tel: 206 543-7829   *Fax:* 206 543-1093
E-mail: psouza@u.washington.edu

Eastern Washington University
Speech-Language Pathology Prgm
Dept of Communication Disorders
310 N Riverpoint Blvd, Box V
Spokane, WA 99202
www.ewu.edu/commdisorders
Prgm Dir: Donald R Fuller, PhD CCC-SLP
Tel: 509 368-6889   *Fax:* 509 368-6791
E-mail: dfuller@mail.ewu.edu

West Virginia

Marshall University
Speech-Language Pathology Prgm
Communication Disorders
400 Hal Greer Blvd
Huntington, WV 25755-2675
Prgm Dir: Kathryn Chezik
Tel: 304 696-2979   *Fax:* 304 696-2986
E-mail: chezik@marshall.edu

West Virginia University
Speech-Language Pathology Prgm
Department of Speech Pathology and Audiology
805 Allen Hall, Box 6122
Morgantown, WV 26506-6122
Prgm Dir: Lynn R Cartwright, EdD
Tel: 304 293-2377   *Fax:* 304 293-7565
E-mail: kjohnso2@wvu.edu

Wisconsin

University of Wisconsin - Eau Claire
Speech-Language Pathology Prgm
Dept of Communication Sciences and Disorders
105 Garfield Ave
Eau Claire, WI 54702-4004
Prgm Dir: Kristine S Retherford, PhD
Tel: 715 836-4186   *Fax:* 715 836-4846
E-mail: retherk@uwec.edu

University of Wisconsin - Madison
Speech-Language Pathology Prgm
Communicative Disorders
475 Goodnight Hall
Madison, WI 53706
Prgm Dir: Julie Washington
Tel: 608 262-7823   *Fax:* 608 262-6466
E-mail: jawashington@wisc.edu

Marquette University
Speech-Language Pathology Prgm
Dept of Speech-Language Pathology and Audiology
PO Box 1881
Milwaukee, WI 53201-1881
Prgm Dir: Steven H Long, PhD
Tel: 414 288-3428   *Fax:* 414 288-3980
E-mail: steven.long@marquette.edu

University of Wisconsin - Milwaukee
Speech-Language Pathology Prgm
Dept of Communication Sciences and Disorders
PO Box 413
Milwaukee, WI 53201-0413
http://cfprod.imt.uwm.edu/chs/ugp/csd/
   graduatestudents.html
Prgm Dir: Marylou Gelfer, PhD
Tel: 414 229-6465   *Fax:* 414 229-2620
E-mail: gelfer@uwm.edu

University of Wisconsin - River Falls
Speech-Language Pathology Prgm
Communicative Disorders
401 S Third St
River Falls, WI 54022-5001
www.uwrf.edu/comm-dis/
Prgm Dir: Michael Harris, PhD CCC-SLP
Tel: 715 425-0602   *Fax:* 715 425-3800
E-mail: michael.d.harris@uwrf.edu

University of Wisconsin - Stevens Point
Speech-Language Pathology Prgm
Communicative Disorders
1901 4th Ave
Stevens Point, WI 54481-3897
www.uwsp.edu/commD/
Prgm Dir: Gary Cumley, PhD
Tel: 715 346-2328   *Fax:* 715 346-2157
E-mail: gcumley@uwsp.edu

University of Wisconsin - Whitewater
Speech-Language Pathology Prgm
Communicative Disorders
1011 Roseman Bldg, 800 W Main St
Whitewater, WI 53190-1790
Prgm Dir: Pat Casey, PhD
Tel: 414 472-1301   *Fax:* 414 472-5210
E-mail: caseyp@uww.edu

Wyoming

University of Wyoming
Speech-Language Pathology Prgm
Division of Communication Disorders
Dept 3311, 1000 E University Ave
Laramie, WY 82071
www.uwyo.edu/comdis
Prgm Dir: Mary Hardin-Jones, PhD
Tel: 307 766-6427   *Fax:* 307 766-5584
E-mail: mhardinj@uwyo.edu

Speech-Language Pathologist

Programs*	Class Capacity	Begins	Length (months)	Award	Res. Tuition	Non-res. Tuition	Stipend	Offers:‡ 1	2	3	4
Alabama											
University of Alabama (Tuscaloosa)	30	Summer, Fall	24, 16	BS, MA						•	
Arizona											
Arizona State University (Tempe)	35	Aug	24	Dipl, MS, AuD						•	
Arkansas											
University of Arkansas for Medical Sciences (Little Rock)	18	Fall semester	21	MS	$270	$583				•	
University of Central Arkansas (Conway)	40	Aug 15	24, 48	MS, BS	$5,754	$10,254				•	
California											
California State University - Fullerton	27	Spring Fall	30	MA	$3,944	$12,080				•	
California State University - Los Angeles	18	Sep	24	Dipl, MA	$4,800	$10,170			•		
California State University - Sacramento	15	Aug Jan	30	Dipl, BS, MS						•	
Loma Linda University	18	Sep	24	Dipl, BS, MS	$20,000	$20,000					
San Diego State University	40	Aug	24	Cert, MA	$3,704	$8,136			•	•	
University of Redlands	45	Sep	21	MS	$19,111	$19,111	$7,500			•	
Colorado											
University of Northern Colorado (Greeley)	22	Aug	24	MA	$5,118	$14,832		•		•	•
Connecticut											
Southern Connecticut State University (New Haven)	40	Sep	30	Dipl, Cert, MS	$3,242	$7,193		•		•	
University of Connecticut (Storrs)	40	Aug	24	Masters	$10,000	$25,000				•	
District of Columbia											
George Washington University	35	Sep	20	Dipl, MA	$20,000	$0		•		•	
Florida											
Florida State University (Tallahassee)	35	Aug	24	Dipl, MS	$6,500	$21,000	$2,600			•	•
University of South Florida (Tampa)	60	Aug	24	MS	$9,000	$29,000	$10,000	•		•	
Georgia											
Armstrong Atlantic State University (Savannah)		Fall semester	24	MEd	$2,802	$5,019		•			
Idaho											
Idaho State University (Pocatello)	30	Fall	36	MS SLP	$5,860	$14,130					
Illinois											
Eastern Illinois University (Charleston)	200	Fall	36, 21	BS, MS	$7,068	$17,481	$775			•	
Illinois State University (Normal)	40	Aug Jan	24	Dipl, MS	$3,000	$6,000			•	•	
Northwestern University (Evanston)	125	Fall	24, 29	MA	$37,872	$46,752				•	
Saint Xavier University (Chicago)	30	Aug	21	MS	$14,900	$14,900				•	
Southern Illinois University (Edwardsville)	60	Fall semester	6, 11	Dipl, MS					•		
Univ of Illinois at Urbana-Champaign	30	Jun	27	MA, PhD	$7,160	$20,000				•	
Kansas											
Fort Hays State University	15	Aug Jan	48, 24	BS, MS	$3,712	$9,808				•	
University of Kansas (Lawrence)	30	Aug	24	Dipl, Masters	$8,000	$17,000				•	
Kentucky											
Eastern Kentucky University (Richmond)	30	Fall semester	48	MA	$7,545	$21,261		•		•	
Louisiana											
Louisiana State Univ Health Sciences Center (New Orleans)	25	May	24	Dipl, MCD	$3,555	$5,430		•		•	
Louisiana Tech University (Ruston)	40	Sep 1	24	Dipl, MA	$3,900	$10,000		•			
Southeastern Louisiana University (Hammond)	25	Fall Spring	36	Dipl, Cert, MS	$1,490	$1,998		•		•	•
University of Louisiana at Lafayette	24	Aug	16, 30	MS, PhD				•			

*Data are shown only for programs that completed the 2007 AMA Survey of Health Professions Education Programs.
‡Key to Offers: 1: Evening or weekend classes; 2: Non-English instruction; 3: Cultural competence instruction; 4: Distance education component.

Speech-Language Pathologist

Programs*	Class Capacity	Begins	Length (months)	Award	Res. Tuition	Non-res. Tuition	Stipend	Offers:‡ 1	2	3	4
University of Louisiana at Monroe	20	Fall	48, 22	Dipl, BS, MS	$5,039	$13,706	$5,000			•	
Maine											
University of Maine - Orono	20	Sep	48, 24	Dipl, BA, MA	$5,962	$15,844					
Maryland											
Univ of Maryland at College Park	25	Aug	20	MA	$10,250	$17,500	$8,000				
Massachusetts											
Boston University	35	Sep 1	24	MS	$33,330	$0				•	
MGH Institute of Health Professions (Boston)	42	Sep	24	MS	$29,750	$29,750		•		•	•
Michigan											
Wayne State University (Detroit)	36	Fall term	20, 48	MA	$15,600	$32,650				•	
Minnesota											
Minnesota State University - Mankato	25	Aug	20	Dipl, MS	$7,097	$11,184				•	
St Cloud State University	18	Fall	48, 24	BS, MS	$2,522	$5,166		•		•	
University of Minnesota - Duluth	15	Sep	30	Dipl, MA							
Mississippi											
University of Southern Mississippi (Hattiesburg)	35	Fall	15	Dipl, Masters	$2,156	$2,715	$6,000				
Missouri											
Saint Louis University (St Louis)	20	Summer	22	Dipl, MA	$880	$880				•	
Truman State University (Kirksville)	15	Rolling enrollment	24	MA	$3,052	$5,205	$2,000				
University of Missouri - Columbia	15	Fall semester	21	MHS	$287	$454				•	
Nebraska											
University of Nebraska - Kearney	20	Fall semester	24	MS	$3,852	$7,968	$8,200			•	
University of Nebraska - Lincoln	50	Fall	21	MS, PhD	$150	$435		•		•	
University of Nebraska - Omaha	25-	Fall Spring	21	Masters	$3,720	$10,140		•		•	
Nevada											
University of Nevada - Reno				Dipl, MS, PhD							
New Jersey											
Seton Hall University (South Orange)	30	Fall	24	MS	$826	$826					
New Mexico											
New Mexico State University (Las Cruces)	25	Aug	24, 36	MA	$4,544	$14,164				•	
University of New Mexico (Albuquerque)	65	Aug	20, 36	Dipl, MS SLP	$4,973	$14,942		•		•	
New York											
CUNY Brooklyn College	40	Sep 1	30	MS	$6,000	$0				•	
Hofstra University (Hempstead)	35	Sep	24, 48	MA, AuD	$24,000	$24,000		•		•	
Ithaca College	30	Late Aug	21	MS	$13,835	$13,835	$25,000	•		•	
New York Medical College (Valhalla)	24	Fall term	21	Dipl, MS	$25,000	$0				•	
New York University	65	Sep	29	Dipl, BS, MA	$1,048	$0				•	
University at Buffalo - SUNY	75	Aug	24	Masters							
North Carolina											
East Carolina University (Greenville)	25	Fall	21	Dipl, MS, PhD	$2,912	$13,300	$5,000			•	•
North Carolina Central University (Durham)	30	Aug Jan	21	MEd	$6,010	$17,300	$2,500	•	•	•	
University of North Carolina - Greensboro	28	Aug 14	21	MS	$2,842	$11,050	$4,000	•		•	
North Dakota											
Minot State University	Open	Fall semester		BS, MS	$6,000	$0					
Ohio											
Kent State University	35	Sep Apr	24	MA	$8,460	$15,470	$5,500	•			
University of Akron	150	Fall semester	48, 24	Dipl, BA, MA SLP	$10,662	$18,964				•	•
Oklahoma											
Oklahoma State University (Stillwater)	20	Fall	40, 21	Dipl, BS, MS	$141	$416	$4,800	•			•
Pennsylvania											
Duquesne University (Pittsburgh)	25	Aug Sep	23	MS						•	
Edinboro University of Pennsylvania	20	Fall semester	22	Dipl, MA	$6,048	$9,678	$3,780			•	
Indiana University of Pennsylvania	22	Fall semester	36, 21	BSEd, MS	$6,214	$9,944	$2,400	•		•	
La Salle University (Philadelphia)	35	Aug	24	MS	$16,200	$16,200		•		•	
Marywood University (Scranton)	40	Fall semester	24, 60	BS/MS, MS	$650	$650				•	
University of Pittsburgh	98	Aug 28	24, 60	Dipl, MA/MS, PhD	$24,576	$31,920	$17,234	•		•	
South Dakota											
University of South Dakota (Vermillion)	50	Aug Sep	24	MA	$3,006	$5,448				•	
Tennessee											
University of Memphis	45	Fall semester	24, 48	MA, AuD	$9,119	$23,532	$4,500				
Texas											
Abilene Christian University	12	Fall semester	18	Dipl, MS	$521	$521				•	
Our Lady of the Lake University (San Antonio)	24	Summer Fall	24	Dipl, MA	$13,000	$13,000		•		•	
Texas State University - San Marcos	20	Fall semester	21	MSCD, MA						•	
Texas Tech Univ Health Sciences Center (Lubbock)	30	Fall	27	Masters	$8,000	$18,000	$3,000			•	

*Data are shown only for programs that completed the 2007 AMA Survey of Health Professions Education Programs.
‡Key to Offers: 1: Evening or weekend classes; 2: Non-English instruction; 3: Cultural competence instruction; 4: Distance education component.

Speech-Language Pathologist

Programs*	Class Capacity	Begins	Length (months)	Award	Res. Tuition	Non-res. Tuition	Stipend	Offers:‡ 1	2	3	4
Univ of Texas - Pan American (Edinburg)	30	Fall	24	Dipl, MS	$810	$2,772				•	
University of Texas at Austin	32	Fall semester	21, 45	MA, AuD	$8,500	$18,300					
West Texas A&M University (Canyon)	30	Summer Fall	21	Dipl, BS, MS					•		
Utah											
Brigham Young University (Provo)	30	Sep 1	24	MS	$5,000	$8,200	$2,400			•	
University of Utah Health Science Center (Salt Lake City)	30	Fall	21	MS, AuD	$8,000	$12,000				•	
Utah State University (Logan)	30	Fall semester	24, 27	Dipl, MS, MEd						•	•
Vermont											
University of Vermont (Burlington)	15	Aug 20	21	MS	$10,422	$26,306			•	•	
Washington											
Eastern Washington University (Spokane)	70	Sep	24	BA, MS	$4,044	$13,317				•	
Western Washington University (Bellingham)	20	Fall	24	MA	$6,252	$16,215				•	
Wisconsin											
University of Wisconsin - Milwaukee	25	Jun Sep	24	Dipl, MS	$10,500	$27,500				•	
University of Wisconsin - River Falls	14	Sep	21	Dipl, MS, MSE	$6,664	$17,274		•		•	
University of Wisconsin - Stevens Point	45	Sep	24, 48	Dipl, SLP, AuD						•	
Wyoming											
University of Wyoming (Laramie)	20	Aug	24	Dipl, MS	$164	$470				•	•

*Data are shown only for programs that completed the 2007 AMA Survey of Health Professions Education Programs.
‡Key to Offers: 1: Evening or weekend classes; 2: Non-English instruction; 3: Cultural competence instruction; 4: Distance education component.

Surgical Assistant

As defined by the American College of Surgeons, the surgical assistant provides aid in exposure, hemostasis, closure, and other intraoperative technical functions that help the surgeon carry out a safe operation with optimal results for the patient. In addition to intraoperative duties, the surgical assistant also performs preoperative and postoperative duties to better facilitate proper patient care. The surgical assistant to the surgeon during the operation does so under the direction and supervision of that surgeon and in accordance with hospital policy and appropriate laws and regulations.

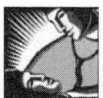

Career Description

In general, surgical assistants have the following responsibilities:
- Determine specific equipment needed per procedure
- Review permit to confirm procedure and special needs
- Select and place of x-rays for reference
- Assist in moving and positioning of patient
- Insert and remove Foley urinary bladder catheter
- Place pneumatic tourniquet
- Confirm procedure with surgeon
- Drape patient within surgeon's guidelines
- Provide retraction of tissue and organs for optimal visualization with regard to tissue type and appropriate retraction instrument and/or technique
- Assist in maintaining hemostasis by direct pressure, use and application of appropriate surgical instrument for the task, placement of ties, placement of suture ligatures, application of chemical hemostatic agents, or other measures as directed by the surgeon
- Use electrocautery mono- and bi-polar
- Clamp, ligate, and cut tissue per surgeon's directive
- Harvest saphenous vein, including skin incision, per surgeon's directive
- Dissect common femoral artery and bifurcate per surgeon's directive
- Maintain integrity of sterile field
- Close all wound layers (facia, subcutaneous and skin) as per surgeon's directive
- Insert drainage tubes per surgeon's directive
- Select and apply wound dressings
- Assist with resuscitation of patient during cardiac arrest or other life-threatening events in the operating room
- Perform any other duties or procedures incident to the surgical procedure deemed necessary and as directed by the surgeon

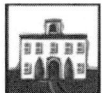

Employment Characteristics

Certified surgical assistants assist in a variety of surgery specialties:
- General surgery
- Orthopaedic surgery
- Neurosurgery
- Spinal surgery
- Otolaryngology
- Obstetrical surgery
- Gynecological surgery
- Craniofacial surgery
- Radial neck surgery
- Genitourinary surgery
- Cardiac surgery
- Thoracic surgery
- Vascular surgery
- Trauma surgery
- Plastic surgery
- Ophthalmologic surgery

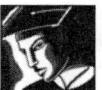

Educational Programs

Length. Current CAAHEP-accredited programs range from 10 months to 22 months. Surgical assisting is a specialty profession that requires specific training over and above a degree in science, nursing, physician assisting, or another health profession.

Prerequisites. Recommended eligibility requirements for admission into a surgical assisting program are:
- Bachelor of Science degree (or higher)
- Associate degree in an allied health field, with 3 years of recent experience
- CST, CNOR, or PA-C, with current certification
- Three years of current operating room scrub and/or assisting experience within the last 5 years
- Military medical training with surgical assistant experience
- Proof of liability insurance
- Current CPR/BLS certification
- Acceptable health and immunization records
- Computer literacy
- Students also must be able to show proof of successful completion of basic science (college level) instruction, including:
- Microbiology
- Pathophysiology
- Pharmacology
- Anatomy and physiology
- Medical terminology

Curriculum. Course content includes:
- Advanced surgical anatomy
- Surgical microbiology
- Surgical pharmacology
- Anesthesia methods and agents
- Bioscience
- Ethical and legal considerations
- Fundamental technical skills
- Complications during surgery
- Interpersonal skills
- Clinical application of computers

Students must possess a working knowledge of operating room fundamentals, including aseptic principles and techniques, before moving on to the advanced levels of the program.

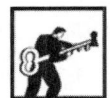

Credentialing

The National Board for Surgical Technology and Surgical Assisting (formerly Liaison Council on Certification for the Surgical Technologist) offers the Certified First Assistant (CST/CFA) credential, and the National Surgical Assistant Association (NSAA) offers a Certified Surgical Assistant (CSA) credential. To be eligible for NBSTSA testing, individuals must be graduates of a CAAHEP- accredited surgical assistant program or a CST with current certification who meets a number of other eligibility requirements.

 **Inquiries**

Careers/Curriculum
Association of Surgical Assistants
6 West Dry Creek Circle, Suite 200
Littleton, CO 80120
800 637-7433 or 303 694-9130
303 694-9169 Fax
www.surgicalassistant.org

National Surgical Assistant Association
2615 Amesbury Road
Winston Salem, NC 27103
888 633-0479
www.nsaa.net

Certification
National Board for Surgical Technology and Surgical Assisting (formerly Liaison Council on Certification for the Surgical Technologist)
6 West Dry Creek Circle, Suite 100
Littleton, CO 80120
800 707-0057
303-325-2536 Fax
www.nbstsa.org

National Surgical Assistant Association
2615 Amesbury Road
Winston Salem, NC 27103
888 633-0479
www.nsaa.net

Program Accreditation
Commission on Accreditation of Allied Health Education Programs (CAAHEP) in collaboration with:
Accreditation Review Committee on Education on Surgical Technology
Subcommittee on Accreditation for Surgical Assisting
6 West Dry Creek Circle, Suite 110
Littleton, CO 80120
303 694-9262
303 741-3655 Fax
E-mail: cindy.collinsworth@arcst.org
www.arcst.org

Surgical Assistant

Indiana

Vincennes University
Surgical Assistant Prgm
1002 N First St
Vincennes, IN 47510
Prgm Dir: Chris Keegan, CST MS
Tel: 812 888-5893   *Fax:* 812 888-4550
E-mail: ckeegan@vinu.edu

Kentucky

Madisonville Community College
Surgical Assistant Prgm
Health Campus
750 N Laffoon St
Madisonville, KY 42431
Prgm Dir: Jeff Bidwell, CSTCSA MA
Tel: 270 824-1740   *Fax:* 270 824-8642
E-mail: jeff.bidwell@kctcs.edu

Michigan

William Beaumont Hospital
Cosponsor: Oakland Community College
Surgical Assistant Prgm
22322 Rutland Dr
Southfield, MI 48075
Prgm Dir: Rebecca Pieknik, CST CSA MS
Tel: 248 898-7685   *Fax:* 248 898-4406
E-mail: rpieknik@beaumonthospitals.com

Tennessee

Meridian Institute of Surgical Assisting
Surgical Assistant Prgm
PO Box 758
Joelton, TN 37080
Prgm Dir: Dennis A Stover, CST SA-C
Tel: 615 299-1416   *Fax:* 615 299-1418
E-mail: meridianinst@aol.com

Nashville State Community College
Surgical Assistant Prgm
120 White Bridge Rd
Nashville, TN 37209
Prgm Dir: T Van Bates, BA CST
Tel: 615 353-3735
E-mail: van.bates@nscc.edu

Texas

South Plains College
Surgical Assistant Prgm
819 Gilbert Dr, Bldg 5
Lubbock, TX 79416
www.southplainscollege.edu
Prgm Dir: Stacey May, CST
Tel: 806 885-3048, Ext 4642   *Fax:* 806 885-5608
E-mail: smay@southplainscollege.edu

Virginia

Eastern Virginia Medical School
Surgical Assistant Prgm
700 W Olney Rd, Ste 1100
Norfolk, VA 23507
Prgm Dir: R Clinton Crews, MPH
Tel: 757 446-6100   *Fax:* 757 446-6179
E-mail: SurgAsst@evms.edu

Surgical Assistant

Programs*	Class Capacity	Begins	Length (months)	Award	Res. Tuition	Non-res. Tuition	Stipend	Offers:‡ 1	2	3	4
Indiana											
Vincennes University	15	Aug	9	Cert	$3,073	$7,671				•	
Kentucky											
Madisonville Community College	25	Aug	9	Cert	$1,840	$5,520		•			
Texas											
South Plains College (Lubbock)	10	Aug	12	Cert	$1,502	$1,854					
Virginia											
Eastern Virginia Medical School (Norfolk)	24	Jul	22	Cert	$10,200	$10,200					

*Data are shown only for programs that completed the 2007 AMA Survey of Health Professions Education Programs.
‡Key to Offers: 1: Evening or weekend classes; 2: Non-English instruction; 3: Cultural competence instruction; 4: Distance education component.

PROGRAMS

Surgical technologists are an integral part of the team of medical practitioners providing surgical care to patients in a variety of settings.

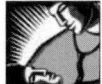

Career Description

Surgical technologists prepare the operating room by selecting and opening sterile supplies. Preoperative duties also include assembling, adjusting, and checking nonsterile equipment to ensure that it is in proper working order. Common duties include operating sterilizers, lights, suction machines, electrosurgical units, and diagnostic equipment.

When patients arrive in the surgical suite, surgical technologists assist in preparing them for surgery by providing physical and emotional support, checking charts, and observing vital signs. They have been educated to properly position the patient on the operating table, assist in connecting and applying surgical equipment and/or monitoring devices, and prepare the incision site. Surgical technologists have primary responsibility for maintaining the sterile field, being constantly vigilant that all members of the team adhere to aseptic technique.

They most often function as the sterile member of the surgical team who passes instruments, sutures, and sponges during surgery. After "scrubbing," they don sterile gown and gloves and prepare the sterile setup for the appropriate procedure. After other members of the sterile team have scrubbed, they assist them with gowning and gloving and with the application of sterile drapes that isolate the operative site.

In order that surgery may proceed smoothly, surgical technologists anticipate the needs of surgeons, passing instruments and providing sterile items in an efficient manner. They share with the circulator the responsibility of accounting for sponges, needles, and instruments before, during, and after surgery.

Surgical technologists may hold retractors or instruments, sponge or suction the operative site, or cut suture materials as directed by the surgeon. They connect drains and tubing and receive and prepare specimens for subsequent pathologic analysis. They are responsible for preparing and applying sterile dressings following the procedure and may assist in the application of nonsterile dressings, including plaster or synthetic casting materials. After surgery, they prepare the operating room for the next patient.

Surgical technologists are most often members of the sterile team but may function in the nonsterile role of circulator. The circulator is not gowned and gloved during the surgical procedure but is available to respond to the needs of the anesthesia provider, keep a written account of the surgical procedure, and participate jointly with the scrubbed person in counting sponges, needles, and instruments before, during, and after surgery. In operating rooms where local anesthetics are administered, they meet the needs of the conscious patient.

Certified surgical technologists with additional specialized education or training also may act in the role of the surgical first assistant. The surgical first assistant provides aid in exposure, hemostasis, and other technical functions under the surgeon's direction that will help the surgeon carry out a safe operation with optimal results for the patient.

Surgical technologists also may provide staffing in postoperative recovery rooms where patients' responses are carefully monitored in the critical phases following general anesthesia.

Employment Characteristics

A majority of surgical technologists work in hospitals, principally in the surgical suite and also in emergency rooms and other settings that call for knowledge of, and ability in, maintaining asepsis, such as materials management and central service. A number work in a wide variety of settings and arrangements, including outpatient surgicenters, private employment by physicians, or as self-employed technologists.

Those who work in hospital and other institutional settings are usually expected to work rotating shifts or to accommodate on-call assignments to ensure adequate staffing for emergency surgical procedures during evening, night, weekend, and holiday hours. Otherwise, surgical technologists follow a standard hospital workday.

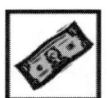

Salary

Salaries vary depending on the experience and education of the individual, the economy of a given region, the responsibilities of the position, and the working hours. According to the US Bureau of Labor Statistics, the median annual salary for surgical technologists was $34,010 in 2004. Refer to Section IV, Table 5 of this *Directory* for more information, or see www.ama-assn.org/go/hpsalary.

Employment Outlook

According to a recent study conducted by the US Bureau of Labor Statistics, the forecast for employment opportunities for surgical technologists is one of rapid growth. Demand for technologists varies among communities and geographic regions. Prospective students are advised to assess the market for graduates within the region in which they would like to work before matriculating in an educational program. Such information is likely to be available through local employment offices, local accredited programs, and hospital councils or hospitals.

Educational Programs

Length. Programs range from 12 to 24 months.

Prerequisites. High school diploma or equivalent.

Curriculum. Accreditation standards require didactic instruction and supervised clinical practice. Subject areas include:

- Medical terminology, professional ethics, and legal aspects of surgical patient care
- Anatomy and physiology, microbiology, anesthesia, and pharmacology
- Sterilization methods and aseptic technique
- Instruments, supplies, and equipment used in surgery
- Surgical patient care and safety precautions
- Operative procedures and biomedical sciences
- Supervised clinical practice in the operating room must include commonly performed procedures in general surgery, obstetrics and gynecology, ophthalmology, otorhinolaryngology, plastic surgery, urology, orthopedics, neurosurgery, thoracic surgery, and cardiovascular and peripheral vascular surgery.

Inquiries

Careers/Curriculum
Association of Surgical Technologists
6 West Dry Creek Circle, Suite 200
Littleton, CO 80120
800 637-7433 or 303 694-9130
303 694-9169 Fax
www.ast.org

Certification/Registration
Inquiries regarding certification as a certified surgical technologist (CST) or a CST certified first assistant (CST/CFA) may be addressed to:

National Board for Surgical Technology and Surgical Assisting (formerly Liaison Council on Certification for the Surgical Technologist)
6 West Dry Creek Circle, Suite 100
Littleton, CO 80120
800 707-0057
303 325-2536 Fax
www.nbstsa.org

Program Accreditation
Commission on Accreditation of Allied Health Education Programs (CAAHEP) in collaboration with:
Accreditation Review Committee on Education in Surgical Technology
6 West Dry Creek Circle, Suite 110
Littleton, CO 80120
303 694-9262
303 741-3655 Fax
E-mail: cindy.collinsworth@arcst.org.

Surgical Technologist

Alabama

James H Faulkner State Community College
Surgical Technology Prgm
1900 Hwy 31 S
Bay Minette, AL 36507
www.faulknerstate.edu
Prgm Dir: Jean Graham, MSN CNOR
Tel: 251 580-2293   *Fax:* 251 580-2199
E-mail: jgraham@faulknerstate.edu

Virginia College
Surgical Technology Prgm
PO Box 19249
Birmingham, AL 35209
Prgm Dir: Nancy H Wright
Tel: 205 271-8250
E-mail: nwright@vc.edu

Calhoun Community College
Surgical Technology Prgm
PO Box 2216
Decatur, AL 35609-2219
Prgm Dir: Grant Wilson, MEd CST
Tel: 256 306-2950   *Fax:* 256 306-2507
E-mail: sgw@calhoun.edu

Flowers Hospital
Surgical Technology Prgm
Home Health Bldg
4370 W Main St, Ste 1
Dothan, AL 36302
Prgm Dir: Elizabeth Andrews, RN BSN CNOR CST
Tel: 334 794-5000, Ext 1129   *Fax:* 334 615-7285
E-mail: stprogram@flowershospital.com

Virginia College
Surgical Technology Prgm
2970 Cottage Hill Rd
Mobile, AL 36606
Prgm Dir: Sharon Jones
Tel: 251 343-7227, Ext 2427   *Fax:* 251 343-7287
E-mail: sjones@vc.edu

Southern Union State Community College
Surgical Technology Prgm
1701 Lafayette Pkwy
Opelika, AL 36801
Prgm Dir: Dot Nichols, BBA RN CNOR
Tel: 334 745-6437, Ext 5536   *Fax:* 334 745-6342
E-mail: dotnichols@suscc.edu

Bevill State Community College
Surgical Technology Prgm
PO Box 800
Sumiton, AL 35148
Prgm Dir: Linda Neumann, RN CNOR
Tel: 205 648-3271, Ext 5569   *Fax:* 205 648-2288
E-mail: lneuman@bscc.edu

Arizona

Mohave Community College
Surgical Technology Prgm
1977 W Acoma Blvd
Lake Havasu City, AZ 86403
Prgm Dir: Sandra Namio, CST CFA
Tel: 928 505-3374   *Fax:* 928 505-3381
E-mail: snamio@imail.mohave.edu

GateWay Community College
Surgical Technology Prgm
108 N 40th St
Phoenix, AZ 85034
Prgm Dir: Susan Wallen, RN MS CNOR CRNFA
Tel: 602 286-8515   *Fax:* 602 392-5244
E-mail: wallen@gatewaycc.edu

Lamson College
Surgical Technology Prgm
1126 N Scottsdale Rd #17
Tempe, AZ 85281
www.lamsoncollege.com
Prgm Dir: Kelly Harris, AAS
Tel: 480 898-7000, Ext 215   *Fax:* 480 967-6645
E-mail: ccrabtree@lamsoncollege.com

Pima Community College
Surgical Technology Prgm
5901 S Calle Santa Cruz
Tucson, AZ 85709-6350
http://cc.pima.edu/CTD/
Prgm Dir: Eric Moorefield
Tel: 520 206-6322   *Fax:* 520 206-6478
E-mail: Eric.Moorefield@pima.edu

Arkansas

Univ of Arkansas Comm Coll - Batesville
Surgical Technology Prgm
PO Box 3350
Batesville, AR 72503
Prgm Dir: Dianne Plemmons, RN MSN
Tel: 870 612-2071   *Fax:* 870 793-4988
E-mail: dplemmons@uaccb.edu

University of Arkansas - Fort Smith
Surgical Technology Prgm
PO Box 3649
Fort Smith, AR 72913
www.uafortsmith.edu
Prgm Dir: Sydney Fulbright, MSN RN CNOR
Tel: 479 788-7855   *Fax:* 479 788-7153
E-mail: sfulbrig@uafortsmith.edu

North Arkansas College
Surgical Technology Prgm
1515 Pioneer Dr
Harrison, AR 72601
Prgm Dir: Charlitta Parton, RN CNOR
Tel: 870 391-3269   *Fax:* 870 391-3250
E-mail: lparton@northark.edu

Baptist Health Schools Little Rock
Surgical Technology Prgm
11900 Colonel Glenn Rd, Ste 1000
Little Rock, AR 72210-2820
www.baptist-health.org
Prgm Dir: Gordon Ward, BSN RN CNOR
Tel: 501 202-7746   *Fax:* 501 202-7712
E-mail: gbward@baptist-health.org

University of Arkansas for Medical Sciences
Surgical Technology Prgm
2200 Fort Roots Dr/Slot 14B/NLR
North Little Rock, AR 72114-1706
www.uams.edu/chrp
Prgm Dir: Gennie Castleberry, BS CST
Tel: 501 257-2354   *Fax:* 501 257-2349
E-mail: castleberrygennier@uams.edu

Southeast Arkansas College
Surgical Technology Prgm
1900 Hazel St
Pine Bluff, AR 71603
Prgm Dir: Clemetine Wesley, RN ORT AAS
Tel: 870 543-5967   *Fax:* 870 543-5912
E-mail: cwesley@seark.edu

Northwest Technical Institute
Surgical Technology Prgm
PO Box 2000
709 S Old Missouri Rd
Springdale, AR 72765
www.nti.tec.ar.us
Prgm Dir: Katie Fritz, CST
Tel: 479 751-8824, Ext 117   *Fax:* 479 751-7780
E-mail: kfritz@nti.tec.ar.us

California

San Joaquin Valley College - Bakersfield
Surgical Technology Prgm
201 New Stine Rd
Bakersfield, CA 93309
Prgm Dir: Patricia Siefkas, ASSc CST
Tel: 661 834-0126, Ext 141   *Fax:* 661 834-1021
E-mail: PatriciaS@sjvc.edu

Southwestern College
Surgical Technology Prgm
900 Otay Lakes Rd
Chula Vista, CA 91910
Prgm Dir: Bill Maddox, MHA BS RN
Tel: 619 421-6700, Ext 5616   *Fax:* 619 482-6439
E-mail: wmaddox@swc.cc.ca.us

Mt Diablo Adult Education
Surgical Technology Prgm
1266 San Carlos Ave
Concord, CA 94518
Prgm Dir: Susan Garske, BA MS
Tel: 925 685-7340, Ext 2734   *Fax:* 925 363-9757

Fresno City College
Surgical Technology Prgm
1101 E University Ave
Fresno, CA 93741
Prgm Dir: Mary Jane McClain, RN CNOR
Tel: 559 244-2643   *Fax:* 559 244-2626
E-mail: maryjane.mcclain@fresnocitycollege.edu

San Joaquin Valley College
Surgical Technology Prgm
295 E Sierra Ave
Fresno, CA 93710
www.sjcv.edu
Prgm Dir: Teri Junge, CST CFA FAST
Tel: 559 448-8282   *Fax:* 559 448-8250
E-mail: terij@sjvc.edu

Glendale Career College
Surgical Technology Prgm
1015 Grandview Ave
Glendale, CA 91201
www.success.edu
Prgm Dir: Connie Bell, CST
Tel: 818 956-4915, Ext 261   *Fax:* 818 243-6028
E-mail: cbell@success.edu

Everest College - Hayward
Surgical Technology Prgm
22336 Main St
Hayward, CA 94541
Prgm Dir: Rechelle A Bowen, CST
Tel: 510 582-9500   *Fax:* 510 582-9645
E-mail: rbowen@cci.edu

Premiere Career College
Surgical Technology Prgm
12901 Ramona Blvd
Irwindale, CA 91706
Prgm Dir: Antonio Torres, BS MEd CST CRCST
Tel: 626 814-2080   *Fax:* 626 814-3242
E-mail: antotorres@netzero.net

Career Colleges of America - Los Angeles
Surgical Technology Prgm
1801 S LaCienega Blvd
Los Angeles, CA 90035
Prgm Dir: Angela Gomez
Tel: 310 287-9901
E-mail: angelag@careercolleges.org

Concorde Career College - North Hollywood
Surgical Technology Prgm
12412 Victory Blvd
North Hollywood, CA 91606
Prgm Dir: Yvonne Williams
Tel: 818 766-8151, Ext 251   *Fax:* 818 766-1587
E-mail: ywilliams@concorde.edu

Glendale Career College - Oceanside Campus
Surgical Technology Prgm
2204 El Camino Real, Ste 315
Oceanside, CA 92054
www.landmarked.com
Prgm Dir: Donna McCasland
Tel: 760 450-0340   *Fax:* 760 450-0396
E-mail: dmccasland@success.edu

Career Networks Institute
Surgical Technology Prgm
986 Town and Country Rd
Orange, CA 92868
Prgm Dir: Mike Kaputikyan, CST
Tel: 714 568-0047, Ext 103
E-mail: mike.kaputikyan@cniworks.com

American College of Health Professions
Surgical Technology Prgm
700 E Redland Blvd, #U227
Redlands, CA 92374
Prgm Dir: Michele Ray, CST
Tel: 909 307-6022   *Fax:* 909 307-6032
E-mail: achpfaculty@msn.com

Everest College - Reseda
Surgical Technology Prgm
18040 Sherman Way
Reseda, CA 91335
Prgm Dir: David Camarena, MD
Tel: 818 774-0550
E-mail: dcamarena@cci.edu

Career Colleges of America - San Bernardino
Surgical Technology Prgm
184 W Club Center Dr
San Bernardino, CA 92408
Prgm Dir: Debbie Bessent
Tel: 909 824-0897   *Fax:* 909 872-1144
E-mail: debbieb@careercolleges.org

Concorde Career College - San Bernardino
Surgical Technology Prgm
201 E Airport Dr, Ste A
San Bernardino, CA 92408
www.concorde.edu
Prgm Dir: Michelle Rey, CST
Tel: 909 884-8891   *Fax:* 909 384-1265
E-mail: mrey@concorde.edu

Skyline College
Surgical Technology Prgm
3300 College Dr
San Bruno, CA 94066
Prgm Dir: Alice Erskine, CST MSN CNOR
Tel: 650 738-4470   *Fax:* 650 738-4179
E-mail: erskine@smccd.edu

Concorde Career College
Surgical Technology Prgm
4393 Imperial Ave
Ste 100
San Diego, CA 92113
www.concorde.edu
Prgm Dir: Niall E Davis, CST
Tel: 619 688-0800, Ext 307   *Fax:* 619 220-4177
E-mail: ndavis@concorde.edu

Naval School of Health Sciences, San Diego
Surgical Technology Prgm
34101 Farenholt Ave
San Diego, CA 92134-5291
Prgm Dir: CDR Thomas A Sweet, NC, USN, MSN CNOR
Tel: 619 532-7831   *Fax:* 619 532-7796
E-mail: tsweet@nshs-sd.med.navy.mil
Notes: US Armed Forces Program

UCSF Medical Center
Surgical Technology Prgm
505 Parnassus Ave
San Francisco, CA 94143
Prgm Dir: Jane Kuhn, MSN
Tel: 415 353-1309   *Fax:* 415 353-1834
E-mail: jane.kuhn@ucsfmedctr.org
Notes: Currently inactive

Newbridge College
Surgical Technology Prgm
1840 E 17th St, Ste 140
Santa Ana, CA 92705
Prgm Dir: Claro Nunez, CST
Tel: 714 550-8000   *Fax:* 714 550-6740
E-mail: cnunez@newbridgecollege.edu

Simi Valley Adult School
Surgical Technology Prgm
3192 Los Angeles Ave
Simi Valley, CA 93065
Prgm Dir: Ronald O Kruzel, BA CST
Tel: 805 579-6200, Ext 249   *Fax:* 805 522-8902
E-mail: ronk@simi.tec.ca.us

Career Colleges of America - South Gate
Surgical Technology Prgm
5612 E Imperial Hwy
South Gate, CA 90802
Prgm Dir: Claro M Nunez, CST
Tel: 562 861-8702, Ext 126   *Fax:* 562 869-7013
E-mail: claron@careercolleges.org

Colorado

Concorde Career College - Aurora
Surgical Technology Prgm
111 N Havana St
Aurora, CO 80010
www.concorde.edu
Prgm Dir: Karyn Songer, CST FAST
Tel: 303 861-1151, Ext 233   *Fax:* 303 839-5478
E-mail: ksonger@concorde.edu

Everest College
Surgical Technology Prgm
9065 Grant St
Thornton, CO 80229
Prgm Dir: Damen L Sanchez
Tel: 303 457-2757   *Fax:* 303 457-4030
E-mail: dsanchez@cci.edu

Connecticut

Bridgeport Hospital
Surgical Technology Prgm
200 Mill Hill Ave
Bridgeport, CT 06610
Prgm Dir: Janet Serra, RN BSN CNOR
Tel: 203 384-3205   *Fax:* 203 384-3046
E-mail: njserr@bpthosp.org

Danbury Hospital
Surgical Technology Prgm
24 Hospital Ave
Danbury, CT 06810
www.danburyhospital.org
Prgm Dir: Mary E Janell, MS RN CNOR
Tel: 203 739-7724   *Fax:* 203 797-0706
E-mail: mary.janell@danhosp.org

Eli Whitney Vocational Technical School
Surgical Technology Prgm
71 Jones Rd
Hamden, CT 06514
Prgm Dir: Karen Dempsey, CNOR BSN MBA
Tel: 203 397-4031, Ext 386   *Fax:* 203 397-4129
E-mail: Karen.Dempsey@po.ct.state.us

PROGRAMS

A I Prince Technical High School
Surgical Technology Prgm
401 Flatbush Ave
Hartford, CT 06106
www.cttech.org/prince
Prgm Dir: Elia Acosta, CST BA MS
Tel: 860 286-9712   *Fax:* 860 286-9715
E-mail: Elia.Acosta@ct.gov

Manchester Community College
Surgical Technology Prgm
MS 17, PO Box 1046
Manchester, CT 06045
Prgm Dir: Richard Clark, CST MA
Tel: 860 512-2715   *Fax:* 860 512-2621
E-mail: rclark@mcc.commnet.edu

Florida

Lee County High Tech Center - North
Surgical Technology Prgm
360 Santa Barbara Blvd N
Cape Coral, FL 33993
Prgm Dir: Dona J Hoyt, RN
Tel: 239 574-4440, Ext 227   *Fax:* 239 458-3721
E-mail: donajh@leeschools.net

Brevard Community College
Surgical Technology Prgm
1519 Clearlake Rd
Cocoa, FL 32922
Prgm Dir: Judith C Schatte, RN CNOR CRNFA
Tel: 321 632-1111, Ext 64123   *Fax:* 321 634-3731
E-mail: schattej@brevardcc.edu

Daytona Beach Community College
Surgical Technology Prgm
PO Box 2811
1200 W International Speedway Blvd
Daytona Beach, FL 32120
Prgm Dir: Dana Earnest, CST
Tel: 386 506-3747   *Fax:* 386 506-3000
E-mail: earnesd@dbcc.edu

Sanford-Brown Institute - Ft Lauderdale
Surgical Technology Prgm
1201 W Cypress Creek Rd
Fort Lauderdale, FL 33309
Prgm Dir: Pierrot Alexis, CST
Tel: 954 308-7396   *Fax:* 954 375-6940
E-mail: palexis@sbftlaud.com

Indian River Community College
Surgical Technology Prgm
3209 Virginia Ave
Fort Pierce, FL 34981
Prgm Dir: Kathy A Gelety, ST RN CNOR
Tel: 772 336-6227   *Fax:* 772 336-6235
E-mail: kgelety@ircc.edu

National School of Technology
Surgical Technology Prgm
Hialeah Campus
4410 W 16th Ave, Ste 52
Hialeah, FL 33012
Prgm Dir: Ingrid Mendez, ST
Tel: 305 558-9500, Ext 146   *Fax:* 305 558-4419
E-mail: imendez@cci.edu

Sheridan Technical Center
Surgical Technology Prgm
5400 Sheridan St
Hollywood, FL 33021
www.sheridantechnical.com
Prgm Dir: Karen Connolly, CST
Tel: 754 321-5480, Ext 3092   *Fax:* 754 321-5467
E-mail: karen.connolly@browardschools.com

Concorde Career Institute - Jacksonville
Surgical Technology Prgm
7960 Arlington Expressway
Ste 120
Jacksonville, FL 32211
www.concorde.edu
Prgm Dir: Luis Melendez, CST CFA
Tel: 904 807-5132   *Fax:* 904 721-9944
E-mail: lmelendez@concorde.edu

Florida Community College - Jacksonville
Surgical Technology Prgm
4501 Capper Rd
Jacksonville, FL 32218
Prgm Dir: Neal Henning
Tel: 904 766-6524   *Fax:* 904 713-4859
E-mail: nhenning@fccj.edu

Palm Beach Community College
Surgical Technology Prgm
4200 S Congress Ave, MS60
Lake Worth, FL 33461
Prgm Dir: Toni Crowley, MS RNFA CNOR
Tel: 561 868-3561   *Fax:* 561 868-3635
E-mail: crowleyt@pbcc.edu

Traviss Career Center
Surgical Technology Prgm
3225 Winter Lake Rd
Lakeland, FL 33803
Prgm Dir: Pamela Troxell, RN BSN CNOR
Tel: 863 499-2700, Ext 299   *Fax:* 863 499-2067
E-mail: pam.troxell@polk-fl.net

Concorde Career Institute
Surgical Technology Prgm
4000 N State Rd 7
Lauderdale Lakes, FL 33319
www.concorde.edu
Prgm Dir: James Bell, CST CFA
Tel: 954 731-8880   *Fax:* 954 485-2961
E-mail: jbell@concorde.edu

Lindsey Hopkins Tech Education Center
Surgical Technology Prgm
750 NW 20th St
Miami, FL 33127
http://lindsey.dadeschools.net
Prgm Dir: Ibia Bustelo, RN BSN CNOR
Tel: 305 324-6070, Ext 8015
E-mail: IBustelo@dadeschools.net

National School of Technology
Surgical Technology Prgm
Kendall Campus
9020 SW 137th Ave
Miami, FL 33186
Prgm Dir: Rosie Sirota
Tel: 305 386-9900   *Fax:* 305 558-4419
E-mail: rsirota@cci.edu

National School of Technology
Surgical Technology Prgm
Miami Campus
111 NW 183rd St
Miami, FL 33169
Prgm Dir: John Mays, CST OSA BSHA
Tel: 305 949-9500   *Fax:* 305 558-4419
E-mail: jmays@cci.edu

Keiser Career College
Surgical Technology Prgm
17395 NW 59th Ave
Miami Lakes, FL 33015
Prgm Dir: Ceilia Gonzalez, BSN CST
Tel: 305 820-5003
E-mail: bgonzalez@keisercareer.edu

Lorenzo Walker Institute of Technology
Surgical Technology Prgm
3702 Estey Ave
Naples, FL 34104
Prgm Dir: Nancy Turmelle, RN CNOR
Tel: 941 430-6900, Ext 2049   *Fax:* 941 430-6922
E-mail: turmelna@collier.k12.fl.us

Okaloosa-Walton College
Surgical Technology Prgm
100 College Blvd
Niceville, FL 32578
www.owc.edu
Prgm Dir: April Carter, MSN
Tel: 850 729-6444   *Fax:* 850 729-6460
E-mail: cartera@owc.edu

Central Florida Community College
Surgical Technology Prgm
PO Box 1388
3001 SW College Rd
Ocala, FL 34478-1388
www.cf.edu
Prgm Dir: Brenda Frazier, MEd RN CNOR CST BSN
Tel: 352 237-2111, Ext 1271   *Fax:* 352 873-5889
E-mail: frazierb@cf.edu

Orlando Tech
Surgical Technology Prgm
301 W Amelia St
Orlando, FL 32801
www.ocps.net
Prgm Dir: Betty Arnett, RMA CST
Tel: 407 246-7060, Ext 4887   *Fax:* 407 317-3372
E-mail: arnettb@ocps.net

Central Florida Institute
Surgical Technology Prgm
30522 US 19th N, Ste 310
Palm Harbor, FL 34684
Prgm Dir: Karen Niles, CST MHS MBA
Tel: 727 786-4707, Ext 240   *Fax:* 727 781-9421
E-mail: kniles@cfinstitute.com

MedVance Institute - Atlantis Campus
Surgical Technology Prgm
1630 S Congress Ave, Ste 300
Palm Springs, FL 33461
Prgm Dir: Nancy K Phelps, CST
Tel: 561 304-3466, Ext 130   *Fax:* 561 304-3471
E-mail: nphelps@medvance.edu

Gulf Coast Community College
Surgical Technology Prgm
5230 W US Hwy 98
Panama City, FL 32401
http://surgtech.gulfcoast.edu
Prgm Dir: Mary E McNaron, RN CNOR CST BSN MS
Tel: 850 769-1551, Ext 3551   *Fax:* 850 747-3246
E-mail: lmcnaron@gulfcoast.edu

Pensacola Junior College
Surgical Technology Prgm
5555 Hwy 98 W
Pensacola, FL 32507
Prgm Dir: Gayle Griffin, BSN RN
Tel: 850 484-2257   *Fax:* 850 484-2326
E-mail: ggriffin@pjc.edu

Virginia College at Penascola
Surgical Technology Prgm
19 W Garden St
Pensacola, FL 32501
Prgm Dir: Barbara Inkel, RN CNOR
Tel: 850 436-8444   *Fax:* 850 436-2677
E-mail: binkel@vc.edu

MedVance Institute - Plantation Campus
Surgical Technology Prgm
4101 NW 3rd Ct, Ste 9
Plantation, FL 33317
Prgm Dir: Bonnie Merschdorf
Tel: 954 587-7100   *Fax:* 954 587-7704
E-mail: bmerschdorf@medvance.edu

Keiser University
Surgical Technology Prgm
10330 South US 1
Port St Lucie, FL 34952
Prgm Dir: Jean Lindo, CST
Tel: 772 398-9990
E-mail: jlindo@keiseruniversity.edu

Sarasota County Technical Institute
Surgical Technology Prgm
4748 Beneva Rd
Sarasota, FL 34233
Prgm Dir: Harlean Satin, MPA RNCNA BC
Tel: 941 924-1365, Ext 372   *Fax:* 941 361-6886
E-mail: harlean_satin@srqit.sarasota.k12.fl.us
Notes: Currently inactive

Keiser Career College
Surgical Technology Prgm
11208 Danka Blvd
St Petersburg, FL 33716
Prgm Dir: Heather Spitz, CST
Tel: 727 576-6500   *Fax:* 727 576-6589
E-mail: hspitz@keisercareer.edu

Pinellas Tech Educ Ctr - Clearwater Campus
Surgical Technology Prgm
901 34th St S
St Petersburg, FL 33711
www.myptec.org
Prgm Dir: Candace Gioia, RN BSN CNOR
Tel: 727 893-2500, Ext 1077   *Fax:* 727 893-2776
E-mail: gioiac@pcsb.org

Concorde Career Institute - Tampa
Surgical Technology Prgm
4202 W Spruce St
Tampa, FL 33607
Prgm Dir: Robin Ward
Tel: 813 314-2478   *Fax:* 813 872-6884
E-mail: rward@concorde.edu

Erwin Technical Center
Surgical Technology Prgm
2010 E Hillsborough Ave
Tampa, FL 33610-8299
Prgm Dir: Deborah Pearson, CST FA-CRCST
Tel: 813 231-1800, Ext 1331   *Fax:* 813 231-1820
E-mail: deborah.pearson@sdhc.k12.fl.us

Florida Metropolitan Univ - Tampa College
Surgical Technology Prgm
3924 Coconut Palm Dr
Tampa, FL 33619
www.fmu.edu
Prgm Dir: Shirlyn Chinnery-Boynes, BS CST
Tel: 813 621-0041, Ext 171   *Fax:* 813 623-5769
E-mail: sboynes@cci.edu

Sanford-Brown Institute
Surgical Technology Prgm
5701 E Hillsborough Ave, Ste 1417
Tampa, FL 33610
Prgm Dir: Joseph Milam, CST CSPDT
Tel: 813 496-2777   *Fax:* 813 630-1309
E-mail: jmilam@sbtampa.com

Georgia

Albany Technical College
Surgical Technology Prgm
1704 S Slappey Blvd
Albany, GA 31701-3514
Prgm Dir: Lori Day, CST
Tel: 229 430-3552   *Fax:* 229 430-5115
E-mail: lday@albanytech.edu

Athens Technical College
Surgical Technology Prgm
800 US Hwy 29 N
Athens, GA 30601-1500
Prgm Dir: Beth Jackson-Streb, CST RN BSN MEd
Tel: 706 355-5072   *Fax:* 706 425-3104
E-mail: bjackson-streb@athenstech.edu

Augusta Technical College
Surgical Technology Prgm
3200 Augusta Tech Dr, 900 Bldg
Augusta, GA 30906
Prgm Dir: Patty Young, RN CNOR
Tel: 706 771-4191   *Fax:* 706 771-4181
E-mail: pyoung@augusta.tec.ga.us

Coastal Georgia Community College
Surgical Technology Prgm
3700 Altama Ave
Brunswick, GA 31520-3644
www.cgcc.edu
Prgm Dir: Joyce K Tate, RN BSN CNOR
Tel: 912 264-7250   *Fax:* 912 262-3283
E-mail: jtate@cgcc.edu

DeKalb Technical College
Surgical Technology Prgm
495 N Indian Creek Dr
Clarkston, GA 30021
www.dekalbtech.edu
Prgm Dir: Frances Offutt, RN ASN
Tel: 404 297-9522, Ext 1159   *Fax:* 404 294-6496
E-mail: offuttf@dekalbtech.edu

Columbus Technical College
Surgical Technology Prgm
928 Manchester Expwy
Columbus, GA 31904-6572
www.columbustech.edu
Prgm Dir: Kellie Byrd, RN BSEd MSN CNOR
Tel: 706 649-1498   *Fax:* 706 641-5284
E-mail: kbyrd@columbustech.edu

Dalton State College
Surgical Technology Prgm
213 N College Dr
Dalton, GA 30720
Prgm Dir: Alice Kirby, RN BSN
Tel: 706 272-2658   *Fax:* 706 272-4563
E-mail: akirby@em.daltonstate.edu

Griffin Technical College
Surgical Technology Prgm
501 Varsity Rd
Griffin, GA 30223
Prgm Dir: Claudia Holley, RN CST
Tel: 770 233-6166   *Fax:* 770 229-3294
E-mail: holleyc@griftec.org

Gwinnett Technical College
Surgical Technology Prgm
5150 Sugarloaf Pkwy
Lawrenceville, GA 30043-5702
www.gwinnetttech.edu
Prgm Dir: T C Parker, CST AAS
Tel: 770 962-7580, Ext 6348   *Fax:* 770 962-1506
E-mail: tcparker@gwinnetttech.edu

Central Georgia Technical College
Surgical Technology Prgm
3300 Macon Tech Dr
Macon, GA 31206
Prgm Dir: Becky P Darley, RN CNOR
Tel: 478 757-3560   *Fax:* 478 757-3575
E-mail: bdarley@centralgatech.edu

Chattahoochee Technical College
Surgical Technology Prgm
980 S Cobb Ave
Marietta, GA 30060
Prgm Dir: Lorraine Wilderman, RN BSN CNOR
Tel: 770 528-4488   *Fax:* 770 528-4584
E-mail: lwilderman@chattcollege.com

Georgia Medical Institute
Surgical Technology Prgm
1600 Terrell Mill Rd
Marietta, GA 30067
Prgm Dir: Barbara Armstrong
Tel: 770 428-6303   *Fax:* 770 428-8415
E-mail: barmstro@cci.edu

Lanier Technical College
Surgical Technology Prgm
2990 Landrum Education Dr
Oakwood, GA 30566
Prgm Dir: Jamey Watson, CST AAT
Tel: 770 531-6421   *Fax:* 770 531-6306
E-mail: jwatson@laniertech.edu

Northwestern Technical College
Surgical Technology Prgm
265 Bicentennial Trail
Rock Spring, GA 30739
Prgm Dir: Mary L Jirsa, RN BSN CNOR
Tel: 706 764-3544   *Fax:* 706 764-3718
E-mail: mjirsa@northwesterntech.edu

Coosa Valley Technical College
Surgical Technology Prgm
1 Maurice Culberson Dr
Rome, GA 30161
Prgm Dir: Tina M Cummings, CST
Tel: 706 295-6100   *Fax:* 706 295-6894
E-mail: tcummings@coosavalleytech.edu

Savannah Technical College
Surgical Technology Prgm
5717 White Bluff Rd
Savannah, GA 31405
Prgm Dir: Brenda L McMillin, CST MA
Tel: 912 303-1816   *Fax:* 912 303-4317
E-mail: bmcmillin@savtec.org

Ogeechee Technical College
Surgical Technology Prgm
1 Joe Kennedy Blvd
Statesboro, GA 30458
Prgm Dir: Deborah Scott, RNC CNOR
Tel: 912 486-7401, Ext 565   *Fax:* 912 486-7604
E-mail: dscott@ogeecheetech.edu

Flint River Technical College
Surgical Technology Prgm
1533 Hwy 19 S
Thomaston, GA 30286
Prgm Dir: Thomas Satterfield, BA CST
Tel: 706 646-6185   *Fax:* 706 646-6163
E-mail: tsatterfield@flintrivertech.org

Southwest Georgia Technical College
Surgical Technology Prgm
15689 US Hwy 19 N
Thomasville, GA 31792
Prgm Dir: Sherrie Holliman, RN MSN RNFA
Tel: 229 225-5205   *Fax:* 229 225-5289
E-mail: sholliman@southwestgatech.edu

Valdosta Technical College
Surgical Technology Prgm
4089 Val Tech Rd
Valdosta, GA 31602
www.valdostatech.edu
Prgm Dir: Dorothy E Cox-Carter, RN BSN
Tel: 229 245-3860   *Fax:* 229 259-5567
E-mail: dcox@valdostatech.edu

Southeastern Technical College
Surgical Technology Prgm
3001 E First St
Vidalia, GA 30474
www.southeasterntech.edu
Prgm Dir: Deborah Smith, RN CNOR
Tel: 912 538-3182   *Fax:* 912 538-3106
E-mail: dsmith@southeasterntech.edu

West Central Technical College
Surgical Technology Prgm
176 Murphy Campus Blvd
Waco, GA 30180
www.westcentraltech.edu
Prgm Dir: Richard T Bailey, RN BSN
Tel: 770 537-6044   *Fax:* 770 537-7992
E-mail: rbailey@westcentraltech.edu

Middle Georgia Technical College
Surgical Technology Prgm
80 Cohen Walker Dr
Warner Robins, GA 31088
www.middlegatech.edu
Prgm Dir: Lorna Cox, CST AAS
Tel: 478 988-6800, Ext 4045   *Fax:* 478 988-6875
E-mail: lcox@middlegatech.edu

Okefenokee Technical College
Surgical Technology Prgm
1701 Carswell Ave
Waycross, GA 31503
www.okefenokeetech.edu
Prgm Dir: Sally M Smith, RN MEd
Tel: 912 287-5839   *Fax:* 912 287-4865
E-mail: smsmith@okefenokeetech.edu

Hawaii

Kapi'olani Community College
Surgical Technology Prgm
4303 Diamond Head Rd
Honolulu, HI 96816
Prgm Dir: Christine Nadamoto, CST RN MS
Tel: 808 734-9305
E-mail: nadamoto@hawaii.edu

Idaho

Boise State University
Surgical Technology Prgm
College of Technology
Boise, ID 83725
Prgm Dir: Mona Bourbonnais
Tel: 208 426-1519   *Fax:* 208 426-3155
E-mail: mbourbonnais@boisestate.edu

Eastern Idaho Technical College
Surgical Technology Prgm
1600 S 25th E
Idaho Falls, ID 83404-5788
Prgm Dir: Becky Chapman, CST
Tel: 208 524-3000, Ext 3427   *Fax:* 208 525-7038
E-mail: bchapman@eitc.edu

College of Southern Idaho
Surgical Technology Prgm
315 Falls Ave, Aspen Bldg #158
PO Box 1238
Twin Falls, ID 83303-1238
Prgm Dir: Janet Milligan, RN CNOR
Tel: 208 732-6706   *Fax:* 208 733-4743
E-mail: jmilligan@csi.edu

Illinois

Parkland College
Surgical Technology Prgm
2400 W Bradley Ave
Champaign, IL 61821
Prgm Dir: Jody Randolph, BSN RN CNOR
Tel: 217 351-2375   *Fax:* 217 373-3830
E-mail: jorandolph@parkland.edu

Malcolm X College
Surgical Technology Prgm
1900 W Van Buren St
Chicago, IL 60612
Prgm Dir: Marietta McDuffy, CST BS MEd
Tel: 312 850-7351   *Fax:* 312 850-7453
E-mail: mmcduffy@ccc.edu

Prairie State College
Surgical Technology Prgm
202 S Halsted St
Chicago Heights, IL 60411
www.prairiestate.edu
Prgm Dir: Susan Chap, BS PA RN
Tel: 708 709-3780   *Fax:* 708 709-3777
E-mail: schap@prairiestate.edu

Richland Community College
Surgical Technology Prgm
1 College Park
Decatur, IL 62521-8512
Prgm Dir: Katherine Lee, MS CST
Tel: 217 875-7200, Ext 763   *Fax:* 217 875-6965
E-mail: klee@richland.edu

Shawnee Community College
Surgical Technology Prgm
East St Louis Higher Education Ctr
601 James R Thompson Blvd
East St Louis, IL 62201
Prgm Dir: Denisa Huff
Tel: 618 874-8714   *Fax:* 618 634-3300
E-mail: dhuff@eslccc.com

Elgin Community College
Surgical Technology Prgm
1700 Spartan Dr
Elgin, IL 60123
www.elgin.edu
Prgm Dir: Maureen Lange, RNC CNOR CNE MS
Tel: 847 214-7303   *Fax:* 847 214-7527
E-mail: mlange@elgin.edu

College of Lake County
Surgical Technology Prgm
19351 W Washington St
Grayslake, IL 60030
Prgm Dir: Soheila Kayoud, CST BA
Tel: 847 543-2776   *Fax:* 847 223-1357
E-mail: skayoud@clcillinois.edu

Southern Illinois Collegiate Common Market
Surgical Technology Prgm
3213 S Park Ave
Herrin, IL 62948
www.siccm.com
Prgm Dir: Pamela Appleton, RN BS CNOR
Tel: 618 942-6902   *Fax:* 618 942-6658
E-mail: appleton@siccm.com

Illinois Central College
Surgical Technology Prgm
Peoria Campus Div
201 SW Adams St
Peoria, IL 61635-0001
www.icc.edu
Prgm Dir: William Hammer, CST MEd
Tel: 309 999-4633   *Fax:* 309 673-9626
E-mail: bhammer@icc.edu

John Wood Community College
Surgical Technology Prgm
1301 S 48th St
Quincy, IL 62305
Prgm Dir: Sandra McKelvie, RN
Tel: 217 641-4550, Ext 4550   *Fax:* 217 224-4208
E-mail: mckelvie@jwcc.edu

Triton College
Surgical Technology Prgm
2000 N Fifth Ave
River Grove, IL 60171
Prgm Dir: Jessica Brown, CST
Tel: 708 456-0300, Ext 3563   *Fax:* 708 583-3336
E-mail: jbrown@triton.edu

Trinity College of Nursing & Health Sciences
Surgical Technology Prgm
2122 25th Ave
Rock Island, IL 61201-1216
Prgm Dir: Farla Champ, MS RN CNOR CST
Tel: 309 779-7768   *Fax:* 309 779-7746
E-mail: champf@trinityqc.com

Rock Valley College
Surgical Technology Prgm
3301 N Mulford Rd
Rockford, IL 61114-5699
Prgm Dir: Paula Malone, RCST/SFA LPN II
Tel: 815 921-3205   *Fax:* 815 921-3249
E-mail: PMalone@RockValleyCollege.edu

Waubonsee Community College
Surgical Technology Prgm
Rte 47 at Waubonsee Dr
Sugar Grove, IL 60554
www.waubonsee.edu
Prgm Dir: Jess Toussaint, MS
Tel: 630 466-2350   *Fax:* 630 466-4119
E-mail: jtoussaint@waubonsee.edu

College of DuPage
Surgical Technology Prgm
550 E Washington St
West Chicago, IL 60185
www.cod.edu
Prgm Dir: Kathy Cabai, CST RN CNOR MSinEd CST
Tel: 630 293-4115, Ext 2601   *Fax:* 630 293-4129
E-mail: cabaik@cod.edu

Indiana

Bloomington Hospital
Surgical Technology Prgm
PO Box 1149
605 W Second St
Bloomington, IN 47402
http://bloomingtonhospital.org
Prgm Dir: Lillian Bartlett, RN BSN CNOR
Tel: 812 335-5571   *Fax:* 812 335-5444
E-mail: lbartlett@bloomingtonhospital.org

Ivy Tech Community College - Columbus
Surgical Technology Prgm
4475 Central Ave
Columbus, IN 47203-1868
Prgm Dir: Susan D Sheets, RN BSN CNOR
Tel: 812 372-9925, Ext 185   *Fax:* 812 372-0311
E-mail: ssheets@ivytech.edu

Ivy Tech Community College - Evansville
Surgical Technology Prgm
3501 First Ave
Evansville, IN 47710
Prgm Dir: Julia Hinkle, RN MHS CNOR BSN
Tel: 812 429-1490   *Fax:* 812 429-9805
E-mail: jhinkle@ivytech.edu

Indiana Business College - Ft Wayne
Surgical Technology Prgm
6413 N Clinton St
Fort Wayne, IN 46825
Prgm Dir: Jill Lobacz, AAS CST
Tel: 260 471-7667
E-mail: jill.lobacz@ibcschools.edu

University of Saint Francis
Surgical Technology Prgm
2701 Spring St
Fort Wayne, IN 46808
www.sf.edu/healthscience/surgtech/
Prgm Dir: Elizabeth Slagle, MS RN CST
Tel: 260 434-7673   *Fax:* 260 434-7697
E-mail: eslagle@sf.edu

Clarian Health Partners Inc
Surgical Technology Prgm
PO Box 1367
Indianapolis, IN 46206-1367
www.clarian.org
Prgm Dir: Terry Myers, RN
Tel: 317 962-1864   *Fax:* 317 962-2102
E-mail: tmyers@clarian.org

Indiana Business College
Surgical Technology Prgm
8150 Brookville Rd
Indianapolis, IN 46239
Prgm Dir: Susan C Fisher, CST CFA
Tel: 317 375-8000   *Fax:* 317 351-1871
E-mail: susan.fisher@ibcschools.edu

Ivy Tech Community College
Surgical Technology Prgm
Central Indiana Region
One W 26th St, PO Box 1763
Indianapolis, IN 46206-1763
Prgm Dir: Wanda L Haver, CST BS ED
Tel: 317 921-4404   *Fax:* 317 921-4753
E-mail: whaver@ivytech.edu

Ivy Tech Community College - Kokomo
Surgical Technology Prgm
700 E Firmin St
Kokomo, IN 46902
www.ivytech.edu
Prgm Dir: Judi Townsend, BSN RN CNOR
Tel: 765 457-0858, Ext 107   *Fax:* 765 457-1036
E-mail: jtownsen@ivytech.edu

Ivy Tech Community College - Lafayette
Surgical Technology Prgm
3101 S Creasy Ln, PO Box 6299
Lafayette, IN 47903
Prgm Dir: Dorothy S Hall, MSN RN CST
Tel: 765 269-5208   *Fax:* 765 269-5248
E-mail: dhall@ivytech.edu

Everest College
Surgical Technology Prgm
707 E 80th Pl, Ste 46410
Merrillville, IN 46410
Prgm Dir: Patricia Rich
Tel: 219 756-6811   *Fax:* 219 756-6812
E-mail: prich@cci.edu

Ivy Tech Community College - Michigan City
Surgical Technology Prgm
3714 Franklin St
Michigan City, IN 46350
www.ivytech.edu
Prgm Dir: Lora Plank, RN CNOR CST
Tel: 219 879-9137, Ext 227   *Fax:* 219 879-9157
E-mail: lplank@ivytech.edu

Ivy Tech Community College - Muncie
Surgical Technology Prgm
4301 S Cowan Rd
Muncie, IN 47302
Prgm Dir: Caryn Humphrey, BSN RN CNOR
Tel: 765 289-2291, Ext 542   *Fax:* 765 289-2292
E-mail: chumphre@ivytech.edu

Vincennes University
Surgical Technology Prgm
1002 N First St, WAB-1
Vincennes, IN 47591
Prgm Dir: Chris Keegan, MS CST
Tel: 812 888-5893   *Fax:* 812 888-4550
E-mail: ckeegan@vinu.edu

Iowa

Kirkwood Community College
Surgical Technology Prgm
6301 Kirkwood Blvd SW
Cedar Rapids, IA 52406
Prgm Dir: Terri Grell, RN BSN CNOR
Tel: 319 398-5566, Ext 5513   *Fax:* 319 398-1293
E-mail: tgrell@kirkwood.cc.ia.us

Mercy College of Health Sciences
Surgical Technology Prgm
928 Sixth Ave
Des Moines, IA 50309-1239
www.mchs.edu
Prgm Dir: Tralanda Davis, CST
Tel: 515 643-6718   *Fax:* 515 643-6686
E-mail: tdavis@mercydesmoines.org

Western Iowa Tech Community College
Surgical Technology Prgm
4647 Stone Ave, PO Box 5199
Sioux City, IA 51106-5199
Prgm Dir: Renee Nemitz, RN CST
Tel: 712 274-8733, Ext 1391   *Fax:* 712 274-6412
E-mail: nemitzra@witcc.edu

Iowa Lakes Community College
Surgical Technology Prgm
1900 N Grand Ave, Ste 8
Spencer, IA 51301-2294
Prgm Dir: Dana Grafft, CST
Tel: 712 262-7141, Ext 6624   *Fax:* 712 262-4047
E-mail: dgrafft@iowalakes.edu

Kansas

Hutchinson Community College
Surgical Technology Prgm
815 N Walnut, Davis Hall
Hutchinson, KS 67501
www.hutchcc.edu
Prgm Dir: Katherine Gill, RN BSN CNOR
Tel: 620 665-4950
E-mail: gillk@hutchcc.edu

Seward County Community College
Surgical Technology Prgm
PO Box 1137
1801 N Kansas Ave
Liberal, KS 67905-1137
Prgm Dir: Carmen Summer, RN BSN CNOR
Tel: 620 626-3078   *Fax:* 620 626-3040
E-mail: carmen.sumner@sccc.edu

Kaw Area Technical School
Surgical Technology Prgm
5724 Huntoon
Topeka, KS 66604
www.kats.tec.ks.us
Prgm Dir: Donna Hess, CST
Tel: 785 228-6340   *Fax:* 785 273-7080
E-mail: dhess@kats.tec.ks.us

Wichita Area Technical College
Surgical Technology Prgm
324 N Emporia St
Wichita, KS 67202-2591
Prgm Dir: Cathy Mattingly, RN
Tel: 316 677-1355   *Fax:* 316 677-1332
E-mail: cmattingly@watc.edu

Kentucky

Ashland Technical College
Surgical Technology Prgm
4818 Roberts Dr
Ashland, KY 41102-9046
Prgm Dir: Jaqueline Cavins, RN BSN CNOR
Tel: 606 929-2005   *Fax:* 606 928-4330
E-mail: jacqueline.cavins@kctcs.edu

Bowling Green Technical College
Surgical Technology Prgm
1845 Loop Dr
Bowling Green, KY 42101
Prgm Dir: Sherry Wells, CST CFA
Tel: 270 901-1079   *Fax:* 270 901-1139
E-mail: sherry.wells@kctcs.edu

National College
Surgical Technology Prgm
7627 Ewing Blvd
Florence, KY 41042
www.national-college.edu
Prgm Dir: Dalla Woodrome
Tel: 859 525-6510   *Fax:* 859 525-8961
E-mail: drwoodrome@national-college.edu

Bluegrass Community and Technical College
Surgical Technology Prgm
308 Vo-Tech Rd
Lexington, KY 40511-2626
Prgm Dir: Kevin R Craycraft, CST
Tel: 859 296-5600   *Fax:* 859 246-2504
E-mail: kevinr.craycraft@kctcs.edu

Jefferson Community and Technical College
Surgical Technology Prgm
800 W Chestnut St
Louisville, KY 40203
Prgm Dir: Richard McClure, CST
Tel: 502 213-4236   *Fax:* 502 213-4502
E-mail: richard.mcclure@kctcs.edu

National College
Surgical Technology Prgm
4205 Dixie Hwy
Louisville, KY 40216
www.national-college.edu
Prgm Dir: Kellie Johnson, CST
Tel: 502 447-7634
E-mail: kejohnson@national-college.edu

Spencerian College
Surgical Technology Prgm
4627 Dixie Hwy
Louisville, KY 40216
Prgm Dir: R Matt Matthews, CST CFA BSN BSEd
Tel: 502 447-1000, Ext 7875   *Fax:* 502 447-4574
E-mail: mmatthews@spencerian.edu

Madisonville Community College
Surgical Technology Prgm
750 Laffoon St
Madisonville, KY 42431
Prgm Dir: Jeff Bidwell, CST CSA MA
Tel: 270 824-1740   *Fax:* 270 824-7069
E-mail: jeff.bidwell@kctcs.edu

Maysville Comm & Tech College
Surgical Technology Prgm
1755 US 68
Maysville, KY 41056
Prgm Dir: Connie L Tucker
Tel: 606 759-7141   *Fax:* 606 759-7176
E-mail: connie.tucker@kctcs.edu

Kentucky Community Technical College
Surgical Technology Prgm
4800 New Hartford Rd
Owensboro, KY 42303
Prgm Dir: Peggy Howard, RN CNOR BSN
Tel: 270 686-4634   *Fax:* 270 686-4662
E-mail: peggy.howard@kctcs.edu

West Kentucky Community & Technical College
Surgical Technology Prgm
Blandville Rd, PO Box 7408
Paducah, KY 42002
Prgm Dir: Debbie Swain, CST
Tel: 270 534-3482   *Fax:* 270 534-3498
E-mail: debbie.swain@kctcs.edu

Southeast Kentucky Comm & Tech College
Surgical Technology Prgm
3300 US Highway 25E S
Pineville, KY 40977
Prgm Dir: Roberta Dean, RN BS MSN
Tel: 606 248-2117   *Fax:* 606 248-2166
E-mail: roberta.dean@kctcs.edu

Somerset Community College
Surgical Technology Prgm
808 Monticello St
Somerset, KY 42501
www.somerset.kctcs.edu
Prgm Dir: Tammy Watters, CST RN
Tel: 606 451-6792, Ext 16792   *Fax:* 606 679-4369
E-mail: tammy.watters@kctcs.edu

Louisiana

MedVance Institute
Surgical Technology Prgm
9255 Interline Ave
Baton Rouge, LA 70809
Prgm Dir: Deborah LaMonica, CST
Tel: 225 248-1015   *Fax:* 225 248-9517
E-mail: dlamonica@medvance.org

Our Lady of the Lake College
Surgical Technology Prgm
7434 Perkins Rd
Baton Rouge, LA 70808
www.ololcollege.edu
Prgm Dir: Alice Comish, RN BSN CNOR
Tel: 225 768-1734   *Fax:* 225 768-0819
E-mail: acomish@ololcollege.edu

Bossier Parish Community College
Surgical Technology Prgm
6220 E Texas St
Bossier City, LA 71111
Prgm Dir: Al Smith, RN BSN MEd
Tel: 318 678-6330   *Fax:* 318 678-6199
E-mail: asmith@bpcc.edu

Louisiana Tech College - Lafayette Campus
Surgical Technology Prgm
1101 Bertrand Dr
PO Box 4909
Lafayette, LA 70506
www.ltc.edu
Prgm Dir: Lorie Lavergne, CST
Tel: 337 262-5962, Ext 238   *Fax:* 337 262-5122
E-mail: lorie.lavergne@ltc.edu

Career Technical College
Surgical Technology Prgm
2319 Louisville Ave
Monroe, LA 71201
www.careertc.com
Prgm Dir: Regena Pardon, CST CFA RN
Tel: 318 998-5602   *Fax:* 318 324-9883
E-mail: rpardon@careertc.com

Delgado Community College
Surgical Technology Prgm
615 City Park Ave
New Orleans, LA 70119-4399
www.dcc.edu
Prgm Dir: Sandra Palmer, MA
Tel: 504 571-1366   *Fax:* 504 568-5494
E-mail: spalme@dcc.edu

Southern Univ at Shreveport
Surgical Technology Prgm
610 Texas St, Ste 333
Shreveport, LA 71101
Prgm Dir: Didaciane G Keys, RN BSN
Tel: 318 678-4638   *Fax:* 318 678-4627
E-mail: dkeys@susla.edu

Louisiana Tech College - Lafourche Campus
Surgical Technology Prgm
1425 Tiger Dr
Thibodaux, LA 70301
www.ltc.edu
Prgm Dir: Delores Gordon, CST
Tel: 985 447-0924, Ext 111   *Fax:* 985 447-0927
E-mail: delores.gordon@ltc.edu

Maine

Eastern Maine Community College
Surgical Technology Prgm
354 Hogan Rd
Bangor, ME 04401
Prgm Dir: Suzanne Brunner
Tel: 207 941-4600   *Fax:* 207 941-4608
E-mail: sbrunner@emcc.edu

Maine Medical Center
Surgical Technology Prgm
School of Surgical Technology
Fort Rd
Portland, ME 04106
Prgm Dir: Diane Fecteau, RN MSA
Tel: 207 662-8030   *Fax:* 207 662-8198
E-mail: fected@mmc.org

Maryland

Baltimore City Community College
Surgical Technology Prgm
2901 Liberty Heights Ave
Baltimore, MD 21215
Prgm Dir: Audretta F Smith, BSN
Tel: 410 462-7722   *Fax:* 410 462-7734
E-mail: asmith@bccc.edu

Community College of Baltimore County - Essex Campus
Surgical Technology Prgm
7201 Rossville Blvd
Baltimore, MD 21237-3899
Prgm Dir: Susan Fisher, CST CFA
Tel: 410 780-6869   *Fax:* 410 780-6856
E-mail: sfisher@ccbcmd.edu

Frederick Community College
Surgical Technology Prgm
7932 Opossumtown Pike
Frederick, MD 21702
Prgm Dir: Nancy N Dankanich, RN BSN MA
Tel: 301 846-2506   *Fax:* 301 846-2498
E-mail: ndankanich@frederick.edu

Montgomery College
Surgical Technology Prgm
900 Hungerford Dr
Rockville, MD 20850
Prgm Dir: Patrice Upshaw, RN MSN
Tel: 301 562-5541   *Fax:* 301 650-1335
E-mail: patrice.upshaw@montgomerycollege.edu

Chesapeake College
Surgical Technology Prgm
PO Box 8
Wye Mills, MD 21632
Prgm Dir: Lisa T Szewczyk, CST
Tel: 410 770-3511, Ext 712   *Fax:* 410 770-3764
E-mail: lszewczyk@chesapeake.edu

Massachusetts

Bunker Hill Community College
Surgical Technology Prgm
175 Hawthorne St
Chelsea Campus
Chelsea, MA 02150-2917
Prgm Dir: Jane S Roman, RN MEd CNOR
Tel: 617 228-3363   *Fax:* 617 228-2106
E-mail: Jroman@bhcc.mass.edu

North Shore Community College
Surgical Technology Prgm
1 Ferncroft Rd
PO Box 3340
Danvers, MA 01923-0840
www.northshore.edu
Prgm Dir: Anne Baras, BSN CNOR MS
Tel: 978 762-4000, Ext 1503   *Fax:* 978 762-4181
E-mail: abaras@northshore.edu

Massachusetts Bay Community College
Surgical Technology Prgm
19 Flagg Dr
Framingham, MA 01700
Prgm Dir: Patricia Caggiano, RN MS CNOR
Tel: 508 875-5300
E-mail: pcaggiano@massbay.edu

Charles H McCann Technical School
Surgical Technology Prgm
70 Hodges Cross Rd
North Adams, MA 01247
Prgm Dir: Tom Lescarbeau, CST CFA AS
Tel: 413 663-5383, Ext 180   *Fax:* 413 664-9424
E-mail: tlescarbeau@mccanntech.org

Quincy College
Surgical Technology Prgm
1495 Hanock St, 4th Fl Heritage Bldg
Quincy, MA 02169
Prgm Dir: Catherine DeLorey
Tel: 617 984-1718   *Fax:* 617 984-1792
E-mail: cdelorey@quincycollege.edu

Springfield Technical Community College
Surgical Technology Prgm
One Armory Sq
Springfield, MA 01105
Prgm Dir: Paula Hutchinson
Tel: 413 755-4887   *Fax:* 413 733-0688
E-mail: phutchinson@stcc.edu

Quinsigamond Community College
Surgical Technology Prgm
670 W Boylston St
Worcester, MA 01606-2092
Prgm Dir: Deborah A Coleman, MSN
Tel: 508 854-2734   *Fax:* 508 854-2704
E-mail: dcoleman@qcc.mass.edu

Michigan

Baker College of Cadillac
Surgical Technology Prgm
9600 E 13th St
Cadillac, MI 49601
Prgm Dir: Mary Gauthier, CST RN
Tel: 231 775-8458   *Fax:* 231 779-9157
E-mail: mary.gauthier@baker.edu

Baker College of Clinton Township
Surgical Technology Prgm
34950 Little Mack Ave
Clinton Township, MI 48035
www.baker.edu
Prgm Dir: Lynda Custer, CST MA Ed
Tel: 586 790-2802   *Fax:* 586 791-6611
E-mail: lynda.custer@baker.edu

Macomb Community College
Surgical Technology Prgm
44575 Garfield Rd
Clinton Township, MI 48038-1139
Prgm Dir: Elizabeth Ness, CST BA
Tel: 586 286-2192   *Fax:* 586 286-2098
E-mail: nesse@macomb.edu

Henry Ford Community College
Surgical Technology Prgm
5101 Evergreen Rd
Dearborn, MI 48128
Prgm Dir: Dorothy C Rothgery, MA CST/CFA
Tel: 313 317-6598 *Fax:* 313 317-6569
E-mail: drothger@hfcc.net

Wayne County Community College District
Surgical Technology Prgm
801 W Fort St
Detroit, MI 48226
Prgm Dir: Damus Golida, CST
Tel: 313 496-2680, Ext 2680 *Fax:* 313 961-9648
E-mail: dgolid1@wcccd.edu

Baker College of Flint
Surgical Technology Prgm
1050 W Bristol Rd
Flint, MI 48507-5508
https://www.baker.edu/departments/healthsci/main.cfm
Prgm Dir: Julia A Jackson, CST MEd FAST
Tel: 810 766-4151 *Fax:* 810 766-2055
E-mail: Julia.Jackson@baker.edu

Baker College of Jackson
Surgical Technology Prgm
2800 Springport Rd
Jackson, MI 49202
www.baker.edu
Prgm Dir: Paula Hayes, CST BBA
Tel: 517 841-4535 *Fax:* 517 789-6302
E-mail: Paula.Hayes@baker.edu

Kalamazoo Valley Community College
Surgical Technology Prgm
6767 West O Ave
PO Box 4070
Kalamazoo, MI 49003-4070
www.kvcc.edu
Prgm Dir: James Taylor, MA
Tel: 269 488-4208 *Fax:* 269 488-4458
E-mail: jtaylor@kvcc.edu

Lansing Community College
Surgical Technology Prgm
3400 Human Health and Public Service
PO Box 40010
Lansing, MI 48901-7210
www.lcc.edu
Prgm Dir: Joseph Long, CST BA MPA FAST EdD
Tel: 517 483-1432 *Fax:* 517 483-1508
E-mail: longj9@lcc.edu

Northern Michigan University
Surgical Technology Prgm
1401 Presque Isle Ave
Marquette, MI 49855
Prgm Dir: Sandra Kontio, CST
Tel: 906 227-1669 *Fax:* 906 227-1309

Baker College of Muskegon
Surgical Technology Prgm
1903 Marquette Ave
Muskegon, MI 49442
Prgm Dir: Ruth Deters, RN BAHA CST
Tel: 616 777-5277 *Fax:* 616 777-5291
E-mail: ruth.deters@baker.edu

Baker College of Port Huron
Surgical Technology Prgm
3403 Lapeer Rd
Port Huron, MI 48060
www.baker.edu
Prgm Dir: Donna McFadden, RN CNOR
Tel: 810 982-9005
E-mail: donna.mcfadden@baker.edu

Oakland Community College
Cosponsor: William Beaumont Hospital
Surgical Technology Prgm
3601 W 13 Mile Rd
Royal Oak, MI 48073
Prgm Dir: Rebecca Pieknik, MS CST CSA
Tel: 248 898-7685 *Fax:* 248 898-4406
E-mail: rpieknik@beaumonthospitals.com

Delta College
Surgical Technology Prgm
1961 Delta Rd
University Center, MI 48710
www.delta.edu
Prgm Dir: Margrethe May, CST MS
Tel: 989 686-9505 *Fax:* 989 667-2230
E-mail: mmay@delta.edu

Minnesota

Anoka Technical College
Surgical Technology Prgm
1355 W Hwy 10
Anoka, MN 55303
www.anokatech.edu
Prgm Dir: Rita M Schutz, RN
Tel: 763 576-4974 *Fax:* 763 576-4715
E-mail: rschutz@anokatech.edu

Lake Superior College
Surgical Technology Prgm
2101 Trinity Rd
Duluth, MN 55811
Prgm Dir: Candace S Melde, RN
Tel: 218 733-5906 *Fax:* 218 723-4921
E-mail: c.melde@lsc.mnscu.edu

Northland Community & Technical College
Surgical Technology Prgm
2022 Central Ave NE
East Grand Forks, MN 56721
Prgm Dir: Ruth LeTexier, BSN
Tel: 218 773-4623 *Fax:* 218 773-4502
E-mail: ruth.letexier@northlandcollege.edu

St Mary's University of Minnesota
Surgical Technology Prgm
2500 Park Ave
Minneapolis, MN 55404-4403
Prgm Dir: Becky Brodine
Tel: 612 728-5162, Ext 162 *Fax:* 612 728-5167
E-mail: bbrodin@smumn.edu

Rochester Community & Technical College
Surgical Technology Prgm
851 30th Ave SE
Rochester, MN 55904
www.rctc.edu
Prgm Dir: Jane Kruger, RN BSN CNOR
Tel: 507 280-3118 *Fax:* 507 280-3180
E-mail: jane.kruger@roch.edu

St Cloud Technical College
Surgical Technology Prgm
1540 Northway Dr
St Cloud, MN 56303
www.sctc.edu
Prgm Dir: Terry Wilson, MEd RN
Tel: 320 308-5921 *Fax:* 320 308-5971
E-mail: twilson@sctc.edu

Mississippi

East Central Community College
Surgical Technology Prgm
PO Box 129
Decatur, MS 39327
Prgm Dir: Melanie Gilmore
Tel: 601 635-2111, Ext 294 *Fax:* 601 635-4031
E-mail: mgilmore@eccc.edu

Holmes Community College
Surgical Technology Prgm
1060 Avent Dr
Grenada, MS 38901
www.holmescc.edu
Prgm Dir: Jessica Elliott, CST
Tel: 662 227-2310 *Fax:* 662 227-2296
E-mail: jelliott@holmescc.edu

Pearl River Community College
Surgical Technology Prgm
5448 US Hwy 49 S
Hattiesburg, MS 39401
Prgm Dir: Debbie Hinton, BS CST
Tel: 601 554-5542 *Fax:* 601 554-5548
E-mail: dhinton@prcc.edu

Hinds Community College
Surgical Technology Prgm
1750 Chadwick Dr
Jackson, MS 39204
Prgm Dir: Teresa Jones, RN
Tel: 601 371-3513 *Fax:* 601 371-3529
E-mail: tajones@hindscc.edu

Mississippi Gulf Coast Community College
Surgical Technology Prgm
PO Box 77
11203 Old Hwy 63 S
Lucedale, MS 39452
http://mgccc.edu
Prgm Dir: Karen Howell, RN MS CNOR
Tel: 601 766-6430 *Fax:* 601 947-4899
E-mail: karen.howell@mgccc.edu

Itawamba Community College
Surgical Technology Prgm
2176 S Eason Blvd
Tupelo, MS 38804
Prgm Dir: Tonya Tice, RN
Tel: 662 620-5121 *Fax:* 662 620-5077
E-mail: tltice@iccms.edu

Missouri

Southeast Missouri Hospital College of Nursing and Health Sciences
Surgical Technology Prgm
2001 William St
Cape Girardeau, MO 63703
Prgm Dir: Susan Jackson, BSN CNOR
Tel: 573 334-6825, Ext 28 *Fax:* 573 339-7805
E-mail: sjackson@sehosp.org

Columbia Public Schools
Surgical Technology Prgm
1818 W Worley St
Columbia, MO 65203-6100
Prgm Dir: Jane Klick, RN CNOR
Tel: 573 886-2276 *Fax:* 573 886-2080
E-mail: jklick@columbia.k12.mo.us

Sanford-Brown College - Hazelwood Campus
Surgical Technology Prgm
75 Village Square
Hazelwood, MO 63042
Prgm Dir: Amy Gray, MD CST
Tel: 314 687-2940 *Fax:* 314 731-0550
E-mail: agray@sbc-hazelwood.com

Franklin Tech Ctr/Missouri Southern St Univ
Surgical Technology Prgm
3950 E Newman Rd
Joplin, MO 64801
Prgm Dir: Gayla Roper, CST
Tel: 417 625-9723 *Fax:* 417 659-4408
E-mail: roper-g@mssu.edu

Metropolitan Community College - Penn Valley
Surgical Technology Prgm
2700 E 18th St
Kansas City, MO 64127
Prgm Dir: Carolyn A Parks, RN BAN CNOR
Tel: 816 482-5073   *Fax:* 816 482-5110
E-mail: Carolyn.Parks@mcckc.edu

Rolla Technical Center
Surgical Technology Prgm
500 Forum Dr
Rolla, MO 65401
Prgm Dir: Tammy Mangold, MEd CST/CFA
Tel: 573 458-0160, Ext 16535   *Fax:* 573 458-0164
E-mail: tmangold@rolla.k12.mo.us

Ozarks Technical Community College
Surgical Technology Prgm
1001 E Chestnut Expressway
Springfield, MO 65802
www.otc.edu/degrees/alldhlth/surgtec/
Prgm Dir: Arlene Chriswell, RN BSN MSBA CNOR
Tel: 417 447-8845   *Fax:* 417 447-8806
E-mail: chriswea@otc.edu

Hillyard Technical Center
Surgical Technology Prgm
3434 Faraon St
St Joseph, MO 64506
Prgm Dir: Linda Ann VanDyke, CST CFA
Tel: 816 671-4170
E-mail: linda.vandyke@sjsd.k12.mo.us

St Louis Community College - Forest Park
Surgical Technology Prgm
5600 Oakland Ave
St Louis, MO 63110
Prgm Dir: Diane Gerardot, MA CST
Tel: 314 644-9340   *Fax:* 314 951-9412
E-mail: dgerardot@stlcc.edu

South Central Career Center
Surgical Technology Prgm
1009 Jackson St
West Plains, MO 65775
Prgm Dir: Mary Waterhouse, RN AND
Tel: 417 256-8883   *Fax:* 417 256-5786
E-mail: mwaterhouse@mail.wphs.k12.mo.us

Montana

Montana State Univ - Great Falls Coll of Tech
Surgical Technology Prgm
2100 16th Ave S
Great Falls, MT 59406-6010
Prgm Dir: Diona Davis, CST CFA
Tel: 406 771-4358   *Fax:* 406 771-4317
E-mail: ddavis@msugf.edu

Flathead Valley Community College
Surgical Technology Prgm
777 Grandview Dr
Kalispell, MT 59901
Prgm Dir: Erin Howardson, CST
Tel: 406 751-6994   *Fax:* 406 756-0317
E-mail: eahowardson@yahoo.com

University of Montana
Surgical Technology Prgm
College of Technology
909 South Ave W
Missoula, MT 59801
Prgm Dir: Debbie Fillmore
Tel: 406 396-5157   *Fax:* 406 243-7899
E-mail: deborah.fillmore@umontana.edu

Nebraska

Southeast Community College
Surgical Technology Prgm
8800 O St
Lincoln, NE 68520
Prgm Dir: Kathleen Uribe, MA CST
Tel: 402 437-2785   *Fax:* 402 437-2404
E-mail: kuribe@southest.edu

Nebraska Methodist College
Surgical Technology Prgm
515 S 26th St
Omaha, NE 68105
Prgm Dir: Patricia Boettger, RN CNOR CRNFA
Tel: 402 354-6528   *Fax:* 402 354-6550
E-mail: pat.boettger@methodistcollege.edu

Nevada

Western Nevada Community College
Surgical Technology Prgm
2201 W College Pkwy
Carson City, NV 89703
Prgm Dir: Duane Sorensen, CST
Tel: 775 445-3248   *Fax:* 775 887-3021
E-mail: dsorense@wncc.edu

College of Southern Nevada
Surgical Technology Prgm
6375 W Charleston Blvd
Las Vegas, NV 89146
Prgm Dir: Eugene Lewis, CST
Tel: 702 651-5945   *Fax:* 702 651-5501
E-mail: eugene.lewis@csn.edu

Nevada Career Institute
Surgical Technology Prgm
3025 E Desert Inn Rd, Ste A
Las Vegas, NV 89121
www.landmarked.com
Prgm Dir: Donna McCasland, LPN CST
Tel: 702 893-4725, Ext 231   *Fax:* 702 893-3881
E-mail: dmccasland@success.edu

New Hampshire

Concord Hospital
Surgical Technology Prgm
250 Pleasant St
Concord, NH 03301
Prgm Dir: Colleen Rutherford, RN MS CNOR
Tel: 603 225-2711, Ext 3891   *Fax:* 603 228-7306
E-mail: crutherf@crhc.org

Dartmouth Hitchcock Medical Center
Surgical Technology Prgm
One Medical Center Dr
Lebanon, NH 03756-0001
Prgm Dir: Carol Majewski
Tel: 603 650-8134
E-mail: carol.a.majewski@hitchcock.org

New Hampshire Comm Tech College - Stratham
Surgical Technology Prgm
277 Portsmouth Ave
Stratham, NH 03885-2297
Prgm Dir: Sandra Carlson, RN BSN CNOR
Tel: 603 775-2367   *Fax:* 603 772-1198
E-mail: scarlson@nhctc.edu

New Jersey

Atlantic Cape Community College
Surgical Technology Prgm
Worthington Atlantic City Center
1535 Bacharach Blvd
Atlantic City, NJ 08401
www.atlantic.edu
Prgm Dir: Karen Sherback, CST
Tel: 609 343-4819
E-mail: ksherbac@atlantic.edu

Sanford-Brown Institute
Surgical Technology Prgm
675 US Hwy 1
Iselin, NJ 08830
Prgm Dir: Carol Conover
Tel: 732 623-5786   *Fax:* 866 614-2413
E-mail: cconover@sb-nj.com

Sussex County Community College
Surgical Technology Prgm
1 College Hill Rd
Newton, NJ 07860
Prgm Dir: Barbara J Cook, BA CMA
Tel: 973 300-2263   *Fax:* 973 300-2303
E-mail: bcook@sussex.edu

Bergen Community College
Surgical Technology Prgm
400 Paramus Rd
Paramus, NJ 07652
Prgm Dir: Joan Ann Verderame, MA RN
Tel: 201 447-7944, Ext 7921   *Fax:* 201 612-3876
E-mail: jverderame@bergen.edu

New Mexico

Central New Mexico Community College
Surgical Technology Prgm
525 Buena Vista SE
Albuquerque, NM 87106
Prgm Dir: Elizabeth L Alongi, RN BSN CNOR
Tel: 505 224-4166   *Fax:* 505 224-4120
E-mail: ealongi@cnm.edu

New York

Long Island University - Brooklyn Campus
Surgical Technology Prgm
Center for Health Science Technologies
School of Health Professions
Brooklyn, NY 11201
Prgm Dir: Karen Chambers, CST
Tel: 718 488-3438, Ext 3438   *Fax:* 718 780-4575
E-mail: karen.chambers@liu.edu

SUNY Downstate Medical Center
Surgical Technology Prgm
440 Lenox Rd
Brooklyn, NY 11203
Prgm Dir: Tomas Wharton, MD
Tel: 718 270-2983   *Fax:* 718 270-8114
E-mail: twharton@downstate.edu

Trocaire College
Surgical Technology Prgm
360 Choate Ave
Buffalo, NY 14220-2094
Prgm Dir: Linda Kerwin, RN MSN MA
Tel: 716 826-1200, Ext 1254   *Fax:* 716 828-6107
E-mail: kerwinl@trocaire.edu

Nassau Community College
Surgical Technology Prgm
One Education Dr
Dept AHS
Garden City, NY 11530
www.ncc.edu
Prgm Dir: Caroline Kaufmann, Asst Prof RN CNOR
Tel: 516 572-7918 *Fax:* 516 572-7565
E-mail: caroline.kaufmann@ncc.edu

Bronx Lebanon Hospital
Surgical Technology Prgm
Health Care Institute
275 7th Ave, 16th Flr
New York, NY 10001
www.cwe.org
Prgm Dir: Smyrna E Clause, RN MS
Tel: 212 647-1900, Ext 275 *Fax:* 212 647-1916
E-mail: sclause@cwe.org

New York University Medical Center
Surgical Technology Prgm
660 1st Ave, 2nd Fl
New York, NY 10016
www.surgtech.com
Prgm Dir: Zaida Jacoby, RN MA MEd
Tel: 212 263-6644 *Fax:* 212 263-0600
E-mail: zaida.jacoby@med.nyu.edu

Western Suffolk BOCES
Surgical Technology Prgm
152 Laurel Hill Rd
Northport, NY 11768
Prgm Dir: Kathleen Baker, RN BSN MSEd
Tel: 631 261-3727 *Fax:* 631 623-4908
E-mail: kbaker@wsboces.org

Ulster County Board of Cooperative Ed Service
Surgical Technology Prgm
PO Box 601, Rte 9W
Port Ewen, NY 12466
www.mhric.org
Prgm Dir: Marita Kitchell, EdMS SAS BSN
Tel: 845 331-5050, Ext 2232 *Fax:* 845 339-8797
E-mail: mkitchel@mhric.org

Niagara County Community College
Surgical Technology Prgm
3111 Saunders Settlement Rd
Sanborn, NY 14132
Prgm Dir: Gemma Fournier, RN CST
Tel: 716 614-6417 *Fax:* 716 614-6879
E-mail: fournier@niagaracc.suny.edu

Stony Brook University
Surgical Technology Prgm
School of Nursing
Health Sciences Center, Level 2
Stony Brook, NY 11794-8240
Prgm Dir: Ora James Bouey, RN
Tel: 631 444-2644 *Fax:* 631 444-7763
E-mail: ora.bouey@stonybrook.edu

Onondaga Community College
Surgical Technology Prgm
4941 Onondaga Rd
Syracuse, NY 13215
Prgm Dir: Mary Pat M Annable, RN MSN CNOR
Tel: 315 498-2463 *Fax:* 315 498-2751
E-mail: annablem@sunyocc.edu

North Carolina

Asheville-Buncombe Technical Comm College
Surgical Technology Prgm
340 Victoria Rd
Asheville, NC 28801
www.abtech.edu
Prgm Dir: Robin B Keith, CST RN BSN CNOR
Tel: 828 254-1921, Ext 892 *Fax:* 828 251-6355
E-mail: rkeith@abtech.edu

South College - Asheville
Surgical Technology Prgm
1567 Patton Ave
Asheville, NC 28803
Prgm Dir: Tara Luhrs
Tel: 828 252-2486
E-mail: tluhrs@southcollegenc.com

Miller-Motte College
Surgical Technology Prgm
2205 Walnut St
Cary, NC 27511
Prgm Dir: Cynthia Woolford, CST
Tel: 919 532-7171, Ext 7006 *Fax:* 919 532-7151
E-mail: cgibbons@miller-motte.edu

Carolinas College of Health Sciences
Surgical Technology Prgm
1200 Blythe Rd, PO Box 32861
Charlotte, NC 28232-2861
Prgm Dir: Rebecca M Cuthbertson, BSN
Tel: 704 355-1547 *Fax:* 704 355-5967
E-mail: rcuthbertson@carolinas.org

Central Piedmont Community College
Surgical Technology Prgm
Central Campus, PO Box 35009
Terrell Bldg 511
Charlotte, NC 28235
www.cpcc.edu
Prgm Dir: Eugene Pease, RN MSN CNOR
Tel: 704 330-6265 *Fax:* 704 330-6677
E-mail: gene.pease@cpcc.edu

Cabarrus College of Health Sciences
Surgical Technology Prgm
401 Medical Park Dr
Concord, NC 28025
http://cabarruscollege.edu
Prgm Dir: Karen H Galloway, RN CNOR PhD
Tel: 704 783-1555, Ext 3503 *Fax:* 704 783-1764
E-mail: kgallowa@northeastmedical.org

Durham Technical Community College
Surgical Technology Prgm
1637 Lawson St
Durham, NC 27703
Prgm Dir: Tammy Holden, CST
Tel: 919 686-3690 *Fax:* 919 686-3705
E-mail: holdent@durhamtech.edu

College of The Albemarle
Surgical Technology Prgm
1208 N Road St, PO Box 2327
Elizabeth City, NC 27906-2327
www.albemarle.edu
Prgm Dir: Irene M Jack, CST AGE
Tel: 252 335-0821, Ext 2995 *Fax:* 252 335-2011
E-mail: irenejack@albemarle.edu

Fayetteville Technical Community College
Surgical Technology Prgm
PO Box 35236
Fayetteville, NC 28303
www.faytechcc.edu
Prgm Dir: Terry Herring, MS CST/CFA
Tel: 910 678-8358
E-mail: herringt@faytechcc.edu

Blue Ridge Community College
Surgical Technology Prgm
100 College Dr
Flat Rock, NC 28731-9624
Prgm Dir: Debra Houdek, RN BSN MSN CST FNP
Tel: 828 694-1831 *Fax:* 828 692-2441
E-mail: debrah@blueridge.edu

Catawba Valley Community College
Surgical Technology Prgm
2550 Hwy 70 SE
Hickory, NC 28602
Prgm Dir: Carol Harrison, RN
Tel: 704 327-7000, Ext 4332 *Fax:* 704 327-7301
E-mail: charriso@cvcc.cc.nc.us

Coastal Carolina Community College
Surgical Technology Prgm
444 Western Blvd
Jacksonville, NC 28546-6877
Prgm Dir: Karen Gurney, RN
Tel: 910 938-6274 *Fax:* 910 938-6806
E-mail: gurneyk@coastal.cc.nc.us

Guilford Technical Community College
Surgical Technology Prgm
601 High Point Rd, PO Box 309
Jamestown, NC 27282-0309
Prgm Dir: Arthur A Makin, BS CST
Tel: 336 334-4822, Ext 2764 *Fax:* 336 454-3554
E-mail: aamakin@gtcc.edu

Lenoir Community College
Surgical Technology Prgm
PO Box 188
Kinston, NC 28502-0188
www.lenoircc.edu
Prgm Dir: Jimi Spears, RN ADN ST
Tel: 252 527-6223, Ext 802 *Fax:* 252 233-6893
E-mail: jspears@lenoircc.edu

Robeson Community College
Surgical Technology Prgm
5160 Fayetteville Rd
Lumberton, NC 28360
Prgm Dir: Ernest V Singley, Jr, CST
Tel: 910 272-3405 *Fax:* 910 272-3328
E-mail: esingley@robeson.cc.nc.us

Sandhills Community College
Surgical Technology Prgm
2200 Airport Rd
Pinehurst, NC 28374
Prgm Dir: Brenda Luck
Tel: 910 695-3838 *Fax:* 910 692-2756
E-mail: luckb@sandhills.edu

South Piedmont Community College
Surgical Technology Prgm
PO Box 126
Polkton, NC 28135
Prgm Dir: Carol Courtney, BSN
Tel: 704 272-7635, Ext 280 *Fax:* 704 272-8904
E-mail: ccourtney@spcc.edu

Wake Technical Community College
Surgical Technology Prgm
9109 Fayetteville Rd
Raleigh, NC 27603
www.waketech.edu
Prgm Dir: Martha Shurtleff, RN MSN CNOR
Fax: 919 250-4329
E-mail: mashurtl@waketech.edu

Cleveland Community College
Surgical Technology Prgm
137 S Post Rd
Shelby, NC 28152
Prgm Dir: Wanda Leonard, CST
Tel: 704 484-6615 *Fax:* 704 484-5304
E-mail: leonardw@cleveland.cc.nc.us

Edgecombe Community College
Surgical Technology Prgm
2009 W Wilson St
Tarboro, NC 27886
Prgm Dir: Linda Harrison, CST F-AST
Tel: 252 823-5166, Ext 232 *Fax:* 252 823-6817
E-mail: harrisonl@edgecombe.edu

Rockingham Community College
Surgical Technology Prgm
PO Box 38
Wentworth, NC 27375
Prgm Dir: Mary Margaret Martin, RN BSN CNOR
APRN-BC
Tel: 336 342-4261, Ext 2259 *Fax:* 336 634-1253
E-mail: martinm@rockinghamcc.edu

Miller-Motte College
Surgical Technology Prgm
5000 Market St
Wilmington, NC 28405
www.mmtcwilmington.net
Prgm Dir: Glenn Grady, MEd BSMT(ASCP) CMA
Tel: 910 392-4660, Ext 2015   *Fax:* 910 799-6224
E-mail: ggrady@miller-motte.edu

Wilson Technical Community College
Surgical Technology Prgm
902 Herring Ave
Wilson, NC 27893
www.wilsontech.edu
Prgm Dir: Lynanne Boyette, RN
Tel: 252 246-1323   *Fax:* 252 246-1411
E-mail: lboyette@wilsontech.edu

North Dakota

Bismarck State College
Surgical Technology Prgm
PO Box 5587
Bismarck, ND 58506-5587
www.bismarckstate.edu
Prgm Dir: Jean Hinton, RN CNOR CST
Tel: 701 224-5722   *Fax:* 701 255-0167
E-mail: Jean.Hinton@bsc.nodak.edu

Ohio

University of Akron
Surgical Technology Prgm
Polsky Bldg Rm 124 H
Akron, OH 44325-3702
www.commtech.uakron.edu/current/departments/allied
   health
Prgm Dir: Sherry Gamble, RN MSN CNOR
Tel: 330 972-6514   *Fax:* 330 972-2016
E-mail: slg@uakron.edu

Univ of Cincinnati - Clermont College
Surgical Technology Prgm
4200 Clermont College Dr
Batavia, OH 45103
Prgm Dir: Linda M Baker-Numrich, RN BS CNOR
Tel: 513 732-5331   *Fax:* 513 732-5304
E-mail: bakerlm@email.uc.edu

Collins Career Center
Surgical Technology Prgm
11627 State Route 243
Chesapeake, OH 45619
Prgm Dir: Katherine Hall, RN
Tel: 740 867-6641, Ext 520   *Fax:* 740 867-9626
E-mail: kehall@collins-cc.k12.oh.us

Cincinnati State Tech & Comm College
Surgical Technology Prgm
3520 Central Pkwy
Cincinnati, OH 45223
Prgm Dir: Wanda Dantzler, RN MEd BSN CNOR CRCST
Tel: 513 569-1673   *Fax:* 513 569-1659
E-mail: wanda.dantzler@cincinnatistate.edu

Cuyahoga Community College
Surgical Technology Prgm
2900 Community College Ave
HCS 126-H
Cleveland, OH 44115-3196
www.tri-c.edu/surgical
Prgm Dir: Beth Stokes, BFA AAS CST
Tel: 216 987-6146, Ext 6146   *Fax:* 216 987-4366
E-mail: beth.stokes@tri-c.edu

Columbus State Community College
Surgical Technology Prgm
550 E Spring St, PO Box 1609
Columbus, OH 43216-1609
Prgm Dir: Dennis Murphy, BS CST
Tel: 614 287-2514, Ext 2514   *Fax:* 614 287-3854
E-mail: dmurphy@cscc.edu

Mt Carmel College of Nursing
Surgical Technology Prgm
127 S Davis Ave
Columbus, OH 43222
Prgm Dir: Linda Atkinson, RN AD
Tel: 614 234-1388   *Fax:* 614 234-2875
E-mail: latkinson@mchs.com

Miami-Jacobs Career College
Surgical Technology Prgm
110 N Patterson Blvd
Dayton, OH 45402
www.miamijacobs.edu
Prgm Dir: Michael Batterson, CST
Tel: 937 461-5174, Ext 136   *Fax:* 937 461-3384
E-mail: michael.batterson@miamijacobs.edu

Sinclair Community College
Surgical Technology Prgm
444 W Third St
Rm 1012 Surgical Technology
Dayton, OH 45402-1460
www.sinclair.edu
Prgm Dir: Susan Willin-Mulay, RN MSN MBA CNOR
Tel: 937 512-2850   *Fax:* 937 512-2058
E-mail: susan.willin-mulay@sinclair.edu

Lorain County Community College
Surgical Technology Prgm
1005 N Abbe Rd
Elyria, OH 44035
Prgm Dir: Patricia Sedlak, RN BSN CNOR RNFA
Tel: 800 995-5222, Ext 7159   *Fax:* 440 366-4116
E-mail: psedlak@lorainccc.edu

Lakeland Community College
Surgical Technology Prgm
7700 Clocktower Dr
Kirtland, OH 44094
Prgm Dir: Nancymarie Phillips, RN BA BSN MEd CNOR
   RNFA
Tel: 440 525-7016   *Fax:* 440 525-4733
E-mail: nphillips@lakelandcc.edu

Apollo Career Center
Surgical Technology Prgm
3325 Shawnee Rd
Lima, OH 45806
Prgm Dir: Barbara E Cook, RN BSN CNOR
Tel: 419 999-5618   *Fax:* 419 998-2994
E-mail: ap_cook@noacsc.org

Scioto County Joint Vocational School
Surgical Technology Prgm
951 Vern Riffe Dr
Lucasville, OH 45648
www.scjvs.com
Prgm Dir: Jean Turner, CST CFA
Tel: 740 259-5526, Ext 1123   *Fax:* 740 259-8312
E-mail: jturner_sj@scoca-k12.org

EHOVE Ghrist Adult Career Center
Surgical Technology Prgm
316 W Mason Rd
Milan, OH 44846
http://ehove.net
Prgm Dir: Beth Lucas, CST AAS
Tel: 419 499-8173   *Fax:* 419 499-8173
E-mail: blucas@ehove-jvs.k12.oh.us

Central Ohio Technical College
Surgical Technology Prgm
1179 University Dr
Newark, OH 43055-1797
Prgm Dir: Jacob Benjamin
Tel: 740 366-1351, Ext 229   *Fax:* 740 366-9275
E-mail: benjamin.17@osu.edu

Buckeye Hills Career Center
Surgical Technology Prgm
351 Buckeye Hills Rd
Rio Grande, OH 45674
Prgm Dir: Sue Gilliam, RN CNOR
Tel: 740 245-5334, Ext 252   *Fax:* 740 245-9465
E-mail: bj_sgilliam@seovec.org

Owens Community College
Surgical Technology Prgm
PO Box 10,000, Oregon Rd
Toledo, OH 43699
Prgm Dir: Kristine Flickinger, RN BA CNOR
Tel: 567 661-7000, Ext 7310   *Fax:* 567 661-7665
E-mail: kristine_flickinger@owens.edu

Choffin Career & Technical Center
Cosponsor: Youngstown City Schools
Surgical Technology Prgm
200 E Wood St
Youngstown, OH 44503
Prgm Dir: Carole DuBose, LPN CST
Tel: 330 744-8763   *Fax:* 330 744-8705
E-mail: youn_cgd@access-k12.org

Oklahoma

Southern Oklahoma Technology Center
Surgical Technology Prgm
2610 Sam Noble Pkwy
Ardmore, OK 73401
Prgm Dir: Tracie Kelch, RN
Tel: 580 220-6273   *Fax:* 580 220-6534
E-mail: tkelch@sotc.org

Canadian Valley Technology Center
Surgical Technology Prgm
1401 Michigan Ave
Chickasha, OK 73018
www.cvtech.org
Prgm Dir: Anita Followwill, RN
Tel: 405 224-7220, Ext 583   *Fax:* 405 222-7511
E-mail: afollowwill@cvtech.org

Central Technology Center
Surgical Technology Prgm
3 Court Circle
Drumright, OK 74030
Prgm Dir: LaDonna Gear
Tel: 918 352-2551, Ext 289   *Fax:* 918 352-2441
E-mail: ladonnag@ctechok.org

Autry Technology Center
Surgical Technology Prgm
1201 W Willow
Enid, OK 73703
Prgm Dir: Kim McFarland
Tel: 405 242-2750, Ext 127   *Fax:* 405 233-8262
E-mail: kmcfarland@autrytech.com

Great Plains Technology Center
Surgical Technology Prgm
4500 W Lee Blvd
Lawton, OK 73505
Prgm Dir: Ann Tahah, LPN
Tel: 580 250-5574   *Fax:* 580 250-5583
E-mail: atahah@gptech.org

Oklahoma Health Academy
Surgical Technology Prgm
1939 N Moore Ave
Moore, OK 73160
Prgm Dir: Kirk Webster, MSEd
Tel: 405 912-2777   *Fax:* 405 912-2770
E-mail: jkwebster@oklahomahealthacademy.org

Moore Norman Technology Center
Surgical Technology Prgm
4701 12th Ave NW
PO Box 4701
Norman, OK 73069
http://mntechnology.com
Prgm Dir: Kim Shannon, RN
Tel: 405 364-5763, Ext 6525 *Fax:* 405 447-6289
E-mail: kshannon@mntechnology.com

Heritage College
Surgical Technology Prgm
7100 I-35 Service Rd
Oklahoma City, OK 73149
Prgm Dir: Courtney Powers
Tel: 405 631-3399 *Fax:* 405 631-6711
E-mail: courtneyp@heritage-education.com

Metro Technology Centers
Surgical Technology Prgm
Health Careers Center
1720 Springlake Dr
Oklahoma City, OK 73111
Prgm Dir: Vicki Bushey, CST
Tel: 405 424-8324, Ext 620 *Fax:* 405 424-9403
E-mail: vbushey@metrotech.org

Platt College - Oklahoma City
Surgical Technology Prgm
309 S Ann Arbor
Oklahoma City, OK 73128
Prgm Dir: Terri Taylor, CST
Tel: 405 946-7799 *Fax:* 405 943-2150
E-mail: terrrit@plattcollege.org

Community Care College
Surgical Technology Prgm
4242 S Sheridan
Tulsa, OK 74145
Prgm Dir: Pamela Buff, CST
Tel: 918 610-0027, Ext 229 *Fax:* 918 610-0029
E-mail: pbuff@communitycarecollege.com

Platt College - Tulsa
Surgical Technology Prgm
3801 S Sheridan
Tulsa, OK 74145
Prgm Dir: Pam Buff, CST
Tel: 918 663-9000 *Fax:* 918 622-1240
E-mail: pamb@plattcollege.org

Tulsa Technology Center
Surgical Technology Prgm
3420 S Memorial Dr
Tulsa, OK 74145-1390
Prgm Dir: Carol Dollar, RN BSN
Tel: 918 828-1036 *Fax:* 918 828-5239
E-mail: carol.dollar@tulsatech.org

Wes Watkins Technology Center District 25
Surgical Technology Prgm
7892 Hwy 9
Wetumka, OK 74883
www.wwtech.org
Prgm Dir: Natalie Kennedy, CST
Tel: 405 452-5500, Ext 291 *Fax:* 405 452-3561
E-mail: nkennedy@wwtech.org

Oregon

Mt Hood Community College
Surgical Technology Prgm
26000 SE Stark St
Gresham, OR 97030
Prgm Dir: Jacqueline Morfitt, RN CNOR
Tel: 503 491-7179 *Fax:* 503 491-6047
E-mail: morfittj@mhcc.edu

Concorde Career Institute - Portland
Surgical Technology Prgm
1425 NE Irving St, Bldg 300
Portland, OR 97232
Prgm Dir: Jonathan Lee
Tel: 503 248-6139 *Fax:* 503 281-6739
E-mail: jlee@concorde.edu

Pennsylvania

Northampton Community College
Surgical Technology Prgm
3835 Green Pond Rd
Bethlehem, PA 18020
Prgm Dir: Judith Rex, RNC MSN
Tel: 610 861-5094 *Fax:* 610 332-6556
E-mail: jrex@northampton.edu

St Luke's Hospital
Surgical Technology Prgm
801 Ostrum St
Bethlehem, PA 18015
Prgm Dir: Barbara Benfield, LPN CST
Tel: 610 954-4466 *Fax:* 610 954-6097

Mount Aloysius College
Surgical Technology Prgm
7373 Admiral Peary Hwy
Cresson, PA 16630-1999
Prgm Dir: Amanda Minor, CST BS
Tel: 814 886-6340 *Fax:* 814 886-2978
E-mail: aminor@mtaloy.edu

Great Lakes Institute of Technology
Surgical Technology Prgm
5100 Peach St
Erie, PA 16509
Prgm Dir: Brian Lock, II, RN PhD
Tel: 814 864-6666, Ext 233 *Fax:* 814 868-1717
E-mail: brianl@glit.edu

Harrisburg Area Community College - Harrisburg
Surgical Technology Prgm
349 Wiconisco St
One HACC Dr
Harrisburg, PA 17110
www.hacc.edu
Prgm Dir: Amy Kennedy, RN MSN CNOR
Tel: 717 221-1321 *Fax:* 717 909-4010
E-mail: alkenned@hacc.edu

Conemaugh Memorial Medical Center
Surgical Technology Prgm
1086 Franklin St
Johnstown, PA 15905
http://intranet.conemaugh.org
Prgm Dir: Patricia Pavlikowski, MA RN CNOR CST
Tel: 814 534-9772 *Fax:* 814 534-9945
E-mail: Ppavlik@conemaugh.org/education/

Harrisburg Area Community College - Lancaster
Surgical Technology Prgm
Lancaster Campus
1641 Old Philadelphia Pike
Lancaster, PA 17602
www.hacc.edu
Prgm Dir: Amy Kennedy, RN MSN CNOR
Tel: 717 358-2871 *Fax:* 717 358-2865
E-mail: alkenned@hacc.edu

Lancaster Gen Coll of Nursing & Hlth Sciences
Surgical Technology Prgm
410 N Lime St
Lancaster, PA 17602
www.LancasterGeneral.org
Prgm Dir: Christina Baumer, RN PhD CNOR CHES
Tel: 717 544-4912, Ext 76984 *Fax:* 717 290-5970
E-mail: clbaumer@lancastergeneralcollege.edu

Delaware County Community College
Surgical Technology Prgm
901 S Media Line Rd
Media, PA 19063-1094
www.dccc.edu
Prgm Dir: Jane Rothrock, DNSc RN CNOR FAAN
Tel: 610 359-5286 *Fax:* 610 359-7350
E-mail: drjaner2@comcast.net

Comm College of Allegheny County
Surgical Technology Prgm
595 Beatty Rd
Monroeville, PA 15146
Prgm Dir: Linda C Radzvin
Tel: 724 325-6779 *Fax:* 412 325-6799
E-mail: lradzvin@ccac.edu

Western School of Health & Business - Monroeville
Surgical Technology Prgm
1 Monroeville Center
Ste 125
Monroeville, PA 15146
Prgm Dir: Rachelle Graft-Hall, RN BSN
Tel: 412 373-9038, Ext 227 *Fax:* 412 373-2544
E-mail: rhall@western-school.com

Luzerne County Community College
Surgical Technology Prgm
1333 S Prospect St
Nanticoke, PA 18634
Prgm Dir: Elizabeth Senczakowicz
Tel: 800 377-5222, Ext 506 *Fax:* 570 740-0553
E-mail: esenczakowicz@luzerne.edu

Connelley Technical Institute
Surgical Technology Prgm
1501 Bedford Ave
Pittsburgh, PA 15219
Prgm Dir: G A Candie Gagne, CST CRCST MS
Tel: 412 338-3720 *Fax:* 412 338-3742
E-mail: candiegagne@comcast.net

Montgomery County Community College
Surgical Technology Prgm
101 College Dr
Pottstown, PA 19464
www.mc3.edu
Prgm Dir: Bessie Lindberg, CST
Tel: 610 718-1806
E-mail: blindber@mc3.edu

Reading Hospital & Medical Center
Surgical Technology Prgm
School of Health Sciences
PO Box 16052
Reading, PA 19612
Prgm Dir: Bonita McCoy, RN MEd CNOR
Tel: 610 988-8546 *Fax:* 610 988-5004
E-mail: mccoyb@readinghospital.org

McCann School of Business and Technology
Surgical Technology Prgm
1147 N Fourth St
Sunbury, PA 17601
Prgm Dir: Josette Crebs, RN CNOR
Tel: 570 286-3058 *Fax:* 570 286-4723
E-mail: jcrebs@mccannschool.com

Pennsylvania College of Technology
Surgical Technology Prgm
1 College Ave
Williamsport, PA 17701
Prgm Dir: Thomas J Campana, MD FACS
Tel: 570 320-2400, Ext 7744
E-mail: tcampana@pct.edu

Westmoreland County Community College
Surgical Technology Prgm
400 Armbrust Rd
Youngwood, PA 15697-1895
Prgm Dir: Patricia E Mihalcin, RN PhD
Tel: 724 925-4028 *Fax:* 724 925-4293
E-mail: mihalcinp@wccc-pa.edu

Rhode Island

New England Institute of Technology
Surgical Technology Prgm
2500 Post Rd
Warwick, RI 02886-2266
Prgm Dir: Lisa Reed, RN MS CNOR
Tel: 401 739-5000, Ext 3485   *Fax:* 401 739-7738
E-mail: lreed@neit.edu

South Carolina

Technical College of the Lowcountry
Surgical Technology Prgm
PO Box 1288
Beaufort, SC 29901
Prgm Dir: Julio A Acosta
Tel: 843 470-8415
E-mail: jacosta@tcl.edu

Midlands Technical College
Surgical Technology Prgm
PO Box 2408
Columbia, SC 29202
Prgm Dir: Kathy Patnaude, CST AOT
Tel: 803 822-3438   *Fax:* 803 822-3417
E-mail: patnaudek@midlandstech.edu

Florence-Darlington Technical College
Surgical Technology Prgm
PO Box 100548
Florence, SC 29501-0548
www.fdtc.edu
Prgm Dir: Neva B Lawson, CST FA RN
Tel: 843 661-8149   *Fax:* 843 292-0851
E-mail: neva.lawson@fdtc.edu

Horry - Georgetown Technical College
Surgical Technology Prgm
4003 S Fraser St
Georgetown, SC 29440
www.hgtc.edu
Prgm Dir: Dolores Aurand
Tel: 843 520-1435   *Fax:* 843 546-1437
E-mail: dolores.aurand@hgtc.edu

Aiken Technical College
Surgical Technology Prgm
2276 Jefferson Davis Hwy
PO Box 696
Graniteville, SC 29829
www.atc.edu
Prgm Dir: Amoret O'Rourke, RN BSN MSA
Tel: 803 593-9954, Ext 1648   *Fax:* 803 593-3106
E-mail: orourkea@atc.edu

Greenville Technical College
Surgical Technology Prgm
PO Box 5616
Greenville, SC 29606-8616
www.greenvilletech.com
Prgm Dir: Orrie Burdine, RN CNOR
Tel: 864 250-8298, Ext 8298   *Fax:* 864 250-8549
E-mail: Orrie.Burdine@gvltec.edu

Piedmont Technical College
Surgical Technology Prgm
PO Box 1467, Emerald Rd
Greenwood, SC 29646
Prgm Dir: Susan Boggs, RN BSN CNOR
Tel: 864 941-8535   *Fax:* 864 941-8684
E-mail: boggs.s@ptc.edu

Miller-Motte Technical College
Surgical Technology Prgm
8085 Rivers Ave
North Charleston, SC 29406
www.miller-motte.net
Prgm Dir: Lise Cayer, CST FA
Tel: 843 574-0101, Ext 55   *Fax:* 843 266-3424
E-mail: lcayer@miller-motte.net

Tri-County Technical College
Surgical Technology Prgm
PO Box 587
Pendleton, SC 29670-0587
Prgm Dir: Louise Vandiver, CST
Tel: 864 646-8361, Ext 1401   *Fax:* 864 646-1892
E-mail: lvandive@tctc.edu

York Technical College
Surgical Technology Prgm
452 S Anderson Rd
Rock Hill, SC 29730
Prgm Dir: Liz Boatwright, CST
Tel: 803 981-7071   *Fax:* 803 981-7216
E-mail: boatwright@yorktech.com

Spartanburg Community College
Surgical Technology Prgm
PO Drawer 4386
Spartanburg, SC 29305
Prgm Dir: Emily W Rogers, BS RN CNOR CST
Tel: 864 592-4870   *Fax:* 864 592-4881
E-mail: rogerse@sccsc.edu

Central Carolina Technical College
Surgical Technology Prgm
506 N Guignard Dr
Bldg 600
Sumter, SC 29150
www.cctech.edu
Prgm Dir: Lynn Shorter, CST
Tel: 803 778-1961, Ext 214
E-mail: shortersl@cctech.edu

South Dakota

Presentation College
Surgical Technology Prgm
1500 N Main St
Aberdeen, SD 57401
www.presentation.edu
Prgm Dir: Christina Rice, CST CET
Tel: 605 229-8415   *Fax:* 605 229-8518
E-mail: christina.rice@presentation.edu

Western Dakota Technical Institute
Surgical Technology Prgm
800 Mickelson Dr
Rapid City, SD 57703
Prgm Dir: Lynn Seime
Tel: 605 394-4034, Ext 307   *Fax:* 605 394-1789
E-mail: lseime@wdti.tec.sd.us

Southeast Technical Institute
Surgical Technology Prgm
2320 N Career Ave
Sioux Falls, SD 57107
Prgm Dir: Ruby A Castardo, BS Social Work CST
Tel: 605 367-4774   *Fax:* 605 367-6108
E-mail: ruby.castardo@southeasttech.com

Tennessee

Northeast State Technical Comm College
Surgical Technology Prgm
PO Box 246, 2425 Hwy 75
Blountville, TN 37617-0246
Prgm Dir: Laurie M Bollman, CST AS
Tel: 423 279-3681   *Fax:* 423 477-4859
E-mail: lmbollman@northeaststate.edu

Chattanooga State Technical Comm College
Surgical Technology Prgm
4501 Amnicola Hwy
Chattanooga, TN 37406-1097
Prgm Dir: Lucy Hampton, BSN RN CNOR
Tel: 423 697-4491   *Fax:* 423 697-2413
E-mail: lucy.hampton@chattanoogastate.edu

Miller-Motte Technical College - Chattanooga
Surgical Technology Prgm
6020 Shallowford Rd
Chattanooga, TN 37421
Prgm Dir: Kimberly Hudgins Laster
Tel: 423 510-9675   *Fax:* 423 510-1985
E-mail: klaster@miller-motte.com

Miller-Motte Technical College - Clarksville
Surgical Technology Prgm
1820 Business Park Dr
Clarksville, TN 37040
www.miller-motte.com
Prgm Dir: Diana Holter, AS BS
Tel: 931 553-0071
E-mail: dholter@miller-motte.com

MedVance Institute
Surgical Technology Prgm
1025 Highway 111
Cookeville, TN 38501
Prgm Dir: Rita Reagan, CST
Tel: 931 526-3660, Ext 244   *Fax:* 931 372-2603
E-mail: rreagan@medvance.org

Tennessee Technology Center - Crossville
Surgical Technology Prgm
910 Miller Ave
PO Box 2959
Crossville, TN 38557
Prgm Dir: Willie Green, CST
Tel: 931 484-7502, Ext 119   *Fax:* 931 484-8911
E-mail: willie.green@mail.tec.tn.us

Tennessee Technology Center - Dickson
Surgical Technology Prgm
740 Hwy 46 South
Dickson, TN 37055
www.ttcdickson.edu
Prgm Dir: Laura Travis, RN BSN
Tel: 615 441-6220, Ext 110   *Fax:* 615 441-6223
E-mail: laura.travis@ttcdickson.edu

Dyersburg State Community College
Surgical Technology Prgm
1510 Lake Rd
Dyersburg, TN 38024
Prgm Dir: Laura Dudley, BSN
Tel: 731 286-3390   *Fax:* 731 288-7744
E-mail: dudley@dscc.edu

Tennessee Technology Center - Hohenwald
Surgical Technology Prgm
813 W Main St
Hohenwald, TN 38462
www.hohenwald.tec.tn.us
Prgm Dir: Rick Brewer
Tel: 931 796-5351, Ext 125   *Fax:* 931 796-4892
E-mail: Rbrewer@hohenwald.tec.tn.us

Tennessee Technology Center - Jackson
Surgical Technology Prgm
2468 Technology Center Dr
Jackson, TN 38301
Prgm Dir: Barbara Avent, BSN
Tel: 731 424-0691, Ext 120   *Fax:* 731 424-0807
E-mail: bavent@jackson.tec.tn.us

Fort Sanders Regional Medical Center
Surgical Technology Prgm
9352 Park W Blvd
PO Box 22993
Knoxville, TN 37916
Prgm Dir: Mary Rippy, RN BSAOM CNOR
Tel: 865 541-5151   *Fax:* 865 694-5804
E-mail: mrippy@covhlth.com

Tennessee Technology Center - Knoxville
Surgical Technology Prgm
1100 Liberty St
Knoxville, TN 37919
Prgm Dir: Dorothy McGhee, RN ASN
Tel: 423 546-5567, Ext 122   *Fax:* 423 971-4474
E-mail: dmcghee@knoxville.tec.tn.us

Tennessee Technology Center - McMinnville
Surgical Technology Prgm
241 Vo-Tech Dr
McMinnville, TN 37110
Prgm Dir: Patricia Merlo, BS RN
Tel: 931 473-5587, Ext 243   *Fax:* 931 473-6380
E-mail: pmerlo@mcminnville.tec.tn.us

Concorde Career College - Memphis
Surgical Technology Prgm
5100 Poplar Ave, Ste 132
Memphis, TN 38137
www.concordecareercolleges.com
Prgm Dir: Chris Lee, CST AAS
Tel: 901 761-9494, Ext 242   *Fax:* 901 761-3293
E-mail: clee@concorde.edu

Tennessee Technology Center - Memphis
Surgical Technology Prgm
550 Alabama Ave
Memphis, TN 38105-3799
Prgm Dir: Elizabeth Oxner
Tel: 901 543-6164   *Fax:* 901 543-6126
E-mail: eoxner@ttcmemphis.edu

Tennessee Technology Center - Murfreesboro
Surgical Technology Prgm
1303 Old Fort Pkwy
Murfreesboro, TN 37129
Prgm Dir: Mike Ford, AD RN
Tel: 615 898-8010, Ext 146   *Fax:* 615 893-4194
E-mail: mford@ttcmurfreesboro.edu

Nashville State Community College
Surgical Technology Prgm
120 White Bridge Rd
Nashville, TN 37209
Prgm Dir: Van Bates, BA CST
Tel: 615 353-3329   *Fax:* 615 353-3376
E-mail: van.bates@nscc.edu

Tennessee Technology Center - Paris
Surgical Technology Prgm
312 S Wilson St
Paris, TN 38242
Prgm Dir: Alice McCutcheon, RN
Tel: 731 644-7365, Ext 140   *Fax:* 731 644-7368
E-mail: amccutcheon@paris.tec.tn.us

Texas

Cisco Junior College
Surgical Technology Prgm
717 E Industrial Blvd
Abilene, TX 79602
www.cisco.cc.tx.us
Prgm Dir: Kelly Meyer, BS
Tel: 325 794-4400, Ext 4441   *Fax:* 254 442-5100
E-mail: kelly.meyer@cjc.edu

Amarillo College
Surgical Technology Prgm
PO Box 447
Amarillo, TX 79178
www.actx.edu
Prgm Dir: Lisa Holdaway, RN CST
Tel: 806 356-3663   *Fax:* 806 354-6076
E-mail: holdaway-le@actx.edu

Concorde Career Institute - Arlington
Surgical Technology Prgm
601 Ryan Plaza Dr
Ste 200
Arlington, TX 76011
www.concorde.edu
Prgm Dir: Benjamin McCrory, Jr, CST
Tel: 817 792-2518   *Fax:* 817 461-3443
E-mail: bmccrory@concorde.edu

Austin Community College
Surgical Technology Prgm
3401 Webberville Rd
Austin, TX 78702
www.austincc.edu/health
Prgm Dir: Pedro Barrera, III, CST
Tel: 512 223-5804   *Fax:* 512 223-5901
E-mail: pbarrera@austincc.edu

Virginia College at Austin
Surgical Technology Prgm
6301 E Hwy 290
Austin, TX 78723
www.vc.edu
Prgm Dir: Javier Espinales, MEd CST
Tel: 512 279-2807   *Fax:* 512 317-3502
E-mail: jespinales@vc.edu

St Joseph Regional Health Center
Surgical Technology Prgm
2801 Franciscan Dr
Bryan, TX 77802-2544
Prgm Dir: Steve Heacock
Tel: 979 776-5902   *Fax:* 979 776-2981
E-mail: sheacock@st-joseph.org

North Central Texas College
Surgical Technology Prgm
1500 N Corinth St
Corinth, TX 76208-5408
www.nctc.edu
Prgm Dir: Judie Rodgers, RN BS CST
Tel: 940 498-6260   *Fax:* 940 498-6444
E-mail: jrodgers@nctc.edu

Del Mar College
Surgical Technology Prgm
101 Baldwin and Ayers Sts
Corpus Christi, TX 78404
Prgm Dir: Elena Mendieta, MS RN
Tel: 512 698-1105   *Fax:* 512 886-1598
E-mail: emendie@delmar.edu

El Centro College
Surgical Technology Prgm
801 Main St
Dallas, TX 75202-3604
Prgm Dir: Cindy Calcaterra, MBA RN CNOR
Tel: 214 860-2281   *Fax:* 214 860-2268
E-mail: CCalcaterra@dcccd.edu

Career Centers of Texas
Surgical Technology Prgm
8360 Burnham Rd, Ste 100
El Paso, TX 79907
Prgm Dir: Steven Wherrey, CST
Tel: 915 595-1935   *Fax:* 915 595-6619
E-mail: swherrey@cct-ep.com

El Paso Community College
Surgical Technology Prgm
PO Box 20500
El Paso, TX 79998
www.epcc.edu
Prgm Dir: Cynthia Rivera, RN BSN
Tel: 915 831-4086   *Fax:* 915 831-4114
E-mail: CynthiaR@epcc.edu

Galveston College
Surgical Technology Prgm
4015 Ave Q
Galveston, TX 77550
Prgm Dir: Suzanna Martinez, CST
Tel: 409 944-1493, Ext 493   *Fax:* 409 762-9367
E-mail: sumartin@gc.edu

Texas State Technical College - Harlingen
Surgical Technology Prgm
1902 N Loop 499
Harlingen, TX 78550
www.harlingen.tstc.edu/surgtech
Prgm Dir: Robert Sanchez, BSN CST RN
Tel: 956 364-4805   *Fax:* 956 364-5160
E-mail: robert.sanchez@harlingen.tstc.edu

Academy of Health Care Professions
Surgical Technology Prgm
240 Northwest Mall
Houston, TX 77092
Prgm Dir: Terry Rogers, CST AAS
Tel: 713 424-3100, Ext 3132   *Fax:* 713 425-3193
E-mail: trogers@academyofhealth.com

Houston Community College
Surgical Technology Prgm
1900 Pressler
Houston, TX 77030
www.hccs.edu
Prgm Dir: Christine Castillo-Sainz, RN BA
Tel: 713 718-7362   *Fax:* 713 718-7653
E-mail: christine.castillo@hccs.edu

MedVance Institute
Surgical Technology Prgm
6220 Westpark, Ste 180
Houston, TX 77057
Prgm Dir: Shawn Kelly, CST BSBM
Tel: 713 266-6594   *Fax:* 713 782-5873
E-mail: Shawn.kelly@medvance.edu

Sanford-Brown Institute - Houston
Surgical Technology Prgm
10500 Forum Place Dr #200
Houston, TX 77036
Prgm Dir: Linda Hill
Tel: 832 214-5291   *Fax:* 713 779-2408
E-mail: lhill@sbhouston.com

Tarrant County College - Northeast Campus
Surgical Technology Prgm
828 Harwood Rd
Hurst, TX 76054
Prgm Dir: Don Braziel, CST BS
Tel: 817 515-6160   *Fax:* 817 515-6700
E-mail: donnie.braziel@tccd.edu

Trinity Valley Community College
Surgical Technology Prgm
Hlth Science Ctr, 800 Hwy 243 W
Kaufman, TX 75142
www.tvcc.edu/healthscience/surgtech.htm
Prgm Dir: Nancy L Couch, RN CNOR
Tel: 972 932-4309, Ext 29   *Fax:* 972 932-5010
E-mail: ncouch@tvcc.edu

Kilgore College
Surgical Technology Prgm
1100 Broadway
Kilgore, TX 75662
www.kilgore.edu
Prgm Dir: Lane J Barnett, MSN RN CNOR
Tel: 903 983-8163   *Fax:* 903 988-7596
E-mail: lbarnett@kilgore.edu

South Plains College
Surgical Technology Prgm
Reese Center
819 Gilbert Dr
Lubbock, TX 79416
Prgm Dir: Stacey May, AAS ST
Tel: 806 885-3048, Ext 4642   *Fax:* 806 885-5608
E-mail: smay@southplainscollege.edu

Paris Junior College
Surgical Technology Prgm
2400 Clarksville St
Paris, TX 75460
www.parisjc.edu
Prgm Dir: Norman Gilbert, CFA SA
Tel: 903 782-0734   *Fax:* 903 782-0733
E-mail: ngilbert@parisjc.edu

San Jacinto College Central
Surgical Technology Prgm
8060 Spencer Hwy, PO Box 2007
Pasadena, TX 77505-2007
Prgm Dir: Diane DeYoung, MEd RN
Tel: 713 478-2759   *Fax:* 713 478-2754
E-mail: diane.deyoung@sjcd.edu

Lamar State College - Port Arthur
Surgical Technology Prgm
PO Box 310
Port Arthur, TX 77641-0310
www.lamarpa.edu
Prgm Dir: Brandon Buckner, CST
Tel: 409 984-6367   *Fax:* 409 984-6005
E-mail: brandon.buckner@lamarpa.edu

Howard College
Surgical Technology Prgm
3501 N US Hwy 67
San Angelo, TX 76905
Prgm Dir: Kay Millican, RN MSN FNP
Tel: 915 481-8300, Ext 233
E-mail: kmillican@howardcollege.edu

Baptist Health System
Surgical Technology Prgm
School of Health Professions
8400 Datapoint Dr
San Antonio, TX 78229
www.wshp.edu
Prgm Dir: Christallia Starks, RN MSN CRCST
Tel: 210 297-9166   *Fax:* 210 297-0941
E-mail: cstarks@baptisthealthsystem.com

St Philip's College
Surgical Technology Prgm
1801 Martin Luther King Dr
San Antonio, TX 78203-2098
http://accd.edu/spc
Prgm Dir: Lana Seay, RN BSOE
Tel: 210 531-3418   *Fax:* 210 531-3459
E-mail: lseay@accd.edu

Temple College
Surgical Technology Prgm
2600 S First St
Temple, TX 76504
Prgm Dir: Carol A Reinking, RN MS CNOR
Tel: 254 298-8652   *Fax:* 254 298-8278
E-mail: carol.reinking@templejc.edu

Tyler Junior College
Surgical Technology Prgm
PO Box 9020
1530 SSW Loop 323
Tyler, TX 75711
www.tjc.edu
Prgm Dir: Sherry Seaton, RN BSN CNOR
Tel: 903 510-2962   *Fax:* 903 510-2948
E-mail: ssea@tjc.edu

Wharton County Junior College
Surgical Technology Prgm
911 Boling Hwy
Wharton, TX 77488
Prgm Dir: Melissa Wade, LVN
Tel: 979 532-6310   *Fax:* 979 532-6489
E-mail: melissaw@wcjc.edu

Vernon College
Surgical Technology Prgm
4105 Maplewood Ave
Wichita Falls, TX 76308
Prgm Dir: Jeff Feix, LVN CST/CFA
Tel: 940 696-8752, Ext 3266   *Fax:* 940 696-3244
E-mail: jfeix@vernoncollege.edu

Utah

Davis Applied Technology College
Surgical Technology Prgm
550 East 300 South
Kaysville, UT 84037
www.datc.edu
Prgm Dir: Pamela June Carter, RN BSN MEd CNOR
Tel: 801 593-2330   *Fax:* 801 593-2400
E-mail: pjcarter@datc.edu

Stevens-Henager College
Surgical Technology Prgm
1890 S 1350 West
PO Box 9428
Ogden, UT 84401
Prgm Dir: Lee Berger, CST
Tel: 801 394-7791, Ext 1031   *Fax:* 801 621-0853
E-mail: berger_lee@yahoo.com

AmeriTech College
Surgical Technology Prgm
1675 N Freedom Blvd, Ste 3B
Provo, UT 84604
Prgm Dir: Adrian Dominguez, CST
Tel: 801 377-2900, Ext 207   *Fax:* 801 375-3077
E-mail: adominguez@ameritech.edu

Intermountain Healthcare
Surgical Technology Prgm
LDS Hospital
8th Ave and C Street
Salt Lake City, UT 84143
Prgm Dir: Carolyn H Scheese, CST RN BSN MS
Tel: 801 408-3240   *Fax:* 801 408-5240
E-mail: carolyn.scheese@intermountainmail.org

Dixie State College of Utah
Surgical Technology Prgm
225 South 700 East St
St George, UT 84770
www.dixie.edu
Prgm Dir: Jeanne Mortenson, RN BSN CNOR
Tel: 435 652-7567   *Fax:* 435 652-7873
E-mail: jmortenson@dixie.edu

Salt Lake Community College
Surgical Technology Prgm
9301 S Wights Fort Rd
West Jordan, UT 84088
Prgm Dir: Mia Carsey, CST BS
Tel: 801 256-5922   *Fax:* 801 256-5930
E-mail: mia.carsey@slcc.edu

Virginia

Piedmont Virginia Community College
Surgical Technology Prgm
501 College Dr
Charlottesville, VA 22902
Prgm Dir: Ann Smith, RN MSN CNOR
Tel: 434 961-5239   *Fax:* 434 961-5441
E-mail: asmith@pvcc.edu

Miller-Motte Technical College
Surgical Technology Prgm
1011 Creekside Lane
Lynchburg, VA 24502
Prgm Dir: Sandra Henderson
Tel: 434 239-5222
E-mail: shenderson@miller-motte.com

Riverside School of Health Careers
Surgical Technology Prgm
316 Main St
Newport News, VA 23601
Prgm Dir: Carolyn M Branson, CNOR CST RN BS
Tel: 757 240-2214   *Fax:* 757 240-2201
E-mail: carol.branson@rivhs.com

Naval School of Health Sciences
Surgical Technology Prgm
1001 Holcomb Rd, Building 104
Portsmouth, VA 23708-5200
http://www-nshspts.med.navy.mil/
Prgm Dir: John Kane, CDR
Tel: 757 953-6434   *Fax:* 757 953-7380
E-mail: john.kane@med.navy.mil

J Sargeant Reynolds Community College
Surgical Technology Prgm
700 E Jackson St
Richmond, VA 23285-5622
Prgm Dir: Ed DeGennaro
Tel: 804 786-1375   *Fax:* 804 768-5298
E-mail: edegennaro@jsr.vccs.edu
Notes: Currently inactive

Washington

Bellingham Technical College
Surgical Technology Prgm
3028 Lindbergh Ave
Bellingham, WA 98225
Prgm Dir: Lorrie Zwiers, RN CNOR
Tel: 360 752-8415   *Fax:* 360 676-2798
E-mail: lzwiers@btc.ctc.edu

Clover Park Technical College
Surgical Technology Prgm
4500 Steilacoom Blvd SW
Lakewood, WA 98499
Prgm Dir: Kezia Clark, ST
Tel: 253 589-5530   *Fax:* 253 589-5866
E-mail: kezia.clark@cptc.edu

Renton Technical College
Surgical Technology Prgm
3000 NE Fourth St
Renton, WA 98056
www.rtc.edu
Prgm Dir: Rosemary Thurston, RN
Tel: 425 235-7812   *Fax:* 425 235-5836
E-mail: rthurston@rtc.edu

Seattle Central Community College
Surgical Technology Prgm
1701 Broadway
Seattle, WA 98122
Prgm Dir: Annejeannette Serba, RN CNOR
Tel: 206 587-6950   *Fax:* 206 587-6337
E-mail: aserba@sccd.ctc.edu

Spokane Community College
Surgical Technology Prgm
N 1810 Greene St
Spokane, WA 99207
Prgm Dir: Jeannie Hurd, RN BS CNOR
Tel: 509 533-7303   *Fax:* 509 533-8621
E-mail: jhurd@scc.spokane.edu

Yakima Valley Community College
Surgical Technology Prgm
PO Box 22520
Yakima, WA 98907-2520
Prgm Dir: Libby A McRae, CST
Tel: 509 574-6845   *Fax:* 509 574-6811
E-mail: lmcrae@yvcc.edu

West Virginia

Carver Career Center
Surgical Technology Prgm
4799 Midland Dr
Charleston, WV 25306
Prgm Dir: Letitia Hodovan, CNOR
Tel: 304 348-1965, Ext 110   *Fax:* 304 348-1932

Monongalia County Tech Education Center
Cosponsor: Monongalia County Board of Education
Surgical Technology Prgm
1000 Mississippi St
Morgantown, WV 26501
Prgm Dir: Lynda Overking, RN BSN MS
Tel: 304 291-9240, Ext 22   *Fax:* 304 291-9247
E-mail: loverkin@access.k12.wv.us

Southern West Virginia Comm & Tech College
Surgical Technology Prgm
PO Box 2900
Dempsey Branch Rd
Mount Gay, WV 25637
Prgm Dir: Judith Curry, RN BSN
Tel: 304 792-7098, Ext 113   *Fax:* 304 792-7043
E-mail: judyc@southern.wvnet.edu

West Virginia University - Parkersburg
Surgical Technology Prgm
300 Campus Dr
Parkersburg, WV 26104
Prgm Dir: Margaret Ponce, RN
Tel: 304 424-8300   *Fax:* 304 424-8315
E-mail: peggy.ponce@mail.wvu.edu

West Virginia Northern Community College
Surgical Technology Prgm
15th and Jacob Sts
Wheeling, WV 26003
Prgm Dir: Teresa Ramsey
Tel: 304 233-5900, Ext 5510   *Fax:* 304 233-5837
E-mail: tramsey@northern.wvnet.edu

Wisconsin

Chippewa Valley Technical College
Surgical Technology Prgm
620 W Clairemont Ave
Eau Claire, WI 54701-6162
Prgm Dir: David Yount
Tel: 715 858-1897   *Fax:* 715 833-6431
E-mail: dyount@cvtc.edu

Northeast Wisconsin Technical College
Surgical Technology Prgm
2740 W Mason St, PO Box 19042
Green Bay, WI 54307-9042
www.nwtc.edu
Prgm Dir: Cynthia McDonald, CST BSN MS CNOR
Tel: 920 498-5540   *Fax:* 920 491-2660
E-mail: cindy.mcdonald@nwtc.edu

Gateway Technical College
Surgical Technology Prgm
3520 30th Ave
Kenosha, WI 53144-1690
Prgm Dir: Kristina Vines, CST
Tel: 262 564-2748   *Fax:* 262 564-2299
E-mail: vinesk@gtc.edu

Western Technical College
Surgical Technology Prgm
304 N Sixth St, PO Box C-908
La Crosse, WI 54602-0908
Prgm Dir: Joan Miksis, CST RN BSN
Tel: 608 785-9193   *Fax:* 608 785-9087
E-mail: miksisj@wwtc.edu

Madison Area Technical College
Surgical Technology Prgm
Center for Health and Safety Education
3550 Anderson St
Madison, WI 53704
www.matcmadison.edu
Prgm Dir: Kathy Moninger, RN
Tel: 608 246-6280   *Fax:* 608 246-6013
E-mail: kmoninger@matcmadison.edu

Mid-State Technical College
Surgical Technology Prgm
2600 W Fifth St
Marshfield, WI 54449
www.mstc.edu
Prgm Dir: Kelly Altmann, RN BSN CNOR
Tel: 715 387-2538, Ext 7030   *Fax:* 715 389-2864
E-mail: Kelly.altmann@mstc.edu

Milwaukee Area Technical College
Surgical Technology Prgm
700 W State St
Milwaukee, WI 53233
www.matc.edu
Prgm Dir: Patricia Stapleton, RN MSN
Tel: 414 297-7151   *Fax:* 414 297-8955
E-mail: stapletp@matc.edu

Waukesha County Technical College
Surgical Technology Prgm
800 Main St
Pewaukee, WI 53072
Prgm Dir: Sharon A Corrao, RN BSN MEd CNOR CST
Tel: 262 691-5407   *Fax:* 262 691-5241
E-mail: scorrao@wctc.edu

Northcentral Technical College
Surgical Technology Prgm
1000 Campus Dr
Wausau, WI 54401
Prgm Dir: Julie Osness-Thorson, RN MSN
Tel: 715 675-3331, Ext 4497   *Fax:* 715 675-9776
E-mail: osness@ntc.edu

Wyoming

Laramie County Community College
Surgical Technology Prgm
1400 E College Dr
Cheyenne, WY 82007
www.lccc.wy.edu
Prgm Dir: Katherine Snyder, CST FAST BS
Tel: 307 778-1155   *Fax:* 307 778-1395
E-mail: ksnyder@lccc.wy.edu

Surgical Technologist

Programs*	Class Capacity	Begins	Length (months)	Award	Res. Tuition	Non-res. Tuition	Stipend	Offers:‡ 1	2	3	4
Alabama											
James H Faulkner State Community College (Bay Minette)	25	Aug	18, 24	Cert, AAS	$93	$164					
Arizona											
Lamson College (Tempe)	48	Every 4 wks	16	Dipl, Assoc	$22,353	$22,353		•			
Pima Community College (Tucson)	12	Jan	12	Cert	$9,360	$9,360					
Arkansas											
Baptist Health Schools Little Rock	24	Jul	12	Dipl	$5,700	$8,445					
North Arkansas College (Harrison)	9	Aug	9, 24	Cert, AAS	$1,590	$2,710					•
Northwest Technical Institute (Springdale)	20	Aug	11	Dipl	$3,940	$3,940					
University of Arkansas - Fort Smith	18	Aug	18	AAS	$1,830	$6,840					•
University of Arkansas for Medical Sciences (North Little Rock)	16	Aug	10, 20	Cert, AS	$6,554	$14,111					
California											
Concorde Career College (San Diego)	24	Jan May Oct	13	Dipl	$21,100	$21,110					
Concorde Career College - North Hollywood	24	Jan Apr Jul Oct	13	Dipl	$21,125	$21,125					
Concorde Career College - San Bernardino	72	Apr Jul Dec	13	Dipl	$21,121	$21,121					
Glendale Career College	30	Every 12 wks	16	Dipl	$21,700	$21,700		•			
Glendale Career College - Oceanside Campus	20	Open	17	Dipl	$22,075	$22,075					
San Joaquin Valley College (Fresno)	16	Oct	16	AS	$24,200	$24,200					
Skyline College (San Bruno)	25	Aug	10	Cert, AS	$600	$6,360					•
Colorado											
Concorde Career College - Aurora	24	3x/yr	13	Cert	$22,891	$22,891					
Connecticut											
A I Prince Technical High School (Hartford)	18	Aug	10	Cert	$2,700	$0					
Danbury Hospital	12	Sep	12	Dipl	$3,000	$3,000					
Florida											
Central Florida Community College (Ocala)	25	Aug	11	Cert	$2,500	$9,900					
Concorde Career Institute (Lauderdale Lakes)	24	Oct Dec Apr	13	Dipl	$20,578	$20,578					
Concorde Career Institute - Jacksonville	24	Feb Jul Oct	12	Dipl	$20,350	$20,350					

*Data are shown only for programs that completed the 2007 AMA Survey of Health Professions Education Programs.
‡Key to Offers: 1: Evening or weekend classes; 2: Non-English instruction; 3: Cultural competence instruction; 4: Distance education component.

Surgical Technologist

Programs*	Class Capacity	Begins	Length (months)	Award	Res. Tuition	Non-res. Tuition	Stipend	Offers:‡ 1	2	3	4
Concorde Career Institute - Tampa	24	Feb May Jun Sep Aug Oct	12	Dipl	$19,854	$19,854		•			
Daytona Beach Community College	20	Aug	10	Cert	$2,316	$9,157					
Florida Metropolitan Univ - Tampa College		Quarterly	24	AS	$12,096	$12,096		•			
Gulf Coast Community College (Panama City)	20	Jan	12	Cert	$4,081	$12,182				•	•
Indian River Community College (Fort Pierce)	20	Jun	12	Cert	$3,000	$6,000				•	
Keiser University (Port St Lucie)	24	Every 4 wks	20	AS	$11,832	$11,832		•		•	
Lee County High Tech Center - North (Cape Coral)	20	Jan	12	Cert	$2,314	$9,256					
Lindsey Hopkins Tech Education Center (Miami)	16	Jul Mar	15	Cert	$2,800	$6,000					
MedVance Institute - Atlantis Campus (Palm Springs)	30	Jun Dec	15	Dipl	$26,000	$26,000					
Okaloosa-Walton College (Niceville)	14	Aug	12	Cert	$4,477	$11,627				•	
Orlando Tech	15	Summer Fall	13	Cert	$4,600	$12,000					
Pinellas Tech Educ Ctr - Clearwater Campus (St Petersburg)	20	Aug	10	Cert	$1,776	$7,124				•	
Sheridan Technical Center (Hollywood)	26	Jun	12	Cert	$2,554	$10,201					
Georgia											
Chattahoochee Technical College (Marietta)	25	Jun	18	Dipl	$1,956	$3,612				•	
Coastal Georgia Community College (Brunswick)	12	May	15	Cert	$3,600	$13,124					
Columbus Technical College	50	Apr Oct	18, 24	Dipl, AAS	$4,464	$8,928					
DeKalb Technical College (Clarkston)	15	Jul	18	Dipl	$1,876	$6,340					
Gwinnett Technical College (Lawrenceville)	30	Jul	15	Dipl	$3,600	$7,000				•	
Middle Georgia Technical College (Warner Robins)	16	Jan	12	Dipl	$2,326	$4,653					•
Okefenokee Technical College (Waycross)	15	Fall quarter	24, 15	Dipl, AAS	$2,592	$0					
Southeastern Technical College (Vidalia)	18	Jul	18	Dipl	$2,265	$5,530				•	
Valdosta Technical College	25	Jul	15	Dipl	$1,845	$3,405					
West Central Technical College (Waco)	12	Sep	12	Dipl	$3,400	$0					
Illinois											
College of DuPage (West Chicago)	30	Jan	12	Cert, AAS	$5,926	$12,000					
Elgin Community College	24	Jan	12	Cert	$3,528	$15,090					
Illinois Central College (Peoria)	20	Aug	17, 22	Cert, AAS	$3,675	$4,900					
Prairie State College (Chicago Heights)	20	Aug	11	Cert	$3,042	$7,630					
Richland Community College (Decatur)	30	Aug	21	Cert, AAS	$7,993	$19,940					
Rock Valley College (Rockford)	17	Aug	12	Cert	$3,515	$9,154					
Southern Illinois Collegiate Common Market (Herrin)	24	Aug	12	Cert	$1,803	$1,916					
Trinity College of Nursing & Health Sciences (Rock Island)	16	Jun	11	Cert, AAS	$8,395	$8,395				•	
Waubonsee Community College (Sugar Grove)	25	Aug	12	Cert	$2,792	$7,654		•			•
Indiana											
Bloomington Hospital	12	Feb	11	Cert	$6,000	$6,000				•	
Clarian Health Partners Inc (Indianapolis)	24	Aug	11	Cert	$3,951	$3,951					
Ivy Tech Community College - Kokomo	12	Aug	24	AS	$2,984	$6,069				•	•
Ivy Tech Community College - Michigan City	32	Aug	24	AAS	$3,378	$6,873		•			
University of Saint Francis (Fort Wayne)	22	Aug	20	AS	$19,570	$19,570		•	•	•	•
Vincennes University	20	Aug	11, 24	Cert, AS, AA	$4,552	$11,365				•	•
Iowa											
Mercy College of Health Sciences (Des Moines)	20	Sep	11	Cert, AS	$16,965	$16,965					
Western Iowa Tech Community College (Sioux City)	24	Aug	9, 18	Dipl, AAS	$3,007	$4,526		•		•	
Kansas											
Hutchinson Community College	18	Aug	10	Cert	$2,747	$4,223					
Kaw Area Technical School (Topeka)	12	Aug 10 (app)	10	Cert	$4,043	$17,466				•	
Kentucky											
Bluegrass Community and Technical College (Lexington)	20	Aug	16, 24	Dipl, AAS	$109	$327					
Madisonville Community College	18	Aug	10	Dipl, Assoc	$109	$370					•
National College (Florence)	24	Jun Dec	24	AS	$8,976	$8,976					
National College (Louisville)	24	Mar Jun Sep Dec	24	AS	$8,976	$8,976					
Somerset Community College	12	Aug	24	AAS	$3,815	$11,445					
West Kentucky Community & Technical College (Paducah)	16	Aug	11	Dipl, AAS	$1,185	$3,595					
Louisiana											
Bossier Parish Community College (Bossier City)	16	Jun	18	Dipl	$860	$1,930				•	
Career Technical College (Monroe)	17	Jan Apr Jul Oct	9, 24	AOS	$185	$0		•			
Delgado Community College (New Orleans)	25	Jan Aug	14	Cert	$1,236	$3,376					
Louisiana Tech College - Lafayette Campus	30	Jan	24	AAS	$1,115	$1,905				•	
Louisiana Tech College - Lafourche Campus (Thibodaux)	12	Jan Aug	15	AAS	$1,552	$2,636					
Our Lady of the Lake College (Baton Rouge)	20	Jun	12	AD							
Massachusetts											
North Shore Community College (Danvers)	20	Sep-May	9	Cert	$4,800	$6,888					
Michigan											
Baker College of Clinton Township	20	Jun	24	AAS	$8,680	$8,680		•		•	

*Data are shown only for programs that completed the 2007 AMA Survey of Health Professions Education Programs.
‡Key to Offers: 1: Evening or weekend classes; 2: Non-English instruction; 3: Cultural competence instruction; 4: Distance education component.

Programs*	Class Capacity	Begins	Length (months)	Award	Res. Tuition	Non-res. Tuition	Stipend	Offers:‡ 1	2	3	4
Baker College of Flint	20	Jun	24	AAS	$18,375	$18,375				•	
Baker College of Jackson	20	Sep	24	AAS	$7,285	$0					
Baker College of Port Huron	12	Jun	12	AAS	$5,400	$5,400		•			
Delta College (University Center)	15	Aug	20	Cert, AAS	$2,508	$3,597				•	
Kalamazoo Valley Community College	16	Aug	10	Cert	$2,135	$4,760					
Lansing Community College	24	Aug	18	AAS	$5,700	$8,000					
Northern Michigan University (Marquette)	16	Aug	24	Assoc	$8,431	$0					
Oakland Community College (Royal Oak)	25	Sep	24	AAS	$3,490	$6,435				•	
Minnesota											
Anoka Technical College	30	Aug Jan	13	Dipl, AAS	$8,102	$16,203		•			
Rochester Community & Technical College	25	Aug	18	AAS	$9,594	$17,978		•		•	
St Cloud Technical College	24	Jun Aug	12, 19	Dipl, AAS	$4,589	$4,589		•		•	
Mississippi											
Holmes Community College (Grenada)	15	Aug	12, 24	Cert, AAS	$1,806	$4,356				•	
Mississippi Gulf Coast Community College (Lucedale)	15	Jan	12	Dipl, Cert	$2,703	$5,406					
Missouri											
Franklin Tech Ctr/Missouri Southern St Univ (Joplin)	20	Aug	9	Cert	$8,500	$8,500					
Ozarks Technical Community College (Springfield)	20	Aug	9, 18	Cert, AAS	$4,085	$5,375				•	
St Louis Community College - Forest Park	25	Aug	12	Dipl, Cert	$4,298	$7,106				•	
Nevada											
College of Southern Nevada (Las Vegas)	15	Sep	10	Cert	$1,857	$5,795					
Nevada Career Institute (Las Vegas)	30	Every 12 wks	17	Dipl	$22,075	$22,075					
New Hampshire											
Concord Hospital	9	Sep	12	Cert	$5,000	$5,000					
New Jersey											
Atlantic Cape Community College (Atlantic City)	12	Jan	11	Cert	$10,160	$0					
New York											
Bronx Lebanon Hospital (New York)	15	Sep	10	Cert				•			
Nassau Community College (Garden City)	64	Sep	24	AAS	$1,655	$3,310		•			•
New York University Medical Center	30	Sep Mar	12	Cert	$10,000	$10,000		•			
Stony Brook University	20	Jan	11	Cert	$9,500	$9,500				•	
Ulster County Board of Cooperative Ed Service (Port Ewen)	15	Sep	10	Cert	$7,100	$7,100					
Western Suffolk BOCES (Northport)	12	Mar Sep	10	Cert	$0	$9,525				•	
North Carolina											
Asheville-Buncombe Technical Comm College	16	Aug	12	Dipl	$1,896	$10,536				•	•
Cabarrus College of Health Sciences (Concord)	20	Aug	9, 18	Dipl, AS	$9,900	$9,900				•	
Catawba Valley Community College (Hickory)	20	Aug	12	Dipl	$1,800	$9,000				•	
Central Piedmont Community College (Charlotte)	24	Aug	22	AS	$1,556	$7,316		•		•	•
College of The Albemarle (Elizabeth City)	20	Aug	12	Dipl	$1,500	$8,400				•	
Durham Technical Community College	24	Aug	12	Dipl	$1,896	$10,536				•	•
Edgecombe Community College (Tarboro)	15	Aug	12	Dipl	$339	$2,046				•	
Fayetteville Technical Community College	15	Aug	12, 24	Dipl, AAS	$1,986	$10,626					•
Lenoir Community College (Kinston)	28	Aug	12	Dipl	$1,341	$6,975					
Miller-Motte College (Cary)	30	Jan Apr Jul Oct	18	AS	$14,848	$14,848					
Miller-Motte College (Wilmington)	30	Jan Jul	24	AAS	$12,800	$12,800					
Wake Technical Community College (Raleigh)	16	Aug	12	Dipl	$1,800	$8,000				•	
Wilson Technical Community College	20	Aug	12	Dipl	$1,950	$10,559					
North Dakota											
Bismarck State College	24	Aug	20	AAS	$4,055	$9,465				•	
Ohio											
Choffin Career & Technical Center (Youngstown)	25	Aug	10	Cert	$6,500	$6,500				•	
Columbus State Community College	30	Sep (Autumn)	12, 18	Cert, AS	$4,460	$9,576		•	•	•	
Cuyahoga Community College (Cleveland)	24	Aug	21, 12	Cert, AAS	$80	$106		•		•	
EHOVE Ghrist Adult Career Center (Milan)	30	Aug (FT) Dec (PT)	9, 14	Cert	$7,665	$7,665					
Miami-Jacobs Career College (Dayton)	24	Jul	24	AS	$13,920	$13,920		•			
Scioto County Joint Vocational School (Lucasville)	15	Jan	11	Cert	$6,984	$0					
Sinclair Community College (Dayton)	24	Sep	20	AAS	$2,407	$4,547				•	
University of Akron	22	Aug	22	AAS	$8,140	$8,752				•	
Oklahoma											
Canadian Valley Technology Center (Chickasha)	15	Open entry	18	Dipl	$1,755	$24,804				•	•
Community Care College (Tulsa)	80	Jan 7	13, 20	Dipl, AAS	$16,673	$16,673					
Moore Norman Technology Center	20	Aug	9	Dipl	$2,300	$2,700					
Tulsa Technology Center	18	Aug Nov Jan	9, 12	Cert	$3,000	$3,000		•			
Wes Watkins Technology Center District 25 (Wetumka)	14	Aug	10	Cert						•	
Oregon											
Concorde Career Institute - Portland	24	Apr Aug Dec	12	Dipl	$22,079	$22,079					

*Data are shown only for programs that completed the 2007 AMA Survey of Health Professions Education Programs.

‡Key to Offers: 1: Evening or weekend classes; 2: Non-English instruction; 3: Cultural competence instruction; 4: Distance education component.

Surgical Technologist

Programs*	Class Capacity	Begins	Length (months)	Award	Res. Tuition	Non-res. Tuition	Stipend	Offers:‡ 1	2	3	4
Pennsylvania											
Conemaugh Memorial Medical Center (Johnstown)	14	Aug 27	12	Cert, AS	$13,476	$27,376				•	
Delaware County Community College (Media)	16	Sep	12	AAS	$5,100	$9,500				•	
Harrisburg Area Community College - Harrisburg	10	Aug	21	Cert, Assoc	$1,020	$1,920				•	
Harrisburg Area Community College - Lancaster	8	Jan	21	Cert, Assoc	$1,920	$1,920				•	
Lancaster Gen Coll of Nursing & Hlth Sciences	16	Aug	12, 24	Dipl, AD	$19,480	$19,480		•		•	•
Luzerne County Community College (Nanticoke)	20		14	AAS	$5,432	$6,784				•	
Montgomery County Community College (Pottstown)	20	Sep (Fall semester)	12, 16	Cert, AAS	$5,056	$5,056					
Mount Aloysius College (Cresson)	25	Aug	24	Dipl, AS	$15,390	$15,390				•	
Reading Hospital & Medical Center	10	Aug	10	Dipl	$4,500	$4,500				•	
St Luke's Hospital (Bethlehem)	16	Aug	11	Cert	$7,300	$0					
South Carolina											
Aiken Technical College (Graniteville)	20	Aug	12	Dipl	$4,785	$13,404					
Central Carolina Technical College (Sumter)	20	May	12	Dipl	$6,050	$7,100				•	
Florence-Darlington Technical College	24	Aug	12	Dipl	$6,544	$7,056				•	
Greenville Technical College	35	Aug	12	Dipl	$1,500	$1,625		•		•	
Horry - Georgetown Technical College	24	Aug	12	Cert	$3,600	$4,650					
Miller-Motte Technical College (North Charleston)	20	Jan	18, 24	Assoc	$6,840	$6,840					
Spartanburg Community College	25	Aug	12, 24	Dipl, AS	$4,731	$5,910					
York Technical College (Rock Hill)	20	Aug	12	Dipl	$4,554	$8,886					
South Dakota											
Presentation College (Aberdeen)	12	Aug	18	AS	$12,300	$12,300					
Southeast Technical Institute (Sioux Falls)	35	Aug	12	Dipl	$5,057	$5,297		•		•	
Tennessee											
Concorde Career College - Memphis	24	Feb Jun Sep Dec	12	Dipl	$20,318	$20,318		•			
Miller-Motte Technical College - Clarksville	24	Jan Oct	24	AAS	$21,408	$0					
Tennessee Technology Center - Dickson	16	Sep	12	Dipl	$2,058	$2,058				•	
Tennessee Technology Center - Hohenwald	25	Jan	12	Dipl	$3,620	$3,620					
Tennessee Technology Center - Memphis	30	May Sep	12	Dipl	$2,058	$2,058					
Texas											
Amarillo College	25	Aug	10, 24	Dipl, Cert, AAS	$1,900	$3,677					
Austin Community College	16	Aug Jan	16, 24	Cert, AAS	$2,618	$11,944				•	
Baptist Health System (San Antonio)	15	Jan Aug	12	Cert	$6,320	$6,320		•		•	
Cisco Junior College (Abilene)	12	Aug	12	Cert	$2,985	$3,444					
Concorde Career Institute - Arlington	24	Feb Oct Dec	12	Dipl	$19,150	$19,150					
El Centro College (Dallas)	30	Aug	15	Cert	$1,788	$3,078		•		•	
El Paso Community College	12	Jun	12, 24	Cert, AAS	$3,500	$5,000				•	
Houston Community College	35	Aug	12	Cert	$3,500	$4,000					
Kilgore College	12	Jun	18, 24	Cert, AAS	$5,940	$8,050					
Lamar State College - Port Arthur	24	Jul	12, 24	Cert, AAS	$2,352	$11,466					
North Central Texas College (Corinth)	24	Aug	12	Cert	$1,930	$3,025					
Paris Junior College	12	Aug	19	Cert	$1,292	$2,006					
South Plains College (Lubbock)	40	Aug	12	Cert, AAS	$3,660	$3,940				•	
St Philip's College (San Antonio)	25	Aug	12	Cert	$2,500	$6,000					
Tarrant County College - Northeast Campus (Hurst)	30	Aug	11	Cert	$3,800	$5,700					
Texas State Technical College - Harlingen	30	Sep	12	AAS	$6,205	$14,605					
Trinity Valley Community College (Kaufman)	12	Aug	12, 24	Cert, AAS	$1,846	$2,366				•	
Tyler Junior College	15	Aug	9, 21	Cert, AAS	$3,702	$5,414	$1,500			•	
Virginia College at Austin	25	Jan Jul	24	AAS	$15,680	$15,680					
Utah											
Davis Applied Technology College (Kaysville)	30	Open enrollment	15	Cert	$1,450	$3,969				•	
Dixie State College of Utah (St George)	10	Aug	9	Cert	$943	$3,517				•	
Intermountain Healthcare (Salt Lake City)	13	Varies	6	Cert	$400	$400		•		•	
Virginia											
Naval School of Health Sciences (Portsmouth)	50	Jan May Sep	6	Cert							
Riverside School of Health Careers (Newport News)	15	Aug	11	Dipl	$7,385	$7,385				•	
Washington											
Renton Technical College	36	Sep Jan	11, 24	Cert, AAS-ST, AASTST	$4,780	$4,780				•	
Yakima Valley Community College	8	Sep	27	Dipl, AAS	$2,449	$0				•	•
West Virginia											
Carver Career Center (Charleston)	15	Aug	10	Cert	$1,438	$1,438				•	
Southern West Virginia Comm & Tech College (Mount Gay)	20	Aug	18	Dipl, AS	$1,634	$2,732				•	
Wisconsin											
Madison Area Technical College	20	Jun	12	Dipl	$3,782	$0		•		•	•

*Data are shown only for programs that completed the 2007 AMA Survey of Health Professions Education Programs.
‡Key to Offers: 1: Evening or weekend classes; 2: Non-English instruction; 3: Cultural competence instruction; 4: Distance education component.

Surgical Technologist

	Class Capacity	Begins	Length (months)	Award	Res. Tuition	Non-res. Tuition	Stipend	Offers:‡ 1	2	3	4
Mid-State Technical College (Marshfield)	20	Jun	12	Dipl	$3,314	$17,350		•			
Milwaukee Area Technical College	16	Aug Jan	18	AAS	$3,268	$18,320					•
Northeast Wisconsin Technical College (Green Bay)	26	Jun Aug	12	Dipl	$3,863	$19,106		•			•
Wyoming											
Laramie County Community College (Cheyenne)	12	Aug	20	AAS	$2,004	$4,860					

*Data are shown only for programs that completed the 2007 AMA Survey of Health Professions Education Programs.
‡Key to Offers: 1: Evening or weekend classes; 2: Non-English instruction; 3: Cultural competence instruction; 4: Distance education component.

Therapeutic Recreation Specialist

Therapeutic recreation uses treatment, education, and recreation services to help people with illnesses, disabilities, and other conditions develop and use their leisure in ways that enhance their health, functional abilities, independence, and quality of life.

Therapeutic recreation services contribute to the broad spectrum of health care through treatment (recreational therapy), education, and providing recreational opportunities, all of which are instrumental to improving and maintaining physical, cognitive, emotional, and social functioning, preventing secondary health conditions, and enhancing independent living skills and the overall quality of life.

Recreational therapy services use various interventions to treat physical, cognitive, emotional, and social conditions associated with illness, injury, or chronic disabilities. Recreational therapy includes an education component, which enables individuals to become more informed and active partners in their health care by using activity to cope with the stress of illness and disability. Furthermore, these services assist individuals with managing their disabilities so they may achieve and maintain optimal levels of independence, productivity, and well-being and enter/re-enter the mainstream of community life.

Therapeutic recreation services also include the provision of recreational opportunities (eg, wheelchair sports, exercise and fitness programs, social activities) that can minimize health care costs by allowing individuals with disabilities mechanisms to prevent declines in their physical, cognitive, social, and emotional health, thereby reducing the need for medical services.

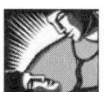

Career Description

The day-to-day work experience of therapeutic recreation specialists can vary dramatically, depending on the setting and clients they serve. All therapeutic recreation specialists, however, conduct assessments of physical, mental, emotional, and social functioning to determine the client's needs, interests, and abilities. The therapeutic recreation specialist works with the client, family, and others to design and implement an individualized treatment, education, or program plan, depending on the setting.

Professional therapeutic recreation services are divided into three specific service areas, which represent a comprehensive continuum approach based on individual needs:

Treatment is intended to improve functional skills for individuals with disabilities who require treatment or remediation of functional skills as a prerequisite to their involvement in meaningful leisure experiences.

Leisure education provides persons in clinical, residential, and community settings—including individuals with disabilities—opportunities to attain skills, knowledge, and attitudes of leisure involvement.

Recreation participation provides opportunities for voluntary involvement in recreation interests and activities. Specialized recreation participation programs are provided when assistance and/or adapted recreation equipment are needed or when appropriate community recreation opportunities are not available.

During a typical day, a therapeutic recreation specialist will be responsible for one or more group activities. These might include a stress management group, a high or low ropes course activity, a community outing, a family activity, an exercise group, or a leisure education group. The therapeutic recreation specialist might also meet with individual clients to conduct an assessment, develop a leisure discharge plan, or plan evening and weekend activities. Charting client progress and communicating with professionals in other disciplines and clients' family members are also part of a typical day.

A therapeutic recreation specialist working in a community recreation agency also conducts assessments to determine client needs and interests and is responsible for adapting activities as needed and for providing adaptive equipment to enable individuals with disabilities or limitations to participate. In addition, the therapeutic recreation specialist provides in-service training for recreation staff who have individuals with disabilities in their programs to orient them to the needs of these individuals and to promote general sensitivity. The therapeutic recreation specialist will generally seek to include clients in existing recreation programs, activities, and classes when possible.

An important responsibility for a therapeutic recreation specialist in both community and clinical settings is to serve as an advocate on behalf of individuals with disabilities. This includes addressing such issues as limited transportation resources, inaccessible facilities, and legislation that affects people with disabilities or limitations. A therapeutic recreation specialist frequently serves on advisory committees and consults with outside agencies to ensure that resources and services are provided for people with disabilities.

One of the most attractive qualities of the therapeutic recreation profession is the opportunity for variety and diversity. The many changes in the health care delivery system have provided—and will continue to offer—an array of challenges and opportunities for continued growth in therapeutic recreation. In addition, the opportunity to positively affect the quality of life of an individual with a disability or limitation is extremely rewarding.

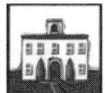

Employment Characteristics

In clinical settings, such as hospitals and rehabilitation centers, therapeutic recreation specialists treat and rehabilitate individuals with specific medical problems, usually in cooperation with physicians, nurses, psychologists, social workers, and physical and occupational therapists. In long-term care facilities, residential facilities, and community recreation departments, they use leisure activities, individual as well as group-oriented, to improve general health and well-being, but also may treat medical problems. A bachelor's degree in therapeutic recreation (or in recreation with an option in therapeutic recreation) is the usual requirement for an entry-level position in a hospital and in other clinical positions.

Therapeutic recreation specialists assess patients, based on information from medical records, medical staff, family, and patients themselves. They then develop and implement therapeutic recreation programs consistent with patients' needs and interests. For instance, a patient having trouble socializing may be helped to play games with others, or a client with right-side paralysis may be helped to use the left arm to throw a ball or swing a racket.

Therapeutic recreation specialists observe and document patients' participation, reactions, and progress. These records are used by the interdisciplinary team and others to monitor progress, to justify changes or end therapeutic recreation services, and for billing, if applicable.

Community-based therapeutic recreation specialists work in park and recreation departments, special education programs, or programs for older adults or people with disabilities. In these programs, therapeutic recreation specialists help clients become involved in leisure activities and provide them with opportunities for exercise, mental stimulation, creativity, and fun.

Therapeutic recreation specialists often lift and carry equipment as well as implement activities. They generally work a 40-hour week, which may include some evenings, weekends, and holidays.

Therapeutic recreation specialists should be comfortable working with people with disabilities and be patient, tactful, and persuasive. Ingenuity and imagination are helpful in adapting activities to individual needs.

Therapeutic recreation specialists held about 39,000 jobs in 1998. About 38% were in hospitals and 26% were in nursing and personal care facilities. Others were in community mental health centers, adult day care programs, correctional facilities, residential facilities, community programs for people with disabilities, and substance abuse centers. About one out of three therapeutic recreation specialists was self-employed, generally contracting with long-term care facilities or community agencies to develop and oversee programs.

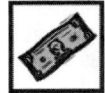

Salary

As of 2004, salary for therapeutic recreation specialists with the CTRS credential averaged $30,000 (starting), $39,000 (overall average), and $60,000 to $70,000 (upper ranges).

Refer to Section IV, Table 5 of this *Directory* for more information, or see www.ama-assn.org/go/hpsalary.

Employment Outlook

Employment of therapeutic recreation specialists is expected to grow as fast as the average for all occupations through the year 2008, because of anticipated expansion in long-term care, physical and psychiatric rehabilitation, and services for people with disabilities. The US Bureau of Labor Statistics projects that there are approximately 39,000 positions in therapeutic recreation. Nonetheless, the total number of job openings will be relatively low because the occupation is small.

Health care facilities will provide a growing number of jobs in hospital-based adult day care and outpatient programs and units offering short-term mental health and alcohol or drug abuse services; rehabilitation, home health care, transitional programs, and psychiatric facilities will provide additional jobs.

The rapidly growing number of older people is expected to spur job growth for therapeutic recreation specialists and paraprofessionals in long-term care facilities, retirement communities, assisted living facilities, adult day care programs, and social service agencies. Continued growth is also expected in community residential facilities, as well as adult day care programs for people with disabilities.

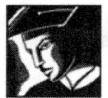

Educational Programs

Length. A major in therapeutic recreation or recreation with an option in therapeutic recreation entails completion of a bachelor's degree, including a minimum of 18 semester or 24 quarter units in therapeutic recreation and general recreation content coursework; completion of supportive courses to include a minimum of 18 semester units or 27

quarter units; and completion of a minimum 480-hour, 12-consecutive-week internship/field placement experience in a clinical, residential, or community-based therapeutic recreation program.

Curriculum. In addition to therapeutic recreation courses in clinical practice, program design, management, and professional issues, students study human anatomy, physiology, abnormal psychology, medical and psychiatric terminology, human development, characteristics of illness and disabilities, and the concepts of inclusion and normalization. Additional courses cover professional ethics, assessment and referral procedures, and the use of adaptive and medical equipment. In addition, 360 hours of internship under the supervision of a certified therapeutic recreation specialist are required.

Licensure, Certification, and Registration

A few states regulate the therapeutic recreation profession through licensure, certification, or registration of titles. Applicants for licensure must pass a state examination. Licensure is required in Utah. For more information, contact

Division of Occupational and Professional Licensure
160 East 300 South
Salt Lake City, UT 84145-0801
801 530-6628

National certification is available through the National Council for Therapeutic Recreation Certification (NCTRC), which awards the title of Certified Therapeutic Recreation Specialist (CTRS).

Through registration, qualified individuals are listed on an official roster maintained by a governmental or nongovernmental agency. Information regarding registration requirements may be obtained from state recreation and park associations.

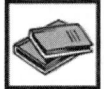

Career Planning Publications

The *2002 SPRE Curriculum Catalog* (published by the Society for Park and Recreation Educators) provides valuable information on curricula and faculty in the parks, recreation, and leisure studies profession. Degree levels offered and accreditation status are indicated for each program. Each listing includes the location and mailing address for the program, enrollment data, a description of the character of the campus and community, and a detailed listing of the faculty and specialties.

The NRPA Career Center can be accessed at www.nrpa.org.

Preparing for a Career in Therapeutic Recreation describes the continuum of services within therapeutic recreation and includes a listing of colleges and universities that offer therapeutic recreation programs, including those accredited by the NRPA Council on Accreditation.

Inquiries

Careers
National Therapeutic Recreation Society
22377 Belmont Ridge Road
Ashburn, VA 20148-4501
703 858-2151
800 626-NRPA—membership information and other services
703 858-0794 Fax
E-mail: ntrs@nrpa.org

American Therapeutic Recreation Association
1414 Prince Street, Suite 204
Alexandria, VA 22314
703 683-9420
703 683-9431 Fax

Certification
National Council for Therapeutic Recreation Certification
7 Elmwood Drive
New City, NY 10956
845 639-1439
845 639-1471 Fax
E-mail: nctrc@nctrc.org
www.nctrc.org

Program Accreditation
National Recreation and Park Association
Council on Accreditation
22377 Belmont Ridge Road
Ashburn, VA 20148-4501
703 858-2150
703 858-0794 Fax
E-Mail: coa@nrpa.org
www.nrpa.org

Therapeutic Recreation Specialist

California

California State University - Chico
Therapeutic Recreation Specialist Prgm
Dept of Recreation and Parks Mgmt
YOLO, Rm 173
Chico, CA 95929-0560
Prgm Dir: James Fletcher, PhD
Tel: 530 898-4635 *Fax:* 530 898-6557
E-mail: jfletcher@csuchico.edu

California State University - Long Beach
Therapeutic Recreation Specialist Prgm
Dept of Recreation and Leisure Studies
1250 Bellflower Blvd
Long Beach, CA 90840-4903
Prgm Dir: Maridith Janssen, EdD RTC/CTRS
Tel: 562 985-4071, Ext 4079 *Fax:* 562 985-8154
E-mail: mjanssen@csulb.edu

District of Columbia

Gallaudet University
Therapeutic Recreation Specialist Prgm
Dept of Physical Educ and Recreation
800 Florida Ave NE
Washington, DC 20002
Prgm Dir: Edward Ronald Dreher, PhD
Tel: 202 651-5591 *Fax:* 202 651-5861
E-mail: edward.dreher@gallaudet.edu

Florida

University of Florida
Therapeutic Recreation Specialist Prgm
Dept of Recreation, Parks and Tourism
Rm 300 Florida Gym, PO Box 118208
Gainesville, FL 32611-8208
Prgm Dir: Stephen Holland
Tel: 352 392-4042 *Fax:* 352 392-7588
E-mail: sholland@hhp.ufl.edu
Notes: Currently inactive

Georgia

Georgia Southern University
Therapeutic Recreation Specialist Prgm
Dept of Hospitality, Tourism and Family & Consumer
　　Sciences
PO Box 8034
Statesboro, GA 30460-8077
Prgm Dir: Henry Eisenhart, PhD
Tel: 912 681-5345 *Fax:* 912 681-0276
E-mail: henry_e@georgiasouthern.edu

Illinois

Southern Illinois University Carbondale
Therapeutic Recreation Specialist Prgm
Dept of Health Educ and Recreation
Pulliam Hall 307/Postal Code 4632
Carbondale, IL 62901
www.siu.edu
Prgm Dir: David Birch, PhD
Tel: 618 453-4331 *Fax:* 618 453-1829
E-mail: dabirch@siu.edu

Eastern Illinois University
Therapeutic Recreation Specialist Prgm
Recreation Administration
600 Lincoln Ave
Charleston, IL 61920
Prgm Dir: William Higelmire, EdD CTRS
Tel: 217 581-6344 *Fax:* 217 581-7804
E-mail: cfwfh@eiu.edu

Western Illinois University
Therapeutic Recreation Specialist Prgm
Recreation, Park and Tourism Admin
400 Currens Hall
Macomb, IL 61455
Prgm Dir: Dale Adkins, PhD
Tel: 309 298-1967 *Fax:* 309 298-2967
E-mail: KD-Adkins1@wiu.edu

Illinois State University
Therapeutic Recreation Specialist Prgm
Recreation and Park Admin Prgm
McCormick Hall Rm 101, CB 5121
Normal, IL 61790-5121
Prgm Dir: Barbara E Schlatter, PhD
Tel: 309 438-5608 *Fax:* 309 438-5561
E-mail: beschla@ilstu.edu

Indiana

Indiana University - Bloomington
Therapeutic Recreation Specialist Prgm
Department of Recreation, Park, and Tourism Studies
HPER Building 133
Bloomington, IN 47405
Prgm Dir: Lynn Jamieson, ReD
Tel: 812 855-4711 *Fax:* 812 855-3998
E-mail: lyjamies@indiana.edu

Iowa

University of Northern Iowa
Therapeutic Recreation Specialist Prgm
Leisure, Youth and Human Services Div
School of HPELS/217 WRC
Cedar Falls, IA 50614-0161
Prgm Dir: Joe Wilson, EdD
Tel: 319 273-2313 *Fax:* 319 273-5958
E-mail: Joe.Wilson@uni.edu

University of Iowa
Therapeutic Recreation Specialist Prgm
Leisure Studies Program
LSP 408 Jefferson Bldg
Iowa City, IA 52242-1111
www.uiowa.edu/~interdi/leisure/
Prgm Dir: Kenneth Mobily, PhD
Tel: 319 335-0172 *Fax:* 319 335-3884
E-mail: ken-mobily@uiowa.edu

Kansas

Pittsburg State University
Therapeutic Recreation Specialist Prgm
1701 S Broadway
Pittsburg, KS 66762-7557
Prgm Dir: Charles Killingsworth, EdD
Tel: 620 235-4665 *Fax:* 620 235-4520
E-mail: ckilling@pittstate.edu

Kentucky

Eastern Kentucky University
Therapeutic Recreation Specialist Prgm
Department of Recreation and Park Administration
Begley 405
Richmond, KY 40475
www.recreation.eku.edu
Prgm Dir: Charlie Everett, EdD
Tel: 859 622-1833 *Fax:* 859 622-2971
E-mail: charlie.everett@eku.edu

PROGRAMS

Louisiana

Grambling State University
Therapeutic Recreation Specialist Prgm
Leisure Studies/Recreation Career Prgm
GSU Box 4244
Grambling, LA 71245
www.gram.edu
Prgm Dir: Willie F Daniel
Tel: 318 274-2294 *Fax:* 318 274-6053
E-mail: danielw@gram.edu

Massachusetts

Springfield College
Therapeutic Recreation Specialist Prgm
Dept of Recreation and Leisure Services
263 Alden St, Locklin Hall
Springfield, MA 01109-3797
Prgm Dir: Matthew J Pantera, EdD
Tel: 413 748-3749 *Fax:* 413 748-3685
E-mail: mpantera@spfldcol.edu

Michigan

Central Michigan University
Therapeutic Recreation Specialist Prgm
Dept of Recreation and Park Admin
Mount Pleasant, MI 48859
Prgm Dir: Roger Coles, EdD CPRP
Tel: 517 774-3858 *Fax:* 517 774-2161
E-mail: roger.l.coles@cmich.edu

Minnesota

University of Minnesota - Minneapolis
Therapeutic Recreation Specialist Prgm
Division of Recreation, Park and Leisure Studies
100 Cooke Hall, 1900 University Ave SE
Minneapolis, MN 55455
Prgm Dir: Keith Russell, PhD
Tel: 612 626-4280 *Fax:* 612 626-7700
E-mail: krussell@umn.edu

Mississippi

University of Southern Mississippi
Therapeutic Recreation Specialist Prgm
School of Human Performance and Recreation
Box 5142
Hattiesburg, MS 39406-5142
Prgm Dir: Rick Green, PhD
Tel: 601 266-5576 *Fax:* 601 266-4445
E-mail: rick.green@usm.edu

Missouri

University of Missouri - Columbia
Therapeutic Recreation Specialist Prgm
Dept of Parks, Recreation and Tourism
105k Anheuser Busch Nat Res Bldg
Columbia, MO 65211-7230
Prgm Dir: C Randal Vessell, PhD
Tel: 573 882-9515 *Fax:* 573 882-9526
E-mail: VessellC@missouri.edu

New Hampshire

University of New Hampshire
Therapeutic Recreation Specialist Prgm
Dept of Recreation Management and Policy
108 Hewitt Hall
Durham, NH 03824
Prgm Dir: Janet Sable, PhD CTRS
Tel: 603 862-3401 *Fax:* 603 862-2722
E-mail: Jrsable@cisunix.unh.edu

New York

SUNY College at Cortland
Therapeutic Recreation Specialist Prgm
Recreation and Leisure Studies Dept
PO Box 2000
Cortland, NY 13045
www.cortland.edu/rec
Prgm Dir: Lynn S Anderson, CTRS
Tel: 607 753-4941 *Fax:* 607 753-5982
E-mail: rls@cortland.edu

Ithaca College
Therapeutic Recreation Specialist Prgm
Dept of Therapeutic Recreation and Leisure
36 Hill Center
Ithaca, NY 14850
Prgm Dir: Linda Heyne, PhD
Tel: 607 274-3050 *Fax:* 607 274-1943
E-mail: lheyne@ithaca.edu

North Carolina

University of North Carolina - Greensboro
Therapeutic Recreation Specialist Prgm
Dept of Recreation, Tourism, and Hospitality
   Management
420 HHP Building
Greensboro, NC 27402-6170
www.uncg.edu/rth/
Prgm Dir: Stuart J Schleien, PhD CTRS CPRP
Tel: 336 334-5327 *Fax:* 336 334-3238
E-mail: sjs@uncg.edu

University of North Carolina - Wilmington
Therapeutic Recreation Specialist Prgm
Parks and Recreation Mgmt Curriculum
601 S College Rd
Wilmington, NC 28403-3297
Prgm Dir: Terry Kinney, PhD
Tel: 910 962-7570 *Fax:* 910 962-7073
E-mail: kinneyt@uncw.edu

Winston-Salem State University
Therapeutic Recreation Specialist Prgm
Dept of Human Performance and Sport Science
Old Nursing Building
Winston-Salem, NC 27110
http://wssu.edu
Prgm Dir: Cynthia Stanley, PhD LRT CTRS
Tel: 336 750-2588 *Fax:* 336 750-2591
E-mail: stanleyc@wssu.edu

Ohio

University of Toledo
Therapeutic Recreation Specialist Prgm
Dept of Pub Hlth and Rehab Serv, Hlth Ed Ctr
2801 W Bancroft St, 252 Health Ed Ctr
Toledo, OH 43606
Prgm Dir: Bruce Groves, PhD
Tel: 419 530-4353 *Fax:* 419 530-4759
E-mail: bruce.groves2@utoledo.edu

Oklahoma

Oklahoma State University
Therapeutic Recreation Specialist Prgm
Dept of Leisure Studies
103 Colvin Center
Stillwater, OK 74078
Prgm Dir: Jerry Jordan, CTRS
Tel: 405 744-9424 *Fax:* 405 744-6507
E-mail: jerry.jordan@okstate.edu

Pennsylvania

Temple University
Therapeutic Recreation Specialist Prgm
Sport and Recreation Management
412-C Vivacqua Hall
Philadelphia, PA 19122
Prgm Dir: Ira Shapiro
Tel: 215 204-6295 *Fax:* 215 204-8705
E-mail: ira.shapiro@temple.edu

Slippery Rock University of Pennsylvania
Therapeutic Recreation Specialist Prgm
Dept of Parks and Recreation/Environmental Education
101 Eisenberg
Slippery Rock, PA 16057
Prgm Dir: Bruce G Boliver
Tel: 724 738-2068 *Fax:* 724 738-2938
E-mail: bruce.boliver@sru.edu

South Carolina

Clemson University
Therapeutic Recreation Specialist Prgm
Parks, Recreation and Tourism Mgmt
276 Lehotsky Hall
Clemson, SC 29634-0735
Prgm Dir: Brett A Wright, PhD
Tel: 864 656-3036 *Fax:* 864 656-2226
E-mail: wright@clemson.edu

Tennessee

University of Tennessee - Knoxville
Therapeutic Recreation Specialist Prgm
1914 Andy Holt Ave
Knoxville, TN 37996-2710
Prgm Dir: Gene Hayes, PhD
Tel: 865 974-1288 *Fax:* 865 974-8981
E-mail: ghayes1@utk.edu

Texas

Texas State University - San Marcos
Therapeutic Recreation Specialist Prgm
601 University Dr
Jowers Center
San Marcos, TX 78666
Prgm Dir: Tom Gustafson, PhD
Tel: 512 245-2972 *Fax:* 512 245-8678
E-mail: tg08@txstate.edu

Utah

Brigham Young University
Therapeutic Recreation Specialist Prgm
Recreation Mgmt and Youth Leadership
273 Richards Bldg
Provo, UT 84602
Prgm Dir: Patti Freeman, PhD
Tel: 801 422-1286 *Fax:* 801 378-7461
E-mail: patti_freeman@byu.edu

University of Utah
Therapeutic Recreation Specialist Prgm
Dept of Parks, Recreation, and Tourism
250 S 1850 E, HPER N-226
Salt Lake City, UT 84112-0920
Prgm Dir: Gary D Ellis, PhD
Tel: 801 581-4511 *Fax:* 801 581-4930
E-mail: gary.ellis@health.utah.edu

Virginia

Longwood University
Therapeutic Recreation Specialist Prgm
Dept of Health, Recreation and Kinesiology
201 High St
Farmville, VA 23909-1899
Prgm Dir: Glenda Taylor, PhD
Tel: 434 395-2545   *Fax:* 434 395-2380
E-mail: taylorgp@longwood.edu

**George Mason University School of
Recreation, Health, and Tourism**
Therapeutic Recreation Specialist Prgm
Parks, Recreation and Leisure Studies Program
10900 University Blvd, MS 4E5
Manassas, VA 20110
Prgm Dir: Brenda Wiggins, PhD
Tel: 703 993-2068   *Fax:* 703 993-2025
E-mail: bwiggins@gmu.edu

Radford University
Therapeutic Recreation Specialist Prgm
Dept of Recreation Parks and Tourism
Box 6963
Radford, VA 24142
Prgm Dir: Ed Udd, PhD
Tel: 540 831-7720   *Fax:* 540 831-6487
E-mail: eudd@radford.edu

Washington

Eastern Washington University
Therapeutic Recreation Specialist Prgm
Recreation and Leisure Studies
Dept of PEHR
Cheney, WA 99004
Prgm Dir: Susan Beam
Tel: 509 359-2341   *Fax:* 509 359-4833
E-mail: Susan.Beam@mail.ewu.edu

Wisconsin

University of Wisconsin - La Crosse
Therapeutic Recreation Specialist Prgm
Recreation Mgmt and Therapeutic Recreation
128 Wittich Hall
La Crosse, WI 54601
Prgm Dir: George Arimond, PhD
Tel: 608 785-8155   *Fax:* 608 785-8206
E-mail: arimond.geor@uwlax.edu

Therapeutic Recreation Specialist

Programs*	Class Capacity	Begins	Length (months)	Award	Res. Tuition	Non-res. Tuition	Stipend	Offers:‡ 1	2	3	4
California											
California State University - Long Beach	142	Sep Jan	30	Cert, BA, MA	$3,200	$7,200		•		•	
Florida											
University of Florida (Gainesville)	50	Aug Jan May	48	BS	$1,926	$7,842					
Georgia											
Georgia Southern University (Statesboro)	30	Aug Jan May	48	BS	$2,350	$9,290				•	
Illinois											
Southern Illinois University Carbondale	60	Aug	30, 24	BS, MS	$4,000	$6,400	$9,990	•		•	
Iowa											
University of Iowa (Iowa City)	60	Aug	24	BS, MA	$6,294	$19,466		•			•
University of Northern Iowa (Cedar Falls)	25	Aug Jan	12, 24	Cert, BA	$5,387	$12,705				•	
Kentucky											
Eastern Kentucky University (Richmond)			48	BS	$1,896	$5,232					•
Louisiana											
Grambling State University	300	Aug Jan	40	BS	$3,622	$8,972		•		•	
Michigan											
Central Michigan University (Mount Pleasant)	25	Aug Jan	12, 30	BS, MA	$6,390	$14,850				•	
New York											
SUNY College at Cortland	40	Aug Jan	48, 18	BS, MS/MSE	$5,300	$11,200		•		•	•
North Carolina											
University of North Carolina - Greensboro	60	Aug Jan	48	BS, MS	$2,028	$13,296		•		•	
Winston-Salem State University	100	Aug Jan	36	BS	$2,805	$11,444		•		•	
Oklahoma											
Oklahoma State University (Stillwater)	40	Aug	48	BS, MS	$1,716	$3,811		•			
Virginia											
Longwood University (Farmville)	40	Aug	48	BS	$6,233	$9,600		•		•	

*Data are shown only for programs that completed the 2007 AMA Survey of Health Professions Education Programs.
‡Key to Offers: 1: Evening or weekend classes; 2: Non-English instruction; 3: Cultural competence instruction; 4: Distance education component.

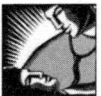

Career Description

Veterinarians play a major role in the health care of pets, livestock, and zoo, sporting, and laboratory animals. Some veterinarians use their skills to protect humans against diseases carried by animals and conduct clinical research on human and animal health problems. Others work in basic research, broadening the scope of fundamental theoretical knowledge, and in applied research, developing new ways to use knowledge.

Veterinarians diagnose animal health problems; vaccinate against diseases, such as distemper and rabies; medicate animals suffering from infections or illnesses; treat and dress wounds; set fractures; perform surgery; and advise owners about animal feeding, behavior, and breeding.

Veterinarians who treat animals use medical equipment such as stethoscopes, surgical instruments, and diagnostic equipment, including radiographic and ultrasound equipment. Veterinarians working in research use a full range of sophisticated laboratory equipment.

Most veterinarians perform clinical work in private practices. More than 50 percent of these veterinarians predominately or exclusively treat small animals. Small-animal practitioners usually care for companion animals, such as dogs and cats, but also treat birds, reptiles, rabbits, and other animals that can be kept as pets. About one fourth of all veterinarians work in mixed animal practices, where they see pigs, goats, sheep, and some nondomestic animals in addition to companion animals.

A small number of private-practice veterinarians work exclusively with large animals, mostly horses or cows; some also care for various kinds of food animals. These veterinarians usually drive to farms or ranches to provide veterinary services for herds or individual animals. Much of this work involves preventive care to maintain the health of the animals. These veterinarians test for and vaccinate against diseases and consult with farm or ranch owners and managers regarding animal production, feeding, and housing issues. They also treat and dress wounds, set fractures, and perform surgery, including cesarean sections on birthing animals. Veterinarians euthanize animals when necessary. Other veterinarians care for zoo, aquarium, or laboratory animals.

In addition to self-employment in a solo or group practice and working as salaried employees of another practice, veterinarians are employed by the federal government, state and local governments, colleges of veterinary medicine, medical schools, research laboratories, animal food companies, and pharmaceutical companies. A few veterinarians work for zoos, but most veterinarians caring for zoo animals are private practitioners who contract with the zoos to provide services, usually on a part-time basis. In addition, many veterinarians hold faculty positions in colleges and universities.

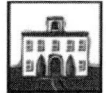

Employment Characteristics

Veterinarians often work long hours. Those in group practices may take turns being on call for evening, night, or weekend work; solo practitioners may work extended and weekend hours, responding to emergencies or squeezing in unexpected appointments. The work setting often can be noisy.

Veterinarians in large-animal practice spend time driving between their office and farms or ranches. They work outdoors in all kinds of weather and may have to treat animals or perform surgery under unsanitary conditions. When working with animals that are frightened or in pain, veterinarians risk being bitten, kicked, or scratched.

Veterinarians working in nonclinical areas, such as public health and research, have working conditions similar to those of other professionals in those lines of work. In these cases, veterinarians enjoy clean, well-lit offices or laboratories and spend much of their time dealing with people rather than animals.

Some veterinarians are involved in food safety. Veterinarians who are livestock inspectors check animals for transmissible diseases, advise owners on the treatment of their animals and may quarantine animals. Veterinarians who are meat, poultry, or egg product inspectors examine slaughtering and processing plants, check live animals and carcasses for disease, and enforce government regulations regarding food purity and sanitation.

Veterinarians can contribute to human as well as animal health. A number of veterinarians work with physicians and scientists as they research ways to prevent and treat various human health problems. For example, veterinarians contributed greatly in conquering malaria and yellow fever, solved the mystery of botulism, produced an anticoagulant used to treat some people with heart disease, and defined and developed surgical techniques for humans, such as hip and knee joint replacements and limb and organ transplants. Today, some determine the effects of drug therapies, antibiotics, or new surgical techniques by testing them on animals.

At its 2007 annual meeting, the American Medical Association (AMA) House of Delegates voted to adopt new policy supporting more educational and research collaborations between the medical and veterinary professions to help with assessing, treating, and preventing cross-species disease transmission. Benefits of current collaborative efforts include rabies control efforts and foodborne illness evaluations. "Many infectious diseases can infect both humans and animals," said AMA Board Member Duane M. Cady, MD. "New infections continue to emerge and with threats of cross-species disease transmission and pandemic in our global health environment, the time has come for the human and veterinary medical professions to work closer together for the greater protection of the public health in the 21st Century."

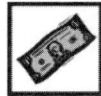

Salary

Median annual earnings of veterinarians were $66,590 in 2004. The middle 50 percent earned between $51,420 and $88,060. The lowest 10 percent earned less than $39,020, and the highest 10 percent earned more than $118,430.

According to a survey by the American Veterinary Medical Association, average starting salaries of veterinary medical college graduates in 2004 varied by type of practice as follows:

- Small animals, predominantly $50,878
- Small animals, exclusively $50,703
- Large animals, exclusively $50,403
- Private clinical practice $49,635
- Large animals, predominantly $48,529
- Mixed animals $47,704
- Equine (horses) $38,628

The average annual salary for veterinarians in the federal government in nonsupervisory, supervisory, and managerial positions was $78,769 in 2005.

Refer to Section IV, Table 5 of this *Directory* for more information, or see www.ama-assn.org/go/hpsalary.

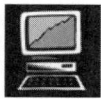

Employment Outlook

Currently more than 86,000 veterinarians actively practice in the United States. Employment of veterinarians is expected to increase as fast as average for all occupations through 2014. Despite this average growth, very good job opportunities are expected because the 28 schools of veterinary medicine, even at full capacity, produce a limited number of graduates each year. At the same time, admission to veterinary school is highly competitive.

Most veterinarians practice in animal hospitals or clinics and care primarily for companion animals. Recent trends indicate particularly strong interest in cats as pets. Faster growth of the cat population is expected to increase the demand for feline medicine and veterinary services, while demand for veterinary care for dogs should grow at a more modest pace.

As pets are increasingly viewed as a member of the family, pet owners will be more willing to spend on advanced veterinary medical care, creating further demand for veterinarians. More pet owners even purchase pet insurance, increasing the likelihood that a considerable amount of money will be spent on veterinary care for their pets. More pet owners also will take advantage of nontraditional veterinary services, such as preventive dental care.

New graduates continue to be attracted to companion-animal medicine because they prefer to deal with pets and to live and work near heavily populated areas. This situation will not necessarily limit the ability of veterinarians to find employment or to set up and maintain a practice in a particular area. Rather, beginning veterinarians may take positions requiring evening or weekend work to accommodate the extended hours of operation that many practices are offering. Some veterinarians take salaried positions in retail stores offering veterinary services. Self-employed veterinarians usually have to work intensively for several years to build a sufficient client base.

The number of jobs for large-animal veterinarians is likely to grow more slowly than that for veterinarians in private practice who care for companion animals. Nevertheless, job prospects may be better for veterinarians who specialize in farm animals than for companion-animal practitioners because of low earnings in the former specialty and because many veterinarians do not want to work in rural or isolated areas.

Continued support for public health and food safety, national disease control programs, and biomedical research on human health problems will contribute to the demand for veterinarians, although positions in these areas of interest are few in number. Homeland security also may provide opportunities for veterinarians involved in efforts to minimize animal diseases and prevent them from entering the country. Veterinarians with training in food safety, animal health and welfare, and public health and epidemiology should have the best opportunities for a career in the federal government.

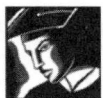

Educational Programs

Award, Length. Graduates earn a Doctor of Veterinary Medicine (DVM or VMD) degree from a 4-year program at an accredited college of veterinary medicine.

Prerequisites. Prerequisites for admission vary. For example, many colleges do not require a bachelor's degree for entrance, but all require a significant number of credit hours—ranging from 45 to 90 semester hours—at the undergraduate level. Nonetheless, most of the students admitted have completed an undergraduate program, and those without a bachelor's degree face a difficult task gaining admittance. Competition for admission to veterinary school is keen. The number of accredited veterinary colleges has remained largely the same since 1983, whereas the number of applicants has risen significantly. Only about one in three applicants was accepted in 2004; approximately 80 percent of entering students are female.

Students interested in a career in veterinary medicine should perform well in general science and biology in junior high school and pursue a strong science, mathematics, and biology program in high school. Before applying to veterinary college/school, students must successfully complete university-level preveterinary undergraduate course work. Each college or school of veterinary medicine establishes its own preveterinary requirements, but typically these include demonstrating basic language and communication skills and completion of courses in the social sciences, humanities, mathematics, biology, chemistry, and physics.

In addition to satisfying preveterinary course requirements, applicants must submit test scores from the Graduate Record Examination (GRE), the Veterinary College Admission Test (VCAT), or the Medical College Admission Test (MCAT), depending on the preference of the college to which they are applying. Currently, 22 schools require the GRE, 4 require the VCAT, and 2 accept the MCAT.

In admittance decisions, some veterinary medical colleges place heavy consideration on a candidate's veterinary and animal experience. Formal experience, such as work with veterinarians or scientists in clinics, agribusiness, research, or some area of health science, is particularly advantageous. Less formal experience, such as working with animals on a farm or ranch or at a stable or animal shelter, also is helpful. Students must demonstrate ambition and an eagerness to work with animals.

Prospective veterinarians must have good manual dexterity, as well as an inquiring mind, keen powers of observation, and aptitude and interest in the biological sciences. Veterinarians must maintain a lifelong interest in scientific learning They should have an affinity for animals and the ability to get along with their owners and express compassion. Veterinarians who intend to go into private practice should possess excellent communication, managerial, leadership, and business skills, because they will need to manage their practice and employees successfully and promote, market, and sell their services.

Curriculum. Veterinary medical colleges typically require classes in organic and inorganic chemistry, physics, biochemistry, general biology, animal biology, animal nutrition, genetics, vertebrate embryology, cellular biology, microbiology, zoology, and systemic physiology. Some programs require calculus; some require only statistics, college algebra and trigonometry, or precalculus. Most veterinary medical colleges also require core courses, including some in English or literature, the social sciences, and the humanities. Increasingly, courses in practice management and career development are becoming a standard part of the curriculum, to provide a foundation of general business knowledge for new graduates.

Advanced Training. Veterinary specialties—such as pathology, internal medicine, dentistry, nutrition, ophthalmology, surgery, radiology, preventive medicine, and laboratory animal medicine—are usually in the form of a 2-year internship. Interns receive a small salary but usually find that their internship experience leads to a higher beginning salary relative to those of other starting veterinarians. Veterinarians who seek board certification in a specialty also must complete a 3- to 4-year residency program that provides intensive training in specialties such as internal medicine, oncology, radiology, surgery, dermatology, anesthesiology, neurology, cardiology, ophthalmology, and exotic small-animal medicine.

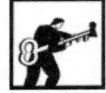

Licensure

All states and the District of Columbia require that veterinarians be licensed before they can practice. The only exemptions are for veterinarians working for some federal agencies and some state governments. Licensing is controlled by the states and is not strictly uniform, although all states require the successful completion of the DVM degree—or equivalent education—and a passing grade on a national board examination. The Educational Commission for Foreign Veterinary Graduates (ECFVG) grants certification to individuals trained outside the United States who demonstrate that they meet specified requirements for the English language and for clinical proficiency. ECFVG certification fulfills the educational requirement for licensure in all states. Applicants for licensure satisfy the examination requirement by passing the North American Veterinary Licensing Exam (NAVLE), an 8-hour computer-based examination consisting of 360 multiple-choice questions covering all aspects of veterinary medicine. Administered by the National Board of Veterinary Medical Examiners (NBVME), the NAVLE includes visual materials designed to test diagnostic skills and constituting 10 percent of the total examination.

The majority of states also require candidates to pass a state jurisprudence examination covering state laws and regulations. Some states do additional testing on clinical competency as well. There are few reciprocal agreements between states, making it difficult for a veterinarian to practice in a different state without first taking that state's examination.

Nearly all states have continuing education requirements for licensed veterinarians. Requirements differ by state and may involve attending a class or otherwise demonstrating knowledge of recent medical and veterinary advances.

Inquiries

Education, Careers, Resources
American Veterinary Medical Association
1931 North Meacham Road, Suite 100
Schaumburg, IL 60173-4360
www.avma.org

Association of American Veterinary Medical Colleges
1101 Vermont Avenue NW, Suite 710
Washington, DC 20005
www.aavmc.org

Licensure
National Board of Veterinary Medical Examiners
PO Box 1356
Bismarck, ND 58502
http://www.nbvme.org/

Program Accreditation
American Veterinary Medical Association, Council on Education
1931 North Meacham Road, Suite 100
Schaumburg, IL 60173-4360
www.avma.org/education/cvea/about_accred.asp

Note: Adapted in part from the Bureau of Labor Statistics, US Department of Labor, *Occupational Outlook Handbook*, 2006-07 Edition, Veterinarians, on the Internet at www.bls.gov/oco/ocos076.htm (visited September 06, 2007).

Veterinarian

Alabama

Auburn University
Veterinary Medicine Prgm
College of Veterinary Medicine
104 J E Greene Hall
Auburn University, AL 36849
www.vetmed.auburn.edu

Tuskegee University
Veterinary Medicine Prgm
School of Veterinary Medicine
Tuskegee, AL 36088
http://tuskegee.edu

California

University of California - Davis
Veterinary Medicine Prgm
Davis, CA 95616
www.vetmed.ucdavis.edu

Western Univ of Health Sciences
Veterinary Medicine Prgm
College of Veterinary Medicine
309 E Second St - College Plaza
Pomona, CA 91766
www.westernu.edu/cvm.html

Colorado

Colorado State University
Veterinary Medicine Prgm
College of Veterinary Medicine
Fort Collins, CO 80523
www.cvmbs.colostate.edu

Florida

University of Florida
Veterinary Medicine Prgm
College of Veterinary Medicine
PO Box 100125
Gainesville, FL 32610
www.vetmed.ufl.edu

Georgia

University of Georgia
Veterinary Medicine Prgm
College of Veterinary Medicine
Athens, GA 30602
www.vet.uga.edu

Illinois

Univ of Illinois at Urbana-Champaign
Veterinary Medicine Prgm
College of Veterinary Medicine
2001 S Lincoln Ave
Urbana, IL 61802
www.cvm.uiuc.edu

Indiana

Purdue University
Veterinary Medicine Prgm
School of Veterinary Medicine
1240 Lynn Hall
West Lafayette, IN 47907
www.vet.purdue.edu

Iowa

Iowa State University
Veterinary Medicine Prgm
College of Veterinary Medicine
Ames, IA 50011
www.vetmed.iastate.edu

Kansas

Kansas State University
Veterinary Medicine Prgm
College of Veterinary Medicine
Manhattan, KS 66506
www.vet.ksu.edu

Louisiana

Louisiana State University
Veterinary Medicine Prgm
School of Veterinary Medicine
Baton Rouge, LA 70803
www.vetmed.lsu.edu

Massachusetts

Tufts University
Veterinary Medicine Prgm
School of Veterinary Medicine
200 Westboro Rd
North Grafton, MA 01536
www.tufts.edu/vet

Michigan

Michigan State University
Veterinary Medicine Prgm
College of Veterinary Medicine
G-100 Veterinary Medical Center
East Lansing, MI 48824
http://cvm.msu.edu

Minnesota

University of Minnesota - Minneapolis
Veterinary Medicine Prgm
College of Veterinary Medicine
1365 Gortner Ave
St Paul, MN 55108
www.cvm.umn.edu

Mississippi

Mississippi State University
Veterinary Medicine Prgm
College of Veterinary Medicine
Mississippi State, MS 39762
www.cvm.msstate.edu

Missouri

University of Missouri - Columbia
Veterinary Medicine Prgm
College of Veterinary Medicine
Columbia, MO 65211
www.cvm.missouri.edu

New York

Cornell University
Veterinary Medicine Prgm
College of Veterinary Medicine
Ithaca, NY 14853
www.vet.cornell.edu

North Carolina

North Carolina State University
Veterinary Medicine Prgm
College of Veterinary Medicine
4700 Hillsborough St
Raleigh, NC 27606
www.cvm.ncsu.edu

Ohio

Ohio State University
Veterinary Medicine Prgm
College of Veterinary Medicine
1900 Coffey Rd
Columbus, OH 43210
www.vet.ohio-state.edu

Oklahoma

Oklahoma State University
Veterinary Medicine Prgm
College of Veterinary Medicine
Stillwater, OK 74078
www.cvm.okstate.edu

Ontario, Canada

University of Guelph
Veterinary Medicine Prgm
Ontario Veterinary College
Guelph, ON N1G 2W1
www.ovc.uoguelph.ca/

Oregon

Oregon State University
Veterinary Medicine Prgm
College of Veterinary Medicine
Corvallis, OR 97331
www.vet.orst.edu

Pennsylvania

University of Pennsylvania
Veterinary Medicine Prgm
School of Veterinary Medicine
3800 Spruce St
Philadelphia, PA 19104
www.vet.upenn.edu

Prince Edward Island, Canada

University of Prince Edward Island
Veterinary Medicine Prgm
Atlantic Veterinary College
550 University Ave
Charlottetown, PEI, Canada C1A 4P3
www.upei.ca/~avc

Quebec, Canada

University de Montreal
Veterinary Medicine Prgm
College of Veterinary Medicine
CP 5000
Montreal, QC H3C 3J7
www.medvet.umontreal.ca

Saskatchewan, Canada

University of Saskatchewan
Veterinary Medicine Prgm
Western College of Veterinary Medicine
52 Campus Dr
Saskatoon, SK S7N 0W3
www.usask.ca/wcvm

Tennessee

Univ of Tennessee Medical Ctr at Knoxville
Veterinary Medicine Prgm
College of Veterinary Medicine
2407 River Dr
Knoxville, TN 37996
www.vet.utk.edu

Texas

Texas A&M University
Veterinary Medicine Prgm
College of Veterinary Medicine and Biomedical Sciences
College Station, TX 77843
www.cvm.tamu.edu

Virginia

Virginia Polytechnic Inst & State Univ
Veterinary Medicine Prgm
Virginia-Maryland Regional College of Veterinary
    Medicine
Blacksburg, VA 24061
www.vetmed.vt.edu

Washington

Washington State University
Veterinary Medicine Prgm
College of Veterinary Medicine
Pullman, WA 99164
www.vetmed.wsu.edu

Wisconsin

University of Wisconsin - Madison
Veterinary Medicine Prgm
School of Veterinary Medicine
2015 Linden Dr W
Madison, WI 53706
www.vetmed.wisc.edu

Veterinary Technologist and Technician

Career Description

Owners of pets and other animals today expect state-of-the-art veterinary care. To provide this service, veterinarians use the skills of veterinary technologists and technicians, who perform many of the same duties for a veterinarian that a nurse would for a physician, including routine laboratory and clinical procedures. Although specific job duties vary by employer, there often is little difference between the tasks carried out by technicians and by technologists, despite some differences in formal education and training. As a result, most workers in this occupation are called technicians.

Veterinary technologists and technicians typically conduct clinical work in a private practice under the supervision of a veterinarian—often performing various medical tests along with treating and diagnosing medical conditions and diseases in animals. For example, they may perform laboratory tests such as urinalysis and blood counts, assist with dental prophylaxis, prepare tissue samples, take blood samples, or assist veterinarians in a variety of tests and analyses in which they often utilize various items of medical equipment, such as test tubes and diagnostic equipment. While most of these duties are performed in a laboratory setting, many are not. For example, some veterinary technicians obtain and record patients' case histories, expose and develop x rays, and provide specialized nursing care. In addition, experienced veterinary technicians may discuss a pet's condition with its owners and train new clinic personnel. Veterinary technologists and technicians assisting small-animal practitioners usually care for companion animals, such as cats and dogs, but can perform a variety of duties with mice, rats, sheep, pigs, cattle, monkeys, birds, fish, and frogs. Very few veterinary technologists work in mixed animal practices where they care for both small companion animals and larger, nondomestic animals.

Besides working in private clinics and animal hospitals, veterinary technologists and technicians may work in research facilities, where they may administer medications orally or topically, prepare samples for laboratory examinations, and record information on an animal's genealogy, diet, weight, medications, food intake, and clinical signs of pain and distress. Some may be required to sterilize laboratory and surgical equipment and provide routine postoperative care. At research facilities, veterinary technologists typically work under the guidance of veterinarians, physicians, and other laboratory technicians. Some veterinary technologists vaccinate newly admitted animals and occasionally are required to euthanize seriously ill, severely injured, or unwanted animals.

While the goal of most veterinary technologists and technicians is to promote animal health, some contribute to human health as well. Veterinary technologists occasionally assist veterinarians as they work with other scientists in medical-related fields such as gene therapy and cloning. Some find opportunities in biomedical research, wildlife medicine, the military, livestock management, or pharmaceutical sales.

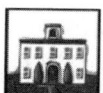

Employment Characteristics

People who love animals get satisfaction from working with and helping them. Some of the work, however, may be unpleasant, physically and emotionally demanding, and sometimes dangerous. At times, veterinary technicians must clean cages and lift, hold, or restrain animals, risking exposure to bites or scratches. These workers must take precautions when treating animals with germicides or insecticides. The work setting can be noisy.

Veterinary technologists and technicians who witness abused animals or who euthanize unwanted, aged, or hopelessly injured animals may experience emotional stress. Those working for humane societies and animal shelters often deal with the public, some of whom might react with hostility to any implication that the owners are neglecting or abusing their pets. Such workers must maintain a calm and professional demeanor while they enforce the laws regarding animal care. In some animal hospitals, research facilities, and animal shelters, a veterinary technician is on duty 24 hours a day, which means that some may work night shifts. Most full-time veterinary technologists and technicians work about 40 hours a week, although some work 50 or more hours a week.

Veterinary technologists and technicians held about 60,000 jobs in 2004. Most worked in veterinary services. The remainder worked in boarding kennels, animal shelters, stables, grooming salons, zoos, and local, state, and federal agencies.

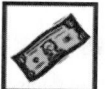

Salary

Median hourly earnings of veterinary technologists and technicians were $11.99 in May 2004. The middle 50 percent earned between $9.88 and $14.56. The bottom 10 percent earned less than $8.51, and the top 10 percent earned more than $17.12.

Refer to Section IV, Table 5 of this *Directory* for more information, or see www.ama-assn.org/go/hpsalary.

Employment Outlook

Employment of veterinary technologists and technicians is expected to grow much faster than average for all occupations through the year 2014. Job openings also will stem from the need to replace veterinary technologists and technicians who leave the occupation over the 2004-14 period. Keen competition is expected for veterinary technologist and technician jobs in zoos, due to expected slow growth in zoo capacity, low turnover among workers, the limited number of positions, and the fact that the occupation attracts many candidates.

Pet owners are becoming more affluent and more willing to pay for advanced care because many of them consider their pet to be part of the family. This growing affluence and view of pets will spur employment growth for veterinary technologists and technicians. The number of dogs used as companion pets, which also drives employment growth, is expected to increase more slowly during the projection period than in the previous decade. However, the rapidly growing number of cats as companion pets is expected to boost the demand for feline medicine and services, offsetting any reduced demand for veterinary care for dogs. The availability of advanced veterinary services, such as preventive dental care and surgical procedures, may provide opportunities for workers specializing in those areas. Additional jobs for veterinary technologists and technicians will be available in:

- Biomedical facilities
- Diagnostic laboratories

- Wildlife facilities
- Humane societies
- Animal control facilities
- Drug or food manufacturing companies
- Food safety inspection facilities

Furthermore, demand for these workers will stem from the desire to replace veterinary assistants with more highly skilled technicians and technologists in animal clinics and hospitals, shelters, kennels, and humane societies.

Employment of veterinary technicians and technologists is relatively stable during periods of economic recession. Layoffs are less likely to occur among veterinary technologists and technicians than in some other occupations because animals will continue to require medical care.

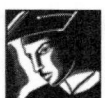

Educational Programs

Award, Length. Most entry-level veterinary technicians have a 2-year degree, usually an associate's degree, from an accredited community college program in veterinary technology. Veterinary technology programs, in contrast, culminate in a 4-year bachelor's degree.

Prerequisites. Persons interested in careers as veterinary technologists and technicians should take as many high school science, biology, and math courses as possible. Science courses taken beyond high school, in an associate's or bachelor's degree program, should emphasize practical skills in a clinical or laboratory setting. Because veterinary technologists and technicians often deal with pet owners, communication skills are very important. In addition, technologists and technicians should be able to work well with others, because teamwork with veterinarians is common. Organizational ability and attention to detail also are important.

On-the-job Training. Technologists and technicians usually begin work as trainees in routine positions under a veterinarian's direct supervision. Entry-level workers whose training or educational background encompasses extensive hands-on experience with a variety of laboratory equipment, including diagnostic and medical equipment, usually require a shorter period of on-the-job training. As they gain experience, technologists and technicians take on more responsibility and carry out more assignments under only general veterinary supervision. Some eventually may become supervisors.

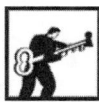

Licensure, Certification, Registration

Graduation from a veterinary technology program accredited by the American Veterinary Medical Association (AVMA) allows students to take the credentialing exam in any state in the country. Each state regulates veterinary technicians and technologists differently; however, all states require them to pass a credentialing exam following coursework. Passing the state exam assures the public that the technician or technologist has sufficient knowledge to work in a veterinary clinic or hospital. Candidates are tested for competency through an examination that includes oral, written, and practical portions and that is regulated by the state Board of Veterinary Examiners or the appropriate state agency. Depending on the state, candidates may become registered, licensed, or certified. Most states, however, use the National Veterinary Technician (NVT) exam. Prospects usually can have their passing scores transferred from one state to another, so long as both states utilize the same exam.

Employers recommend American Association for Laboratory Animal Science (AALAS) certification for those seeking employment in a research facility. AALAS offers certification for three levels of technician competence, with a focus on three principal areas—animal husbandry, facility management, and animal health and welfare. Those seeking certification must satisfy a combination of education and experience requirements prior to taking an exam. Work experience must be directly related to the maintenance, health, and well-being of laboratory animals and must be gained in a laboratory animal facility as defined by AALAS. The levels of certification, from lowest to highest, are Assistant Laboratory Animal Technician (ALAT), Laboratory Animal Technician (LAT), and Laboratory Animal Technologist (LATG).

Inquiries

Education, Careers, Resources
American Veterinary Medical Association
1931 North Meacham Road, Suite 100
Schaumburg, IL 60173-4360
www.avma.org

Certification
American Association for Laboratory Animal Science
9190 Crestwyn Hills Drive
Memphis, TN 38125
www.aalas.org

Program Accreditation
American Veterinary Medical Association
Committee on Veterinary Technician Education and Activities
1931 North Meacham Road, Suite 100
Schaumburg, IL 60173-4360
www.avma.org/education/cvea/about_accred.asp
www.avma.org/education/cvea/cvtea_process.asp#

Note: Adapted in part from the Bureau of Labor Statistics, US Department of Labor, *Occupational Outlook Handbook*, 2006-07 Edition, Veterinary Technologists and Technicians, on the Internet at www.bls.gov/oco/ocos183.htm (visited October 23, 2007).

Veterinary Technologist and Technician

Alabama

Jefferson State Community College
Veterinary Technology Distance Learning Program
2601 Carson Rd
Birmingham, AL 35215
www.jeffstateonline.com/vet_tech/

Arizona

Mesa Community College
Veterinary Technology/Animal Health Program
1833 W Southern Ave
Mesa, AZ 85202
www.mc.maricopa.edu

Kaplan College
Veterinary Technology Prgm
13610 N Black Canyon Hwy
Phoenix, AZ 85029
www.longtechnicalcollege.com

Penn Foster College
Veterinary Tech Distance Education Program
14624 N Scottsdale Rd, Ste 310
Scottsdale, AZ 85254
www.pennfostercollege.edu

Pima Community College
Veterinary Technology Prgm
8181 E Irvington Rd
Tucson, AZ 85709
www.pima.edu

California

Western Career College - Citrus
Veterinary Technology Prgm
7301 Greenback Ln, Ste A
Citrus Heights, CA 95621
www.westerncollege.edu

Foothill Community College
Veterinary Technology Prgm
12345 El Monte Rd
Los Altos Hills, CA 94022
www.foothill.fhda.edu

Yuba Community College
Veterinary Technology Prgm
2088 N Beale Rd
Marysville, CA 95901
www.yccd.edu/yuba/vettech/

Western Career College - Pleasant Hill
Veterinary Technology Prgm
380 Civic Dr, Ste 300
Pleasant Hill, CA 94523
www.westerncollege.com/ph_campus.asp

California State Polytechnic University
Veterinary Technology Prgm
College of Agriculture
Animal Health Technology Program
Pomona, CA 91768
www.csupomona.edu

Cosumnes River Community College
Veterinary Technology Prgm
8401 Center Pkwy
Sacramento, CA 95823

Western Career College - Sacramento
Veterinary Technology Prgm
8909 Folsom Blvd
Sacramento, CA 95826
www.westerncollege.com/ph_campus.asp

Hartnell College
Veterinary Technology Prgm
Animal Health Technology Program
156 Homestead Ave
Salinas, CA 93901
www.hartnell.cc.ca.us

Western Career College - San Jose
Veterinary Technician Education Program
6201 San Ignacio Ave
San Jose, CA 95119
www.westerncollege.edu

Western Career College - San Leandro
Veterinary Technology Prgm
Veterinary Technology Program
170 Bayfair Mall
San Leandro, CA 94578
www.westerncollege.com/ph_campus.asp

Western Career College
Veterinary Technician Education Program
1313 W Robinhood Dr
Stockton, CA 95207
www.westerncollege.com

Mt San Antonio College
Animal Health Technology Program
1100 N Grand Ave
Walnut, CA 91789
www.mtsac.edu

Los Angeles Pierce College
Veterinary Technology Prgm
6201 Winnetka Ave
Woodland Hills, CA 91371
www.macrohead.com/rvt

Colorado

Bel-Rea Institute of Animal Technology
Veterinary Technology Prgm
1681 S Dayton St
Denver, CO 80231
www.bel-rea.com

Community College of Denver
Veterinary Technology Prgm
1070 Alton Way
Denver, CO 80230
www.ccd.rightchoice.org

Front Range Comm College
Veterinary Research Technology Program
4616 S Shields
Fort Collins, CO 80526
www.frcc.cc.co.us

Colorado Mountain College
Veterinary Technology Prgm
Spring Valley Campus
Glenwood Springs, CO 81601
www.coloradomtn.edu

Connecticut

Quinnipiac University
Veterinary Technology Prgm
Mt Carmel Ave
Hamden, CT 06518
www.quinnipiac.edu

Northwestern Connecticut Comm College
Veterinary Technology Prgm
Park Place E
Winsted, CT 06098
www.nwctc.commnet.edu/vettech/

Delaware

Delaware Technical & Community College - Owens Campus
Veterinary Technology Prgm
PO Box 610 Route 18
Georgetown, DE 19947
www.dtcc.edu

Florida

Brevard Community College
Veterinary Technology Prgm
1519 Clearlake Rd
Cocoa, FL 32922
www.brevard.cc.fl.us

Miami Dade College
Veterinary Technology Prgm
Medical Center Campus
Miami, FL 33127
www.mdcc.edu/medical/aht/vettech

St Petersburg College
Veterinary Technology Prgm
Box 13489
St Petersburg, FL 33733
www.spcollege.edu/hec/vt

Georgia

Athens Technical College
Veterinary Technology Prgm
800 US Hwy 29 N
Athens, GA 30601
www.athenstech.edu

Fort Valley State University
Veterinary Technology Prgm
1005 State University Dr
Fort Valley, GA 31030
www.fvsu.edu

Gwinnett Technical College
Veterinary Technology Prgm
5150 Sugarloaf Prkwy
Lawrenceville, GA 30043
www.gwinnetttechnicalcollege.com

Ogeechee Technical College
Veterinary Technology Prgm
1 Joe Kennedy Blvd
Statesboro, GA 30458

Idaho

College of Southern Idaho
Veterinary Technology Prgm
315 Falls Ave
Twin Falls, ID 83303
www.csi.id.us

Illinois

Parkland College
Veterinary Technology Prgm
2400 W Bradley Ave
Champaign, IL 61821
www.parkland.edu

Joliet Junior College
Veterinary Technology Prgm
Agriculture Sciences Dept
1215 Houbolt Rd
Joliet, IL 60431
www.jjc.cc.il.us

Indiana

International Business Coll - Ft Wayne
Veterinary Technology Prgm
The Vet Tech Instutite
5699 Coventry Lane
Fort Wayne, IN 46804
www.vettechinstitute.edu/camp_wayne.php

Purdue University
Veterinary Technology Prgm
School of Veterinary Medicine
West Lafayette, IN 47907
www.vet.purdue.edu/vettech/

Iowa

Des Moines Area Community College
Veterinary Technology Prgm
2805 SW Snyder Dr, Ste 505
Ankeny, IA 50023
www.dmacc.edu

Kirkwood Community College
Veterinary Technology Prgm
Animal Health
6301 Kirkwood Blvd SW
Cedar Rapids, IA 52406
www.kirkwood.edu

Iowa Western Community College
Veterinary Technology Prgm
2700 College Rd
Council Bluffs, IA 51502
http://iwcc.cc.ia.us/programs/departments/
veterinary-tech.asp

Kansas

Colby Community College
Veterinary Technology Prgm
1255 S Range
Colby, KS 67701
www.colbycc.edu

Kentucky

Morehead State University
Veterinary Technology Prgm
25 MSU Farm Dr
Morehead, KY 40351
www.morehead-st.edu

Murray State University
Veterinary Technology Prgm
Animal Health
Dept of Agriculture
Murray, KY 42071
www.mursuky.edu

Louisiana

Delgado Community College
Veterinary Technology Prgm
615 City Park Ave
Bldg 4, Rm 301
New Orleans, LA 70119
www.dcc.edu/

Northwestern State University
Veterinary Technology Prgm
Dept of Life Sciences
New Orleans, LA 71497
www.nsula.edu

Maine

University College of Bangor
Veterinary Technology Prgm
85 Texas Ave
Bangor, ME 04401
www.uma.maine.edu/bangor

Maryland

Community College of Baltimore County - Essex Campus
Veterinary Technology Prgm
7201 Rossville Blvd
Baltimore, MD 21237
www.ccbcmd.edu

Massachusetts

North Shore Community College
Veterinary Technology Prgm
1 Ferncroft Rd
Danvers, MA 01923
www.northshore.edu

Holyoke Community College
Veterinary Technician Program
303 Homestead Ave
Holyoke, MA 01040
www.hcc.mass.edu

Becker College
Veterinary Technology Prgm
964 Main St
Leicester, MA 01524
www.beckercollege.com

Mt Ida College
Veterinary Technology Prgm
777 Dedham St
Newton, MA 02459
www.mountida.edu

Michigan

Baker College of Cadillac
Veterinary Technology Prgm
9600 E 13th St
Cadillac, MI 49601
www.baker.edu

Macomb Community College
Veterinary Technology Prgm
44575 Garfield Rd
Clinton Township, MI 48044
www.macomb.cc.mi.us

Michigan State University
Veterinary Technology Prgm
College of Veterinary Medicine
A-10 Veterinary Medical Center
East Lansing, MI 48824
www.cvm.msu.edu/vettech

Baker College of Flint
Veterinary Technology Prgm
1050 W Bristol Rd
Flint, MI 48507
www.baker.edu

Baker College of Jackson
Veterinary Technology Prgm
2800 Springport Rd
Jackson, MI 49202
www.baker.edu

Baker College of Muskegon
Veterinary Technology Prgm
1903 Marquette Ave
Muskegon, MI 49442
www.baker.edu

Baker College of Port Huron
Veterinary Technology Prgm
3403 Lapeer Rd
Port Huron, MI 48060
www.baker.edu

Minnesota

Minnesota School of Business - Blaine
Veterinary Technology Prgm
3680 Pheasant Ridge Dr NE
Blaine, MN 55449
www.msbcollege.edu

Duluth Business University
Veterinary Technology Prgm
4724 Mike Colalillo Dr
Duluth, MN 55807
www.dbumn.edu

Argosy University - Twin Cities
Veterinary Technology Prgm
Veterinary Technician Program
1515 Central Parkway
Eagan, MN 55121
www.argosy.edu

Minneapolis Business College - Plymouth
Veterinary Technology Prgm
1455 County Rd, 101 North
Plymouth, MN 55447
www.msbcollege.edu

Rochester Community & Technical College
Veterinary Technology Prgm
Animal Health Technology Program
851 30th Ave SE
Rochester, MN 55904
www.rctc.edu

Minnesota School of Business - Shakopee
Veterinary Technology Prgm
1200 Shakopee Town Square
Shakopee, MN 55379
www.msbcollege.edu

Minnesota School of Business - Waite Park
Veterinary Technology Prgm
1201 2nd St South
Waite Park, MN 56387
www.msbcollege.edu

Ridgewater College - Willmar Campus
Veterinary Technology Prgm
2101 15th Ave, NW
Willmar, MN 56201
www.ridgewater.mnscu.edu

Globe University - Woodbury
Veterinary Technology Prgm
8089 Globe Dr
Woodbury, MN 55125
www.globecollege.edu

Mississippi

Hinds Community College
Veterinary Technology Prgm
1100 PMB 11160
Raymond, MS 39154
www.hindscc.edu/Departments/Agriculture/
VeterinaryTech.aspx

Northwest Mississippi Community College
Veterinary Technology Prgm
4975 Hwy 51 N
Senatobia, MS 38668
www.northwestms.edu

Missouri

Jefferson College
Veterinary Technology Prgm
1000 Viking Dr
Hillsboro, MO 63050
www.jeffco.edu

Maple Woods Community College
Veterinary Technology Prgm
2601 NE Barry Rd
Kansas City, MO 64156
www.mcckc.edu

Crowder College
Veterinary Technology Prgm
601 LaClede Ave
Neosho, MO 64850
www.crowder.edu

Nebraska

Nebraska College of Technical Agriculture
Veterinary Technology Prgm
RR3 Box 23A
Curtis, NE 69025
www.ncta.unl.edu

Northeast Community College
Veterinary Technology Prgm
801 E Benjamin Ave
Norfolk, NE 68702
www.northeastcollege.com

Vatterott College - Omaha Campus
Veterinary Technology Prgm
11818 I Street
Omaha, NE 68137
www.vatterott-college.com

Nevada

College of Southern Nevada
Veterinary Technology Prgm
6375 W Charleston Blvd
Las Vegas, NV 89146
www.ccsn.nevada.edu

Pima Medical Institute
Veterinary Technology Prgm
3333 E Flamingo Rd
Las Vegas, NV 89121
www.pmi.edu

Truckee Meadows Community College
Veterinary Technology Prgm
7000 Dandini Blvd
Reno, NV 89512

New Hampshire

New Hampshire Comm Tech College - Stratham
Veterinary Technology Prgm
277 Portsmouth Ave
Stratham, NH 03885
www.nhctc.edu

New Jersey

Camden County College
Veterinary Technology Prgm
Animal Science Technology Program
PO Box 200
Blackwood, NJ 08012
www.camdencc.edu

Northern NJ Consortium
Veterinary Technician Prgm
Consortium for Veterinary Technician Education
400 Paramus Rd
Paramus, NJ 07652

New Mexico

Central New Mexico Community College
Veterinary Technology Prgm
525 Buena Vista SE
Albuquerque, NM 87106

San Juan College
Veterinary Technology Prgm
Distance Learning Program
4601 College Blvd
Farmington, NM 87402
www.sjc.cc.nm.us/pages/1.asp

New York

Alfred State College - SUNY
Veterinary Technology Prgm
Agriculture Science Building
Alfred, NY 14801
www.alfredstate.edu

Suffolk County Community College - Grant Campus
Veterinary Technology Prgm
Western Campus
Brentwood, NY 11717
www.sunysuffolk.edu

Medaille College
Veterinary Technology Prgm
18 Agassiz Cr
Buffalo, NY 14214
www.medaille.edu

SUNY at Canton
Veterinary Science Technology Prgm
School of Science, Health, and Professional Studies
Canton, NY 13617
www.canton.edu

SUNY - Delhi
Veterinary Technology Prgm
156 Farnsworth Hall
Delhi, NY 13753
www.delhi.edu

Mercy College
Veterinary Technology Prgm
555 Broadway
Dobbs Ferry, NY 10522
www.mercy.edu/acadivisions/natscivettech/VetTech.cfm

LaGuardia Community College
Veterinary Technology Prgm
31-10 Thomson Ave
Long Island City, NY 11101
www.lagcc.cuny.edu

SUNY Ulster
Veterinary Technology Prgm
Cottekill Rd
Stone Ridge, NY 12484
www.sunyulster.edu

North Carolina

Asheville-Buncombe Technical Comm College
Veterinary Medical Technology Prgm
340 Victoria Rd
Asheville, NC 28801
www.abtech.edu/ah/vet

Gaston College - Dallas
Veterinary Medical Technology Program
201 Hwy 321 S
Dallas, NC 28034
www.gaston.cc.nc.us

Central Carolina Community College
Veterinary Medical Technology Program
1105 Kelley Dr
Sanford, NC 27330
www.ccarolina.cc.nc.us

North Dakota

North Dakota State University
Veterinary Technology Prgm
Van Es Laboratories
Fargo, ND 58105
http://vettech.ndsu.nodak.edu

Ohio

UC Raymond Walters College - Blue Ash
Veterinary Technology Prgm
9555 Plainfield Rd
Blue Ash, OH 45236
www.rwc.uc.edu

Bradford School
Veterinary Technology Prgm
2469 Stelzer Rd
Columbus, OH 43219
www.bradfordschoolcolumbus.edu

Columbus State Community College
Veterinary Technology Prgm
550 E Spring St
Columbus, OH 43216
www.cscc.edu

Cuyahoga Community College
Veterinary Technology Prgm
11000 Pleasant Valley Rd
Parma, OH 44130
www.tri-c.cc.oh.us

Stautzenberger College - Strongsville
Veterinary Technology Prgm
12925 Pearl Rd
Strongsville, OH 44136
www.sctoday.edu/strongsville/veterinary.php

Stautzenberger College
Veterinary Technology Prgm
5355 Southwyck
Toledo, OH 43614
www.stautzen.com

Oklahoma

Oklahoma State University
Veterinary Technology Prgm
900 N Portland Ave
Oklahoma City, OK 73107
www.osuokc.edu

Murray State College
Veterinary Technology Prgm
One Murray Campus
Tishomingo, OK 73460
www.msc.cc.ok.us

Tulsa Community College
Veterinary Technology Prgm
7505 W 41st St
Tulsa, OK 74107
www.tulsacc.edu

Ontario, Canada

University of Guelph
Veterinary Technology Prgm
Ridgetown College
Main St E
Ridgetown, ON N0P 2C0
www.ridgetownc.on.ca

Oregon

Portland Community College
Veterinary Technology Prgm
PO Box 19000
Portland, OR 97219
www.pcc.edu

Pennsylvania

Lehigh Carbon Community College
Cosponsor: Northampton Community College
Veterinary Technology Prgm
3835 Green Pond Rd
Bethlehem, PA 18020
www.lccc.edu

Harcum College
Veterinary Technology Prgm
750 Montgomery Ave
Bryn Mawr, PA 19010
www.harcum.edu

Wilson College
Veterinary Technology Prgm
1015 Philadelphia Ave
Chambersburg, PA 17201
www.wilson.edu

Manor College
Veterinary Technology Prgm
700 Fox Chase Rd
Jenkintown, PA 19046
www.manorvettech.com

Vet Tech Institute
Veterinary Technology Prgm
125 Seventh St
Pittsburgh, PA 15222
www.vettechinstitute.com

Western School of Health & Business - Pittsburgh
Veterinary Technology Prgm
421 7th Ave
Pittsburgh, PA 15219
www.westernschool.com

Johnson College
Veterinary Science Technology Prgm
3427 N Main Ave
Scranton, PA 18508
www.johnsoncollege.com

Puerto Rico

University of Puerto Rico
Veterinary Technology Prgm
Medical Sciences Campus
San Juan, PR 00936
www.cprsweb.rcm.upr.edu

South Carolina

Trident Technical College
Veterinary Technology Prgm
1001 S Live Oak Dr
Moncks Corner, SC 29461
www.tridenttech.edu

Newberry College
Veterinary Technology Prgm
2100 College St
Newberry, SC 29108
www.newberry.edu

Tri-County Technical College
Veterinary Technology Prgm
PO Box 587
Pendleton, SC 29670
www.tctc.edu

South Dakota

National American University
Veterinary Technology Prgm
321 Kansas City St
Rapid City, SD 57701
www.national.edu/veterinary_tech.html

Tennessee

Columbia State Community College
Veterinary Technology Prgm
PO Box 1315
Columbia, TN 38401
www.coscc.cc.tn.us

Lincoln Memorial University
Veterinary Technology Prgm
Cumberland Gap Pkwy
Harrogate, TN 37752
www.lmunet.edu

Texas

Sul Ross State University
Veterinary Technology Prgm
School of Agriculture and Natural Resource Sciences
PO Box C-114
Alpine, TX 79830
www.sulross.edu

Cedar Valley College
Veterinary Technology Prgm
3030 N Dallas Ave
Lancaster, TX 75134
www.ollie.dcccd.edu/vettech

Midland College
Veterinary Technology Prgm
3600 N Garfield
Midland, TX 79705
www.midland.edu

Palo Alto College
Veterinary Technology Prgm
1400 W Villaret Blvd
San Antonio, TX 78224
www.accd.edu

Tomball College - NHMCCD
Veterinary Technology Prgm
30555 Tomball Pkwy
Tomball, TX 77375
www.tc.nhmccd.cc.tx.us

McLennan Community College
Veterinary Technology Prgm
1400 College Dr
Waco, TX 76708
www.mclennan.edu./departments/workforce/vtech/

Utah

Utah Career College
Veterinary Technology Prgm
1902 West 7800 South
West Jordan, UT 84088
www.utahcollege.com

Vermont

Vermont Technical College
Veterinary Technology Prgm
Randolph Center, VT 05061
www.vtc.vcs.edu

Virginia

Northern Virginia Community College
Veterinary Technology Prgm
Loudoun Campus
1000 Harry Flood Byrd Hwy
Sterling, VA 20164
www.nv.cc.va.us

Blue Ridge Community College
Veterinary Technology Prgm
Box 80
Weyers Cave, VA 24486
www.br.cc.va.us

Washington

Pierce College
Veterinary Technology Prgm
9401 Farwest Dr SW
Lakewood, WA 98498
www.pierce.ctc.edu

Yakima Valley Community College
Veterinary Technology Prgm
PO Box 22520
Yakima, WA 98907
www.yvcc.edu

West Virginia

Fairmont State Univ
Cosponsor: Pierpont Community & Technical College
Veterinary Technology Prgm
1201 Locust Ave
Fairmont, WV 26554
www.fscwv.edu

Wisconsin

Madison Area Technical College
Veterinary Technology Prgm
3550 Anderson
Madison, WI 53704
www.madions.tec.wi.us/matc

Wyoming

Eastern Wyoming College
Veterinary Technology Prgm
3200 West C St
Torrington, WY 82240
http://ewc.wy.edu

Section II

Institutions Sponsoring Accredited Programs

Alabama

Andalusia

Lurleen B Wallace Junior College
Seth Hammett, MBA, President
PO Box 1418
Andalusia, AL 36420
205 222-6591
Type: Junior or Comm Coll
Control: State, County, or Local Govt
• Emergency Med Tech-Paramedic Prgm

Auburn University

Auburn University
Edward Richardson, President
107 Sanford Hall
Auburn University, AL 36849
334 844-4650
Type: 4-year Coll or Univ
Control: State, County, or Local Govt
• Audiologist Prgm
• Counseling Prgm
• Dietetics-Didactic Prgm
• Nursing Prgm
• Pharmacy Prgm
• Psychology Prgm
• Rehabilitation Counseling Prgm
• Speech-Language Pathology Prgm
• Veterinary Medicine Prgm

Bay Minette

James H Faulkner State Community College
Gary L Branch, President
1900 Hwy 31 S
Bay Minette, AL 36507-2619
334 580-2100
Type: Junior or Comm Coll
Control: State, County, or Local Govt
• Dental Assisting Prgm
• Surgical Technology Prgm

Birmingham

Carraway Methodist Medical Center
Cathy Fickes, Administrator
1600 N 26th St
Birmingham, AL 35234
205 226-6000
Type: Hosp or Med Ctr: 300-499 Beds
Control: Nonprofit (Private or Religious)
• Radiography Prgm

Jefferson State Community College
Judy M Merritt, PhD, President
2601 Carson Rd
Birmingham, AL 35215
205 856-7777
Type: Junior or Comm Coll
Control: State, County, or Local Govt
• Clin Lab Technician/Med Lab Technician Prgm
• Physical Therapist Assistant Prgm
• Radiography Prgm
• Veterinary Technology Prgm

Samford University
Thomas E Corts, PhD, President
800 Lakeshore Dr
Birmingham, AL 35229
205 870-5727
Type: 4-year Coll or Univ
Control: Nonprofit (Private or Religious)
• Athletic Training Prgm
• Dietetics-Didactic Prgm
• Exercise Science Prgm
• Nursing Prgm
• Pharmacy Prgm

University of Alabama at Birmingham
Carol Garrison, PhD, President
AB 1070
Birmingham, AL 35294-0110
205 934-4636
Type: 4-year Coll or Univ
Control: State, County, or Local Govt
• Clin Lab Scientist/Med Technologist Prgm
• Cytotechnology Prgm
• Dietetic Internship Prgm
• Emergency Med Tech-Paramedic Prgm
• Health Information Admin Prgm
• Nuclear Medicine Technology Prgm
• Nursing Prgm
• Occupational Therapy Prgm
• Optometry Prgm
• Physical Therapy Prgm
• Radiation Therapy Prgm
• Radiography Prgm
• Rehabilitation Counseling Prgm
• Respiratory Therapist (Advanced) Prgm
• Surgical Physician Assistant Prgm

Decatur

Calhoun Community College
Marilyn Beck, EdD, President
PO Box 2216 Hwy 31 N
Decatur, AL 35609
256 306-2500
Type: Junior or Comm Coll
Control: State, County, or Local Govt
• Dental Assisting Prgm
• Emergency Med Tech-Paramedic Prgm
• Surgical Technology Prgm

Dothan

Flowers Hospital
L Keith Granger, BS, President
PO Box 6907
Dothan, AL 36302
334 793-5000
Type: Hosp or Med Ctr: 100-299 Beds
Control: For Profit
• Surgical Technology Prgm

George C Wallace Community College
Linda Young, EdD, President
1141 Wallace Dr
Dothan, AL 36303
800 543-2426
Type: Junior or Comm Coll
Control: State, County, or Local Govt
• Emergency Med Tech-Paramedic Prgm
• Medical Assistant Prgm
• Pharmacy Technician Prgm
• Physical Therapist Assistant Prgm
• Radiography Prgm
• Respiratory Therapist (Advanced) Prgm

Florence

University of North Alabama
Florence, AL 35632
Type: 4-year Coll or Univ
Control: State, County, or Local Govt
• Nursing Prgm

Gadsden

Gadsden State Community College
Renee D Culverhouse, BA JD, President
PO Box 227
1001 George Wallace Dr
Gadsden, AL 35902-0227
256 549-8221
Type: Junior or Comm Coll
Control: State, County, or Local Govt
• Clin Lab Technician/Med Lab Technician Prgm
• Emergency Med Tech-Paramedic Prgm
• Radiography Prgm

Hanceville

Wallace State Community College
Vicki Hawsey, EdD, President
Commerce Bldg
PO Box 2000
Hanceville, AL 35077-2000
256 352-8130
Type: Junior or Comm Coll
Control: State, County, or Local Govt
• Clin Lab Technician/Med Lab Technician Prgm
• Dental Assisting Prgm
• Dental Hygiene Prgm
• Diagnostic Med Sonography Prgm
• Emergency Med Tech-Paramedic Prgm
• Health Information Tech Prgm
• Medical Assistant Prgm
• Occupational Therapy Asst Prgm (2)
• Physical Therapist Assistant Prgm
• Radiography Prgm
• Respiratory Therapist (Advanced) Prgm

Huntsville

Crestwood Medical Center
One Hospital Dr SE
Huntsville, AL 35801
Type: Acad Health Ctr/Med Sch
Control: Nonprofit (Private or Religious)
• Radiography Prgm

Huntsville Hospital
David Spillers, MHA, CEO
101 Sivley Rd
Huntsville, AL 35801
256 265-8123
Type: Hosp or Med Ctr: 500> Beds
Control: State, County, or Local Govt
• Radiography Prgm

Oakwood College
Benjamin F Reaves, President
Huntsville, AL 35896
205 726-7000
Type: 4-year Coll or Univ
Control: Nonprofit (Private or Religious)
• Dietetic Internship Prgm
• Dietetics-Didactic Prgm

Univ of Alabama at Birmingham - Huntsville
Frank A Franz, MD, President
301 Sparkman Dr
Huntsville, AL 35899-1911
256 890-6150
Type: 4-year Coll or Univ
Control: State, County, or Local Govt
• Nursing Prgm

Jacksonville

Jacksonville State University
Harold J McGee, President
Jacksonville, AL 36265
205 782-5781
Type: 4-year Coll or Univ
Control: State, County, or Local Govt
• Dietetics-Didactic Prgm
• Nursing Prgm

Livingston

University of West Alabama
Richard Holland, PhD, President
Station 1
Livingston, AL 35470
205 652-3527
Type: 4-year Coll or Univ
Control: State, County, or Local Govt
• Athletic Training Prgm

Mobile

Bishop State Community College
Yvonne Kennedy, PhD, President
351 N Broad St
Mobile, AL 36603-5898
205 690-6416
Type: Junior or Comm Coll
Control: State, County, or Local Govt
• Health Information Tech Prgm
• Physical Therapist Assistant Prgm

Institute of Ultrasound Diagnostics
Smyth R Gill, BA, CFO
1230 Montlimar Dr, Ste A
Mobile, AL 36609
251 460-2485
Type: Vocational or Tech Sch
Control: For Profit
• Diagnostic Med Sonography Prgm

Spring Hill College
Mobile, AL 36608
Type: 4-year Coll or Univ
Control: Nonprofit (Private or Religious)
• Nursing Prgm

University of Mobile
Mark R Foley, PhD, President
5735 College Pkwy
Mobile, AL 36663-0220
251 442-2201
Type: 4-year Coll or Univ
Control: State, County, or Local Govt
• Athletic Training Prgm
• Nursing Prgm

University of South Alabama
V Gordon Moulton, MBA, President
307 N University Blvd
Mobile, AL 36688-0002
251 460-6111
Type: 4-year Coll or Univ
Control: State, County, or Local Govt
• Allopathic Medicine Prgm
• Audiologist Prgm
• Clin Lab Scientist/Med Technologist Prgm
• Emergency Med Tech-Paramedic Prgm
• Nursing Prgm
• Occupational Therapy Prgm
• Physical Therapy Prgm
• Physician Assistant Prgm
• Radiography Prgm
• Respiratory Therapist (Advanced) Prgm
• Speech-Language Pathology Prgm

Virginia College
Madeline Little, President, South Region
5901 Airport Blvd
Mobile, AL 36608
251 343-7227
Type: Vocational or Tech Sch
Control: For Profit
• Surgical Technology Prgm (2)

Montevallo

University of Montevallo
Robert M McChesney, President
Station 6001
Montevallo, AL 35115
205 665-6000
Type: 4-year Coll or Univ
Control: State, County, or Local Govt
• Counseling Prgm
• Dietetics-Didactic Prgm
• Speech-Language Pathology Prgm

Montgomery

Alabama State University
Joe A Lee, PhD, President
915 S Jackson St
Montgomery, AL 36101-0271
334 229-4202
Type: 4-year Coll or Univ
Control: State, County, or Local Govt
• Health Information Admin Prgm
• Occupational Therapy Prgm
• Physical Therapy Prgm

Auburn University Montgomery
Guin Nance, PhD, Chancellor
PO Box 244023
Montgomery, AL 36124
334 244-3602
Type: 4-year Coll or Univ
Control: State, County, or Local Govt
• Clin Lab Scientist/Med Technologist Prgm
• Cytotechnology Prgm
• Nursing Prgm

Baptist Medical Center South
Russ Tyner, BA MHA, CEO
301 Brown Springs Rd
Montgomery, AL 36117
334 273-4400
Type: Hosp or Med Ctr: 300-499 Beds
Control: Nonprofit (Private or Religious)
• Clin Lab Scientist/Med Technologist Prgm
• Diagnostic Med Sonography Prgm
• Radiography Prgm

H Council Trenholm State Technical College
Sam Munnerlyn, MA, Interim President
1225 Air Base Blvd
Montgomery, AL 36108
334 420-4200
Type: Vocational or Tech Sch
Control: State, County, or Local Govt
• Dental Assisting Prgm
• Dental Lab Technician Prgm
• Emergency Med Tech-Paramedic Prgm
• Medical Assistant Prgm

Huntingdon College
J Cameron West, Th M M Div, President
1500 E Fairview Ave
Montgomery, AL 36106
334 833-4409
Type: 4-year Coll or Univ
Control: Nonprofit (Private or Religious)
• Athletic Training Prgm

South University
Victor Biebighauser, BA, President
5355 Vaughn Rd
Montgomery, AL 36116-1120
334 395-8800
Type: 4-year Coll or Univ
Control: For Profit
• Medical Assistant Prgm
• Physical Therapist Assistant Prgm

Muscle Shoals

Northwest-Shoals Community College
Humphrey Lee, EdD, President
PO Box 2545
Muscle Shoals, AL 35662
256 331-5200
Type: Junior or Comm Coll
Control: State, County, or Local Govt
• Emergency Med Tech-Paramedic Prgm

Normal

Alabama A&M University
Robert R Jennings, EdD, President
PO Box 1357
Normal, AL 35762
205 851-5000
Type: 4-year Coll or Univ
Control: State, County, or Local Govt
• Dietetics-Didactic Prgm
• Rehabilitation Counseling Prgm
• Speech-Language Pathology Prgm

Opelika

Southern Union State Community College
Susan E Salatto, MACT, President
1701 LaFayette Pkwy
Opelika, AL 36801
334 745-6437
Type: Junior or Comm Coll
Control: State, County, or Local Govt
• Emergency Med Tech-Paramedic Prgm
• Radiography Prgm
• Surgical Technology Prgm

Rainsville

Northeast Alabama Community College
David Campbell, PhD, President
PO Box 159
Rainsville, AL 35986-0159
256 228-6001
Type: Junior or Comm Coll
Control: State, County, or Local Govt
• Emergency Med Tech-Paramedic Prgm

Sumiton

Bevill State Community College
Harold Wade, EdD, President
PO Box 800
Sumiton, AL 35148-0800
205 648-3271
Type: Junior or Comm Coll
Control: State, County, or Local Govt
• Emergency Med Tech-Paramedic Prgm
• Surgical Technology Prgm

Troy

Troy University
Jack Hawkins, Jr, PhD, Chancellor
University Ave
Troy, AL 36082
334 670-3200
Type: 4-year Coll or Univ
Control: State, County, or Local Govt
• Athletic Training Prgm
• Counseling Prgm (2)
• Rehabilitation Counseling Prgm

Tuscaloosa

DCH Regional Medical Center
Bryan N Kindred, MBA, President/CEO
809 University Blvd E
Tuscaloosa, AL 35401
205 759-7177
Type: Hosp or Med Ctr: 500> Beds
Control: State, County, or Local Govt
• Radiography Prgm

Shelton State Community College
JoAnn Jordan, EdD, Interim President
9500 Old Greensboro Rd
Tuscaloosa, AL 35405
205 391-2472
Type: Junior or Comm Coll
Control: State, County, or Local Govt
• Emergency Med Tech-Paramedic Prgm
• Respiratory Therapist (Advanced) Prgm

University of Alabama
Robert Witt, PhD, President
PO Box 870100
Tuscaloosa, AL 35487
205 348-5100
Type: 4-year Coll or Univ
Control: State, County, or Local Govt
• Allopathic Medicine Prgm
• Athletic Training Prgm
• Counseling Prgm
• Dentistry Prgm
• Dietetics-Coordinated Prgm
• Dietetics-Didactic Prgm
• Medical Librarian Prgm
• Music Therapy Prgm
• Nursing Prgm
• Psychology Prgm (2)
• Rehabilitation Counseling Prgm
• Speech-Language Pathology Prgm

Tuskegee

Tuskegee University
Benjamin F Payton, PhD, President
308 Kresge Ctr
Tuskegee, AL 36088-1677
334 727-8501
Type: 4-year Coll or Univ
Control: Nonprofit (Private or Religious)
• Clin Lab Scientist/Med Technologist Prgm
• Dietetics-Didactic Prgm
• Occupational Therapy Prgm
• Veterinary Medicine Prgm

Alaska

Anchorage

University of Alaska Anchorage
Fran Ulmer, JD, Intermim Chancellor
3211 Providence Dr
ADM 217
Anchorage, AK 99508
907 786-1437
Type: 4-year Coll or Univ
Control: State, County, or Local Govt
• Clin Lab Scientist/Med Technologist Prgm
• Clin Lab Technician/Med Lab Technician Prgm
• Dental Assisting Prgm
• Dental Hygiene Prgm
• Dietetic Internship Prgm
• Massage Therapy Prgm
• Medical Assistant Prgm

Fairbanks

University of Alaska - Fairbanks
Steve Jones, PhD, Chancellor
320 Signers Hall
Fairbanks, AK 99775-7500
907 474-7112
Type: 4-year Coll or Univ
Control: State, County, or Local Govt
• Medical Assistant Prgm

Juneau

University of Alaska Southeast
John Pugh, Chancellor
11120 Glacier Hwy
Juneau, AK 99801-8691
907 796-6457
Type: 4-year Coll or Univ
Control: State, County, or Local Govt
• Health Information Tech Prgm

Alberta, Canada

Calgary

University of Calgary
Calgary, AB T2N 4N1
Type: Acad Health Ctr/Med Sch
Control: State, County, or Local Government
• Allopathic Medicine Prgm

INSTITUTIONS

Edmonton

University of Alberta
Indira Samarasekera, PhD, President
Edmonton, AB T6G 2M7
Control: Nonprofit (Private or Religious)
• Allopathic Medicine Prgm
• Medical Librarian Prgm

Arizona

Chandler

Chandler-Gilbert Community College
Maria L Hesse, EdD, President
2626 East Pecos Road
Chandler, AZ 85225
480 732-7075
Type: Acad Health Ctr/Med Sch
Control: For Profit
• Dietetic Technician-AD Prgm

Coolidge

Central Arizona College
Kathleen Arns, PhD, President
Woodruff at Overfield Rd
Coolidge, AZ 85228
602 426-4444
Type: Junior or Comm Coll
Control: State, County, or Local Govt
• Dietetic Technician-AD Prgm

Flagstaff

Northern Arizona University
Haeger John, PhD, President
PO Box 4092
Flagstaff, AZ 86011
928 523-3232
Type: 4-year Coll or Univ
Control: State, County, or Local Govt
• Athletic Training Prgm
• Counseling Prgm
• Dental Hygiene Prgm
• Nursing Prgm
• Physical Therapy Prgm
• Speech-Language Pathology Prgm

Glendale

Midwestern University - Glendale Campus
Kathleen H Goeppinger, PhD, President and CEO
19555 N 59th Ave
Glendale, AZ 85308
623 572-3400
Type: Acad Health Ctr/Med Sch
Control: Nonprofit (Private or Religious)
• Occupational Therapy Prgm
• Osteopathic Medicine Prgm
• Perfusion Prgm
• Pharmacy Prgm
• Physician Assistant Prgm
• Podiatric Medicine Prgm

Kingman

Mohave Community College
Thomas C Henry, PhD, Chancellor
1971 Jagerson Ave
Kingman, AZ 86401
928 757-0800
Type: Junior or Comm Coll
Control: State, County, or Local Govt
• Dental Hygiene Prgm
• Surgical Technology Prgm

Mesa

AT Still University of Health Sciences
James J McGovern, PhD, President
5850 E Still Circle
Mesa, AZ 85206
480 219-6000
Type: Acad Health Ctr/Med Sch
Control: Nonprofit (Private or Religious)
• Dentistry Prgm
• Occupational Therapy Prgm
• Osteopathic Medicine Prgm
• Physical Therapy Prgm
• Physician Assistant Prgm

Mesa Community College
Wayne Giles, EdD, President
1833 W Southern Ave
Mesa, AZ 85205
480 461-7299
Type: Junior or Comm Coll
Control: State, County, or Local Govt
• Dental Assisting Prgm
• Dental Hygiene Prgm
• Veterinary Technology Prgm

Phoenix

Apollo College
Ralph Bilbao, EdD, Executive Director
2701 W Bethany Home Rd
Phoenix, AZ 85017
602 433-1333
Type: Vocational or Tech Sch
Control: For Profit
• Radiography Prgm

Argosy University
Phoenix, AZ 85021
Type: 4-year Coll or Univ
Control: State, County, or Local Govt
• Psychology Prgm

Arizona Department of Health Services
Susan Gerard, Director
150 N 18th Ave, Ste 310
Phoenix, AZ 85007
602 542-1001
Control: State, County, or Local Govt
• Dietetic Internship Prgm

GateWay Community College
Eugene Giovannini, EdD, President
108 N 40th St
Phoenix, AZ 85034
602 286-8000
Type: Junior or Comm Coll
Control: State, County, or Local Govt
• Diagnostic Med Sonography Prgm
• Nuclear Medicine Technology Prgm
• Physical Therapist Assistant Prgm
• Radiography Prgm
• Respiratory Therapist (Advanced) Prgm
• Surgical Technology Prgm

Grand Canyon University
Gil Stafford, PhD, President
PO Box 111097
Phoenix, AZ 85061-1097
602 249-3300
Type: 4-year Coll or Univ
Control: Nonprofit (Private or Religious)
• Athletic Training Prgm
• Nursing Prgm

Kaplan College
Debra Thibodeaux, MBA, Executive Director
13610 N Black Canyon Hwy 104
Phoenix, AZ 85029
602 548-1955
Type: Vocational or Tech Sch
Control: For Profit
• Medical Assistant Prgm
• Respiratory Therapist (Advanced) Prgm
• Veterinary Technology Prgm

Paradise Valley Community College
Mary Kay Kickels, President
18401 N 32nd St
Phoenix, AZ 85032
602 787-6610
Type: Acad Health Ctr/Med Sch
Control: For Profit
• Dietetic Technician-AD Prgm

Paradise Valley Unified School District
20621 N 32nd St
Phoenix, AZ 85032
602 493-2600
Control: State, County, or Local Govt
• Dietetic Internship Prgm

Phoenix College
Anna Solley, EdD, President
1202 W Thomas Rd
Phoenix, AZ 85013
602 285-7364
Type: Junior or Comm Coll
Control: State, County, or Local Govt
• Dental Assisting Prgm
• Dental Hygiene Prgm
• Health Information Tech Prgm
• Nursing Prgm

Southwestern DI Consortium
Poenix Indian Medical Center
Phoenix, AZ 85016
Control: Nonprofit (Private or Religious)
• Dietetic Internship Prgm

University of Phoenix
Laura Palmer Noone, PhD JD, President
4615 E Elwood St
PO Box 52076
Phoenix, AZ 85040
480 966-9577
Type: 4-year Coll or Univ
Control: For Profit
• Counseling Prgm
• Nursing Prgm

Prescott

Yavapai County Health Department
930 Division St
Prescott, AZ 86301
602 771-3122
Control: State, County, or Local Govt
• Dietetic Internship Prgm

Scottsdale

Penn Foster College
Richard W Ferrin, PhD, President
14300 N Northsight Blvd
Scottsdale, Az 85254
480 947-6644
Type: 4-year Coll or Univ
Control: State, County, or Local Govt
• Veterinary Technology Prgm

Tempe

Arizona State University
Michael M Crow, PhD, President
Box 872203
Tempe, AZ 85287-2203
480 965-5606
Type: 4-year Coll or Univ
Control: State, County, or Local Govt
• Audiologist Prgm
• Clin Lab Scientist/Med Technologist Prgm
• Counseling Prgm
• Dietetic Internship Prgm
• Dietetics-Didactic Prgm
• Music Therapy Prgm
• Nursing Prgm
• Psychology Prgm
• Speech-Language Pathology Prgm

Lamson College
Donna Green, MS, Campus President
1126 N Scottsdale Rd #17
Tempe, AZ 85281
480 898-7000
Type: Junior or Comm Coll
Control: For Profit
• Surgical Technology Prgm

Maricopa County Dept of Public Health
Office of Nutrition Services
1414 W Broadway Ste 237
Tempe, AZ 85282
602 966-3090
Control: State, County, or Local Govt
• Dietetic Internship Prgm

Rio Salado College
Linda M Thor, President
2323 W 14th St
Tempe, AZ 85281-6950
480 517-8000
Type: Junior or Comm Coll
Control: State, County, or Local Govt
• Dental Hygiene Prgm

Tucson

Carondelet St Mary's Hospital
Morrisons Custom Management Company
1601 W St Mary's Rd
Tucson, AZ 85745
520 622-5833
Control: Nonprofit (Private or Religious)
• Dietetic Internship Prgm

Desert Institute of the Healing Arts
Tucson, AZ 85705
Type: Acad Health Ctr/Med Sch
Control: For Profit
• Massage Therapy Prgm

Pima Community College
Roy Flores, PhD, Chancellor
4905 E Broadway
Tucson, AZ 85709-1005
520 206-4747
Type: Junior or Comm Coll
Control: State, County, or Local Govt
• Dental Assisting Prgm
• Dental Hygiene Prgm
• Dental Lab Technician Prgm
• Histotechnician Prgm
• Pharmacy Technician Prgm
• Radiography Prgm
• Respiratory Therapist (Advanced) Prgm
• Surgical Technology Prgm
• Veterinary Technology Prgm

Pima Medical Institute
Richard L Luebke, Jr, BS, President
3350 E Grant Rd #200
Tucson, AZ 85716
520 326-1600
Type: Vocational or Tech Sch
Control: For Profit
• Radiography Prgm (2)
• Respiratory Therapist (Advanced) Prgm (2)

Pima Medical Institute - Denver
Richard L Luebke, Sr, President
3350 E Grant Rd #200
Tucson, AZ 85716
520 326-1600
Type: Vocational or Tech Sch
Control: For Profit
• Ophthalmic Med Technician Prgm
• Radiography Prgm
• Respiratory Therapist (Advanced) Prgm

University Medical Center
Susan Bristol, MS RD CNSD, Clinical Nutrition
  Managr
PO Box 245088
1501 N Campbell Ave
Tucson, AZ 85724
480 727-3278
Type: Hosp or Med Ctr: 100-299 Beds
Control: Nonprofit (Private or Religious)
• Dietetics-Didactic Prgm

University of Arizona
Robert Shelton, PhD, President
Adminstration Bldg Rm 712
Tucson, AZ 85721-0066
520 621-5511
Type: Acad Health Ctr/Med Sch
Control: State, County, or Local Govt
• Allopathic Medicine Prgm
• Audiologist Prgm
• Dietetic Internship Prgm
• Medical Librarian Prgm
• Orientation and Mobility Specialist Prgm
• Perfusion Prgm
• Pharmacy Prgm
• Psychology Prgm
• Rehabilitation Counseling Prgm
• Speech-Language Pathology Prgm
• Teacher of the Visually Impaired Prgm

Yuma

Arizona Western College
Don Schoening, PhD, President
PO Box 929
Yuma, AZ 85366-0929
Type: 4-year Coll or Univ
Control: State, County, or Local Govt
• Radiography Prgm

Arkansas

Arkadelphia

Henderson State University
Charles Dunn, PhD, President
HSU Box 7532
Arkadelphia, AR 71999-0001
870 230-5091
Control: State, County, or Local Govt
• Athletic Training Prgm
• Dietetics-Didactic Prgm
• Nursing Prgm

Ouachita Baptist University
Andrew Westmoreland, EdD, President
410 Ouachita Ct
OBU Box 3753
Arkadelphia, AR 71998
870 245-5000
Type: 4-year Coll or Univ
Control: Nonprofit (Private or Religious)
• Athletic Training Prgm
• Dietetics-Didactic Prgm

Batesville

Univ of Arkansas Comm Coll - Batesville
Anthony G Kinkel, EdD, Chancellor
PO Box 3350
Batesville, AR 72501
870 793-7581
Type: Consortium
Control: State, County, or Local Govt
• Emergency Med Tech-Paramedic Prgm
• Surgical Technology Prgm

Beebe

Arkansas State University - Beebe
Eugene McKay, PhD, Chancellor
PO Box 1000
Beebe, AR 72012
501 882-8356
Type: Junior or Comm Coll
Control: State, County, or Local Govt
• Clin Lab Technician/Med Lab Technician Prgm

Bentonville

NorthWest Arkansas Community College
Rebecca Paneitz, PhD, President
One College Dr
Bentonville, AR 72712-5091
479 619-4251
Type: Junior or Comm Coll
Control: State, County, or Local Govt
• Emergency Med Tech-Paramedic Prgm
• Physical Therapist Assistant Prgm
• Respiratory Therapist (Advanced) Prgm

Blytheville

Arkansas Northeastern College
Robin Myers, EdD, President
PO Box 1109
Blytheville, AR 72316
870 762-1020
Type: Junior or Comm Coll
Control: State, County, or Local Govt
• Dental Assisting Prgm
• Emergency Med Tech-Paramedic Prgm

Conway

University of Central Arkansas
Lu Hardin, JD, President
Wingo Hall, Ste 207
201 Donaghey Ave
Conway, AR 72035
501 450-3170
Type: 4-year Coll or Univ
Control: State, County, or Local Govt
• Athletic Training Prgm
• Dietetic Internship Prgm
• Dietetics-Didactic Prgm
• Nursing Prgm
• Occupational Therapy Prgm
• Physical Therapy Prgm
• Speech-Language Pathology Prgm

El Dorado

South Arkansas Community College
Thomas Alan Rasco, EdD, President and CEO
PO Box 7010
300 S West Ave
El Dorado, AR 71731-7010
870 862-8131
Type: Junior or Comm Coll
Control: State, County, or Local Govt
• Clin Lab Technician/Med Lab Technician Prgm
• Occupational Therapy Asst Prgm
• Physical Therapist Assistant Prgm
• Radiography Prgm

Fayetteville

University of Arkansas
John White, PhD, Chancellor
Adminstration Bldg
Fayetteville, AR 72701
479 575-4148
Type: 4-year Coll or Univ
Control: State, County, or Local Govt
• Athletic Training Prgm
• Counseling Prgm
• Dietetics-Didactic Prgm
• Nursing Prgm
• Rehabilitation Counseling Prgm
• Speech-Language Pathology Prgm

Forrest City

East Arkansas Community College
Coy Grace, President
1700 Newcastle Rd
Forrest City, AR 72335
870 633-4480
Type: Junior or Comm Coll
Control: State, County, or Local Govt
• Emergency Med Tech-Paramedic Prgm

Fort Smith

University of Arkansas - Fort Smith
Paul Beran, PhD, Chancellor
5201 Grand Ave
PO Box 3649
Fort Smith, AR 72913
479 788-7004
Type: 4-year Coll or Univ
Control: State, County, or Local Govt
• Dental Hygiene Prgm
• Radiography Prgm
• Surgical Technology Prgm

Harrison

North Arkansas College
Jeffery R. Olson, PhD, President
1515 Pioneer Dr
Harrison, AR 72601-5599
870 391-3200
Type: Junior or Comm Coll
Control: State, County, or Local Govt
• Clin Lab Technician/Med Lab Technician Prgm
• Emergency Med Tech-Paramedic Prgm
• Radiography Prgm
• Surgical Technology Prgm

Helena

Phillips Community College/U of Arkansas
Steven Murray, EdD, Chancellor
PO Box 785
1000 Campus Dr
Helena, AR 72342
870 338-6474
Type: Junior or Comm Coll
Control: State, County, or Local Govt
• Clin Lab Technician/Med Lab Technician Prgm
• Phlebotomy Prgm

Hope

Univ of Arkansas Comm Coll - Hope
Welch Charles, EdD, Chancellor
PO Box 140
2500 S Main
Hope, AR 71801
870 777-5722
Type: Junior or Comm Coll
Control: State, County, or Local Govt
• Respiratory Therapist (Entry-Level) Prgm

Hot Springs

National Park Community College
Sally Carder, PhD, President
101 College Dr
Hot Springs, AR 71913-9174
501 760-4222
Type: Junior or Comm Coll
Control: State, County, or Local Govt
• Clin Lab Technician/Med Lab Technician Prgm
• Emergency Med Tech-Paramedic Prgm
• Health Information Tech Prgm
• Radiography Prgm

Little Rock

Baptist Health Schools Little Rock
Russell D Harrington, Jr, FACHE, President
11900 Colonel Glenn Rd #1000
Little Rock, AR 72210
501 202-2274
Type: Hosp or Med Ctr: 500> Beds
Control: Nonprofit (Private or Religious)
• Clin Lab Scientist/Med Technologist Prgm
• Histotechnician Prgm
• Nuclear Medicine Technology Prgm
• Occupational Therapy Asst Prgm
• Radiography Prgm
• Surgical Technology Prgm

Central Arkansas Radiation Therapy Inst
Janice Burford, CEO, President
PO Box 55050
Little Rock, AR 72215
501 664-8573
Type: Nonhosp HC Facil, BB, or Lab
Control: Nonprofit (Private or Religious)
• Radiation Therapy Prgm

Saint Vincent Health System
Peter Banko, CEO
Two St Vincent Circle
Little Rock, AR 72205-5499
501 552-3910
Type: Consortium
Control: Nonprofit (Private or Religious)
• Radiography Prgm

University of Arkansas at Little Rock
Joel Anderson, Chancellor
2801 S University Ave
Little Rock, AR 72204
501 569-3000
Type: 4-year Coll or Univ
Control: State, County, or Local Govt
• Allopathic Medicine Prgm
• Orientation and Mobility Specialist Prgm
• Rehabilitation Counseling Prgm
• Vision Rehabilitation Therapy Prgm

University of Arkansas for Medical Sciences
I Dodd Wilson, MD, Chancellor
4301 W Markham Slot 541
Little Rock, AR 72205
501 686-5680
Type: Acad Health Ctr/Med Sch
Control: State, County, or Local Govt
- Audiologist Prgm
- Clin Lab Scientist/Med Technologist Prgm
- Cytotechnology Prgm
- Dental Hygiene Prgm
- Diagnostic Med Sonography Prgm
- Dietetic Internship Prgm
- Emergency Med Tech-Paramedic Prgm
- Genetic Counseling Prgm
- Health Information Tech Prgm
- Nuclear Medicine Technology Prgm
- Nursing Prgm
- Ophthalmic Med Technologist Prgm
- Perfusion Prgm
- Psychology Prgm
- Radiography Prgm (3)
- Respiratory Therapist (Advanced) Prgm (2)
- Speech-Language Pathology Prgm
- Surgical Technology Prgm

Magnolia

Southern Arkansas University
David F Rankin, PhD CFA, President
100 E University
Magnolia, AR 71753-5000
870 235-4001
Type: 4-year Coll or Univ
Control: State, County, or Local Govt
- Athletic Training Prgm

Monticello

U of Arkansas-Monticello Coll of Tech-McGehee
H Jack Lassiter, PhD, Chancellor
346 University Dr
PO Box 3596
Monticello, AR 71656
870 460-1020
Type: 4-year Coll or Univ
Control: State, County, or Local Govt
- Emergency Med Tech-Paramedic Prgm

North Little Rock

Pulaski Technical College
Dan Bakke, EdD, President
3000 W Scenic Rd
North Little Rock, AR 72118
501 812-2216
Type: Junior or Comm Coll
Control: State, County, or Local Govt
- Dental Assisting Prgm

Ozark

Arkansas Tech University - Ozark Campus
Jo Alice Blondin, PhD, Chancellor
1701 Helberg Lane
Ozark, AR 72949
479 667-2117
Type: 4-year Coll or Univ
Control: Nonprofit (Private or Religious)
- Emergency Med Tech-Paramedic Prgm

Pine Bluff

Southeast Arkansas College
Phil E Shirley, PhD, President
1900 Hazel St
Pine Bluff, AR 71603
870 543-5907
Type: Junior or Comm Coll
Control: State, County, or Local Govt
- Emergency Med Tech-Paramedic Prgm
- Radiography Prgm
- Respiratory Therapist (Advanced) Prgm
- Surgical Technology Prgm

University of Arkansas at Pine Bluff
Lawrence A Davis, Chancellor
1200 N University Dr
Pine Bluff, AR 71601
501 575-8470
Type: 4-year Coll or Univ
Control: State, County, or Local Govt
- Dietetics-Didactic Prgm

Pocahontas

Black River Technical College
Richard Gaines, MS, Director
PO Box 468
Pocahontas, AR 72455
870 248-4000
Type: Vocational or Tech Sch
Control: State, County, or Local Govt
- Dietetic Technician-AD Prgm
- Emergency Med Tech-Paramedic Prgm
- Respiratory Therapist (Entry-Level) Prgm

Russellville

Arkansas Tech University
Robert Charles Brown, PhD, President
Administration 210
1605 Coliseum Dr
Russellville, AR 72801
479 968-0237
Type: 4-year Coll or Univ
Control: State, County, or Local Govt
- Health Information Admin Prgm
- Medical Assistant Prgm

Searcy

Harding University
David B Burks, President
915 E Market Ave
Searcy, AR 72149-2256
501 279-4000
Type: 4-year Coll or Univ
Control: Nonprofit (Private or Religious)
- Athletic Training Prgm
- Dietetics-Didactic Prgm
- Physician Assistant Prgm

Springdale

Northwest Technical Institute
George Burch, EdD, President
PO Box 2000
709 S Old Missouri Rd
Springdale, AR 72765
479 751-8824
Type: Vocational or Tech Sch
Control: State, County, or Local Govt
- Surgical Technology Prgm

State University

Arkansas State University
Robert Potts, PhD, Chancellor
Administration, PO Box 600
State University, AR 72467-0010
870 972-3030
Type: 4-year Coll or Univ
Control: State, County, or Local Govt
- Athletic Training Prgm
- Clin Lab Scientist/Med Technologist Prgm
- Clin Lab Technician/Med Lab Technician Prgm
- Counseling Prgm
- Diagnostic Med Sonography Prgm
- Physical Therapist Assistant Prgm
- Physical Therapy Prgm
- Radiation Therapy Prgm
- Radiography Prgm
- Rehabilitation Counseling Prgm
- Speech-Language Pathology Prgm

British Columbia, Canada

Burnaby

Simon Fraser University
Burnaby, BC V5A 1S6
Type: 4-year Coll or Univ
Control: State, County, or Local Govt
- Psychology Prgm

Langley

Trinity Western University
7600 Glover Rd
Langley, BC V2Y 1Y1
604 888-7511
Type: 4-year Coll or Univ
Control: Nonprofit (Private or Religious)
- Counseling Prgm

Vancouver

British Columbia's Children's Hospital
4480 Oak St
Vancouver, BC V6N 3V4
604 875-2111
Type: Hosp or Med Ctr: 100-299 Beds
Control: State, County, or Local Govt
- Orthoptist Prgm

University of British Columbia
Stephen J Toope, PhD, President
T325-Third Floor-Koerner Pavillion
2211 Westbrook Mall
Vancouver, BC V6T 1Z1
Type: 4-year Coll or Univ
Control: State, County, or Local Govt
• Allopathic Medicine Prgm
• Genetic Counseling Prgm
• Medical Librarian Prgm
• Psychology Prgm

Victoria

University of Victoria
Victoria, BC V8W 3P5
Type: 4-year Coll or Univ
Control: State, County, or Local Govt
• Psychology Prgm

California

Alameda

College of Alameda
George Herring, President
555 Atlantic Ave
Alameda, CA 94501
510 522-7221
Type: Junior or Comm Coll
Control: State, County, or Local Govt
• Dental Assisting Prgm

Alhambra

Everest College - Alhambra
Melody Rider, BA, School President
2215 Mission Rd
Alhambra, CA 91803
626 979-4940
Type: Vocational or Tech Sch
Control: For Profit
• Medical Assistant Prgm

Anaheim

Everest College
Cheryl K Smith, BS, School President
511 N Brookhurst St, Ste 300
Anaheim, CA 92801
714 953-6500
Type: Vocational or Tech Sch
Control: For Profit
• Medical Assistant Prgm (2)

North Orange County Community College
Jerome Hunter, PhD, Chancellor
1830 W Romneya Dr
Anaheim, CA 92801
714 808-4797
Type: 4-year Coll or Univ
Control: State, County, or Local Govt
• Pharmacy Technician Prgm

Antioch

Western Career College
Tim Gienapp, BS DC, Executive Director
2157 Country Hills Dr
Antioch, CA 94509
925 522-7749
Type: Vocational or Tech Sch
Control: For Profit
• Medical Assistant Prgm (3)
• Pharmacy Technician Prgm (4)
• Veterinary Technology Prgm (2)

Aptos

Cabrillo College
Brian King, PhD, President/Superintendent
6500 Soquel Dr
Aptos, CA 95003
831 479-6306
Type: Junior or Comm Coll
Control: State, County, or Local Govt
• Dental Hygiene Prgm
• Medical Assistant Prgm
• Radiography Prgm

Arcata

Humboldt State University
Rollin C Richmond, PhD, President
1 Harpst St
Arcata, CA 95521
707 826-3311
Type: 4-year Coll or Univ
Control: State, County, or Local Govt
• Athletic Training Prgm
• Nursing Prgm

Azusa

Azusa Pacific University
Jon R Wallace, DBA, President
901 E Alosta Ave
Azusa, CA 91702
626 812-3031
Type: 4-year Coll or Univ
Control: Nonprofit (Private or Religious)
• Athletic Training Prgm
• Nursing Prgm
• Physical Therapy Prgm
• Psychology Prgm

Bakersfield

Bakersfield College
William Andrews, EdD, President
1801 Panorama Dr
Bakersfield, CA 93305
661 395-4211
Type: Junior or Comm Coll
Control: State, County, or Local Govt
• Emergency Med Tech-Paramedic Prgm
• Radiography Prgm

California State University - Bakersfield
Thomas Arciniega, PhD, President
9001 Stockdale Hwy
Bakersfield, CA 93311
805 833-2241
Type: 4-year Coll or Univ
Control: State, County, or Local Govt
• Nursing Prgm

Clinica Sierra Vista
1430 Truxtun Ave, Ste 120
Bakersfield, CA 93301-3834
Type: Acad Health Ctr/Med Sch
Control: Nonprofit (Private or Religious)
• Dietetic Internship Prgm

Belmont

Notre Dame de Namur University
Jack Oblack, President
Ralston Ave
Belmont, CA 94002
415 593-1601
Type: 4-year Coll or Univ
Control: Nonprofit (Private or Religious)
• Art Therapy Prgm

Berkeley

The Wright Insitute
Berkeley, CA 94704
Type: Acad Health Ctr/Med Sch
Control: For Profit
• Psychology Prgm

TPMG Regional Laboratory
Berkeley, CA 94710
Type: Hosp or Med Ctr: 100-299 Beds
Control: Nonprofit (Private or Religious)
• Histotechnician Prgm

University of California - Berkeley
Robert Berdahl, Chancellor
Berkeley, CA 94720
510 642-6000
Type: 4-year Coll or Univ
Control: State, County, or Local Govt
• Dietetics-Didactic Prgm
• Optometry Prgm
• Psychology Prgm

Burlingame

Mills-Peninsula Health Services
Robert W Merwin, MS, CEO
1501 Trousdale Dr
Burlingame, CA 94010
650 696-5678
Type: Hosp or Med Ctr: 300-499 Beds
Control: Nonprofit (Private or Religious)
• Radiography Prgm

Carson

California State University - Dominguez Hills
Boice Bowman, EdD, Interim President
1000 E Victoria St
Carson, CA 90747
310 243-3301
Type: 4-year Coll or Univ
Control: State, County, or Local Govt
• Clin Lab Scientist/Med Technologist Prgm
• Nursing Prgm
• Occupational Therapy Prgm
• Orthotist/Prosthetist Prgm

Chico

California State University - Chico
Manuel A Esteban, President
Chico, CA 95929-0222
916 898-5871
Type: 4-year Coll or Univ
Control: State, County, or Local Govt
• Dietetic Internship Prgm
• Dietetics-Didactic Prgm
• Nursing Prgm
• Speech-Language Pathology Prgm
• Therapeutic Recreation Specialist Prgm

Chula Vista

Pima Medical Institute
Richard L Luebke, Jr, CEO
780 Bay Blvd, Ste 101
Chula Vista, CA 91910
619 425-3200
Type: Vocational or Tech Sch
Control: Nonprofit (Private or Religious)
• Radiography Prgm
• Respiratory Therapist (Advanced) Prgm

Southwestern College
Neil Yoneji, MS, Interim Supt/President
900 Otay Lakes Rd
Chula Vista, CA 91910
619 482-6301
Type: Junior or Comm Coll
Control: State, County, or Local Govt
• Dental Hygiene Prgm
• Emergency Med Tech-Paramedic Prgm
• Surgical Technology Prgm

Citrus Heights

Western Career College - Citrus
Greg Nathanson, BA, President
7301 Greenback Lane, Ste A
Citrus Heights, CA 95621
916 722-8200
Type: 4-year Coll or Univ
Control: State, County, or Local Govt
• Medical Assistant Prgm
• Pharmacy Technician Prgm
• Veterinary Technology Prgm

Colton

Arrowhead Regional Medical Center
June Griffith-Collison, Director
400 N Pepper Ave
Colton, CA 92324-1819
909 580-6160
Type: Hosp or Med Ctr: 300-499 Beds
Control: State, County, or Local Govt
• Radiography Prgm

Commerce

Los Angeles County Paramedic Training Inst
Cathy Chidester, MSN, Assistant Director
5555 Ferguson Dr, Ste 220
Commerce, CA 90022
323 890-7545
Type: Junior or Comm Coll
Control: State, County, or Local Govt
• Emergency Med Tech-Paramedic Prgm

Concord

Mt Diablo Adult Education
Joanne Durkee, Director of Adult Educ
1266 San Carlos Ave
Concord, CA 94518
925 685-7340
Type: Vocational or Tech Sch
Control: Nonprofit (Private or Religious)
• Surgical Technology Prgm

Costa Mesa

Career Networks Institute
Jim Buffington, BA, President
3420 Bristol St, Ste 209
Costa Mesa, CA 92626
714 568-1566
Type: Vocational or Tech Sch
Control: For Profit
• Surgical Technology Prgm

Orange Coast College
Robert Dees, MA, President
2701 Fairview Rd
Costa Mesa, CA 92628-5005
714 432-5712
Type: Junior or Comm Coll
Control: State, County, or Local Govt
• Cardiovascular Technology Prgm
• Dental Assisting Prgm
• Diagnostic Med Sonography Prgm
• Dietetic Technician-AD Prgm
• Electroneurodiagnostic Tech Prgm
• Medical Assistant Prgm
• Polysomnographic Technology Prgm
• Radiography Prgm
• Respiratory Therapist (Advanced) Prgm

Vanguard University
Murray Dempster, PhD, President
55 Fair Dr
Costa Mesa, CA 92626
714 556-3610
Type: 4-year Coll or Univ
Control: Nonprofit (Private or Religious)
• Athletic Training Prgm

Culver City

West Los Angeles College
Frank Quiambao, President
9000 Overland Ave
Culver City, CA 90230
310 287-4200
Type: Junior or Comm Coll
Control: State, County, or Local Govt
• Dental Hygiene Prgm

Cupertino

De Anza College
Martha Kanter, PhD, President
21250 Stevens Creek Blvd
Cupertino, CA 95014
408 864-8705
Type: Junior or Comm Coll
Control: State, County, or Local Govt
• Clin Lab Technician/Med Lab Technician Prgm

Cypress

Cypress College
Michael Kasler, PhD, President
9200 Valley View St
Cypress, CA 90630
714 484-7000
Type: Junior or Comm Coll
Control: State, County, or Local Govt
• Dental Assisting Prgm
• Dental Hygiene Prgm
• Diagnostic Med Sonography Prgm
• Health Information Tech Prgm
• Radiography Prgm

Duarte

City of Hope
Virgina Opipare, MD, EVP and COO
1500 E Duarte Rd
Duarte, CA 91010
626 359-8111
Type: Hosp or Med Ctr: 300-499 Beds
Control: Nonprofit (Private or Religious)
• Radiation Therapy Prgm

El Cajon

Grossmont College
Sunita Cooke, PhD, President
8800 Grossmont College Dr
El Cajon, CA 92020
619 644-7100
Type: Junior or Comm Coll
Control: State, County, or Local Govt
• Cardiovascular Technology Prgm
• Occupational Therapy Asst Prgm
• Respiratory Therapist (Advanced) Prgm

Encino

Phillips Graduate Institute
Lisa Porche-Burke, PhD, President
5445 Balboa Blvd
Encino, CA 91316-1509
818 386-5600
Control: Nonprofit (Private or Religious)
• Art Therapy Prgm

Eureka

College of the Redwoods
Casey Crabill, President
Tompkins Hill Rd
Eureka, CA 95501
707 445-6700
Type: Junior or Comm Coll
Control: State, County, or Local Govt
• Dental Assisting Prgm

North Coast Emergency Medical Services
Larry Karsteadt, MS, Executive Director
3340 Glenwood St
Eureka, Ca 95501
707 445-2081
Type: Vocational or Tech Sch
Control: State, County, or Local Govt
• Emergency Med Tech-Paramedic Prgm

Foster City

California EMS Academy Inc
Nancy L Black, RN MS, President
1098 Foster City Blvd
Ste 106 PMB 708
Foster City, CA 94404
866 577-9197
Type: Vocational or Tech Sch
Control: State, County, or Local Govt
• Emergency Med Tech-Paramedic Prgm

Fremont

Ohlone College
Douglas Treadway, PhD,
   Superintendent/President
43600 Mission Blvd
PO Box 3909
Fremont, CA 94539
510 659-6200
Type: Junior or Comm Coll
Control: State, County, or Local Govt
• Physical Therapist Assistant Prgm
• Respiratory Therapist (Advanced) Prgm

Fresno

Alliant International University
Fresno, CA 93727
Type: 4-year Coll or Univ
Control: Nonprofit (Private or Religious)
• Psychology Prgm (7)

California State University - Fresno
John D Welty, EdD, President
5241 N Maple Ave
Fresno, CA 93740-0080
559 278-2423
Type: 4-year Coll or Univ
Control: State, County, or Local Govt
• Athletic Training Prgm
• Counseling Prgm
• Dietetic Internship Prgm
• Dietetics-Didactic Prgm
• Nursing Prgm
• Physical Therapy Prgm
• Rehabilitation Counseling Prgm
• Speech-Language Pathology Prgm

Fresno City College
Ned Doffoney, PhD, President
1101 E University Ave
Fresno, CA 93741
559 442-8244
Type: Junior or Comm Coll
Control: State, County, or Local Govt
• Dental Hygiene Prgm
• Emergency Med Tech-Paramedic Prgm
• Health Information Tech Prgm
• Radiography Prgm
• Respiratory Therapist (Advanced) Prgm
• Surgical Technology Prgm

Fresno County Paramedic Program
Brad Maggy, MPA, Interim Director
1221 Fulton Mall
Fresno, CA 93721
559 445-3200
Type: Junior or Comm Coll
Control: State, County, or Local Govt
• Emergency Med Tech-Paramedic Prgm

Fullerton

California State University - Fullerton
Milton A Gordon, PhD, President
PO Box 6810
Fullerton, CA 92834-6810
714 278-3456
Type: 4-year Coll or Univ
Control: State, County, or Local Govt
• Athletic Training Prgm
• Nursing Prgm
• Speech-Language Pathology Prgm

Southern California College of Optometry
Lesley Walls, OD MD, President
2575 Yorba Linda Blvd
Fullerton, CA 92831
714 870-7226
Type: Junior or Comm Coll
Control: Nonprofit (Private or Religious)
• Optometry Prgm

Gardena

Everest College - Gardena
Bill Wherritt, President
1045 W Redondo Beach Blvd, Ste 275
Gardena, CA 90247
310 527-7105
Type: Vocational or Tech Sch
Control: For Profit
• Medical Assistant Prgm

Glendale

Glendale Career College
Serjik Kesachekian, MBA, Regional Campus
   Director
1015 Grandview Ave
Glendale, CA 91201
818 956-4915
Type: Vocational or Tech Sch
Control: For Profit
• Surgical Technology Prgm (2)

Glendale Memorial Hospital and Health Center
1420 S Central Ave
Glendale, CA 91204
818 502-2334
Control: Nonprofit (Private or Religious)
• Dietetic Internship Prgm

Glendora

Citrus College
Michael J Viera, PhD, President/Superintendent
1000 W Foothill
Glendora, CA 91740
818 963-0323
Control: State, County, or Local Govt
• Dental Assisting Prgm

Hayward

California State University - East Bay
Norma S Rees, President
25800 Carlos Bee Blvd
Hayward, CA 94542
510 881-3086
Type: 4-year Coll or Univ
Control: State, County, or Local Govt
• Speech-Language Pathology Prgm

Chabot College
Robert E Carlson, EdD, President
25555 Hesperian Blvd
PO Box 5001
Hayward, CA 94545-5001
510 786-6640
Type: Junior or Comm Coll
Control: State, County, or Local Govt
• Dental Hygiene Prgm
• Health Information Tech Prgm
• Medical Assistant Prgm

Everest College - Hayward
Hector Albizo, President
22336 Main St
Hayward, CA 94541
510 582-9500
Type: Vocational or Tech Sch
Control: For Profit
• Surgical Technology Prgm

Imperial

Imperial Valley Community College
Paul Pai, EdD, President
380 E Aten Rd
Imperial, CA 92251
760 355-6219
Type: Junior or Comm Coll
Control: State, County, or Local Govt
• Emergency Med Tech-Paramedic Prgm

Irvine

Concordia Univesity - Irvine
Jacob Preus, STM ThD, President
1530 Concordia West
Irvine, CA 92612
949 854-8002
Type: 4-year Coll or Univ
Control: Nonprofit (Private or Religious)
• Athletic Training Prgm

University of CA - Irvine School of Medicine
Michael V Drake, MD, Chancellor
510 Administration
Campus Dr
Irvine, CA 92697
949 824-5111
Type: Acad Health Ctr/Med Sch
Control: State, County, or Local Govt
• Allopathic Medicine Prgm
• Genetic Counseling Prgm

Irwindale

Premiere Career College
Fe Ludovico-Aragon, MD, Executive Director
12901 Ramona Blvd
Irwindale, CA 91706
626 814-2080
Type: Vocational or Tech Sch
Control: For Profit
• Surgical Technology Prgm

Public Health Foundation Enterprises
WIC Program
12781 Schabarum Ave
Irwindale, CA 91706-6802
818 856-6376
Control: Nonprofit (Private or Religious)
• Dietetic Internship Prgm

Kentfield

College of Marin
Frances White, PhD, Superintendent/President
835 College Ave
Kentfield, CA 94904
415 457-8811
Type: Junior or Comm Coll
Control: State, County, or Local Govt
• Dental Assisting Prgm

La Jolla

National University
La Jolla, CA 92037
Type: 4-year Coll or Univ
Control: Nonprofit (Private or Religious)
• Nursing Prgm

University of California - San Diego
Marye Anne Fox, PhD, Chancellor
9500 Gilman Dr MC 0005
La Jolla, CA 92093-0657
858 534-3135
Type: Acad Health Ctr/Med Sch
Control: State, County, or Local Government
• Pharmacy Prgm

La Mirada

Biola University
La Mirada, CA 90639
Type: 4-year Coll or Univ
Control: State, County, or Local Govt
• Psychology Prgm (3)

La Puente

Hacienda LaPuente Adult Education
Alan Kern, MA, Adult School Director
Willow Campus
14101 E Nelson Ave
La Puente, CA 91746-2640
626 933-3915
Type: Consortium
Control: Nonprofit (Private or Religious)
• Dental Assisting Prgm
• Respiratory Therapist (Entry-Level) Prgm

La Verne

University of La Verne
Stephen Morgan, EdD, President
1950 Third St
La Verne, CA 91750
909 593-4900
Type: 4-year Coll or Univ
Control: State, County, or Local Govt
• Athletic Training Prgm
• Psychology Prgm

Lake Forest

California Paramedic Institute
Rich Wiederhold, Executive Director
23141 Lake Center Dr
Lake Forest, CA 92630
Type: Acad Health Ctr/Med Sch
Control: Nonprofit (Private or Religious)
• Emergency Med Tech-Paramedic Prgm

Lancaster

Antelope Valley College
Steve Buffalo, PhD, President
3041 W Ave K, Admin Bldg
Lancaster, CA 93534
805 943-3241
Type: 4-year Coll or Univ
Control: State, County, or Local Govt
• Emergency Med Tech-Paramedic Prgm

Livermore

Northern California Training Institute
Floyd Graves, VP Admin & Support Serv
7575 Southfront Rd
Livermore, CA 94550
800 827-0111
Type: Vocational or Tech Sch
Control: For Profit
• Emergency Med Tech-Paramedic Prgm (3)

Loma Linda

Loma Linda University
Richard H Hart, MD Dr PH, Chancellor, CEO
Office of the Chancellor
Magan Hall, Rm 111
Loma Linda, CA 92350-0001
909 558-4540
Type: Acad Health Ctr/Med Sch
Control: Nonprofit (Private or Religious)
• Allopathic Medicine Prgm
• Clin Lab Scientist/Med Technologist Prgm
• Cytotechnology Prgm
• Dental Hygiene Prgm
• Dentistry Prgm
• Diagnostic Med Sonography Prgm
• Dietetic Technician-AD Prgm
• Dietetics-Coordinated Prgm (2)
• Health Information Admin Prgm
• Nursing Prgm
• Occupational Therapy Asst Prgm
• Occupational Therapy Prgm
• Pharmacy Prgm
• Phlebotomy Prgm
• Physical Therapist Assistant Prgm
• Physical Therapy Prgm
• Physician Assistant Prgm
• Psychology Prgm (2)
• Radiation Therapy Prgm
• Radiography Prgm
• Respiratory Therapist (Advanced) Prgm
• Speech-Language Pathology Prgm

Long Beach

American University of Health Sciences
Kim Dang, PhD, President/Owner
3501 Atlantic Ave
Long Beach, CA 90807
562 988-2278
Type: 4-year Coll or Univ
Control: For Profit
• Pharmacy Technician Prgm

California State University - Long Beach
F King Alexander, PhD, President
1250 Bellflower Blvd SS/AD 300
Long Beach, CA 90840-0115
562 985-4121
Type: 4-year Coll or Univ
Control: State, County, or Local Govt
• Athletic Training Prgm
• Dietetic Internship Prgm
• Dietetics-Didactic Prgm
• Kinesiotherapy Prgm
• Nursing Prgm
• Phlebotomy Prgm
• Physical Therapy Prgm
• Radiation Therapy Prgm
• Speech-Language Pathology Prgm
• Therapeutic Recreation Specialist Prgm

Long Beach City College
E Jan Kehoe, PhD, Superintendent/President
4901 E Carson St
Long Beach, CA 90808
562 938-4121
Type: Junior or Comm Coll
Control: State, County, or Local Govt
• Dietetic Technician-AD Prgm

Los Altos Hills

Foothill Community College
Penny Patz, PhD, Interim President
12345 El Monte Rd
Los Altos Hills, CA 94022
650 949-7200
Type: Junior or Comm Coll
Control: State, County, or Local Govt
• Dental Assisting Prgm
• Dental Hygiene Prgm
• Diagnostic Med Sonography Prgm
• Emergency Med Tech-Paramedic Prgm
• Pharmacy Technician Prgm
• Radiography Prgm
• Respiratory Therapist (Advanced) Prgm
• Veterinary Technology Prgm

Los Angeles

American Career College
David A Pyle, President
4021 Rosewood Ave 101
Los Angeles, CA 90004
Type: Vocational or Tech Sch
Control: For Profit
• Pharmacy Technician Prgm

California State University - Los Angeles
James M Rosser, President
5151 State University Dr
Los Angeles, CA 90032
323 343-4690
Type: 4-year Coll or Univ
Control: State, County, or Local Govt
• Audiologist Prgm
• Counseling Prgm
• Dietetics-Coordinated Prgm
• Dietetics-Didactic Prgm
• Orientation and Mobility Specialist Prgm
• Rehabilitation Counseling Prgm
• Speech-Language Pathology Prgm

Center for Child Development/Disabilities/UAP
Walter W Noce, Jr, MPH, President, CEO
4650 Sunset Blvd
Los Angeles, CA 90027
213 669-2301
Type: Hosp or Med Ctr: 300-499 Beds
Control: Nonprofit (Private or Religious)
• Dietetic Internship Prgm

Charles R Drew Univ of Med & Science
Susan Kelly, MD, President/COO
1731 E 120th St
Los Angeles, CA 90059
323 563-4800
Type: 4-year Coll or Univ
Control: Nonprofit (Private or Religious)
• Health Information Tech Prgm
• Pharmacy Technician Prgm
• Physician Assistant Prgm
• Radiography Prgm

Childrens Hospital Los Angeles
4650 Sunset Blvd
Los Angeles, CA 90027
Type: Hosp or Med Ctr: 300-499 Beds
Control: Nonprofit (Private or Religious)
• Orthoptist Prgm

East Los Angeles Education and Career Center
2100 Marengo St
Los Angeles, CA 90033
213 223-1283
Type: Vocational or Tech Sch
Control: State, County, or Local Govt
• Radiography Prgm

Everest College - Los Angeles
Mariam Mohammadi, MET, President
3640 Wilshire Blvd, Ste 500
Los Angeles, CA 90010
213 388-9950
Type: Vocational or Tech Sch
Control: For Profit
• Medical Assistant Prgm

Greater LA Cytotechnology Training Consortium
Sheldon King, MD, Interim Med Ctr Dir
Administration 17-165 CHS
10833 Le Conte Ave
Los Angeles, CA 90024-1730
310 825-5041
Type: Consortium
Control: State, County, or Local Govt
• Cytotechnology Prgm

Jules Stein Eye Institute, UCLA
Bartly J Mondino, MD, Director
100 Stein Plaza
Los Angeles, CA 90095
Type: Acad Health Ctr/Med Sch
Control: Nonprofit (Private or Religious)
• Ophthalmic Assistant Prgm

Los Angeles City College
Jamillah Moore, PhD, Interim President
855 N Vermont Ave
Los Angeles, CA 90029
323 953-4000
Type: Junior or Comm Coll
Control: State, County, or Local Govt
• Dental Lab Technician Prgm
• Dietetic Technician-AD Prgm
• Radiography Prgm

Los Angeles County+USC Healthcare Network
Douglas D Bagley, MS, Interim Exec Dir
1200 N State St, Rm 112
Los Angeles, CA 90033
213 226-6501
Type: Hosp or Med Ctr: 500> Beds
Control: State, County, or Local Govt
• Dietetic Internship Prgm

Loyola Marymount University
Robert B Lawton, SJ, President
1 LMU Dr
Los Angeles, CA 90045
310 338-2700
Type: 4-year Coll or Univ
Control: Nonprofit (Private or Religious)
• Art Therapy Prgm

Mount St Mary's College
Jacqueline Powers Doud, PhD, President
Chalon Campus
12001 Chalon Rd
Los Angeles, CA 90049-1599
310 954-4000
Type: 4-year Coll or Univ
Control: Nonprofit (Private or Religious)
• Nursing Prgm
• Physical Therapy Prgm

UCLA Center for Prehospital Care
Michael Karpf, MD, Vice Provost
17-165 CHS 10833 LeConte Ave
Los Angeles, CA 90095
310 824-5041
Type: Acad Health Ctr/Med Sch
Control: State, County, or Local Govt
• Emergency Med Tech-Paramedic Prgm

University of California - Los Angeles
Albert Carnesale, Chancellor
Box 951405, Murphy Hall 2147
Los Angeles, CA 90095-1405
Type: 4-year Coll or Univ
Control: State, County, or Local Govt
• Allopathic Medicine Prgm
• Dentistry Prgm
• Medical Librarian Prgm
• Nursing Prgm
• Psychology Prgm

University of Southern California
Steven B. Sample, PhD, President
University Park Campus
ADM-110
Los Angeles, CA 90089-0012
213 740-2111
Type: 4-year Coll or Univ
Control: Nonprofit (Private or Religious)
• Allopathic Medicine Prgm
• Dental Hygiene Prgm
• Dentistry Prgm
• Occupational Therapy Prgm
• Pharmacy Prgm
• Physical Therapy Prgm
• Physician Assistant Prgm
• Psychology Prgm

VA Greater Los Angeles Healthcare System
Kenneth J Clark, MA JD, Director
11301 Wilshire Blvd
Los Angeles, CA 90073
310 268-3132
Type: Dept of Veterans Affairs
Control: Fed Govt
• Dietetic Internship Prgm

Malibu

Pepperdine University
David Davenport, President
24255 Pacific Coast Hwy
Malibu, CA 90263
310 456-4000
Type: 4-year Coll or Univ
Control: Nonprofit (Private or Religious)
• Dietetics-Didactic Prgm
• Psychology Prgm

Marysville

Yuba Community College
Paul Mendoza, President
2088 N Beale Rd
Marysville, CA 95901
916 741-6716
Type: Junior or Comm Coll
Control: State, County, or Local Govt
• Radiography Prgm
• Veterinary Technology Prgm

Merced

Merced College
Benjamin Duran, PhD, President/Superintendent
3600 M St
Merced, CA 95348-2898
209 384-6101
Type: Junior or Comm Coll
Control: State, County, or Local Govt
• Diagnostic Med Sonography Prgm
• Radiography Prgm

Mission Viejo

Saddleback College
Dixie Bullock, RN MN, President
28000 Marguerite Pkwy
Mission Viejo, CA 92692
949 582-4500
Type: Junior or Comm Coll
Control: State, County, or Local Govt
• Emergency Med Tech-Paramedic Prgm

Modesto

Modesto Junior College
Richard Rose, PhD, President
435 College Ave
Modesto, CA 95350-9977
209 575-6067
Type: Junior or Comm Coll
Control: State, County, or Local Govt
• Dental Assisting Prgm
• Medical Assistant Prgm
• Respiratory Therapist (Advanced) Prgm

Monterey

Monterey Peninsula College
Kirk Avery, Superintendant/Pres
980 Fremont Ave
Monterey, CA 93940
408 646-4010
Type: Junior or Comm Coll
Control: State, County, or Local Govt
• Dental Assisting Prgm

Monterey Park

East Los Angeles College
Ernest H Moreno, MA, President
1301 Avenida Cesar Chavez
Monterey Park, CA 91754
323 265-8662
Type: Junior or Comm Coll
Control: State, County, or Local Govt
• Health Information Tech Prgm
• Respiratory Therapist (Advanced) Prgm

Moorpark

Moorpark College
Eva Conrad, PhD, President
7075 Campus Rd
Moorpark, CA 93021
805 378-1400
Type: Junior or Comm Coll
Control: State, County, or Local Govt
• Radiography Prgm

Moreno Valley

Riverside County Regional Medical Center
Salvatore Rotella, PhD, President
Moreno Valley Campus
16130 Lasselle St
Moreno Valley, CA 92551-2045
951 571-6166
Type: Acad Health Ctr/Med Sch
Control: State, County, or Local Govt
• Physician Assistant Prgm

Napa

Napa State Hospital
2100 Napa Vallejo Hwy
Napa, CA 94558
707 253-5428
Control: Nonprofit (Private or Religious)
• Dietetic Internship Prgm

Napa Valley College
Diane Carey, PhD, President/Superintendent
2277 Napa Vallejo Hwy
Napa, CA 94558
707 253-3360
Type: Junior or Comm Coll
Control: State, County, or Local Govt
• Respiratory Therapist (Advanced) Prgm

North Hollywood

Maric College
Mark Newman, MA, President
6180 Laurel Canyon Blvd
Suite 101
North Hollywood, CA 91606
818 763-2563
Type: Vocational or Tech Sch
Control: For Profit
• Radiography Prgm
• Respiratory Therapist (Advanced) Prgm

Northridge

California State University - Northridge
Jolene Koester, PhD, President
18111 Nordhoff St
Northridge, CA 91330
818 677-2121
Type: 4-year Coll or Univ
Control: State, County, or Local Govt
• Athletic Training Prgm
• Audiologist Prgm
• Counseling Prgm
• Dietetic Internship Prgm
• Dietetics-Didactic Prgm
• Genetic Counseling Prgm
• Music Therapy Prgm
• Nursing Prgm
• Physical Therapy Prgm
• Radiography Prgm
• Speech-Language Pathology Prgm

Norwalk

Cerritos College
Noelia Vela, EdD, President/Superintendent
11110 E Alondra Blvd
Norwalk, CA 90650
562 860-2451
Type: Junior or Comm Coll
Control: State, County, or Local Govt
• Dental Assisting Prgm
• Dental Hygiene Prgm
• Pharmacy Technician Prgm
• Physical Therapist Assistant Prgm

Oakland

Holy Names University
Oakland, CA 94619
Type: 4-year Coll or Univ
Control: Nonprofit (Private or Religious)
• Nursing Prgm

Merritt College
Evelyn Wesley, PhD, President
12500 Campus Dr
Oakland, CA 94619
510 436-2414
Type: Junior or Comm Coll
Control: State, County, or Local Govt
• Dietetic Technician-AD Prgm
• Radiography Prgm

Samuel Merritt College
Sharon Diaz, MS RN, President
450 30th St
Ste 2840
Oakland, CA 94609-3108
510 869-6512
Type: Acad Health Ctr/Med Sch
Control: Nonprofit (Private or Religious)
• Nursing Prgm
• Occupational Therapy Prgm
• Physical Therapy Prgm
• Physician Assistant Prgm
• Podiatric Medicine Prgm

Orange

Chapman University
James L Doti, PhD, President
One University Dr
Orange, CA 92866
714 997-6611
Type: 4-year Coll or Univ
Control: Nonprofit (Private or Religious)
• Athletic Training Prgm
• Music Therapy Prgm
• Physical Therapy Prgm

Univ of California Irvine Med Ctr
Mark Laret, Executive Director
UCI Medical Ctr
101 City Dr S
Orange, CA 92868-3298
714 456-5678
Type: Acad Health Ctr/Med Sch
Control: State, County, or Local Govt
• Clin Lab Scientist/Med Technologist Prgm

Oroville

Butte College
Diana Van Der Ploeg, PhD, President
3536 Butte Campus Dr
Oroville, CA 95965
530 895-2484
Type: Junior or Comm Coll
Control: State, County, or Local Govt
• Emergency Med Tech-Paramedic Prgm
• Respiratory Therapist (Advanced) Prgm

Oxnard

Oxnard College
Steven F Arvizu, PhD, President
4000 S Rose Ave
Oxnard, CA 93033-6699
805 986-5800
Type: Junior or Comm Coll
Control: State, County, or Local Govt
• Dental Hygiene Prgm

Palo Alto

Pacific Graduate School of Psychology
Palo Alto, CA 94303
Type: Acad Health Ctr/Med Sch
Control: For Profit
• Psychology Prgm (2)

VA Palo Alto Health Care System
Elizabeth Joyce Freeman, Director
3801 Miranda Ave
Palo Alto, CA 94304
650 493-5000
Type: Hosp or Med Ctr: 500> Beds
Control: Nonprofit (Private or Religious)
• Nuclear Medicine Technology Prgm

Pasadena

Fuller Theological Seminary
Pasadena, CA 91101
Type: Acad Health Ctr/Med Sch
Control: For Profit
• Psychology Prgm (2)

Pasadena City College
Paulette Purfumo, PhD, President
1570 E Colorado Blvd
Pasadena, CA 91106
626 585-7123
Type: Junior or Comm Coll
Control: State, County, or Local Govt
• Dental Assisting Prgm
• Dental Hygiene Prgm
• Dental Lab Technician Prgm
• Medical Assistant Prgm
• Radiography Prgm

Patton

Patton State Hospital
3102 E Highland Ave
Patton, CA 92369
909 425-7297
Control: Nonprofit (Private or Religious)
• Dietetic Internship Prgm

Petaluma

Sonoma College
Joe Keats, Chief Executive Officer
1304 Southpoint Blvd, Ste 280
Petaluma, CA 94954
707 283-0800
Type: Vocational or Tech Sch
Control: For Profit
• Physical Therapist Assistant Prgm

Pleasant Hill

Diablo Valley College
Judy Walters, President
321 Golf Club Rd
Pleasant Hill, CA 94523
510 685-1230
Type: Junior or Comm Coll
Control: State, County, or Local Govt
• Dental Assisting Prgm
• Dental Hygiene Prgm

John F Kennedy University
Pleasant Hill, CA 94523
Type: 4-year Coll or Univ
Control: Nonprofit (Private or Religious)
• Psychology Prgm

Pomona

California State Polytechnic University
Bob H Suzuki, President
3801 W Temple Ave
Pomona, CA 91768
909 869-2000
Type: 4-year Coll or Univ
Control: State, County, or Local Govt
• Dietetic Internship Prgm
• Dietetics-Didactic Prgm
• Veterinary Technology Prgm

DeVry University - Pomona Campus
Rose Dishman, Regional Vice President
901 Corporate Center Dr
Pomona, CA 91768
909 868-4180
Type: 4-year Coll or Univ
Control: State, County, or Local Govt
• Health Information Tech Prgm

Western Univ of Health Sciences
Philip Pumerantz, PhD, President
309 E Second St
Pomona, CA 91766-1854
909 469-5200
Type: Acad Health Ctr/Med Sch
Control: Nonprofit (Private or Religious)
• Osteopathic Medicine Prgm
• Pharmacy Prgm
• Physical Therapy Prgm
• Physician Assistant Prgm
• Veterinary Medicine Prgm

Porterville

Porterville Development Center
Porterville, CA 93258
209 782-2753
Control: Nonprofit (Private or Religious)
• Dietetic Internship Prgm

Rancho Cucamonga

Chaffey College
Henry Shannon, PhD, Superintendent/President
5885 Haven Ave
Rancho Cucamonga, CA 91737
909 941-2100
Type: Junior or Comm Coll
Control: State, County, or Local Govt
• Dental Assisting Prgm
• Dietetic Technician-AD Prgm
• Radiography Prgm

Rancho Mirage

Eisenhower Medical Center
Andrew Deems, President/CEO
39000 Bob Hope Dr
Rancho Mirage, CA 92270
619 340-3911
Type: Hosp or Med Ctr: 100-299 Beds
Control: Nonprofit (Private or Religious)
• Clin Lab Scientist/Med Technologist Prgm

Redding

Shasta College
Gary Lewis, Superintendent/President
PO Box 496006
Redding, CA 96049-6006
530 225-4600
Type: Junior or Comm Coll
Control: State, County, or Local Govt
• Dental Hygiene Prgm

Redlands

American College of Health Professions
Michele Brooks, President/CEO
700 E Redlands Blvd, U227
Redlands, CA 92373
909 307-6022
Type: Vocational or Tech Sch
Control: For Profit
• Surgical Technology Prgm

University of Redlands
Stuart Dorsey, President
PO Box 3080
1200 E Colton Ave
Redlands, CA 92373-0999
909 793-2121
Type: 4-year Coll or Univ
Control: Nonprofit (Private or Religious)
• Speech-Language Pathology Prgm

Redwood City

Canada College
Tom Mohr, President
4200 Farm Hill Blvd
Redwood City, CA 94061
650 306-3283
Type: Junior or Comm Coll
Control: State, County, or Local Govt
• Radiography Prgm

Reedley

Central Valley WIC Dietetic Internship
1560 E Manning Ave
Reedley, CA 93654
Type: Acad Health Ctr/Med Sch
Control: Fed Govt
• Dietetic Internship Prgm

Reseda

Everest College - Reseda
Steven R Schilling, BA MA, President
18040 Sherman Way
Reseda, CA 91335
818 774-0550
Type: Vocational or Tech Sch
Control: For Profit
• Surgical Technology Prgm

Richmond

Kaiser Permanente Sch of Allied Hlth Sciences
Gwenette S Jackson, BA CRT, School
  Administrator
938 Marina Way South
Richmond, CA 94804
510 307-2412
Type: Vocational or Tech Sch
Control: Nonprofit (Private or Religious)
• Diagnostic Med Sonography Prgm
• Nuclear Medicine Technology Prgm
• Radiation Therapy Prgm
• Radiography Prgm

Riverside

Riverside Comm Coll - Moreno Valley Campus
Salvatore G Rotella, PhD, President
4800 Magnolia Ave
Riverside, CA 92506-1299
909 222-8000
Type: Junior or Comm Coll
Control: State, County, or Local Govt
• Dental Hygiene Prgm
• Emergency Med Tech-Paramedic Prgm

Rohnert Park

Sonoma State University
1801 E Cotati Ave
Rohnert Park, CA 94928-3609
707 664-2880
Type: 4-year Coll or Univ
Control: State, County, or Local Govt
• Counseling Prgm

Sacramento

American River College
David Viar, EdD, President
4700 College Oak Dr
Sacramento, CA 95841
916 484-8211
Type: Junior or Comm Coll
Control: State, County, or Local Govt
• Emergency Med Tech-Paramedic Prgm
• Respiratory Therapist (Advanced) Prgm

California State University - Sacramento
Alexander Gonzalez, PhD, President
CSUS 6000 J St
Sacramento, CA 95819
916 278-7737
Type: 4-year Coll or Univ
Control: State, County, or Local Govt
• Athletic Training Prgm
• Audiologist Prgm
• Dietetic Internship Prgm
• Dietetics-Didactic Prgm
• Nursing Prgm
• Physical Therapy Prgm
• Rehabilitation Counseling Prgm
• Speech-Language Pathology Prgm

Charles A Jones Skills & Business Ed Center
Kirk Williams, CEO, Principal
5451 Lemon Hill Ave
Sacramento, CA 95824-1529
Type: Acad Health Ctr/Med Sch
Control: State, County, or Local Govt
• Pharmacy Technician Prgm

Cosumnes River Community College
Francisco Rodriguez, PhD, President
8401 Center Pkwy
Sacramento, CA 95823
916 688-7321
Type: Junior or Comm Coll
Control: State, County, or Local Govt
• Dietetic Technician-AD Prgm
• Health Information Tech Prgm
• Medical Assistant Prgm
• Veterinary Technology Prgm

Sacramento City College
Deborah J Travis, MBA, Interim President
3835 Freeport Blvd
Sacramento, CA 95822-1386
916 558-2100
Type: Junior or Comm Coll
Control: State, County, or Local Govt
• Dental Assisting Prgm
• Dental Hygiene Prgm
• Occupational Therapy Asst Prgm
• Physical Therapist Assistant Prgm

UC Davis Medical Center
2315 Stockton Blvd
Sacramento, CA 95817
Type: Acad Health Ctr/Med Sch
Control: State, County, or Local Govt
• Dietetic Internship Prgm

Univ of California Davis Health System
Ann Rice, Hospital CEO
2315 Stockton Blvd
Sacramento, CA 95817
916 453-0750
Type: Acad Health Ctr/Med Sch
Control: State, County, or Local Govt
• Clin Lab Scientist/Med Technologist Prgm

University of California - Davis
Claire Pomeroy, MD, Dean
School of Medicine
4610 X Street, Ste 3101
Sacramento, CA 95817
916 734-3578
Type: Acad Health Ctr/Med Sch
Control: State, County, or Local Govt
• Allopathic Medicine Prgm
• Dietetics-Didactic Prgm
• Physician Assistant Prgm
• Veterinary Medicine Prgm

Western Career College - Sacramento
Greg Nathanson, BA, President
7801 Folsom Blvd, Ste 210
Sacramento, CA 95826-9823
916 388-2800
Type: Vocational or Tech Sch
Control: For Profit
• Dental Hygiene Prgm
• Medical Assistant Prgm
• Pharmacy Technician Prgm
• Veterinary Technology Prgm

Salinas

Hartnell College
Edward J Valeau, EdD, President
156 Homestead Ave
Salinas, CA 93901
831 755-6700
Type: Junior or Comm Coll
Control: State, County, or Local Govt
• Clin Lab Technician/Med Lab Technician Prgm
• Veterinary Technology Prgm

San Bernardino

California State University - San Bernardino
Anthony H Evans, President
5500 University Pkwy
San Bernardino, CA 92407
909 880-5000
Type: 4-year Coll or Univ
Control: State, County, or Local Govt
• Dietetics-Didactic Prgm
• Nursing Prgm
• Rehabilitation Counseling Prgm

Everest College - San Bernardino
217 E Club Center Dr
San Bernardino, CA 92408
Type: Vocational or Tech Sch
Control: For Profit
• Medical Assistant Prgm

San Bruno

Skyline College
Victoria Morrow, PhD, President
3300 College Dr
San Bruno, CA 94066
650 738-4111
Type: Junior or Comm Coll
Control: State, County, or Local Govt
• Respiratory Therapist (Advanced) Prgm
• Surgical Technology Prgm

San Diego

California College San Diego
Carl Barney, CEO
2820 Camino del Rio S
San Diego, CA 92108
619 295-5785
Type: 4-year Coll or Univ
Control: For Profit
• Respiratory Therapist (Advanced) Prgm
• Respiratory Therapist (Entry-Level) Prgm

Concorde Career College
Timothy Vogeley, MBA, Campus President
4393 Imperial Ave
Ste 100
San Diego, CA 92113
619 688-0800
Type: Vocational or Tech Sch
Control: For Profit
• Medical Assistant Prgm (2)
• Respiratory Therapist (Advanced) Prgm
• Respiratory Therapist (Entry-Level) Prgm
• Surgical Technology Prgm (3)

Mueller College of Holistic Massage Therapies
Jeff Welsh, PhD MA HHP, President and CEO
4607 Park Blvd
San Diego, CA 92116
619 291-9811
Type: Vocational or Tech Sch
Control: For Profit
• Massage Therapy Prgm

Naval School of Health Sciences, San Diego
FC Crosby, CAPT MSC USN, Commanding Officer
34101 Farenholt Ave
San Diego, CA 92134-5291
619 532-7700
Type: Dept of Defense
Control: Fed Govt
• Cardiovascular Technology Prgm
• Clin Lab Technician/Med Lab Technician Prgm
• Radiography Prgm
• Surgical Technology Prgm

Point Loma Nazarene University
Bob Brower, PhD, President
3900 Lomaland Dr
San Diego, CA 92106
619 849-2216
Type: Acad Health Ctr/Med Sch
Control: For Profit
• Athletic Training Prgm
• Dietetics-Didactic Prgm
• Nursing Prgm

San Diego Mesa College
Rita Cepeda, EdD, President
7250 Mesa College Dr
San Diego, CA 92111
619 388-2755
Type: Junior or Comm Coll
Control: State, County, or Local Govt
• Dental Assisting Prgm
• Health Information Tech Prgm
• Medical Assistant Prgm
• Physical Therapist Assistant Prgm
• Radiography Prgm

San Diego State University
Stephen L Weber, PhD, President
5500 Campanile Dr
San Diego, CA 92182-1518
619 594-7746
Type: 4-year Coll or Univ
Control: State, County, or Local Govt
• Athletic Training Prgm
• Audiologist Prgm
• Dietetic Internship Prgm
• Dietetics-Didactic Prgm
• Kinesiotherapy Prgm
• Nursing Prgm
• Psychology Prgm
• Rehabilitation Counseling Prgm
• Speech-Language Pathology Prgm

Univ of California San Diego Med Ctr
Richard Liekweg, Director
200 W Arbor Dr, H-910C
San Diego, CA 92103-8970
619 543-6654
Type: Hosp or Med Ctr: 300-499 Beds
Control: State, County, or Local Govt
• Allopathic Medicine Prgm
• Diagnostic Med Sonography Prgm
• Nursing Prgm

VA San Diego Healthcare System
3350 La Jolla Village Dr
San Diego, CA 92161
619 552-8585
Control: Fed Govt
• Dietetic Internship Prgm

San Fernando

Northeast Valley Health Corporation
1172 N Maclay Ave
San Fernando, CA 91340
Control: Nonprofit (Private or Religious)
• Dietetic Internship Prgm

San Francisco

California Institute of Integral Studies
San Francisco, CA 94103
Type: Acad Health Ctr/Med Sch
Control: Nonprofit (Private or Religious)
• Psychology Prgm

City College of San Francisco
Philip R Day, Jr, PhD, Chancellor
50 Phelan Ave
San Francisco, CA 94112
415 239-3000
Type: Junior or Comm Coll
Control: State, County, or Local Govt
• Dental Assisting Prgm
• Emergency Med Tech-Paramedic Prgm
• Health Information Tech Prgm
• Medical Assistant Prgm
• Radiation Therapy Prgm
• Radiography Prgm

Everest College - San Francisco
Barbara Woosley, MA, President
814 Mission St
San Francisco, CA 94103
415 777-2500
Type: Vocational or Tech Sch
Control: For Profit
• Medical Assistant Prgm

Heald College
Nolan Miura, MBA, President/CEO
670 Howard St
San Francisco, CA 94105
415 808-1400
Type: Vocational or Tech Sch
Control: For Profit
• Dental Assisting Prgm (3)
• Medical Assistant Prgm (9)

San Francisco State University
Robert A Corrigan, PhD, President
1600 Holloway Ave
San Francisco, CA 94132
415 338-1381
Type: 4-year Coll or Univ
Control: State, County, or Local Govt
• Audiologist Prgm
• Clin Lab Scientist/Med Technologist Prgm
• Counseling Prgm
• Dietetic Internship Prgm
• Dietetics-Didactic Prgm
• Nursing Prgm
• Orientation and Mobility Specialist Prgm
• Rehabilitation Counseling Prgm
• Speech-Language Pathology Prgm

UCSF Medical Center
Mark Laret, MA, CEO
500 Parnassus Ave
San Francisco, CA 94143
415 353-2733
Type: Hosp or Med Ctr: 300-499 Beds
Control: State, County, or Local Govt
• Surgical Technology Prgm

University of California - San Francisco
Hailet Debas, MD, Chancellor
Box 0402
San Francisco, CA 94143
415 476-2401
Type: Acad Health Ctr/Med Sch
Control: State, County, or Local Govt
• Allopathic Medicine Prgm
• Dentistry Prgm
• Dietetic Internship Prgm
• Nursing Prgm
• Pharmacy Prgm
• Physical Therapy Prgm

San Jose

San Jose City College
Chui Tsang, President
2100 Moorpark Ave
San Jose, CA 95128
408 298-2181
Control: State, County, or Local Govt
• Dental Assisting Prgm

San Jose State University
Don W Kassing, MBA, President
Tower Hall 206
One Washington Square
San Jose, CA 95192-0002
408 924-1177
Type: 4-year Coll or Univ
Control: State, County, or Local Govt
• Athletic Training Prgm
• Clin Lab Scientist/Med Technologist Prgm
• Dietetic Internship Prgm
• Dietetics-Didactic Prgm
• Medical Librarian Prgm
• Nursing Prgm
• Occupational Therapy Prgm
• Speech-Language Pathology Prgm

Western Career College - San Jose
Steve Shishani, MA, Executive Director
6201 San Ignacio Ave
San Jose, CA 95119
408 360-0840
Type: Vocational or Tech Sch
Control: For Profit
• Medical Assistant Prgm
• Pharmacy Technician Prgm
• Veterinary Technology Prgm

WestMed College
Veronica Shepardson, RN, School Director
1330 S Bascom Ave, Ste G
San Jose, CA 95128
408 977-0723
Type: Vocational or Tech Sch
Control: For Profit
• Emergency Med Tech-Paramedic Prgm

San Leandro

Western Career College - San Leandro
Greg Nathanson, President
15555 E 14th St, Ste 500
San Leandro, CA 94578-9930
510 276-3888
Type: Vocational or Tech Sch
Control: For Profit
- Medical Assistant Prgm
- Pharmacy Technician Prgm
- Veterinary Technology Prgm

San Luis Obispo

California Polytechnic State University
Warren J Baker, President
San Luis Obispo, CA 93407
805 756-1111
Type: 4-year Coll or Univ
Control: State, County, or Local Govt
- Dietetic Internship Prgm
- Dietetics-Didactic Prgm

Central California School of Continuing Edu
Gene R Appleby, Administrator
3195 McMillan #F
San Luis Obispo, CA 93401
805 543-9123
Type: Vocational or Tech Sch
Control: For Profit
- Radiography Prgm

San Marcos

Palomar Community College
Robert Deegan, EdD, Superintendent/President
1140 W Mission Rd
San Marcos, CA 92069
760 744-1150
Type: Junior or Comm Coll
Control: State, County, or Local Govt
- Dental Assisting Prgm
- Emergency Med Tech-Paramedic Prgm

San Mateo

College of San Mateo
Peter J Landsberger, President
1700 W Hillsdale Blvd
San Mateo, CA 94402
415 574-6161
Type: Junior or Comm Coll
Control: State, County, or Local Govt
- Dental Assisting Prgm

Hospital Consortium Education Network
Francine Serafin-Dickson, MBA RN, Executive
    Director
222 W 39th Ave
Ste 3A09, San Mateo Medical Center
San Mateo, CA 94403
650 573-3930
Type: Consortium
Control: Nonprofit (Private or Religious)
- Emergency Med Tech-Paramedic Prgm

San Pablo

Contra Costa College
D Candy Rose, President
2600 Mission Bell Dr
San Pablo, CA 94806
510 235-7800
Control: State, County, or Local Govt
- Dental Assisting Prgm

San Rafael

Dominican University of California
Joseph R Fink, PhD, President
50 Acacia Ave
San Rafael, CA 94901-2298
415 485-3200
Type: 4-year Coll or Univ
Control: State, County, or Local Govt
- Nursing Prgm
- Occupational Therapy Prgm

Santa Ana

Newbridge College
J Ramon Villanueva, School Director
1840 E 17th St, Ste 140
Santa Ana, CA 92705
714 550-8000
Type: Vocational or Tech Sch
Control: For Profit
- Surgical Technology Prgm

Santa Ana College
Erlinda Martinez, EdD, President
1530 W 17th St
Santa Ana, CA 92706-3398
714 564-6975
Type: Junior or Comm Coll
Control: State, County, or Local Govt
- Occupational Therapy Asst Prgm
- Pharmacy Technician Prgm

Santa Barbara

Fielding Graduate University
Santa Barbara, CA 93105
Type: 4-year Coll or Univ
Control: Nonprofit (Private or Religious)
- Psychology Prgm

Santa Barbara City College
John Romo, Supt/President
721 Cliff Dr
Santa Barbara, CA 93109-2394
805 965-0581
Type: Junior or Comm Coll
Control: State, County, or Local Govt
- Health Information Tech Prgm
- Radiography Prgm

Santa Barbara Cottage Hospital
James L Ash, President/CEO
PO Box 689 Pueblo at Bath Sts
Santa Barbara, CA 93102
805 569-7290
Type: Hosp or Med Ctr: 300-499 Beds
Control: Nonprofit (Private or Religious)
- Clin Lab Scientist/Med Technologist Prgm

Santa Cruz

Emergency Training Services Inc
David Barbin, BS, CEO
3050 Paul Sweet Rd
Santa Cruz, CA 95065
831 476-8813
Type: Vocational or Tech Sch
Control: For Profit
- Emergency Med Tech-Paramedic Prgm

Santa Rosa

Santa Rosa Junior College
Robert F Agrella, EdD, Superintendent/President
1501 Mendocino Ave
Santa Rosa, CA 95401
707 527-4431
Type: Junior or Comm Coll
Control: State, County, or Local Govt
- Dental Assisting Prgm
- Dental Hygiene Prgm
- Emergency Med Tech-Paramedic Prgm
- Radiography Prgm

Saratoga

West Valley Community College District
Phil Hartley, PhD, President
14000 Fruitvale Ave
Saratoga, CA 95070
408 867-2200
Type: Junior or Comm Coll
Control: State, County, or Local Govt
- Medical Assistant Prgm

Simi Valley

Simi Valley Adult School
Sondra Jones, MA, Director
3192 Los Angeles Ave
Simi Valley, CA 93065
805 579-6200
Type: Vocational or Tech Sch
Control: State, County, or Local Govt
- Respiratory Therapist (Entry-Level) Prgm
- Surgical Technology Prgm

South Gate

Career Colleges of America
Jeff Meisel, CEO
5612 E Imperial Hwy
South Gate, CA 90280
562 861-8702
Type: Vocational or Tech Sch
Control: For Profit
- Surgical Technology Prgm (3)

Stanford

Stanford University School of Medicine
Phillip Pizzo, MD, Dean
School of Medicine Rm M121
Stanford, CA 94305-5302
415 723-6436
Type: Acad Health Ctr/Med Sch
Control: Nonprofit (Private or Religious)
- Allopathic Medicine Prgm
- Physician Assistant Prgm

INSTITUTIONS

Stockton

Emergency Medical Sciences Training Institute
Craig Stroup, BS EMT-P, Program Director
343 E Main St #906
Stockton, CA 95202
209 461-5550
Type: Vocational or Tech Sch
Control: Nonprofit (Private or Religious)
• Emergency Med Tech-Paramedic Prgm

San Joaquin General Hospital
Richard Aldred, Hospital Director
PO Box 1020
Stockton, CA 95201
209 468-6600
Type: Hosp or Med Ctr: 100-299 Beds
Control: State, County, or Local Govt
• Radiography Prgm

University of the Pacific
Donald De Rosa, President
3601 Pacific Ave
Stockton, CA 95211
209 946-2222
Type: 4-year Coll or Univ
Control: For Profit
• Athletic Training Prgm
• Dentistry Prgm
• Music Therapy Prgm
• Pharmacy Prgm
• Physical Therapy Prgm
• Speech-Language Pathology Prgm

Sylmar

Olive View/UCLA Medical Center
Melinda D Anderson, CEO
14445 Olive View Dr, Rm 2C155
Sylmar, CA 91342-1495
818 364-4224
Type: Hosp or Med Ctr: 100-299 Beds
Control: State, County, or Local Govt
• Dietetic Internship Prgm

Taft

Taft College
Darnell Roe, EdD, President/Superintendent
29 Emmons Park Dr
Box 1437
Taft, CA 93268
661 763-7700
Type: Junior or Comm Coll
Control: State, County, or Local Govt
• Dental Hygiene Prgm

Thousand Oaks

California Lutheran University
Howard Wennes, PhD, Interim President
60 W Olsen Rd, MC-1300
Thousand Oaks, CA 91360
805 493-3100
Type: 4-year Coll or Univ
Control: Nonprofit (Private or Religious)
• Athletic Training Prgm

Torrance

El Camino College
Thomas M Fallo, Superintendent/President
16007 Crenshaw Blvd
Torrance, CA 90506
310 532-3670
Type: Junior or Comm Coll
Control: State, County, or Local Govt
• Radiography Prgm
• Respiratory Therapist (Entry-Level) Prgm

LA County Harbor UCLA Medical Center
Tecla Mickoseff, MBA, Acting Hosp Admin
1000 W Carson St Box 1
Torrance, CA 90509-2910
310 222-2101
Type: Hosp or Med Ctr: 500> Beds
Control: State, County, or Local Govt
• Nuclear Medicine Technology Prgm
• Radiography Prgm

Southern California Regional Occupational Ctr
Christine Hoffman, EdD, Superintendent
2300 Crenshaw Blvd
Torrance, CA 90501
310 224-4220
Type: Vocational or Tech Sch
Control: State, County, or Local Govt
• Medical Assistant Prgm

Turlock

California State University - Stanislaus
David P Dauwalder, PhD, Provost/VP
801 W Monte Vista Ave
Turlock, CA 95382
209 667-3203
Type: 4-year Coll or Univ
Control: State, County, or Local Govt
• Nursing Prgm

Ukiah

Mendocino Community College
Marylyn G Brock, EdD, President
1000 Hensley Creek Rd
Ukiah, CA 95482
707 468-3071
Type: Junior or Comm Coll
Control: State, County, or Local Govt
• Emergency Med Tech-Paramedic Prgm

Vallejo

Touro University Mare Island
Bernard Laner, President
1310 Johnson Ln
Vallejo, CA 94592
707 638-5442
Type: 4-year Coll or Univ
Control: State, County, or Local Govt
• Osteopathic Medicine Prgm
• Pharmacy Prgm
• Physician Assistant Prgm

Valley Glen

Los Angeles Valley College
Tyree Weider, EdD, President
5800 Fulton Ave
Valley Glen, CA 91401-4096
818 947-2321
Type: Junior or Comm Coll
Control: State, County, or Local Govt
• Respiratory Therapist (Advanced) Prgm

Ventura

Ventura College
Larry Claderon, EdD, President
School of Prehospital & Emergency Med
4667 Telegraph Rd
Ventura, CA 93003
805 654-6460
Type: Junior or Comm Coll
Control: State, County, or Local Govt
• Emergency Med Tech-Paramedic Prgm

Victorville

Victor Valley Community College District
Patricia Spencer, PhD, President/Superintendent
18422 Bear Valley Rd
Victorville, CA 92392-5849
760 245-4271
Type: Junior or Comm Coll
Control: State, County, or Local Govt
• Emergency Med Tech-Paramedic Prgm
• Respiratory Therapist (Advanced) Prgm

Visalia

San Joaquin Valley College
Mark Perry, President
3828 W Caldwell Ave
Visalia, CA 93277
559 734-9000
Type: Junior or Comm Coll
Control: For Profit
• Dental Hygiene Prgm
• Physician Assistant Prgm
• Respiratory Therapist (Advanced) Prgm (3)
• Surgical Technology Prgm (2)

Walnut

Mt San Antonio College
Christopher C O'Hearn, MA MEd, President/CEO
1100 N Grand Ave
Walnut, CA 91789
909 594-5611
Type: Junior or Comm Coll
Control: State, County, or Local Govt
• Emergency Med Tech-Paramedic Prgm
• Histotechnician Prgm
• Radiography Prgm
• Respiratory Therapist (Advanced) Prgm
• Veterinary Technology Prgm

West Covina

East San Gabriel Valley ROP
Laurel Adler, EdD, Superintendent
1501 W Del Norte Ave
West Covina, CA 91790
626 472-5121
Type: Vocational or Tech Sch
Control: State, County, or Local Govt
• Medical Assistant Prgm

North-West College
Marsha Fuerst, President/CEO
2121 W Garvey Ave N
West Covina, CA 91790
626 960-5046
Type: Vocational or Tech Sch
Control: For Profit
• Pharmacy Technician Prgm (4)

Woodland Hills

Los Angeles Pierce College
Robert Garber, President
6201 Winnetka Ave
Woodland Hills, CA 91371
818 719-6408
Type: 4-year Coll or Univ
Control: State, County, or Local Govt
• Veterinary Technology Prgm

Yucaipa

Crafton Hills College
Gloria Macias Harrison, MA, President
11711 Sand Canyon Rd
Yucaipa, CA 92399
909 389-3200
Type: Junior or Comm Coll
Control: State, County, or Local Govt
• Emergency Med Tech-Paramedic Prgm
• Respiratory Therapist (Advanced) Prgm
• Respiratory Therapist (Entry-Level) Prgm

Colorado

Alamosa

Adams State College
Richard Wueste, JD, President
208 Edgemont Blvd
Richardson Hall 210
Alamosa, CO 81102-0001
719 587-7341
Type: 4-year Coll or Univ
Control: State, County, or Local Govt
• Counseling Prgm
• Nursing Prgm

Aurora

Concorde Career College - Aurora
Barbara Kearns, MA, Campus President
111 N Havana St
Aurora, CO 80010
303 861-1151
Type: Vocational or Tech Sch
Control: For Profit
• Radiography Prgm
• Surgical Technology Prgm

Rocky Vista Univ Coll of Osteopathic Medicine
3449 Chambers Rd, Ste B
Aurora, CO 80011
Type: Acad Health Ctr/Med Sch
Control: Nonprofit (Private or Religious)
• Osteopathic Medicine Prgm

T H Pickens Technical Center
Art Bogardus, PhD, Executive Director
Career and Technical Education
500 Airport Blvd
Aurora, CO 80011
303 344-4910
Type: Vocational or Tech Sch
Control: State, County, or Local Govt
• Dental Assisting Prgm
• Respiratory Therapist (Advanced) Prgm
• Respiratory Therapist (Entry-Level) Prgm

U of Colorado (Denver) Health Sciences Center
Bruce Schroffel, MS, President
131001 E 17th Pl, Ste C-1015
F-417 PO Box 6508
Aurora, CO 80045-0508
303 724-5773
Type: Acad Health Ctr/Med Sch
Control: State, County, or Local Govt
• Counseling Prgm
• Dentistry Prgm
• Diagnostic Med Sonography Prgm
• Genetic Counseling Prgm
• Physical Therapy Prgm
• Physician Assistant Prgm

Boulder

Naropa University
Thomas Coburn, PhD, President
2130 Arapahoe Ave
Boulder, CO 80302
303 444-0202
Type: 4-year Coll or Univ
Control: Nonprofit (Private or Religious)
• Art Therapy Prgm
• Dance/Movement Therapy Prgm

University of Colorado at Boulder
Campus Box 409
Boulder, CO 80309-0409
303 492-6445
Type: 4-year Coll or Univ
Control: State, County, or Local Government
• Audiologist Prgm
• Psychology Prgm
• Speech-Language Pathology Prgm

Colorado Springs

Centura Health/Penrose-St Francis Hlth Serv
Rick O'Connell, MBA, CEO
Penrose Hospital, Member Centura Health
2222 N Nevada Ave, PO Box 7021
Colorado Springs, CO 80907-7021
719 776-5111
Type: Hosp or Med Ctr: 300-499 Beds
Control: Nonprofit (Private or Religious)
• Clin Lab Scientist/Med Technologist Prgm
• Dietetic Internship Prgm

Everest College
Larry Jackson, MA BA, President
1815 Jet Wing Dr
Colorado Springs, CO 80916
719 638-6580
Type: Junior or Comm Coll
Control: For Profit
• Medical Assistant Prgm (3)
• Surgical Technology Prgm

IntelliTec Medical Institute
2345 N Academy Blvd
Colorado Springs, CO 80909
Type: Hosp or Med Ctr: 100-299 Beds
Control: Nonprofit (Private or Religious)
• Dental Assisting Prgm

Memorial Hospital
Richard Eitel, MBA, Exec Director
1400 East Boulder
175 S Union Suite 240
Colorado Springs, CO 80909
719 365-5000
Type: Hosp or Med Ctr: 300-499 Beds
Control: State, County, or Local Govt
• Radiography Prgm

Pikes Peak Community College
Edwin Ray, PhD, VP of Educational Service
5765 S Academy Blvd
Colorado Springs, CO 80906
719 502-3100
Type: Junior or Comm Coll
Control: State, County, or Local Govt
• Dental Assisting Prgm
• Emergency Med Tech-Paramedic Prgm

University of Colorado at Colorado Springs
Pam Shockley Zalabat, PhD, Chancellor
1420 Austin Bluffs Pkwy
Colorado Springs, CO 80933-7150
719 262-3000
Type: 4-year Coll or Univ
Control: State, County, or Local Govt
• Counseling Prgm
• Dietetics-Didactic Prgm
• Nursing Prgm

Denver

Bel-Rea Institute of Animal Technology
Nolan Rucker, BS MS DVM, Dean of Education
1681 S Dayton St
Denver, CO 80231
Control: Nonprofit (Private or Religious)
• Veterinary Technology Prgm

Centura Health-St Anthony Hospitals
George Zara, CEO, St Anthony Hospitals
4231 W 16th Ave
Denver, CO 80204
303 629-4350
Type: Hosp or Med Ctr: 500> Beds
Control: Nonprofit (Private or Religious)
• Emergency Med Tech-Paramedic Prgm
• Radiography Prgm

INSTITUTIONS

Colorado Center for Med Laboratory Science
Anne Warhover, MD, President/CEO
501 S Cherry St #1100
Denver, CO 80246
303 953-3600
Type: Acad Health Ctr/Med Sch
Control: Nonprofit (Private or Religious)
• Clin Lab Scientist/Med Technologist Prgm

Community College of Aurora
Les Moroye, MA, Assoc VP
9235 E 10th Dr, Rm 118
Denver, CO 80230
303 340-7119
Type: Junior or Comm Coll
Control: State, County, or Local Govt
• Emergency Med Tech-Paramedic Prgm

Community College of Denver
Barbara Casey, JD, President
PO Box 173363
Denver, CO 80217
303 556-2600
Type: Junior or Comm Coll
Control: State, County, or Local Govt
• Dental Hygiene Prgm
• Medical Assistant Prgm
• Radiography Prgm
• Veterinary Technology Prgm

Denver Health Medical Center
Patricia Gabow, MD, CEO
660 Bannock St Mail Code 0278
Denver, CO 80204
303 436-6611
Type: Hosp or Med Ctr: 300-499 Beds
Control: State, County, or Local Govt
• Emergency Med Tech-Paramedic Prgm

Emily Griffith Opportunity School
Sharon Johnson
1250 Welton St
Denver, CO 80204
303 575-4721
Type: Vocational or Tech Sch
Control: State, County, or Local Govt
• Dental Assisting Prgm

Heritage College
Richard Shepard, BS, President
4704 Harlan St #100
Denver, CO 80212
720 855-6014
Type: Vocational or Tech Sch
Control: For Profit
• Surgical Technology Prgm

Johnson & Wales University
7150 Montview Blvd
Denver, CO 80220
Control: Nonprofit (Private or Religious)
• Dietetics-Didactic Prgm

Massage Therapy Institute of Colorado
Mark Manton, Director
1441 York St, Ste 301
Denver, CO 80206
303 329-6345
Type: Acad Health Ctr/Med Sch
Control: For Profit
• Massage Therapy Prgm

Metropolitan State College of Denver
Raymond Kieft, EdD, Interim President
Campus Box 1
PO Box 173362
Denver, CO 80217-3362
303 556-3022
Type: 4-year Coll or Univ
Control: State, County, or Local Govt
• Athletic Training Prgm

Regis University
Michael J Sheeran, SJ, President
3333 Regis Blvd
Denver, CO 80221-1099
303 458-4190
Type: 4-year Coll or Univ
Control: Nonprofit (Private or Religious)
• Health Information Admin Prgm
• Nursing Prgm
• Physical Therapy Prgm

University of Colorado at Denver
Mark Heckler, Provost
Campus Box 168
PO Box 173364
Denver, CO 80217-3364
303 556-2400
Type: 4-year Coll or Univ
Control: State, County, or Local Govt
• Allopathic Medicine Prgm
• Dental Hygiene Prgm
• Nursing Prgm
• Pharmacy Prgm
• Psychology Prgm (2)

Westwood College
Tony Caggiano, Campus President
7350 N Broadway
Denver, CO 80221-3653
800 992-5050
Type: Vocational or Tech Sch
Control: For Profit
• Medical Assistant Prgm

Durango

Fort Lewis College
Brad Bartel, PhD, President
1000 Rim Dr
Durango, CO 81301-3999
970 247-7100
Type: 4-year Coll or Univ
Control: State, County, or Local Govt
• Athletic Training Prgm

Eaton

Academy of Natural Therapy
123 Elm Ave
PO Box 237
Eaton, CO 80615
Type: Vocational or Tech Sch
Control: For Profit
• Massage Therapy Prgm

Englewood

HealthONE EMS
Mary White, President
501 E Hampden
Englewood, CO 80110
303 788-6484
Type: Hosp or Med Ctr: 300-499 Beds
Control: For Profit
• Emergency Med Tech-Paramedic Prgm

Tri-County Health Department
7000 E Bellview Ave, Ste 301
Englewood, CO 80111-1628
303 220-9200
Type: State, County, or Local Govt
• Dietetic Internship Prgm

Fort Collins

Colorado State University
Larry Penley, PhD, President
102 Administration Bldg
Fort Collins, CO 80523
970 491-6211
Type: 4-year Coll or Univ
Control: State, County, or Local Govt
• Counseling Prgm
• Dietetic Internship Prgm
• Dietetics-Coordinated Prgm
• Music Therapy Prgm
• Occupational Therapy Prgm
• Veterinary Medicine Prgm

Fort Morgan

Morgan Community College
John R McKay, PhD, President
17800 Rd 20
Fort Morgan, CO 80701-4399
970 867-3081
Type: Junior or Comm Coll
Control: State, County, or Local Govt
• Physical Therapist Assistant Prgm

Glenwood Springs

Colorado Mountain College
Bob Spuhler, PhD, President
831 Grand Ave
Glenwood Springs, CO 81601
970 945-8366
Type: Junior or Comm Coll
Control: State, County, or Local Govt
• Emergency Med Tech-Paramedic Prgm
• Veterinary Technology Prgm

Grand Junction

Mesa State College
Timothy Foster, JD, President
1100 North Ave
Grand Junction, CO 81501
970 248-1498
Type: 4-year Coll or Univ
Control: State, County, or Local Govt
• Athletic Training Prgm
• Nursing Prgm
• Radiography Prgm

Greeley

University of Northern Colorado
Kay Norton, JD, President
Carter Hall 4000
Greeley, CO 80639
970 351-2121
Type: 4-year Coll or Univ
Control: State, County, or Local Govt
• Athletic Training Prgm
• Audiologist Prgm
• Counseling Prgm
• Dietetic Internship Prgm
• Dietetics-Didactic Prgm
• Nursing Prgm
• Orientation and Mobility Specialist Prgm
• Rehabilitation Counseling Prgm
• Speech-Language Pathology Prgm

Lakewood

Red Rocks Community College
Cliff Richardson, PhD, President
13300 W Sixth Ave
Lakewood, CO 80228-1255
303 914-6600
Type: Junior or Comm Coll
Control: State, County, or Local Govt
• Medical Assistant Prgm
• Physician Assistant Prgm
• Radiography Prgm

Littleton

Arapahoe Community College
Berton Glandon, PhD, President
5900 S Santa Fe Dr
PO Box 9002
Littleton, CO 80160-9002
303 797-5701
Type: Junior or Comm Coll
Control: State, County, or Local Govt
• Clin Lab Technician/Med Lab Technician Prgm
• Health Information Tech Prgm
• Medical Assistant Prgm
• Pharmacy Technician Prgm
• Physical Therapist Assistant Prgm

Denver Seminary
Craig Williford, PhD
6399 S Santa Fe Dr
Littleton, CO 80120
303 761-2482
Control: Nonprofit (Private or Religious)
• Counseling Prgm

Pueblo

Colorado State University - Pueblo
Joe Garcia, PhD, President
Adm 301 - 2200 Bonforte Blvd
Pueblo, CO 81001
719 549-2306
Type: 4-year Coll or Univ
Control: State, County, or Local Govt
• Athletic Training Prgm

Parkview Medical Center
C W Smith, MBA, President/CEO
400 W 16th St
Pueblo, CO 81003
719 584-4573
Type: Hosp or Med Ctr: 100-299 Beds
Control: Nonprofit (Private or Religious)
• Clin Lab Scientist/Med Technologist Prgm

Pueblo Community College
John Garvin, EdD, President
900 W Orman Ave
Pueblo, CO 81004-1499
719 549-3213
Type: Junior or Comm Coll
Control: State, County, or Local Govt
• Dental Assisting Prgm
• Dental Hygiene Prgm
• Emergency Med Tech-Paramedic Prgm
• Occupational Therapy Asst Prgm
• Physical Therapist Assistant Prgm
• Respiratory Therapist (Advanced) Prgm

Rangley

Colorado Northwestern Community College
John Boyd, President
500 Kennedy Dr
Rangley, CO 81648
970 675-2261
Type: Junior or Comm Coll
Control: State, County, or Local Govt
• Dental Hygiene Prgm

Westminster

Front Range Comm College
Karen Reinertson, PhD, President
3645 W 112th Ave
Westminster, CO 80030
303 404-5422
Type: Junior or Comm Coll
Control: Nonprofit (Private or Religious)
• Dental Assisting Prgm
• Dietetic Technician-AD Prgm
• Medical Assistant Prgm
• Pharmacy Technician Prgm
• Veterinary Technology Prgm

Connecticut

Branford

Branford Hall Career Institute
Gary Camp, CEO
One Summit Pl
Branford, CT 06405
203 488-2525
Type: Vocational or Tech Sch
Control: For Profit
• Medical Assistant Prgm

Bridgeport

Bridgeport Hospital
Robert Trefry, President
267 Grant St
Bridgeport, CT 06610
203 384-3464
Type: Hosp or Med Ctr: 500> Beds
Control: Nonprofit (Private or Religious)
• Surgical Technology Prgm

Housatonic Community College
Anita Gliniecki, MSN, President
900 Lafayette Blvd
Bridgeport, CT 06604-4704
203 332-5224
Type: Junior or Comm Coll
Control: State, County, or Local Govt
• Occupational Therapy Asst Prgm

St Vincent's College
John K Fisher, EdD, President
2800 Main St
Bridgeport, CT 06606
203 576-5578
Type: Junior or Comm Coll
Control: Nonprofit (Private or Religious)
• Medical Assistant Prgm
• Radiography Prgm

U of Bridgeport/Fones Sch of Dental Hygiene
Neil Albert Salonen, President
30 Hazel St
Bridgeport, CT 06601
203 576-4000
Type: 4-year Coll or Univ
Control: Nonprofit (Private or Religious)
• Dental Hygiene Prgm

Danbury

Danbury Hospital
Frank Kelly, President/CEO
24 Hospital Ave
Danbury, CT 06810
203 739-7210
Type: Hosp or Med Ctr: 300-499 Beds
Control: Nonprofit (Private or Religious)
• Clin Lab Scientist/Med Technologist Prgm
• Dietetic Internship Prgm
• Radiography Prgm
• Surgical Technology Prgm

Western Connecticut State University
181 White St
Danbury, CT 06810-6885
203 837-8200
Type: 4-year Coll or Univ
Control: State, County, or Local Govt
• Counseling Prgm
• Nursing Prgm

Danielson

Quinebaug Valley Community College
Dianne E Williams, BS MS, President
742 Upper Maple St
Danielson, CT 06239
860 774-1160
Type: Junior or Comm Coll
Control: State, County, or Local Govt
• Medical Assistant Prgm

East Hartford

Goodwin College
Mark E Scheinberg, BA, President
745 Burnside Ave
East Hartford, CT 06108
860 528-4111
Type: Junior or Comm Coll
Control: Nonprofit (Private or Religious)
• Histotechnician Prgm
• Medical Assistant Prgm

Enfield

Porter and Chester Institute - Enfield
Henry Kamerzel, Executive Director
138 Weymouth Rd
Enfield, CT 06082
203 741-2561
Type: Vocational or Tech Sch
Control: For Profit
• Dental Assisting Prgm

Fairfield

Fairfield University
1073 N Benson Rd
Fairfield, CT 06430-5195
203 254-4000
Type: 4-year Coll or Univ
Control: State, County, or Local Govt
• Counseling Prgm
• Nursing Prgm

Sacred Heart University
Anthony J Cernera, PhD, President
5151 Park Ave
Fairfield, CT 06825
203 371-7999
Type: 4-year Coll or Univ
Control: Nonprofit (Private or Religious)
• Athletic Training Prgm
• Nursing Prgm
• Occupational Therapy Prgm
• Physical Therapy Prgm

Farmington

Tunxis Community College
Cathryn L Addy, PhD, President
271 Scott Swamp Rd
Farmington, CT 06032-3187
860 255-3500
Type: Junior or Comm Coll
Control: State, County, or Local Govt
• Dental Assisting Prgm
• Dental Hygiene Prgm

University of Connecticut Health Center
Peter Deckers, MD, EVP Health Affairs
263 Farmington Ave
Farmington, CT 06030
860 679-2594
Type: Acad Health Ctr/Med Sch
Control: State, County, or Local Govt
• Cytotechnology Prgm

Hamden

Eli Whitney Vocational Technical School
E Paulett Moore, Director
71 Jones Rd
Hamden, CT 06514
203 397-4031
Type: Vocational or Tech Sch
Control: State, County, or Local Govt
• Dental Assisting Prgm
• Surgical Technology Prgm

Quinnipiac University
John L Lahey, PhD, President
275 Mt Carmel Ave
Hamden, CT 06518-1908
203 582-3344
Type: 4-year Coll or Univ
Control: Nonprofit (Private or Religious)
• Athletic Training Prgm
• Occupational Therapy Prgm
• Pathologists' Assistant Prgm
• Perfusion Prgm
• Physical Therapy Prgm
• Physician Assistant Prgm
• Radiography Prgm
• Respiratory Therapist (Advanced) Prgm
• Veterinary Technology Prgm

Stone Academy
William Mangini, School Director
1315 Dixwell Ave
Hamden, CT 06514
203 288-7474
Type: Vocational or Tech Sch
Control: For Profit
• Medical Assistant Prgm

Hartford

A I Prince Technical High School
William Chaffin, PhD, Principal
401 Flatbush Ave
Hartford, CT 06106
860 951-7112
Type: Vocational or Tech Sch
Control: State, County, or Local Govt
• Dental Assisting Prgm
• Surgical Technology Prgm

Capital Community College
Calvin Woodland, EdD PsyD, President
950 Main St
Hartford, CT 06103
860 906-5000
Type: Junior or Comm Coll
Control: State, County, or Local Govt
• Emergency Med Tech-Paramedic Prgm
• Medical Assistant Prgm
• Radiography Prgm

Hartford Hospital
John J Meehan, MHA, President/CEO
80 Seymour St
PO Box 5037
Hartford, CT 06102-5037
860 545-2100
Type: Hosp or Med Ctr: 500> Beds
Control: Nonprofit (Private or Religious)
• Clin Lab Scientist/Med Technologist Prgm
• Radiation Therapy Prgm
• Radiography Prgm

St Francis Hospital & Medical Center
David D'Eramo, PhD, President
114 Woodland St
Hartford, CT 06105
860 714-4900
Type: Hosp or Med Ctr: 500> Beds
Control: Nonprofit (Private or Religious)
• Diagnostic Med Sonography Prgm

Manchester

Manchester Community College
Jonathan Daube, EdD, President
Great Path Mail Station 1
PO Box 1046
Manchester, CT 06045-1046
860 512-3100
Type: Junior or Comm Coll
Control: State, County, or Local Govt
• Occupational Therapy Asst Prgm
• Respiratory Therapist (Advanced) Prgm
• Surgical Technology Prgm

Middletown

Middlesex Community College
Wilfredo Nieves, EdD, President
100 Training Hill Rd
Middletown, CT 06457
860 343-5701
Type: Junior or Comm Coll
Control: State, County, or Local Govt
• Ophthalmic Dispensing Optician Prgm
• Radiography Prgm

New Britain

Central Connecticut State University
Jack Miller, EdD, President
1615 Stanley St
New Britain, CT 06050-4010
860 832-3003
Type: 4-year Coll or Univ
Control: State, County, or Local Govt
• Athletic Training Prgm
• Nursing Prgm
• Rehabilitation Counseling Prgm

Lincoln Tech Institute
Craig Avery, BS, Regional Exec Director
200 John Downey Dr
New Britain, CT 06051
860 225-8641
Type: Vocational or Tech Sch
Control: For Profit
• Medical Assistant Prgm

New Haven

Albertus Magnus College
Julia M McNamara, PhD
700 Prospect St
New Haven, CT 06511
203 773-8529
Type: 4-year Coll or Univ
Control: Nonprofit (Private or Religious)
• Art Therapy Prgm

Gateway Community College
Dorsey Kendrick, PhD, President
60 Sargent Dr
New Haven, CT 06511
203 285-2060
Type: Junior or Comm Coll
Control: State, County, or Local Govt
• Dietetic Technician-AD Prgm
• Nuclear Medicine Technology Prgm
• Radiation Therapy Prgm
• Radiography Prgm

Southern Connecticut State University
Cheryl Norton, PhD, President
501 Crescent St
New Haven, CT 06515
203 397-4234
Type: 4-year Coll or Univ
Control: State, County, or Local Govt
• Athletic Training Prgm
• Audiologist Prgm
• Counseling Prgm
• Medical Librarian Prgm
• Nursing Prgm (2)
• Speech-Language Pathology Prgm

Yale University School of Medicine
Robert Alpern, MD, Dean
333 Cedar St
New Haven, CT 06510
203 785-4672
Type: Acad Health Ctr/Med Sch
Control: Nonprofit (Private or Religious)
• Allopathic Medicine Prgm
• Physician Assistant Prgm
• Psychology Prgm

Yale-New Haven Hospital
20 York St GBB
New Haven, CT 06504
203 785-5074
Control: Nonprofit (Private or Religious)
• Dietetic Internship Prgm

New London

Ridley-Lowell Business & Technical Institute
Wilfred T Weymouth, MS, President
470 Bank St
New London, CT 06320
860 443-7441
Type: Vocational or Tech Sch
Control: For Profit
• Medical Assistant Prgm

Newington

Connecticut Center for Massage Therapy
Stephen Kitts, Executive Director
75 Kitts Lane
Newington, CT 06111
860 667-1886
Type: Vocational or Tech Sch
Control: For Profit
• Massage Therapy Prgm (3)

Hanger Orthopedic Group
Ivan Sabel, President/CEO
181 Patricia M Genova Dr
Newington, CT 06111
860 667-5304
Control: For Profit
• Orthotist/Prosthetist Prgm

Norwalk

Norwalk Community College
David Levinson, PhD, President
188 Richards Ave
Norwalk, CT 06854-1655
203 857-7003
Type: Junior or Comm Coll
Control: State, County, or Local Govt
• Medical Assistant Prgm

Norwalk Hospital/Norwalk Community College
David W Osborne, MS, CEO
Maple St
Norwalk, CT 06856
203 852-2211
Type: Hosp or Med Ctr: 100-299 Beds
Control: Nonprofit (Private or Religious)
• Respiratory Therapist (Advanced) Prgm

Southington

Briarwood College
Lynn Brooks, JD, President
2279 Mt Vernon Rd
Southington, CT 06489
860 628-4751
Type: Vocational or Tech Sch
Control: For Profit
• Dental Assisting Prgm
• Dietetic Technician-AD Prgm
• Health Information Tech Prgm
• Medical Assistant Prgm
• Occupational Therapy Asst Prgm

Stamford

Stamford Hospital
Brian G Grissler, MA, President/CEO
Shelburne Rd PO Box 9317
Stamford, CT 06904-9317
203 276-7000
Type: Hosp or Med Ctr: 300-499 Beds
Control: Nonprofit (Private or Religious)
• Radiography Prgm

Storrs

University of Connecticut
Philip H Austin, President
Storrs, CT 06269
860 486-2000
Type: 4-year Coll or Univ
Control: State, County, or Local Govt
• Allopathic Medicine Prgm
• Athletic Training Prgm
• Audiologist Prgm
• Cytogenetic Technology Prgm
• Dentistry Prgm
• Dietetic Internship Prgm
• Dietetics-Coordinated Prgm
• Dietetics-Didactic Prgm
• Pharmacy Prgm
• Physical Therapy Prgm
• Psychology Prgm
• Speech-Language Pathology Prgm

Waterbury

Naugatuck Valley Community College
Richard L Sanders, EdD, President
750 Chase Pkwy
Waterbury, CT 06708
203 575-8044
Type: Junior or Comm Coll
Control: State, County, or Local Govt
• Physical Therapist Assistant Prgm
• Radiography Prgm
• Respiratory Therapist (Advanced) Prgm

West Hartford

Fox Institute of Business
Christopher Coutts, President
99 South St
West Hartford, CT 06110
860 947-2299
Type: Vocational or Tech Sch
Control: For Profit
• Medical Assistant Prgm

Saint Joseph College
Winifred E Coleman, President
1678 Asylum Ave
West Hartford, CT 06117
203 232-4571
Type: 4-year Coll or Univ
Control: Nonprofit (Private or Religious)
• Dietetic Internship Prgm
• Dietetics-Coordinated Prgm
• Dietetics-Didactic Prgm
• Nursing Prgm

University of Hartford
Walter Harrison, PhD, President
200 Bloomfield Ave
West Hartford, CT 06117-1599
860 768-4417
Type: 4-year Coll or Univ
Control: Nonprofit (Private or Religious)
• Clin Lab Scientist/Med Technologist Prgm
• Nursing Prgm
• Physical Therapy Prgm
• Psychology Prgm
• Radiography Prgm
• Respiratory Therapist (Advanced) Prgm

West Haven

University of New Haven
Lawrence J Denardis, President
300 Orange Ave
West Haven, CT 06516
203 932-7000
Type: 4-year Coll or Univ
Control: Nonprofit (Private or Religious)
• Dental Hygiene Prgm
• Dietetics-Didactic Prgm

Wethersfield

Porter and Chester Institute - Wethersfield
Raymond Clark, Executive Director
125 Silas Deane Hwy
Wethersfield, CT 06109
203 529-2519
Type: Vocational or Tech Sch
Control: For Profit
• Medical Assistant Prgm

Willimantic

Windham Community Memorial Hospital
Richard Brvenik, MA FACHE, President/CEO
112 Mansfield Ave
Willimantic, CT 06226
860 456-6800
Type: Hosp or Med Ctr: 100-299 Beds
Control: Nonprofit (Private or Religious)
• Radiography Prgm

INSTITUTIONS

Windham Regional Vocational Tech School
210 Birch St
Willimantic, CT 06226
203 456-3789
Type: Vocational or Tech Sch
Control: State, County, or Local Govt
• Dental Assisting Prgm

Winsted

Northwestern Connecticut Comm College
Barbara Douglass, PhD, President
Park Place E
Winsted, CT 06098
860 738-6410
Type: Junior or Comm Coll
Control: State, County, or Local Govt
• Medical Assistant Prgm
• Veterinary Technology Prgm

Delaware

Dagsboro

National Massage Therapy Institute
Dagsboro, DE 19939
Type: Acad Health Ctr/Med Sch
Control: For Profit
• Massage Therapy Prgm

Dover

Delaware State University
William B Delauder, President
Dover, DE 19901
302 739-4924
Type: 4-year Coll or Univ
Control: State, County, or Local Govt
• Dietetics-Didactic Prgm
• Nursing Prgm

Delaware Technical & Community College
Daniel Simpson, MS, VP, Asst Campus Director
100 Campus Dr
Dover, DE 19904
302 857-1126
Type: Junior or Comm Coll
Control: State, County, or Local Govt
• Clin Lab Technician/Med Lab Technician Prgm
• Dental Hygiene Prgm
• Diagnostic Med Sonography Prgm
• Emergency Med Tech-Paramedic Prgm
• Histotechnician Prgm
• Medical Assistant Prgm
• Nuclear Medicine Technology Prgm
• Occupational Therapy Asst Prgm (2)
• Physical Therapist Assistant Prgm (2)
• Radiography Prgm (2)
• Respiratory Therapist (Advanced) Prgm (2)
• Veterinary Technology Prgm

New Castle

Wilmington College
320 Dupont Hwy
New Castle, DE 19720-6491
302 328-9401
Type: 4-year Coll or Univ
Control: State, County, or Local Govt
• Counseling Prgm
• Nursing Prgm

Newark

University of Delaware
David P Roselle, PhD, President
104A Hullihen Hall
Newark, DE 19716
302 831-2111
Type: 4-year Coll or Univ
Control: Nonprofit (Private or Religious)
• Athletic Training Prgm
• Clin Lab Scientist/Med Technologist Prgm
• Dietetic Internship Prgm
• Dietetics-Didactic Prgm
• Nursing Prgm
• Physical Therapy Prgm
• Psychology Prgm

District of Columbia

Washington

American University
Washington, DC 20016
Type: 4-year Coll or Univ
Control: State, County, or Local Govt
• Psychology Prgm

Armed Forces Institute of Pathology
Washington, DC 20306
Control: Fed Govt
• Histotechnician Prgm

Catholic University of America
Br Patrick F Ellis, FSC, President
103 Executive Bldg
Washington, DC 20064
202 319-5100
Type: 4-year Coll or Univ
Control: Nonprofit (Private or Religious)
• Medical Librarian Prgm
• Nursing Prgm
• Psychology Prgm

Gallaudet University
I King Jordan, PhD, President
800 Florida Ave NE
Washington, DC 20002
202 651-5329
Type: 4-year Coll or Univ
Control: Nonprofit (Private or Religious)
• Audiologist Prgm
• Counseling Prgm
• Psychology Prgm
• Speech-Language Pathology Prgm
• Therapeutic Recreation Specialist Prgm

George Washington University
John F Williams, MD EdD, VP, Provost Hlth
    Affairs
2121 I Street NW, Ste 701
Washington, DC 20052
202 994-1000
Type: 4-year Coll or Univ
Control: Nonprofit (Private or Religious)
• Allopathic Medicine Prgm
• Art Therapy Prgm
• Athletic Training Prgm
• Clin Lab Scientist/Med Technologist Prgm
• Counseling Prgm
• Diagnostic Med Sonography Prgm
• Emergency Med Tech-Paramedic Prgm
• Physical Therapy Prgm
• Physician Assistant Prgm
• Psychology Prgm (2)
• Rehabilitation Counseling Prgm
• Speech-Language Pathology Prgm

Georgetown University Medical Center
Sam Wiesel, MD, Exec VP Hlth Sciences
120 Bldg D, 4000 Reservoir Dr NW
Washington, DC 20007
202 687-4601
Type: Acad Health Ctr/Med Sch
Control: Nonprofit (Private or Religious)
• Allopathic Medicine Prgm
• Nursing Prgm
• Ophthalmic Med Technician Prgm

Howard University
H Patrick Swygert, JD, President
Mordecai Wyatt Johnson Admin Bldg
2400 Sixth St NW
Washington, DC 20059
202 806-2500
Type: 4-year Coll or Univ
Control: Nonprofit (Private or Religious)
• Allopathic Medicine Prgm
• Audiologist Prgm
• Clin Lab Scientist/Med Technologist Prgm
• Dental Hygiene Prgm
• Dentistry Prgm
• Dietetics-Coordinated Prgm
• Genetic Counseling Prgm
• Music Therapy Prgm
• Nursing Prgm
• Occupational Therapy Prgm
• Pharmacy Prgm
• Physical Therapy Prgm
• Physician Assistant Prgm
• Psychology Prgm
• Radiation Therapy Prgm
• Speech-Language Pathology Prgm

Potomac Massage Training Institute
Demara Stamler, Executive Director
5028 Wisconsin Ave NW, LL
Washington, DC 20016-4118
202 686-7046
Type: Vocational or Tech Sch
Control: Nonprofit (Private or Religious)
• Massage Therapy Prgm

University of the District of Columbia
Timothy L Jenkins, Jr, President
4200 Connecticut Ave NW
Washington, DC 20008
202 274-5100
Type: 4-year Coll or Univ
Control: State, County, or Local Govt
• Dietetics-Didactic Prgm
• Radiography Prgm
• Respiratory Therapist (Advanced) Prgm
• Speech-Language Pathology Prgm

Walter Reed Army Medical Center
Patricia D. Horoho, MD COL MC, Healthcare Sys
  Commander
6900 Georgia Ave, NW
Bulding 2, Command Suite
Washington, DC 20307-5001
202 782-6104
Type: Dept of Defense
Control: Fed Govt
• Clin Lab Scientist/Med Technologist Prgm
• Perfusion Prgm
• Specialist in BB Tech Prgm

Washington Hospital Center
James Caldas, MHSA, President, CEO
110 Irving St NW
Washington, DC 20010
202 877-6101
Type: Hosp or Med Ctr: 500> Beds
Control: Nonprofit (Private or Religious)
• Clin Lab Scientist/Med Technologist Prgm
• Radiography Prgm

Florida

Avon Park

South Florida Community College
Norman L Stephens, Jr, EdD, President
600 W College Dr
Avon Park, FL 33825-9399
863 453-6661
Type: Junior or Comm Coll
Control: State, County, or Local Govt
• Dental Assisting Prgm
• Dental Hygiene Prgm

Bay Pines

Bay Pines VA Medical Center
Bay Pines, FL 33744
Type: Hosp or Med Ctr: 300-499 Beds
Control: Nonprofit (Private or Religious)
• Dietetic Internship Prgm

Boca Raton

Florida Atlantic University
Frank T Brogan, MEd, President
777 Glades Rd
Boca Raton, FL 33431
561 297-3450
Type: 4-year Coll or Univ
Control: State, County, or Local Govt
• Counseling Prgm
• Nursing Prgm
• Rehabilitation Counseling Prgm
• Speech-Language Pathology Prgm

West Boca Medical Center
Richard Gold, CEO
21644 State Rd 7
Boca Raton, FL 33428
561 488-8000
Type: Hosp or Med Ctr: 100-299 Beds
Control: For Profit
• Radiography Prgm

Boynton Beach

Bethesda Memorial Hospital
Robert Hill, MHA, President
2815 S Seacrest Blvd
Boynton Beach, FL 33435
561 737-7733
Type: Hosp or Med Ctr: 300-499 Beds
Control: Nonprofit (Private or Religious)
• Radiography Prgm

Bradenton

Lake Erie Coll of Osteopathic Medicine
5000 Lakewood Ranch Blvd
Bradenton, FL 34211
Type: Acad Health Ctr/Med Sch
Control: Nonprofit (Private or Religious)
• Osteopathic Medicine Prgm

Manatee Community College
Sarah H Pappas, EdD, President
5840 26th St W
PO Box 1849
Bradenton, FL 34207-7046
941 752-5201
Type: Junior or Comm Coll
Control: State, County, or Local Govt
• Dental Hygiene Prgm
• Occupational Therapy Asst Prgm
• Physical Therapist Assistant Prgm
• Radiography Prgm

Manatee Technical Institute
Mary Cantrell, PhD, Director
5603 34th St W
Bradenton, FL 34210
941 751-7900
Type: Vocational or Tech Sch
Control: State, County, or Local Govt
• Dental Assisting Prgm
• Emergency Med Tech-Paramedic Prgm
• Medical Assistant Prgm

Cape Coral

21st Cent Oncology Inc Sch-Rad Therapy Tech
Daniel E Dosoretz, MD ABR, CEO
1419 SE 8th Terrace
Cape Coral, FL 33990
941 489-3420
Type: Nonhosp HC Facil, BB, or Lab
Control: For Profit
• Radiation Therapy Prgm

Lee County High Tech Center - North
Michael Schiffer, MEd, Director
360 Santa Barbara Blvd N
Cape Coral, FL 33993-2479
239 574-4440
Type: Vocational or Tech Sch
Control: State, County, or Local Govt
• Surgical Technology Prgm

Clearwater

Florida Metropolitan Univ - Pinellas Campus
John Buck, BME, President
2471 McMullen Booth Rd, Ste 200
Clearwater, FL 34619
727 725-2688
Type: 4-year Coll or Univ
Control: For Profit
• Medical Assistant Prgm

Pinellas Tech Educ Ctr - Clearwater Campus
Warren Laux, EdD, Director
6100 - 154th Ave N
Clearwater, FL 33760
727 538-7161
Type: Vocational or Tech Sch
Control: State, County, or Local Govt
• Surgical Technology Prgm

Cocoa

Brevard Community College
James A. Drake, PhD, District President
1519 Clearlake Rd
Cocoa, FL 32922
321 433-7000
Type: Junior or Comm Coll
Control: State, County, or Local Govt
• Clin Lab Technician/Med Lab Technician Prgm
• Dental Assisting Prgm
• Dental Hygiene Prgm
• Emergency Med Tech-Paramedic Prgm
• Medical Assistant Prgm
• Radiography Prgm
• Surgical Technology Prgm
• Veterinary Technology Prgm

Coral Gables

University of Miami
Donna Shalala, PhD, President
University Station
PO Box 248006
Coral Gables, FL 33124
305 284-5155
Type: 4-year Coll or Univ
Control: Nonprofit (Private or Religious)
• Athletic Training Prgm
• Music Therapy Prgm
• Nursing Prgm
• Physical Therapy Prgm
• Psychology Prgm

Davie

McFatter Technical Center
Mark Thomas, MS, Director
6500 Nova Dr
Davie, FL 33317
754 321-5700
Type: Vocational or Tech Sch
Control: For Profit
• Dental Lab Technician Prgm
• Medical Assistant Prgm
• Pharmacy Technician Prgm

Daytona Beach

Daytona Beach Community College
Kent D Sharples, EdD, President
PO Box 2811
Daytona Beach, FL 32120-2811
386 506-3200
Type: Junior or Comm Coll
Control: State, County, or Local Govt
- Dental Assisting Prgm
- Dental Hygiene Prgm
- Emergency Med Tech-Paramedic Prgm
- Health Information Tech Prgm
- Medical Assistant Prgm
- Occupational Therapy Asst Prgm
- Physical Therapist Assistant Prgm
- Respiratory Therapist (Advanced) Prgm
- Surgical Technology Prgm

Halifax Medical Center
Dan Lang, MHA, Chief Operating Officer
303 N Clyde Morris Blvd
PO Box 2830
Daytona Beach, FL 32114
386 254-4065
Type: Hosp or Med Ctr: 500> Beds
Control: Nonprofit (Private or Religious)
- Radiation Therapy Prgm
- Radiography Prgm

Deland

Stetson University
H Douglas Lee, BD ThM PhD, President
421 N Woodland Blvd, Unit 8258
Deland, FL 32720-3701
386 822-7250
Type: 4-year Coll or Univ
Control: Nonprofit (Private or Religious)
- Counseling Prgm

Eustis

Lake Technical Center
Steve Hand, MEd, Director
2001 Kurt St
Eustis, FL 32726
352 742-6486
Type: Vocational or Tech Sch
Control: State, County, or Local Govt
- Emergency Med Tech-Paramedic Prgm

Fern Park

Americare School of Nursing
Gerald Newman, ABA, President
7275 Estapano Circle
Fern Park, FL 32730
407 673-7406
Type: Vocational or Tech Sch
Control: For Profit
- Dental Assisting Prgm

Fort Lauderdale

Broward Community College
J David Armstrong, Jr, PhD, President
111 E Las Olas Blvd
Fort Lauderdale, FL 33301
954 201-7401
Type: Junior or Comm Coll
Control: State, County, or Local Govt
- Dental Assisting Prgm
- Dental Hygiene Prgm
- Diagnostic Med Sonography Prgm
- Emergency Med Tech-Paramedic Prgm
- Health Information Tech Prgm
- Medical Assistant Prgm
- Physical Therapist Assistant Prgm
- Respiratory Therapist (Advanced) Prgm

Keiser Career College
Carole Fuller, BPS, President
1900 W Commerical Blvd
Fort Lauderdale, FL 33309
954 776-4476
Type: Junior or Comm Coll
Control: For Profit
- Surgical Technology Prgm (2)

Keiser University
Peter Crocitto, MBA BS, Executive Vice
  Chancellor
1500 NW 49th St
Fort Lauderdale, FL 33309
954 776-4456
Type: 4-year Coll or Univ
Control: For Profit
- Clin Lab Technician/Med Lab Technician Prgm
- Diagnostic Med Sonography Prgm
- Occupational Therapy Asst Prgm
- Physical Therapist Assistant Prgm
- Radiography Prgm (2)
- Surgical Technology Prgm

Keiser University - Daytona Beach
Arthur Keiser, PhD, Chief Executive Officer
1900 Business Park Blvd
Bldg 2
Fort Lauderdale, FL 33309
954 776-4456
Type: 4-year Coll or Univ
Control: For Profit
- Diagnostic Med Sonography Prgm
- Medical Assistant Prgm
- Radiography Prgm

Nova Southeastern University
Ray Ferrero, JSD, President
3301 College Ave
Fort Lauderdale, FL 33314-7796
954 262-7575
Type: 4-year Coll or Univ
Control: Nonprofit (Private or Religious)
- Anesthesiologist Asst Prgm
- Athletic Training Prgm
- Audiologist Prgm
- Dentistry Prgm
- Diagnostic Med Sonography Prgm
- Nursing Prgm
- Occupational Therapy Prgm
- Optometry Prgm
- Osteopathic Medicine Prgm
- Pharmacy Prgm
- Physical Therapy Prgm
- Physician Assistant Prgm (3)
- Psychology Prgm (2)
- Speech-Language Pathology Prgm

Fort Myers

Edison College
Kenneth P Walker, PhD, President
8099 College Pkwy SW
PO Box 60210
Fort Myers, FL 33906-6210
239 941-9211
Type: Junior or Comm Coll
Control: State, County, or Local Govt
- Cardiovascular Technology Prgm
- Dental Assisting Prgm
- Dental Hygiene Prgm
- Emergency Med Tech-Paramedic Prgm
- Radiography Prgm
- Respiratory Therapist (Advanced) Prgm

Florida Gulf Coast University
Richard Pegnetter, PhD, President
10501 FGCU Blvd S
Fort Myers, FL 33965-6565
239 590-1055
Type: 4-year Coll or Univ
Control: State, County, or Local Govt
- Athletic Training Prgm
- Counseling Prgm
- Nursing Prgm
- Occupational Therapy Prgm
- Physical Therapy Prgm

International College
Terry P McMahan, JD, President
8695 College Pkwy, Ste 217
Fort Myers, FL 33919
941 482-0019
Type: 4-year Coll or Univ
Control: Nonprofit (Private or Religious)
- Health Information Tech Prgm
- Medical Assistant Prgm

Fort Pierce

Indian River Community College
Edwin R Massey, PhD, President
3209 Virginia Ave
Fort Pierce, FL 34981-5599
772 462-7201
Type: Junior or Comm Coll
Control: State, County, or Local Govt
• Clin Lab Technician/Med Lab Technician Prgm
• Dental Assisting Prgm
• Dental Hygiene Prgm
• Dental Lab Technician Prgm
• Emergency Med Tech-Paramedic Prgm
• Health Information Tech Prgm
• Medical Assistant Prgm
• Physical Therapist Assistant Prgm
• Radiography Prgm
• Respiratory Therapist (Advanced) Prgm
• Surgical Technology Prgm

Gainesville

Florida School of Massage
Gainesville, FL 32608
Type: Acad Health Ctr/Med Sch
Control: For Profit
• Massage Therapy Prgm

Santa Fe Community College
Jackson Sasser, PhD, President
3000 NW 83rd St
Gainesville, FL 32606-6200
352 395-5164
Type: Junior or Comm Coll
Control: State, County, or Local Govt
• Cardiovascular Technology Prgm
• Dental Assisting Prgm
• Dental Hygiene Prgm
• Emergency Med Tech-Paramedic Prgm
• Health Information Tech Prgm
• Nuclear Medicine Technology Prgm
• Radiography Prgm

University of Florida
Bernard Machen, DDS PhD, President
PO Box 113150
Gainesville, FL 32611-3150
352 392-1311
Type: 4-year Coll or Univ
Control: State, County, or Local Govt
• Allopathic Medicine Prgm
• Athletic Training Prgm
• Audiologist Prgm
• Counseling Prgm (3)
• Dentistry Prgm
• Dietetic Internship Prgm
• Dietetics-Didactic Prgm
• Nursing Prgm
• Occupational Therapy Prgm
• Ophthalmic Med Technologist Prgm
• Orthoptist Prgm
• Pharmacy Prgm
• Physical Therapy Prgm
• Physician Assistant Prgm
• Psychology Prgm
• Rehabilitation Counseling Prgm
• Speech-Language Pathology Prgm
• Therapeutic Recreation Specialist Prgm
• Veterinary Medicine Prgm

Hollywood

Sheridan Technical Center
D Robert Boegli, Director
5400 Sheridan St
Hollywood, FL 33021
754 321-2007
Type: Vocational or Tech Sch
Control: State, County, or Local Govt
• Surgical Technology Prgm

Jacksonville

Florida Community College - Jacksonville
Steven R Wallace, PhD, President
501 W State St
Jacksonville, FL 32202
904 632-3000
Type: Junior or Comm Coll
Control: State, County, or Local Govt
• Clin Lab Technician/Med Lab Technician Prgm
• Dental Hygiene Prgm
• Dietetic Technician-AD Prgm
• Emergency Med Tech-Paramedic Prgm
• Health Information Tech Prgm
• Histotechnician Prgm
• Physical Therapist Assistant Prgm
• Respiratory Therapist (Advanced) Prgm
• Surgical Technology Prgm

Jacksonville University
Jacksonville, FL 32211
Type: 4-year Coll or Univ
Control: State, County, or Local Govt
• Nursing Prgm

Mayo Clinic Jacksonville
Michael B Wood, MD, President
4500 San Pablo Rd
Jacksonville, FL 32224
Type: Hosp or Med Ctr: 300-499 Beds
Control: Nonprofit (Private or Religious)
• Radiography Prgm

Shands Jacksonville
Jim Burkhart, Interim COO
655 W Eighth St
Jacksonville, FL 32209
904 244-0000
Type: Hosp or Med Ctr: 500> Beds
Control: Nonprofit (Private or Religious)
• Clin Lab Scientist/Med Technologist Prgm
• Radiography Prgm

St Luke's Hosp/Mayo Clinic Jacksonville
4201 Belfort Rd
Jacksonville, FL 32216-1431
904 296-3733
Control: Nonprofit (Private or Religious)
• Dietetic Internship Prgm

St Vincent's Medical Center
John J Maher, MBA MHA, President
1800 Barrs St
Jacksonville, FL 32204
904 308-4001
Type: Hosp or Med Ctr: 500> Beds
Control: Nonprofit (Private or Religious)
• Clin Lab Scientist/Med Technologist Prgm
• Diagnostic Med Sonography Prgm
• Nuclear Medicine Technology Prgm
• Radiography Prgm

University of North Florida
John Delaney, JD, President
Office of the President
1 University Dr
Jacksonville, FL 32224-2645
904 620-2500
Type: 4-year Coll or Univ
Control: State, County, or Local Govt
• Athletic Training Prgm
• Counseling Prgm
• Dietetic Internship Prgm
• Dietetics-Didactic Prgm
• Nursing Prgm
• Physical Therapy Prgm
• Rehabilitation Counseling Prgm

Lake City

Lake City Community College
Charles Hall, EdD, President
149 SE College Place
Lake City, FL 32025
386 754-4200
Type: Junior or Comm Coll
Control: State, County, or Local Govt
• Emergency Med Tech-Paramedic Prgm
• Pharmacy Technician Prgm
• Physical Therapist Assistant Prgm

Lake Worth

Palm Beach Community College
Dennis P Gallon, PhD, President
4200 Congress Ave
Lake Worth, FL 33461-4796
561 868-3350
Type: Junior or Comm Coll
Control: State, County, or Local Govt
• Dental Assisting Prgm
• Dental Hygiene Prgm
• Diagnostic Med Sonography Prgm
• Emergency Med Tech-Paramedic Prgm
• Medical Assistant Prgm
• Radiography Prgm
• Respiratory Therapist (Advanced) Prgm
• Surgical Technology Prgm

Lakeland

Florida Career Institute
Pamela J Corrigan, RN MEd, CEO
4222 S Florida Ave
Lakeland, FL 33813
863 646-1400
Type: Vocational or Tech Sch
Control: For Profit
• Medical Assistant Prgm

Florida Metropolitan Univ - Lakeland Campus
Edmund K Gross, EdD, President
995 E Memorial Blvd, Ste 110
Lakeland, FL 33801
941 686-1444
Type: 4-year Coll or Univ
Control: For Profit
• Medical Assistant Prgm

Florida Southern College
Anne Kerr, PhD, President
111 Lake Hollingsworth Dr
Lakeland, FL 33801-5698
863 680-4100
Type: 4-year Coll or Univ
Control: Nonprofit (Private or Religious)
• Athletic Training Prgm
• Nursing Prgm

Lakeland Regional Medical Center
Jack T Stephens, President/CEO
1324 Lakeland Hills Blvd
PO Box 95448
Lakeland, FL 33804
863 687-1100
Type: Hosp or Med Ctr: 500> Beds
Control: Nonprofit (Private or Religious)
• Radiography Prgm

Traviss Career Center
Kenneth Lloyd, PhD
3225 Winter Lake Rd
Lakeland, FL 33803
863 449-2700
Type: Vocational or Tech Sch
Control: State, County, or Local Govt
• Dental Assisting Prgm
• Surgical Technology Prgm

Lauderdale Lakes

Sanford-Brown Institute - Ft Lauderdale
1201 W Cypress Creek Rd
Lauderdale Lakes, FL 33309
954 733-8900
Type: Vocational or Tech Sch
Control: For Profit
• Surgical Technology Prgm

Leesburg

Lake-Sumter Community College
Charles Mojock, PhD, President
9501 US Hwy 441
Leesburg, FL 34788
352 365-3523
Type: Junior or Comm Coll
Control: State, County, or Local Govt
• Health Information Tech Prgm

Maitland

Florida College of Natural Health
Dale Weiberg, Campus Director
2600 Lake Lucian Dr
Maitland, FL 33126
407 261-0319
Type: Vocational or Tech Sch
Control: For Profit
• Massage Therapy Prgm (4)

Melbourne

Florida Institute of Technology
Melbourne, FL 32901
Type: Acad Health Ctr/Med Sch
Control: For Profit
• Psychology Prgm

Florida Metropolitan Univ - Melbourne Campus
Mark Judge, President
2401 N Harbor City Blvd
Melbourne, FL 32935
321 253-2929
Type: 4-year Coll or Univ
Control: For Profit
• Medical Assistant Prgm
• Pharmacy Technician Prgm

Keiser University - Melbourne Campus
Colleen Rupp, MBA, Campus President
900 S Babcock St
Melbourne, FL 32901
321 409-4800
Type: 4-year Coll or Univ
Control: For Profit
• Occupational Therapy Asst Prgm
• Radiography Prgm

Miami

Carlos Albizu University
Miami, FL 33172
Type: 4-year Coll or Univ
Control: Nonprofit (Private or Religious)
• Psychology Prgm

Educating Hands School of Massage
Iris Burman
120 SW 8th St
Miami, FL 33130
305 285-6991
Type: Vocational or Tech Sch
Control: For Profit
• Massage Therapy Prgm

Florida International University
Modesto Maidique, PhD, President
Office of Academic Affairs
University Park Campus
Miami, FL 33199
305 348-2111
Type: 4-year Coll or Univ
Control: State, County, or Local Govt
• Counseling Prgm
• Dietetics-Coordinated Prgm
• Dietetics-Didactic Prgm
• Health Information Admin Prgm
• Occupational Therapy Prgm
• Physical Therapy Prgm
• Speech-Language Pathology Prgm

Jackson Mem Medical Center
Marvin O'Quinn, MHA, President and CEO
Jackson Health System
1611 NW 12th Ave
Miami, FL 33136
305 585-6754
Type: Hosp or Med Ctr: 500> Beds
Control: State, County, or Local Govt
• Nuclear Medicine Technology Prgm
• Radiography Prgm

Lindsey Hopkins Tech Education Center
Rosa Borgen, MS, Principal
750 NW 20th St
Miami, FL 33127
305 324-6070
Type: Vocational or Tech Sch
Control: State, County, or Local Govt
• Dental Assisting Prgm
• Surgical Technology Prgm

Miami Dade College
Eduardo J Padron, PhD, College President
Wolfson Campus
300 NE 2nd Ave
Miami, FL 33132-2296
305 237-3316
Type: Junior or Comm Coll
Control: State, County, or Local Govt
• Clin Lab Technician/Med Lab Technician Prgm
• Dental Hygiene Prgm
• Diagnostic Med Sonography Prgm
• Emergency Med Tech-Paramedic Prgm
• Health Information Tech Prgm
• Histotechnician Prgm
• Ophthalmic Dispensing Optician Prgm
• Physical Therapist Assistant Prgm
• Physician Assistant Prgm
• Radiation Therapy Prgm
• Radiography Prgm
• Respiratory Therapist (Advanced) Prgm
• Veterinary Technology Prgm

Robert Morgan Educational Center
Greg Zawyer, MS, Principal
18180 SW 122nd Ave
Miami, FL 33177
305 253-9920
Type: Vocational or Tech Sch
Control: State, County, or Local Govt
• Dental Assisting Prgm
• Medical Assistant Prgm

Sanford-Brown Institute
David T Ruggieri, President
4400 Biscayne Blvd
Miami, FL 33137
800 445-6108
Type: Vocational or Tech Sch
Control: For Profit
• Surgical Technology Prgm

University of Miami School of Medicine
Bernard J Fogel, MD, Vice Pres/Dean
1600 NW 10th Ave R-699
Miami, FL 33136
305 585-6545
Type: Acad Health Ctr/Med Sch
Control: Nonprofit (Private or Religious)
• Allopathic Medicine Prgm

Miami Shores

Barry University
Linda M Bevilacqua, OP, President
11300 NE 2nd Ave
Miami Shores, FL 33161-6695
305 899-3010
Type: 4-year Coll or Univ
Control: Nonprofit (Private or Religious)
• Athletic Training Prgm
• Counseling Prgm
• Histotechnology Prgm
• Nursing Prgm
• Occupational Therapy Prgm
• Perfusion Prgm
• Physician Assistant Prgm
• Podiatric Medicine Prgm

Naples

Lorenzo Walker Institute of Technology
Jeanette Johnson, MS, Principal
3702 Estey Ave
Naples, FL 34104
239 377-0906
Type: Vocational or Tech Sch
Control: State, County, or Local Govt
• Dental Assisting Prgm
• Medical Assistant Prgm
• Surgical Technology Prgm

New Port Richey

Pasco County Health Department
10841 Little Rd
New Port Richey, FL 34654-2533
813 869-3900
Control: State, County, or Local Govt
• Dietetic Internship Prgm

Pasco-Hernando Community College
Katherine M Johnson, EdD, President
10230 Ridge Rd
New Port Richey, FL 34654-5199
727 847-2727
Type: Junior or Comm Coll
Control: State, County, or Local Govt
• Dental Hygiene Prgm
• Emergency Med Tech-Paramedic Prgm

Niceville

Okaloosa-Walton College
James R Richburg, EdD, President
100 College Blvd
Niceville, FL 32578-1295
850 729-5360
Type: Junior or Comm Coll
Control: State, County, or Local Govt
• Dental Assisting Prgm
• Surgical Technology Prgm

North Miami Beach

National School of Technology
Martin Knobel, B Ed MS, CEO
12000 Biscayne Blvd #302
North Miami Beach, FL 33181
305 893-0005
Type: Vocational or Tech Sch
Control: For Profit
• Surgical Technology Prgm (3)

Ocala

Central Florida Community College
Charles Dassance, PhD, President
3001 SW College Rd
PO Box 1388
Ocala, FL 34474
352 854-2322
Type: Junior or Comm Coll
Control: State, County, or Local Govt
• Dental Assisting Prgm
• Emergency Med Tech-Paramedic Prgm
• Health Information Tech Prgm
• Physical Therapist Assistant Prgm
• Surgical Technology Prgm

Community Technical & Adult Education Center
Samuel Lauff Jr, MA, Administrator
1014 SW 7th Rd
Ocala, FL 34474
352 671-7200
Type: Vocational or Tech Sch
Control: State, County, or Local Govt
• Medical Assistant Prgm

Marion County School of Radiologic Tech
Deborah Jenkins, MEd, Administrator
1014 SW 7th Rd
Ocala, FL 34474-3172
352 671-7200
Type: Vocational or Tech Sch
Control: State, County, or Local Govt
• Radiography Prgm

Orlando

Florida Hospital
Lars Houmann, PhD, CEO
601 E Rollins St
Orlando, FL 32803
407 303-1531
Type: Hosp or Med Ctr: 500> Beds
Control: Nonprofit (Private or Religious)
• Phlebotomy Prgm

Florida Hospital College of Health Sciences
David E Greenlaw, DMiN, President
671 Winyah Dr
Orlando, FL 32803
407 303-7747
Type: 4-year Coll or Univ
Control: Nonprofit (Private or Religious)
• Nuclear Medicine Technology Prgm
• Occupational Therapy Asst Prgm
• Radiography Prgm

Florida Metro Univ - North Orlando Campus
Ouida B Kirby, BS, President
5421 Diplomat Circle
Orlando, FL 32810
407 628-5870
Type: 4-year Coll or Univ
Control: For Profit
• Medical Assistant Prgm

Florida Metro Univ - Orlando College South
J Gary Adcox, PhD, President
9200 SouthPark Center Loop
Orlando, FL 32819
407 851-2525
Type: 4-year Coll or Univ
Control: For Profit
• Medical Assistant Prgm

Orlando Tech
Ferol Lynne Voltaggio, MEd, Senior Director
301 W Amelia St
Orlando, FL 32801
407 246-7060
Type: Vocational or Tech Sch
Control: State, County, or Local Govt
• Dental Assisting Prgm
• Surgical Technology Prgm

University of Central Florida
John C Hitt, PhD, President
308 Millican Hall
4000 Central Florida Blvd
Orlando, FL 32816-0002
407 823-1823
Type: 4-year Coll or Univ
Control: State, County, or Local Govt
• Athletic Training Prgm
• Clin Lab Scientist/Med Technologist Prgm
• Counseling Prgm
• Health Information Admin Prgm
• Nursing Prgm
• Physical Therapy Prgm
• Psychology Prgm
• Radiography Prgm
• Respiratory Therapist (Advanced) Prgm
• Speech-Language Pathology Prgm

Valencia Community College
Sanford C Shugart, PhD, President
PO Box 3028
Orlando, FL 32802-3028
407 299-5000
Type: Junior or Comm Coll
Control: State, County, or Local Govt
• Dental Hygiene Prgm
• Diagnostic Med Sonography Prgm
• Emergency Med Tech-Paramedic Prgm
• Radiography Prgm
• Respiratory Therapist (Advanced) Prgm

Osprey

Sarasota District Schools
101 Old Venice Rd
Osprey, FL 34229-9023
Control: State, County, or Local Govt
• Dietetic Internship Prgm

Palatka

St Johns River Community College
R L McLendon, Jr, PhD, President
5001 St Johns Ave
Palatka, FL 32177
386 312-4113
Type: Junior or Comm Coll
Control: State, County, or Local Govt
• Health Information Tech Prgm

Palm Harbor

Central Florida Institute
Alfred A McCloy, MBA, President
30522 US 19 N, Ste 200
Palm Harbor, FL 34684
727 786-4707
Type: Vocational or Tech Sch
Control: For Profit
• Cardiovascular Technology Prgm
• Surgical Technology Prgm

INSTITUTIONS

Panama City

Gulf Coast Community College
James Kerley, PhD, President
5230 W US Hwy 98
Panama City, FL 32401-1041
850 769-1551
Type: Junior or Comm Coll
Control: State, County, or Local Govt
• Dental Assisting Prgm
• Dental Hygiene Prgm
• Emergency Med Tech-Paramedic Prgm
• Physical Therapist Assistant Prgm
• Radiography Prgm
• Respiratory Therapist (Advanced) Prgm
• Surgical Technology Prgm

Pensacola

Pensacola Junior College
G Thomas Delaino, PhD, President
1000 College Blvd
Pensacola, FL 32501
850 484-1700
Type: Junior or Comm Coll
Control: State, County, or Local Govt
• Dental Assisting Prgm
• Dental Hygiene Prgm
• Dietetic Technician-AD Prgm
• Emergency Med Tech-Paramedic Prgm
• Health Information Tech Prgm
• Medical Assistant Prgm
• Physical Therapist Assistant Prgm
• Radiography Prgm
• Surgical Technology Prgm

University of West Florida
John Cavanaugh, PhD, President
11000 University Pkwy
Pensacola, FL 32514-5750
904 474-2202
Type: 4-year Coll or Univ
Control: State, County, or Local Govt
• Athletic Training Prgm
• Clin Lab Scientist/Med Technologist Prgm
• Nursing Prgm

Virginia College at Penascola
Bruce G Capps, BS, President
19 W Garden St
Pensacola, FL 32501
850 916-9868
Type: Vocational or Tech Sch
Control: For Profit
• Surgical Technology Prgm

Port Charlotte

Charlotte Technical Center
Judith Willis, Director
18300 Toledo Blade Blvd
Port Charlotte, FL 33948-3399
941 255-7500
Type: Vocational or Tech Sch
Control: State, County, or Local Govt
• Dental Assisting Prgm

Sanford

Seminole Community College
E Ann McGee, EdD, President
100 Weldon Blvd
Sanford, FL 32773
407 708-4722
Type: Junior or Comm Coll
Control: State, County, or Local Govt
• Emergency Med Tech-Paramedic Prgm
• Medical Assistant Prgm
• Physical Therapist Assistant Prgm
• Respiratory Therapist (Advanced) Prgm

Sarasota

Sarasota County Technical Institute
Bruce Andersen, MA, Director
4748 Beneva Rd
Sarasota, FL 34233-1798
813 924-1365
Type: Vocational or Tech Sch
Control: State, County, or Local Govt
• Emergency Med Tech-Paramedic Prgm
• Medical Assistant Prgm
• Surgical Technology Prgm

Sarasota Memorial Hospital
1700 S Tamiami Trail
Sarasota, FL 34239-3555
813 917-1080
Control: Nonprofit (Private or Religious)
• Dietetic Internship Prgm

Sarasota School of Massage Therapy
Joe Lubow, BS LMT, Director
1932 Ringling Blvd
Sarasota, FL 34236
941 957-0577
Type: Vocational or Tech Sch
Control: For Profit
• Massage Therapy Prgm

St Augustine

First Coast Technical Institute
Christine Cothron, President
2980 Collins Ave
St Augustine, FL 32095-1919
904 824-4401
Type: Vocational or Tech Sch
Control: State, County, or Local Govt
• Medical Assistant Prgm

Univ of St Augustine for Health Sciences
Stanley V Paris, PhD PT FAPTA, President
1 University Blvd
St Augustine, FL 32086
904 826-0084
Type: Junior or Comm Coll
Control: For Profit
• Occupational Therapy Prgm
• Physical Therapy Prgm

St Petersburg

Bayfront Medical Center
Sue S Brody, MHA, President/CEO
701 Sixth St S
St Petersburg, FL 33701
813 893-6085
Type: Hosp or Med Ctr: 500> Beds
Control: Nonprofit (Private or Religious)
• Clin Lab Scientist/Med Technologist Prgm

Pinellas Tech Educ Ctr - St Petersburg
Dennis Jauch, EdD, Chief Operating Officer
901 34th St S
St Petersburg, FL 33711-2298
727 893-2500
Type: Vocational or Tech Sch
Control: State, County, or Local Govt
• Dental Assisting Prgm
• Medical Assistant Prgm
• Pharmacy Technician Prgm

St Petersburg College
Sandra W Pepicello, PhD RN, Provost, Health
  Educ Ctr
PO Box 13489
St Petersburg, FL 33733
727 341-3664
Type: 4-year Coll or Univ
Control: State, County, or Local Govt
• Clin Lab Technician/Med Lab Technician Prgm
• Dental Hygiene Prgm
• Emergency Med Tech-Paramedic Prgm
• Health Information Tech Prgm
• Nursing Prgm
• Physical Therapist Assistant Prgm
• Respiratory Therapist (Advanced) Prgm
• Veterinary Technology Prgm

Transfusion Med Acad Ctr FL Blood Svcs
German F Leparc, MD, Chief Medical Officer
10100 Dr Martin Luther King Jr St N
St Petersburg, FL 33716-3806
727 568-5433
Type: Nonhosp HC Facil, BB, or Lab
Control: Nonprofit (Private or Religious)
• Specialist in BB Tech Prgm

Tallahassee

Core Institute
George Kousaleos, MassT, Executive Director
223 W Carolina St
Tallahassee, FL 32301
850 222-8673
Type: Acad Health Ctr/Med Sch
Control: For Profit
• Massage Therapy Prgm

Florida A&M University
Larry Robinson, PhD, President
400 Lee Hall
Tallahassee, FL 32307-3100
850 599-3225
Type: 4-year Coll or Univ
Control: State, County, or Local Govt
• Health Information Admin Prgm
• Occupational Therapy Prgm
• Pharmacy Prgm
• Physical Therapy Prgm
• Respiratory Therapist (Advanced) Prgm

Florida Department of Education
325 W Gaines St, Rm 1032
Tallahassee, FL 32399-0400
Type: Acad Health Ctr/Med Sch
Control: State, County, or Local Govt
• Dietetic Internship Prgm

Florida State University
TK Wetherell, PhD, President
211 WES
Tallahassee, FL 32306
850 644-2525
Type: 4-year Coll or Univ
Control: State, County, or Local Govt
• Allopathic Medicine Prgm
• Art Therapy Prgm
• Athletic Training Prgm
• Counseling Prgm
• Dietetic Internship Prgm
• Dietetics-Didactic Prgm
• Medical Librarian Prgm
• Music Therapy Prgm
• Nursing Prgm
• Orientation and Mobility Specialist Prgm
• Psychology Prgm
• Rehabilitation Counseling Prgm
• Speech-Language Pathology Prgm
• Teacher of the Visually Impaired Prgm
• Vision Rehabilitation Therapy Prgm

Lively Technical Center
Jean Ferguson, MS, Principal
500 N Appleyard Dr
Tallahassee, FL 32304
904 487-7401
Type: Vocational or Tech Sch
Control: State, County, or Local Govt
• Medical Assistant Prgm

Tallahassee Community College
William Law, PhD, President
444 Appleyard Dr
Tallahassee, FL 32304
850 201-8660
Type: Junior or Comm Coll
Control: State, County, or Local Govt
• Dental Assisting Prgm
• Dental Hygiene Prgm
• Emergency Med Tech-Paramedic Prgm
• Respiratory Therapist (Advanced) Prgm

Tampa

Argosy University
Tampa, FL 33614
Type: 4-year Coll or Univ
Control: State, County, or Local Govt
• Psychology Prgm

Concorde Career Institute
Donna Hallam, MA, Campus President
4204 W Spruce St
Tampa, FL 33607
813 874-0094
Type: Vocational or Tech Sch
Control: For Profit
• Surgical Technology Prgm (3)

Erwin Technical Center
Michael D Donohue, MEd, Principal
2010 E Hillsborough Ave
Tampa, FL 33610-8299
813 231-1800
Type: Vocational or Tech Sch
Control: State, County, or Local Govt
• Clin Lab Technician/Med Lab Technician Prgm
• Dental Assisting Prgm
• Electroneurodiagnostic Tech Prgm
• Medical Assistant Prgm
• Surgical Technology Prgm

Florida Metro U - Tampa Coll - Hillsborough
Thomas M Barlow, President
3319 W Hillsborough Ave
Tampa, FL 33614
813 879-6000
Type: 4-year Coll or Univ
Control: For Profit
• Medical Assistant Prgm

Florida Metropolitan Univ - Tampa College
Stan Banks, II, BS, President
3924 Coconut Palm Dr
Tampa, FL 33619
813 621-0041
Type: 4-year Coll or Univ
Control: For Profit
• Medical Assistant Prgm
• Surgical Technology Prgm

Henry W Brewster Technical Center
Janice Carter Collier, Prinicpal
2222 N Tampa St
Tampa, FL 33602
Type: Vocational or Tech Sch
Control: State, County, or Local Govt
• Pharmacy Technician Prgm

Hillsborough Community College
Gwendolyn Stephenson, PhD, President
PO Box 31127
39 Columbia Dr (Davis Island)
Tampa, FL 33631-3127
813 253-7050
Type: Junior or Comm Coll
Control: State, County, or Local Govt
• Dental Assisting Prgm
• Dental Hygiene Prgm
• Diagnostic Med Sonography Prgm
• Emergency Med Tech-Paramedic Prgm
• Nuclear Medicine Technology Prgm
• Ophthalmic Dispensing Optician Prgm
• Radiation Therapy Prgm
• Radiography Prgm
• Respiratory Therapist (Advanced) Prgm

James A Haley Veteran's Hospital
13000 N Bruce B Downs Blvd
Tampa, FL 33612-4745
813 972-2000
Control: Fed Govt
• Dietetic Internship Prgm

Tampa General Hospital
Ron Hytoff, MD, President, CEO
PO Box 1289
Tampa, FL 33601
813 251-7383
Type: Hosp or Med Ctr: 500> Beds
Control: Nonprofit (Private or Religious)
• Clin Lab Scientist/Med Technologist Prgm

University of South Florida
Judith Genshaft, PhD, President
ADM 241
Tampa, FL 33620
813 974-2791
Type: 4-year Coll or Univ
Control: State, County, or Local Govt
• Allopathic Medicine Prgm
• Athletic Training Prgm
• Audiologist Prgm
• Counseling Prgm
• Medical Librarian Prgm
• Nursing Prgm
• Physical Therapy Prgm
• Psychology Prgm
• Rehabilitation Counseling Prgm
• Speech-Language Pathology Prgm

University of Tampa
Ronald Vaughn, PhD, President
401 W Kennedy Blvd
Tampa, FL 33606
813 253-6201
Type: 4-year Coll or Univ
Control: Nonprofit (Private or Religious)
• Athletic Training Prgm

West Palm Beach

MedVance Institute
Deborah K Schwarzberg, PhD, President
KIMC Investments LP - Esperante Ste 200
222 Lakeview Ave
West Palm Beach, FL 33401
561 832-3535
Control: For Profit
• Radiography Prgm (3)
• Surgical Technology Prgm (2)

Palm Beach Atlantic University
David W Clark, PhD, President
PO Box 24708
West Palm Beach, FL 33416-4708
561 803-2302
Type: 4-year Coll or Univ
Control: Nonprofit (Private or Religious)
• Athletic Training Prgm
• Nursing Prgm
• Pharmacy Prgm

South University
Tracey Schoonmaker, President
1760 N Congress Ave
West Palm Beach, FL 33409
561 697-9200
Type: 4-year Coll or Univ
Control: For Profit
• Medical Assistant Prgm
• Nursing Prgm
• Physical Therapist Assistant Prgm

INSTITUTIONS

Winter Haven

Polk Community College
Eileen Holden, PhD, President
999 Ave H NE
Winter Haven, FL 33881-4299
863 297-1098
Type: Junior or Comm Coll
Control: State, County, or Local Govt
- Emergency Med Tech-Paramedic Prgm
- Health Information Tech Prgm
- Occupational Therapy Asst Prgm
- Physical Therapist Assistant Prgm
- Radiography Prgm

Winter Park

Central Florida College
Roger Bradley, President
1573 W Fairbanks Ave
Winter Park, FL 32789
407 843-3984
Type: Vocational or Tech Sch
Control: For Profit
- Medical Assistant Prgm

Rollins College
1000 Holt Ave
Winter Park, FL 32789-4499
407 646-2000
Type: 4-year Coll or Univ
Control: Nonprofit (Private or Religious)
- Counseling Prgm

Winter Park Tech
Eleanor Cain, Director
901 Webster Ave
Winter Park, FL 32789
407 647-6366
Type: Vocational or Tech Sch
Control: State, County, or Local Govt
- Medical Assistant Prgm

Georgia

Acworth

North Metro Technical College
Steve Dougherty, MA, President
5198 Ross Rd
Acworth, GA 30102
770 975-4126
Type: Vocational or Tech Sch
Control: State, County, or Local Govt
- Medical Assistant Prgm
- Radiography Prgm

Albany

Albany Technical College
Anthony Parker, PhD, President
1704 S Slappey Blvd
Albany, GA 31701-3514
229 430-3500
Type: Vocational or Tech Sch
Control: State, County, or Local Govt
- Dental Assisting Prgm
- Medical Assistant Prgm
- Radiography Prgm
- Surgical Technology Prgm

Darton College
Peter J Sireno, EdD, President
2400 Gillionville Rd
Albany, GA 31707
229 317-6905
Type: Junior or Comm Coll
Control: State, County, or Local Govt
- Clin Lab Technician/Med Lab Technician Prgm
- Dental Hygiene Prgm
- Health Information Tech Prgm
- Histotechnician Prgm
- Occupational Therapy Asst Prgm
- Physical Therapist Assistant Prgm
- Respiratory Therapist (Advanced) Prgm

Athens

Athens Technical College
Flora Tydings, EdD, President
800 US Hwy 29 N
Athens, GA 30601
706 355-5000
Type: Vocational or Tech Sch
Control: State, County, or Local Govt
- Dental Assisting Prgm
- Dental Hygiene Prgm
- Physical Therapist Assistant Prgm
- Radiography Prgm
- Respiratory Therapist (Advanced) Prgm
- Surgical Technology Prgm
- Veterinary Technology Prgm

University of Georgia
Michael F Adams, PhD, President
Administration Bldg
Athens, GA 30602
706 542-1214
Type: 4-year Coll or Univ
Control: State, County, or Local Govt
- Athletic Training Prgm
- Counseling Prgm
- Dietetic Internship Prgm
- Dietetics-Didactic Prgm
- Music Therapy Prgm
- Pharmacy Prgm
- Psychology Prgm
- Speech-Language Pathology Prgm
- Veterinary Medicine Prgm

Atlanta

Argosy University
Atlanta, GA 30328
Type: 4-year Coll or Univ
Control: State, County, or Local Govt
- Psychology Prgm

Atlanta Technical College
Brenda W Jones, PhD, President
1560 Metropolitan Parkway SW
Atlanta, GA 30310
404 225-4400
Type: 4-year Coll or Univ
Control: State, County, or Local Govt
- Dental Assisting Prgm
- Dental Lab Technician Prgm
- Medical Assistant Prgm

Div of Pub Hlth/Georgia Dept of Hum Res
2 Peachtree St NE
Atlanta, GA 30303-3141
404 657-2884
Control: State, County, or Local Govt
- Dietetic Internship Prgm

Emory University
James W Wagner, PhD, President
408 Administration Bldg
Atlanta, GA 30322
404 727-6012
Type: Acad Health Ctr/Med Sch
Control: Nonprofit (Private or Religious)
- Allopathic Medicine Prgm
- Anesthesiologist Asst Prgm
- Nursing Prgm
- Ophthalmic Med Technologist Prgm
- Physical Therapy Prgm
- Physician Assistant Prgm
- Psychology Prgm
- Radiography Prgm

Emory University Hospital
John D Henry, Sr, FACHE, CEO
1364 Clifton Rd NE, Rm B216
Atlanta, GA 30322
404 712-4881
Type: Hosp or Med Ctr: 500> Beds
Control: Nonprofit (Private or Religious)
- Dietetic Internship Prgm

Georgia Institute of Technology
Wayne G Clough, PhD, President
225 North Ave NW
Atlanta, GA 30332-0325
404 894-5051
Type: 4-year Coll or Univ
Control: State, County, or Local Govt
- Orthotist/Prosthetist Prgm

Georgia Medical Institute
Anthony Galang, BS, President
1706 Northeast Expwy
Atlanta, GA 30329
404 327-8787
Type: Vocational or Tech Sch
Control: For Profit
- Surgical Technology Prgm

Georgia State University
Carl V Patton, PhD, President
PO Box 3999
300 Alumni Hall
Atlanta, GA 30302-3999
404 651-2560
Type: 4-year Coll or Univ
Control: State, County, or Local Govt
- Counseling Prgm
- Dietetic Internship Prgm
- Dietetics-Coordinated Prgm
- Dietetics-Didactic Prgm
- Nursing Prgm
- Physical Therapy Prgm
- Psychology Prgm
- Rehabilitation Counseling Prgm
- Respiratory Therapist (Advanced) Prgm
- Speech-Language Pathology Prgm

Grady Health System
Otis L. Story, Sr, MA MS FACHE, President/CEO
80 Jesse Hill Jr Dr, SE
PO Box 26189
Atlanta, GA 30303-3050
404 616-4252
Type: Hosp or Med Ctr: 500> Beds
Control: State, County, or Local Govt
• Diagnostic Med Sonography Prgm
• Radiation Therapy Prgm
• Radiography Prgm

Morehouse School of Medicine
John E Maupin, Jr, DDS MBA, President
720 Westview Dr SW
Atlanta, GA 30310
Type: Acad Health Ctr/Med Sch
Control: Nonprofit (Private or Religious)
• Allopathic Medicine Prgm

Sanford-Brown Institute
Glenn W Alderson, BA, Executive Director
1140 Hammond Dr, Ste 1150
Atlanta, GA 30328
770 350-0009
Type: Vocational or Tech Sch
Control: For Profit
• Diagnostic Med Sonography Prgm

Augusta

Augusta Area Dietetic Internship
Larry Read, CEO, Univ Hlth Care Syst
University Hospital
1350 Walton Way (10)
Augusta, GA 30901-2629
706 774-8045
Type: Hosp or Med Ctr: 300-499 Beds
Control: Nonprofit (Private or Religious)
• Dietetic Internship Prgm

Augusta Technical College
Terry D Elam, MEd, President
3200 Augusta Tech Dr
Augusta, GA 30906
706 771-4005
Type: Vocational or Tech Sch
Control: State, County, or Local Govt
• Dental Assisting Prgm
• Medical Assistant Prgm
• Occupational Therapy Asst Prgm
• Respiratory Therapist (Advanced) Prgm
• Surgical Technology Prgm

Harry T Harper Jr Sch of Cardiac & Vas Tech
Larry Read, MA, President/CEO
1350 Walton Way
Augusta, GA 30901
706 774-8045
Type: Acad Health Ctr/Med Sch
Control: Nonprofit (Private or Religious)
• Cardiovascular Technology Prgm

Medical College of Georgia
Daniel Rahn, MD, President
1120 15th St, Rm AA-312
Augusta, GA 30912-0079
706 721-2301
Type: Acad Health Ctr/Med Sch
Control: State, County, or Local Govt
• Allopathic Medicine Prgm
• Clin Lab Scientist/Med Technologist Prgm
• Dental Hygiene Prgm
• Dentistry Prgm
• Diagnostic Med Sonography Prgm
• Health Information Admin Prgm
• Medical Illustrator Prgm
• Nuclear Medicine Technology Prgm
• Nursing Prgm
• Occupational Therapy Prgm
• Physical Therapy Prgm
• Physician Assistant Prgm
• Radiation Therapy Prgm
• Respiratory Therapist (Advanced) Prgm

Savannah River College
Darryl H Kerr, BS, President
2528 Centerwest Pkwy Bldg A
Augusta, GA 30909
706 738-5046
Type: Junior or Comm Coll
Control: For Profit
• Medical Assistant Prgm

University Hospital
Donald C Bray, MS, President/CEO
1350 Walton Way
Augusta, GA 30901
706 722-9011
Type: Hosp or Med Ctr: 500> Beds
Control: Nonprofit (Private or Religious)
• Radiography Prgm

Brunswick

Coastal Georgia Community College
Dorothy L Lord, PhD, President
3700 Altama Ave
Brunswick, GA 31520-3644
912 264-7201
Type: Junior or Comm Coll
Control: State, County, or Local Govt
• Clin Lab Technician/Med Lab Technician Prgm
• Radiography Prgm
• Surgical Technology Prgm

Carrollton

University of West Georgia
Beheruz N Sethna, President
Carrollton, GA 30118-0001
770 836-6500
Type: 4-year Coll or Univ
Control: State, County, or Local Govt
• Counseling Prgm
• Nursing Prgm

Clarkesville

North Georgia Technical College
Ruth Nichols, EdD, President
PO Box 65
1500 Hwy 197 N
Clarkesville, GA 30523
706 754-7701
Type: Vocational or Tech Sch
Control: State, County, or Local Govt
• Clin Lab Technician/Med Lab Technician Prgm
• Medical Assistant Prgm (2)

Clarkston

DeKalb Technical College
Robin Hoffman, PhD, President
495 N Indian Creek Dr
Clarkston, GA 30021
404 297-9522
Type: Vocational or Tech Sch
Control: State, County, or Local Govt
• Clin Lab Technician/Med Lab Technician Prgm
• Medical Assistant Prgm
• Ophthalmic Dispensing Optician Prgm
• Surgical Technology Prgm

Cochran

Middle Georgia College
Richard Federinko, PhD, President
1100 Second St SE
Cochran, GA 31014-1599
478 934-3011
Type: Junior or Comm Coll
Control: State, County, or Local Govt
• Occupational Therapy Asst Prgm

Columbus

Columbus State University
Frank D Brown, PhD, President
4225 University Ave
Columbus, GA 31907-5645
706 568-2211
Type: 4-year Coll or Univ
Control: State, County, or Local Govt
• Counseling Prgm

Columbus Technical College
J Robert Jones, EdS, President
928 Manchester Expwy
Columbus, GA 31904-6572
706 649-1837
Type: Vocational or Tech Sch
Control: State, County, or Local Govt
• Dental Assisting Prgm
• Dental Hygiene Prgm
• Medical Assistant Prgm
• Radiography Prgm
• Surgical Technology Prgm

Dahlonega

North Georgia College & State University
David Potter, PhD, President
Prince Memorial Hall
Dahlonega, GA 30597
706 864-1993
Type: 4-year Coll or Univ
Control: State, County, or Local Govt
• Athletic Training Prgm
• Physical Therapy Prgm

Dalton

Dalton State College
James A Burran, PhD, President
650 College Dr
Dalton, GA 30720-3778
706 272-4438
Type: 4-year Coll or Univ
Control: State, County, or Local Govt
• Clin Lab Technician/Med Lab Technician Prgm
• Medical Assistant Prgm
• Phlebotomy Prgm
• Radiography Prgm
• Surgical Technology Prgm

Decatur

DeKalb Medical Center
Eric Norwood, MHA, CEO
2701 N Decatur Rd
Decatur, GA 30033
404 501-5206
Type: Hosp or Med Ctr: 300-499 Beds
Control: Nonprofit (Private or Religious)
• Radiography Prgm

DeVry University - Atlanta
250 N Arcadia Ave
Decatur, GA 30030-2198
Type: 4-year Coll or Univ
Control: State, County, or Local Govt
• Health Information Tech Prgm

Georgia Perimeter College
Jacquelyn M Belcher, President
3251 Panthersville Rd
Decatur, GA 30034
404 244-2365
Type: Junior or Comm Coll
Control: State, County, or Local Govt
• Dental Hygiene Prgm

Douglas

East Central Technical College
Ray Perren, DSL, President
706 West Baker Hwy
Douglas, GA 31533
229 468-2078
Type: Vocational or Tech Sch
Control: State, County, or Local Govt
• Medical Assistant Prgm

Dublin

Heart of Georgia Technical College
Randall L Peters, MA, President
560 Pinehill Rd
Dublin, GA 31021
478 275-6590
Type: Vocational or Tech Sch
Control: State, County, or Local Govt
• Medical Assistant Prgm
• Radiography Prgm
• Respiratory Therapist (Advanced) Prgm

Fort Valley

Fort Valley State University
Larry E Rivers, PhD, President
1005 State University Dr
Fort Valley, GA 31030-4313
478 825-6315
Type: 4-year Coll or Univ
Control: State, County, or Local Govt
• Dietetics-Didactic Prgm
• Rehabilitation Counseling Prgm
• Veterinary Technology Prgm

Gainesville

Brenau University
Ed L Schrader, PhD, President
500 Washington SE
Gainesville, GA 30501
770 534-6110
Type: 4-year Coll or Univ
Control: Nonprofit (Private or Religious)
• Nursing Prgm
• Occupational Therapy Prgm

Griffin

Griffin Technical College
Robert Arnold, EdD, CEO
501 Varsity Rd
Griffin, GA 30223
770 228-7365
Type: Vocational or Tech Sch
Control: State, County, or Local Govt
• Medical Assistant Prgm
• Radiography Prgm
• Respiratory Therapist (Advanced) Prgm
• Surgical Technology Prgm

Jasper

Appalachian Technical College
Sanford Chandler, PhD, President
100 Campus Dr
Jasper, GA 30143
706 253-4500
Type: Vocational or Tech Sch
Control: State, County, or Local Govt
• Medical Assistant Prgm

Kennesaw

Kennesaw State University
Betty L Siegel, President
1000 Chastain Rd
Kennesaw, GA 30144-5591
770 423-6000
Type: 4-year Coll or Univ
Control: State, County, or Local Govt
• Cytogenetic Technology Prgm
• Nursing Prgm

LaGrange

West Georgia Technical College
Daryl Gilley, PhD, President
303 Fort Dr
LaGrange, GA 30240
706 845-4323
Type: Vocational or Tech Sch
Control: State, County, or Local Govt
• Medical Assistant Prgm
• Radiography Prgm

Lawrenceville

Gwinnett Technical College
Sharon Rigsby, ABJ MEd, President
5150 Sugarloaf Pkwy
Lawrenceville, GA 30043
770 962-7580
Type: Junior or Comm Coll
Control: State, County, or Local Govt
• Dental Assisting Prgm
• Emergency Med Tech-Paramedic Prgm
• Medical Assistant Prgm
• Physical Therapist Assistant Prgm
• Radiography Prgm
• Respiratory Therapist (Advanced) Prgm
• Surgical Technology Prgm
• Veterinary Technology Prgm

Macon

Central Georgia Technical College
Ronald D Natale, PhD, President
3300 Macon Tech Dr
Macon, GA 31206
912 757-3400
Type: Vocational or Tech Sch
Control: State, County, or Local Govt
• Clin Lab Technician/Med Lab Technician Prgm
• Dental Hygiene Prgm
• Surgical Technology Prgm

Macon State College
David Bell, PhD, President
100 College Station Dr
Macon, GA 31206-5145
478 471-2700
Type: 4-year Coll or Univ
Control: State, County, or Local Govt
• Health Information Admin Prgm
• Health Information Tech Prgm
• Respiratory Therapist (Advanced) Prgm

Mercer University
William D Underwood, President
Macon, GA 31207
Type: Acad Health Ctr/Med Sch
Control: Nonprofit (Private or Religious)
• Allopathic Medicine Prgm
• Nursing Prgm
• Pharmacy Prgm
• Physician Assistant Prgm

Marietta

Chattahoochee Technical College
Harlon D Crimm, EdD, President
980 S Cobb Dr
Marietta, GA 30060
770 528-4500
Type: Vocational or Tech Sch
Control: State, County, or Local Govt
• Medical Assistant Prgm
• Surgical Technology Prgm

Life University
Sid E Williams, President
1269 Barclay Cir
Marietta, GA 30060
404 424-0554
Type: 4-year Coll or Univ
Control: Nonprofit (Private or Religious)
• Dietetic Internship Prgm
• Dietetics-Didactic Prgm

Milledgeville

Georgia College & State University
Dorothy Leland, President
Milledgeville, GA 31061
478 445-4444
Type: 4-year Coll or Univ
Control: State, County, or Local Govt
• Athletic Training Prgm
• Music Therapy Prgm

Morrow

Clayton State University
Thomas K Harden, EdD, President
2000 Clayton State Blvd
Morrow, GA 30260
678 466-4300
Type: 4-year Coll or Univ
Control: State, County, or Local Govt
• Dental Hygiene Prgm
• Medical Assistant Prgm
• Nursing Prgm

Moultrie

Moultrie Technical College
Tina Anderson, EdD, President
800 Veterans Pkwy N
Moultrie, GA 31788
229 891-7000
Type: Vocational or Tech Sch
Control: State, County, or Local Govt
• Medical Assistant Prgm
• Radiography Prgm

Oakwood

Lanier Technical College
Michael Moye, EdD, President
2990 Landrum Education Dr
Oakwood, GA 30566-0058
770 531-6304
Type: Vocational or Tech Sch
Control: State, County, or Local Govt
• Clin Lab Technician/Med Lab Technician Prgm
• Dental Assisting Prgm
• Dental Hygiene Prgm
• Medical Assistant Prgm
• Radiography Prgm
• Surgical Technology Prgm

Riverdale

Southern Regional Medical Center
11 Upper Riverdale Rd SW
Riverdale, GA 30274-2600
770 991-8053
Control: Nonprofit (Private or Religious)
• Dietetic Internship Prgm

Rock Spring

Northwestern Technical College
Ray Brooks, EdD, President
PO Box 569
265 Bicentennial Trail
Rock Spring, GA 30739
706 764-3530
Type: Vocational or Tech Sch
Control: State, County, or Local Govt
• Medical Assistant Prgm
• Occupational Therapy Asst Prgm
• Surgical Technology Prgm

Rome

Coosa Valley Technical College
Craig McDaniel, EdD, President
One Maurice Culberson Dr
Rome, GA 30161
706 295-6927
Type: Vocational or Tech Sch
Control: State, County, or Local Govt
• Dental Assisting Prgm
• Diagnostic Med Sonography Prgm
• Medical Assistant Prgm
• Nuclear Medicine Technology Prgm
• Radiation Therapy Prgm
• Radiography Prgm
• Respiratory Therapist (Advanced) Prgm
• Surgical Technology Prgm

Georgia Highlands College
Randy Pierce, President
3175 Cedartown Hwy SE
Rome, GA 30161
706 802-5000
Type: Junior or Comm Coll
Control: State, County, or Local Govt
• Dental Hygiene Prgm

Savannah

Armstrong Atlantic State University
Thomas Jones, PhD, President
11935 Abercorn St
Savannah, GA 31419-1997
912 927-5258
Type: 4-year Coll or Univ
Control: State, County, or Local Govt
• Clin Lab Scientist/Med Technologist Prgm
• Dental Hygiene Prgm
• Nuclear Medicine Technology Prgm
• Nursing Prgm
• Physical Therapy Prgm
• Radiation Therapy Prgm
• Radiography Prgm
• Respiratory Therapist (Advanced) Prgm
• Speech-Language Pathology Prgm

Savannah Technical College
C B Rathburn, PhD, President
5717 White Bluff Rd
Savannah, GA 31405-5521
912 443-3026
Type: Vocational or Tech Sch
Control: State, County, or Local Govt
• Dental Assisting Prgm
• Medical Assistant Prgm
• Surgical Technology Prgm

South University
John South, Chancellor
709 Mall Blvd
Savannah, GA 31406
912 201-8000
Type: 4-year Coll or Univ
Control: For Profit
• Anesthesiologist Asst Prgm
• Medical Assistant Prgm
• Pharmacy Prgm
• Physical Therapist Assistant Prgm
• Physician Assistant Prgm

Smyrna

Medix School
Duncan Anderson, President
2108 Cobb Pkwy
Smyrna, GA 30080
770 980-0002
Type: Vocational or Tech Sch
Control: For Profit
• Dental Assisting Prgm
• Medical Assistant Prgm

Statesboro

Georgia Southern University
Bruce F Grube, PhD, President
PO Box 8033
Marvin Pittman Admin Bldg
Statesboro, GA 30460-8033
912 681-5211
Type: 4-year Coll or Univ
Control: State, County, or Local Govt
• Athletic Training Prgm
• Dietetics-Didactic Prgm
• Nursing Prgm
• Therapeutic Recreation Specialist Prgm

Ogeechee Technical College
Dawn Cartee, PhD, President
One Joe Kennedy Blvd
Statesboro, GA 30458
912 681-5500
Type: Vocational or Tech Sch
Control: State, County, or Local Govt
• Dental Assisting Prgm
• Diagnostic Med Sonography Prgm
• Health Information Tech Prgm
• Magnetic Resonance Prgm
• Medical Assistant Prgm
• Ophthalmic Dispensing Optician Prgm
• Pharmacy Technician Prgm
• Radiography Prgm
• Surgical Technology Prgm
• Veterinary Technology Prgm

Suwanee

Georgia Campus - PA Coll of Osteopathic Med
625 Old Peachtree Rd
Suwanee, GA 30024
Type: Acad Health Ctr/Med Sch
Control: Nonprofit (Private or Religious)
• Osteopathic Medicine Prgm

Swainsboro

Swainsboro Technical College
Glenn Deibert, EdD, President
346 Kite Rd
Swainsboro, GA 30401
478 289-2250
Type: Vocational or Tech Sch
Control: State, County, or Local Govt
• Medical Assistant Prgm

Thomaston

Flint River Technical College
Kathy Love, PhD, President
1533 Hwy 19 S
Thomaston, GA 30286
706 646-6148
Type: Junior or Comm Coll
Control: State, County, or Local Govt
• Surgical Technology Prgm

Thomasville

Southwest Georgia Technical College
Glenn Deibert, EdD, President
15689 US Hwy 19 N
Thomasville, GA 31792
229 225-5069
Type: Junior or Comm Coll
Control: State, County, or Local Govt
• Clin Lab Technician/Med Lab Technician Prgm
• Medical Assistant Prgm
• Pharmacy Technician Prgm
• Respiratory Therapist (Advanced) Prgm
• Surgical Technology Prgm

Thomas University
Gary Bonvillian, PhD, President
Forbes Bldg
1501 Millpond Rd
Thomasville, GA 31792
229 226-1621
Type: 4-year Coll or Univ
Control: Nonprofit (Private or Religious)
• Clin Lab Scientist/Med Technologist Prgm
• Rehabilitation Counseling Prgm

Valdosta

Valdosta State University
Ronald M Zaccari, PhD, President
West Hall
Valdosta, GA 31698
229 333-5952
Type: 4-year Coll or Univ
Control: State, County, or Local Govt
• Athletic Training Prgm
• Dental Hygiene Prgm
• Nursing Prgm
• Speech-Language Pathology Prgm

Valdosta Technical College
Robert Abene, PhD-Ed, President
4089 Valtech Rd
PO Box 928
Valdosta, GA 31602
229 333-2119
Type: Vocational or Tech Sch
Control: State, County, or Local Govt
• Clin Lab Technician/Med Lab Technician Prgm
• Dental Assisting Prgm
• Dental Hygiene Prgm
• Pharmacy Technician Prgm
• Radiography Prgm
• Surgical Technology Prgm

Vidalia

Southeastern Technical College
Cathryn T Meehan, EdD, President
3001 E First St
Vidalia, GA 30474
912 538-3100
Type: Vocational or Tech Sch
Control: State, County, or Local Govt
• Clin Lab Technician/Med Lab Technician Prgm
• Medical Assistant Prgm
• Pharmacy Technician Prgm
• Radiography Prgm
• Surgical Technology Prgm

Waco

West Central Technical College
Skip Sullivan, PhD, President
176 Murphy Campus Blvd
Waco, GA 30182
770 537-7940
Type: Vocational or Tech Sch
Control: For Profit
• Clin Lab Technician/Med Lab Technician Prgm
• Dental Hygiene Prgm
• Medical Assistant Prgm
• Radiography Prgm
• Surgical Technology Prgm

Warner Robins

Middle Georgia Technical College
Ivan Allen, EdD, President
80 Cohen Walker Dr
Warner Robins, GA 31088
478 988-6833
Type: Vocational or Tech Sch
Control: State, County, or Local Govt
• Dental Assisting Prgm
• Dental Hygiene Prgm
• Nuclear Medicine Technology Prgm
• Radiography Prgm
• Surgical Technology Prgm

Waycross

Okefenokee Technical College
Gail Thaxton, EdD, President
1701 Carswell Ave
Waycross, GA 31503
912 287-5828
Type: Vocational or Tech Sch
Control: State, County, or Local Govt
• Clin Lab Technician/Med Lab Technician Prgm
• Radiography Prgm
• Surgical Technology Prgm

Guam

GMF Barrigada

Guam Community College
Herominiano Delos Santos, EdD, President
PO Box 23069
GMF Barrigada, GU 96921
671 735-5636
Type: Junior or Comm Coll
Control: State, County, or Local Govt
• Medical Assistant Prgm

Hawaii

Honolulu

Argosy University
Honolulu, HI 96813
Type: Acad Health Ctr/Med Sch
Control: For Profit
• Psychology Prgm

Heald College - Honolulu Campus
Evelyn A Schemmel, BS, Executive Director
1500 Kapiolani Blvd
Honolulu, HI 96814
808 955-1500
Type: Junior or Comm Coll
Control: For Profit
• Medical Assistant Prgm

Kapi'olani Community College
Leon Richards, PhD, Chancellor
4303 Diamond Head Rd
Ilima Bldg, Rm 213
Honolulu, HI 96816-4421
808 734-9565
Type: Junior or Comm Coll
Control: State, County, or Local Govt
- Clin Lab Technician/Med Lab Technician Prgm
- Medical Assistant Prgm
- Occupational Therapy Asst Prgm
- Phlebotomy Prgm
- Physical Therapist Assistant Prgm
- Radiography Prgm
- Respiratory Therapist (Advanced) Prgm
- Surgical Technology Prgm

University of Hawaii
Denise Konan, PhD, Interim Chancellor
Hawaii 202C, 2500 Campus Rd
Honolulu, HI 96822
808 956-7651
Type: Acad Health Ctr/Med Sch
Control: State, County, or Local Govt
- Allopathic Medicine Prgm
- Athletic Training Prgm
- Clin Lab Scientist/Med Technologist Prgm
- Counseling Prgm
- Dental Hygiene Prgm
- Dietetics-Didactic Prgm
- Medical Librarian Prgm
- Nursing Prgm
- Psychology Prgm
- Rehabilitation Counseling Prgm
- Speech-Language Pathology Prgm

Kahului

Maui Community College
310 Kaahumana Ave
Kahului, HI 96732
808 984-3500
Type: Junior or Comm Coll
Control: State, County, or Local Govt
- Dental Assisting Prgm

Idaho

Boise

Apollo College - Boise
Chuck Ericson, Executive Director
1200 N Liberty St
Boise, ID 83704
208 377-8080
Type: Vocational or Tech Sch
Control: For Profit
- Dental Assisting Prgm
- Dental Hygiene Prgm

Boise State University
Robert Kustra, PhD, President
1910 University Dr
Boise, ID 83725-1000
208 426-1491
Type: 4-year Coll or Univ
Control: State, County, or Local Govt
- Athletic Training Prgm
- Counseling Prgm
- Dental Assisting Prgm
- Diagnostic Med Sonography Prgm
- Health Information Tech Prgm
- Radiography Prgm
- Respiratory Therapist (Advanced) Prgm
- Surgical Technology Prgm

Idaho Falls

Eastern Idaho Technical College
William Robertson, MEd, President
1600 South 2500 East
Idaho Falls, ID 83404-5788
208 524-3000
Type: Vocational or Tech Sch
Control: State, County, or Local Govt
- Medical Assistant Prgm
- Surgical Technology Prgm

Lewiston

Lewis-Clark State College
Dene Thomas, PhD, President
500 8th Ave
Lewiston, ID 83501
208 792-2216
Type: Vocational or Tech Sch
Control: State, County, or Local Govt
- Medical Assistant Prgm
- Nursing Prgm

Moscow

University of Idaho
Timothy White, PhD, President
PO Box 443151
Moscow, ID 83844-3151
208 885-6365
Type: 4-year Coll or Univ
Control: State, County, or Local Govt
- Athletic Training Prgm
- Counseling Prgm
- Dietetics-Coordinated Prgm
- Rehabilitation Counseling Prgm

Nampa

Northwest Nazarene University
Richard A Hagood, President
623 Holly St
Nampa, ID 83686-5897
208 467-8011
Type: 4-year Coll or Univ
Control: State, County, or Local Govt
- Counseling Prgm
- Nursing Prgm

Pocatello

Idaho State University
Arthur Vailas, PhD, President
Campus Box 8310
Pocatello, ID 83209-8063
208 282-2171
Type: 4-year Coll or Univ
Control: State, County, or Local Govt
- Audiologist Prgm
- Clin Lab Scientist/Med Technologist Prgm
- Counseling Prgm
- Dental Hygiene Prgm
- Dental Lab Technician Prgm
- Dietetic Internship Prgm
- Dietetics-Didactic Prgm
- Emergency Med Tech-Paramedic Prgm
- Health Information Tech Prgm
- Medical Assistant Prgm
- Nursing Prgm
- Occupational Therapy Prgm
- Pharmacy Prgm
- Physical Therapist Assistant Prgm
- Physical Therapy Prgm
- Physician Assistant Prgm
- Psychology Prgm
- Speech-Language Pathology Prgm

Twin Falls

College of Southern Idaho
Jerry Beck, EdD, President
315 Falls Ave
PO Box 1238
Twin Falls, ID 83303-1238
208 732-6728
Type: Junior or Comm Coll
Control: State, County, or Local Govt
- Emergency Med Tech-Paramedic Prgm
- Medical Assistant Prgm
- Radiography Prgm
- Surgical Technology Prgm
- Veterinary Technology Prgm

Illinois

Aurora

Aurora University
Rebecca L Sherrick, PhD, President
347 S Gladstone Ave
Aurora, IL 60506-4892
630 844-5476
Type: 4-year Coll or Univ
Control: Nonprofit (Private or Religious)
- Athletic Training Prgm
- Nursing Prgm

INSTITUTIONS

Belleville

Southwestern Illinois College
Elmer Kirchoff, PhD, President
2500 Carlyle Ave
Belleville, IL 62221-5899
800 222-5131
Type: Junior or Comm Coll
Control: State, County, or Local Govt
- Clin Lab Technician/Med Lab Technician Prgm
- Health Information Tech Prgm
- Medical Assistant Prgm
- Physical Therapist Assistant Prgm
- Radiography Prgm
- Respiratory Therapist (Advanced) Prgm

Bloomington

Illinois Wesleyan University
Bloomington, IL 61702
Type: 4-year Coll or Univ
Control: Nonprofit (Private or Religious)
- Nursing Prgm

Bourbonnais

Olivet Nazarene University
John C Bowling, EdD, President
One University Ave
Bourbonnais, IL 60914
815 939-5011
Type: 4-year Coll or Univ
Control: Nonprofit (Private or Religious)
- Athletic Training Prgm
- Dietetics-Didactic Prgm
- Nursing Prgm

Carbondale

Southern Illinois University Carbondale
Fernando Trevino, PhD, Chancellor
116 Anthony Hall, MC 6801
Carbondale, IL 62901
618 453-2341
Type: 4-year Coll or Univ
Control: State, County, or Local Govt
- Athletic Training Prgm
- Counseling Prgm
- Dental Hygiene Prgm
- Diagnostic Med Sonography Prgm
- Dietetic Internship Prgm
- Dietetics-Didactic Prgm
- Medical Dosimetry Prgm
- Physical Therapist Assistant Prgm
- Physician Assistant Prgm
- Psychology Prgm
- Rehabilitation Counseling Prgm
- Respiratory Therapist (Advanced) Prgm
- Speech-Language Pathology Prgm
- Therapeutic Recreation Specialist Prgm

Carterville

John A Logan College
Robert Mees, PhD, President
700 Logan College Rd
Carterville, IL 62918
618 985-2828
Type: Junior or Comm Coll
Control: Nonprofit (Private or Religious)
- Dental Assisting Prgm
- Dental Hygiene Prgm
- Diagnostic Med Sonography Prgm

Centralia

Kaskaskia College
James Underwood, EdD, President
27210 College Rd
Centralia, IL 62801
618 545-3000
Type: Junior or Comm Coll
Control: State, County, or Local Govt
- Dental Assisting Prgm
- Physical Therapist Assistant Prgm
- Radiography Prgm
- Respiratory Therapist (Advanced) Prgm

Champaign

Parkland College
Thomas Ramage, EdD, President
2400 W Bradley Ave
Champaign, IL 61821-1899
217 351-2231
Type: Junior or Comm Coll
Control: State, County, or Local Govt
- Dental Hygiene Prgm
- Occupational Therapy Asst Prgm
- Radiography Prgm
- Respiratory Therapist (Advanced) Prgm
- Surgical Technology Prgm
- Veterinary Technology Prgm

Univ of Illinois at Urbana-Champaign
Richard Herman, PhD, Chancellor
317 Swanlund Admin
MC 304
Champaign, IL 61801
217 333-6290
Type: 4-year Coll or Univ
Control: State, County, or Local Govt
- Athletic Training Prgm
- Audiologist Prgm
- Dietetic Internship Prgm
- Dietetics-Didactic Prgm
- Medical Librarian Prgm
- Psychology Prgm
- Rehabilitation Counseling Prgm
- Speech-Language Pathology Prgm
- Veterinary Medicine Prgm

Charleston

Eastern Illinois University
William Perry, PhD, President
600 Lincoln Ave
Charleston, IL 61920
217 581-2011
Type: 4-year Coll or Univ
Control: State, County, or Local Govt
- Athletic Training Prgm
- Counseling Prgm
- Dietetic Internship Prgm
- Dietetics-Didactic Prgm
- Speech-Language Pathology Prgm
- Therapeutic Recreation Specialist Prgm

Chicago

Adler School of Professional Psychology
Ray Crossman, PhD, President
65 E Wacker Pl, Ste 2100
Chicago, IL 60601-7203
312 201-5900
Control: Nonprofit (Private or Religious)
- Art Therapy Prgm
- Psychology Prgm

Advocate Illinois Masonic Medical Center
Susan Nordstrom-Lopez, Chief Executive
836 W Wellington Ave
Chicago, IL 60657
773 296-7081
Type: Hosp or Med Ctr: 500> Beds
Control: Nonprofit (Private or Religious)
- Radiography Prgm

Advocate Trinity Hospital
Anthony Munroe, EdD, Chief Executive Officer
2320 E 93rd St
Chicago, IL 60617
773 967-5000
Type: Hosp or Med Ctr: 100-299 Beds
Control: Nonprofit (Private or Religious)
- Radiography Prgm

Argosy University
Chicago, IL 60654
Type: 4-year Coll or Univ
Control: Nonprofit (Private or Religious)
- Psychology Prgm (2)

Chicago School of Massage Therapy
Jason Scholte, President
17 N State, 5th Fl
Chicago, IL 60602
312 753-7900
Type: Vocational or Tech Sch
Control: For Profit
- Massage Therapy Prgm (2)

Chicago School of Professional Psychology
Chicago, IL 60610
Type: Acad Health Ctr/Med Sch
Control: Nonprofit (Private or Religious)
- Psychology Prgm

Chicago State University
Elnora D Daniel, PhD, President
9501 S King Dr
Chicago, IL 60628-1598
773 995-2400
Type: 4-year Coll or Univ
Control: State, County, or Local Govt
• Counseling Prgm
• Health Information Admin Prgm
• Occupational Therapy Prgm

Columbia College
Warrick L Carter, PhD, President
600 S Michigan
Chicago, IL 60605-9988
Type: 4-year Coll or Univ
Control: State, County, or Local Govt
• Dance/Movement Therapy Prgm

DePaul University
Rev John Richardson, President
25 E Jackson Blvd
Chicago, IL 60604
312 341-8000
Type: 4-year Coll or Univ
Control: Nonprofit (Private or Religious)
• Nursing Prgm
• Psychology Prgm

DeVry University
Jim Treleaven, President
3300 N Campbell Ave
Chicago, IL 60618
773 697-2080
Type: 4-year Coll or Univ
Control: State, County, or Local Govt
• Health Information Tech Prgm (2)

Illinois College of Optometry
Arol Augsburger, OD MS, President
3241 S Michigan Ave
Chicago, IL 60616
312 949-7400
Type: Junior or Comm Coll
Control: Nonprofit (Private or Religious)
• Optometry Prgm

Illinois Institute of Technology
Lewis M Collens, President
3300 S Federal St
Chicago, IL 60616
312 567-3000
Type: 4-year Coll or Univ
Control: Nonprofit (Private or Religious)
• Psychology Prgm
• Rehabilitation Counseling Prgm

Kaplan University
Chicago, IL 60607
Type: 4-year Coll or Univ
Control: Nonprofit (Private or Religious)
• Nursing Prgm

Kennedy-King College
Wayne Watson, President
6800 S Wentworth Ave
Chicago, IL 60621
773 602-5229
Type: Junior or Comm Coll
Control: State, County, or Local Govt
• Dental Hygiene Prgm

Loyola University of Chicago
John J Piderit, President
820 N Michigan Ave
Chicago, IL 60611
312 915-6000
Type: 4-year Coll or Univ
Control: Nonprofit (Private or Religious)
• Dietetic Internship Prgm
• Nursing Prgm
• Psychology Prgm

Malcolm X College
Zerrie D Campbell, MS MA, President
1900 W Van Buren St
Chicago, IL 60612
312 850-7037
Type: Junior or Comm Coll
Control: State, County, or Local Govt
• Pharmacy Technician Prgm
• Physician Assistant Prgm
• Radiography Prgm
• Respiratory Therapist (Advanced) Prgm
• Surgical Technology Prgm

North Park University
David L Parkyn, President
3225 W Foster Ave
Chicago, IL 60625
773 244-5710
Type: 4-year Coll or Univ
Control: State, County, or Local Govt
• Athletic Training Prgm
• Nursing Prgm

Northeastern Illinois University
5500 N St Louis Ave
Chicago, IL 60625-4699
773 583-4050
Type: 4-year Coll or Univ
Control: State, County, or Local Govt
• Counseling Prgm
• Rehabilitation Counseling Prgm

Northwestern Memorial Hospital
Dean Harrison, MBA, President and CEO
251 E Huron St
Feinberg 3-710
Chicago, IL 60611
312 926-3007
Type: Hosp or Med Ctr: 500> Beds
Control: Nonprofit (Private or Religious)
• Diagnostic Med Sonography Prgm
• Nuclear Medicine Technology Prgm
• Radiation Therapy Prgm

Olive Harvey College
Valerie R Roberson, PhD, Interim President
10001 W Woodlawn Ave
Chicago, IL 60628
773 291-6313
Type: 4-year Coll or Univ
Control: State, County, or Local Govt
• Respiratory Therapist (Advanced) Prgm

Robert Morris College
Michael Viollt, President
401 S State St
Chicago, IL 60605
312 935-6600
Type: 4-year Coll or Univ
Control: Nonprofit (Private or Religious)
• Medical Assistant Prgm (7)

Roosevelt University
Charles R Middleton, PhD, President
430 S Michigan Ave
Chicago, IL 60605-1394
312 341-3500
Type: 4-year Coll or Univ
Control: Nonprofit (Private or Religious)
• Counseling Prgm
• Psychology Prgm

Rush University
Larry J Goodman, MD, President
1725 W Harrison St, Ste 364
Chicago, IL 60612
312 942-7073
Type: Acad Health Ctr/Med Sch
Control: Nonprofit (Private or Religious)
• Allopathic Medicine Prgm
• Clin Lab Scientist/Med Technologist Prgm
• Diagnostic Med Sonography Prgm
• Nursing Prgm
• Occupational Therapy Prgm
• Perfusion Prgm
• Specialist in BB Tech Prgm

Rush University Medical Center
Larry Goodman, MD, President and CEO
1725 W Harrison St, Ste 364
Chicago, IL 60612
312 942-7073
Type: Acad Health Ctr/Med Sch
Control: Nonprofit (Private or Religious)
• Audiologist Prgm
• Dietetic Internship Prgm
• Speech-Language Pathology Prgm

Saint Xavier University
Richard A Yanikoski, President
3700 W 103rd St
Chicago, IL 60655
312 298-3561
Type: 4-year Coll or Univ
Control: Nonprofit (Private or Religious)
• Nursing Prgm
• Speech-Language Pathology Prgm

School of the Art Institute of Chicago
Carol Becker, PhD, Dean of Faculty
37 S Wabash Ave
Chicago, IL 60603
312 899-1236
Type: 4-year Coll or Univ
Control: Nonprofit (Private or Religious)
• Art Therapy Prgm

Spanish Coalition for Jobs Inc
Mary Gonzalez-Koening, President
2011 W Pershing Rd
Chicago, IL 60609
773 247-0707
Type: Vocational or Tech Sch
Control: Nonprofit (Private or Religious)
• Medical Assistant Prgm

St Augustine College
Z Clara Brennan, PhD, President
1333-45 W Argyle St
Chicago, IL 60640
773 878-8756
Type: Junior or Comm Coll
Control: Nonprofit (Private or Religious)
• Respiratory Therapist (Entry-Level) Prgm

INSTITUTIONS

University of Chicago
Chicago, IL 60637
Type: Acad Health Ctr/Med Sch
Control: Nonprofit (Private or Religious)
• Allopathic Medicine Prgm

University of Illinois at Chicago
R Michael Tanner, PhD, Provost
University Hall
601 S Morgan St M/C 105
Chicago, IL 60612-7128
312 413-3450
Type: 4-year Coll or Univ
Control: State, County, or Local Govt
• Allopathic Medicine Prgm
• Dentistry Prgm
• Dietetics-Coordinated Prgm
• Dietetics-Didactic Prgm
• Health Information Admin Prgm
• Medical Illustrator Prgm
• Nursing Prgm
• Occupational Therapy Prgm
• Pharmacy Prgm
• Physical Therapy Prgm
• Psychology Prgm

Westwood College
Lou Pagano, MS, Executive Director
8501 W Higgins Rd
Chicago, IL 60631
847 928-1710
Type: Vocational or Tech Sch
Control: For Profit
• Medical Assistant Prgm

Wright College
Charles P Guengerich, PhD, President
4300 N Narragansett Ave
Chicago, IL 60634
773 777-7900
Type: Junior or Comm Coll
Control: State, County, or Local Govt
• Occupational Therapy Asst Prgm
• Radiography Prgm

Chicago Heights

Prairie State College
Paul J McCarthy, PhD, President
202 S Halsted
Chicago Heights, IL 60411
708 709-3500
Type: Junior or Comm Coll
Control: State, County, or Local Govt
• Dental Hygiene Prgm
• Surgical Technology Prgm

Cicero

Morton College
Brent Knight, PhD, President
3801 S Central Ave
Cicero, IL 60804
708 656-8000
Type: Junior or Comm Coll
Control: State, County, or Local Govt
• Massage Therapy Prgm
• Physical Therapist Assistant Prgm

Danville

Danville Area Community College
Alice M Jacobs, PhD, President
2000 E Main St
Danville, IL 61832
217 443-8848
Type: Junior or Comm Coll
Control: State, County, or Local Govt
• Health Information Tech Prgm
• Radiography Prgm

Lakeview College of Nursing
Danville, IL 61832
Type: Acad Health Ctr/Med Sch
Control: Nonprofit (Private or Religious)
• Nursing Prgm

Decatur

Millikin University
Douglas E Zemke, President
1184 W Main
Decatur, IL 62522
800 373-7733
Type: 4-year Coll or Univ
Control: Nonprofit (Private or Religious)
• Athletic Training Prgm
• Nursing Prgm

Richland Community College
Gayle Saunders, PhD, President
1 College Park
Decatur, IL 62521-8512
217 875-7200
Type: Junior or Comm Coll
Control: State, County, or Local Govt
• Surgical Technology Prgm

Deerfield

Trinity International University
Gregory L Waybright, PhD, President
2065 Half Day Rd
Deerfield, IL 60015
Type: 4-year Coll or Univ
Control: State, County, or Local Govt
• Athletic Training Prgm

DeKalb

Northern Illinois University
John Peters, PhD, President
Altgeld Hall
DeKalb, IL 60115
815 753-9501
Type: 4-year Coll or Univ
Control: State, County, or Local Govt
• Athletic Training Prgm
• Audiologist Prgm
• Clin Lab Scientist/Med Technologist Prgm
• Counseling Prgm
• Dietetic Internship Prgm
• Dietetics-Didactic Prgm
• Nursing Prgm
• Orientation and Mobility Specialist Prgm
• Physical Therapy Prgm
• Psychology Prgm
• Rehabilitation Counseling Prgm
• Speech-Language Pathology Prgm
• Teacher of the Visually Impaired Prgm
• Vision Rehabilitation Therapy Prgm

Des Plaines

Oakton Community College
Margaret B Lee, PhD, President
1600 E Golf Rd
Des Plaines, IL 60016
847 635-1732
Type: Junior or Comm Coll
Control: State, County, or Local Govt
• Clin Lab Technician/Med Lab Technician Prgm
• Health Information Tech Prgm
• Physical Therapist Assistant Prgm

Dixon

Sauk Valley Community College
George J Mihel, EdD, President
173 IL Rte 2
Dixon, IL 61021-9110
815 288-5511
Type: Junior or Comm Coll
Control: State, County, or Local Govt
• Radiography Prgm

Downers Grove

Midwestern University
Kathleen H Goepplinger, PhD, President
555 31st St
Downers Grove, IL 60515-1235
630 515-7300
Type: Acad Health Ctr/Med Sch
Control: Nonprofit (Private or Religious)
• Occupational Therapy Prgm
• Osteopathic Medicine Prgm
• Pharmacy Prgm
• Physical Therapy Prgm
• Physician Assistant Prgm

East Peoria

Illinois Central College
John S Erwin, President
One College Dr
East Peoria, IL 61635-0001
309 694-5431
Type: Junior or Comm Coll
Control: State, County, or Local Govt
• Clin Lab Technician/Med Lab Technician Prgm
• Dental Hygiene Prgm
• Occupational Therapy Asst Prgm
• Physical Therapist Assistant Prgm
• Radiography Prgm
• Respiratory Therapist (Advanced) Prgm
• Surgical Technology Prgm

Edwardsville

Southern Illinois University
Vaughn Vandegrift, PhD, Chancellor
Box 1151
Edwardsville, IL 62026
618 650-2475
Type: 4-year Coll or Univ
Control: State, County, or Local Govt
• Allopathic Medicine Prgm
• Art Therapy Prgm
• Dentistry Prgm
• Nursing Prgm
• Pharmacy Prgm
• Speech-Language Pathology Prgm

Elgin

Elgin Community College
David Sam, PhD, President
1700 Spartan Dr
Elgin, IL 60123-7193
847 697-1000
Type: Junior or Comm Coll
Control: State, County, or Local Govt
• Clin Lab Technician/Med Lab Technician Prgm
• Dental Assisting Prgm
• Surgical Technology Prgm

Elmhurst

Elmhurst College
Elmhurst, IL 60126
Type: 4-year Coll or Univ
Control: Nonprofit (Private or Religious)
• Nursing Prgm

Evanston

Evanston Northwestern Healthcare - Evanston
Raymond Grady, President/CEO
Hospitals and Clinics, Evanston Hospital
2650 Ridge Ave
Evanston, IL 60201
847 570-2005
Type: Acad Health Ctr/Med Sch
Control: Nonprofit (Private or Religious)
• Clin Lab Scientist/Med Technologist Prgm

Northwestern University
Henry S Bienen, PhD, President
2299 Sheridan Rd
Evanston, IL 60201
708 491-7456
Type: 4-year Coll or Univ
Control: Nonprofit (Private or Religious)
• Allopathic Medicine Prgm
• Audiologist Prgm
• Genetic Counseling Prgm
• Orthotist/Prosthetist Prgm
• Physical Therapy Prgm
• Psychology Prgm (2)
• Speech-Language Pathology Prgm

St Francis Hospital
Jeffrey Murphy, CEO
355 Ridge Ave
Evanston, IL 60202
847 492-4000
Type: Hosp or Med Ctr: 300-499 Beds
Control: Nonprofit (Private or Religious)
• Radiography Prgm

Galesburg

Carl Sandburg College
Thomas A Schmidt, MBA, President
2400 Tom L Wilson Blvd
Galesburg, IL 61401
309 344-2518
Type: Junior or Comm Coll
Control: State, County, or Local Govt
• Dental Hygiene Prgm

Glen Ellyn

College of DuPage
Sunil Chand, PhD, President
425 Fawell Blvd
Glen Ellyn, IL 60137-6599
630 942-2200
Type: Junior or Comm Coll
Control: State, County, or Local Govt
• Dental Hygiene Prgm
• Diagnostic Med Sonography Prgm
• Health Information Tech Prgm
• Nuclear Medicine Technology Prgm
• Physical Therapist Assistant Prgm
• Radiography Prgm
• Surgical Technology Prgm

Godfrey

Lewis & Clark Community College
Dale T Chapman, EdD, President
5800 Godfrey Rd
Godfrey, IL 62035-2466
618 468-2000
Type: Junior or Comm Coll
Control: State, County, or Local Govt
• Dental Assisting Prgm
• Dental Hygiene Prgm
• Occupational Therapy Asst Prgm

Grayslake

College of Lake County
DeRionne Pollard, PhD, VP of Educational Affairs
19351 W Washington St
Grayslake, IL 60030
847 543-2201
Type: Junior or Comm Coll
Control: State, County, or Local Govt
• Dental Hygiene Prgm
• Health Information Tech Prgm
• Phlebotomy Prgm
• Radiography Prgm
• Surgical Technology Prgm

Harvey

Ingalls Memorial Hospital
One Ingalls Dr
Harvey, IL 60426
708 333-2300
Control: Nonprofit (Private or Religious)
• Dietetic Internship Prgm

Herrin

Southern Illinois Collegiate Common Market
Mary J. Sullivan, PhD, Executive Director
3213 S Park Ave
Herrin, IL 62948
618 942-6902
Type: Consortium
Control: State, County, or Local Govt
• Clin Lab Technician/Med Lab Technician Prgm
• Health Information Tech Prgm
• Occupational Therapy Asst Prgm
• Surgical Technology Prgm

Hines

Edward Hines Jr VA Hospital
Nathan Geraths, Director
Fifth Ave and Roosevelt Rd
PO Box 5000
Hines, IL 60141
708 216-2153
Type: Dept of Veterans Affairs
Control: Fed Govt
• Clin Lab Scientist/Med Technologist Prgm
• Dietetic Internship Prgm
• Nuclear Medicine Technology Prgm

Jacksonville

MacMurray College
Jacksonville, IL 62650
Type: 4-year Coll or Univ
Control: Nonprofit (Private or Religious)
• Nursing Prgm

Joliet

Joliet Junior College
Gena Proulx, PhD, President
1215 Houbolt Rd
Joliet, IL 60431
815 280-2207
Type: Junior or Comm Coll
Control: State, County, or Local Govt
• Veterinary Technology Prgm

University of St Francis
Connie Bauer, PhD, Provost
500 Wilcox St
Joliet, IL 60435
815 740-3369
Type: 4-year Coll or Univ
Control: Nonprofit (Private or Religious)
• Nursing Prgm

Kankakee

Kankakee Community College
Jerry Weber, PhD, President
100 College Drive
Kankakee, IL 60901-0888
815 802-8112
Type: Junior or Comm Coll
Control: State, County, or Local Govt
• Clin Lab Technician/Med Lab Technician Prgm
• Respiratory Therapist (Advanced) Prgm

Lebanon

McKendree University
James M Dennis, PhD, President
701 College Rd
Lebanon, IL 62254-1299
618 537-6936
Type: 4-year Coll or Univ
Control: Nonprofit (Private or Religious)
• Athletic Training Prgm

Lincoln

Midwest Technical Institute
Brian Huff, President
405 N Limit St
PO Box 506
Lincoln, IL 62656
217 735-3105
Type: Vocational or Tech Sch
Control: For Profit
• Medical Assistant Prgm

Lisle

Benedictine University
William J Carroll, President
5700 College Rd
Lisle, IL 60532
708 960-1500
Type: 4-year Coll or Univ
Control: Nonprofit (Private or Religious)
• Dietetic Internship Prgm
• Dietetics-Didactic Prgm

Lombard

National University of Health Sciences
James F Winterstein, DC, President
200 E Roosevelt Rd
Lombard, IL 60148
630 889-6604
Type: Acad Health Ctr/Med Sch
Control: Nonprofit (Private or Religious)
• Massage Therapy Prgm

Macomb

McDonough District Hospital
Stephen R Hopper, MS, President
525 E Grant St
Macomb, IL 61455
309 833-4101
Type: Hosp or Med Ctr: 100-299 Beds
Control: State, County, or Local Govt
• Radiography Prgm

Western Illinois University
Al Goldfarb, PhD, President
209 Sherman Hall
1 University Circle
Macomb, IL 61455
309 298-1824
Type: 4-year Coll or Univ
Control: State, County, or Local Govt
• Athletic Training Prgm
• Counseling Prgm
• Dietetics-Didactic Prgm
• Music Therapy Prgm
• Speech-Language Pathology Prgm
• Therapeutic Recreation Specialist Prgm

Malta

Kishwaukee College
Thomas Choice, PhD, President
21193 Malta Rd
Malta, IL 60150
815 825-2086
Type: Junior or Comm Coll
Control: State, County, or Local Govt
• Massage Therapy Prgm
• Radiography Prgm

Mattoon

Lake Land College
Scott Lensink, MBA, interim President
5001 Lake Land Blvd
Mattoon, IL 61938-9366
217 234-5253
Type: Junior or Comm Coll
Control: State, County, or Local Govt
• Dental Hygiene Prgm
• Physical Therapist Assistant Prgm

Maywood

Loyola University Medical Center
Anthony Barbato, MD, Executive Vice President
2160 S First Ave
Maywood, IL 60153
708 216-9000
Type: Hosp or Med Ctr: 500> Beds
Control: Nonprofit (Private or Religious)
• Allopathic Medicine Prgm
• Emergency Med Tech-Paramedic Prgm

Moline

Black Hawk College
Keith Miller, PhD, President
6600 34th Ave
Moline, IL 61265-5899
309 796-1311
Type: Junior or Comm Coll
Control: State, County, or Local Govt
• Physical Therapist Assistant Prgm

Naperville

North Central College
Harold R Wilde, PhD, President
30 N Brainard
Naperville, IL 60540
630 637-5454
Type: 4-year Coll or Univ
Control: Nonprofit (Private or Religious)
• Athletic Training Prgm

Normal

Bloomington-Normal School of Radiography
Mike Johnson, MBA RT(R), Chair, Board of
  Directors
900 Franklin Ave
Normal, IL 61761
309 452-2834
Type: Hosp or Med Ctr: 100-299 Beds
Control: Nonprofit (Private or Religious)
• Radiography Prgm

Illinois State University

C Alvin Bowman, PhD, President
1000 President's Office
418 Hovey Hall
Normal, IL 61790-1000
309 438-5677
Type: 4-year Coll or Univ
Control: State, County, or Local Govt
• Athletic Training Prgm
• Audiologist Prgm
• Clin Lab Scientist/Med Technologist Prgm
• Dietetic Internship Prgm
• Dietetics-Didactic Prgm
• Health Information Admin Prgm
• Music Therapy Prgm
• Nursing Prgm
• Speech-Language Pathology Prgm
• Therapeutic Recreation Specialist Prgm

North Aurora

Everest College
Robert Van Elsen, BS, Campus President
150 S Lincoln Way, Ste 100
North Aurora, IL 60542
630 896-2140
Type: Vocational or Tech Sch
Control: For Profit
• Medical Assistant Prgm (3)

North Chicago

Rosalind Franklin Univ of Medicine & Science
K Michael Welch, MBChB FRCP, President/CEO
3333 Green Bay Rd
North Chicago, IL 60064
847 578-3000
Type: Acad Health Ctr/Med Sch
Control: Nonprofit (Private or Religious)
• Allopathic Medicine Prgm
• Clin Lab Scientist/Med Technologist Prgm
• Pathologists' Assistant Prgm
• Physical Therapy Prgm
• Physician Assistant Prgm
• Podiatric Medicine Prgm
• Psychology Prgm

Oak Park

West Suburban College of Nursing
Oak Park, IL 60302
Type: Acad Health Ctr/Med Sch
Control: Nonprofit (Private or Religious)
• Nursing Prgm

Oglesby

Illinois Valley Community College
Jean Goodnow, President
815 N Orlando Smith Ave
Oglesby, IL 61348-9691
815 224-2720
Type: Junior or Comm Coll
Control: State, County, or Local Govt
• Dental Assisting Prgm

Olney

Olney Central College
Jackie Davis, EdD, President
305 N West St
Olney, IL 62450
618 395-7777
Type: Junior or Comm Coll
Control: State, County, or Local Govt
• Radiography Prgm

Palatine

Harper College
Robert Breuder, PhD, President
1200 W Algonquin Rd
Palatine, IL 60067
847 925-6000
Type: Junior or Comm Coll
Control: State, County, or Local Govt
• Dental Hygiene Prgm
• Dietetic Technician-AD Prgm
• Medical Assistant Prgm

Palos Heights

Trinity Christian College
Palos Heights, IL 60463
Type: 4-year Coll or Univ
Control: Nonprofit (Private or Religious)
• Nursing Prgm

Palos Hills

Moraine Valley Community College
Vernon Crawley, PhD, President/CEO
9000 W College Pkwy
Palos Hills, IL 60465
708 974-5201
Type: Junior or Comm Coll
Control: State, County, or Local Govt
• Health Information Tech Prgm
• Medical Assistant Prgm
• Phlebotomy Prgm
• Radiography Prgm
• Respiratory Therapist (Advanced) Prgm

Peoria

Bradley University
David Broski, President
1501 W Bradley Ave
Peoria, IL 61625
309 676-7611
Type: 4-year Coll or Univ
Control: Nonprofit (Private or Religious)
• Counseling Prgm
• Dietetics-Didactic Prgm
• Physical Therapy Prgm

Midstate College
R Dale Bunch, President
411 W Northmoor Rd
Peoria, IL 61614
309 692-4092
Type: Junior or Comm Coll
Control: For Profit
• Medical Assistant Prgm

OSF St Francis Medical Center
Keith Steffen, Administrator
530 NE Glen Oak Ave
Peoria, IL 61637
309 655-2020
Type: Hosp or Med Ctr: 500> Beds
Control: Nonprofit (Private or Religious)
• Clin Lab Scientist/Med Technologist Prgm
• Dietetic Internship Prgm
• Histotechnician Prgm
• Radiography Prgm

Quincy

Blessing Hospital
Maureen Kahn, RN MHA, President/CEO
Broadway at 11th St
PO Box 7005
Quincy, IL 62305
217 223-8400
Type: Hosp or Med Ctr: 300-499 Beds
Control: Nonprofit (Private or Religious)
• Clin Lab Technician/Med Lab Technician Prgm
• Nursing Prgm
• Pharmacy Technician Prgm
• Radiography Prgm

John Wood Community College
William M Simpson, EdD, President
1301 S 48th St
Quincy, IL 62305
217 224-6500
Type: Junior or Comm Coll
Control: State, County, or Local Govt
• Surgical Technology Prgm

River Forest

Concordia University
Manfred Booa, PhD, Acting President
7400 Augusta
River Forest, IL 60305-1499
708 771-8300
Type: Vocational or Tech Sch
Control: Nonprofit (Private or Religious)
• Counseling Prgm

Dominican University
Donna M Carroll, President
7900 W Division
River Forest, IL 60305
708 366-2490
Type: 4-year Coll or Univ
Control: Nonprofit (Private or Religious)
• Dietetics-Coordinated Prgm
• Dietetics-Didactic Prgm
• Medical Librarian Prgm

River Grove

Triton College
Patricia Granados, EdD, President
2000 N Fifth Ave
River Grove, IL 60171
708 456-0300
Type: Junior or Comm Coll
Control: State, County, or Local Govt
• Diagnostic Med Sonography Prgm
• Nuclear Medicine Technology Prgm
• Ophthalmic Med Technician Prgm
• Radiography Prgm
• Respiratory Therapist (Advanced) Prgm
• Surgical Technology Prgm

Rock Island

Trinity College of Nursing & Health Sciences
Carol Dwyer, RN MSN MM, President
2122 25th Ave
Rock Island, IL 61201
309 779-2256
Type: 4-year Coll or Univ
Control: Nonprofit (Private or Religious)
• Emergency Med Tech-Paramedic Prgm
• Nursing Prgm
• Radiography Prgm
• Surgical Technology Prgm

Rockford

OSF St Anthony Medical Center
David Schertz, Administrator
5666 E State St
Rockford, IL 61108
815 226-2000
Type: Hosp or Med Ctr: 100-299 Beds
Control: Nonprofit (Private or Religious)
• Clin Lab Scientist/Med Technologist Prgm
• Nursing Prgm

Rock Valley College
Jack J. Becherer, EdD, President
3301 N Mulford Rd
Rockford, IL 61114-5699
815 654-4260
Type: Junior or Comm Coll
Control: State, County, or Local Govt
• Dental Hygiene Prgm
• Respiratory Therapist (Advanced) Prgm
• Surgical Technology Prgm

Rockford Business College
James Devaney, PhD, CEO
730 N Church
Rockford, IL 61103
815 965-8616
Type: Vocational or Tech Sch
Control: For Profit
• Medical Assistant Prgm

Rockford Memorial Hospital
Gary Kaatz, MS, President
2400 N Rockton Ave
Rockford, IL 61103
815 971-5000
Type: Hosp or Med Ctr: 300-499 Beds
Control: Nonprofit (Private or Religious)
• Radiography Prgm

Swedish American Hospital
William Gorski, MD, President/CEO
1401 E State St
Rockford, IL 61104-2298
815 968-4400
Type: Hosp or Med Ctr: 300-499 Beds
Control: Nonprofit (Private or Religious)
• Radiation Therapy Prgm
• Radiography Prgm

Romeoville

Lewis University
Brother James Gaffney, FSC, President
One University Pkwy
Romeoville, IL 60446
815 838-0500
Type: 4-year Coll or Univ
Control: State, County, or Local Govt
• Athletic Training Prgm
• Nursing Prgm

Rosemont

Northwestern Business College
Lawrence W Schumacher, BA, President
9700 W Higgins Rd, Ste 750
Rosemont, IL 60018
847 318-8550
Type: Junior or Comm Coll
Control: For Profit
• Health Information Tech Prgm
• Medical Assistant Prgm (3)

South Holland

South Suburban College
George Dammer, MS, President
15800 S State St
South Holland, IL 60473-1262
708 596-2000
Type: Junior or Comm Coll
Control: State, County, or Local Govt
• Diagnostic Med Sonography Prgm
• Medical Assistant Prgm
• Occupational Therapy Asst Prgm
• Pharmacy Technician Prgm
• Phlebotomy Prgm
• Radiography Prgm

Springfield

Lincoln Land Community College
Charlotte Warren, PhD, President
5250 Shepherd Rd
PO Box 19256
Springfield, IL 62794-9256
217 786-2273
Type: Junior or Comm Coll
Control: State, County, or Local Govt
• Occupational Therapy Asst Prgm
• Radiography Prgm

St John's Hospital
Richard Carlson, FACHE, Exec Vice President
800 E Carpenter
Springfield, IL 62769
217 544-6464
Type: Consortium
Control: Nonprofit (Private or Religious)
• Clin Lab Scientist/Med Technologist Prgm
• Electroneurodiagnostic Tech Prgm
• Respiratory Therapist (Advanced) Prgm

University of Illinois at Springfield
Richard Ringeisen, PhD, Chancellor
One University Plaza
Springfield, IL 62703
217 786-6634
Type: 4-year Coll or Univ
Control: State, County, or Local Govt
• Clin Lab Scientist/Med Technologist Prgm
• Counseling Prgm

Sugar Grove

Waubonsee Community College
Christine J Sobek, EdD, President
Rte 47 at Waubonsee Dr
Sugar Grove, IL 60554
630 466-7900
Type: Junior or Comm Coll
Control: State, County, or Local Govt
• Medical Assistant Prgm
• Surgical Technology Prgm

Ullin

Shawnee Community College
Terry G Ludwig, PhD, President
8364 Shawnee College Rd
Ullin, IL 62992
618 634-3221
Type: Junior or Comm Coll
Control: State, County, or Local Govt
• Surgical Technology Prgm

University Park

Governors State University
Elaine Maimon, PhD, President
1 University Pkwy
University Park, IL 60466
708 534-4130
Type: 4-year Coll or Univ
Control: State, County, or Local Govt
• Counseling Prgm
• Occupational Therapy Prgm
• Physical Therapy Prgm
• Speech-Language Pathology Prgm

Wheaton

Wheaton College
Wheaton, IL 60187
Type: 4-year Coll or Univ
Control: State, County, or Local Govt
• Psychology Prgm

Indiana

Alexandria

Alexandria School of Scientific Therapeutics
Herbert Hobbs, CEO
809 S Harrison
PO Box 287
Alexandria, IN 46001
765 724-9152
Type: Acad Health Ctr/Med Sch
Control: For Profit
• Massage Therapy Prgm

Anderson

Anderson University
James L Edwards, PhD, President
1100 E 5th St
Anderson, IN 46012
765 641-4011
Type: 4-year Coll or Univ
Control: Nonprofit (Private or Religious)
• Athletic Training Prgm
• Nursing Prgm

Beech Grove

St Francis Hospital & Health Centers
Robert J Brody, MHA, President/CEO
1600 Albany St
Beech Grove, IN 46107
317 783-8220
Type: Hosp or Med Ctr: 500> Beds
Control: Nonprofit (Private or Religious)
• Clin Lab Scientist/Med Technologist Prgm
• Emergency Med Tech-Paramedic Prgm

Bloomington

Bloomington Hospital
Nancy Carlstedt, MS, President
PO Box 1149
Bloomington, IN 47402
812 336-6821
Type: Hosp or Med Ctr: 300-499 Beds
Control: Nonprofit (Private or Religious)
• Surgical Technology Prgm

Indiana University - Bloomington
Adam Herbert, PhD, President
President's Office, Bryan Hall
Bloomington, IN 47405
812 855-4613
Type: 4-year Coll or Univ
Control: State, County, or Local Govt
• Athletic Training Prgm
• Audiologist Prgm
• Counseling Prgm
• Dietetics-Didactic Prgm
• Optometric Technician Prgm
• Optometry Prgm
• Psychology Prgm
• Speech-Language Pathology Prgm
• Therapeutic Recreation Specialist Prgm

Columbus

Columbus Area Career Connection/Ivy Tech St
Christy Ross, BS CDA, Instructor, Director
230 S Marr Rd
Columbus, IN 47201
812 376-4202
Type: Vocational or Tech Sch
Control: Nonprofit (Private or Religious)
• Dental Assisting Prgm

Columbus Regional Hospital
Douglas J Leonard, Vice President
2400 E 17th St
Columbus, IN 47201
812 376-5439
Type: Hosp or Med Ctr: 300-499 Beds
Control: State, County, or Local Govt
• Radiography Prgm

Elkhart

Elkhart General Hospital
Greg Lintjer, President
600 E Blvd
Elkhart, IN 46514
574 293-8961
Type: Hosp or Med Ctr: 300-499 Beds
Control: State, County, or Local Govt
• Emergency Med Tech-Paramedic Prgm

Evansville

University of Evansville
Stephen G Jennings, President
1800 Lincoln Ave
Evansville, IN 47722
812 488-2151
Type: 4-year Coll or Univ
Control: Nonprofit (Private or Religious)
• Athletic Training Prgm
• Music Therapy Prgm
• Physical Therapist Assistant Prgm
• Physical Therapy Prgm

University of Southern Indiana
H Ray Hoops, PhD, President
8600 University Blvd
Evansville, IN 47712-3534
812 464-1756
Type: 4-year Coll or Univ
Control: State, County, or Local Govt
• Dental Assisting Prgm
• Dental Hygiene Prgm
• Nursing Prgm
• Occupational Therapy Asst Prgm
• Occupational Therapy Prgm
• Radiography Prgm
• Respiratory Therapist (Advanced) Prgm

Fort Wayne

Fort Wayne School of Radiography
Kirk Ray, MD, CEO
St Joseph Hospital
700 Broadway
Fort Wayne, IN 46802
260 425-3990
Type: Hosp or Med Ctr: 100-299 Beds
Control: For Profit
• Radiography Prgm

Indiana Univ - Purdue Univ Ft Wayne
Michael A Wartell, PhD, Chancellor
2101 Coliseum Blvd E
Fort Wayne, IN 46805
260 481-6103
Type: 4-year Coll or Univ
Control: State, County, or Local Govt
• Dental Assisting Prgm
• Dental Hygiene Prgm
• Dental Lab Technician Prgm
• Music Therapy Prgm

International Business Coll - Ft Wayne
Jim C Zillman, President
5699 Coventry Ln
Fort Wayne, IN 46804
260 459-4500
Type: 4-year Coll or Univ
Control: For Profit
• Medical Assistant Prgm
• Veterinary Technology Prgm

Parkview Hospital
Sue Ehinger, MD, COO
2200 Randallia Dr
Fort Wayne, IN 46805
260 373-3606
Type: Hosp or Med Ctr: 500> Beds
Control: Nonprofit (Private or Religious)
• Clin Lab Scientist/Med Technologist Prgm

University of Saint Francis
Sr M Elise Kriss, OSF PhD, President
2701 Spring St
Fort Wayne, IN 46808
260 434-3101
Type: 4-year Coll or Univ
Control: Nonprofit (Private or Religious)
• Nursing Prgm
• Physical Therapist Assistant Prgm
• Physician Assistant Prgm
• Radiography Prgm
• Surgical Technology Prgm

Franklin

Franklin College
Jay Moseley, PhD, President
Old Main
Franklin, IN 46131
317 738-8010
Type: 4-year Coll or Univ
Control: State, County, or Local Govt
• Athletic Training Prgm

Gary

Indiana University Northwest
Bruce Bergland, PhD, Chancellor
3400 Broadway
Gary, IN 46408
219 980-6700
Type: 4-year Coll or Univ
Control: State, County, or Local Govt
• Clin Lab Technician/Med Lab Technician Prgm
• Dental Assisting Prgm
• Dental Hygiene Prgm
• Health Information Tech Prgm
• Nursing Prgm
• Phlebotomy Prgm
• Radiation Therapy Prgm
• Radiography Prgm
• Respiratory Therapist (Advanced) Prgm

Methodist Hospitals Inc
Claude Watts, President/CEO
Northlake Campus
600 Grant St
Gary, IN 46402
219 886-4602
Type: Hosp or Med Ctr: 500> Beds
Control: Nonprofit (Private or Religious)
• Emergency Med Tech-Paramedic Prgm

Goshen

Goshen College
Goshen, IN 46526
Type: 4-year Coll or Univ
Control: Nonprofit (Private or Religious)
• Nursing Prgm

Granger

Davenport University
Jean Redinger, MA, Campus Executive Director
7121 Grape Rd
Granger, IN 46530
574 277-8447
Type: 4-year Coll or Univ
Control: Nonprofit (Private or Religious)
• Medical Assistant Prgm (2)

Greencastle

DePauw University
Robert G Bottoms, President
313 S Locust
Administration Bldg
Greencastle, IN 46135
765 658-4055
Type: 4-year Coll or Univ
Control: Nonprofit (Private or Religious)
• Athletic Training Prgm

Greenfield

Hancock Regional Hospital
Bobby Keen, PhD, President and CEO
801 N State St
Greenfield, IN 46140
317 462-0457
Type: Hosp or Med Ctr: 100-299 Beds
Control: For Profit
• Radiography Prgm

Hammond

St Margaret Mercy Healthcare Centers
Tom Gryzbek, President/CEO
Mercy Healthcare Ctrs
5454 Hohman Ave
Hammond, IN 46320
219 932-2300
Type: Hosp or Med Ctr: 300-499 Beds
Control: Nonprofit (Private or Religious)
• Clin Lab Scientist/Med Technologist Prgm

Indianapolis

Butler University/Clarian Health
Bobby Fong, PhD, President
4600 Sunset Ave
Indianapolis, IN 46208-3485
317 940-9900
Type: 4-year Coll or Univ
Control: Nonprofit (Private or Religious)
• Counseling Prgm
• Pharmacy Prgm
• Physician Assistant Prgm

Clarian Health Partners Inc
Daniel F Evans, JD, President/CEO
PO Box 1367
Indianapolis, IN 46206-1367
317 962-5900
Type: Hosp or Med Ctr: 500> Beds
Control: Nonprofit (Private or Religious)
• Clin Lab Scientist/Med Technologist Prgm
• Electroneurodiagnostic Tech Prgm
• Emergency Med Tech-Paramedic Prgm
• Pharmacy Technician Prgm
• Respiratory Therapist (Advanced) Prgm
• Surgical Technology Prgm

Community Health Network
William E Corley, President
1500 N Ritter Ave
Indianapolis, IN 46219
317 355-5529
Type: Hosp or Med Ctr: 500> Beds
Control: For Profit
• Radiography Prgm

Indiana Blood Center
Byron Buhner, AB MS, President/CEO
3450 N Meridian St
Indianapolis, IN 46208
317 916-5001
Type: Hosp or Med Ctr: 300-499 Beds
Control: Nonprofit (Private or Religious)
• Specialist in BB Tech Prgm

Indiana Business College
Kenneth J Konesco, President
550 E Washington St
Indianapolis, IN 46204
Type: Vocational or Tech Sch
Control: For Profit
• Medical Assistant Prgm (9)
• Surgical Technology Prgm (2)

Indiana Univ-Purdue U-Indianapolis
Charles R Bantz, Chancellor
425 University Blvd
Cavanaugh Hall 441
Indianapolis, IN 46202
Type: 4-year Coll or Univ
Control: State, County, or Local Govt
• Music Therapy Prgm
• Psychology Prgm

Indiana University
Charles Bantz, PhD, Chancellor
Administrative Building, Rm 104
355 N Lansing St
Indianapolis, IN 46202-2896
317 274-4417
Type: 4-year Coll or Univ
Control: State, County, or Local Govt
• Allopathic Medicine Prgm
• Clin Lab Scientist/Med Technologist Prgm
• Cytotechnology Prgm
• Dental Assisting Prgm
• Dental Hygiene Prgm
• Dentistry Prgm
• Dietetic Internship Prgm
• Genetic Counseling Prgm
• Health Information Admin Prgm
• Histotechnician Prgm
• Medical Librarian Prgm
• Nuclear Medicine Technology Prgm
• Nursing Prgm
• Occupational Therapy Prgm
• Pathologists' Assistant Prgm
• Physical Therapy Prgm
• Radiation Therapy Prgm
• Radiography Prgm
• Respiratory Therapist (Advanced) Prgm

International Business Coll - Indianapolis
Eric Stovall, President
7205 Shadeland Station
Indianapolis, IN 46256
317 841-6400
Type: Vocational or Tech Sch
Control: For Profit
• Medical Assistant Prgm

Ivy Tech Community College
Thomas J Snyder, MBA, President
50 W Fall Creek Pkwy North Dr
Indianapolis, IN 46208
317 921-4860
Type: Junior or Comm Coll
Control: State, County, or Local Govt
• Clin Lab Technician/Med Lab Technician Prgm
  (2)
• Dental Assisting Prgm (3)
• Emergency Med Tech-Paramedic Prgm (3)
• Medical Assistant Prgm (16)
• Phlebotomy Prgm
• Physical Therapist Assistant Prgm (2)
• Radiography Prgm (3)
• Respiratory Therapist (Advanced) Prgm (6)
• Surgical Technology Prgm (7)

Kaplan College
Barri Shirk, BA MS, Executive Directror
7302 Woodland Dr
Indianapolis, IN 46278-1736
317 299-6001
Type: Vocational or Tech Sch
Control: For Profit
• Dental Assisting Prgm
• Medical Assistant Prgm

Marian College
Daniel A Felicetti, PhD, President
3200 Cold Spring Rd
Indianapolis, IN 46222
317 929-0237
Type: 4-year Coll or Univ
Control: Nonprofit (Private or Religious)
• Nursing Prgm

University of Indianapolis
Beverly Pitts, PhD, President
1400 E Hanna Ave
Indianapolis, IN 46227
317 788-3211
Type: 4-year Coll or Univ
Control: Nonprofit (Private or Religious)
• Athletic Training Prgm
• Nursing Prgm
• Occupational Therapy Prgm
• Physical Therapist Assistant Prgm
• Physical Therapy Prgm
• Psychology Prgm

Kokomo

Indiana University - Kokomo
Ruth J Person, PhD, Chancellor
2300 S Washington St
Kokomo, IN 46902
765 453-2000
Type: 4-year Coll or Univ
Control: State, County, or Local Govt
• Nursing Prgm
• Radiography Prgm

St Vincent Health/St Joseph Hospital
Darcy Burthay, MSN RN, President
1907 W Sycamore St
Kokomo, IN 46901
317 452-5611
Type: Consortium
Control: Nonprofit (Private or Religious)
• Radiography Prgm

Madison

King's Daughters' Hospital & Health Services
Roger J Allman, MHA, President/CEO
One King's Daughters Dr, PO Box 447
Madison, IN 47250
812 265-5211
Type: Hosp or Med Ctr: 100-299 Beds
Control: Nonprofit (Private or Religious)
• Radiography Prgm

Marion

Indiana Wesleyan University
James Barnes, EdD, President
4201 S Washington St
Marion, IN 46953
765 677-2100
Type: 4-year Coll or Univ
Control: Nonprofit (Private or Religious)
• Athletic Training Prgm
• Counseling Prgm
• Nursing Prgm

Merrillville

Everest College
Mary Klinefelter, President
707 E 80th Pl, Ste 200
Merrillville, IN 46410
219 756-6811
Type: Vocational or Tech Sch
Control: State, County, or Local Govt
• Surgical Technology Prgm

Muncie

Ball Memorial Hospital
Brent Batman, MHA, President
2401 University Ave
Muncie, IN 47303-3499
765 747-3393
Type: Hosp or Med Ctr: 300-499 Beds
Control: Nonprofit (Private or Religious)
• Clin Lab Scientist/Med Technologist Prgm
• Radiography Prgm

Ball State University
Jo Ann Gora, PhD, President
Administration Bldg 101
Muncie, IN 47306
317 285-5555
Type: 4-year Coll or Univ
Control: State, County, or Local Govt
• Athletic Training Prgm
• Audiologist Prgm
• Counseling Prgm
• Dietetic Internship Prgm
• Dietetics-Didactic Prgm
• Nursing Prgm
• Radiography Prgm
• Rehabilitation Counseling Prgm
• Speech-Language Pathology Prgm

New Albany

Indiana University Southeast
New Albany, IN 47150
Type: 4-year Coll or Univ
Control: State, County, or Local Govt
• Nursing Prgm

North Manchester

Manchester College
Parker C Marden, PhD, President
Box 176
North Manchester, IN 46962
219 982-5050
Type: 4-year Coll or Univ
Control: Nonprofit (Private or Religious)
• Athletic Training Prgm

Richmond

Reid Hospital & Health Care Services
Barry S MacDowell, MHA, President
1401 Chester Blvd
Richmond, IN 47374
765 983-3122
Type: Hosp or Med Ctr: 100-299 Beds
Control: Nonprofit (Private or Religious)
• Radiography Prgm

South Bend

Brown Mackie College
Connie S Adelman, BGS, Campus President
1030 E Jefferson Blvd
South Bend, IN 46617-3123
574 237-0774
Type: Vocational or Tech Sch
Control: For Profit
• Medical Assistant Prgm (2)
• Occupational Therapy Asst Prgm (2)
• Physical Therapist Assistant Prgm

Indiana University South Bend
Una Mae Reck, PhD, Chancellor
1700 Mishawaka Ave, Box 7111
South Bend, IN 46634
574 237-4220
Type: 4-year Coll or Univ
Control: State, County, or Local Govt
• Counseling Prgm
• Dental Assisting Prgm
• Dental Hygiene Prgm
• Nursing Prgm
• Radiography Prgm

St Mary of the Woods

St Mary of the Woods College
Joan Lescinski, President
St Mary of the Woods, IN 47876
812 535-5154
Type: 4-year Coll or Univ
Control: Nonprofit (Private or Religious)
• Music Therapy Prgm

Terre Haute

Indiana State University
Lloyd Benjamin, PhD, President
Condit House
Terre Haute, IN 47809
812 237-4000
Type: 4-year Coll or Univ
Control: State, County, or Local Govt
• Athletic Training Prgm
• Counseling Prgm
• Dietetics-Coordinated Prgm
• Psychology Prgm
• Speech-Language Pathology Prgm

Valparaiso

Valparaiso University
Valparaiso, IN 46383
Type: 4-year Coll or Univ
Control: Nonprofit (Private or Religious)
• Nursing Prgm

Vincennes

Good Samaritan Hospital
Matt Bailey, MHA, President and CEO
520 S Seventh St
Vincennes, IN 47591
812 885-3195
Type: Hosp or Med Ctr: 100-299 Beds
Control: State, County, or Local Govt
• Clin Lab Scientist/Med Technologist Prgm
• Radiography Prgm

Vincennes University
Richard E Helton, PhD, President
1002 First St N
Vincennes, IN 47591
812 888-4201
Type: 4-year Coll or Univ
Control: State, County, or Local Govt
• Health Information Tech Prgm
• Physical Therapist Assistant Prgm
• Surgical Assistant Prgm
• Surgical Technology Prgm

West Lafayette

Purdue University
France A. Cordova, PhD, President
Hovde Hall
West Lafayette, IN 47907
765 494-9708
Type: 4-year Coll or Univ
Control: State, County, or Local Govt
• Athletic Training Prgm
• Audiologist Prgm
• Counseling Prgm
• Dietetics-Coordinated Prgm
• Dietetics-Didactic Prgm
• Nursing Prgm
• Pharmacy Prgm
• Psychology Prgm
• Speech-Language Pathology Prgm
• Veterinary Medicine Prgm
• Veterinary Technology Prgm

Iowa

Ames

Iowa State University
Gregory Geoffroy, PhD, President
2035 President
117 Beardshear
Ames, IA 50011
515 294-2042
Type: 4-year Coll or Univ
Control: State, County, or Local Govt
• Athletic Training Prgm
• Dietetic Internship Prgm
• Dietetics-Didactic Prgm
• Veterinary Medicine Prgm

Anamosa

Carlson College of Massage Therapy
Ruth Carlson
11809 County Rd X28
Box 28
Anamosa, IA 52205
319 462-3402
Type: Acad Health Ctr/Med Sch
Control: For Profit
• Massage Therapy Prgm

Ankeny

Des Moines Area Community College
Robert Denson, JD, President
Bldg 22
2006 S Ankeny Blvd
Ankeny, IA 50023
515 964-6638
Type: Junior or Comm Coll
Control: State, County, or Local Govt
• Clin Lab Technician/Med Lab Technician Prgm
• Dental Assisting Prgm
• Dental Hygiene Prgm
• Medical Assistant Prgm
• Respiratory Therapist (Advanced) Prgm
• Veterinary Technology Prgm

Bettendorf

Scott Community College
Thomas Coley, PhD, President
500 Belmont Rd
Bettendorf, IA 52722
563 441-4061
Type: Junior or Comm Coll
Control: State, County, or Local Govt
• Dental Assisting Prgm
• Electroneurodiagnostic Tech Prgm
• Health Information Tech Prgm
• Radiography Prgm

Calmar

Northeast Iowa Community College
Penelope Wills, PhD, President
1625 Hwy 150 S
PO Box 400
Calmar, IA 52132
563 562-3263
Type: Junior or Comm Coll
Control: State, County, or Local Govt
• Dental Assisting Prgm
• Health Information Tech Prgm
• Radiography Prgm
• Respiratory Therapist (Advanced) Prgm

Cedar Falls

University of Northern Iowa
Benjamin Allen, PhD, President
Seerley Hall
Cedar Falls, IA 50614-0002
319 273-2566
Type: 4-year Coll or Univ
Control: State, County, or Local Govt
• Athletic Training Prgm
• Counseling Prgm
• Speech-Language Pathology Prgm
• Therapeutic Recreation Specialist Prgm

INSTITUTIONS

Cedar Rapids

Coe College
James Phifer, PhD, President
1220 First Ave NE
Cedar Rapids, IA 52402
319 399-8686
Type: 4-year Coll or Univ
Control: Nonprofit (Private or Religious)
• Athletic Training Prgm
• Nursing Prgm

Kirkwood Community College
Mick Starcevich, EdD, President
6301 Kirkwood Blvd SW
PO Box 2068
Cedar Rapids, IA 52406-9973
319 398-5501
Type: Junior or Comm Coll
Control: State, County, or Local Govt
• Dental Assisting Prgm
• Dental Hygiene Prgm
• Dental Lab Technician Prgm
• Electroneurodiagnostic Tech Prgm
• Emergency Med Tech-Paramedic Prgm
• Health Information Tech Prgm
• Medical Assistant Prgm
• Occupational Therapy Asst Prgm
• Physical Therapist Assistant Prgm
• Respiratory Therapist (Advanced) Prgm
• Surgical Technology Prgm
• Veterinary Technology Prgm

Mount Mercy College
Cedar Rapids, IA 52402
Type: 4-year Coll or Univ
Control: Nonprofit (Private or Religious)
• Nursing Prgm

St Luke's Hospital
Ted Townsand, MD, President/CEO
PO Box 3026
1026 A Avenue NE
Cedar Rapids, IA 52406-3026
319 369-7309
Type: Hosp or Med Ctr: 300-499 Beds
Control: Nonprofit (Private or Religious)
• Clin Lab Scientist/Med Technologist Prgm
• Radiography Prgm

Council Bluffs

Iowa Western Community College
Dan Kinney, PhD, President
2700 College Rd Box 4-C
Council Bluffs, IA 51502-3004
712 325-3200
Type: Junior or Comm Coll
Control: State, County, or Local Govt
• Dental Assisting Prgm
• Dental Hygiene Prgm
• Medical Assistant Prgm
• Veterinary Technology Prgm

Jennie Edmundson Memorial Hospital
David M Holcomb, MHA, CEO
933 E Pierce St
Council Bluffs, IA 51501
712 328-6239
Type: Hosp or Med Ctr: 100-299 Beds
Control: Nonprofit (Private or Religious)
• Radiography Prgm

Davenport

Institute of Therapeutic Massage & Wellness
Dan Howes, PhD
1730 Wilkes Ave
Davenport, IA 52804
563 445-1055
Type: Vocational or Tech Sch
Control: For Profit
• Massage Therapy Prgm

Kaplan University, Davenport Campus
John Neal, PhD, Exec Dir/Campus President
1801 E Kimberly Rd, Ste 1
Davenport, IA 52807
563 355-3500
Type: Vocational or Tech Sch
Control: For Profit
• Medical Assistant Prgm

St Ambrose University
Edward Rogalski, PhD, President
518 W Locust St
Davenport, IA 52803
563 333-6212
Type: 4-year Coll or Univ
Control: Nonprofit (Private or Religious)
• Nursing Prgm
• Occupational Therapy Prgm
• Physical Therapy Prgm

Decorah

Luther College
Richard L Torgerson, PhD, President
700 College Dr
Decorah, IA 52101
563 387-1001
Type: 4-year Coll or Univ
Control: Nonprofit (Private or Religious)
• Athletic Training Prgm
• Nursing Prgm

Des Moines

Des Moines University
Terry Branstad, DSC, President
3440 Grand Ave
Des Moines, IA 50312
515 271-1500
Type: 4-year Coll or Univ
Control: Nonprofit (Private or Religious)
• Osteopathic Medicine Prgm
• Physical Therapy Prgm
• Physician Assistant Prgm
• Podiatric Medicine Prgm

Drake University
David Maxwell, President
25th St and University Ave
Des Moines, IA 50311
515 271-2011
Type: 4-year Coll or Univ
Control: Nonprofit (Private or Religious)
• Pharmacy Prgm
• Rehabilitation Counseling Prgm

Grand View College
Des Moines, IA 50316
Type: 4-year Coll or Univ
Control: Nonprofit (Private or Religious)
• Nursing Prgm

Iowa Methodist Med Ctr/Iowa Hlth - Des Moines
Eric Crowell, MS MHA, President and CEO
1200 Pleasant St
Des Moines, IA 50309-1453
515 241-6201
Type: Hosp or Med Ctr: 500> Beds
Control: Nonprofit (Private or Religious)
• Radiography Prgm

Mercy College of Health Sciences
Barbara Quijano Decker, JD, President
928 Sixth Ave
Des Moines, IA 50309
515 643-6601
Type: 4-year Coll or Univ
Control: Nonprofit (Private or Religious)
• Diagnostic Med Sonography Prgm
• Medical Assistant Prgm
• Nuclear Medicine Technology Prgm
• Nursing Prgm
• Radiography Prgm
• Surgical Technology Prgm

Mercy Medical Center
David Vellinga, CEO
1111 6th Ave
Des Moines, IA 50314
515 247-4278
Type: Hosp or Med Ctr: 500> Beds
Control: Nonprofit (Private or Religious)
• Clin Lab Scientist/Med Technologist Prgm
• Cytotechnology Prgm
• Emergency Med Tech-Paramedic Prgm

Vatterott College - Des Moines Campus
Pamela Belll, President
6100 Thornton Ave
Ste 290
Des Moines, IA 50321
515 309-9000
Type: Vocational or Tech Sch
Control: For Profit
• Dental Assisting Prgm

Dubuque

Clarke College
Joanne Burrows, PhD, President
1550 Clarke Dr
Dubuque, IA 52001-3198
563 588-6300
Type: 4-year Coll or Univ
Control: Nonprofit (Private or Religious)
• Athletic Training Prgm
• Nursing Prgm
• Physical Therapy Prgm

Loras College
James E Collins, President
1450 Alta Vista
Dubuque, IA 52004-0178
563 588-7647
Type: 4-year Coll or Univ
Control: State, County, or Local Govt
• Athletic Training Prgm

Estherville

Iowa Lakes Community College
Mike Hupfer, BSE JD, President
19 S 7th St
Estherville, IA 51334-2295
712 362-0438
Type: Junior or Comm Coll
Control: State, County, or Local Govt
• Medical Assistant Prgm
• Surgical Technology Prgm

Fayette

Upper Iowa University
Alan Walker, PhD, President
605 Washington St
PO Box 1857
Fayette, IA 52142
563 425-5201
Type: 4-year Coll or Univ
Control: Nonprofit (Private or Religious)
• Athletic Training Prgm

Fort Dodge

Iowa Central Community College
Robert A Paxton, PhD, President
330 Ave M
Fort Dodge, IA 50501
515 576-7201
Type: Junior or Comm Coll
Control: State, County, or Local Govt
• Clin Lab Technician/Med Lab Technician Prgm
• Medical Assistant Prgm
• Radiography Prgm

Indianola

Simpson College
John Byrd, President
701 North C St
Hillman Hall
Indianola, IA 50125
515 961-1611
Type: 4-year Coll or Univ
Control: State, County, or Local Govt
• Athletic Training Prgm

Iowa City

University of Iowa
Sally Mason, PhD, President
101 Jessup Hall
Iowa City, IA 52242
319 335-3549
Type: 4-year Coll or Univ
Control: State, County, or Local Govt
• Allopathic Medicine Prgm
• Athletic Training Prgm
• Audiologist Prgm
• Counseling Prgm
• Dentistry Prgm
• Medical Librarian Prgm
• Music Therapy Prgm
• Nursing Prgm
• Pharmacy Prgm
• Physical Therapy Prgm
• Physician Assistant Prgm
• Psychology Prgm
• Rehabilitation Counseling Prgm
• Speech-Language Pathology Prgm
• Therapeutic Recreation Specialist Prgm

University of Iowa Hospitals & Clinics
Donna Katen-Bahensky, CEO
200 Hawkins Dr 1353 JCP
Iowa City, IA 52242-1059
319 356-3155
Type: Hosp or Med Ctr: 500> Beds
Control: State, County, or Local Govt
• Diagnostic Med Sonography Prgm
• Dietetic Internship Prgm
• Emergency Med Tech-Paramedic Prgm
• Nuclear Medicine Technology Prgm
• Orthoptist Prgm
• Perfusion Prgm
• Radiation Therapy Prgm
• Radiography Prgm

Lamoni

Graceland University
John Menzies, PhD, President
1 University Place
Lamoni, IA 50140
641 784-5111
Type: 4-year Coll or Univ
Control: Nonprofit (Private or Religious)
• Athletic Training Prgm

Marshalltown

Marshalltown Community College
Tim A Wynes, JD, President
3702 S Center St
Marshalltown, IA 50158
515 752-4643
Type: Junior or Comm Coll
Control: State, County, or Local Govt
• Dental Assisting Prgm

Mason City

Mercy Medical Center - North Iowa
James Fitzpatrick, CHE, President/CEO
1000 Fourth St SW
Mason City, IA 50401
800 637-2994
Type: Hosp or Med Ctr: 300-499 Beds
Control: Nonprofit (Private or Religious)
• Radiography Prgm

North Iowa Area Community College
Michael Morrison, PhD, President
500 College Dr
Mason City, IA 50401
515 421-4200
Type: Junior or Comm Coll
Control: State, County, or Local Govt
• Medical Assistant Prgm
• Physical Therapist Assistant Prgm

Orange City

Northwestern College
Bruce Murphy, PhD, President
101 7th St SW
Orange City, IA 51041-1996
712 707-7100
Type: 4-year Coll or Univ
Control: Nonprofit (Private or Religious)
• Athletic Training Prgm

Ottumwa

Indian Hills Community College
Jim Lindenmayer, PhD, President
525 Grandview Ave, Building 1
Ottumwa, IA 52501
641 683-5185
Type: Junior or Comm Coll
Control: State, County, or Local Govt
• Health Information Tech Prgm
• Physical Therapist Assistant Prgm
• Radiography Prgm

Pella

Central College
David Roe, PhD, President
812 University Box 6300
Pella, IA 50219
641 628-5269
Type: 4-year Coll or Univ
Control: Nonprofit (Private or Religious)
• Athletic Training Prgm

Sheldon

Northwest Iowa Community College
William Giddings, PhD, President
603 W Park St
Sheldon, IA 51201
712 324-5061
Type: Junior or Comm Coll
Control: State, County, or Local Govt
• Health Information Tech Prgm

Sioux Centetr

Dordt College
Carl E Zylstra, PhD, President
498 4th Ave NE
Sioux Center, IA 51250
712 722-6002
Type: 4-year Coll or Univ
Control: Nonprofit (Private or Religious)
• Nursing Prgm

Sioux City

Mercy Medical Center - Sioux City
Paul Dougherty, President/CEO
801 Fifth St
Sioux City, IA 51101
712 279-2018
Type: Hosp or Med Ctr: 100-299 Beds
Control: Nonprofit (Private or Religious)
• Clin Lab Scientist/Med Technologist Prgm

St Luke's College
Peter Thoreen, MBA, President, CEO
2720 Stone Park Blvd
Sioux City, IA 51104
712 279-3500
Type: Vocational or Tech Sch
Control: Nonprofit (Private or Religious)
• Clin Lab Scientist/Med Technologist Prgm
• Radiography Prgm
• Respiratory Therapist (Advanced) Prgm

Western Iowa Tech Community College
Robert Dunker, PhD, President
4647 Stone Ave
PO Box 5199
Sioux City, IA 51102-5199
712 274-6400
Type: Junior or Comm Coll
Control: State, County, or Local Govt
• Dental Assisting Prgm
• Physical Therapist Assistant Prgm
• Surgical Technology Prgm

Storm Lake

Buena Vista University
Fredrick V Moore, President
610 W Fourth St
Storm Lake, IA 50588
712 749-2103
Type: 4-year Coll or Univ
Control: State, County, or Local Govt
• Athletic Training Prgm

Waterloo

Allen College
Jerry Durham, PhD, Chancellor
1825 Logan Ave
Waterloo, IA 50703
319 226-2015
Type: 4-year Coll or Univ
Control: Nonprofit (Private or Religious)
• Nursing Prgm
• Radiography Prgm

Covenant Medical Center
Jack Dusenbery, CEO/Administrator
3421 W Ninth
Waterloo, IA 50702
319 272-7302
Type: Hosp or Med Ctr: 300-499 Beds
Control: Nonprofit (Private or Religious)
• Radiography Prgm

Hawkeye Community College
Greg Schmitz, MA, President
1501 E Orange Rd
PO Box 8015
Waterloo, IA 50704-8015
319 296-4200
Type: Junior or Comm Coll
Control: State, County, or Local Govt
• Clin Lab Technician/Med Lab Technician Prgm
• Dental Assisting Prgm
• Dental Hygiene Prgm
• Respiratory Therapist (Advanced) Prgm

Waverly

Wartburg College
Jack Ohle, President
902 12th St NW
Waverly, IA 50677
319 352-0979
Type: 4-year Coll or Univ
Control: Nonprofit (Private or Religious)
• Music Therapy Prgm

West Burlington

Southeastern Community College
Beverly Simone, President
1500 W Agency Rd
PO Box 180
West Burlington, IA 52655-0180
319 752-2731
Type: Junior or Comm Coll
Control: State, County, or Local Govt
• Medical Assistant Prgm
• Respiratory Therapist (Advanced) Prgm

Kansas

Arkansas City

Cowley County Community College
Patrick J McAtee, PhD, President
PO Box 1147
Arkansas City, KS 67005
800 593-2222
Type: Junior or Comm Coll
Control: State, County, or Local Govt
• Emergency Med Tech-Paramedic Prgm

Atchison

Benedictine College
Daniel Carey, PhD, President
1020 N Second St
Atchison, KS 66002-1499
913 367-5340
Type: 4-year Coll or Univ
Control: State, County, or Local Govt
• Athletic Training Prgm

Coffeyville

Coffeyville Community College
Howard G Bass, PhD, President
400 W 11th St
Coffeyville, KS 67337
620 251-7700
Type: Junior or Comm Coll
Control: State, County, or Local Govt
• Emergency Med Tech-Paramedic Prgm

Colby

Colby Community College
Lynn Krider, PhD, President
1255 S Range
Colby, KS 67701
785 462-3984
Type: Junior or Comm Coll
Control: State, County, or Local Govt
• Physical Therapist Assistant Prgm
• Veterinary Technology Prgm

Emporia

Emporia State University
Michael Lane, PhD, President
1200 Commercial St, Box 4001
Emporia, KS 66801
620 341-5551
Type: 4-year Coll or Univ
Control: State, County, or Local Govt
• Art Therapy Prgm
• Athletic Training Prgm
• Counseling Prgm
• Medical Librarian Prgm
• Rehabilitation Counseling Prgm

Flint Hills Technical College
Dean Hollenbeck, PhD, President
3301 W 18th Ave
Emporia, KS 66801
620 343-4600
Type: Vocational or Tech Sch
Control: State, County, or Local Govt
• Dental Assisting Prgm
• Emergency Med Tech-Paramedic Prgm

Garden City

Garden City Community College
Carol Ballantyne, PhD, President
801 Campus Dr
Garden City, KS 67846
620 276-9602
Type: Junior or Comm Coll
Control: State, County, or Local Govt
• Emergency Med Tech-Paramedic Prgm

Goodland

Northwest Kansas Technical College
Kenneth Clouse, MS, President
1209 Harrison St
PO Box 668
Goodland, KS 67735-0668
785 890-3641
Type: Vocational or Tech Sch
Control: State, County, or Local Govt
• Medical Assistant Prgm

Great Bend

Barton County Community College
Carl Heilman, PhD, President
245 NE 30th Rd
Great Bend, KS 67530-9283
620 792-2701
Type: Junior or Comm Coll
Control: State, County, or Local Govt
• Clin Lab Technician/Med Lab Technician Prgm
• Emergency Med Tech-Paramedic Prgm

Hays

Fort Hays State University
Lawrence Gould, PhD, Provost
600 Park St
Hays, KS 67601
785 628-4000
Type: 4-year Coll or Univ
Control: State, County, or Local Govt
• Athletic Training Prgm
• Nursing Prgm
• Radiography Prgm
• Speech-Language Pathology Prgm

Hillsboro

Tabor College
Larry W Nikkel, MPH, President
400 S Jefferson
Hillsboro, KS 67063
620 947-3121
Type: 4-year Coll or Univ
Control: Nonprofit (Private or Religious)
• Athletic Training Prgm
• Nursing Prgm

Hutchinson

Hutchinson Community College
Edward E Berger, EdD, President
1300 N Plum St
Hutchinson, KS 67501
620 665-3505
Type: Junior or Comm Coll
Control: State, County, or Local Govt
• Health Information Tech Prgm
• Radiography Prgm
• Surgical Technology Prgm

Kansas City

Bethany Med Ctr/Kansas City Kansas Comm Coll
Shirley Wendel, PhD, Consortial Comm Chair
7250 State Ave
Kansas City, KS 66112
913 288-7126
Type: Consortium
Control: State, County, or Local Govt
• Respiratory Therapist (Advanced) Prgm
• Respiratory Therapist (Entry-Level) Prgm

Kansas City Kansas Community College
Thomas R Burke, PhD, President
7250 State Ave
PO Box 12951
Kansas City, KS 66112-9978
913 288-7123
Type: Junior or Comm Coll
Control: State, County, or Local Govt
• Emergency Med Tech-Paramedic Prgm
• Physical Therapist Assistant Prgm

University of Kansas Medical Center
Barbara Atkinson, MD, Exec Vice Chancellor
3901 Rainbow Blvd
3015 Murphy Administration Bldg MS 1049
Kansas City, KS 66160
913 588-1433
Type: Acad Health Ctr/Med Sch
Control: State, County, or Local Govt
• Allopathic Medicine Prgm
• Clin Lab Scientist/Med Technologist Prgm
• Cytotechnology Prgm
• Diagnostic Med Sonography Prgm (2)
• Diagnostic Molecular Scientist Prgm
• Dietetic Internship Prgm
• Health Information Admin Prgm
• Nuclear Medicine Technology Prgm
• Occupational Therapy Prgm
• Physical Therapy Prgm
• Respiratory Therapist (Advanced) Prgm

Lawrence

University of Kansas
Robert E Hemenway, Chancellor
3031 Dole Ctr
Lawrence, KS 66045
785 864-0630
Type: 4-year Coll or Univ
Control: State, County, or Local Govt
• Athletic Training Prgm
• Audiologist Prgm
• Music Therapy Prgm
• Nursing Prgm
• Pharmacy Prgm
• Psychology Prgm (2)
• Speech-Language Pathology Prgm

Liberal

Seward County Community College
Duane Dunn, EdD, President
PO Box 1137
Liberal, KS 67905
620 624-1951
Type: Junior or Comm Coll
Control: State, County, or Local Govt
• Clin Lab Technician/Med Lab Technician Prgm
• Respiratory Therapist (Advanced) Prgm
• Surgical Technology Prgm

Manhattan

Kansas State University
Jon Wefald, President
Anderson Hall
Manhattan, KS 66506-5301
913 532-6221
Type: 4-year Coll or Univ
Control: State, County, or Local Govt
• Athletic Training Prgm
• Dietetics-Coordinated Prgm
• Dietetics-Didactic Prgm
• Speech-Language Pathology Prgm
• Veterinary Medicine Prgm

North Newton

Bethel College
E LaVerne Epp, JD, President
300 E 27th St
North Newton, KS 67117
316 283-2500
Type: 4-year Coll or Univ
Control: Nonprofit (Private or Religious)
• Athletic Training Prgm
• Nursing Prgm

Olathe

Mid-America Nazarene University
Edwin H Robinson, President
2030 E College Way
Olathe, KS 66062
913 782-3750
Type: 4-year Coll or Univ
Control: State, County, or Local Govt
• Athletic Training Prgm
• Nursing Prgm

Overland Park

BMSI Institute
C Michael Pizzuto, NCBTMB, Director
8665 W 96th, Ste 300
Overland Park, KS 66212
913 649-3322
Type: Acad Health Ctr/Med Sch
Control: For Profit
• Massage Therapy Prgm

Johnson County Community College
Larry Tyree, EdD, Interim President
12345 College Blvd
Overland Park, KS 66210-1299
913 469-8500
Type: Junior or Comm Coll
Control: State, County, or Local Govt
• Dental Hygiene Prgm
• Emergency Med Tech-Paramedic Prgm
• Respiratory Therapist (Advanced) Prgm

Parsons

Labette Community College
George Knox, EdD, President
200 S 14th St
Parsons, KS 67357
620 421-6700
Type: Junior or Comm Coll
Control: State, County, or Local Govt
• Radiography Prgm
• Respiratory Therapist (Advanced) Prgm

INSTITUTIONS

Pittsburg

Pittsburg State University
Thomas Bryant
1701 S Broadway
Pittsburg, KS 66762-7500
316 231-7000
Type: 4-year Coll or Univ
Control: State, County, or Local Govt
• Counseling Prgm
• Nursing Prgm
• Therapeutic Recreation Specialist Prgm

Salina

Kansas Wesleyan University
Phillip P Kerstetter, PhD, President
100 E Claflin Ave
Salina, KS 67401-6198
785 827-5541
Type: 4-year Coll or Univ
Control: Nonprofit (Private or Religious)
• Athletic Training Prgm

Salina Area Technical School
Duane Custer, Director
2562 Centennial Rd
Salina, KS 67401
785 309-3108
Type: Vocational or Tech Sch
Control: State, County, or Local Govt
• Dental Assisting Prgm

Sterling

Sterling College
Bruce Douglas, PhD, President
125 W Cooper
Sterling, KS 67579
620 278-4213
Type: 4-year Coll or Univ
Control: State, County, or Local Govt
• Athletic Training Prgm

Topeka

Baker University
Kathleen L Harr, DNSc RN, Chief Nurse
    Administrator
1500 SW Tenth St
Topeka, KS 66604
785 354-5853
Type: 4-year Coll or Univ
Control: Nonprofit (Private or Religious)
• Nursing Prgm

Kaw Area Technical School
Richard Hoffman, BS MS, General Director
5724 Huntoon
Topeka, KS 66604
785 228-6300
Type: Vocational or Tech Sch
Control: State, County, or Local Govt
• Surgical Technology Prgm

Washburn University
Jerry Farley, PhD, President
1700 SW College
Topeka, KS 66621
785 670-1556
Type: 4-year Coll or Univ
Control: State, County, or Local Govt
• Athletic Training Prgm
• Diagnostic Med Sonography Prgm
• Health Information Tech Prgm
• Nursing Prgm
• Physical Therapist Assistant Prgm
• Radiography Prgm
• Respiratory Therapist (Advanced) Prgm

Wichita

Newman University
Noreen Carrocci, PhD, President/CEO
3100 McCormick Ave
Wichita, KS 67213-2097
316 942-4291
Type: 4-year Coll or Univ
Control: Nonprofit (Private or Religious)
• Nursing Prgm
• Occupational Therapy Asst Prgm
• Radiography Prgm
• Respiratory Therapist (Advanced) Prgm

Wichita Area Technical College
Peter Gustaf, BS MS EMAB, President
301 S Grove
Wichita, KS 67201
316 677-9500
Type: Vocational or Tech Sch
Control: State, County, or Local Govt
• Clin Lab Technician/Med Lab Technician Prgm
• Dental Assisting Prgm
• Medical Assistant Prgm
• Surgical Technology Prgm

Wichita State University
Donald Beggs, PhD, President
1845 N Fairmont
Wichita, KS 67260-0001
316 978-3001
Type: 4-year Coll or Univ
Control: State, County, or Local Govt
• Audiologist Prgm
• Clin Lab Scientist/Med Technologist Prgm
• Dental Hygiene Prgm
• Nursing Prgm
• Physical Therapy Prgm
• Physician Assistant Prgm
• Psychology Prgm
• Speech-Language Pathology Prgm

Winfield

Southwestern College
W R Merriman, Jr, PhD, President
100 College St
Winfield, KS 67156
620 229-6223
Type: 4-year Coll or Univ
Control: Nonprofit (Private or Religious)
• Athletic Training Prgm
• Nursing Prgm

Kentucky

Ashland

Ashland Technical College
Stu Taylor, School Director
4818 Roberts Dr
Ashland, KY 41102-9046
606 929-2055
Type: Vocational or Tech Sch
Control: State, County, or Local Govt
• Surgical Technology Prgm

King's Daughters' Medical Center
Fred Jackson, President
2201 Lexington Ave
Ashland, KY 41101
606 327-4000
Type: Hosp or Med Ctr: 300-499 Beds
Control: Nonprofit (Private or Religious)
• Radiography Prgm

Berea

Berea College
Larry D Shinn, President
Berea, KY 40404
606 986-9341
Type: 4-year Coll or Univ
Control: Nonprofit (Private or Religious)
• Nursing Prgm

Bowling Green

Bowling Green Technical College
Nathan Hodges, EdD, President
1845 Loop Dr
Bowling Green, KY 42101
270 901-1162
Type: Junior or Comm Coll
Control: State, County, or Local Govt
• Diagnostic Med Sonography Prgm
• Radiography Prgm
• Respiratory Therapist (Advanced) Prgm
• Surgical Technology Prgm

Western Kentucky University
Gary A Ransdell, PhD, President
Wetherby Administration Bldg 135
Bowling Green, KY 42101-3576
270 745-4346
Type: 4-year Coll or Univ
Control: State, County, or Local Govt
• Counseling Prgm
• Dental Hygiene Prgm
• Dietetics-Didactic Prgm
• Health Information Tech Prgm
• Nursing Prgm
• Speech-Language Pathology Prgm

Columbia

Lindsey Wilson College
210 Lindsey Wilson St
Columbia, KY 42728-1298
502 384-2126
Type: 4-year Coll or Univ
Control: Nonprofit (Private or Religious)
• Counseling Prgm

Edgewood

St Elizabeth Medical Center
Joseph Gross, FACHE, President/CEO
One Medical Village Dr
Edgewood, KY 41017
606 344-2111
Type: Hosp or Med Ctr: 500> Beds
Control: Nonprofit (Private or Religious)
• Clin Lab Scientist/Med Technologist Prgm

Elizabethtown

Elizabethtown Community & Technical College
Thelma White, PhD, President
620 College Street Rd
Elizabethtown, KY 42701
270 769-2371
Type: Junior or Comm Coll
Control: State, County, or Local Govt
• Radiography Prgm

Grayson

Kentucky Christian University
Grayson, KY 41143
Type: 4-year Coll or Univ
Control: Nonprofit (Private or Religious)
• Nursing Prgm

Hazard

Hazard Community & Technical College
Kathy Smoot, PhD, Interim President
One Community College Dr, Hwy 15 S
Hazard, KY 41701
606 436-5721
Type: Junior or Comm Coll
Control: State, County, or Local Govt
• Physical Therapist Assistant Prgm
• Radiography Prgm

Henderson

Henderson Community College
Patrick Lake, EdD, President
2660 S Green St
Henderson, KY 42420
270 827-1867
Type: Junior or Comm Coll
Control: State, County, or Local Govt
• Dental Hygiene Prgm
• Medical Assistant Prgm

Highland Heights

Northern Kentucky University
James Votruba, PhD, President
Office of the President, Admin Ctr 800B
Highland Heights, KY 41099-2104
606 572-5123
Type: 4-year Coll or Univ
Control: State, County, or Local Govt
• Athletic Training Prgm
• Radiography Prgm
• Respiratory Therapist (Advanced) Prgm

Lexington

Bluegrass Community and Technical College
Larry Durrence, EdD, Interim President
470 Cooper Dr, Oswald Bldg
Rm 209
Lexington, KY 40506-0235
859 246-6501
Type: Junior or Comm Coll
Control: State, County, or Local Govt
• Dental Assisting Prgm
• Dental Hygiene Prgm
• Dental Lab Technician Prgm
• Medical Assistant Prgm
• Radiography Prgm
• Respiratory Therapist (Advanced) Prgm
• Surgical Technology Prgm

St Joseph Healthcare
Gene Woods, MHA, President/CEO
One St Joseph Dr
Lexington, KY 40504
859 313-1000
Type: Hosp or Med Ctr: 300-499 Beds
Control: Nonprofit (Private or Religious)
• Radiography Prgm

Sullivan University - Lexington
James Ploskonka, PhD, Executive Director
2355 Harrodsburg Rd
Lexington, KY 40504
606 276-4357
Type: 4-year Coll or Univ
Control: For Profit
• Medical Assistant Prgm

Univ of Kentucky Hospital
Murray Clark, PhD, Assoc VP, Med Ctr
N106 Chandler Medical Center
Lexington, KY 40536-0293
859 323-2044
Type: Acad Health Ctr/Med Sch
Control: Nonprofit (Private or Religious)
• Dietetic Internship Prgm
• Radiation Therapy Prgm

University of Kentucky
Lee Todd, PhD, President
Administration Bldg
Lexington, KY 40506
859 257-9000
Type: 4-year Coll or Univ
Control: State, County, or Local Govt
• Allopathic Medicine Prgm
• Clin Lab Scientist/Med Technologist Prgm
• Dentistry Prgm
• Dietetic Internship Prgm
• Dietetics-Coordinated Prgm
• Dietetics-Didactic Prgm
• Medical Librarian Prgm
• Nursing Prgm
• Pharmacy Prgm
• Physical Therapy Prgm
• Physician Assistant Prgm
• Psychology Prgm
• Rehabilitation Counseling Prgm
• Speech-Language Pathology Prgm

Louisville

Bellarmine University
Doris Tegart, PhD, VP, Academic Affairs
2001 Newburg Rd
Louisville, KY 40205
502 452-8000
Type: 4-year Coll or Univ
Control: Nonprofit (Private or Religious)
• Clin Lab Scientist/Med Technologist Prgm
• Nursing Prgm
• Physical Therapy Prgm

James Graham Brown Cancer Center
Patty Melvin, Vice President, Planning
529 S Jackson St
Louisville, KY 40202
502 562-4585
Type: Hosp or Med Ctr: 500> Beds
Control: For Profit
• Radiation Therapy Prgm

Jefferson Community and Technical College
Anthony Newberry, PhD, President
109 E Broadway
Louisville, KY 40202
502 213-5333
Type: Junior or Comm Coll
Control: State, County, or Local Govt
• Health Information Tech Prgm
• Medical Assistant Prgm
• Nuclear Medicine Technology Prgm
• Occupational Therapy Asst Prgm
• Physical Therapist Assistant Prgm
• Radiography Prgm
• Respiratory Therapist (Advanced) Prgm
• Surgical Technology Prgm

Norton Healthcare
Stephen A Williams, BA MHA, President
PO box 35070
Louisville, KY 40202
502 629-8791
Type: Hosp or Med Ctr: 300-499 Beds
Control: Nonprofit (Private or Religious)
• Cardiovascular Technology Prgm

Spalding University
Joann Ronney, JD, President
851 S Fourth St
Louisville, KY 40203-2188
502 585-9911
Type: 4-year Coll or Univ
Control: Nonprofit (Private or Religious)
• Nursing Prgm
• Occupational Therapy Prgm
• Psychology Prgm

Spencerian College
Jan M Gordon, MEd, Executive Director
4627 Dixie Hwy
Louisville, KY 40216
502 447-1000
Type: Vocational or Tech Sch
Control: For Profit
• Cardiovascular Technology Prgm
• Medical Assistant Prgm (2)
• Radiography Prgm
• Surgical Technology Prgm

University of Louisville
James Ramsey, PhD, President
Grawmeyer Hall
Health Sciences Center
Louisville, KY 40292
502 852-5417
Type: Acad Health Ctr/Med Sch
Control: State, County, or Local Govt
- Allopathic Medicine Prgm
- Art Therapy Prgm
- Audiologist Prgm
- Dental Hygiene Prgm
- Dentistry Prgm
- Music Therapy Prgm
- Nursing Prgm
- Psychology Prgm
- Speech-Language Pathology Prgm

Madisonville

HCC/MCC Consortium
Judith Rhoads, EdD, President
2000 College Dr
Madisonville, KY 42431
270 824-8562
Type: Consortium
Control: State, County, or Local Govt
- Clin Lab Technician/Med Lab Technician Prgm

Madisonville Community College
Judith Rhoads, EdD, President
2000 College Dr
Madisonville, KY 42431
270 824-8562
Type: Junior or Comm Coll
Control: State, County, or Local Govt
- Occupational Therapy Asst Prgm
- Physical Therapist Assistant Prgm
- Radiography Prgm
- Respiratory Therapist (Advanced) Prgm
- Surgical Assistant Prgm
- Surgical Technology Prgm

Morehead

Maysville Comm & Tech College
Kenneth J Brown, Director
609 Viking Dr
Morehead, KY 40351
606 783-1538
Type: Vocational or Tech Sch
Control: State, County, or Local Govt
- Medical Assistant Prgm
- Respiratory Therapist (Entry-Level) Prgm
- Surgical Technology Prgm

Morehead State University
Wayne Andrews, PhD, President
201 Howell McDowell Admin Bldg
Morehead, KY 40351
606 783-2022
Type: 4-year Coll or Univ
Control: State, County, or Local Govt
- Diagnostic Med Sonography Prgm
- Dietetics-Didactic Prgm
- Nursing Prgm
- Radiography Prgm
- Veterinary Technology Prgm

Mt Vernon

Laurel Technical College - Rockcastle
Donna Hopkins, MA, Principal
PO Box 275
Mt Vernon, KY 40456
606 676-9065
Type: Vocational or Tech Sch
Control: State, County, or Local Govt
- Respiratory Therapist (Entry-Level) Prgm

Murray

Murray State University
Randy Dunn, EdD, President
President's Office
218 Wells Hall
Murray, KY 42071
270 762-3763
Type: 4-year Coll or Univ
Control: State, County, or Local Govt
- Athletic Training Prgm
- Dietetic Internship Prgm
- Dietetics-Didactic Prgm
- Nursing Prgm
- Speech-Language Pathology Prgm
- Veterinary Technology Prgm

Owensboro

Kentucky Community Technical College
Jackie Addington, PhD, President/CEO
4800 New Hartford Rd
Owensboro, KY 42303
270 686-4400
Type: Junior or Comm Coll
Control: State, County, or Local Govt
- Surgical Technology Prgm

Owensboro Community & Technical College
Jacqueline Addington, PhD, President
4800 New Hartford Rd
Owensboro, KY 42303-1899
270 686-4400
Type: Junior or Comm Coll
Control: State, County, or Local Govt
- Radiography Prgm

Owensboro Medical Health System
Jeffery Barber, CEO
811 E Parrish Ave
PO Box 20007
Owensboro, KY 42303
502 688-2100
Type: Hosp or Med Ctr: 300-499 Beds
Control: Nonprofit (Private or Religious)
- Clin Lab Scientist/Med Technologist Prgm

Paducah

West Kentucky Community & Technical College
Barbara Veazey, PhD RN, President/CEO
PO Box 7380
4810 Alben Barkley Dr
Paducah, KY 42002-7380
270 534-3082
Type: Junior or Comm Coll
Control: State, County, or Local Govt
- Dental Assisting Prgm
- Diagnostic Med Sonography Prgm
- Medical Assistant Prgm
- Physical Therapist Assistant Prgm
- Radiography Prgm
- Respiratory Therapist (Advanced) Prgm
- Respiratory Therapist (Entry-Level) Prgm
- Surgical Technology Prgm

Pikeville

Pikeville College
Harold H Smith, President
214 Sycamore St
Pikeville, KY 41501-119
606 432-9200
Control: Nonprofit (Private or Religious)
- Osteopathic Medicine Prgm

Pineville

Southeast Kentucky Comm & Tech College
W Bruce Ayers, President
3300 US 25E S
Pineville, KY 40977
606 248-2118
Type: Junior or Comm Coll
Control: State, County, or Local Govt
- Clin Lab Technician/Med Lab Technician Prgm
- Radiography Prgm
- Respiratory Therapist (Advanced) Prgm
- Respiratory Therapist (Entry-Level) Prgm
- Surgical Technology Prgm

Prestonsburg

Big Sandy Community & Technical College
George D Edwards, PhD, President/CEO
1 Bert T Combs Dr
Prestonsburg, KY 41653
888 641-4132
Type: Junior or Comm Coll
Control: State, County, or Local Govt
- Dental Hygiene Prgm
- Respiratory Therapist (Advanced) Prgm

Richmond

Eastern Kentucky University
Doug Whitlock, PhD, President
Coates Admin Bldg Rm 107
521 Lancaster Ave
Richmond, KY 40475
859 622-2194
Type: 4-year Coll or Univ
Control: State, County, or Local Govt
- Athletic Training Prgm
- Clin Lab Scientist/Med Technologist Prgm
- Clin Lab Technician/Med Lab Technician Prgm
- Counseling Prgm
- Dietetic Internship Prgm
- Dietetics-Didactic Prgm
- Emergency Med Tech-Paramedic Prgm
- Health Information Admin Prgm
- Medical Assistant Prgm
- Nursing Prgm
- Occupational Therapy Prgm
- Speech-Language Pathology Prgm
- Therapeutic Recreation Specialist Prgm

Somerset

Somerset Community College
Jo Marshall, PhD, President
808 Monticello St
Somerset, KY 42501
606 679-8501
Type: Junior or Comm Coll
Control: State, County, or Local Govt
- Clin Lab Technician/Med Lab Technician Prgm
- Physical Therapist Assistant Prgm
- Radiography Prgm
- Surgical Technology Prgm

St Catharine

St Catharine College
William D Huston, MA, President
2735 Bardstown Rd
St Catharine, KY 40061
859 336-5082
Type: Junior or Comm Coll
Control: Nonprofit (Private or Religious)
- Diagnostic Med Sonography Prgm
- Radiography Prgm

Lebanon

Byblos

Lebanese American Univ School of Pharmacy
Joseph G Jabbra, PhD, President
PO Box 36
Byblos, Lebanon
Type: 4-year Coll or Univ
Control: For Profit
- Pharmacy Prgm

Louisiana

Alexandria

Louisiana State University - Alexandria
J Robert Cavanaugh, Chancellor
8100 Hwy 71 S
Alexandria, LA 71302-9121
318 445-3672
Type: 4-year Coll or Univ
Control: State, County, or Local Govt
- Clin Lab Technician/Med Lab Technician Prgm
- Pharmacy Technician Prgm

Rapides Regional Medical Center
A C Buchanan, BS MS, President
211 Fourth St
PO Box 30101
Alexandria, LA 71301
318 473-3150
Type: Hosp or Med Ctr: 300-499 Beds
Control: For Profit
- Clin Lab Scientist/Med Technologist Prgm
- Phlebotomy Prgm

Baton Rouge

Baton Rouge General Medical Center
William Holman, President/CEO
3600 Florida St
PO Box 2511-70821
Baton Rouge, LA 70806
225 387-7000
Type: Hosp or Med Ctr: 300-499 Beds
Control: Nonprofit (Private or Religious)
- Radiography Prgm

Blue Cliff College - Baton Rouge
Kathie Lea Love
6160 Perkins Rd, Ste 200
Baton Rouge, LA 70808-4191
225 757-3770
Type: Vocational or Tech Sch
Control: For Profit
- Massage Therapy Prgm

Louisiana State Univ and A&M College
William E Davis, Chancellor
Baton Rouge, LA 70803
504 388-3202
Type: 4-year Coll or Univ
Control: State, County, or Local Govt
- Audiologist Prgm
- Speech-Language Pathology Prgm

Louisiana State University
Eric Hovland, DDS MBA, Dean
8000 GSRI Rd
Bldg 3110
Baton Rouge, LA 70820
225 334-1816
Type: 4-year Coll or Univ
Control: State, County, or Local Govt
- Athletic Training Prgm
- Counseling Prgm
- Dental Hygiene Prgm
- Dental Lab Technician Prgm
- Dentistry Prgm
- Dietetics-Didactic Prgm
- Medical Librarian Prgm
- Psychology Prgm
- Veterinary Medicine Prgm

Louisiana Tech College
Margaret Montgomery-Richard, Chancellor
150 3rd St
Baton Rouge, LA 70801
337 262-5962
Type: Vocational or Tech Sch
Control: State, County, or Local Govt
- Clin Lab Technician/Med Lab Technician Prgm
- Respiratory Therapist (Entry-Level) Prgm
- Surgical Technology Prgm (2)

MedVance Institute
John Hopkins, CEO
9255 Interline Ave
Baton Rouge, LA 70809
225 248-1015
Type: Vocational or Tech Sch
Control: For Profit
- Clin Lab Technician/Med Lab Technician Prgm
- Radiography Prgm
- Surgical Technology Prgm

Our Lady of the Lake College
Sandra Harper, PhD, President
7434 Perkins Rd
Baton Rouge, LA 70808
225 768-1710
Type: 4-year Coll or Univ
Control: Nonprofit (Private or Religious)
- Clin Lab Scientist/Med Technologist Prgm
- Clin Lab Technician/Med Lab Technician Prgm
- Physical Therapist Assistant Prgm
- Physician Assistant Prgm
- Radiography Prgm
- Respiratory Therapist (Entry-Level) Prgm
- Surgical Technology Prgm

Southern Univ and A&M College
Edward Jackson, PhD, Chancellor
Baton Rouge, LA 70813
225 771-5020
Type: 4-year Coll or Univ
Control: State, County, or Local Govt
- Dietetic Internship Prgm
- Dietetics-Didactic Prgm
- Nursing Prgm
- Rehabilitation Counseling Prgm
- Speech-Language Pathology Prgm

Bossier City

Bossier Parish Community College
Tom Carleton, MA, Chancellor
6220 E Texas St
Bossier City, LA 71111
318 678-6014
Type: Junior or Comm Coll
Control: State, County, or Local Govt
- Emergency Med Tech-Paramedic Prgm
- Medical Assistant Prgm
- Pharmacy Technician Prgm
- Phlebotomy Prgm
- Physical Therapist Assistant Prgm
- Respiratory Therapist (Advanced) Prgm
- Respiratory Therapist (Entry-Level) Prgm
- Surgical Technology Prgm

INSTITUTIONS

Eunice

Louisiana State University - Eunice
William J Nunez III, PhD, Interim Chancellor
PO Box 1129
Eunice, LA 70535
318 457-7311
Type: Junior or Comm Coll
Control: State, County, or Local Govt
• Diagnostic Med Sonography Prgm
• Radiography Prgm
• Respiratory Therapist (Entry-Level) Prgm

Grambling

Grambling State University
Horace Judson, President
Grambling, LA 71245
318 247-3811
Type: 4-year Coll or Univ
Control: State, County, or Local Govt
• Therapeutic Recreation Specialist Prgm

Hammond

North Oaks Medical Center
James E Cathey, Jr, CEO
15790 Paul Vega MD Dr
Hammond, LA 70403
985 345-2700
Type: Hosp or Med Ctr: 300-499 Beds
Control: State, County, or Local Govt
• Dietetic Internship Prgm
• Radiography Prgm

Southeastern Louisiana University
Randay Moffett, EdD, President
SLU 10784
Hammond, LA 70402
985 549-2280
Type: 4-year Coll or Univ
Control: State, County, or Local Govt
• Athletic Training Prgm
• Counseling Prgm
• Speech-Language Pathology Prgm

Houma

L E Fletcher Technical Community College
F Travis Lavigne Jr, BS MS, Chancellor
310 Saint Charles St
Houma, LA 70360-2863
Type: Vocational or Tech Sch
Control: Nonprofit (Private or Religious)
• Phlebotomy Prgm

Lafayette

Lafayette General Medical Center
John J Burdin, Jr, MHA, President
1214 Coolidge Ave
PO Box 52009 OCS
Lafayette, LA 70505
318 289-7381
Type: Hosp or Med Ctr: 100-299 Beds
Control: Nonprofit (Private or Religious)
• Radiography Prgm

University of Louisiana at Lafayette
Ray Authement, PhD, President
UL Drawer 41008
Lafayette, LA 70504
337 482-6203
Type: 4-year Coll or Univ
Control: State, County, or Local Govt
• Athletic Training Prgm
• Dietetic Internship Prgm
• Dietetics-Didactic Prgm
• Health Information Admin Prgm
• Speech-Language Pathology Prgm

Lake Charles

Lake Charles Mem Hosp Sch of Med Tech
Elton Williams, CPA, President
1701 Oak Park Blvd
Lake Charles, LA 70601
337 494-3200
Type: Hosp or Med Ctr: 300-499 Beds
Control: Nonprofit (Private or Religious)
• Clin Lab Scientist/Med Technologist Prgm

McNeese State University
Robert D Hebert, PhD, President
Box 93300
Lake Charles, LA 70609
337 475-5556
Type: 4-year Coll or Univ
Control: State, County, or Local Govt
• Clin Lab Scientist/Med Technologist Prgm
• Dietetic Internship Prgm
• Dietetics-Didactic Prgm
• Radiography Prgm

Monroe

Career Technical College
Rick Nail, College Director
2319 Louisville Ave
Monroe, LA 71201
318 323-2889
Type: Vocational or Tech Sch
Control: State, County, or Local Govt
• Medical Assistant Prgm
• Radiography Prgm
• Surgical Technology Prgm

St Francis Medical Center
Wester Scott, MHA, President/CEO
309 Jackson St
Monroe, LA 71201
318 327-4141
Type: Hosp or Med Ctr: 300-499 Beds
Control: Nonprofit (Private or Religious)
• Clin Lab Scientist/Med Technologist Prgm

University of Louisiana at Monroe
James E Cofer, Sr, EdD, President
700 University Ave, NE Station
Monroe, LA 71209-0430
318 342-1010
Type: 4-year Coll or Univ
Control: State, County, or Local Govt
• Counseling Prgm
• Dental Hygiene Prgm
• Exercise Physiology Prgm
• Exercise Science Prgm
• Nursing Prgm
• Occupational Therapy Asst Prgm
• Pharmacy Prgm
• Radiography Prgm
• Speech-Language Pathology Prgm

Natchitoches

Northwestern State University
Randall J Webb, EdD, President
Natchitoches, LA 71497
318 357-5701
Type: 4-year Coll or Univ
Control: State, County, or Local Govt
• Counseling Prgm
• Nursing Prgm
• Radiography Prgm
• Veterinary Technology Prgm

New Orleans

Delgado Community College
Alex Johnson, PhD, Chancellor
615 City Park Ave
New Orleans, LA 70119
504 762-3000
Type: Junior or Comm Coll
Control: State, County, or Local Govt
• Clin Lab Technician/Med Lab Technician Prgm
• Diagnostic Med Sonography Prgm
• Dietetic Technician-AD Prgm
• Emergency Med Tech-Paramedic Prgm
• Health Information Tech Prgm
• Nuclear Medicine Technology Prgm
• Occupational Therapy Asst Prgm
• Ophthalmic Assistant Prgm
• Pharmacy Technician Prgm
• Phlebotomy Prgm
• Physical Therapist Assistant Prgm
• Radiation Therapy Prgm
• Radiography Prgm
• Respiratory Therapist (Advanced) Prgm
• Surgical Technology Prgm
• Veterinary Technology Prgm

Louisiana State Univ Health Sciences Center
Larry H Hollier, MD, Chancellor
433 Bolivar St
New Orleans, LA 70112-2223
504 568-4800
Type: Acad Health Ctr/Med Sch
Control: State, County, or Local Govt
• Allopathic Medicine Prgm
• Cardiovascular Technology Prgm
• Clin Lab Scientist/Med Technologist Prgm
• Nursing Prgm
• Occupational Therapy Prgm
• Ophthalmic Med Technologist Prgm
• Physical Therapy Prgm
• Rehabilitation Counseling Prgm
• Respiratory Therapist (Advanced) Prgm
• Speech-Language Pathology Prgm

Loyola University New Orleans
Kevin Wildes, SJ, President
6363 St Charles Ave
New Orleans, LA 70118
504 865-2011
Type: 4-year Coll or Univ
Control: Nonprofit (Private or Religious)
• Counseling Prgm
• Music Therapy Prgm

Medical Center of Louisiana
Dwayne Thomas, PhD
2021 Perdido St
New Orleans, LA 70112
504 903-3000
Type: Hosp or Med Ctr: 300-499 Beds
Control: State, County, or Local Govt
• Specialist in BB Tech Prgm

Our Lady of Holy Cross College
Rev Anthony DeConcilliis, PhD, President
4123 Woodland Dr
New Orleans, LA 70131-7399
504 394-7744
Type: 4-year Coll or Univ
Control: Nonprofit (Private or Religious)
• Counseling Prgm
• Radiography Prgm
• Respiratory Therapist (Advanced) Prgm

Touro Infirmary
Gary M Stein, MA, President
1401 Foucher St
New Orleans, LA 70115
504 897-8244
Type: Hosp or Med Ctr: 100-299 Beds
Control: Nonprofit (Private or Religious)
• Dietetic Internship Prgm

Tulane University
Eamon M Kelly, President
New Orleans, LA 70118
504 865-5000
Type: 4-year Coll or Univ
Control: Nonprofit (Private or Religious)
• Allopathic Medicine Prgm
• Dietetic Internship Prgm

University of New Orleans
Timothy P Ryan, PhD, Chancellor
Lake Front
New Orleans, LA 70148-0001
504 280-6000
Type: 4-year Coll or Univ
Control: State, County, or Local Govt
• Counseling Prgm

Xavier Univ of Louisiana College of Pharmacy
Wayne Harris, BS MS PhD, Professor & Dean
1 Drexel Dr
New Orleans, LA 70125
504 520-7421
Type: Acad Health Ctr/Med Sch
Control: Nonprofit (Private or Religious)
• Pharmacy Prgm

Pineville

Louisiana College
Joe Aguillard, President
Alexandria Hall, Rm 125
Pineville, LA 71359
318 487-7401
Type: 4-year Coll or Univ
Control: State, County, or Local Govt
• Athletic Training Prgm
• Nursing Prgm

Ruston

Louisiana Tech University
Daniel D Reneau, PhD, President
PO Box 3168
Ruston, LA 71272
318 257-3785
Type: 4-year Coll or Univ
Control: State, County, or Local Govt
• Audiologist Prgm
• Dietetic Internship Prgm
• Dietetics-Didactic Prgm
• Health Information Admin Prgm
• Health Information Tech Prgm
• Speech-Language Pathology Prgm

Shreveport

Louisiana State U Hlth Sci Ctr - Shreveport
John McDonald, MD, Chancellor and Dean
1501 Kings Hwy
Shreveport, LA 71130
318 675-6141
Type: Acad Health Ctr/Med Sch
Control: State, County, or Local Govt
• Allopathic Medicine Prgm
• Clin Lab Scientist/Med Technologist Prgm
• Occupational Therapy Prgm
• Physical Therapy Prgm
• Physician Assistant Prgm
• Respiratory Therapist (Advanced) Prgm
• Speech-Language Pathology Prgm

Overton Brooks VA Medical Center
George Moore, MHA, Director
510 E Stoner Ave
Shreveport, LA 71101-4295
318 424-6037
Type: Hosp or Med Ctr: 100-299 Beds
Control: Fed Govt
• Clin Lab Scientist/Med Technologist Prgm

Southern Univ at Shreveport
Ray Belton, PhD, Chancellor
3050 Martin Luther King Jr Dr
Shreveport, LA 71107-8032
318 674-3300
Type: Junior or Comm Coll
Control: State, County, or Local Govt
• Clin Lab Technician/Med Lab Technician Prgm
• Dental Hygiene Prgm
• Health Information Tech Prgm
• Radiography Prgm
• Respiratory Therapist (Advanced) Prgm
• Surgical Technology Prgm

Thibodaux

Nicholls State University
Stephen Hulbert, EdD, President
PO Box 2001
Thibodaux, LA 70310
504 448-4003
Type: 4-year Coll or Univ
Control: State, County, or Local Govt
• Athletic Training Prgm
• Cytotechnology Prgm
• Dietetic Internship Prgm
• Dietetics-Didactic Prgm
• Nursing Prgm
• Respiratory Therapist (Advanced) Prgm
• Respiratory Therapist (Entry-Level) Prgm

Maine

Auburn

Central Maine Community College
Scott E Knapp, PhD, President
1250 Turner St
Auburn, ME 04210-6498
207 755-5100
Type: Vocational or Tech Sch
Control: State, County, or Local Govt
• Clin Lab Technician/Med Lab Technician Prgm

Augusta

University College of Bangor
Richard Randall, MA, President
University of Maine-Augusta
46 University Dr
Augusta, ME 04330
207 621-3000
Type: 4-year Coll or Univ
Control: State, County, or Local Govt
• Dental Assisting Prgm
• Dental Hygiene Prgm
• Veterinary Technology Prgm

University of Maine
Charles Lyons, DEd, President
46 University Dr
Augusta, ME 04330
207 621-3403
Type: 4-year Coll or Univ
Control: State, County, or Local Govt
• Nursing Prgm

Bangor

Beal College
Allen Stehle, BS, President
99 Farm Road
Bangor, ME 04401
207 947-4591
Type: Junior or Comm Coll
Control: For Profit
• Medical Assistant Prgm

Eastern Maine Community College
Joyce B Hedlund, EdD, President
354 Hogan Rd
Bangor, ME 04401
207 974-4691
Type: Junior or Comm Coll
Control: State, County, or Local Govt
• Radiography Prgm
• Surgical Technology Prgm

Eastern Maine Medical Center
Debbie Johnson, President, CEO
489 State St
Bangor, ME 04401
207 973-7051
Type: Hosp or Med Ctr: 300-499 Beds
Control: Nonprofit (Private or Religious)
• Clin Lab Scientist/Med Technologist Prgm

Husson College
William H Beardsly, PhD, President
One College Circle
206 Peabody Hall
Bangor, ME 04401-2999
207 973-7138
Type: 4-year Coll or Univ
Control: Nonprofit (Private or Religious)
• Nursing Prgm
• Occupational Therapy Prgm
• Physical Therapy Prgm

Biddeford

University of New England
Danielle Ripich, PhD, President
11 Hills Beach Rd
Biddeford, ME 04005-9599
207 283-0171
Type: 4-year Coll or Univ
Control: Nonprofit (Private or Religious)
• Athletic Training Prgm
• Dental Hygiene Prgm
• Occupational Therapy Prgm
• Osteopathic Medicine Prgm
• Physical Therapy Prgm
• Physician Assistant Prgm

Fairfield

Kennebec Valley Community College
Barbara W Woodlee, EdD, President
92 Western Ave
Fairfield, ME 04937-1367
207 453-5129
Type: Junior or Comm Coll
Control: State, County, or Local Govt
• Health Information Tech Prgm
• Medical Assistant Prgm
• Occupational Therapy Asst Prgm
• Physical Therapist Assistant Prgm
• Radiography Prgm
• Respiratory Therapist (Advanced) Prgm

Lewiston

Central Maine Medical Center
Peter Chalke, MHA, President
300 Main St
Lewiston, ME 04240
207 795-2700
Type: Hosp or Med Ctr: 100-299 Beds
Control: Nonprofit (Private or Religious)
• Nuclear Medicine Technology Prgm
• Radiography Prgm

Orono

University of Maine - Orono
Robert Kennedy, PhD, President
5703 Alumni Hall, Rm 200
Orono, ME 04469
207 581-1512
Type: 4-year Coll or Univ
Control: State, County, or Local Govt
• Athletic Training Prgm
• Dietetic Internship Prgm
• Dietetics-Didactic Prgm
• Nursing Prgm
• Psychology Prgm
• Speech-Language Pathology Prgm

Portland

Maine Medical Center
Vincent Conti, President
22 Bramhall St
Portland, ME 04102
207 871-2491
Type: Hosp or Med Ctr: 500> Beds
Control: Nonprofit (Private or Religious)
• Surgical Technology Prgm

Mercy Hospital
Eileen F Skinner, MHACHE, President
144 State St
Portland, ME 04029
207 879-3000
Type: Hosp or Med Ctr: 100-299 Beds
Control: Nonprofit (Private or Religious)
• Radiography Prgm

University of Southern Maine
Joseph Wood, PhD, Interim President
96 Falmouth St PO Box 9300
Portland, ME 04104-9300
207 780-4480
Type: 4-year Coll or Univ
Control: State, County, or Local Govt
• Athletic Training Prgm
• Counseling Prgm
• Nursing Prgm
• Occupational Therapy Prgm
• Rehabilitation Counseling Prgm

Presque Isle

University of Maine - Presque Isle
Don Zillman, PhD, President
181 Main St
22 Preble Hall
Presque Isle, ME 04769
207 768-9525
Type: 4-year Coll or Univ
Control: State, County, or Local Govt
• Athletic Training Prgm
• Clin Lab Technician/Med Lab Technician Prgm

South Portland

Southern Maine Community College
James Ortiz, Eed, President
Fort Rd
South Portland, ME 04106
207 741-5500
Type: Junior or Comm Coll
Control: State, County, or Local Govt
• Dietetic Technician-AD Prgm
• Radiation Therapy Prgm
• Radiography Prgm
• Respiratory Therapist (Advanced) Prgm

Standish

Saint Joseph's College of Maine
Standish, ME 04084
Type: 4-year Coll or Univ
Control: Nonprofit (Private or Religious)
• Nursing Prgm

Waldoboro

Downeast School of Massage
Nancy W Dail, BA LMT NCTMB, Director
99 Moose Meadow Lane
Waldoboro, ME 04572
207 832-5531
Type: Acad Health Ctr/Med Sch
Control: For Profit
• Massage Therapy Prgm

Manitoba, Canada

Winnipeg

Massage Therapy College of Manitoba
Garth Beddome, BA RMT, Director
Winnipeg, MB R3G 1C3
204 772-8999
Type: Acad Health Ctr/Med Sch
Control: For Profit
• Massage Therapy Prgm

University of Manitoba
770 Bannatyne Ave
Winnipeg, MB R3E 0W3
Control: Nonprofit (Private or Religious)
• Allopathic Medicine Prgm
• Psychology Prgm

Maryland

Arnold

Anne Arundel Community College
Martha R Smith, PhD, President
101 College Pkwy
Arnold, MD 21012-1875
410 777-2222
Type: Junior or Comm Coll
Control: State, County, or Local Govt
• Emergency Med Tech-Paramedic Prgm
• Medical Assistant Prgm
• Pharmacy Technician Prgm
• Physician Assistant Prgm
• Radiography Prgm

Baltimore

Chesapeake Area Consortium for Higher Educ
101 College Pkwy
Arnold, MD 21012
Type: Consortium
Control: Nonprofit (Private or Religious)
• Physical Therapist Assistant Prgm

Baltimore

Baltimore City Community College
Richard Turner, DME, President
2901 Liberty Heights Ave
Baltimore, MD 21215-7893
410 462-7799
Type: Junior or Comm Coll
Control: State, County, or Local Govt
• Dental Hygiene Prgm
• Dietetic Technician-AD Prgm
• Health Information Tech Prgm
• Physical Therapist Assistant Prgm
• Respiratory Therapist (Advanced) Prgm
• Surgical Technology Prgm

Coppin State University
Sadie Gregory, Interim President
2500 W North Ave
Baltimore, MD 21216
410 951-3838
Type: 4-year Coll or Univ
Control: State, County, or Local Govt
• Rehabilitation Counseling Prgm

Greater Baltimore Medical Center
Lawerence Merlis, MBA, President
6701 N Charles St
Baltimore, MD 21204
443 849-2121
Type: Hosp or Med Ctr: 300-499 Beds
Control: Nonprofit (Private or Religious)
• Orthoptist Prgm
• Radiography Prgm

Johns Hopkins Bayview Medical Center
4940 Eastern Ave
Baltimore, MD 21224-2735
Type: Acad Health Ctr/Med Sch
Control: Nonprofit (Private or Religious)
• Dietetic Internship Prgm
• Dietetics-Coordinated Prgm

Johns Hopkins Hospital
Ronald R Peterson, MHA, President
733 N Broadway, BRB 104
Baltimore, MD 21287
410 955-9540
Type: Hosp or Med Ctr: 500> Beds
Control: Nonprofit (Private or Religious)
• Cytotechnology Prgm
• Diagnostic Med Sonography Prgm
• Nuclear Medicine Technology Prgm
• Radiography Prgm
• Specialist in BB Tech Prgm

Johns Hopkins School of Medicine
Edward D Miller, Jr, MD, President, CEO
100 Medical Admin Bldg
720 N Rutland Ave
Baltimore, MD 21205
410 955-3180
Type: Acad Health Ctr/Med Sch
Control: Nonprofit (Private or Religious)
• Allopathic Medicine Prgm
• Medical Illustrator Prgm

Johns Hopkins University
Baltimore, MD 21205
Type: 4-year Coll or Univ
Control: Nonprofit (Private or Religious)
• Genetic Counseling Prgm
• Nursing Prgm

Loyola College of Maryland
Brian Linnane, SJ PhD, President
4501 N Charles St
Baltimore, MD 21210
410 617-2000
Type: 4-year Coll or Univ
Control: Nonprofit (Private or Religious)
• Counseling Prgm (2)
• Psychology Prgm
• Speech-Language Pathology Prgm

Morgan State University
Earl S Richardson, EdD, President
Coldspring Ln and Hillen Rd
Baltimore, MD 21239
410 319-3200
Type: 4-year Coll or Univ
Control: State, County, or Local Govt
• Clin Lab Scientist/Med Technologist Prgm
• Dietetics-Didactic Prgm

University of Maryland
David J Ramsay, DM DPhil, President
515 Lombard Bldg
Second Fl
Baltimore, MD 21201
410 706-7131
Type: Acad Health Ctr/Med Sch
Control: State, County, or Local Govt
• Allopathic Medicine Prgm
• Clin Lab Scientist/Med Technologist Prgm
• Dental Hygiene Prgm
• Dentistry Prgm
• Genetic Counseling Prgm
• Medical Librarian Prgm
• Pathologists' Assistant Prgm
• Physical Therapy Prgm
• Rehabilitation Counseling Prgm

University of Maryland Baltimore County
John Martello, PhD, Pres CEO, Training Centers
UMBC South Campus, Technology Center
1450 S Rolling Rd
Baltimore, MD 21227
443 543-5400
Type: 4-year Coll or Univ
Control: State, County, or Local Govt
• Diagnostic Med Sonography Prgm
• Emergency Med Tech-Paramedic Prgm
• Pharmacy Prgm
• Psychology Prgm

University of Maryland Medical System
22 S Greene St
Baltimore, MD 21201-1544
410 328-2561
Control: State, County, or Local Govt
• Dietetic Internship Prgm

Baltimore County

Community College of Baltimore County
Sandra Kurtinitis, PhD, President
7201 Rossville Blvd
Baltimore County, MD 21237-3898
410 780-6322
Type: Junior or Comm Coll
Control: State, County, or Local Govt
• Emergency Med Tech-Paramedic Prgm
• Occupational Therapy Asst Prgm
• Radiation Therapy Prgm
• Radiography Prgm
• Respiratory Therapist (Advanced) Prgm
• Surgical Technology Prgm
• Veterinary Technology Prgm

Bel Air

Harford Community College
James F LaCalle, EdD, President
401 Thomas Run Rd
Bel Air, MD 21015
410 836-4200
Type: Junior or Comm Coll
Control: State, County, or Local Govt
• Histotechnician Prgm

Bethesda

National Institutes of Health
10 Center Dr
Bethesda, MD 20892
301 496-3311
Control: Fed Govt
• Dietetic Internship Prgm

NIH Clinical Center Blood Bank
Walter L Jones, Deputy Director
NIH/CC/DTM Bldg 10 Rm IC-711
10 Ctr Dr MSC 1184
Bethesda, MD 20892-1184
301 496-4506
Type: Hosp or Med Ctr: 300-499 Beds
Control: Fed Govt
• Specialist in BB Tech Prgm

Uniformed Serv Univ of the Hlth Sci
Bethesda, MD 20814
Type: Acad Health Ctr/Med Sch
Control: Federal Government
• Allopathic Medicine Prgm
• Psychology Prgm

College Park

Univ of Maryland at College Park
William E Kirwan, President
College Park, MD 20742
301 405-1000
Type: 4-year Coll or Univ
Control: State, County, or Local Govt
• Audiologist Prgm
• Counseling Prgm
• Dietetic Internship Prgm
• Dietetics-Didactic Prgm
• Psychology Prgm
• Speech-Language Pathology Prgm

INSTITUTIONS

Columbia

Howard Community College
Kathleen Heatherington, PhD, President
10901 Little Patuxent Parkway
Columbia, MD 21044
410 772-4820
Type: Junior or Comm Coll
Control: State, County, or Local Govt
• Cardiovascular Technology Prgm
• Emergency Med Tech-Paramedic Prgm

Sodexho Health Care Services, Mid Atlantic
Columbia, MD 21044
Type: Acad Health Ctr/Med Sch
Control: For Profit
• Dietetic Internship Prgm

Cumberland

Allegany College of Maryland
Donald L Alexander, EdD, President
12401 Willowbrook Rd SE
Cumberland, MD 21502-2596
301 784-5270
Type: Junior or Comm Coll
Control: State, County, or Local Govt
• Clin Lab Technician/Med Lab Technician Prgm
• Dental Hygiene Prgm
• Massage Therapy Prgm
• Medical Assistant Prgm
• Occupational Therapy Asst Prgm
• Physical Therapist Assistant Prgm
• Radiography Prgm
• Respiratory Therapist (Advanced) Prgm

Frederick

Frederick Community College
Patricia Stanley, EdD, President
7932 Opossumtown Pike
Frederick, MD 21702
301 846-2400
Type: Junior or Comm Coll
Control: State, County, or Local Govt
• Respiratory Therapist (Advanced) Prgm
• Surgical Technology Prgm

Frostburg

Frostburg State University
Catherine R Gira, PhD, President
101 Braddock Rd
Frostburg, MD 21532
301 687-4111
Type: 4-year Coll or Univ
Control: State, County, or Local Govt
• Athletic Training Prgm

Hagerstown

Hagerstown Community College
Guy Altieri, EdD, President
11400 Robinwood Dr
Hagerstown, MD 21742-6590
301 790-2800
Type: Junior or Comm Coll
Control: State, County, or Local Govt
• Radiography Prgm

Kaplan College
W Christopher Motz, MEd, President
18618 Crestwood Dr
Hagerstown, MD 21742
301 739-2670
Type: Junior or Comm Coll
Control: For Profit
• Health Information Tech Prgm
• Medical Assistant Prgm (2)
• Phlebotomy Prgm

Largo

Prince George's Community College
Charlene Dukes, PhD, President
301 Largo Rd
Largo, MD 20774
301 322-0400
Type: Junior or Comm Coll
Control: State, County, or Local Govt
• Health Information Tech Prgm
• Nuclear Medicine Technology Prgm
• Radiography Prgm
• Respiratory Therapist (Advanced) Prgm

Linthicum

Baltimore School of Massage
Richard Rynders, Campus Director
517 Progress Dr, Ste A - L
Linthicum, MD 21090
410 636-7929
Type: Vocational or Tech Sch
Control: For Profit
• Massage Therapy Prgm

New Market

Associates in Emergency Care
Renee Joyce, RN BSN, Administrator
5628 Wellspring Court
New Market, MD 20872
301 856-6548
Type: Vocational or Tech Sch
Control: For Profit
• Emergency Med Tech-Paramedic Prgm

North East

Cecil Community College
W Stephen Pannill, EdD, President
One Seahawk Dr
North East, MD 21901
410 287-6060
Type: Junior or Comm Coll
Control: State, County, or Local Govt
• Medical Assistant Prgm

Princess Anne

University of Maryland Eastern Shore
Thelma B Thompson, PhD, President
Princess Anne, MD 21853
410 651-2200
Type: 4-year Coll or Univ
Control: State, County, or Local Govt
• Dietetic Internship Prgm
• Dietetics-Didactic Prgm
• Physical Therapy Prgm
• Physician Assistant Prgm
• Rehabilitation Counseling Prgm

Rockville

Montgomery College
Brian K Johnson, EdD, President
Central Admin Office
900 Hungerford
Rockville, MD 20850
240 567-5264
Type: Junior or Comm Coll
Control: State, County, or Local Govt
• Diagnostic Med Sonography Prgm
• Health Information Tech Prgm
• Physical Therapist Assistant Prgm
• Radiography Prgm
• Surgical Technology Prgm

Salisbury

Salisbury University
Janet Dudley-Eshbach, PhD, President
1101 Camden Ave
Holloway Hall
Salisbury, MD 21801
410 543-6012
Type: 4-year Coll or Univ
Control: State, County, or Local Govt
• Athletic Training Prgm
• Clin Lab Scientist/Med Technologist Prgm
• Exercise Science Prgm
• Nursing Prgm
• Respiratory Therapist (Advanced) Prgm

Wor-Wic Community College
Murray K Hoy, PhD, President
32000 Campus Dr
Salisbury, MD 21801
410 334-2800
Type: Junior or Comm Coll
Control: State, County, or Local Govt
• Radiography Prgm

Silver Spring

Holy Cross Hospital
Kevin Sexton, MHA, President and CEO
1500 Forest Glen Rd
Silver Spring, MD 20910
301 754-7000
Type: Hosp or Med Ctr: 500> Beds
Control: Nonprofit (Private or Religious)
• Radiography Prgm

Takoma Park

Columbia Union College
Randall Wisbey, PhD, President
7600 Flower Ave
Takoma Park, MD 20912
301 891-4128
Type: 4-year Coll or Univ
Control: Nonprofit (Private or Religious)
• Respiratory Therapist (Advanced) Prgm

Washington Adventist Hospital
Brian Breckenridge, President
7600 Carroll Ave
Takoma Park, MD 20912
301 891-7600
Type: Hosp or Med Ctr: 300-499 Beds
Control: Nonprofit (Private or Religious)
• Radiography Prgm

Towson

Medix School
Sean London, Director
700 York Rd
Towson, MD 21204
410 337-5155
Type: Vocational or Tech Sch
Control: For Profit
• Dental Assisting Prgm
• Medical Assistant Prgm

Towson University
Robert Caret, PhD, President
8000 York Rd
Towson, MD 21252-0001
410 704-2356
Type: 4-year Coll or Univ
Control: State, County, or Local Govt
• Athletic Training Prgm
• Audiologist Prgm
• Nursing Prgm
• Occupational Therapy Prgm
• Physician Assistant Prgm
• Speech-Language Pathology Prgm

Westminster

Carroll Community College
Faye Pappallardo
1601 Washington Rd
Westminster, MD 21157
410 386-8255
Type: Junior or Comm Coll
Control: State, County, or Local Govt
• Physical Therapist Assistant Prgm

Wye Mills

Chesapeake College
Stuart M Bounds, EdD, President
PO Box 8
Wye Mills, MD 21679
410 822-5400
Type: Junior or Comm Coll
Control: State, County, or Local Govt
• Radiography Prgm
• Surgical Technology Prgm

Massachusetts

Amherst

University of Massachusetts - Amherst
John Lombardi, Chancellor
Amherst, MA 01003
413 545-0111
Type: 4-year Coll or Univ
Control: State, County, or Local Govt
• Audiologist Prgm
• Dietetic Internship Prgm
• Dietetics-Didactic Prgm
• Nursing Prgm
• Psychology Prgm
• Speech-Language Pathology Prgm

Auburndale

Lasell College
Thomas E J De Witt, PhD, President
1844 Commonwealth Ave
Auburndale, MA 02466
617 243-2000
Type: 4-year Coll or Univ
Control: Nonprofit (Private or Religious)
• Athletic Training Prgm

Bedford

Middlesex Community College
Carole A Cowan, EdD, President
Springs Rd
Bedford, MA 01730
978 656-3370
Type: Junior or Comm Coll
Control: State, County, or Local Govt
• Dental Assisting Prgm
• Dental Hygiene Prgm
• Dental Lab Technician Prgm
• Diagnostic Med Sonography Prgm
• Medical Assistant Prgm
• Radiography Prgm

Beverly

Endicott College
Richard Wylie, EdD, President
376 Hale St
Beverly, MA 01915
978 232-2000
Type: 4-year Coll or Univ
Control: Nonprofit (Private or Religious)
• Athletic Training Prgm

Boston

Bay State College
Howard E Horton, Esq, President
122 Commonwealth Ave
Boston, MA 02116
617 217-9000
Type: Junior or Comm Coll
Control: For Profit
• Physical Therapist Assistant Prgm

Berklee College of Music
Roger Brown, President
1140 Boylston St
Boston, MA 02215
617 266-1400
Type: 4-year Coll or Univ
Control: Nonprofit (Private or Religious)
• Music Therapy Prgm

Beth Israel Deaconess Medical Center
David Dolins, President
Meissner Bldg - Room G-21
1 Deaconess Rd
Boston, MA 02215-5399
617 667-2203
Type: Hosp or Med Ctr: 500> Beds
Control: Nonprofit (Private or Religious)
• Dietetic Internship Prgm

Boston University
Robert Brown, President
1 Sherborn St
Boston, MA 02215
617 353-2000
Type: 4-year Coll or Univ
Control: Nonprofit (Private or Religious)
• Allopathic Medicine Prgm
• Athletic Training Prgm
• Dentistry Prgm
• Genetic Counseling Prgm
• Physical Therapy Prgm
• Psychology Prgm
• Rehabilitation Counseling Prgm
• Speech-Language Pathology Prgm

Boston University/Sargent College
Robert A Brown, PhD, President
One Sherborn St
Boston, MA 02215-1605
617 353-2000
Type: 4-year Coll or Univ
Control: Nonprofit (Private or Religious)
• Dietetic Internship Prgm
• Dietetics-Coordinated Prgm
• Dietetics-Didactic Prgm
• Occupational Therapy Prgm

Brigham & Women's Hospital
Gary Gottleib, MD, CEO
75 Francis St
Boston, MA 02115-6195
617 732-5595
Type: Hosp or Med Ctr: 500> Beds
Control: Nonprofit (Private or Religious)
• Dietetic Internship Prgm

Bunker Hill Community College
Mary L Fifield, PhD, President
250 New Rutherford Ave
Boston, MA 02129-2925
617 228-2400
Type: Junior or Comm Coll
Control: State, County, or Local Govt
• Diagnostic Med Sonography Prgm
• Radiography Prgm
• Surgical Technology Prgm

Emerson College
Jacqueline W Liebergott, President
100 Beacon St
Boston, MA 02116
617 578-8500
Control: Nonprofit (Private or Religious)
• Speech-Language Pathology Prgm

Emmanuel College
Boston, MA 02115
Type: 4-year Coll or Univ
Control: Nonprofit (Private or Religious)
• Nursing Prgm

Fisher College
Charles Perkins, JD, President
118 Beacon St
Boston, MA 02116
617 236-8800
Type: Junior or Comm Coll
Control: Nonprofit (Private or Religious)
• Health Information Tech Prgm

INSTITUTIONS

Frances Stern Nutrition Center
Thomas O'Donnell, MD, President
750 Washington St
PO Box 451
Boston, MA 02111
617 636-7655
Type: Hosp or Med Ctr: 300-499 Beds
Control: Nonprofit (Private or Religious)
• Dietetic Internship Prgm

Harvard Medical School
Boston, MA 02118
Type: Acad Health Ctr/Med Sch
Control: Nonprofit (Private or Religious)
• Allopathic Medicine Prgm
• Dentistry Prgm

Mass College of Pharmacy & Health Sciences
Charles F Monahan, Jr, BS ScD (Hon), President
179 Longwood Ave
Boston, MA 02115
617 732-2880
Type: 4-year Coll or Univ
Control: Nonprofit (Private or Religious)
• Dental Hygiene Prgm
• Nuclear Medicine Technology Prgm
• Nursing Prgm
• Pharmacy Prgm (2)
• Physician Assistant Prgm
• Radiation Therapy Prgm
• Radiography Prgm

Massachusetts General Hospital
J Robert Buchanan, MD, General Director
32 Fruit St
Boston, MA 02114
617 726-2101
Type: Hosp or Med Ctr: 500> Beds
Control: Nonprofit (Private or Religious)
• Dietetic Internship Prgm

Massachusetts Sch of Prof Psychology Inc
Boston, MA 02125
Type: Acad Health Ctr/Med Sch
Control: For Profit
• Psychology Prgm

MGH Institute of Health Professions
Janis Bellack, PhD RN FAAN, President
Charlestown Navy Yard
36 First Ave
Boston, MA 02129-4557
617 726-2947
Control: Nonprofit (Private or Religious)
• Physical Therapy Prgm
• Radiography Prgm
• Speech-Language Pathology Prgm

New England College of Optometry
Elizabeth Chen, MBA, President
424 Beacon St
Boston, MA 02115
Type: Junior or Comm Coll
Control: Nonprofit (Private or Religious)
• Optometry Prgm

Northeastern University
Joseph E Aoun, PhD, President
Office of the President
716 Columbus Pl
Boston, MA 02115
617 373-2101
Type: 4-year Coll or Univ
Control: Nonprofit (Private or Religious)
• Athletic Training Prgm
• Audiologist Prgm
• Clin Lab Scientist/Med Technologist Prgm
• Nursing Prgm
• Pharmacy Prgm
• Physical Therapy Prgm
• Physician Assistant Prgm
• Respiratory Therapist (Advanced) Prgm
• Speech-Language Pathology Prgm

Roxbury Community College
Terrence Gomes, EdD, President
1234 Columbus Ave
Boston, MA 02120
617 427-0060
Type: Junior or Comm Coll
Control: State, County, or Local Govt
• Radiography Prgm

Simmons College
Daniel Cheever, Jr, EdD, President
300 The Fenway
Boston, MA 02115
617 521-2000
Type: 4-year Coll or Univ
Control: Nonprofit (Private or Religious)
• Dietetic Internship Prgm
• Dietetics-Didactic Prgm
• Medical Librarian Prgm
• Nursing Prgm
• Physical Therapy Prgm

Suffolk University
David J Sargent, PhD, President
Beacon Hill
Boston, MA 02108-2770
617 573-8000
Type: 4-year Coll or Univ
Control: State, County, or Local Govt
• Psychology Prgm
• Radiation Therapy Prgm

University of Massachusetts - Boston
Keith Motley, Chancellor
100 Morrissey Blvd
Boston, MA 02125
617 287-5000
Type: 4-year Coll or Univ
Control: State, County, or Local Govt
• Allopathic Medicine Prgm
• Nursing Prgm
• Psychology Prgm
• Rehabilitation Counseling Prgm

Braintree

Clark University
Robert Payne, PhD, Vice President
725 Granite Plaza
Braintree, MA 02184
781 794-3400
Type: 4-year Coll or Univ
Control: Nonprofit (Private or Religious)
• Medical Assistant Prgm
• Psychology Prgm

Bridgewater

Bridgewater State College
Adrian Tinsley, PhD, President
Bridgewater, MA 02325
508 697-1201
Type: 4-year Coll or Univ
Control: State, County, or Local Govt
• Athletic Training Prgm

Brockton

Massasoit Community College
Charles Wall, PhD, President
1 Massasoit Blvd
Brockton, MA 02301
508 588-9100
Type: Junior or Comm Coll
Control: State, County, or Local Govt
• Dental Assisting Prgm
• Medical Assistant Prgm
• Radiography Prgm
• Respiratory Therapist (Advanced) Prgm

Cambridge

Lesley University
Joseph Moore, President
29 Everett St
Cambridge, MA 02138
617 868-9600
Type: 4-year Coll or Univ
Control: Nonprofit (Private or Religious)
• Art Therapy Prgm
• Dance/Movement Therapy Prgm
• Music Therapy Prgm

Mount Auburn Hospital
Francis P Lynch, President
330 Mt Auburn St
Cambridge, MA 02238
617 492-3500
Type: Hosp or Med Ctr: 300-499 Beds
Control: Nonprofit (Private or Religious)
• Dietetic Internship Prgm

Chestnut Hill

Boston College
Chestnut Hill, MA 02467
Type: 4-year Coll or Univ
Control: Nonprofit (Private or Religious)
• Nursing Prgm

Chicopee

Elms College
Chicopee, MA 01013
Type: 4-year Coll or Univ
Control: Nonprofit (Private or Religious)
• Nursing Prgm

Porter and Chester Institute - Chicopee
Henry Kamerzel, VP and Executive Director
134 Dulong Circle
Chicopee, MA 01022
413 593-3339
Type: Vocational or Tech Sch
Control: For Profit
• Medical Assistant Prgm

Danvers

North Shore Community College
Wayne M Burton, EdD, President
One Ferncroft Rd, PO Box 3340
Danvers, MA 01923-0840
978 762-4000
Type: Junior or Comm Coll
Control: State, County, or Local Govt
- Medical Assistant Prgm
- Occupational Therapy Asst Prgm
- Physical Therapist Assistant Prgm
- Radiography Prgm
- Respiratory Therapist (Advanced) Prgm
- Surgical Technology Prgm
- Veterinary Technology Prgm

Dorchester

Caritas Labouré College
Joseph McNabb, PhD, President
2120 Dorchester Ave
Dorchester, MA 02124-5698
617 296-8300
Type: Junior or Comm Coll
Control: Nonprofit (Private or Religious)
- Dietetic Technician-AD Prgm
- Electroneurodiagnostic Tech Prgm
- Health Information Tech Prgm
- Radiation Therapy Prgm

Fall River

Bristol Community College
John J Sbrega, PhD, President
777 Elsbree St
Fall River, MA 02720
508 678-2811
Type: Junior or Comm Coll
Control: State, County, or Local Govt
- Clin Lab Technician/Med Lab Technician Prgm
- Dental Hygiene Prgm
- Health Information Tech Prgm
- Medical Assistant Prgm
- Occupational Therapy Asst Prgm

Fitchburg

Fitchburg State College
Michael P Riccards, PhD, President
160 Pearl St
Fitchburg, MA 01420
508 665-3112
Type: 4-year Coll or Univ
Control: State, County, or Local Govt
- Nursing Prgm

Framingham

Framingham State College
Paul F Weller, President
100 State St
Framingham, MA 01701
508 620-1220
Type: 4-year Coll or Univ
Control: State, County, or Local Govt
- Dietetics-Coordinated Prgm
- Dietetics-Didactic Prgm

Gardner

Mt Wachusett Community College
Daniel M Asquino, PhD, President
444 Green St
Gardner, MA 01440
978 632-6600
Type: Junior or Comm Coll
Control: State, County, or Local Govt
- Medical Assistant Prgm
- Physical Therapist Assistant Prgm

Greenfield

Stillpoint Program - Greenfield Comm Coll
270 Main St
Greenfield, MA 01301
Type: Acad Health Ctr/Med Sch
Control: For Profit
- Massage Therapy Prgm

Haverhill

Northern Essex Community College
David F Hartleb, JD, President
100 Elliott Way
Haverhill, MA 01830
978 556-3855
Type: Junior or Comm Coll
Control: State, County, or Local Govt
- Dental Assisting Prgm
- Medical Assistant Prgm
- Polysomnographic Technology Prgm
- Radiography Prgm
- Respiratory Therapist (Advanced) Prgm

Holyoke

Holyoke Community College
William Messner, EdD, President
303 Homestead Ave
Holyoke, MA 01040
413 538-7000
Type: Junior or Comm Coll
Control: State, County, or Local Govt
- Ophthalmic Assistant Prgm
- Pharmacy Technician Prgm
- Radiography Prgm
- Veterinary Technology Prgm

Longmeadow

Bay Path College
Carol A Leary, PhD, President
588 Longmeadow St
Longmeadow, MA 01106
413 565-1241
Type: 4-year Coll or Univ
Control: Nonprofit (Private or Religious)
- Occupational Therapy Prgm

Lowell

University of Massachusetts - Lowell
Martin Meehan, JD, Chancellor
One University Ave
Lowell, MA 01854
978 934-4000
Type: 4-year Coll or Univ
Control: State, County, or Local Govt
- Clin Lab Scientist/Med Technologist Prgm
- Nursing Prgm
- Physical Therapy Prgm

Medford

Tufts University
Lawrence Bacow, PhD, President
Ballou Hall
Medford, MA 02155-7084
617 627-3300
Type: 4-year Coll or Univ
Control: Nonprofit (Private or Religious)
- Allopathic Medicine Prgm
- Dentistry Prgm
- Occupational Therapy Prgm
- Veterinary Medicine Prgm

Milton

Curry College
Kenneth K Quigley Jr, President
1071 Blue Hill Ave
Milton, MA 02186
617 333-0500
Type: 4-year Coll or Univ
Control: Nonprofit (Private or Religious)
- Nursing Prgm

Newton Centre

Mt Ida College
Carol Matteson, PhD, President
School of Business
777 Dedham St
Newton Centre, MA 02459
617 928-4500
Type: 4-year Coll or Univ
Control: Nonprofit (Private or Religious)
- Dental Hygiene Prgm
- Veterinary Technology Prgm

North Adams

Charles H McCann Technical School
James J Brosnan, CAGS, Superintendent
70 Hodges Cross Rd
North Adams, MA 01247
413 663-5383
Type: Vocational or Tech Sch
Control: State, County, or Local Govt
- Dental Assisting Prgm
- Medical Assistant Prgm
- Surgical Technology Prgm

INSTITUTIONS

North Andover

Merrimack College
Richard Santagati, MS DCS, President
315 Turnpike St
North Andover, MA 01845
978 837-5111
Type: 4-year Coll or Univ
Control: Nonprofit (Private or Religious)
• Athletic Training Prgm

North Dartmouth

University of Massachusetts - Dartmouth
Jean MacCormack, EdD, Chancellor
Office of the Chancellor
North Dartmouth, MA 02747-2300
508 999-8004
Type: 4-year Coll or Univ
Control: State, County, or Local Govt
• Clin Lab Scientist/Med Technologist Prgm

Paxton

Anna Maria College
Bernard Parker, President
Sunset Ln
Paxton, MA 01612-1198
508 849-3335
Type: 4-year Coll or Univ
Control: Nonprofit (Private or Religious)
• Music Therapy Prgm

Pittsfield

Berkshire Community College
Paul Raverta, President
1350 West St
Pittsfield, MA 01201
413 499-4660
Type: Junior or Comm Coll
Control: State, County, or Local Govt
• Physical Therapist Assistant Prgm
• Respiratory Therapist (Advanced) Prgm

Berkshire Medical Center
Helen Downey, Chief Operating Officer
725 North St
Pittsfield, MA 01201
413 447-2144
Type: Hosp or Med Ctr: 300-499 Beds
Control: Nonprofit (Private or Religious)
• Clin Lab Scientist/Med Technologist Prgm
• Cytotechnology Prgm

Quincy

Quincy College
G Jeremiah Ryan, President
34 Coddington St
Quincy, MA 02169
617 984-1776
Type: Junior or Comm Coll
Control: State, County, or Local Govt
• Surgical Technology Prgm

Salem

Salem State College
Patricia Maguire Meservey, PhD, President
352 Lafayette St
Salem, MA 01970-5353
978 542-6134
Type: 4-year Coll or Univ
Control: State, County, or Local Govt
• Athletic Training Prgm
• Nuclear Medicine Technology Prgm
• Nursing Prgm
• Occupational Therapy Prgm

South Easton

Southeastern Technical Institute
Luis Lopes, EdS, Superintendent
250 Foundry St
South Easton, MA 02375
508 238-1860
Type: Vocational or Tech Sch
Control: Nonprofit (Private or Religious)
• Dental Assisting Prgm
• Medical Assistant Prgm

Springfield

American International College
Vincent M Maniaci, EdD, President
1000 State St
Springfield, MA 01109-3189
413 205-3202
Type: 4-year Coll or Univ
Control: Nonprofit (Private or Religious)
• Occupational Therapy Prgm
• Physical Therapy Prgm

Springfield College
Richard B Flynn, EdD, President
Marsh Memorial
263 Alden St
Springfield, MA 01109
413 748-3241
Type: 4-year Coll or Univ
Control: Nonprofit (Private or Religious)
• Art Therapy Prgm
• Athletic Training Prgm
• Occupational Therapy Prgm
• Physical Therapy Prgm
• Physician Assistant Prgm
• Rehabilitation Counseling Prgm
• Therapeutic Recreation Specialist Prgm

Springfield Technical Community College

Ira Rubenzahl, PhD, President
One Armory Square, Ste 1
PO Box 9000
Springfield, MA 01102-9000
413 755-4906
Type: Junior or Comm Coll
Control: State, County, or Local Govt
• Clin Lab Technician/Med Lab Technician Prgm
• Clinical Assisting Prgm
• Dental Assisting Prgm
• Dental Hygiene Prgm
• Diagnostic Med Sonography Prgm
• Massage Therapy Prgm
• Nuclear Medicine Technology Prgm
• Occupational Therapy Asst Prgm
• Physical Therapist Assistant Prgm
• Radiography Prgm
• Respiratory Therapist (Advanced) Prgm
• Surgical Technology Prgm

Waltham

Brandeis University
Jehuda Reinharz, President
South St
Waltham, MA 02454-9110
781 736-2000
Type: 4-year Coll or Univ
Control: Nonprofit (Private or Religious)
• Genetic Counseling Prgm

Sodexho Health Care Services
153 Second Ave
Waltham, MA 02254-3730
800 926-7429
Control: For Profit
• Dietetic Internship Prgm (2)

Watertown

Cortiva Institute - Muscular Therapy Inst
Mary Ann DiRoberts, President
103 Morse St
Watertown, MA 02472
617 668-1000
Type: Acad Health Ctr/Med Sch
Control: For Profit
• Massage Therapy Prgm

Wellesley Hills

Massachusetts Bay Community College
Carole Berotte Joseph, PhD, President
Wellesley Hills Campus
50 Oakland St
Wellesley Hills, MA 02481
781 230-3100
Type: Junior or Comm Coll
Control: State, County, or Local Govt
• Physical Therapist Assistant Prgm
• Radiography Prgm
• Surgical Technology Prgm

West Barnstable

Cape Cod Community College
Kathleen Schatzberg, EdD, President
2240 Iyanough Rd
West Barnstable, MA 02668-1599
508 362-2131
Type: Junior or Comm Coll
Control: State, County, or Local Govt
- Dental Hygiene Prgm
- Medical Assistant Prgm

Westfield

Westfield State College
Barry Maloney, MPE, Interim President
Office of the President
577 Western Ave
Westfield, MA 01086-1630
413 572-5203
Type: 4-year Coll or Univ
Control: State, County, or Local Govt
- Athletic Training Prgm
- Exercise Science Prgm

Weston

Regis College
Mary Jane England, PhD, President
235 Wellsley St
Weston, MA 02493
781 768-7000
Type: 4-year Coll or Univ
Control: State, County, or Local Govt
- Radiography Prgm

Worcester

Assumption College
Joseph H Hagan, President
500 Salisbury St
Worcester, MA 01615
508 767-7000
Type: 4-year Coll or Univ
Control: Nonprofit (Private or Religious)
- Rehabilitation Counseling Prgm

Becker College
Franklin M Loew, PhD, President
61 Sever St Box 15071
Worcester, MA 01615-0071
508 791-9241
Type: 4-year Coll or Univ
Control: Nonprofit (Private or Religious)
- Physical Therapist Assistant Prgm
- Veterinary Technology Prgm

Quinsigamond Community College
Gail Carberry, EdD, President
670 W Boylston St
Worcester, MA 01606-2092
508 854-4203
Type: Junior or Comm Coll
Control: State, County, or Local Govt
- Dental Assisting Prgm
- Dental Hygiene Prgm
- Medical Assistant Prgm
- Occupational Therapy Asst Prgm
- Radiography Prgm
- Respiratory Therapist (Advanced) Prgm
- Surgical Technology Prgm

The Salter School
Charlene Keefe, BS, President
155 Ararat St
Worcester, MA 01606-3450
508 853-1074
Type: Vocational or Tech Sch
Control: For Profit
- Medical Assistant Prgm

UMass Memorial Medical Center
John O'Brien, MD, CEO, Clinical Systems
One Biotech Park, 365 Plantation St
Worcester, MA 01655
508 856-4114
Type: Hosp or Med Ctr: 500> Beds
Control: Nonprofit (Private or Religious)
- Nuclear Medicine Technology Prgm
- Radiation Therapy Prgm

Worcester State College
Janelle Ashley, PhD, President
486 Chandler St
Worcester, MA 01602-2597
508 929-8020
Type: 4-year Coll or Univ
Control: State, County, or Local Govt
- Occupational Therapy Prgm
- Speech-Language Pathology Prgm

Michigan

Albion

Albion College
Peter T Mitchell, PhD, President
203 Ferguson Bldg
Albion, MI 49224
517 629-0210
Type: 4-year Coll or Univ
Control: Nonprofit (Private or Religious)
- Athletic Training Prgm

Allen Park

Baker College of Allen Park
4500 Enterprise Dr
Allen Park, MI 48101
313 425-3700
Type: 4-year Coll or Univ
Control: State, County, or Local Govt
- Health Information Tech Prgm

Allendale

Grand Valley State University
Thomas J Haas, PhD, President
One Campus Dr
Allendale, MI 49401-9403
616 331-2182
Type: 4-year Coll or Univ
Control: State, County, or Local Govt
- Athletic Training Prgm
- Clin Lab Scientist/Med Technologist Prgm
- Nursing Prgm
- Occupational Therapy Prgm
- Physical Therapy Prgm
- Physician Assistant Prgm
- Radiation Therapy Prgm

Alma

Alma College
Saundra Tracy, PhD, President
614 W Superior St
Alma, MI 48801
989 463-7146
Type: 4-year Coll or Univ
Control: Nonprofit (Private or Religious)
- Athletic Training Prgm

Alpena

Alpena Community College
Olin Joynton, PhD, President
666 Johnson St
Alpena, MI 49707
989 358-7246
Type: Junior or Comm Coll
Control: State, County, or Local Govt
- Medical Assistant Prgm

Ann Arbor

Ann Arbor Institute of Massage Therapy
Jocelyn Granger, NCBTMB, Director
180 Jackson Plaza
Suite 100
Ann Arbor, MI 48103
734 677-4430
Type: Acad Health Ctr/Med Sch
Control: For Profit
- Massage Therapy Prgm

Huron Valley Ambulance
Dale J Berry, EMT-P, President, CEO
1200 State Circle
Ann Arbor, MI 48108
734 477-6262
Type: Vocational or Tech Sch
Control: Nonprofit (Private or Religious)
- Emergency Med Tech-Paramedic Prgm

University of Michigan
Mary Sue Coleman, PhD, President
2074 Fleming Adm Bldg
503 Thompson St
Ann Arbor, MI 48109-1340
734 764-6270
Type: 4-year Coll or Univ
Control: State, County, or Local Govt
- Allopathic Medicine Prgm
- Athletic Training Prgm
- Dental Hygiene Prgm
- Dentistry Prgm
- Dietetic Internship Prgm
- Dietetics-Didactic Prgm
- Genetic Counseling Prgm
- Medical Librarian Prgm
- Nursing Prgm
- Pharmacy Prgm
- Psychology Prgm

University of Michigan Hospitals & Health Ctr
1500 E Medical Ctr Dr
Ann Arbor, MI 48109-0056
313 936-5199
Control: State, County, or Local Govt
- Dietetic Internship Prgm

W K Kellogg Eye Center
1000 Wall St
Ann Arbor, MI 48105
Control: Nonprofit (Private or Religious)
• Orthoptist Prgm

Washtenaw Community College
Larry Whitworth, EdD, President
PO Box D-1
Ann Arbor, MI 48106-0610
734 973-3491
Type: Junior or Comm Coll
Control: State, County, or Local Govt
• Dental Assisting Prgm
• Pharmacy Technician Prgm
• Radiography Prgm

Auburn Hills

Baker College of Auburn Hills
Jeffrey M Love, President
1500 University Dr
Auburn Hills, MI 48326-2642
248 340-0600
Type: 4-year Coll or Univ
Control: Nonprofit (Private or Religious)
• Medical Assistant Prgm

Battle Creek

Kellogg Community College
G Edward Haring, PhD, President
450 North Ave
Battle Creek, MI 49017
269 965-3931
Type: Junior or Comm Coll
Control: State, County, or Local Govt
• Clin Lab Technician/Med Lab Technician Prgm
• Dental Hygiene Prgm
• Physical Therapist Assistant Prgm
• Radiography Prgm

Benton Harbor

Lake Michigan College
Randall Miller, EdD, President
2755 E Napier Ave
Benton Harbor, MI 49022-1899
269 927-8100
Type: Junior or Comm Coll
Control: State, County, or Local Govt
• Dental Assisting Prgm
• Radiography Prgm

Berrien Springs

Andrews University
Niels-Erik Andreasen, PhD, President
Berrien Springs, MI 49104
269 471-3100
Type: 4-year Coll or Univ
Control: Nonprofit (Private or Religious)
• Clin Lab Scientist/Med Technologist Prgm
• Counseling Prgm
• Dietetic Internship Prgm
• Dietetics-Didactic Prgm
• Physical Therapy Prgm

Big Rapids

Ferris State University
David Eisler, PhD, President
1201 S State St
CSS 301
Big Rapids, MI 49307-2737
616 592-2500
Type: 4-year Coll or Univ
Control: State, County, or Local Govt
• Clin Lab Scientist/Med Technologist Prgm
• Clin Lab Technician/Med Lab Technician Prgm
• Dental Hygiene Prgm
• Health Information Admin Prgm
• Health Information Tech Prgm
• Nuclear Medicine Technology Prgm
• Optometry Prgm
• Pharmacy Prgm
• Radiography Prgm
• Respiratory Therapist (Advanced) Prgm

Bloomfield Hills

Oakland Community College
Mary S Spangler, PhD, Chancellor
George A Bee Administrative Ctr
2480 Opdyke Rd
Bloomfield Hills, MI 48304-2266
248 341-2115
Type: Junior or Comm Coll
Control: State, County, or Local Govt
• Dental Hygiene Prgm
• Diagnostic Med Sonography Prgm
• Medical Assistant Prgm
• Radiography Prgm
• Respiratory Therapist (Advanced) Prgm
• Surgical Technology Prgm

Cadillac

Baker College of Cadillac
Robert VanDellen, PhD, President
9600 E 13th St
Cadillac, MI 49601
231 775-8458
Type: 4-year Coll or Univ
Control: Nonprofit (Private or Religious)
• Medical Assistant Prgm
• Surgical Technology Prgm
• Veterinary Technology Prgm

Centerville

Glen Oaks Community College
Glenn S Oxender, BS MA, President
62249 Shimmel Rd
Centerville, MI 49032
269 467-9945
Type: Junior or Comm Coll
Control: State, County, or Local Govt
• Medical Assistant Prgm

Clinton Township

Baker College of Clinton Township
Donald Torline, MBA, President
34950 Little Mack Ave
Clinton Township, MI 48035
586 791-6610
Type: 4-year Coll or Univ
Control: For Profit
• Medical Assistant Prgm
• Radiography Prgm
• Surgical Technology Prgm

Dearborn

Henry Ford Community College
Gail Mee, EdD, President
5101 Evergreen Rd
Dearborn, MI 48128-1495
313 845-9218
Type: Junior or Comm Coll
Control: State, County, or Local Govt
• Medical Assistant Prgm
• Pharmacy Technician Prgm
• Physical Therapist Assistant Prgm
• Radiography Prgm
• Respiratory Therapist (Advanced) Prgm
• Surgical Technology Prgm

Detroit

Detroit Dept of Hlth & Wellness Promotions
1151 Taylor St
Detroit, MI 48202-1732
313 876-4090
Control: State, County, or Local Govt
• Dietetic Internship Prgm

DMC University Laboratories
Verdell Tolbert, MT, VP, Laboratory Services
4201 St Antoine Blvd
Detroit, MI 48201
313 745-4539
Type: Acad Health Ctr/Med Sch
Control: Nonprofit (Private or Religious)
• Clin Lab Scientist/Med Technologist Prgm
• Cytotechnology Prgm

Harper University Hospital
Paul Broughton, President
3990 John R St
Detroit, MI 48201-2097
313 745-9375
Type: Hosp or Med Ctr: 500> Beds
Control: Nonprofit (Private or Religious)
• Dietetic Internship Prgm

Henry Ford Hospital
Anthony Armada, MBA, CEO
2799 W Grand Blvd
A-2 Administration
Detroit, MI 48202
313 876-1257
Type: Hosp or Med Ctr: 500> Beds
Control: Nonprofit (Private or Religious)
• Diagnostic Med Sonography Prgm
• Dietetic Internship Prgm

Sinai-Grace Hospital
Conrad Mallett, JD, President
6071 W Outer Dr
Detroit, MI 48235
313 966-3525
Type: Hosp or Med Ctr: 300-499 Beds
Control: Nonprofit (Private or Religious)
• Radiography Prgm

University of Detroit Mercy
Rev Gerard L Stockhausen, SJ PhD, President
4001 W McNichols Rd
PO Box 19900
Detroit, MI 48221
313 993-1455
Type: 4-year Coll or Univ
Control: Nonprofit (Private or Religious)
• Counseling Prgm
• Dental Hygiene Prgm
• Dentistry Prgm
• Nursing Prgm
• Physician Assistant Prgm
• Psychology Prgm

Wayne County Community College District
Curtis L Ivery, PhD, Chancellor
801 W Fort St
Detroit, MI 48226-9975
313 496-2510
Type: Junior or Comm Coll
Control: State, County, or Local Govt
• Dental Assisting Prgm
• Dental Hygiene Prgm
• Dietetic Technician-AD Prgm
• Occupational Therapy Asst Prgm
• Pharmacy Technician Prgm
• Surgical Technology Prgm

Wayne State University
Irvin D Reid, PhD, President
4200 Faculty Admin Bldg
Detroit, MI 48202-3489
313 577-2230
Type: 4-year Coll or Univ
Control: State, County, or Local Govt
• Allopathic Medicine Prgm
• Art Therapy Prgm
• Audiologist Prgm
• Clin Lab Scientist/Med Technologist Prgm
• Counseling Prgm
• Dietetics-Coordinated Prgm
• Genetic Counseling Prgm
• Medical Librarian Prgm
• Nursing Prgm
• Occupational Therapy Prgm
• Pathologists' Assistant Prgm
• Pharmacy Prgm
• Physical Therapy Prgm
• Physician Assistant Prgm
• Psychology Prgm
• Radiation Therapy Prgm
• Radiography Prgm
• Rehabilitation Counseling Prgm
• Speech-Language Pathology Prgm

East Lansing

Michigan State University
Kim Wilcox, PhD, Provost
438 Admin Bldg
East Lansing, MI 48824
517 355-1524
Type: 4-year Coll or Univ
Control: State, County, or Local Govt
• Allopathic Medicine Prgm
• Athletic Training Prgm
• Audiologist Prgm
• Clin Lab Scientist/Med Technologist Prgm
• Dietetic Internship Prgm
• Dietetics-Didactic Prgm
• Music Therapy Prgm
• Nursing Prgm
• Osteopathic Medicine Prgm
• Psychology Prgm
• Rehabilitation Counseling Prgm
• Speech-Language Pathology Prgm
• Teacher of the Visually Impaired Prgm
• Veterinary Medicine Prgm
• Veterinary Technology Prgm

Ferndale

Medright Incorporated
Gail Lucas, Program Director
427 Allen
Ferndale, MI 48220
248 547-0834
Type: Acad Health Ctr/Med Sch
Control: For Profit
• Phlebotomy Prgm

Flint

Baker College Center of Graduate Studies
Michael Heberling, PhD, President
1116 W Bristol Rd
Flint, MI 48507-5508
810 766-2033
Control: Nonprofit (Private or Religious)
• Occupational Therapy Prgm

Baker College of Flint
Julianne T Princinsky, EdD, President
1050 W Bristol Rd
Flint, MI 48507-5508
810 766-4036
Type: Junior or Comm Coll
Control: Nonprofit (Private or Religious)
• Health Information Tech Prgm
• Medical Assistant Prgm
• Physical Therapist Assistant Prgm
• Polysomnographic Technology Prgm
• Surgical Technology Prgm
• Veterinary Technology Prgm

Hurley Medical Center
Patrick Wardell, President/CEO
One Hurley Plaza
Flint, MI 48503
810 257-9237
Type: Hosp or Med Ctr: 300-499 Beds
Control: State, County, or Local Govt
• Clin Lab Scientist/Med Technologist Prgm
• Dietetic Internship Prgm
• Radiography Prgm

Mott Community College
M Richard Shaink, President
1401 E Court St
Flint, MI 48503
810 762-0200
Type: Junior or Comm Coll
Control: State, County, or Local Govt
• Dental Assisting Prgm
• Dental Hygiene Prgm
• Occupational Therapy Asst Prgm
• Physical Therapist Assistant Prgm
• Respiratory Therapist (Advanced) Prgm

University of Michigan - Flint
Juan Mestas, MA PhD, Chancellor
303 E Kearsley St
Flint, MI 48502-2186
810 762-3000
Type: 4-year Coll or Univ
Control: State, County, or Local Govt
• Nursing Prgm
• Physical Therapy Prgm
• Radiation Therapy Prgm

Grand Rapids

Aquinas College
Harry J Knopke, PhD, President
1607 Robinson Rd SE
Grand Rapids, MI 49506-1799
616 632-2880
Type: 4-year Coll or Univ
Control: Nonprofit (Private or Religious)
• Athletic Training Prgm

Calvin College
Gaylen Byker, President
Office of the President
Spoelhof Center 390
Grand Rapids, MI 49546
616 526-6100
Type: 4-year Coll or Univ
Control: Nonprofit (Private or Religious)
• Nursing Prgm

Davenport University
Randolph Flechsig, PhD, President
415 E Fulton St
Grand Rapids, MI 49503
616 451-3511
Type: 4-year Coll or Univ
Control: Nonprofit (Private or Religious)
• Health Information Tech Prgm
• Medical Assistant Prgm (4)

Grand Rapids Community College
Juan Olivarez, PhD, President
143 Bostwick Ave NE
Grand Rapids, MI 49503-3295
616 234-3901
Type: Junior or Comm Coll
Control: State, County, or Local Govt
• Dental Assisting Prgm
• Dental Hygiene Prgm
• Occupational Therapy Asst Prgm
• Radiography Prgm

Hancock

Finlandia University
Robert Ubbelohde, President
Quincy 601
Hancock, MI 49930-1882
906 482-6300
Type: Junior or Comm Coll
Control: Nonprofit (Private or Religious)
• Nursing Prgm
• Physical Therapist Assistant Prgm

Harrison

Mid Michigan Community College
Carol C Churchill, MA, President
1375 S Clare Ave
Harrison, MI 48625
517 386-6642
Type: Junior or Comm Coll
Control: State, County, or Local Govt
• Medical Assistant Prgm
• Phlebotomy Prgm
• Radiography Prgm

Holland

Hope College
James Bultman, EdD, President
PO Box 9000
Holland, MI 49422-9000
616 395-7780
Type: 4-year Coll or Univ
Control: Nonprofit (Private or Religious)
• Athletic Training Prgm
• Nursing Prgm

Jackson

Baker College of Jackson
Patricia Kaufman, PhD, President
2800 Springport Rd
Jackson, MI 49202
517 789-6123
Type: 4-year Coll or Univ
Control: Nonprofit (Private or Religious)
• Medical Assistant Prgm
• Radiation Therapy Prgm
• Surgical Technology Prgm
• Veterinary Technology Prgm

Jackson Community College
Daniel J Phelan, PhD, President
2111 Emmons Rd
Jackson, MI 49201-8399
517 787-0800
Type: Junior or Comm Coll
Control: State, County, or Local Govt
• Diagnostic Med Sonography Prgm
• Medical Assistant Prgm

Kalamazoo

Kalamazoo Valley Community College
Marilyn J Schlack, EdD, President
Texas Township Campus
6767 West O Ave, PO Box 4070
Kalamazoo, MI 49003-4070
269 488-4434
Type: Junior or Comm Coll
Control: State, County, or Local Govt
• Dental Hygiene Prgm
• Medical Assistant Prgm
• Respiratory Therapist (Advanced) Prgm
• Surgical Technology Prgm

Western Michigan University
John Dunn, EdD, President
3600 Siebert Admin Bldg
Kalamazoo, MI 49008-5130
269 387-2351
Type: 4-year Coll or Univ
Control: State, County, or Local Govt
• Athletic Training Prgm
• Audiologist Prgm
• Counseling Prgm
• Dietetic Internship Prgm
• Dietetics-Didactic Prgm
• Music Therapy Prgm
• Nursing Prgm
• Occupational Therapy Prgm
• Orientation and Mobility Specialist Prgm
• Physician Assistant Prgm
• Psychology Prgm
• Rehabilitation Counseling Prgm
• Speech-Language Pathology Prgm
• Vision Rehabilitation Therapy Prgm

Lansing

Lansing Community College
Judith Cardenas, PhD, Interim President
521 N Washington Sq
PO Box 40010
Lansing, MI 48901
517 483-1852
Type: Junior or Comm Coll
Control: State, County, or Local Govt
• Dental Hygiene Prgm
• Diagnostic Med Sonography Prgm
• Emergency Med Tech-Paramedic Prgm
• Histotechnician Prgm
• Radiography Prgm
• Surgical Technology Prgm

Livonia

Madonna University
Mary Francilene, President
36600 Schoolcraft Rd
Livonia, MI 48150
313 591-5000
Type: 4-year Coll or Univ
Control: Nonprofit (Private or Religious)
• Dietetics-Didactic Prgm
• Nursing Prgm

Schoolcraft College
Conway A Jeffress, PhD, President
18600 Haggerty Rd
Livonia, MI 48152-2696
734 462-4400
Type: Junior or Comm Coll
Control: State, County, or Local Govt
• Health Information Tech Prgm
• Medical Assistant Prgm

Marquette

Marquette General Health System
William Nemacheck, CEO
420 W Magnetic St
Marquette, MI 49855
906 225-4774
Type: Hosp or Med Ctr: 300-499 Beds
Control: Nonprofit (Private or Religious)
• Radiography Prgm

Northern Michigan University
Leslie Wong, PhD, President
1401 Presque Isle Ave
Marquette, MI 49855
906 227-2242
Type: 4-year Coll or Univ
Control: State, County, or Local Govt
• Athletic Training Prgm
• Clin Lab Scientist/Med Technologist Prgm
• Clin Lab Technician/Med Lab Technician Prgm
• Cytogenetic Technology Prgm
• Diagnostic Molecular Scientist Prgm
• Nursing Prgm
• Surgical Technology Prgm

Monroe

Monroe County Community College
David Nixon, MA, President
1555 S Raisinville Rd
Monroe, MI 48161
734 384-4166
Type: Junior or Comm Coll
Control: State, County, or Local Govt
• Respiratory Therapist (Advanced) Prgm
• Respiratory Therapist (Entry-Level) Prgm

Mt Pleasant

Central Michigan University
Michael Rao, PhD, President
106 Warriner Hall
Mt Pleasant, MI 48859
989 774-3131
Type: 4-year Coll or Univ
Control: State, County, or Local Govt
• Athletic Training Prgm
• Audiologist Prgm
• Dietetic Internship Prgm
• Dietetics-Didactic Prgm
• Physical Therapy Prgm
• Physician Assistant Prgm
• Psychology Prgm
• Speech-Language Pathology Prgm
• Therapeutic Recreation Specialist Prgm

Muskegon

Baker College of Muskegon
Rick E Amidon, PhD, President
1903 Marquette Ave
Muskegon, MI 49442-9982
231 777-5247
Type: 4-year Coll or Univ
Control: Nonprofit (Private or Religious)
- Medical Assistant Prgm
- Occupational Therapy Asst Prgm
- Physical Therapist Assistant Prgm
- Radiography Prgm
- Surgical Technology Prgm
- Veterinary Technology Prgm

Muskegon Community College
David Rule, PhD, President
221 S Quarterline Rd
Muskegon, MI 49442
616 777-0303
Type: Junior or Comm Coll
Control: State, County, or Local Govt
- Respiratory Therapist (Advanced) Prgm

Owosso

Baker College of Owosso
Denise Bannan, PhD, President, CEO
1020 S Washington St
Owosso, MI 48867
989 729-3350
Type: 4-year Coll or Univ
Control: Nonprofit (Private or Religious)
- Clin Lab Technician/Med Lab Technician Prgm
- Medical Assistant Prgm
- Phlebotomy Prgm
- Radiography Prgm

Port Huron

Baker College of Port Huron
Connie Harrison, PhD, President
3403 Lapeer Rd
Port Huron, MI 48060
810 989-2120
Type: 4-year Coll or Univ
Control: Nonprofit (Private or Religious)
- Dental Hygiene Prgm
- Surgical Technology Prgm
- Veterinary Technology Prgm

Lakewood School of Therapeutic Massage
Nancy Levitt, Director
1102 6th St
Port Huron, MI 48060
810 987-3959
Type: Acad Health Ctr/Med Sch
Control: For Profit
- Massage Therapy Prgm

Port Huron Hospital
Brian Connolly, MBA, President
1221 Pine Grove
Port Huron, MI 48061-5011
810 987-5000
Type: Hosp or Med Ctr: 100-299 Beds
Control: Nonprofit (Private or Religious)
- Radiography Prgm

Rochester

Oakland University
Gary D Russi, PhD, President
North Foundation Hall
Rochester, MI 48063
313 370-3500
Type: 4-year Coll or Univ
Control: State, County, or Local Govt
- Counseling Prgm
- Nursing Prgm
- Physical Therapy Prgm

Royal Oak

William Beaumont Hospital
Kenneth Matzick, President, CEO
3601 W 13 Mile Rd
Royal Oak, MI 48073
248 551-0681
Type: Hosp or Med Ctr: 500> Beds
Control: Nonprofit (Private or Religious)
- Clin Lab Scientist/Med Technologist Prgm
- Histotechnician Prgm
- Histotechnology Prgm
- Nuclear Medicine Technology Prgm
- Radiation Therapy Prgm
- Radiography Prgm
- Surgical Assistant Prgm

Sault Ste Marie

Lake Superior State University
Betty Youngblood, PhD, President
650 W Easterday Ave
Sault Ste Marie, MI 49783
906 635-2202
Type: 4-year Coll or Univ
Control: State, County, or Local Govt
- Athletic Training Prgm

Sidney

Montcalm Community College
Donald Burns, PhD, President
2800 College Dr
Sidney, MI 48885
517 328-1221
Type: Junior or Comm Coll
Control: State, County, or Local Govt
- Medical Assistant Prgm

Southfield

National Institute of Technology
Marchelle (Mickey) Weaver, BA, President
26111 Evergreen Rd
Ste 201
Southfield, MI 48076
248 799-9933
Type: Vocational or Tech Sch
Control: For Profit
- Medical Assistant Prgm

Providence Hospital
Diane Radloff, MHA, CEO, Providence Oper Unit
16001 W Nine Mile Rd
Southfield, MI 48075
248 849-3000
Type: Hosp or Med Ctr: 300-499 Beds
Control: Nonprofit (Private or Religious)
- Diagnostic Med Sonography Prgm
- Radiography Prgm

Spring Arbor

Spring Arbor University
Spring Arbor, MI 49283
Type: 4-year Coll or Univ
Control: State, County, or Local Govt
- Nursing Prgm

Traverse City

Northwestern Michigan College
Timothy Nelson, MA, President
1701 E Front St
Traverse City, MI 49686
616 995-1010
Type: Junior or Comm Coll
Control: State, County, or Local Govt
- Dental Assisting Prgm

Troy

Carnegie Institute
Gloria J McEachern-Wiggins, CMA,
   President/CEO
550 Stephenson Hwy, Ste 100-110
Troy, MI 48083
248 589-1078
Type: Vocational or Tech Sch
Control: For Profit
- Cardiovascular Technology Prgm
- Electroneurodiagnostic Tech Prgm
- Medical Assistant Prgm

University Center

Delta College
Jean Goodnow, PhD, President
1961 Delta Rd
University Center, MI 48710
989 686-9201
Type: Junior or Comm Coll
Control: State, County, or Local Govt
- Dental Assisting Prgm
- Dental Hygiene Prgm
- Diagnostic Med Sonography Prgm
- Physical Therapist Assistant Prgm
- Radiography Prgm
- Respiratory Therapist (Advanced) Prgm
- Surgical Technology Prgm

Saginaw Valley State University
Eric R Gilbertson, JD, President
7400 Bay Rd
University Center, MI 48710-0001
989 964-4145
Type: 4-year Coll or Univ
Control: State, County, or Local Govt
- Athletic Training Prgm
- Nursing Prgm
- Occupational Therapy Prgm

INSTITUTIONS

Warren

Macomb Community College
Albert L Lorenzo, PhD, President
14500 E Twelve Mile Rd
Building D-300
Warren, MI 48088-3896
586 445-7241
Type: Junior or Comm Coll
Control: State, County, or Local Govt
• Medical Assistant Prgm
• Occupational Therapy Asst Prgm
• Physical Therapist Assistant Prgm
• Respiratory Therapist (Advanced) Prgm
• Surgical Technology Prgm
• Veterinary Technology Prgm

St John Health
Elliot Joseph, MHSA, President CEO
28000 Dequindre Rd
Warren, MI 48092
586 753-0710
Type: Hosp or Med Ctr: 500> Beds
Control: Nonprofit (Private or Religious)
• Clin Lab Scientist/Med Technologist Prgm
• Radiography Prgm

Ypsilanti

Eastern Michigan University
Donald Loppknow, PhD, Provist, EVP
202 Welch Hall
Ypsilanti, MI 48197-2239
734 487-2211
Type: 4-year Coll or Univ
Control: State, County, or Local Govt
• Athletic Training Prgm
• Clin Lab Scientist/Med Technologist Prgm
• Counseling Prgm
• Dietetics-Coordinated Prgm
• Music Therapy Prgm
• Nursing Prgm
• Occupational Therapy Prgm
• Orthotist/Prosthetist Prgm
• Psychology Prgm
• Speech-Language Pathology Prgm

Minnesota

Alexandria

Alexandria Technical College
Kevin Kopischke, PhD, President
1601 Jefferson St
Alexandria, MN 56308
320 762-0221
Type: Vocational or Tech Sch
Control: State, County, or Local Govt
• Clin Lab Technician/Med Lab Technician Prgm

Anoka

Anoka Technical College
Anne Weyandt, BA JD, President
1355 W Hwy 10
Anoka, MN 55303-1590
763 576-4709
Type: Vocational or Tech Sch
Control: State, County, or Local Govt
• Health Information Tech Prgm
• Medical Assistant Prgm
• Occupational Therapy Asst Prgm
• Surgical Technology Prgm

Austin

Riverland Community College
Gary Rhodes, PhD, President
1600 8th Ave NW
Austin, MN 55912
507 433-0508
Type: Junior or Comm Coll
Control: State, County, or Local Govt
• Radiography Prgm

Bemidji

Bemidji State University
Jeanine E Gangeness, RN MS, Chief Nurse
    Administrator
1500 Birchmont Dr NE
105 Deputy Hall
Bemidji, MN 56601
Type: 4-year Coll or Univ
Control: State, County, or Local Govt
• Nursing Prgm

Northwest Technical College - Bemidji
Jon E Quistgaard, PhD, President
905 Grant Ave SE
Bemidji, MN 56601
218 333-6600
Type: Vocational or Tech Sch
Control: State, County, or Local Govt
• Dental Assisting Prgm

Bloomington

Normandale Community College
Joseph Opatz, PhD, President
9700 France Ave S
Bloomington, MN 55431
952 487-8200
Type: Junior or Comm Coll
Control: State, County, or Local Govt
• Dental Hygiene Prgm
• Dietetic Technician-AD Prgm

Northwestern Health Science University
Alfred Traina, DC
2501 W 84th St
Bloomington, MN 55431
Type: Acad Health Ctr/Med Sch
Control: For Profit
• Massage Therapy Prgm

Brainerd

Central Lakes College
Sally J Ihne, President
300 Quince St
Brainerd, MN 56401
218 828-2525
Control: For Profit
• Dental Assisting Prgm

Brooklyn Park

Hennepin Technical College
Ronald Kraft, Interim President
9000 Brooklyn Blvd
Brooklyn Park, MN 55445
763 488-2414
Type: Vocational or Tech Sch
Control: State, County, or Local Govt
• Dental Assisting Prgm

North Hennepin Community College
Yvette Jackson, PhD, Interim President
7411 85th Ave N
Brooklyn Park, MN 55445
612 424-0820
Type: Junior or Comm Coll
Control: State, County, or Local Govt
• Clin Lab Technician/Med Lab Technician Prgm

Coon Rapids

Anoka Ramsey Community College
Patrick M Johns, PhD, President
11200 Mississippi Blvd NW
Coon Rapids, MN 55433
763 422-3435
Type: Junior or Comm Coll
Control: State, County, or Local Govt
• Physical Therapist Assistant Prgm

Crookston

University of Minnesota - Crookston
Donald G Sargeant, Chancellor
Crookston, MN 56716
218 281-6510
Type: 4-year Coll or Univ
Control: State, County, or Local Govt
• Dietetic Technician-AD Prgm

Crystal

Herzing College
John Slama, MA (Admin), President
5700 W Broadway
Crystal, MN 55428
763 535-3000
Type: Vocational or Tech Sch
Control: For Profit
• Dental Assisting Prgm
• Dental Hygiene Prgm
• Medical Assistant Prgm

Duluth

College of St Scholastica
Larry Goodwin, PhD, President
1200 Kenwood Ave
Duluth, MN 55811
218 723-6033
Type: 4-year Coll or Univ
Control: Nonprofit (Private or Religious)
• Health Information Admin Prgm
• Nursing Prgm
• Occupational Therapy Prgm
• Physical Therapy Prgm

Duluth Business University
James R Gessner, President
4724 Mike Colalillo Dr
Duluth, MN 55807
218 722-4000
Type: Vocational or Tech Sch
Control: For Profit
• Medical Assistant Prgm
• Veterinary Technology Prgm

Lake Superior College
Kathleen Nelson, EdD, President
2101 Trinity Rd
Duluth, MN 55811-3399
218 723-7667
Type: Junior or Comm Coll
Control: State, County, or Local Govt
• Clin Lab Technician/Med Lab Technician Prgm
• Dental Hygiene Prgm
• Medical Assistant Prgm
• Physical Therapist Assistant Prgm
• Radiography Prgm
• Respiratory Therapist (Advanced) Prgm
• Surgical Technology Prgm

University of Minnesota - Duluth
Kathryn A Martin, Chancellor
Duluth, MN 55812
218 726-8000
Type: 4-year Coll or Univ
Control: State, County, or Local Govt
• Athletic Training Prgm
• Speech-Language Pathology Prgm

Eagan

Argosy University - Twin Cities
Scott Tjaden, PsyD, Campus President
1515 Central Pkwy
Eagan, MN 55121
651 846-3407
Type: 4-year Coll or Univ
Control: For Profit
• Clin Lab Technician/Med Lab Technician Prgm
• Dental Hygiene Prgm
• Diagnostic Med Sonography Prgm
• Histotechnician Prgm
• Medical Assistant Prgm
• Psychology Prgm
• Radiation Therapy Prgm
• Radiography Prgm
• Veterinary Technology Prgm

Edina

Fairview University
Gordon Alexander, MD, President
6545 France Ave S
Edina, MN 55435
952 836-3537
Type: Hosp or Med Ctr: 300-499 Beds
Control: Nonprofit (Private or Religious)
• Radiation Therapy Prgm
• Radiography Prgm

Fergus Falls

Greater Minnesota Paramedic Consortium
Beth Domholdt, VP of Student Services
PO Box 1014
214 East Junius Ave
Fergus Falls, MN 56537
218 998-2739
Type: Junior or Comm Coll
Control: State, County, or Local Govt
• Emergency Med Tech-Paramedic Prgm

Minnesota State Community and Technical Coll
Ann Valentine, PhD, President
1414 College Way
Fergus Falls, MN 56537
218 736-1501
Type: Junior or Comm Coll
Control: State, County, or Local Govt
• Clin Lab Technician/Med Lab Technician Prgm

Hibbing

Hibbing Community College
Ken Simberg, MS, President
1515 E 25th St
Hibbing, MN 55746
218 262-7200
Type: Vocational or Tech Sch
Control: State, County, or Local Govt
• Clin Lab Technician/Med Lab Technician Prgm
• Dental Assisting Prgm

Inver Grove Heights

Inver Hills Community College
Cheryl Frank, PhD, President
2500 E 80th St
Inver Grove Heights, MN 55076
651 460-8641
Type: Junior or Comm Coll
Control: State, County, or Local Govt
• Emergency Med Tech-Paramedic Prgm

Mankato

Minnesota State University - Mankato
Richard Davenport, PhD, President
301 Wigley Adminstration Building
Mankato, MN 56001-8400
507 389-2463
Type: 4-year Coll or Univ
Control: State, County, or Local Govt
• Athletic Training Prgm
• Counseling Prgm
• Dental Hygiene Prgm
• Dietetics-Didactic Prgm
• Nursing Prgm
• Rehabilitation Counseling Prgm
• Speech-Language Pathology Prgm

Minneapolis

Augsburg College
William V Frame, PhD, President
2211 Riverside Ave, CB 131
Minneapolis, MN 55454
612 330-1212
Type: 4-year Coll or Univ
Control: Nonprofit (Private or Religious)
• Music Therapy Prgm
• Nursing Prgm
• Physician Assistant Prgm

Fairview Health Services
David Page, President
2450 Riverside Ave
Minneapolis, MN 55455
612 672-6000
Type: Hosp or Med Ctr: 500> Beds
Control: Nonprofit (Private or Religious)
• Clin Lab Scientist/Med Technologist Prgm

Hennepin County Medical Center
Lynn Abrahamsen, Administrator
701 Park Ave S
Minneapolis, MN 55415
612 873-2340
Type: Hosp or Med Ctr: 300-499 Beds
Control: State, County, or Local Govt
• Clin Lab Scientist/Med Technologist Prgm

Minneapolis Community & Technical Coll
Phil Davis, President
1501 Hennepin Ave S
Minneapolis, MN 55403
612 659-6300
Type: Vocational or Tech Sch
Control: State, County, or Local Govt
• Dental Assisting Prgm
• Polysomnographic Technology Prgm

Park Nicolett Orthoptic Fellowship
2001 Blasdell Ave
Minneapolis, MN 55406
952 933-8000
Type: Acad Health Ctr/Med Sch
Control: Nonprofit (Private or Religious)
• Orthoptist Prgm

University of Minnesota - Minneapolis
Robert Bruininks, PhD, President
202 Morrill Hall
100 Church St SE
Minneapolis, MN 55455
612 625-1616
Type: 4-year Coll or Univ
Control: State, County, or Local Govt
- Allopathic Medicine Prgm
- Audiologist Prgm
- Clin Lab Scientist/Med Technologist Prgm
- Dental Hygiene Prgm
- Dentistry Prgm
- Genetic Counseling Prgm
- Music Therapy Prgm
- Nursing Prgm
- Occupational Therapy Prgm
- Orthoptist Prgm
- Pharmacy Prgm
- Physical Therapy Prgm
- Psychology Prgm
- Speech-Language Pathology Prgm
- Therapeutic Recreation Specialist Prgm
- Veterinary Medicine Prgm

University of Minnesota Med Ctr - Fairview
Mark Eustis, President
Fairview Health Services
2450 Riverside Ave
Minneapolis, MN 55454
612 672-6000
Type: Hosp or Med Ctr: 300-499 Beds
Control: Nonprofit (Private or Religious)
- Dietetic Internship Prgm

Veterans Affairs Medical Center
Steven Kleinglass, FACHE, Director
One Veteran's Dr, Mail Rte 114
Minneapolis, MN 55417
612 725-2000
Type: Dept of Veterans Affairs
Control: Fed Govt
- Dietetic Internship Prgm
- Radiography Prgm

Moorhead

Concordia College - Moorhead
Paul J Dovre, President
Moorhead, MN 56562
218 299-3947
Type: 4-year Coll or Univ
Control: Nonprofit (Private or Religious)
- Dietetic Internship Prgm
- Dietetics-Didactic Prgm
- Nursing Prgm

Minnesota State Comm & Tech Coll - Moorhead
Ann Valentine, PhD, President
1900 28th Ave S
Moorhead, MN 56560
888 696-7282
Type: Vocational or Tech Sch
Control: State, County, or Local Govt
- Dental Assisting Prgm
- Dental Hygiene Prgm
- Health Information Tech Prgm
- Pharmacy Technician Prgm

Minnesota State University - Moorhead
211C Lommen Hall
Moorhead, MN 56563
Type: 4-year Coll or Univ
Control: State, County, or Local Govt
- Athletic Training Prgm
- Counseling Prgm
- Nursing Prgm
- Speech-Language Pathology Prgm

North Mankato

South Central College
Keith Stover, MA, President
1920 Lee Blvd
PO Box 1920
North Mankato, MN 56002-1920
507 389-7207
Type: Junior or Comm Coll
Control: State, County, or Local Govt
- Clin Lab Technician/Med Lab Technician Prgm
- Dental Assisting Prgm
- Emergency Med Tech-Paramedic Prgm

Northfield

Minnesota Intercollegiate Nursing Consortium
Northfield, MN 55057
Type: Acad Health Ctr/Med Sch
Control: Nonprofit (Private or Religious)
- Nursing Prgm

Richfield

Minnesota School of Business
Terry L Myhre, President
1401 W 76th St, Ste 500
Richfield, MN 55423-3846
612 861-2000
Type: Vocational or Tech Sch
Control: For Profit
- Medical Assistant Prgm (2)
- Veterinary Technology Prgm (3)

Robbinsdale

North Memorial Medical Center
David Cress, MHA, CEO President
3300 N Oakdale
Robbinsdale, MN 55422
612 520-5000
Type: Hosp or Med Ctr: 300-499 Beds
Control: Nonprofit (Private or Religious)
- Radiography Prgm

Rochester

Mayo Clinic
200 1st St SW
Rochester, MN 55905
Type: Hosp or Med Ctr: 300-499 Beds
Control: Nonprofit (Private or Religious)
- Cytogenetic Technology Prgm

Mayo School of Health Sciences
Denis A Cortese, MD, President/CEO
200 First St SW
Rochester, MN 55905
507 284-2663
Type: Acad Health Ctr/Med Sch
Control: Nonprofit (Private or Religious)
- Allopathic Medicine Prgm
- Cytotechnology Prgm
- Diagnostic Med Sonography Prgm
- Electroneurodiagnostic Tech Prgm
- Nuclear Medicine Technology Prgm
- Physical Therapy Prgm
- Radiation Therapy Prgm
- Radiography Prgm
- Respiratory Therapist (Advanced) Prgm

Rochester Community & Technical College
Donald Supalla, MS, President
851 30th Ave SE
Rochester, MN 55904-4999
507 285-7215
Type: Junior or Comm Coll
Control: State, County, or Local Govt
- Dental Assisting Prgm
- Dental Hygiene Prgm
- Emergency Med Tech-Paramedic Prgm
- Health Information Tech Prgm
- Surgical Technology Prgm
- Veterinary Technology Prgm

St Mary's Hospital
1216 2nd St SW
Rochester, MN 55902-1906
507 255-5221
Control: Nonprofit (Private or Religious)
- Dietetic Internship Prgm

Rosemount

Dakota County Technical College
Ron Thomas, PhD, College President
1300 E 145th St
Rosemount, MN 55068-2999
612 423-2200
Type: Vocational or Tech Sch
Control: State, County, or Local Govt
- Dental Assisting Prgm
- Medical Assistant Prgm

Roseville

Minneapolis Business College
David Whitman, MA, President
1711 W County Rd B
Ste 100N
Roseville, MN 55113
651 636-7406
Type: Vocational or Tech Sch
Control: For Profit
- Medical Assistant Prgm
- Veterinary Technology Prgm

Rasmussen Colleges
Kristi A Waite, President
1700 W Hwy 36, Ste 830
Roseville, MN 55133
651 636-3305
Type: Junior or Comm Coll
Control: For Profit
- Health Information Tech Prgm (2)

St Cloud

St Cloud Hospital
Craig Broman, President
1406 Sixth Ave N
St Cloud, MN 56303
320 255-5666
Type: Hosp or Med Ctr: 300-499 Beds
Control: Nonprofit (Private or Religious)
• Radiography Prgm

St Cloud State University
Earl Potter, President
720 Fourth Ave S
St Cloud, MN 56301
320 255-2240
Type: 4-year Coll or Univ
Control: State, County, or Local Govt
• Athletic Training Prgm
• Counseling Prgm
• Nursing Prgm
• Rehabilitation Counseling Prgm
• Speech-Language Pathology Prgm

St Cloud Technical College
Joyce Helens, MS, President
1540 Northway Dr
St Cloud, MN 56303
320 308-5017
Type: Vocational or Tech Sch
Control: State, County, or Local Govt
• Cardiovascular Technology Prgm
• Dental Assisting Prgm
• Dental Hygiene Prgm
• Diagnostic Med Sonography Prgm
• Emergency Med Tech-Paramedic Prgm
• Surgical Technology Prgm

St Joseph

College of St Benedict/St John's University
Colman O'Connell, President
37 S College Ave
St Joseph, MN 56374
612 363-5011
Type: 4-year Coll or Univ
Control: Nonprofit (Private or Religious)
• Dietetics-Didactic Prgm
• Nursing Prgm

St Louis Park

Methodist Hospital
David Wessner, CEO
6500 Excelsior Blvd
St Louis Park, MN 55426
612 993-3601
Type: Hosp or Med Ctr: 300-499 Beds
Control: Nonprofit (Private or Religious)
• Radiography Prgm

St Paul

Bethel University
George K Brushaber, PhD, President
3900 Bethel Dr
St Paul, MN 55112
651 638-6230
Type: 4-year Coll or Univ
Control: Nonprofit (Private or Religious)
• Athletic Training Prgm
• Nursing Prgm

College of St Catherine
Andrea J Lee, IHM, President
2004 Randolph Ave
St Paul, MN 55105-1794
651 690-6525
Type: 4-year Coll or Univ
Control: Nonprofit (Private or Religious)
• Diagnostic Med Sonography Prgm
• Dietetics-Didactic Prgm
• Health Information Tech Prgm
• Occupational Therapy Asst Prgm
• Occupational Therapy Prgm
• Phlebotomy Prgm
• Physical Therapist Assistant Prgm
• Physical Therapy Prgm
• Radiography Prgm
• Respiratory Therapist (Advanced) Prgm

Metropolitan State University
St Paul, MN 55106
Type: 4-year Coll or Univ
Control: State, County, or Local Govt
• Nursing Prgm

Regions Hospital
Brock D Nelson, President/CEO
640 Jackson St
St Paul, MN 55101
651 254-2189
Type: Hosp or Med Ctr: 300-499 Beds
Control: Nonprofit (Private or Religious)
• Ophthalmic Med Technician Prgm
• Ophthalmic Med Technologist Prgm

Saint Paul College
Donovan Schwichtenberg, PhD, President
235 Marshall Ave
St Paul, MN 55102
651 846-1364
Type: Junior or Comm Coll
Control: State, County, or Local Govt
• Clin Lab Technician/Med Lab Technician Prgm
• Respiratory Therapist (Advanced) Prgm

University of Minnesota - St Paul
1334 Eckles Ave
St Paul, MN 55108
612 624-9278
Type: 4-year Coll or Univ
Control: State, County, or Local Govt
• Dietetic Internship Prgm
• Dietetics-Didactic Prgm

St Peter

Gustavus Adolphus College
James Peterson, PhD, President
800 W College Ave
St Peter, MN 56082
507 933-7537
Type: 4-year Coll or Univ
Control: Nonprofit (Private or Religious)
• Athletic Training Prgm

Thief River Falls

Northland Community & Technical College
Anne Temte, PhD, President
1101 Hwy 1 E
Thief River Falls, MN 56721-2702
218 681-0701
Type: Junior or Comm Coll
Control: State, County, or Local Govt
• Cardiovascular Technology Prgm
• Clin Lab Technician/Med Lab Technician Prgm
• Emergency Med Tech-Paramedic Prgm
• Medical Assistant Prgm
• Occupational Therapy Asst Prgm
• Pharmacy Technician Prgm
• Radiography Prgm
• Respiratory Therapist (Advanced) Prgm
• Respiratory Therapist (Entry-Level) Prgm
• Surgical Technology Prgm

White Bear Lake

Century College
Larry Litecky, PhD, President
3300 Century Ave
White Bear Lake, MN 55110
651 779-3342
Type: Junior or Comm Coll
Control: State, County, or Local Govt
• Dental Assisting Prgm
• Dental Hygiene Prgm
• Emergency Med Tech-Paramedic Prgm
• Medical Assistant Prgm
• Orthotist/Prosthetist Prgm
• Pharmacy Technician Prgm
• Radiography Prgm

Willmar

Rice Memorial Hospital
Lawrence Massa, CEO
301 Becker Ave SW
Willmar, MN 56201
320 235-4543
Type: Hosp or Med Ctr: 100-299 Beds
Control: State, County, or Local Govt
• Radiography Prgm

Ridgewater College - Willmar Campus
Douglas Allen, President
PO Box 1097
Willmar, MN 56201-1097
320 222-5220
Type: Vocational or Tech Sch
Control: State, County, or Local Govt
• Health Information Tech Prgm
• Medical Assistant Prgm
• Veterinary Technology Prgm

Winona

St Mary's University of Minnesota
Louis DeThomasis, PhD, President
700 Terrace Heights #30
Winona, MN 55987
507 457-1503
Type: 4-year Coll or Univ
Control: Nonprofit (Private or Religious)
• Nuclear Medicine Technology Prgm
• Surgical Technology Prgm

Winona State University
Judith Ramaley, PhD, President
PO Box 5838
Winona, MN 55987-5838
507 457-5003
Type: 4-year Coll or Univ
Control: State, County, or Local Govt
• Athletic Training Prgm
• Counseling Prgm
• Nursing Prgm

Woodbury

Globe University
Terry Myhre
8089 Globe Drive
7166 10th St N
Woodbury, MN 55125
651 730-5100
Type: 4-year Coll or Univ
Control: For Profit
• Medical Assistant Prgm
• Veterinary Technology Prgm

Worthington

Minnesota West Comm & Tech College
Ron Wood, PhD, President
1450 Collegeway
Worthington, MN 56187
507 372-3400
Type: Vocational or Tech Sch
Control: State, County, or Local Govt
• Clin Lab Technician/Med Lab Technician Prgm
• Dental Assisting Prgm
• Medical Assistant Prgm

Mississippi

Booneville

Northeast Mississippi Community College
Johnny Allen, PhD, President
Cunningham Blvd
Booneville, MS 38829
601 728-7751
Type: Junior or Comm Coll
Control: State, County, or Local Govt
• Clin Lab Technician/Med Lab Technician Prgm
• Dental Hygiene Prgm
• Medical Assistant Prgm
• Radiography Prgm
• Respiratory Therapist (Advanced) Prgm

Cleveland

Delta State University
John Hilpert, PhD, President
Box A-1
Cleveland, MS 38733-0002
601 846-3000
Type: 4-year Coll or Univ
Control: State, County, or Local Govt
• Athletic Training Prgm
• Counseling Prgm
• Dietetics-Coordinated Prgm
• Nursing Prgm

Clinton

Mississippi College
Royce Lee, PhD, President
200 W College St
Clinton, MS 39058-0001
601 925-3000
Type: 4-year Coll or Univ
Control: Nonprofit (Private or Religious)
• Counseling Prgm

Columbus

Mississippi University for Women
Clyda S Rent, President
PO Box W-1340
Columbus, MS 39701
601 329-4750
Type: 4-year Coll or Univ
Control: State, County, or Local Govt
• Music Therapy Prgm
• Nursing Prgm
• Speech-Language Pathology Prgm

Decatur

East Central Community College
Phil A Suthpin, EdD, President
PO Box 129
Decatur, MS 39327
601 635-2111
Type: Junior or Comm Coll
Control: State, County, or Local Govt
• Emergency Med Tech-Paramedic Prgm
• Surgical Technology Prgm

Ellisville

Jones County Junior College
Jesse Smith, EdD, President
900 S Court St
Ellisville, MS 39437
601 477-4100
Type: Junior or Comm Coll
Control: State, County, or Local Govt
• Emergency Med Tech-Paramedic Prgm
• Pharmacy Technician Prgm
• Radiography Prgm

Fulton

Itawamba Community College
David Cole, PhD, President
602 W Hill St
Fulton, MS 38843
662 862-8001
Type: Junior or Comm Coll
Control: State, County, or Local Govt
• Diagnostic Med Sonography Prgm
• Emergency Med Tech-Paramedic Prgm
• Health Information Tech Prgm
• Occupational Therapy Asst Prgm
• Physical Therapist Assistant Prgm
• Radiography Prgm
• Respiratory Therapist (Advanced) Prgm
• Surgical Technology Prgm

Goodman

Holmes Community College
Glenn Boyce, EdD, President
Goodman Campus
PO Box 369
Goodman, MS 39079
601 472-2312
Type: Junior or Comm Coll
Control: State, County, or Local Govt
• Emergency Med Tech-Paramedic Prgm
• Occupational Therapy Asst Prgm
• Surgical Technology Prgm

Hattiesburg

University of Southern Mississippi
Martha D Saunders, PhD, President
118 College Drive, #5001
Hattiesburg, MS 39406-5001
601 266-5001
Type: 4-year Coll or Univ
Control: State, County, or Local Govt
• Athletic Training Prgm
• Audiologist Prgm
• Clin Lab Scientist/Med Technologist Prgm
• Counseling Prgm
• Dietetic Internship Prgm
• Dietetics-Didactic Prgm
• Kinesiotherapy Prgm
• Medical Librarian Prgm
• Nursing Prgm
• Psychology Prgm
• Speech-Language Pathology Prgm
• Therapeutic Recreation Specialist Prgm

William Carey College
James W Edwards, PhD, President
Tuscan Ave
Hattiesburg, MS 39401-9913
601 582-6223
Type: 4-year Coll or Univ
Control: Nonprofit (Private or Religious)
• Music Therapy Prgm

Jackson

Jackson State University
James E Lyons, Sr, President
1440 JR Lynch St
Jackson, MS 39217
601 968-2100
Type: 4-year Coll or Univ
Control: State, County, or Local Govt
• Psychology Prgm
• Rehabilitation Counseling Prgm
• Speech-Language Pathology Prgm

Mississippi Baptist Medical Center
Gerald Cotton, Exec Director
1225 N State St
Jackson, MS 39202
601 968-5130
Type: Hosp or Med Ctr: 500> Beds
Control: Nonprofit (Private or Religious)
• Clin Lab Scientist/Med Technologist Prgm

Mississippi School of Therapeutic Massage
Zercon Smith, Owner
5140 Galaxie Dr
Jackson, MS 39206
601 362-3624
Type: Acad Health Ctr/Med Sch
Control: For Profit
• Massage Therapy Prgm

St Dominic-Jackson Memorial Hospital
969 Lakeland Dr
Jackson, MS 39216-4699
601 364-6935
Control: Nonprofit (Private or Religious)
• Dietetic Internship Prgm

University of Mississippi Medical Center
Daniel W Jones, MD, Vice Chancellor
2500 N State St
Jackson, MS 39216-4505
601 984-1010
Type: Acad Health Ctr/Med Sch
Control: State, County, or Local Govt
• Clin Lab Scientist/Med Technologist Prgm
• Cytotechnology Prgm
• Dental Hygiene Prgm
• Dentistry Prgm
• Emergency Med Tech-Paramedic Prgm
• Health Information Admin Prgm
• Nuclear Medicine Technology Prgm
• Nursing Prgm
• Occupational Therapy Prgm
• Physical Therapy Prgm
• Radiography Prgm

Lorman

Alcorn State University
Rudolph E Waters, Interim President
Lorman, MS 39096
601 877-6100
Type: 4-year Coll or Univ
Control: State, County, or Local Govt
• Dietetics-Didactic Prgm

Meridian

Meridian Community College
Scott Elliott, PhD, President
910 Hwy 19 N
Meridian, MS 39307
601 484-8618
Type: Junior or Comm Coll
Control: State, County, or Local Govt
• Clin Lab Technician/Med Lab Technician Prgm
• Dental Hygiene Prgm
• Health Information Tech Prgm
• Physical Therapist Assistant Prgm
• Radiography Prgm
• Respiratory Therapist (Advanced) Prgm

Mississippi State

Mississippi State University
Donald W Zacharias, President
Mississippi State, MS 39762
601 325-2131
Type: 4-year Coll or Univ
Control: State, County, or Local Govt
• Counseling Prgm
• Dietetic Internship Prgm
• Dietetics-Didactic Prgm
• Rehabilitation Counseling Prgm
• Veterinary Medicine Prgm

Moorhead

Mississippi Delta Community College
Larry G Bailey, PhD, President
PO Box 668
Moorhead, MS 38761
601 246-6300
Type: Junior or Comm Coll
Control: State, County, or Local Govt
• Clin Lab Technician/Med Lab Technician Prgm
• Dental Hygiene Prgm
• Radiography Prgm

Perkinston

Mississippi Gulf Coast Community College
Willis H Lott, EdD, President
PO Box 609
Perkinston, MS 39573
601 928-5211
Type: Junior or Comm Coll
Control: State, County, or Local Govt
• Clin Lab Technician/Med Lab Technician Prgm
• Emergency Med Tech-Paramedic Prgm
• Radiography Prgm
• Respiratory Therapist (Advanced) Prgm
• Surgical Technology Prgm

Poplarville

Pearl River Community College
William Lewis, EdD, President
101 Hwy 11 N
Poplarville, MS 39470
601 403-1201
Type: Junior or Comm Coll
Control: State, County, or Local Govt
• Clin Lab Technician/Med Lab Technician Prgm
• Dental Assisting Prgm
• Dental Hygiene Prgm
• Occupational Therapy Asst Prgm
• Physical Therapist Assistant Prgm
• Radiography Prgm
• Respiratory Therapist (Advanced) Prgm
• Surgical Technology Prgm

Raymond

Hinds Community College
Vernon Clyde Muse, EdD, President
PO Box 1100
501 E Main St
Raymond, MS 39154-1100
601 857-3230
Type: Junior or Comm Coll
Control: State, County, or Local Govt
• Clin Lab Technician/Med Lab Technician Prgm
• Dental Assisting Prgm
• Diagnostic Med Sonography Prgm
• Health Information Tech Prgm
• Medical Assistant Prgm
• Physical Therapist Assistant Prgm
• Radiography Prgm
• Respiratory Therapist (Advanced) Prgm
• Surgical Technology Prgm
• Veterinary Technology Prgm

Senatobia

Northwest Mississippi Community College
Gary L Spears, MEd, President
4975 Hwy 51 N
Senatobia, MS 38668
601 562-3227
Type: Junior or Comm Coll
Control: State, County, or Local Govt
• Emergency Med Tech-Paramedic Prgm
• Respiratory Therapist (Advanced) Prgm
• Veterinary Technology Prgm

Tupelo

North Mississippi Medical Center
John Heer, Jr, MS, CEO
830 S Gloster
Tupelo, MS 38801
662 377-3136
Type: Hosp or Med Ctr: 500> Beds
Control: Nonprofit (Private or Religious)
• Clin Lab Scientist/Med Technologist Prgm

University

University of Mississippi
Robert C Khayat, Chancellor
University, MS 38677
601 232-7211
Type: 4-year Coll or Univ
Control: State, County, or Local Govt
• Allopathic Medicine Prgm
• Counseling Prgm
• Dietetics-Didactic Prgm
• Pharmacy Prgm
• Psychology Prgm
• Speech-Language Pathology Prgm

Wesson

Copiah-Lincoln Community College
Howell C Garner, EdD, President
PO Box 649
Wesson, MS 39191-0457
601 643-5101
Type: Junior or Comm Coll
Control: State, County, or Local Govt
• Clin Lab Technician/Med Lab Technician Prgm
• Radiography Prgm
• Respiratory Therapist (Advanced) Prgm

Missouri

Bolivar

Southwest Baptist University
Pat Taylor, President
1600 University Ave
Bolivar, MO 65613-2597
417 328-1500
Type: 4-year Coll or Univ
Control: State, County, or Local Govt
- Athletic Training Prgm
- Physical Therapy Prgm

Canton

Culver-Stockton College
William L Fox, PhD, President
1 College Hill
Canton, MO 63435
217 231-6510
Type: 4-year Coll or Univ
Control: Nonprofit (Private or Religious)
- Athletic Training Prgm

Cape Girardeau

Cape Girardeau Career & Technology Center
Richard Payne, Director CTC
Special School Administrator
1080 S Silver Springs Rd
Cape Girardeau, MO 63703
573 334-0449
Type: Vocational or Tech Sch
Control: State, County, or Local Govt
- Respiratory Therapist (Advanced) Prgm
- Respiratory Therapist (Entry-Level) Prgm

Southeast Missouri Hospital
Tonya Buttry, MSN RNC, President
College of Nursing and Health Sciences
2001 William Street
Cape Girardeau, MO 63703
573 334-6825
Type: Hosp or Med Ctr: 100-299 Beds
Control: Nonprofit (Private or Religious)
- Clin Lab Scientist/Med Technologist Prgm
- Radiography Prgm
- Surgical Technology Prgm

Southeast Missouri State University
Kenneth Dobbins, PhD, President
One University Plaza, Mail Stop 3300
Cape Girardeau, MO 63701
573 651-2222
Type: 4-year Coll or Univ
Control: State, County, or Local Govt
- Athletic Training Prgm
- Counseling Prgm
- Dietetic Internship Prgm
- Dietetics-Didactic Prgm
- Nursing Prgm
- Speech-Language Pathology Prgm

Columbia

Columbia Public Schools
James R Ritter, EdD, Superintendent of Schools
1818 W Worley
Columbia, MO 65203
573 886-2149
Type: Vocational or Tech Sch
Control: State, County, or Local Govt
- Surgical Technology Prgm

Stephens College
Wendy B Libby, PhD, President
Campus Box 2001
1200 E Broadway
Columbia, MO 65215
573 876-7210
Type: 4-year Coll or Univ
Control: Nonprofit (Private or Religious)
- Health Information Admin Prgm

University of Missouri - Columbia
Deaton Brady, PhD, Chancellor
105 Jesse Hall
Columbia, MO 65211
573 882-3387
Type: 4-year Coll or Univ
Control: State, County, or Local Govt
- Allopathic Medicine Prgm
- Diagnostic Med Sonography Prgm
- Dietetics-Coordinated Prgm
- Medical Librarian Prgm
- Nuclear Medicine Technology Prgm
- Nursing Prgm
- Occupational Therapy Prgm
- Physical Therapy Prgm
- Psychology Prgm
- Radiography Prgm
- Rehabilitation Counseling Prgm
- Respiratory Therapist (Advanced) Prgm
- Speech-Language Pathology Prgm
- Therapeutic Recreation Specialist Prgm
- Veterinary Medicine Prgm

Farmington

Mineral Area Regional Medical Center
Bob Moore, FACHE, CEO
1212 Weber Rd
Farmington, MO 63640
573 756-4581
Type: Hosp or Med Ctr: 100-299 Beds
Control: For Profit
- Radiography Prgm

Fayette

Central Methodist University
Marianne E Inman, PhD, President
411 CMC Square
Fayette, MO 65248
660 248-6221
Type: 4-year Coll or Univ
Control: Nonprofit (Private or Religious)
- Athletic Training Prgm
- Nursing Prgm

Fulton

William Woods University
Jahnae Barnett, PhD, President
One University Ave
Fulton, MO 65251
573 592-4216
Type: 4-year Coll or Univ
Control: Nonprofit (Private or Religious)
- Athletic Training Prgm

Hannibal

Hannibal Career & Technical Center
Roger McGregor, Director
4550 McMasters Ave
Hannibal, MO 63401
573 221-4430
Type: Vocational or Tech Sch
Control: State, County, or Local Govt
- Respiratory Therapist (Advanced) Prgm

Hazelwood

Sanford-Brown College - Hazelwood Campus
Chad Freeman, MA, Campus President
75 Village Sq
Hazelwood, MO 63042
314 731-5200
Type: Junior or Comm Coll
Control: For Profit
- Occupational Therapy Asst Prgm
- Surgical Technology Prgm

Hillsboro

Jefferson College
Wayne H Watts, PhD, President
1000 Viking Dr
Hillsboro, MO 63050
Type: Acad Health Ctr/Med Sch
Control: For Profit
- Veterinary Technology Prgm

Independence

Graceland University
Independence, MO 64050
Type: 4-year Coll or Univ
Control: Nonprofit (Private or Religious)
- Nursing Prgm

Jefferson City

Missouri Dept of Health & Senior Service
Office of Administration
1706 E Elm St, PO Box 687
Jefferson City, MO 65102
314 751-8145
Control: State, County, or Local Govt
- Dietetic Internship Prgm

Nichols Career Center
Bert Kimble, EdD, Superintendent
609 Union
Jefferson City, MO 65101
573 659-3012
Type: Vocational or Tech Sch
Control: State, County, or Local Govt
- Dental Assisting Prgm
- Radiography Prgm

Joplin

Franklin Tech Ctr/Missouri Southern St Univ
James Simpson, PhD, School Superintendent
1717 E 15th St
Joplin, MO 64802
417 625-5200
Type: Vocational or Tech Sch
Control: State, County, or Local Govt
• Surgical Technology Prgm

Missouri Southern State University
Terri Agee, Acting President
3950 E Newman Rd
Joplin, MO 64801-1595
417 625-9328
Type: 4-year Coll or Univ
Control: State, County, or Local Govt
• Dental Hygiene Prgm
• Radiography Prgm
• Respiratory Therapist (Advanced) Prgm
• Respiratory Therapist (Entry-Level) Prgm

St John's Regional Medical Center
Gary Rowe, MS, President
2727 McClelland Blvd
Joplin, MO 64804
417 781-2727
Type: Hosp or Med Ctr: 300-499 Beds
Control: Nonprofit (Private or Religious)
• Clin Lab Scientist/Med Technologist Prgm

Kansas City

ARAMARK Healthcare Kansas City
St Joseph Health System
1000 Carondelet Dr
Kansas City, MO 64114-4802
816 943-2146
Control: For Profit
• Dietetic Internship Prgm

Avila University
Thomas Gordon, JD LLM, President
11901 Wornall Rd
Kansas City, MO 64145
816 942-8400
Type: 4-year Coll or Univ
Control: Nonprofit (Private or Religious)
• Nursing Prgm
• Radiography Prgm

Colorado Technical University
Paul Goddard, President
520 E 19th St
Kansas City, MO 64116
816 472-7400
Type: 4-year Coll or Univ
Control: State, County, or Local Govt
• Radiography Prgm

Concorde Career College - Kansas City
Deborah Crow, MS, Campus President
3239 Broadway
Kansas City, MO 64111
816 531-5223
Control: For Profit
• Dental Assisting Prgm
• Respiratory Therapist (Advanced) Prgm
• Respiratory Therapist (Entry-Level) Prgm

Kansas City Univ of Medicine and Bioscience
1750 Independence Ave
Kansas City, MO 64106
Type: Acad Health Ctr/Med Sch
Control: Nonprofit (Private or Religious)
• Osteopathic Medicine Prgm

Maple Woods Community College
Mern Saliman, PhD, President
2601 NE Barry Rd
Kansas City, MO 64156
816 437-3044
Type: 4-year Coll or Univ
Control: State, County, or Local Govt
• Veterinary Technology Prgm

Metropolitan Community College - Penn Valley
Bernard Franklin, PhD, President
3201 SW Trafficway
Kansas City, MO 64111-2764
816 759-4201
Type: Junior or Comm Coll
Control: State, County, or Local Govt
• Dental Assisting Prgm
• Health Information Tech Prgm
• Occupational Therapy Asst Prgm
• Physical Therapist Assistant Prgm
• Radiography Prgm
• Surgical Technology Prgm

Research Medical Center
Kevin Hicks, MBA, CEO
2316 E Meyer Blvd
Kansas City, MO 64132-1199
816 276-4101
Type: Hosp or Med Ctr: 500> Beds
Control: For Profit
• Nuclear Medicine Technology Prgm
• Radiography Prgm

Rockhurst University
Thomas Curran, OSFS, President
1100 Rockhurst Rd
Kansas City, MO 64110-2561
816 501-4250
Type: 4-year Coll or Univ
Control: Nonprofit (Private or Religious)
• Occupational Therapy Prgm
• Physical Therapy Prgm
• Speech-Language Pathology Prgm

Saint Luke's Hospital
G Richard Hastings, CEO
4401 Wornall Rd
Kansas City, MO 64111
816 932-2101
Type: Hosp or Med Ctr: 500> Beds
Control: Nonprofit (Private or Religious)
• Clin Lab Scientist/Med Technologist Prgm
• Nursing Prgm
• Phlebotomy Prgm
• Radiography Prgm

University of Missouri - Kansas City
Guy Bailey, PhD, Chancellor
5115 Oak
Kansas City, MO 64110-2499
816 235-1000
Type: 4-year Coll or Univ
Control: State, County, or Local Govt
• Allopathic Medicine Prgm
• Dental Hygiene Prgm
• Dentistry Prgm
• Music Therapy Prgm
• Nursing Prgm
• Pharmacy Prgm
• Psychology Prgm

Kirksville

Kirksville College of Osteopathic Medicine
800 W Jefferson
Kirksville, MO 63501
Type: Acad Health Ctr/Med Sch
Control: Nonprofit (Private or Religious)
• Osteopathic Medicine Prgm

Truman State University
Barbara Dixon, DMA, President
200 McClain Hall
Kirksville, MO 63501
660 785-4000
Type: 4-year Coll or Univ
Control: State, County, or Local Govt
• Athletic Training Prgm
• Nursing Prgm
• Speech-Language Pathology Prgm

Liberty

William Jewell College
Liberty, MO 64068
Type: 4-year Coll or Univ
Control: Nonprofit (Private or Religious)
• Nursing Prgm

Linn

Linn State Technical College
Donald Claycomb, PhD, President
One Technology Dr
Linn, MO 65051
573 897-5000
Type: Vocational or Tech Sch
Control: State, County, or Local Govt
• Physical Therapist Assistant Prgm

Marshall

Missouri Valley College
Bonnie Humphrey, PhD, President
500 E College St
Marshall, MO 65340
660 831-4108
Type: 4-year Coll or Univ
Control: Nonprofit (Private or Religious)
• Athletic Training Prgm

Maryville

Northwest Missouri State University
Dean L Hubbard, President
Maryville, MO 64468
816 562-1212
Type: 4-year Coll or Univ
Control: State, County, or Local Govt
• Dietetics-Didactic Prgm

Neosho

Crowder College
Alan Marble, President
601 LaClede Ave
Neosho, MO 64850
417 455-5534
Type: Acad Health Ctr/Med Sch
Control: For Profit
• Veterinary Technology Prgm

North Kansas City

North Kansas City Hospital
David Carpenter, MS JD, President and CEO
2800 Clay Edwards Dr
North Kansas City, MO 64116
816 691-2000
Type: Hosp or Med Ctr: 300-499 Beds
Control: State, County, or Local Govt
• Clin Lab Scientist/Med Technologist Prgm

Sanford-Brown College
Dennis Townsend, MEd, Campus President
520 E 19th Ave
North Kansas City, MO 64116
816 472-7400
Control: For Profit
• Radiography Prgm
• Respiratory Therapist (Entry-Level) Prgm

Parkville

Park University
Beverley Byers-Pevitts, PhD, President
8700 NW Riverpark Dr
Parkville, MO 64152
816 741-2000
Type: 4-year Coll or Univ
Control: Nonprofit (Private or Religious)
• Athletic Training Prgm

Point Lookout

College of the Ozarks
Jerry C Davis, President
Point Lookout, MO 65726
417 334-6411
Type: 4-year Coll or Univ
Control: Nonprofit (Private or Religious)
• Dietetics-Didactic Prgm

Poplar Bluff

Three Rivers Community College
John Cooper, EdD, President
2080 Three Rivers Blvd
Poplar Bluff, MO 63901-2393
573 840-9698
Type: Junior or Comm Coll
Control: State, County, or Local Govt
• Clin Lab Technician/Med Lab Technician Prgm

Rolla

Rolla Technical Center
Janece Martin, PhD, Director Vocational Prgms
500 Forum Dr
Rolla, MO 65401
573 458-0160
Type: Vocational or Tech Sch
Control: State, County, or Local Govt
• Radiography Prgm
• Respiratory Therapist (Advanced) Prgm
• Surgical Technology Prgm

Sedalia

State Fair Community College
Marsha Drennon, EdD, President
3201 W 16th St
Sedalia, MO 65301
660 530-5800
Type: Junior or Comm Coll
Control: State, County, or Local Govt
• Dental Hygiene Prgm
• Radiography Prgm

Springfield

Cox College of Nursing and Health Services
Springfield, MO 65802
Control: Nonprofit (Private or Religious)
• Dietetic Internship Prgm
• Nursing Prgm

CoxHealth
Robert H Bezanson, MHA, Administrator
1423 N Jefferson St
Springfield, MO 65802
417 269-3108
Type: Hosp or Med Ctr: 500> Beds
Control: Nonprofit (Private or Religious)
• Clin Lab Scientist/Med Technologist Prgm
• Diagnostic Med Sonography Prgm
• Radiation Therapy Prgm
• Radiography Prgm

Drury University
Todd Parnel, PhD, Interim President
Burnham Hall 102
Springfield, MO 65802
417 873-7201
Type: 4-year Coll or Univ
Control: State, County, or Local Govt
• Music Therapy Prgm

Everest College - Springfield Campus
Gary Myers, MS, President
1010 W Sunshine
Springfield, MO 65807
417 864-7220
Type: Vocational or Tech Sch
Control: For Profit
• Medical Assistant Prgm

Forest Institute of Professional Psychology
Springfield, MO 65807
Type: Acad Health Ctr/Med Sch
Control: For Profit
• Psychology Prgm

Lester E Cox Medical Center South
3820 S National Ave, Ste 100
Springfield, MO 65807
Type: Acad Health Ctr/Med Sch
Control: For Profit
• Radiation Therapy Prgm

Missouri State University
Michael Nietzel, PhD, President
901 S National Ave
Springfield, MO 65897
417 836-8500
Type: 4-year Coll or Univ
Control: State, County, or Local Govt
• Athletic Training Prgm
• Audiologist Prgm
• Dietetics-Didactic Prgm
• Nursing Prgm
• Physical Therapy Prgm
• Physician Assistant Prgm
• Speech-Language Pathology Prgm
• Teacher of the Visually Impaired Prgm

Ozarks Technical Community College
Hal Higdon, PhD, President
1001 E Chestnut Expressway
Springfield, MO 65802
417 447-2602
Type: Junior or Comm Coll
Control: State, County, or Local Govt
• Dental Assisting Prgm
• Dental Hygiene Prgm
• Health Information Tech Prgm
• Occupational Therapy Asst Prgm
• Physical Therapist Assistant Prgm
• Respiratory Therapist (Advanced) Prgm
• Surgical Technology Prgm

St John's Regional Health Center
Robert Brodhead, President
1235 E Cherokee
Springfield, MO 65804
417 820-2709
Type: Hosp or Med Ctr: 500> Beds
Control: Nonprofit (Private or Religious)
• Radiography Prgm

St Charles

Lindenwood University
James Evans, President
209 S Kings Hwy
St Charles, MO 63301
636 949-4900
Type: 4-year Coll or Univ
Control: State, County, or Local Govt
• Athletic Training Prgm

St Charles School of Massage Therapy
Kathleen Crawford, LMT, Director
2440 Executive Dr
St Charles, MO 63303
636 498-0777
Type: Vocational or Tech Sch
Control: For Profit
• Massage Therapy Prgm

St Joseph

Hillyard Technical Center
Robert D Stewart, MS, Director
3434 Faragon St
St Joseph, MO 64506
816 671-4170
Type: Vocational or Tech Sch
Control: Nonprofit (Private or Religious)
• Radiography Prgm
• Surgical Technology Prgm

Missouri Western State University
James Scanlon, President
4525 Downs Dr
St Joseph, MO 64507
816 271-4237
Type: 4-year Coll or Univ
Control: State, County, or Local Govt
• Health Information Tech Prgm
• Nursing Prgm
• Physical Therapist Assistant Prgm

St Louis

Barnes-Jewish Coll of Nursing/Allied Health
Ron Evens, MD, President
306 South Kingshighway Blvd
St Louis, MO 63110
314 454-7054
Type: 4-year Coll or Univ
Control: Nonprofit (Private or Religious)
• Cytotechnology Prgm
• Nursing Prgm

DVA Medical Center
Jefferson Barracks Div
One Jefferson Barracks Dr
St Louis, MO 63125
314 894-6631
Control: Fed Govt
• Dietetic Internship Prgm

Fontbonne University
Dennis Golden, President
6800 Wydown Blvd
St Louis, MO 63105
314 862-3456
Type: 4-year Coll or Univ
Control: Nonprofit (Private or Religious)
• Dietetics-Didactic Prgm
• Speech-Language Pathology Prgm

IHM Health Studies Center
Richard S Kurz, PhD, Chairman
3663 Lindell Blvd
St Louis, MO 63108-3342
314 768-1000
Type: Hosp or Med Ctr: 500> Beds
Control: Nonprofit (Private or Religious)
• Emergency Med Tech-Paramedic Prgm

Maryville University
Mark Lombardi, PhD, President
650 Maryville University Dr
St Louis, MO 63141-7299
314 529-9300
Type: 4-year Coll or Univ
Control: Nonprofit (Private or Religious)
• Music Therapy Prgm
• Nursing Prgm
• Occupational Therapy Prgm
• Physical Therapy Prgm
• Rehabilitation Counseling Prgm

Missouri College
Michael Vander Velde, MA, President
10121 Manchester Rd
St Louis, MO 63122
314 821-7700
Type: Vocational or Tech Sch
Control: For Profit
• Dental Assisting Prgm

Saint Louis University
Joseph Weixlmann, PhD, Provost
221 N Grand Blvd #106
DuBourg Hall Rm 106
St Louis, MO 63103
314 977-3718
Type: Acad Health Ctr/Med Sch
Control: Nonprofit (Private or Religious)
• Allopathic Medicine Prgm
• Clin Lab Scientist/Med Technologist Prgm
• Dietetic Internship Prgm
• Dietetics-Didactic Prgm
• Health Information Admin Prgm
• Nuclear Medicine Technology Prgm
• Nursing Prgm
• Occupational Therapy Prgm
• Physical Therapy Prgm
• Physician Assistant Prgm
• Psychology Prgm
• Radiation Therapy Prgm
• Speech-Language Pathology Prgm

St John's Mercy Medical Center
Denny DeNarvaez, President/CEO
615 S New Ballas Rd
St Louis, MO 63141
314 251-1952
Type: Hosp or Med Ctr: 500> Beds
Control: Nonprofit (Private or Religious)
• Clin Lab Scientist/Med Technologist Prgm
• Radiography Prgm

St Louis College of Pharmacy
Wendy Duncan-Hewitt, PhD, Dean
4588 Parkview Place
St Louis, MO 63110
314 446-8341
Type: Acad Health Ctr/Med Sch
Control: For Profit
• Pharmacy Prgm

St Louis Community College
Zelema Harris, EdD, Interim Chancellor
300 S Broadway
St Louis, MO 63102-2800
314 644-9743
Type: Junior or Comm Coll
Control: State, County, or Local Govt
• Clin Lab Technician/Med Lab Technician Prgm
• Dental Assisting Prgm
• Dental Hygiene Prgm
• Diagnostic Med Sonography Prgm
• Dietetic Technician-AD Prgm
• Occupational Therapy Asst Prgm
• Physical Therapist Assistant Prgm
• Radiography Prgm
• Respiratory Therapist (Advanced) Prgm
• Surgical Technology Prgm

University of Missouri - St Louis
Blanche M Touhill, President
8001 Natural Bridge Rd
St Louis, MO 63121-4499
314 516-5000
Type: 4-year Coll or Univ
Control: State, County, or Local Govt
• Counseling Prgm
• Nursing Prgm
• Optometry Prgm
• Psychology Prgm

Washington University
Mark S Wrighton, PhD, Chancellor
Brookings Dr Campus Box 1192
St Louis, MO 63130-4899
314 935-5100
Type: Acad Health Ctr/Med Sch
Control: Nonprofit (Private or Religious)
• Allopathic Medicine Prgm
• Audiologist Prgm
• Occupational Therapy Prgm
• Physical Therapy Prgm
• Psychology Prgm

St Peters

St Charles Community College
John McGuire, PhD, President
4601 Mid Rivers Mall Dr
PO Box 76975
St Peters, MO 63376-0975
636 922-8380
Type: Junior or Comm Coll
Control: State, County, or Local Govt
• Health Information Tech Prgm
• Occupational Therapy Asst Prgm

Warrensburg

University of Central Missouri
Aaron Podolefsky, PhD, President
Warrensburg, MO 64093
816 543-4111
Type: 4-year Coll or Univ
Control: State, County, or Local Govt
• Athletic Training Prgm
• Audiologist Prgm
• Dietetics-Didactic Prgm
• Nursing Prgm
• Speech-Language Pathology Prgm

West Plains

South Central Career Center
Steve Bryant, MS EdS, Director
610 Olden
West Plains, MO 65775
417 256-6152
Type: Vocational or Tech Sch
Control: State, County, or Local Govt
• Surgical Technology Prgm

INSTITUTIONS

Montana

Billings

Montana State University - Billings
Ronald P Sexton, PhD, Chancellor
1500 University Dr
Billings, MT 59101
406 657-2300
Type: 4-year Coll or Univ
Control: State, County, or Local Govt
• Athletic Training Prgm
• Emergency Med Tech-Paramedic Prgm
• Medical Assistant Prgm
• Rehabilitation Counseling Prgm

Rocky Mountain College
Michael Mace, MBA, President
1511 Poly Dr
Billings, MT 59102
406 657-1015
Type: 4-year Coll or Univ
Control: Nonprofit (Private or Religious)
• Physician Assistant Prgm

Bozeman

Health Works Institute
Ruth Marion, Owner-Director
111 S Grand, Annex 3
Bozeman, MT 59715
406 582-1555
Type: Vocational or Tech Sch
Control: For Profit
• Massage Therapy Prgm

Montana State University
Geoffrey Gamble, President
Bozeman, MT 59717
406 994-0211
Type: 4-year Coll or Univ
Control: State, County, or Local Govt
• Counseling Prgm
• Dietetics-Didactic Prgm
• Nursing Prgm

Great Falls

Benefis Healthcare
John Goodnow, CEO
1101 26th St S
Great Falls, MT 59405
406 455-5000
Type: Hosp or Med Ctr: 300-499 Beds
Control: Nonprofit (Private or Religious)
• Radiography Prgm

Montana State Univ - Great Falls Coll of Tech
Mary Sheehy Moe, EdD, Dean
2100 16th Ave S
Great Falls, MT 59405
406 771-4310
Type: Vocational or Tech Sch
Control: State, County, or Local Govt
• Dental Assisting Prgm
• Dental Hygiene Prgm
• Health Information Tech Prgm
• Medical Assistant Prgm
• Respiratory Therapist (Advanced) Prgm
• Surgical Technology Prgm

Helena

Carroll College
Thomas J Trebon, President
1601 N Benton Ave
Helena, MT 59625
406 447-4402
Type: 4-year Coll or Univ
Control: Nonprofit (Private or Religious)
• Nursing Prgm

Kalispell

Flathead Valley Community College
Jane A Karas, PhD, President
777 Grandview Dr
Kalispell, MT 59901
406 756-3822
Type: Junior or Comm Coll
Control: State, County, or Local Govt
• Medical Assistant Prgm
• Surgical Technology Prgm

Missoula

Univ of Montana-Missoula - College of Tech
Dennis Lerum, Dean
909 S Ave W
Missoula, MT 59801
Type: 4-year Coll or Univ
Control: State, County, or Local Govt
• Pharmacy Technician Prgm

University of Montana
George Dennison, PhD, President
University Hall 109
Missoula, MT 59812
406 243-2311
Type: 4-year Coll or Univ
Control: State, County, or Local Govt
• Athletic Training Prgm
• Counseling Prgm
• Pharmacy Prgm
• Physical Therapy Prgm
• Psychology Prgm
• Respiratory Therapist (Advanced) Prgm
• Surgical Technology Prgm

Pablo

Salish Kootenai College
Joseph F McDonald, PhD, President
PO Box 70
52000 Hwy 93
Pablo, MT 59855
406 675-4800
Type: Junior or Comm Coll
Control: Nonprofit (Private or Religious)
• Dental Assisting Prgm

Nebraska

Curtis

Nebraska College of Technical Agriculture
Weldon Sleight, PhD, Dean
Curtis, NE 69025
308 367-5238
Type: Acad Health Ctr/Med Sch
Control: For Profit
• Veterinary Technology Prgm

Grand Island

Central Community College
LaVern Franzen, PhD, President
PO Box 4903
Grand Island, NE 68802-4903
308 389-6300
Type: Junior or Comm Coll
Control: State, County, or Local Govt
• Clin Lab Technician/Med Lab Technician Prgm
• Dental Assisting Prgm
• Dental Hygiene Prgm
• Health Information Tech Prgm
• Medical Assistant Prgm

Hastings

Mary Lanning Memorial Hospital
W Michael Kearney, MHA, Administrator
715 N St Joseph
Hastings, NE 68901
402 463-4521
Type: Hosp or Med Ctr: 100-299 Beds
Control: Nonprofit (Private or Religious)
• Radiography Prgm

Kearney

University of Nebraska - Kearney
Douglas Kristensen, JD, Chancellor
905 W 25th St
Founders Hall
Kearney, NE 68849
308 865-8208
Type: 4-year Coll or Univ
Control: State, County, or Local Govt
• Athletic Training Prgm
• Counseling Prgm
• Speech-Language Pathology Prgm

Lincoln

BryanLGH College of Health Sciences
Phylis Hollamon, MSN, President
5035 Everett St
Lincoln, NE 68506
402 481-3867
Type: 4-year Coll or Univ
Control: Nonprofit (Private or Religious)
• Cardiovascular Technology Prgm

Hamilton College
Thomas Lardenoit, Director
1821 K St
Lincoln, NE 68508
402 474-5315
Type: Junior or Comm Coll
Control: State, County, or Local Govt
• Medical Assistant Prgm

Nebraska Wesleyan University
Jeanie Watson, PhD, President
5000 St Paul Ave
Lincoln, NE 68504
402 466-2371
Type: 4-year Coll or Univ
Control: Nonprofit (Private or Religious)
• Athletic Training Prgm

Southeast Community College
Jack Huck, PhD, President
301 S 68th St Place
Lincoln, NE 68510
402 323-3415
Type: Junior or Comm Coll
Control: State, County, or Local Govt
• Clin Lab Technician/Med Lab Technician Prgm
• Dental Assisting Prgm
• Dietetic Technician-AD Prgm
• Medical Assistant Prgm
• Radiography Prgm
• Respiratory Therapist (Advanced) Prgm
• Surgical Technology Prgm

Union College
David Smith, EdD, President
3800 S 48th St
Lincoln, NE 68506
402 486-2500
Type: 4-year Coll or Univ
Control: Nonprofit (Private or Religious)
• Nursing Prgm
• Physician Assistant Prgm

University of Nebraska - Lincoln
Harvey Perlman, JD, Chancellor
201 ADM
Lincoln, NE 68588-0419
402 472-2116
Type: 4-year Coll or Univ
Control: State, County, or Local Govt
• Athletic Training Prgm
• Audiologist Prgm
• Dental Hygiene Prgm
• Dietetic Internship Prgm
• Dietetics-Didactic Prgm
• Psychology Prgm
• Speech-Language Pathology Prgm

Norfolk

Northeast Community College
Bill R Path
801 E Benjamin Ave
PO Box 469
Norfolk, NE 68702-0469
Type: Junior or Comm Coll
Control: State, County, or Local Govt
• Physical Therapist Assistant Prgm
• Veterinary Technology Prgm

North Platte

Mid-Plains Community College
Michael Chipps, PhD, President
601 W State Farm Rd
North Platte, NE 69101
308 535-3719
Type: Junior or Comm Coll
Control: State, County, or Local Govt
• Clin Lab Technician/Med Lab Technician Prgm
• Dental Assisting Prgm

Omaha

Alegent Health
Wayne A Sensor, FACHE, President/CEO
1010 N 96th St
Omaha, NE 68122
402 343-4410
Type: Hosp or Med Ctr: 300-499 Beds
Control: Nonprofit (Private or Religious)
• Medical Assistant Prgm
• Radiography Prgm
• Respiratory Therapist (Advanced) Prgm

Clarkson College
DeLois Weekes, EdD, President
101 S 42nd St
Omaha, NE 68131-2739
402 552-3394
Type: 4-year Coll or Univ
Control: Nonprofit (Private or Religious)
• Health Information Tech Prgm
• Physical Therapist Assistant Prgm
• Radiography Prgm

College of Saint Mary
Maryanne Stevens, RSM PhD, President
7000 Mercy Rd
Omaha, NE 68106
402 399-2435
Type: 4-year Coll or Univ
Control: Nonprofit (Private or Religious)
• Health Information Admin Prgm
• Health Information Tech Prgm
• Occupational Therapy Prgm

Creighton University
Rev John P Schlegel, SJ PhD, President
2500 California Plaza
Omaha, NE 68178-0001
402 280-2974
Type: Acad Health Ctr/Med Sch
Control: Nonprofit (Private or Religious)
• Allopathic Medicine Prgm
• Athletic Training Prgm
• Dentistry Prgm
• Emergency Med Tech-Paramedic Prgm
• Nursing Prgm
• Occupational Therapy Prgm
• Pharmacy Prgm
• Physical Therapy Prgm

Hamilton College - Omaha
Michael Ziaisky, BA, President
3350 N 90th St
Omaha, NE 68134
402 572-8500
Type: Junior or Comm Coll
Control: For Profit
• Medical Assistant Prgm

Metropolitan Community College
JoAnn McDowell, EdD, President
PO Box 3777
Omaha, NE 68103
402 457-2415
Type: Junior or Comm Coll
Control: State, County, or Local Govt
• Dental Assisting Prgm
• Respiratory Therapist (Advanced) Prgm

NE Methodist Coll Nursing & Allied Hlth
Dennis Joslin, PhD, President
Josie Harper Campus
720 N 87th St
Omaha, NE 68114
402 354-7257
Type: 4-year Coll or Univ
Control: Nonprofit (Private or Religious)
• Diagnostic Med Sonography Prgm
• Respiratory Therapist (Advanced) Prgm

Nebraska Methodist College
Dennis Joslin, PhD, President
720 N 87th St
Omaha, NE 68114-3426
402 354-7257
Type: 4-year Coll or Univ
Control: Nonprofit (Private or Religious)
• Medical Assistant Prgm
• Nursing Prgm
• Surgical Technology Prgm

Nebraska Methodist Hospital
John M Fraser, President/CEO
8303 Dodge St
Omaha, NE 68114
402 354-4531
Type: Hosp or Med Ctr: 300-499 Beds
Control: Nonprofit (Private or Religious)
• Clin Lab Scientist/Med Technologist Prgm

University of Nebraska - Omaha
Nancy Belck, PhD, Chancellor
EAB 201
Omaha, NE 68182-0108
402 554-3211
Type: 4-year Coll or Univ
Control: State, County, or Local Govt
• Allopathic Medicine Prgm
• Athletic Training Prgm
• Counseling Prgm
• Speech-Language Pathology Prgm

University of Nebraska Medical Center
Harold M Maurer, MD, Chancellor
986605 Nebraska Medical Center
Omaha, NE 68198-6605
402 559-4201
Type: Acad Health Ctr/Med Sch
Control: State, County, or Local Govt
• Clin Lab Scientist/Med Technologist Prgm
• Cytotechnology Prgm
• Dentistry Prgm
• Diagnostic Med Sonography Prgm
• Dietetic Internship Prgm
• Nuclear Medicine Technology Prgm
• Nursing Prgm
• Perfusion Prgm
• Pharmacy Prgm
• Physical Therapy Prgm
• Physician Assistant Prgm
• Radiation Therapy Prgm
• Radiography Prgm

Vatterott College - Omaha Campus
William J Stuckey, MS, President
225 N 80th St
Omaha, NE 68114-3617
402 392-1300
Type: 4-year Coll or Univ
Control: State, County, or Local Govt
• Dental Assisting Prgm
• Veterinary Technology Prgm

INSTITUTIONS

Scottsbluff

Regional West Medical Center
Todd Sorensen, MD, CEO
4021 Ave B
Scottsbluff, NE 69361
308 635-3711
Type: Hosp or Med Ctr: 100-299 Beds
Control: Nonprofit (Private or Religious)
• Radiography Prgm

Western Nebraska Community College
Eileen Ely, PhD, President
1601 E 27th St
Scottsbluff, NE 69361-1899
308 635-6101
Type: Junior or Comm Coll
Control: State, County, or Local Govt
• Health Information Tech Prgm

Nevada

Carson City

Western Nevada Community College
Carol A Lucey, PhD, President
2201 W College Pkwy
Carson City, NV 89703
775 445-4450
Type: Junior or Comm Coll
Control: State, County, or Local Govt
• Surgical Technology Prgm

Henderson

Nevada State College
Henderson, NV 89002
Type: 4-year Coll or Univ
Control: State, County, or Local Govt
• Nursing Prgm

Touro University - Nevada
Jay Sexter, CEO
874 American Pacific Dr
Henderson, NV 89014
702 777-8687
Type: Acad Health Ctr/Med Sch
Control: For Profit
• Nursing Prgm
• Occupational Therapy Prgm
• Osteopathic Medicine Prgm
• Physician Assistant Prgm

University of Southern Nevada
Harry Rosenberg, PharmD PhD, President
11 Sunset Way
Henderson, NV 89014
702 990-4433
Type: Acad Health Ctr/Med Sch
Control: Nonprofit (Private or Religious)
• Pharmacy Prgm

Las Vegas

College of Southern Nevada
Michael D Richards, PhD, Interim President
6375 W Charleston Blvd - W3D
Las Vegas, NV 89146-1139
702 651-5600
Type: Junior or Comm Coll
Control: State, County, or Local Govt
• Clin Lab Technician/Med Lab Technician Prgm
• Dental Assisting Prgm
• Dental Hygiene Prgm
• Diagnostic Med Sonography Prgm
• Emergency Med Tech-Paramedic Prgm
• Health Information Tech Prgm
• Medical Assistant Prgm
• Occupational Therapy Asst Prgm
• Ophthalmic Dispensing Optician Prgm
• Physical Therapist Assistant Prgm
• Respiratory Therapist (Advanced) Prgm
• Surgical Technology Prgm
• Veterinary Technology Prgm

Nevada Career Institute
Joanne Leming, LPN, Regional Campus Director
3025 E Desert Inn Rd, Ste A
Las Vegas, NV 89121
702 893-3300
Type: Vocational or Tech Sch
Control: For Profit
• Surgical Technology Prgm

Pima Medical Institute
Richard Luebke, Sr, President
3333 E Flamingo Rd
Las Vegas, NV 89121
Type: Acad Health Ctr/Med Sch
Control: For Profit
• Radiography Prgm
• Respiratory Therapist (Advanced) Prgm
• Veterinary Technology Prgm

Quest Diagnostics - Las Vegas
John P Schwartz, MBA, President
4230 Burnham Ave
Las Vegas, NV 89119
702 733-7866
Type: Nonhosp HC Facil, BB, or Lab
Control: For Profit
• Cytotechnology Prgm

University of Nevada - Las Vegas
David B Ashley, PhD, President
4505 Maryland Pkwy
PO Box 451001
Las Vegas, NV 89154-1001
702 895-3201
Type: 4-year Coll or Univ
Control: State, County, or Local Govt
• Athletic Training Prgm
• Clin Lab Scientist/Med Technologist Prgm
• Counseling Prgm
• Dentistry Prgm
• Dietetic Internship Prgm
• Dietetics-Didactic Prgm
• Nuclear Medicine Technology Prgm
• Physical Therapy Prgm
• Psychology Prgm
• Radiography Prgm

Reno

Truckee Meadows Community College
Delores Sanford, PhD, Interim President
7000 Dandini Blvd (R-200)
Reno, NV 89512-3999
775 673-7025
Type: Junior or Comm Coll
Control: State, County, or Local Govt
• Dental Assisting Prgm
• Dental Hygiene Prgm
• Dietetic Technician-AD Prgm
• Radiography Prgm
• Veterinary Technology Prgm

University of Nevada - Reno
Milton Glick, PhD, President
Reno, NV 89557-0046
702 784-4805
Type: 4-year Coll or Univ
Control: State, County, or Local Govt
• Allopathic Medicine Prgm
• Counseling Prgm
• Dietetic Internship Prgm
• Dietetics-Didactic Prgm
• Nursing Prgm
• Psychology Prgm
• Speech-Language Pathology Prgm

New Brunswick, Canada

Fredericton

University of New Brunswick
Fredericton, NB E3B 6E4
Type: 4-year Coll or Univ
Control: State, County, or Local Government
• Psychology Prgm

Newfoundland, Canada

St John's

Memorial University of Newfoundland
St John's, NF A1C 5S7
Type: Acad Health Ctr/Med Sch
Control: State, County, or Local Government
• Allopathic Medicine Prgm

New Hampshire

Claremont

New Hampshire Comm Tech Coll - Claremont
Cheryl Groeneveld, PhD, President
1 College Dr
Claremont, NH 03743
603 542-7744
Type: Junior or Comm Coll
Control: State, County, or Local Govt
• Clin Lab Technician/Med Lab Technician Prgm
• Medical Assistant Prgm
• Occupational Therapy Asst Prgm
• Physical Therapist Assistant Prgm
• Respiratory Therapist (Advanced) Prgm

Concord

Concord Hospital
Michael Green, BA MS, CEO
250 Pleasant St
Concord, NH 03301
603 225-2711
Type: Hosp or Med Ctr: 100-299 Beds
Control: Nonprofit (Private or Religious)
• Surgical Technology Prgm

New Hampshire Technical Institute
Lynn Kilchenstein, PhD, President
31 College Dr
Concord, NH 03301-7412
603 271-7737
Type: Junior or Comm Coll
Control: State, County, or Local Govt
• Dental Assisting Prgm
• Dental Hygiene Prgm
• Diagnostic Med Sonography Prgm
• Emergency Med Tech-Paramedic Prgm
• Radiation Therapy Prgm
• Radiography Prgm

Durham

University of New Hampshire
Bonnie Newman, PhD, Interim President
Thompson Hall
Durham, NH 03824-3547
603 862-2450
Type: 4-year Coll or Univ
Control: State, County, or Local Govt
• Athletic Training Prgm
• Clin Lab Scientist/Med Technologist Prgm
• Dietetic Internship Prgm
• Dietetic Technician-AD Prgm
• Dietetics-Didactic Prgm
• Nursing Prgm
• Occupational Therapy Prgm
• Speech-Language Pathology Prgm
• Therapeutic Recreation Specialist Prgm

Hanover

Dartmouth Medical School
Hanover, NH 03755
Type: Acad Health Ctr/Med Sch
Control: Nonprofit (Private or Religious)
• Allopathic Medicine Prgm

Hudson

New Hampshire Institute for Therapeutic Arts
Patrick Ian Cowan, PhD, Executive Director
153 Lowell Rd
Hudson, NH 03051
603 882-3022
Type: Vocational or Tech Sch
Control: For Profit
• Massage Therapy Prgm (2)

Keene

Antioch University New England
Peter Temes, PhD, President
40 Avon St
Keene, NH 03431-3516
603 357-3122
Control: Nonprofit (Private or Religious)
• Dance/Movement Therapy Prgm
• Psychology Prgm

Keene State College
Stanley J Yarosewick, PhD, President
229 Main
Keene, NH 03435
603 358-2000
Type: 4-year Coll or Univ
Control: State, County, or Local Govt
• Athletic Training Prgm
• Dietetic Internship Prgm
• Dietetics-Didactic Prgm

Lebanon

Dartmouth Hitchcock Medical Center
James W Varnum, MBA CHE, CEO
One Medical Center Dr
Lebanon, NH 03756-0001
603 650-5000
Type: Hosp or Med Ctr: 300-499 Beds
Control: Nonprofit (Private or Religious)
• Surgical Technology Prgm

Lebanon College
Donald Wenz, PhD, President, CEO
15 Hanover St
Lebanon, NH 03766
603 448-2445
Type: Junior or Comm Coll
Control: Nonprofit (Private or Religious)
• Radiography Prgm

Manchester

Hesser College
Mary Jo Greco, MAT, President
3 Sundial Ave
Manchester, NH 03103
603 668-6660
Type: Junior or Comm Coll
Control: For Profit
• Medical Assistant Prgm
• Physical Therapist Assistant Prgm

Mass College of Pharmacy & Health Sciences
1260 Elm St
Manchester, NH 03101
Type: Acad Health Ctr/Med Sch
Control: Nonprofit (Private or Religious)
• Physician Assistant Prgm

New England EMS Institute
Doug Dean, CEO
One Elliot Way
Manchester, NH 03103
603 628-2220
Type: Hosp or Med Ctr: 300-499 Beds
Control: Nonprofit (Private or Religious)
• Emergency Med Tech-Paramedic Prgm

New Hampshire Comm Tech College - Manchester
Darlene Miller, EdD, President
1066 Front St
Manchester, NH 03102
603 668-6706
Type: Junior or Comm Coll
Control: State, County, or Local Govt
• Medical Assistant Prgm

Saint Anselm College
Manchester, NH 03102
Type: 4-year Coll or Univ
Control: Nonprofit (Private or Religious)
• Nursing Prgm

New London

Colby-Sawyer College
Thomas Galligan, JD LLM, President
541 Main St
New London, NH 03257
603 526-3737
Type: 4-year Coll or Univ
Control: Nonprofit (Private or Religious)
• Athletic Training Prgm
• Nursing Prgm

Plymouth

Plymouth State University
Sara Jayne Steen, PhD, President
MSC 1
Plymouth, NH 03264
603 535-2211
Type: 4-year Coll or Univ
Control: State, County, or Local Govt
• Athletic Training Prgm

Rindge

Franklin Pierce College
George J Hagerty
20 College Rd
Rindge, NH 03461-0060
800 437-0048
Type: 4-year Coll or Univ
Control: Nonprofit (Private or Religious)
• Physical Therapy Prgm

Stratham

New Hampshire Comm Tech College - Stratham
Catherine Smith, EdD, President
277 Portsmouth Ave
Stratham, NH 03885
603 772-1194
Type: Junior or Comm Coll
Control: State, County, or Local Govt
• Surgical Technology Prgm
• Veterinary Technology Prgm

New Jersey

Blackwood

Camden County College
Raymond A Yannuzzi, PhD, President
College Dr
Blackwood, NJ 08012
856 227-7200
Type: Junior or Comm Coll
Control: State, County, or Local Govt
• Clin Lab Technician/Med Lab Technician Prgm
• Dental Assisting Prgm
• Dental Hygiene Prgm
• Dietetic Technician-AD Prgm
• Health Information Tech Prgm
• Ophthalmic Dispensing Optician Prgm
• Ophthalmic Med Technologist Prgm
• Veterinary Technology Prgm

Bloomfield

Bloomfield College
Bloomfield, NJ 07003
Type: Junior or Comm Coll
Control: Nonprofit (Private or Religious)
• Nursing Prgm

Bridgeton

Cumberland County Technical Education Center
Darlene Barber, Superintendent
601 Bridgeton Ave
Bridgeton, NJ 08302
609 451-9000
Type: Vocational or Tech Sch
Control: State, County, or Local Govt
• Dental Assisting Prgm

Bridgewater

Somerset County Technology Institute
David D'Alonzo, EdM BS, Superintendent
North Bridge St & Vogt Dr
PO Box 6350
Bridgewater, NJ 08807-0350
908 526-8900
Type: Vocational or Tech Sch
Control: State, County, or Local Govt
• Medical Assistant Prgm

Caldwell

Caldwell College
Sister Patrice Werner, OP PhD, President
9 Ryerson Ave
Caldwell, NJ 07006
973 618-3000
Type: Acad Health Ctr/Med Sch
Control: For Profit
• Art Therapy Prgm

Camden

Cooper University Hospital
Christopher Olivia, MD, President
One Cooper Plaza
Camden, NJ 08103
856 342-2000
Type: Hosp or Med Ctr: 300-499 Beds
Control: Nonprofit (Private or Religious)
• Perfusion Prgm
• Radiation Therapy Prgm
• Radiography Prgm

SUNJ Rutgers Camden and UMDNJ
Rutgers University, UM & D
UMDNJ - SHRP/401 Haddon Ave
Camden, NJ 08103-1506
Control: State, County, or Local Govt
• Nursing Prgm
• Physical Therapy Prgm

Cape May Courthouse

Cape May County Technical Institute
William Desmond, Superintendant
188 Crest Haven Rd
Cape May Courthouse, NJ 08210
609 465-2161
Type: Vocational or Tech Sch
Control: State, County, or Local Govt
• Dental Assisting Prgm

Clifton

Dover Business College
Timothy Luing, MBA, President
600 Getty Ave
Clifton, NJ 07011
973 546-0123
Type: Vocational or Tech Sch
Control: For Profit
• Medical Assistant Prgm (2)

Cranford

Union County College
Thomas H Brown, PhD, President
1033 Springfield Ave
Cranford, NJ 07016-1599
908 709-7100
Type: Junior or Comm Coll
Control: State, County, or Local Govt
• Physical Therapist Assistant Prgm

East Rutherford

Sodexho Health Care Services
405 Murray Hill Pkwy, Ste 2010
East Rutherford, NJ 07073
201 507-5600
Control: For Profit
• Dietetic Internship Prgm

Edison

Middlesex County College
Joann LaPerla-Morales, EdD, President
2600 Woodbridge Ave
PO Box 3050
Edison, NJ 08818-3050
908 906-2517
Type: Junior or Comm Coll
Control: State, County, or Local Govt
• Clin Lab Technician/Med Lab Technician Prgm
• Dental Hygiene Prgm
• Dietetic Technician-AD Prgm
• Radiography Prgm

Egg Harbor

National Massage Therapy Institute
6712 Washington Ave, Ste 302
Egg Harbor, NJ 08234
Type: Acad Health Ctr/Med Sch
Control: For Profit
• Massage Therapy Prgm (2)

Englewood

Englewood Hospital & Medical Center
Douglas Duchak, President/CEO
350 Engle St
Englewood, NJ 07631
201 894-3002
Type: Hosp or Med Ctr: 500> Beds
Control: Nonprofit (Private or Religious)
• Radiography Prgm

Ewing

College of New Jersey
Barbara Gittenstein, President
2000 Pennington Rd
Ewing, NJ 08628
609 771-1855
Type: 4-year Coll or Univ
Control: State, County, or Local Govt
• Counseling Prgm
• Nursing Prgm
• Speech-Language Pathology Prgm

Fairfield

The Institute for Health Education
7 Spielman Rd
Fairfield, NJ 07004
973 808-1110
Type: Vocational or Tech Sch
Control: For Profit
• Dental Assisting Prgm

Glassboro

Rowan University
Donald J Farish, PhD JD, President
Bole Hall
201 Mullica Hill Rd
Glassboro, NJ 08028
856 256-4100
Type: 4-year Coll or Univ
Control: State, County, or Local Govt
• Athletic Training Prgm

Hackensack

Academy of Massage Therapy
Joanna Sechuck-Tringali, NCBTMB BS, Executive
  Director
321 Main St, 2nd Fl
Hackensack, NJ 07601
888 268-7898
Type: Vocational or Tech Sch
Control: For Profit
• Massage Therapy Prgm

Iselin

Sanford-Brown Institute
Dennis Mascali, MEd, President
675 US Hwy 1
Iselin, NJ 08830
732 623-5740
Type: Vocational or Tech Sch
Control: For Profit
• Diagnostic Med Sonography Prgm
• Surgical Technology Prgm

Jersey City

Christ Hospital
Peter A Kelly, MBA, President/CEO
176 Palisade Ave
Jersey City, NJ 07306
201 795-8200
Type: Hosp or Med Ctr: 300-499 Beds
Control: Nonprofit (Private or Religious)
• Radiography Prgm

Hudson County Community College
Glen Gabert, PhD, President
70 Sip Ave
Jersey City, NJ 07306
201 360-4001
Type: Junior or Comm Coll
Control: State, County, or Local Govt
• Health Information Tech Prgm
• Medical Assistant Prgm

Saint Peter's College
Jersey City, NJ 07306
Type: 4-year Coll or Univ
Control: Nonprofit (Private or Religious)
• Nursing Prgm

Lawrenceville

Rider University
Mordechai Rozanski, President
2083 Lawrenceville Rd
Lawrenceville, NJ 08648-3099
609 896-5000
Type: 4-year Coll or Univ
Control: Nonprofit (Private or Religious)
• Counseling Prgm

Lincroft

Brookdale Community College
Peter F Burnham, PhD, President
765 Newman Springs Rd
Lincroft, NJ 07738-1522
732 224-2204
Type: Junior or Comm Coll
Control: State, County, or Local Govt
• Radiography Prgm
• Respiratory Therapist (Advanced) Prgm

Livingston

St Barnabas Medical Center
John F Bonamo, MD, Executive Director
Old Short Hill Rd
Livingston, NJ 07039
973 332-5628
Type: Hosp or Med Ctr: 500> Beds
Control: Nonprofit (Private or Religious)
• Radiation Therapy Prgm

Lodi

Felician College
Sr Theresa M Martin, MA, President
262 S Main St
Lodi, NJ 07644
973 778-1190
Type: 4-year Coll or Univ
Control: Nonprofit (Private or Religious)
• Nursing Prgm

Long Branch

Monmouth Medical Center
Frank Vozos, MD, Executive Director
300 Second Ave
Long Branch, NJ 07740
732 923-7367
Type: Hosp or Med Ctr: 500> Beds
Control: Nonprofit (Private or Religious)
• Clin Lab Scientist/Med Technologist Prgm

Mays Landing

Atlantic Cape Community College
John T May, PhD, President
5100 Black Horse Pike
Mays Landing, NJ 08330-9888
609 343-4901
Type: Junior or Comm Coll
Control: State, County, or Local Govt
• Surgical Technology Prgm

Atlantic County Institute of Technology
Philip Guenther, EdD, Superintendent
5080 Atlantic Ave
Mays Landing, NJ 08330
609 625-2249
Type: Vocational or Tech Sch
Control: State, County, or Local Govt
• Dental Assisting Prgm

Morristown

College of St Elizabeth
Jacqueline Burns, President
2 Convent Rd
Morristown, NJ 07960
201 292-6300
Type: 4-year Coll or Univ
Control: Nonprofit (Private or Religious)
• Dietetic Internship Prgm
• Dietetics-Didactic Prgm

Morristown Memorial Hospital
Joanne Conroy, MD, Exec VP, COO
100 Madison Ave
Morristown, NJ 07962-1956
973 971-5450
Type: Hosp or Med Ctr: 500> Beds
Control: Nonprofit (Private or Religious)
• Cardiovascular Technology Prgm
• Clin Lab Scientist/Med Technologist Prgm

Neptune

Jersey Shore University Medical Center
Steve Littleson, FACHE, President
1945 Corlies Ave
Neptune, NJ 07753
732 775-5500
Type: Hosp or Med Ctr: 500> Beds
Control: Nonprofit (Private or Religious)
• Clin Lab Scientist/Med Technologist Prgm

New Brunswick

Rutgers University
Francis L Lawrence, PhD, President
Old Queens
New Brunswick, NJ 08901
732 932-7454
Type: 4-year Coll or Univ
Control: State, County, or Local Govt
• Dietetics-Didactic Prgm
• Medical Librarian Prgm
• Pharmacy Prgm
• Psychology Prgm (2)

Newark

Essex County College
A Zachery Yamba, President
303 University Ave
Newark, NJ 07102
201 877-3021
Type: Hosp or Med Ctr: 100-299 Beds
Control: State, County, or Local Govt
• Ophthalmic Dispensing Optician Prgm
• Physical Therapist Assistant Prgm
• Radiography Prgm

Rutgers - SUNJ
Newark, NJ 07102
Type: Acad Health Ctr/Med Sch
Control: Nonprofit (Private or Religious)
• Nursing Prgm

Univ of Medicine & Dent of New Jersey
William F Owen, Jr, MD, President
65 Bergen St Rm 1535
Newark, NJ 07107
973 972-4400
Type: 4-year Coll or Univ
Control: State, County, or Local Govt
- Allopathic Medicine Prgm
- Cardiovascular Technology Prgm
- Clin Lab Scientist/Med Technologist Prgm
- Cytotechnology Prgm
- Dental Assisting Prgm
- Dental Hygiene Prgm
- Dentistry Prgm
- Diagnostic Med Sonography Prgm
- Dietetic Internship Prgm
- Dietetics-Coordinated Prgm
- Nuclear Medicine Technology Prgm
- Osteopathic Medicine Prgm
- Phlebotomy Prgm
- Physical Therapy Prgm
- Physician Assistant Prgm
- Rehabilitation Counseling Prgm
- Respiratory Therapist (Advanced) Prgm (2)

Newton

Sussex County Community College
Constance Mierendorf, PhD, President
One College Hill
Newton, NJ 07860
973 300-2122
Type: Junior or Comm Coll
Control: State, County, or Local Govt
- Medical Assistant Prgm
- Surgical Technology Prgm

Paramus

Bergen Community College
Jeremiah Ryan, PhD, President/CEO
400 Paramus Rd
Paramus, NJ 07652-1595
201 447-7100
Type: Junior or Comm Coll
Control: State, County, or Local Govt
- Dental Hygiene Prgm
- Diagnostic Med Sonography Prgm
- Medical Assistant Prgm
- Physical Therapist Assistant Prgm
- Radiography Prgm
- Respiratory Therapist (Advanced) Prgm
- Surgical Technology Prgm

Northern NJ Consortium
Judith Winn, PhD, President
Bergen CC
400 Paramus Rd
Paramus, NJ 07652-1595
201 447-7237
Type: Consortium
Control: Nonprofit (Private or Religious)
- Veterinary Medicine Prgm

Paterson

Passaic County Community College
Steven M Rose, EdD, President
One College Blvd
Paterson, NJ 07505-1179
201 684-6300
Type: Junior or Comm Coll
Control: State, County, or Local Govt
- Health Information Tech Prgm
- Radiography Prgm

Pemberton

Burlington County College
Robert C Messina, Jr, PhD, President
601 Pemberton Browns Mills Road
Pemberton, NJ 08068-1599
609 894-9311
Type: Junior or Comm Coll
Control: State, County, or Local Govt
- Dental Hygiene Prgm
- Health Information Tech Prgm
- Radiography Prgm

Pennsauken

Omega Institute
F Burke, Owner
7050 Rte 38 East
Pennsauken, NJ 08109
856 663-4299
Type: Acad Health Ctr/Med Sch
Control: For Profit
- Massage Therapy Prgm

Piscataway

Cortiva Institute Somerset Sch of Massage Therapy
Chris Froelich, President
180 Centennial Ave
Piscataway, NJ 08854
212 277-7729
Type: Vocational or Tech Sch
Control: For Profit
- Massage Therapy Prgm (2)

UMDNJ - Robert Wood Johnson Medical School
Piscataway, NJ 08854
Type: Acad Health Ctr/Med Sch
Control: State, County, or Local Government
- Allopathic Medicine Prgm

Plainfield

Muhlenberg Regional Medical Center
John P McGee, President
Park Ave and Randolph Rd
Plainfield, NJ 07061
732 632-1501
Type: Hosp or Med Ctr: 300-499 Beds
Control: Nonprofit (Private or Religious)
- Diagnostic Med Sonography Prgm
- Nuclear Medicine Technology Prgm
- Radiation Therapy Prgm
- Radiography Prgm

Pomona

Richard Stockton College of New Jersey
Herman J Saatkamp, Jr, PhD, President
PO Box 195
Jim Leeds Rd
Pomona, NJ 08240-0195
609 652-4521
Type: 4-year Coll or Univ
Control: State, County, or Local Govt
- Nursing Prgm
- Occupational Therapy Prgm
- Physical Therapy Prgm

Pompton Lakes

Institute for Therapeutic Massage
Lisa Helbig, LMT, Director
125 Wanaque Ave
Pompton Lakes, NJ 07442
973 839-6131
Type: Acad Health Ctr/Med Sch
Control: For Profit
- Massage Therapy Prgm (5)

Randolph

County College of Morris
Edward J Yaw, EdD, President
214 Center Grove Rd
Randolph, NJ 07869
973 328-5370
Type: Junior or Comm Coll
Control: State, County, or Local Govt
- Radiography Prgm

Ridgewood

The Valley Hospital
Audrey Meyers, MBA, President
223 N Van Dien Ave
Ridgewood, NJ 07450
201 447-8021
Type: Hosp or Med Ctr: 300-499 Beds
Control: Nonprofit (Private or Religious)
- Clin Lab Scientist/Med Technologist Prgm
- Radiography Prgm

Sewell

Gloucester County College
William F Anderson, MS, President
1400 Tanyard Rd
Sewell, NJ 08080
856 415-2196
Type: Junior or Comm Coll
Control: State, County, or Local Govt
- Diagnostic Med Sonography Prgm
- Nuclear Medicine Technology Prgm

Sicklerville

Technical Institute of Camden County
Gary Bennett, EdD, Superintendent
343 Berlin Cross Keys Rd
Berlin 343
Sicklerville, NJ 08081-9709
856 767-7000
Type: Vocational or Tech Sch
Control: State, County, or Local Govt
- Dental Assisting Prgm
- Medical Assistant Prgm

Somers Point

Shore Memorial Hospital
Al Gutierrez, CHE MBA RT(R), President
1 E New York Ave
Somers Point, NJ 08244-2387
609 653-3924
Type: Hosp or Med Ctr: 300-499 Beds
Control: Nonprofit (Private or Religious)
• Radiography Prgm

Somerville

Raritan Valley Community College
G Jeremiah Ryan, President
PO Box 3300
Somerville, NJ 08876
908 526-1200
Type: Junior or Comm Coll
Control: State, County, or Local Govt
• Ophthalmic Dispensing Optician Prgm

South Orange

Seton Hall University
Msgr Robert T Sheeran, STD, President
400 S Orange Ave
South Orange, NJ 07079-2687
973 761-9620
Type: 4-year Coll or Univ
Control: Nonprofit (Private or Religious)
• Athletic Training Prgm
• Nursing Prgm
• Occupational Therapy Prgm
• Physical Therapy Prgm
• Physician Assistant Prgm
• Speech-Language Pathology Prgm

Teaneck

Fairleigh Dickinson University
Francis J Mertz, JD, President
1000 River Rd
Teaneck, NJ 07666
973 692-9170
Type: 4-year Coll or Univ
Control: Nonprofit (Private or Religious)
• Nursing Prgm
• Psychology Prgm

Trenton

Mercer County Community College
Patricia Donohue, PhD, President
PO Box B
Trenton, NJ 08690
609 586-4800
Type: Junior or Comm Coll
Control: State, County, or Local Govt
• Clin Lab Technician/Med Lab Technician Prgm
• Physical Therapist Assistant Prgm
• Radiography Prgm

Mercer County Technical Schools
Kimberly Schneider, EdD, Superintendent
1085 Old Trenton Rd
Trenton, NJ 08690
609 586-2123
Type: Vocational or Tech Sch
Control: State, County, or Local Govt
• Medical Assistant Prgm

St Francis Medical Center
Judith Persichilli, President/CEO
601 Hamilton Ave
Trenton, NJ 08629-1986
609 599-5000
Type: Hosp or Med Ctr: 100-299 Beds
Control: Nonprofit (Private or Religious)
• Radiography Prgm

Union

Kean University
Dawood Farahi, PhD, President
1000 Morris Ave
Union, NJ 07083-0411
908 737-7000
Type: 4-year Coll or Univ
Control: State, County, or Local Govt
• Athletic Training Prgm
• Counseling Prgm
• Health Information Admin Prgm
• Occupational Therapy Prgm
• Speech-Language Pathology Prgm

Upper Montclair

Montclair State University
Susan Cole, PhD, President
Upper Montclair, NJ 07043
973 655-4000
Type: 4-year Coll or Univ
Control: State, County, or Local Govt
• Athletic Training Prgm
• Dietetic Internship Prgm
• Dietetics-Didactic Prgm
• Music Therapy Prgm
• Speech-Language Pathology Prgm

Vineland

Cumberland County College
Roland J Chapdelaine, EdD, President
College Dr PO Box 517
Vineland, NJ 08362-0517
609 691-8600
Type: Junior or Comm Coll
Control: State, County, or Local Govt
• Radiography Prgm

South Jersey Healthcare Regional Med Center
Vineland, NJ 08360
Type: Acad Health Ctr/Med Sch
Control: State, County, or Local Govt
• Dietetic Internship Prgm

Washington

Northwest NJ Consortium Resp Care Educ
Stephen Serman, Chairman Regl Oper Cncl
c/o Warren County Community College
475 Rte 57 W
Washington, NJ 07882
908 835-2314
Type: Consortium
Control: Nonprofit (Private or Religious)
• Respiratory Therapist (Advanced) Prgm

Warren County Community College
William Austin, EdD, President
475 Rte 57 W
Washington, NJ 07882-4343
908 835-9222
Type: Junior or Comm Coll
Control: State, County, or Local Govt
• Medical Assistant Prgm

Wayne

Berdan Institute
Duncan Anderson, CEO
201 Willowbrook Blvd, 2nd Fl
Wayne, NJ 07470
973 837-1818
Type: Vocational or Tech Sch
Control: For Profit
• Dental Assisting Prgm
• Medical Assistant Prgm

William Paterson Univ of New Jersey
Arnold Speert, PhD, President
300 Pompton Rd
Wayne, NJ 07470
973 720-2222
Type: 4-year Coll or Univ
Control: State, County, or Local Govt
• Athletic Training Prgm
• Counseling Prgm
• Nursing Prgm
• Speech-Language Pathology Prgm

West Long Branch

Monmouth University
West Long Branch, NJ 07764
Type: 4-year Coll or Univ
Control: Nonprofit (Private or Religious)
• Nursing Prgm

Westwood

Healing Hands Institute for Massage Therapy
Alice Feuerstein, RN LMT, President
41 Bergenline Ave, 2nd Fl
Westwood, NJ 07675
201 722-0099
Type: Vocational or Tech Sch
Control: For Profit
• Massage Therapy Prgm

Pascack Valley Hospital
Sidney Mitchell, President
Old Hook Rd
Westwood, NJ 07675
201 358-3010
Type: Hosp or Med Ctr: 100-299 Beds
Control: Nonprofit (Private or Religious)
• Radiography Prgm

INSTITUTIONS

New Mexico

Alamogordo

New Mexico State U at Alamogordo
Cheri Jimeno, PhD, Campus Executive Officer
2400 N Scenic Dr
PO Box 477
Alamogordo, NM 88310
505 439-3696
Type: Junior or Comm Coll
Control: State, County, or Local Govt
• Clin Lab Technician/Med Lab Technician Prgm

Albuquerque

Central New Mexico Community College
Kathryn Winograd, EdD, President
525 Buena Vista SE
Albuquerque, NM 87106-4096
505 224-4411
Type: Junior or Comm Coll
Control: State, County, or Local Govt
• Clin Lab Technician/Med Lab Technician Prgm
• Dental Assisting Prgm
• Diagnostic Med Sonography Prgm
• Health Information Tech Prgm
• Respiratory Therapist (Advanced) Prgm
• Surgical Technology Prgm
• Veterinary Technology Prgm

Crystal Mountain Sch of Therapeutic Massage
Linda Delker, MS LMT RMTI, Director
4775 Indian School Rd NE, Ste 102
Albuquerque, NM 87110
505 872-2030
Type: Vocational or Tech Sch
Control: For Profit
• Massage Therapy Prgm

Pima Medical Institute - Albuquerque
Richard L Luebke, Jr, BS, Executive Director
2201 San Pedro NE Blvd
Building 3, Ste 100
Albuquerque, NM 87110
505 881-1234
Type: Vocational or Tech Sch
Control: For Profit
• Radiography Prgm

Southwestern Indian Polytechnic Institute
Carolyn Elgin, President
9169 Coors NW, Box 10146
Albuquerque, NM 87184
505 897-5347
Type: Junior or Comm Coll
Control: Fed Govt
• Ophthalmic Dispensing Optician Prgm

University of New Mexico
David J Schmidly, PhD, President
President's Office
1 University of New Mexico MSC 05 3300
Albuquerque, NM 87131-0001
505 277-2626
Type: Acad Health Ctr/Med Sch
Control: State, County, or Local Govt
• Allopathic Medicine Prgm
• Athletic Training Prgm
• Clin Lab Scientist/Med Technologist Prgm
• Clin Lab Technician/Med Lab Technician Prgm
• Counseling Prgm
• Dental Assisting Prgm
• Dental Hygiene Prgm
• Dietetic Internship Prgm
• Dietetics-Didactic Prgm
• Emergency Med Tech-Paramedic Prgm
• Health Information Tech Prgm
• Nursing Prgm
• Occupational Therapy Prgm
• Pharmacy Prgm
• Physical Therapy Prgm
• Physician Assistant Prgm
• Psychology Prgm
• Speech-Language Pathology Prgm

University of St Francis
4401 Silver Ave SE, Ste B
Albuquerque, NM 87108
505 266-5565
Type: 4-year Coll or Univ
Control: State, County, or Local Govt
• Physician Assistant Prgm

Clovis

Clovis Community College
Jim Turner, Interim President
417 Schepps Blvd
Clovis, NM 88101
505 769-4000
Type: Junior or Comm Coll
Control: State, County, or Local Govt
• Radiography Prgm

Espanola

Northern New Mexico College
Jose Griego, PhD, President
921 Paseo de Onate
Espanola, NM 87532
505 747-2100
Type: 4-year Coll or Univ
Control: State, County, or Local Govt
• Radiography Prgm

Farmington

San Juan College
Carol Spencer, PhD, President
4601 College Blvd
Farmington, NM 87402
505 566-3209
Type: Junior or Comm Coll
Control: State, County, or Local Govt
• Dental Hygiene Prgm
• Health Information Tech Prgm
• Physical Therapist Assistant Prgm
• Veterinary Technology Prgm

Las Cruces

Dona Ana Community College
Margie Huerta, PhD, Campus Executive Officer
Box 30001 Dept 3DA
Las Cruces, NM 88003-0001
505 527-7510
Type: Junior or Comm Coll
Control: State, County, or Local Govt
• Dental Assisting Prgm
• Diagnostic Med Sonography Prgm
• Emergency Med Tech-Paramedic Prgm
• Radiography Prgm
• Respiratory Therapist (Advanced) Prgm

New Mexico State University
Michael Martin, PhD, President
PO Box 30001, MSC 3Z
Las Cruces, NM 88003-0001
505 646-2035
Type: 4-year Coll or Univ
Control: State, County, or Local Govt
• Athletic Training Prgm
• Counseling Prgm
• Dietetics-Didactic Prgm
• Nursing Prgm
• Speech-Language Pathology Prgm
• Teacher of the Visually Impaired Prgm

Portales

Eastern New Mexico University
Everett L Frost, President
Portales, NM 88130
505 562-1011
Type: 4-year Coll or Univ
Control: State, County, or Local Govt
• Emergency Med Tech-Paramedic Prgm
• Medical Assistant Prgm
• Occupational Therapy Asst Prgm
• Respiratory Therapist (Advanced) Prgm
• Speech-Language Pathology Prgm

Santa Fe

Santa Fe Community College
Sheila Ortego, PhD, President
6401 Richards Ave
Santa Fe, NM 87509
505 428-1000
Type: Junior or Comm Coll
Control: State, County, or Local Govt
• Dental Assisting Prgm

Southwestern College
James Nolan, President
PO Box 4788
Santa Fe, NM 87502-4788
505 471-5756
Type: 4-year Coll or Univ
Control: Nonprofit (Private or Religious)
• Art Therapy Prgm

Silver City

Western New Mexico University
John Counts, PhD, President
PO Box 680
Silver City, NM 88062-0680
505 538-6238
Type: 4-year Coll or Univ
Control: State, County, or Local Govt
• Occupational Therapy Asst Prgm

New York

Albany

Albany College of Pharmacy
James Gozzo, President
106 New Scotland Ave
Albany, NY 12208-3492
518 694-7200
Type: 4-year Coll or Univ
Control: Nonprofit (Private or Religious)
• Cytotechnology Prgm
• Pharmacy Prgm

Albany Medical College
John L Buono, MD, Dean
47 New Scotland Ave, MC139
Albany, NY 12158
518 262-3830
Type: Acad Health Ctr/Med Sch
Control: Nonprofit (Private or Religious)
• Allopathic Medicine Prgm
• Physician Assistant Prgm

Bryant & Stratton College - Albany
Michael Gutierrez, Campus Director
1259 Central Ave
Albany, NY 12205
518 437-1802
Type: Vocational or Tech Sch
Control: For Profit
• Medical Assistant Prgm

College of St Rose
Louis C Vaccaro, PhD, President
432 Western Ave
Albany, NY 12203
518 454-5111
Type: 4-year Coll or Univ
Control: Nonprofit (Private or Religious)
• Speech-Language Pathology Prgm

Maria College
Laureen Fitzgerald, RSM MA MS, President
700 New Scotland Ave
Albany, NY 12208-1798
518 438-3111
Type: Junior or Comm Coll
Control: Nonprofit (Private or Religious)
• Occupational Therapy Asst Prgm

SUNY at Albany
Karen R Hitchcock, President
1400 Washington Ave
Albany, NY 12222
518 442-3300
Type: 4-year Coll or Univ
Control: State, County, or Local Govt
• Medical Librarian Prgm
• Psychology Prgm
• Rehabilitation Counseling Prgm

Alfred

Alfred State College - SUNY
John Clark, PhD, President
10 Upper College Dr
Alfred, NY 14802
607 587-4211
Type: 4-year Coll or Univ
Control: State, County, or Local Govt
• Health Information Tech Prgm
• Veterinary Technology Prgm

Alfred University
David Szczerbacki, PhD, Provost
1 Saxon Dr
Alfred, NY 14802
607 871-2137
Type: 4-year Coll or Univ
Control: Nonprofit (Private or Religious)
• Athletic Training Prgm

Amherst

Daemen College
Martin J Anisman, PhD, President
4380 Main St
Amherst, NY 14226-3592
716 829-8210
Type: 4-year Coll or Univ
Control: Nonprofit (Private or Religious)
• Physical Therapy Prgm
• Physician Assistant Prgm

Batavia

Genesee Community College
Stuart Steiner, JD EdD, President
One College Rd
Batavia, NY 14020-9704
585 343-0055
Type: Junior or Comm Coll
Control: State, County, or Local Govt
• Occupational Therapy Asst Prgm
• Physical Therapist Assistant Prgm
• Respiratory Therapist (Advanced) Prgm

Binghamton

Binghamton University
Joyce Ferrario, PhD RN, Chief Nurse
   Administrator
PO Box 6000
Binghamton, NY 13902
Control: State, County, or Local Govt
• Nursing Prgm
• Psychology Prgm

Broome Community College
Laurence D Spraggs, DA, President
Wales Bldg, PO Box 1017
Binghamton, NY 13902
607 778-5000
Type: Junior or Comm Coll
Control: State, County, or Local Govt
• Clin Lab Technician/Med Lab Technician Prgm
• Dental Hygiene Prgm
• Health Information Tech Prgm
• Medical Assistant Prgm
• Physical Therapist Assistant Prgm
• Radiography Prgm

Ridley-Lowell Business & Technical Institute
Wilfred T Weymouth, MS, President
116 Front St
Binghamton, NY 13905
607 724-2941
Type: Vocational or Tech Sch
Control: For Profit
• Medical Assistant Prgm (2)

Brockport

SUNY Brockport
John Halstead, PhD, President
350 New Campus Dr
Brockport, NY 14420-2914
585 395-2211
Type: 4-year Coll or Univ
Control: State, County, or Local Govt
• Athletic Training Prgm
• Counseling Prgm
• Nursing Prgm

Bronx

Bronx Community College
Carolyn Williams, President
University Ave and W 181st St
Bronx, NY 10453
718 289-5151
Type: Junior or Comm Coll
Control: State, County, or Local Govt
• Nuclear Medicine Technology Prgm
• Radiography Prgm

Bronx Lebanon Hospital
Steven Anderman, MBA MS, CEO
1650 Grand Concourse
Bronx, NY 10457
718 518-5586
Type: Hosp or Med Ctr: 500> Beds
Control: Nonprofit (Private or Religious)
• Surgical Technology Prgm

CUNY Herbert H Lehman College
Ricardo R Fernandez, President
Bedford Park Blvd W
Bronx, NY 10468
718 960-8000
Type: 4-year Coll or Univ
Control: State, County, or Local Govt
• Dietetic Internship Prgm
• Dietetics-Didactic Prgm
• Nursing Prgm
• Speech-Language Pathology Prgm

Eugenio Maria De Hostos Community College
475 Grand Concourse
Bronx, NY 10451
Type: Junior or Comm Coll
Control: State, County, or Local Govt
• Dental Hygiene Prgm

Fordham University
Bronx, NY 10458
Type: 4-year Coll or Univ
Control: Nonprofit (Private or Religious)
• Psychology Prgm

Hostos Community College of CUNY
Dolores Fernandez, PhD, President
475 Grand Concourse
Bronx, NY 10451
718 518-4300
Type: Junior or Comm Coll
Control: State, County, or Local Govt
• Radiography Prgm

James J Peters VA Medical Center
130 W Kingsbridge Rd
Bronx, NY 10468-3904
718 579-1640
Control: Fed Govt
• Dietetic Internship Prgm

Bronxville

Sarah Lawrence College
Michele Myers, President
One Mead Way
Bronxville, NY 10708
914 337-0700
Type: 4-year Coll or Univ
Control: Nonprofit (Private or Religious)
• Genetic Counseling Prgm

Brooklyn

ARAMARK Healthcare
Kingsbrook Jewish Medical Ctr
585 Schenectady Ave
Brooklyn, NY 11203
718 604-5757
Control: For Profit
• Dietetic Internship Prgm

ASA Institute of Business & Computer Tech
Alex Shchegol, MS, President
81 Willoughby St
Brooklyn, NY 11201
718 522-9073
Type: Vocational or Tech Sch
Control: For Profit
• Medical Assistant Prgm

CUNY Brooklyn College
Christoph M Kimmich, President
2900 Bedford Ave
Brooklyn, NY 11210
718 951-5000
Type: 4-year Coll or Univ
Control: State, County, or Local Govt
• Dietetic Internship Prgm
• Dietetics-Didactic Prgm
• Speech-Language Pathology Prgm

Kingsborough Comm Coll/The City Univ of NY
Byron McClenney, President
2001 Oriental Blvd
Brooklyn, NY 11235-2398
718 368-5109
Type: Junior or Comm Coll
Control: State, County, or Local Govt
• Physical Therapist Assistant Prgm

Long Island College Hospital
Rita Battle, EVP/CEO
339 Hicks St
Brooklyn, NY 11201
718 780-1137
Type: Hosp or Med Ctr: 500> Beds
Control: Nonprofit (Private or Religious)
• Radiography Prgm

Long Island University
Gale Steven Hynes, JD, Provost
1 University Plaza
Rm M-315
Brooklyn, NY 11201
718 488-3438
Type: 4-year Coll or Univ
Control: Nonprofit (Private or Religious)
• Art Therapy Prgm
• Athletic Training Prgm
• Clin Lab Scientist/Med Technologist Prgm
• Counseling Prgm
• Diagnostic Med Sonography Prgm
• Dietetic Internship Prgm
• Dietetics-Didactic Prgm
• Health Information Admin Prgm
• Medical Librarian Prgm
• Nursing Prgm (2)
• Occupational Therapy Prgm
• Pharmacy Prgm
• Physical Therapy Prgm
• Physician Assistant Prgm
• Psychology Prgm (2)
• Radiography Prgm
• Respiratory Therapist (Advanced) Prgm
• Speech-Language Pathology Prgm (2)
• Surgical Technology Prgm

New York City College of Technology
Russ Hotzler, PhD, President
300 Jay St
Brooklyn, NY 11201-2983
718 260-5400
Type: 4-year Coll or Univ
Control: State, County, or Local Govt
• Dental Hygiene Prgm
• Dental Lab Technician Prgm
• Ophthalmic Dispensing Optician Prgm
• Radiography Prgm

New York Methodist Hospital
Mark J Mundy, MSHA, President
506 Sixth St
Brooklyn, NY 11215
718 780-3101
Type: Hosp or Med Ctr: 500> Beds
Control: Nonprofit (Private or Religious)
• Clin Lab Scientist/Med Technologist Prgm
• Emergency Med Tech-Paramedic Prgm
• Radiation Therapy Prgm
• Radiography Prgm

Pratt Institute
Thomas F Schutte, President
200 Willoughby Ave
Brooklyn, NY 11205
718 636-3600
Type: 4-year Coll or Univ
Control: Nonprofit (Private or Religious)
• Art Therapy Prgm
• Dance/Movement Therapy Prgm
• Medical Librarian Prgm

SUNY Downstate Medical Center
John LaRosa, MD, President
450 Clarkson Ave Box 1
Brooklyn, NY 11203-2098
718 270-2611
Type: Acad Health Ctr/Med Sch
Control: State, County, or Local Govt
• Allopathic Medicine Prgm
• Diagnostic Med Sonography Prgm
• Nursing Prgm
• Occupational Therapy Prgm
• Physical Therapy Prgm
• Physician Assistant Prgm
• Surgical Technology Prgm

Brooklyn Heights

St Francis College
Brooklyn Heights, NY 11201
Type: 4-year Coll or Univ
Control: Nonprofit (Private or Religious)
• Nursing Prgm

Buffalo

Bryant & Stratton College - Buffalo
Jeffrey P Tredo, Campus Director
465 Main St, Ste 400
Buffalo, NY 14203
716 884-9120
Type: 4-year Coll or Univ
Control: For Profit
• Medical Assistant Prgm

Buffalo State, SUNY
Muriel Howard, PhD, President
1300 Elmwood Ave
Buffalo, NY 14222
716 878-4000
Type: 4-year Coll or Univ
Control: State, County, or Local Govt
• Dietetics-Coordinated Prgm
• Dietetics-Didactic Prgm
• Speech-Language Pathology Prgm

Canisius College
Vincent M Cooke, SJ PhD, President
2001 Main St
Buffalo, NY 14208-1098
716 888-2100
Type: 4-year Coll or Univ
Control: Nonprofit (Private or Religious)
• Athletic Training Prgm

D'Youville College
Sr Denise A Roche, GNSH PhD, President
320 Porter Ave
Buffalo, NY 14201-1084
716 829-7673
Type: 4-year Coll or Univ
Control: Nonprofit (Private or Religious)
• Dietetics-Coordinated Prgm
• Nursing Prgm
• Occupational Therapy Prgm
• Physical Therapy Prgm
• Physician Assistant Prgm

Erie Community College
William D Reuter, PhD, President
121 Ellicott St
Buffalo, NY 14203
716 851-1202
Type: Junior or Comm Coll
Control: State, County, or Local Govt
• Clin Lab Technician/Med Lab Technician Prgm
• Dental Hygiene Prgm
• Dental Lab Technician Prgm
• Dietetic Technician-AD Prgm
• Health Information Tech Prgm
• Medical Assistant Prgm
• Occupational Therapy Asst Prgm
• Ophthalmic Dispensing Optician Prgm
• Radiation Therapy Prgm
• Respiratory Therapist (Advanced) Prgm

Medaille College
Richard T Jurasek, PhD, President
18 Agassiz Cr
Rm M115
Buffalo, NY 14214
716 880-2201
Type: 4-year Coll or Univ
Control: For Profit
• Veterinary Technology Prgm

SUNY Educational Opportunity Center
Sherryl Weems, PhD
465 Washington St
Buffalo, NY 14203
716 849-6725
Control: State, County, or Local Govt
• Dental Assisting Prgm

Trocaire College
Paul B Hurley, Jr, PhD, President
360 Choate Ave
Buffalo, NY 14220-2094
716 826-1200
Type: Junior or Comm Coll
Control: Nonprofit (Private or Religious)
• Health Information Tech Prgm
• Medical Assistant Prgm
• Phlebotomy Prgm
• Radiography Prgm
• Surgical Technology Prgm

University at Buffalo - SUNY
John B Simpson, PhD, President
501 Capen Hall
Buffalo, NY 14260-0001
716 645-2901
Type: 4-year Coll or Univ
Control: State, County, or Local Govt
• Athletic Training Prgm
• Audiologist Prgm
• Clin Lab Scientist/Med Technologist Prgm
• Dentistry Prgm
• Dietetic Internship Prgm
• Medical Illustrator Prgm
• Medical Librarian Prgm
• Nuclear Medicine Technology Prgm
• Nursing Prgm
• Occupational Therapy Prgm
• Orthoptist Prgm
• Pharmacy Prgm
• Physical Therapy Prgm
• Psychology Prgm
• Rehabilitation Counseling Prgm
• Speech-Language Pathology Prgm

Villa Maria College of Buffalo
Sr Marcella Marie Garus, President
240 Pine Ridge Rd
Buffalo, NY 14225-3999
716 896-0700
Type: Junior or Comm Coll
Control: Nonprofit (Private or Religious)
• Physical Therapist Assistant Prgm

Canton

SUNY at Canton
Joseph L Kennedy, PhD, President
FOB 616, 34 Cornell Dr
Canton, NY 13617-1096
315 386-7204
Type: Junior or Comm Coll
Control: State, County, or Local Govt
• Dental Hygiene Prgm
• Occupational Therapy Asst Prgm
• Physical Therapist Assistant Prgm
• Veterinary Technology Prgm

Cobleskill

SUNY at Cobleskill
Thomas Haas, PhD, President
Knapp Hall 202, SUNY Cobleskill
Cobleskill, NY 12043
518 255-5111
Type: Vocational or Tech Sch
Control: State, County, or Local Govt
• Histotechnician Prgm

Cooperstown

Bassett Healthcare Center for Rural EMS Educ
William F Streck, MD, CEO
One Atwell Dr
Cooperstown, NY 13326
607 547-3100
Type: Hosp or Med Ctr: 100-299 Beds
Control: Nonprofit (Private or Religious)
• Emergency Med Tech-Paramedic Prgm

Cortland

SUNY College at Cortland
Erik Bitterbaum, PhD, President
PO Box 2000
Cortland, NY 13045
607 753-2201
Type: 4-year Coll or Univ
Control: State, County, or Local Govt
• Athletic Training Prgm
• Therapeutic Recreation Specialist Prgm

Dansville

Nicholas H Noyes Memorial Hospital
James Wissler, CEO
111 Clara Barton St
Dansville, NY 14437
Type: Hosp or Med Ctr: 100-299 Beds
Control: Nonprofit (Private or Religious)
• Phlebotomy Prgm

Delhi

SUNY - Delhi
Candace S Vancko, PhD, President
156 Farnsworth Hall
Delhi, NY 13753
Type: Acad Health Ctr/Med Sch
Control: State, County, or Local Government
• Veterinary Technology Prgm

Dix Hills

Western Suffolk BOCES
Michael Mensch, PhD, COO
507 Deer Park Rd
Dix Hills, NY 11746
631 549-4900
Type: Vocational or Tech Sch
Control: Nonprofit (Private or Religious)
• Diagnostic Med Sonography Prgm
• Surgical Technology Prgm

Dobbs Ferry

Mercy College
Louise Feroe, PhD, President
555 Broadway
Dobbs Ferry, NY 10522
914 674-7307
Type: 4-year Coll or Univ
Control: Nonprofit (Private or Religious)
• Nursing Prgm
• Occupational Therapy Asst Prgm
• Occupational Therapy Prgm
• Physical Therapy Prgm
• Physician Assistant Prgm
• Speech-Language Pathology Prgm
• Veterinary Technology Prgm

Elmira

Arnot Ogden Medical Center
Anthony J Cooper, CHE, President/CEO
600 Roe Ave
Elmira, NY 14905-1676
607 737-4231
Type: Hosp or Med Ctr: 100-299 Beds
Control: Nonprofit (Private or Religious)
• Radiography Prgm

Elmira Business Institute
Brad C Phillips, BS, President
303 N Main St
Elmira, NY 14901
607 733-7177
Type: Vocational or Tech Sch
Control: For Profit
• Medical Assistant Prgm

Farmingdale

Farmingdale State College, SUNY
W. Hubert Keen, PhD, President
2350 Broadhollow Rd
Horton Hall
Farmingdale, NY 11735
631 420-2145
Type: 4-year Coll or Univ
Control: State, County, or Local Govt
• Clin Lab Technician/Med Lab Technician Prgm
• Dental Hygiene Prgm

INSTITUTIONS

Flushing

CUNY Queens College
James Muyskens, PhD, President
65-30 Kissena Blvd
Flushing, NY 11367
718 997-5000
Type: 4-year Coll or Univ
Control: State, County, or Local Govt
• Dietetic Internship Prgm
• Dietetics-Didactic Prgm
• Medical Librarian Prgm

Fredonia

SUNY Fredonia
Dennis L Hefner, PhD, President
Fenton Hall 138
Fredonia, NY 14063
716 673-3456
Type: 4-year Coll or Univ
Control: State, County, or Local Govt
• Music Therapy Prgm
• Speech-Language Pathology Prgm

Garden City

Adelphi University
Robert Scott, President
1 South Ave
Garden City, NY 11530
516 877-3000
Type: 4-year Coll or Univ
Control: Nonprofit (Private or Religious)
• Audiologist Prgm
• Nursing Prgm
• Psychology Prgm
• Speech-Language Pathology Prgm

Nassau Community College
Sean A Fanelli, PhD, President
One Education Dr
Garden City, NY 11530
516 572-7205
Type: Junior or Comm Coll
Control: State, County, or Local Govt
• Clin Lab Technician/Med Lab Technician Prgm
• Physical Therapist Assistant Prgm
• Radiation Therapy Prgm
• Radiography Prgm
• Respiratory Therapist (Advanced) Prgm
• Surgical Technology Prgm

Geneseo

SUNY College of Geneseo
Christopher C Dahl, Interim President
One College Circle
Geneseo, NY 14454
716 245-5211
Type: 4-year Coll or Univ
Control: State, County, or Local Govt
• Speech-Language Pathology Prgm

Glens Falls

Glens Falls Hospital
David Kruczlnicki, CEO
100 Park St
Glens Falls, NY 12801
518 792-3151
Type: Hosp or Med Ctr: 300-499 Beds
Control: Nonprofit (Private or Religious)
• Radiography Prgm

Hempstead

Hofstra University
Stuart Rabinowitz, PhD, President
West Library Wing
Hempstead, NY 11550
516 463-6800
Type: 4-year Coll or Univ
Control: Nonprofit (Private or Religious)
• Art Therapy Prgm
• Athletic Training Prgm
• Audiologist Prgm
• Physician Assistant Prgm
• Rehabilitation Counseling Prgm
• Speech-Language Pathology Prgm

Herkimer

Herkimer County Community College
Ronald F Williams, EdD, President
100 Reservoir Rd
Herkimer, NY 13350
315 866-0300
Type: Junior or Comm Coll
Control: State, County, or Local Govt
• Physical Therapist Assistant Prgm

Hornell

St James Mercy Health
Mary LeRowe, MBA, President/CEO
411 Canisteo St
Hornell, NY 14843
607 324-8110
Type: Hosp or Med Ctr: 100-299 Beds
Control: Nonprofit (Private or Religious)
• Radiography Prgm

Ithaca

Cornell University
Hunter R Rawlings, President
Ithaca, NY 14853
607 255-2000
Type: 4-year Coll or Univ
Control: Nonprofit (Private or Religious)
• Allopathic Medicine Prgm
• Dietetic Internship Prgm
• Dietetics-Didactic Prgm
• Veterinary Medicine Prgm

Ithaca College
Peggy Ryan Williams, EdD, President
953 Danby Rd
Ithaca, NY 14850-7001
607 274-3111
Type: 4-year Coll or Univ
Control: Nonprofit (Private or Religious)
• Athletic Training Prgm
• Occupational Therapy Prgm
• Physical Therapy Prgm
• Speech-Language Pathology Prgm
• Therapeutic Recreation Specialist Prgm

Jamaica

CUNY York College
Marcia Keizs, EdD, President
94-20 Guy R Brewer Blvd
Jamaica, NY 11451-9902
718 262-2350
Type: 4-year Coll or Univ
Control: State, County, or Local Govt
• Occupational Therapy Prgm
• Physician Assistant Prgm

Jamestown

Jamestown Community College
Gregory T DeCinque, PhD, President
525 Falconer St
PO Box 20
Jamestown, NY 14702-0020
716 665-5220
Type: Junior or Comm Coll
Control: State, County, or Local Govt
• Occupational Therapy Asst Prgm

Woman's Christian Association Hospital
Betsy Wright, President/CEO
PO Box 840
Jamestown, NY 14702
716 664-8110
Type: Hosp or Med Ctr: 300-499 Beds
Control: Nonprofit (Private or Religious)
• Clin Lab Scientist/Med Technologist Prgm
• Radiography Prgm

Keuka Park

Keuka College
Joseph Burke, PhD, President
Hegeman Hall
Keuka Park, NY 14478-0098
315 536-5201
Type: 4-year Coll or Univ
Control: Nonprofit (Private or Religious)
• Occupational Therapy Prgm

Long Island City

LaGuardia Community College
Gail Mellow, PhD, President
31-10 Thomson Ave
Long Island City, NY 11101-3083
718 482-5050
Type: Junior or Comm Coll
Control: State, County, or Local Govt
• Dietetic Technician-AD Prgm
• Occupational Therapy Asst Prgm
• Physical Therapist Assistant Prgm
• Veterinary Technology Prgm

Manhasset

North Shore University Hospital
Dennis Dowling, CEO
145 Community Dr
Manhasset, NY 11030
516 465-8130
Type: Hosp or Med Ctr: 500> Beds
Control: Nonprofit (Private or Religious)
• Perfusion Prgm

North Shore-Long Island Jewish Hlth System
Manhasset, NY 11030
Control: Nonprofit (Private or Religious)
• Dietetic Internship Prgm

Middletown

Orange County Community College
William Richards, PhD, President
115 South St
Middletown, NY 10940-6404
845 341-4700
Type: Junior or Comm Coll
Control: State, County, or Local Govt
• Clin Lab Technician/Med Lab Technician Prgm
• Dental Hygiene Prgm
• Occupational Therapy Asst Prgm
• Phlebotomy Prgm
• Physical Therapist Assistant Prgm
• Radiography Prgm

Mineola

Winthrop University Hospital
Daniel Walsh, President, CEO
259 First St
Mineola, NY 11501
516 663-2201
Type: Hosp or Med Ctr: 500> Beds
Control: Nonprofit (Private or Religious)
• Radiography Prgm

Morrisville

SUNY at Morrisville
Frederick W Woodward, President
Morrisville, NY 13408
315 684-6000
Type: 4-year Coll or Univ
Control: State, County, or Local Govt
• Dietetic Technician-AD Prgm

New Paltz

SUNY at New Paltz
Steven Poskanzer, JD, President
1 Hawk Drive
New Paltz, NY 12561
845 257-2121
Type: 4-year Coll or Univ
Control: State, County, or Local Govt
• Music Therapy Prgm
• Nursing Prgm
• Speech-Language Pathology Prgm

New Rochelle

College of New Rochelle
Steve Sweeny, PhD, President
29 Castle Pl
New Rochelle, NY 10805
914 632-5300
Type: 4-year Coll or Univ
Control: Nonprofit (Private or Religious)
• Art Therapy Prgm
• Nursing Prgm

New York

Bellevue Hospital Center
Lynda Curtis, MS, Exec Director
First Ave and 27th St
New York, NY 10016
212 562-4132
Type: Hosp or Med Ctr: 500> Beds
Control: State, County, or Local Govt
• Radiography Prgm

City University of New York, The City College
Gregory Williams, PhD, President
Administration Bldg A-300
138th St and Convent Ave
New York, NY 10031
212 650-7285
Type: Acad Health Ctr/Med Sch
Control: State, County, or Local Govt
• Physician Assistant Prgm
• Psychology Prgm

Columbia University
Lee C Bollinger, JD, President
Morningside Campus
411 Low Library
New York, NY 10027
212 854-9970
Type: Acad Health Ctr/Med Sch
Control: Nonprofit (Private or Religious)
• Allopathic Medicine Prgm
• Dental Assisting Prgm
• Dentistry Prgm
• Nursing Prgm
• Occupational Therapy Prgm
• Physical Therapy Prgm

Columbia University Teachers College
Susan Fuhrman, PhD, President
525 W 120th St
124 Zankel Bldg
New York, NY 10027
212 678-3000
Control: Nonprofit (Private or Religious)
• Dietetic Internship Prgm
• Psychology Prgm
• Speech-Language Pathology Prgm

CUNY Borough of Manhattan Community Coll
Antonio Perez, PhD, President
199 Chambers St
New York, NY 10007
212 346-8800
Type: Junior or Comm Coll
Control: State, County, or Local Govt
• Emergency Med Tech-Paramedic Prgm
• Health Information Tech Prgm
• Respiratory Therapist (Advanced) Prgm

CUNY Hunter College
Jennifer Raab, President
365 Fifth Ave
New York, NY 10021
212 772-4000
Type: 4-year Coll or Univ
Control: State, County, or Local Govt
• Audiologist Prgm
• Dietetic Internship Prgm
• Dietetics-Didactic Prgm
• Nursing Prgm
• Orientation and Mobility Specialist Prgm
• Physical Therapy Prgm
• Rehabilitation Counseling Prgm
• Speech-Language Pathology Prgm
• Vision Rehabilitation Therapy Prgm

Harlem Hospital Center
John Palmer, PhD, Exec Director
506 Lenox Ave
New York, NY 10037
212 939-1340
Type: Hosp or Med Ctr: 500> Beds
Control: State, County, or Local Govt
• Radiography Prgm

Institute of Allied Medical Professions
Thomas Haggerty, MS, President
405 Park Ave, Ste 501
New York, NY 10022-4405
212 758-1410
Type: Vocational or Tech Sch
Control: Nonprofit (Private or Religious)
• Nuclear Medicine Technology Prgm

Interboro Institute
Bruce R Kalisch, President
450 W 56th St
New York, NY 10019
212 399-0091
Type: Junior or Comm Coll
Control: For Profit
• Ophthalmic Dispensing Optician Prgm

Memorial Sloan-Kettering Cancer Ctr
Harold Varmus, MD, President
1275 York Ave
New York, NY 10065
212 639-6561
Type: Hosp or Med Ctr: 500> Beds
Control: Nonprofit (Private or Religious)
• Cytotechnology Prgm
• Radiation Therapy Prgm

Mt Sinai School of Medicine
K Davis, MD, President
One Gustave Levy Pl
New York, NY 10029
Type: Acad Health Ctr/Med Sch
Control: Nonprofit (Private or Religious)
• Allopathic Medicine Prgm
• Genetic Counseling Prgm

New York College of Podiatric Medicinie
Louis L Levin, President
1800 Park Ave
New York, NY 10035
212 410-8000
Type: 4-year Coll or Univ
Control: Nonprofit (Private or Religious)
• Podiatric Medicine Prgm

New York Eye & Ear Infirmary
Joseph P Corcoran, President
310 E 14th St
New York, NY 10003
212 979-4300
Type: Hosp or Med Ctr: 100-299 Beds
Control: Nonprofit (Private or Religious)
• Orthoptist Prgm

New York University
John Sexton, PhD, President
70 Washington Square S
Rm 216
New York, NY 10012-1172
212 998-2345
Type: 4-year Coll or Univ
Control: Nonprofit (Private or Religious)
• Allopathic Medicine Prgm
• Art Therapy Prgm
• Dental Hygiene Prgm
• Dentistry Prgm
• Diagnostic Med Sonography Prgm
• Dietetic Internship Prgm
• Dietetics-Didactic Prgm
• Music Therapy Prgm
• Nursing Prgm
• Occupational Therapy Prgm
• Physical Therapist Assistant Prgm
• Physical Therapy Prgm
• Psychology Prgm
• Speech-Language Pathology Prgm

New York University Medical Center
Theresa Bischoff, EVP Deputy Provost
560 First Ave
New York, NY 10016
212 263-7300
Type: 4-year Coll or Univ
Control: Nonprofit (Private or Religious)
• Surgical Technology Prgm

New York-Presbyterian Hospital
David B Skinner, MD, President/CEO
525 E 68th St
New York, NY 10021
212 746-4000
Type: Hosp or Med Ctr: 500> Beds
Control: Nonprofit (Private or Religious)
• Dietetic Internship Prgm

Pace University - Lenox Hill Hospital
David A Caputo, PhD, President
1 Pace Plaza
New York, NY 10038
212 346-1098
Type: 4-year Coll or Univ
Control: Nonprofit (Private or Religious)
• Physician Assistant Prgm

School of Visual Arts
David Rhodes, President
209 E 23rd St
New York, NY 10010
212 592-2000
Type: Vocational or Tech Sch
Control: Nonprofit (Private or Religious)
• Art Therapy Prgm

St Vincent's Hospital Manhattan SVCMC
Henry Amoroso, FACHE, President
153 W 11th St
New York, NY 10011
212 604-6023
Type: Hosp or Med Ctr: 500> Beds
Control: Nonprofit (Private or Religious)
• Clin Lab Scientist/Med Technologist Prgm
• Nuclear Medicine Technology Prgm

SUNY - State College of Optometry
David A Bowers, MBA
33 W 10th Ave
New York, NY 10036
212 938-4900
Type: Junior or Comm Coll
Control: Nonprofit (Private or Religious)
• Optometry Prgm

The New School
New York, NY 10003
Type: Acad Health Ctr/Med Sch
Control: For Profit
• Psychology Prgm

Touro College
Bernard Lander, PhD, President
Executive Offices
27-33 W 23rd St
New York, NY 10010-4202
212 463-0400
Type: 4-year Coll or Univ
Control: Nonprofit (Private or Religious)
• Occupational Therapy Asst Prgm
• Occupational Therapy Prgm (2)
• Osteopathic Medicine Prgm
• Physical Therapist Assistant Prgm
• Physical Therapy Prgm
• Physician Assistant Prgm (2)
• Speech-Language Pathology Prgm

Weill Med College/Cornell Univ Med Sch
Antonio Gotto, Jr, MD, Dean
1300 York Ave, Rm F-105
New York, NY 10021
212 746-6005
Type: Acad Health Ctr/Med Sch
Control: Nonprofit (Private or Religious)
• Physician Assistant Prgm

Wood Tobe'-Coburn School
Sandi Gruninger, President
8 E 40th St
New York, NY 10016
212 686-9040
Type: Junior or Comm Coll
Control: For Profit
• Medical Assistant Prgm

Yeshiva University
Richard M Joel, JD
500 W 185th St
New York, NY 10033
212 960-5300
Type: 4-year Coll or Univ
Control: State, County, or Local Govt
• Allopathic Medicine Prgm
• Psychology Prgm (2)

Newburgh

Mt St Mary College
Sr Ann Sakac, OP PhD, President
330 Powell Ave
Newburgh, NY 12550
914 561-0800
Type: 4-year Coll or Univ
Control: Nonprofit (Private or Religious)
• Nursing Prgm

Oceanside

Robt J Hochstim Sch Rad/S Nassau Comm Hosp
Joseph Quagliata, MA MSHA MSHyg, President and CEO
One Healthy Way
PO Box 9007
Oceanside, NY 11572
516 632-3939
Type: Hosp or Med Ctr: 300-499 Beds
Control: Nonprofit (Private or Religious)
• Radiography Prgm

Old Westbury

New York Institute of Technology
Edward Guiliano, PhD, President
Northern Blvd PO Box 8000
Old Westbury, NY 11568-8000
516 686-7650
Type: 4-year Coll or Univ
Control: Nonprofit (Private or Religious)
• Dietetics-Didactic Prgm
• Occupational Therapy Prgm
• Osteopathic Medicine Prgm
• Physical Therapy Prgm
• Physician Assistant Prgm

Oneonta

Hartwick College
Oneonta, NY 13820
Type: 4-year Coll or Univ
Control: Nonprofit (Private or Religious)
• Nursing Prgm

SUNY College at Oneonta
Alan B Donovan, President
Oneonta, NY 13820
607 436-3500
Type: 4-year Coll or Univ
Control: State, County, or Local Govt
• Dietetic Internship Prgm
• Dietetics-Didactic Prgm

Orangeburg

Dominican College
Mary Eileen O'Brien, OP PhD, President
470 Western Hwy
Orangeburg, NY 10962-1299
845 848-7801
Type: 4-year Coll or Univ
Control: Nonprofit (Private or Religious)
• Athletic Training Prgm
• Nursing Prgm
• Occupational Therapy Prgm
• Physical Therapy Prgm

Plattsburgh

Champlain Valley Phys Hospital Med Ctr
Mundy Stephens, JD, President
75 Beekman St
Plattsburgh, NY 12901
518 561-2000
Type: Hosp or Med Ctr: 300-499 Beds
Control: Nonprofit (Private or Religious)
• Radiography Prgm

Clinton Community College
Maurice Hickey, PhD, President
Lake Shore Rd Rte 9 S
136 Clinton Point Dr
Plattsburgh, NY 12901
518 562-4100
Type: Junior or Comm Coll
Control: State, County, or Local Govt
• Clin Lab Technician/Med Lab Technician Prgm

SUNY College at Plattsburgh
Horace A Judson, President
Plattsburgh, NY 12901
518 564-2000
Type: 4-year Coll or Univ
Control: State, County, or Local Govt
• Counseling Prgm
• Dietetics-Didactic Prgm
• Nursing Prgm
• Speech-Language Pathology Prgm

Pleasantville

Pace University
Pleasantville, NY 10570
Type: 4-year Coll or Univ
Control: Nonprofit (Private or Religious)
• Nursing Prgm

Port Chester

St Joseph's Medical Center
Kevin Dahill, BS, VP Operations
Port Chester, NY 10701
914 934-3000
Type: Hosp or Med Ctr: 100-299 Beds
Control: Nonprofit (Private or Religious)
• Radiography Prgm

Port Ewen

Ulster County Board of Cooperative Ed Service
Martin Ruglis, SDA, District Superintendent
PO Box 601
Rte GW
Port Ewen, NY 12466
845 331-6680
Type: Vocational or Tech Sch
Control: State, County, or Local Govt
• Surgical Technology Prgm

Potsdam

Clarkson University
Dennis G Brown, President
Potsdam, NY 13699-5557
315 268-6400
Type: 4-year Coll or Univ
Control: Nonprofit (Private or Religious)
• Physical Therapy Prgm

Poughkeepsie

Dutchess Community College
David Conklin, PhD, President
53 Pendell Rd
Poughkeepsie, NY 12601
845 431-8980
Type: Junior or Comm Coll
Control: State, County, or Local Govt
• Clin Lab Technician/Med Lab Technician Prgm
• Emergency Med Tech-Paramedic Prgm

Marist College
Dennis J Murray, PhD, President
3399 North Rd
Graystone
Poughkeepsie, NY 12601
845 575-3000
Type: 4-year Coll or Univ
Control: Nonprofit (Private or Religious)
• Athletic Training Prgm
• Clin Lab Scientist/Med Technologist Prgm

Queens

St John's University
Donald J Harrington, CM, President
8000 Utopia Pkwy
Queens, NY 11439
718 990-8421
Type: 4-year Coll or Univ
Control: Nonprofit (Private or Religious)
• Audiologist Prgm
• Clin Lab Scientist/Med Technologist Prgm
• Counseling Prgm
• Medical Librarian Prgm
• Pharmacy Prgm
• Physician Assistant Prgm
• Psychology Prgm
• Radiography Prgm
• Speech-Language Pathology Prgm

Riverdale

College of Mount St Viencent
Charles L Flynn, Jr, PhD, President
6301 Riverdale Ave
Riverdale, NY 10471
718 405-3267
Type: Acad Health Ctr/Med Sch
Control: For Profit
• Nursing Prgm

Riverhead

Peconic Bay Medical Center
Andrew J Mitchell, MBA FACHE, President
1300 Roanoke Ave
Riverhead, NY 11901
631 548-6000
Type: Hosp or Med Ctr: 100-299 Beds
Control: Nonprofit (Private or Religious)
• Radiography Prgm

Rochester

Bryant & Stratton College - Rochester
Beth Tarquino, MS Ed, Market Director
Henrietta Campus
1225 Jefferson Rd
Rochester, NY 14623-3136
716 292-5627
Type: Vocational or Tech Sch
Control: For Profit
• Medical Assistant Prgm

Monroe Community College
Thomas Flynn, MS, President
1000 E Henrietta Rd
Rochester, NY 14623
585 292-2100
Type: Junior or Comm Coll
Control: State, County, or Local Govt
• Dental Assisting Prgm
• Dental Hygiene Prgm
• Emergency Med Tech-Paramedic Prgm
• Health Information Tech Prgm
• Radiography Prgm

Nazareth College of Rochester
Daan Braveman, PhD, President
4245 East Ave
Rochester, NY 14618-2790
585 586-2525
Type: 4-year Coll or Univ
Control: Nonprofit (Private or Religious)
• Art Therapy Prgm
• Music Therapy Prgm
• Nursing Prgm
• Physical Therapy Prgm
• Speech-Language Pathology Prgm

Rochester Business Institute
Carl A Silvio, BA, President
1630 Portland Ave
Rochester, NY 14621
585 266-0430
Type: Junior or Comm Coll
Control: For Profit
• Medical Assistant Prgm

Rochester General Hospital
Mark Clements, MPHA, President and CEO
1425 Portland Ave
Rochester, NY 14621
585 922-4000
Type: Hosp or Med Ctr: 500> Beds
Control: Nonprofit (Private or Religious)
• Clin Lab Scientist/Med Technologist Prgm
• Phlebotomy Prgm

Rochester Institute of Technology
William Destler, PhD, President
One Lomb Memorial Dr
Rochester, NY 14623
585 475-2394
Type: 4-year Coll or Univ
Control: Nonprofit (Private or Religious)
• Diagnostic Med Sonography Prgm
• Dietetics-Didactic Prgm
• Physician Assistant Prgm

St John Fisher College
Rochester, NY 14618
Type: 4-year Coll or Univ
Control: Nonprofit (Private or Religious)
• Nursing Prgm

INSTITUTIONS

University of Rochester
Joel Seligman, PhD, President
Rochester, NY 14627
Type: Acad Health Ctr/Med Sch
Control: Nonprofit (Private or Religious)
- Allopathic Medicine Prgm
- Counseling Prgm
- Psychology Prgm

Rockville Centre

Mercy Medical Center
Martin Bieber, MBA CPA, President/CEO
PO Box 9024
Rockville Centre, NY 11571
516 705-2525
Type: Hosp or Med Ctr: 300-499 Beds
Control: Nonprofit (Private or Religious)
- Radiography Prgm

Molloy College
Drew Bogner, PhD, President
1000 Hempstead Ave
PO Box 5002
Rockville Centre, NY 11571-5002
516 678-5000
Type: 4-year Coll or Univ
Control: Nonprofit (Private or Religious)
- Cardiovascular Technology Prgm
- Health Information Tech Prgm
- Nuclear Medicine Technology Prgm
- Nursing Prgm
- Respiratory Therapist (Advanced) Prgm

Sanborn

Niagara County Community College
James Klyczek, PhD, President
3111 Saunders Settlement Rd
Sanborn, NY 14132
716 614-6222
Type: Junior or Comm Coll
Control: State, County, or Local Govt
- Medical Assistant Prgm
- Physical Therapist Assistant Prgm
- Radiography Prgm
- Surgical Technology Prgm

Saranac Lake

North Country Community College
Gail Rogers Rice, EdD, President
20 Winona Ave
PO Box 89
Saranac Lake, NY 12983
518 891-2915
Type: Junior or Comm Coll
Control: State, County, or Local Govt
- Radiography Prgm

Selden

Suffolk County Community College
Shirley Robinson Pippins, EdD, President
533 College Rd
Bldg NFL 37
Selden, NY 11784-2899
516 451-4112
Type: Junior or Comm Coll
Control: State, County, or Local Govt
- Dietetic Technician-AD Prgm
- Health Information Tech Prgm (2)
- Occupational Therapy Asst Prgm
- Physical Therapist Assistant Prgm
- Veterinary Technology Prgm

Staten Island

CUNY College of Staten Island
Marlene Springer, PhD, President
2800 Victory Blvd
Staten Island, NY 10314
718 982-2400
Type: 4-year Coll or Univ
Control: State, County, or Local Govt
- Physical Therapy Prgm

Wagner College/Staten Island University
Norman R Smith, EdD, President
631 Howard Ave
Staten Island, NY 10301
718 390-3131
Type: 4-year Coll or Univ
Control: Nonprofit (Private or Religious)
- Physician Assistant Prgm

Stone Ridge

SUNY Ulster
Donald C Katt, EdD, President
Cottekill Rd
Stone Ridge, NY 12484
845 687-5279
Type: Junior or Comm Coll
Control: State, County, or Local Govt
- Emergency Med Tech-Paramedic Prgm
- Veterinary Technology Prgm

Stony Brook

Stony Brook University
Shirley Strum Kenny, PhD, President
Nicolls Rd
Admin Bldg Third Fl
Stony Brook, NY 11794-0701
631 632-6255
Type: 4-year Coll or Univ
Control: State, County, or Local Govt
- Athletic Training Prgm
- Clin Lab Scientist/Med Technologist Prgm
- Cytotechnology Prgm
- Dietetic Internship Prgm
- Occupational Therapy Prgm
- Physical Therapy Prgm
- Physician Assistant Prgm
- Respiratory Therapist (Advanced) Prgm
- Surgical Technology Prgm

SUNY at Stony Brook
Shirley S Kenny, PhD, President
310 Administration Bldg
Stony Brook, NY 11794-0001
631 632-6265
Type: 4-year Coll or Univ
Control: State, County, or Local Govt
- Dentistry Prgm
- Nursing Prgm
- Psychology Prgm

University at Stony Brook
Michael Maffetone, DA, CEO
University Hospital and Medical Center
Health Sciences Center-Level 4, Rm 215
Stony Brook, NY 11794-8410
631 444-2701
Type: 4-year Coll or Univ
Control: State, County, or Local Govt
- Allopathic Medicine Prgm

Suffern

Rockland Community College
Cliff Wood, PhD, President
145 College Rd
Suffern, NY 10901-3699
845 574-4575
Type: Junior or Comm Coll
Control: State, County, or Local Govt
- Occupational Therapy Asst Prgm

Syracuse

Bryant & Stratton College - Syracuse
Michael Sattler, Campus Director
953 James St
Syracuse, NY 13203
315 472-6603
Type: Vocational or Tech Sch
Control: For Profit
- Medical Assistant Prgm

Le Moyne College
Charles Beirne, SJ PhD, President
Le Moyne Heights
Syracuse, NY 13214-1399
315 445-4120
Type: 4-year Coll or Univ
Control: Nonprofit (Private or Religious)
- Nursing Prgm
- Physician Assistant Prgm

Onondaga Community College
Deborah Sydow, PhD, President
4941 Onondaga Rd
Syracuse, NY 13215
315 498-2211
Type: Junior or Comm Coll
Control: State, County, or Local Govt
- Health Information Tech Prgm
- Physical Therapist Assistant Prgm
- Respiratory Therapist (Advanced) Prgm
- Surgical Technology Prgm

SUNY Upstate Medical University
David Smith, MD, President
750 E Adams St
Syracuse, NY 13210
315 464-4513
Type: Acad Health Ctr/Med Sch
Control: State, County, or Local Govt
• Allopathic Medicine Prgm
• Clin Lab Scientist/Med Technologist Prgm
• Cytotechnology Prgm
• Emergency Med Tech-Paramedic Prgm
• Nursing Prgm
• Perfusion Prgm
• Physical Therapy Prgm
• Radiation Therapy Prgm
• Radiography Prgm
• Respiratory Therapist (Advanced) Prgm

Syracuse University
Kenneth A Shaw, Chancellor & President
Syracuse, NY 13244
315 443-1870
Type: 4-year Coll or Univ
Control: Nonprofit (Private or Religious)
• Audiologist Prgm
• Counseling Prgm
• Dietetic Internship Prgm
• Dietetics-Coordinated Prgm
• Dietetics-Didactic Prgm
• Medical Librarian Prgm
• Psychology Prgm
• Rehabilitation Counseling Prgm
• Speech-Language Pathology Prgm

Tarrytown

Marymount College
Brigid Driscoll, President
Tarrytown, NY 10591
914 631-3200
Type: 4-year Coll or Univ
Control: Nonprofit (Private or Religious)
• Dietetics-Didactic Prgm

Troy

Hudson Valley Community College
Drew Matonak, PhD, President
80 Vandenburgh Ave
Troy, NY 12180-6096
518 629-4822
Type: Junior or Comm Coll
Control: State, County, or Local Govt
• Dental Hygiene Prgm
• Diagnostic Med Sonography Prgm
• Emergency Med Tech-Paramedic Prgm
• Respiratory Therapist (Advanced) Prgm

The Sage Colleges
Jeanne H Neff, PhD, President
45 Ferry St
Troy, NY 12180-4115
518 244-2214
Type: 4-year Coll or Univ
Control: Nonprofit (Private or Religious)
• Dietetic Internship Prgm
• Dietetics-Didactic Prgm
• Nursing Prgm
• Occupational Therapy Prgm
• Physical Therapy Prgm

Utica

Faxton - St Luke's Healthcare
Andrew E Peterson, MS, Exec Director
Champlin Ave PO Box 479
Utica, NY 13503-0479
315 798-6001
Type: Hosp or Med Ctr: 300-499 Beds
Control: Nonprofit (Private or Religious)
• Radiography Prgm

Mohawk Valley Community College
Michael I Schafer, EdD, President
Payne Hall 305
1101 Sherman Dr
Utica, NY 13501
315 792-5333
Type: Junior or Comm Coll
Control: State, County, or Local Govt
• Health Information Tech Prgm
• Respiratory Therapist (Advanced) Prgm

St Elizabeth Medical Center
Sr M Johanna Deleys, OSF, President, CEO
2209 Genesee St
Utica, NY 13501
315 798-8123
Type: Hosp or Med Ctr: 100-299 Beds
Control: Nonprofit (Private or Religious)
• Radiography Prgm

SUNY Institute of Tech - Utica/Rome
Peter Spina, PhD, President
PO Box 3050
Utica, NY 13504-3050
315 792-7400
Type: 4-year Coll or Univ
Control: State, County, or Local Govt
• Health Information Admin Prgm
• Nursing Prgm

Utica College
Todd S Hutton, PhD, President
1600 Burrstone Rd
Utica, NY 13502-4892
315 792-3222
Type: 4-year Coll or Univ
Control: Nonprofit (Private or Religious)
• Occupational Therapy Prgm
• Physical Therapy Prgm

Valhalla

New York Medical College
Harry C Barrett, DMin MPH, President, CEO
Sunshine Administration Building
Valhalla, NY 10595
914 993-4000
Type: 4-year Coll or Univ
Control: Nonprofit (Private or Religious)
• Allopathic Medicine Prgm
• Physical Therapy Prgm
• Speech-Language Pathology Prgm

Westchester Community College
Joseph N Hankin, EdD, President
75 Grasslands Rd
Valhalla, NY 10595
914 606-6706
Type: Junior or Comm Coll
Control: State, County, or Local Govt
• Dietetic Technician-AD Prgm
• Radiography Prgm
• Respiratory Therapist (Advanced) Prgm

Yonkers

St John's Riverside Hospital
James Foy, President
967 N Broadway
Yonkers, NY 10701
914 964-4444
Type: Acad Health Ctr/Med Sch
Control: Nonprofit (Private or Religious)
• Cytotechnology Prgm

New Zealand

Palmerston North

Massey University
Steven La Grow, MA EdD COMS, Professor, Head of School
School of Health Sciences
Private Bag 11222
Palmerston North, NZ
646 350-5799
Type: 4-year Coll or Univ
Control: State, County, or Local Govt
• Orientation and Mobility Specialist Prgm

North Carolina

Albemarle

Stanly Community College
Michael R Taylor, EdD, President
141 College Dr
Albemarle, NC 28001-9402
704 982-0121
Type: Junior or Comm Coll
Control: State, County, or Local Govt
• Medical Assistant Prgm
• Respiratory Therapist (Advanced) Prgm

Asheville

Asheville-Buncombe Technical Comm College
K Ray Bailey, MEd, President
340 Victoria Rd
Asheville, NC 28801
828 254-1921
Type: Junior or Comm Coll
Control: State, County, or Local Govt
• Clin Lab Technician/Med Lab Technician Prgm
• Dental Assisting Prgm
• Dental Hygiene Prgm
• Diagnostic Med Sonography Prgm
• Phlebotomy Prgm
• Radiography Prgm
• Surgical Technology Prgm
• Veterinary Technology Prgm

South College - Asheville
Robert Davis, MSL, Executive Director
1567 Patton Ave
Asheville, NC 28806
828 252-2486
Type: 4-year Coll or Univ
Control: For Profit
• Medical Assistant Prgm
• Surgical Technology Prgm

INSTITUTIONS

Banner Elk

Lees-McRae College
David Bushman, PhD, President
PO Box 128
191 Main St
Banner Elk, NC 28604
828 898-8785
Type: 4-year Coll or Univ
Control: Nonprofit (Private or Religious)
• Athletic Training Prgm
• Nursing Prgm

Boiling Springs

Gardner-Webb University
Frank R Campbell, PhD, President
Boiling Springs, NC 28017
Type: 4-year Coll or Univ
Control: State, County, or Local Govt
• Athletic Training Prgm

Boone

Appalachian State University
Kenneth Peacock, PhD, Chancellor
Boone, NC 28608
828 262-2040
Type: 4-year Coll or Univ
Control: State, County, or Local Govt
• Athletic Training Prgm
• Counseling Prgm
• Dietetic Internship Prgm
• Dietetics-Didactic Prgm
• Music Therapy Prgm
• Speech-Language Pathology Prgm

Buies Creek

Campbell University
Jerry M Wallace, PhD, President
PO Box 127
143 Main St
Buies Creek, NC 27506
910 893-1205
Type: 4-year Coll or Univ
Control: Nonprofit (Private or Religious)
• Athletic Training Prgm
• Pharmacy Prgm

Chapel Hill

University of North Carolina
Erskine B Bowles, PhD, President
PO Box 2688
Chapel Hill, NC 27515
919 962-1000
Type: 4-year Coll or Univ
Control: State, County, or Local Govt
• Athletic Training Prgm (4)
• Audiologist Prgm
• Clin Lab Scientist/Med Technologist Prgm
• Counseling Prgm (2)
• Cytotechnology Prgm
• Dental Assisting Prgm
• Dental Hygiene Prgm
• Dietetic Internship Prgm
• Dietetics-Coordinated Prgm
• Dietetics-Didactic Prgm (2)
• Genetic Counseling Prgm
• Medical Librarian Prgm (2)
• Nursing Prgm (3)
• Occupational Therapy Prgm
• Physical Therapy Prgm
• Psychology Prgm (2)
• Radiography Prgm
• Rehabilitation Counseling Prgm
• Speech-Language Pathology Prgm (2)
• Therapeutic Recreation Specialist Prgm (2)

University of North Carolina Hospitals
Todd Peterson, MBA, President
101 Manning Dr
Chapel Hill, NC 27514
919 966-5111
Type: Hosp or Med Ctr: 500> Beds
Control: State, County, or Local Govt
• Allopathic Medicine Prgm
• Dentistry Prgm
• Medical Dosimetry Prgm
• Nuclear Medicine Technology Prgm
• Pharmacy Prgm

Charlotte

Carolinas College of Health Sciences
Ellen Sheppard, MA, President
1200 Blythe Rd
PO Box 32861
Charlotte, NC 28232-2861
704 355-5316
Type: Acad Health Ctr/Med Sch
Control: Nonprofit (Private or Religious)
• Clin Lab Scientist/Med Technologist Prgm
• Phlebotomy Prgm
• Radiography Prgm
• Surgical Technology Prgm

Central Piedmont Community College
P Anthony Zeiss, EdD, President
PO Box 35009
Charlotte, NC 28235
704 330-6566
Type: Junior or Comm Coll
Control: State, County, or Local Govt
• Clin Lab Technician/Med Lab Technician Prgm
• Cytotechnology Prgm
• Dental Assisting Prgm
• Dental Hygiene Prgm
• Health Information Tech Prgm
• Medical Assistant Prgm
• Physical Therapist Assistant Prgm
• Respiratory Therapist (Advanced) Prgm
• Surgical Technology Prgm

King's College
Barbara Rockecharlie, MBA, Director
322 Lamar Ave
Charlotte, NC 28204
704 688-3613
Type: Vocational or Tech Sch
Control: For Profit
• Medical Assistant Prgm

Presbyterian Healthcare
Carl Armato, President/CEO
200 Hawthorne Ln
PO Box 33549
Charlotte, NC 28204
704 384-4942
Type: Hosp or Med Ctr: 500> Beds
Control: Nonprofit (Private or Religious)
• Radiography Prgm

Queens University of Charlotte
Pamela Lewis Davies, EdD, President
1900 Selwyn Ave
Charlotte, NC 28274-0001
704 337-2200
Type: 4-year Coll or Univ
Control: Nonprofit (Private or Religious)
• Music Therapy Prgm
• Nursing Prgm

Univ of North Carolina at Charlotte
Phil Dubois, PhD, Chancellor
9201 University Blvd
Charlotte, NC 28223-0001
704 687-2000
Type: 4-year Coll or Univ
Control: State, County, or Local Govt
• Athletic Training Prgm
• Counseling Prgm
• Nursing Prgm

Clyde

Haywood Community College
Nathan Hodges, EdD, President
Freedlander Dr
Clyde, NC 28721-9454
704 627-4515
Type: Junior or Comm Coll
Control: State, County, or Local Govt
• Medical Assistant Prgm

Concord

Cabarrus College of Health Sciences
Anita A Brown, RN MEd, Chancellor
401 Medical Park Dr
Concord, NC 28025
704 783-1558
Type: Junior or Comm Coll
Control: Nonprofit (Private or Religious)
• Medical Assistant Prgm
• Nursing Prgm
• Occupational Therapy Asst Prgm
• Surgical Technology Prgm

Cullowhee

Western Carolina University
John W Bardo, PhD, Chancellor
HF Robinson Admin Bldg
Cullowhee, NC 28723
704 227-7100
Type: 4-year Coll or Univ
Control: State, County, or Local Govt
• Athletic Training Prgm
• Clin Lab Scientist/Med Technologist Prgm
• Counseling Prgm
• Dietetic Internship Prgm
• Dietetics-Didactic Prgm
• Emergency Med Tech-Paramedic Prgm
• Health Information Admin Prgm
• Nursing Prgm
• Physical Therapy Prgm
• Speech-Language Pathology Prgm

Dallas

Gaston College
Patricia A Skinner, PhD, President
201 Hwy 321 S
Dallas, NC 28034-1499
704 922-6475
Type: Junior or Comm Coll
Control: State, County, or Local Govt
• Dietetic Technician-AD Prgm
• Medical Assistant Prgm
• Veterinary Technology Prgm

Dobson

Surry Community College
G Frank Sells, EdD, President
630 S Main St
Dobson, NC 27017-8432
336 386-3213
Type: Junior or Comm Coll
Control: State, County, or Local Govt
• Medical Assistant Prgm

Durham

Duke University
Richard H Brodhead, PhD, President
1202 Spring Garden St
Durham, NC 27708
Type: 4-year Coll or Univ
Control: State, County, or Local Govt
• Nursing Prgm
• Psychology Prgm

Duke University Medical Center
Victor Dzau, MD, Chancellor
Health Affairs
PO Box 3701 M106A Davison Bldg
Durham, NC 27710
919 684-2255
Type: Acad Health Ctr/Med Sch
Control: Nonprofit (Private or Religious)
• Allopathic Medicine Prgm
• Ophthalmic Med Technician Prgm
• Pathologists' Assistant Prgm
• Physical Therapy Prgm
• Physician Assistant Prgm

Durham Technical Community College
Phail Wynn, Jr, EdD MBA, President
1637 Lawson St
Durham, NC 27703-5023
919 686-3374
Type: Junior or Comm Coll
Control: State, County, or Local Government
• Dental Lab Technician Prgm
• Occupational Therapy Asst Prgm
• Ophthalmic Dispensing Optician Prgm
• Pharmacy Technician Prgm
• Respiratory Therapist (Advanced) Prgm
• Surgical Technology Prgm

North Carolina Central University
James H Ammons, PhD, Chancellor
1801 Fayetteville St
113 Hoey Administration Bldg
Durham, NC 27707
919 530-6104
Type: 4-year Coll or Univ
Control: State, County, or Local Govt
• Athletic Training Prgm
• Dietetic Internship Prgm
• Dietetics-Didactic Prgm
• Medical Librarian Prgm
• Orientation and Mobility Specialist Prgm
• Speech-Language Pathology Prgm

Elizabeth City

College of The Albemarle
Lynne M Bunch, MA, President
PO Box 2327
Elizabeth City, NC 27906-2327
252 335-0821
Type: Junior or Comm Coll
Control: State, County, or Local Govt
• Medical Assistant Prgm
• Surgical Technology Prgm

Elon

Elon University
Leo Lambert, PhD, President
Campus Box 2185
Elon, NC 27244
336 278-7900
Type: 4-year Coll or Univ
Control: Nonprofit (Private or Religious)
• Athletic Training Prgm
• Physical Therapy Prgm

Fayetteville

Fayetteville State University
Fayetteville, NC 28301
Type: 4-year Coll or Univ
Control: State, County, or Local Govt
• Nursing Prgm (2)

Fayetteville Technical Community College
J Larry Keen, EdD, President
PO Box 35236
Fayetteville, NC 28303-0236
910 678-8321
Type: Junior or Comm Coll
Control: State, County, or Local Govt
• Dental Assisting Prgm
• Dental Hygiene Prgm
• Phlebotomy Prgm
• Physical Therapist Assistant Prgm
• Radiography Prgm
• Respiratory Therapist (Advanced) Prgm
• Surgical Technology Prgm

Methodist University
Elton Hendricks, PhD, President
5400 Ramsey St
Fayetteville, NC 28311
910 630-7005
Type: 4-year Coll or Univ
Control: Nonprofit (Private or Religious)
• Athletic Training Prgm
• Physician Assistant Prgm

Flat Rock

Blue Ridge Community College
David W Sink, Jr, EdD, President
College Dr
Flat Rock, NC 28737-9624
828 692-3572
Type: Junior or Comm Coll
Control: State, County, or Local Govt
• Surgical Technology Prgm

Fort Bragg

Joint Special Operations Medical Training Ctr
Jeffrey L. Kingsbury, MD MPH, Dean
CDR, SWMG(A)
AOJK-MED (attn: EMT Coord)
Fort Bragg, NC 28310-5200
910 396-7775
Type: Dept of Defense
Control: Fed Govt
• Emergency Med Tech-Paramedic Prgm

Goldsboro

Wayne Community College
Edward H Wilson, EdD, President
Caller Box 8002
Goldsboro, NC 27530
919 735-5151
Type: Junior or Comm Coll
Control: State, County, or Local Govt
• Dental Assisting Prgm
• Dental Hygiene Prgm
• Medical Assistant Prgm

INSTITUTIONS

Graham

Alamance Community College
Martin H Nadelman, EdD, President
PO Box 8000
Graham, NC 27253-8000
336 578-2002
Type: Junior or Comm Coll
Control: State, County, or Local Govt
- Clin Lab Technician/Med Lab Technician Prgm
- Dental Assisting Prgm
- Medical Assistant Prgm

Grantsboro

Pamlico Community College
Marion Altman, EdD, President
PO Box 185
Grantsboro, NC 28529-0185
252 249-1851
Type: Junior or Comm Coll
Control: State, County, or Local Govt
- Electroneurodiagnostic Tech Prgm
- Medical Assistant Prgm

Greensboro

Greensboro College
Craven E Williams, DMin, President
815 W Market St
Greensboro, NC 27401
336 272-7102
Type: 4-year Coll or Univ
Control: State, County, or Local Govt
- Athletic Training Prgm

Moses Cone Health System
Timothy Rice, MBA, President/CEO
1200 N Elm St
Greensboro, NC 27401-1020
336 832-9500
Type: Hosp or Med Ctr: 500> Beds
Control: Nonprofit (Private or Religious)
- Radiography Prgm

North Carolina A&T State University
Edward B Fort, Chancellor
1601 E Market St
Greensboro, NC 27411
910 334-7500
Type: 4-year Coll or Univ
Control: State, County, or Local Govt
- Counseling Prgm
- Dietetics-Didactic Prgm
- Rehabilitation Counseling Prgm

Greenville

East Carolina University
Steven Ballard, PhD, Chancellor
Spillman Building
Greenville, NC 27858-4353
252 328-6212
Type: 4-year Coll or Univ
Control: State, County, or Local Govt
- Allopathic Medicine Prgm
- Athletic Training Prgm
- Audiologist Prgm
- Clin Lab Scientist/Med Technologist Prgm
- Dietetic Internship Prgm
- Dietetics-Didactic Prgm
- Health Information Admin Prgm
- Music Therapy Prgm
- Occupational Therapy Prgm
- Physical Therapy Prgm
- Physician Assistant Prgm
- Rehabilitation Counseling Prgm
- Speech-Language Pathology Prgm

Pitt Community College
Dennis Massey, PhD, President
PO Drawer 7007
Greenville, NC 27835-7007
252 493-7220
Type: Junior or Comm Coll
Control: State, County, or Local Govt
- Diagnostic Med Sonography Prgm
- Health Information Tech Prgm
- Medical Assistant Prgm
- Occupational Therapy Asst Prgm
- Radiation Therapy Prgm
- Radiography Prgm
- Respiratory Therapist (Advanced) Prgm

Hamlet

Richmond Community College
Diane Honeycutt, EdD, President
PO Box 1189
Hamlet, NC 28345
910 582-7000
Type: Junior or Comm Coll
Control: State, County, or Local Govt
- Medical Assistant Prgm

Henderson

Vance-Granville Community College
Randy Parker, MEd, President
PO Box 917
Popular Creek Rd
Henderson, NC 27536
252 492-2061
Type: Junior or Comm Coll
Control: State, County, or Local Govt
- Medical Assistant Prgm
- Radiography Prgm

Hickory

Catawba Valley Community College
Garrett Hinshaw, EdD, President
2550 Hwy 70 SE
Hickory, NC 28602
828 327-7000
Type: Junior or Comm Coll
Control: State, County, or Local Govt
- Dental Hygiene Prgm
- Emergency Med Tech-Paramedic Prgm
- Health Information Tech Prgm
- Respiratory Therapist (Advanced) Prgm
- Surgical Technology Prgm

Lenoir-Rhyne College
Wayne Powell, PhD, President
Box 7163
Hickory, NC 28603
828 328-7334
Type: 4-year Coll or Univ
Control: Nonprofit (Private or Religious)
- Athletic Training Prgm
- Nursing Prgm
- Occupational Therapy Prgm

High Point

High Point University
Nido Qubein, LLD, President
833 Montlieu Ave
High Point, NC 27262
336 841-9201
Type: 4-year Coll or Univ
Control: Nonprofit (Private or Religious)
- Athletic Training Prgm

Hudson

Caldwell Comm College & Tech Institute
Kenneth A Boham, EdD, President
2855 Hickory Blvd
Hudson, NC 28638-1399
828 726-2200
Type: Junior or Comm Coll
Control: State, County, or Local Govt
- Diagnostic Med Sonography Prgm
- Nuclear Medicine Technology Prgm
- Ophthalmic Assistant Prgm
- Physical Therapist Assistant Prgm
- Radiography Prgm

Jacksonville

Coastal Carolina Community College
Ronald K Lingle, PhD, President
444 Western Blvd
Jacksonville, NC 28546-6877
910 938-6210
Type: Junior or Comm Coll
Control: State, County, or Local Govt
- Clin Lab Technician/Med Lab Technician Prgm
- Dental Assisting Prgm
- Dental Hygiene Prgm
- Surgical Technology Prgm

Jamestown

Guilford Technical Community College
Donald C Cameron, EdD, President
PO Box 309
601 High Point Rd
Jamestown, NC 27282
336 334-4822
Type: Junior or Comm Coll
Control: State, County, or Local Govt
- Dental Assisting Prgm
- Dental Hygiene Prgm
- Medical Assistant Prgm (2)
- Physical Therapist Assistant Prgm
- Surgical Technology Prgm

Kenansville

James Sprunt Community College
Mary T Wood, EdD, President
PO Box 398, James Sprunt Dr
Kenansville, NC 28349
910 296-2450
Type: Junior or Comm Coll
Control: State, County, or Local Govt
- Medical Assistant Prgm

Kinston

Lenoir Community College
Brantley Briley, EdD, President
PO Box 188
231 Hwy 58S
Kinston, NC 28502
252 527-6223
Type: Junior or Comm Coll
Control: State, County, or Local Govt
- Medical Assistant Prgm
- Radiography Prgm
- Surgical Technology Prgm

Lexington

Davidson County Community College
Mary Rittling, EdD, President
PO Box 1287
Lexington, NC 27293-1287
336 249-8186
Type: Junior or Comm Coll
Control: State, County, or Local Govt
- Clin Lab Technician/Med Lab Technician Prgm
- Health Information Tech Prgm
- Medical Assistant Prgm

Lumberton

Robeson Community College
Charles Chrestman, EdD, President
PO Box 1420
Lumberton, NC 28359
910 272-3230
Type: Junior or Comm Coll
Control: State, County, or Local Govt
- Respiratory Therapist (Advanced) Prgm
- Surgical Technology Prgm

Marion

McDowell Technical Community College
Bryan Wilson, EdD, President
54 College Dr
Marion, NC 28752
828 652-0635
Type: Junior or Comm Coll
Control: State, County, or Local Govt
- Health Information Tech Prgm

Mars Hill

Mars Hill College
Dan G Lunsford, EdD, President
PO Box 6748
Mars Hill, NC 28754
828 689-1141
Type: 4-year Coll or Univ
Control: State, County, or Local Govt
- Athletic Training Prgm

Morehead City

Carteret Community College
Joseph T Barwick, PhD, President
3505 Arendell St
Morehead City, NC 28557
252 222-6140
Type: Junior or Comm Coll
Control: State, County, or Local Govt
- Medical Assistant Prgm
- Radiography Prgm
- Respiratory Therapist (Advanced) Prgm

Morganton

Western Piedmont Community College
Jim Burnett, EdD, President
1001 Burkemont Ave
Morganton, NC 28655
704 438-6010
Type: Junior or Comm Coll
Control: State, County, or Local Govt
- Clin Lab Technician/Med Lab Technician Prgm
- Dental Assisting Prgm
- Medical Assistant Prgm

Murphy

Tri-County Community College
Norman Oglesby, PhD, President
2300 Hwy 64 E
Murphy, NC 28906
704 837-6810
Type: Junior or Comm Coll
Control: State, County, or Local Govt
- Medical Assistant Prgm

North Wilkesboro

Wilkes Regional Medical Center
Ted Chapin, MPH, CEO
PO Box 609
North Wilkesboro, NC 28659
336 651-8100
Type: Hosp or Med Ctr: 100-299 Beds
Control: State, County, or Local Govt
- Radiography Prgm

Pinehurst

Sandhills Community College
John R Dempsey, PhD, President
3395 Airport Rd
Pinehurst, NC 28374
910 695-3700
Type: Junior or Comm Coll
Control: State, County, or Local Govt
- Clin Lab Technician/Med Lab Technician Prgm
- Radiography Prgm
- Respiratory Therapist (Advanced) Prgm
- Surgical Technology Prgm

Polkton

South Piedmont Community College
John McKay, EdD, President
PO Box 126
Polkton, NC 28135
704 272-7635
Type: Junior or Comm Coll
Control: State, County, or Local Govt
- Medical Assistant Prgm
- Surgical Technology Prgm

Raleigh

Meredith College
John E Weems, President
Raleigh, NC 27607
919 829-8600
Type: 4-year Coll or Univ
Control: Nonprofit (Private or Religious)
- Dietetic Internship Prgm
- Dietetics-Didactic Prgm

North Carolina State University
James Oblinger, PhD, Chancellor
Holladay Hall A, Box 7001
Raleigh, NC 27695
919 515-2191
Type: 4-year Coll or Univ
Control: State, County, or Local Govt
- Counseling Prgm
- Veterinary Medicine Prgm

Shaw University
Clarence G Newsome, PhD, President
118 E South St
Raleigh, NC 27601
919 546-8330
Type: 4-year Coll or Univ
Control: Nonprofit (Private or Religious)
- Kinesiotherapy Prgm

Wake Technical Community College
Stephen Scott, EdD, President
9101 Fayetteville Rd
Raleigh, NC 27603
919 662-3400
Type: Junior or Comm Coll
Control: State, County, or Local Govt
- Clin Lab Technician/Med Lab Technician Prgm
- Dental Assisting Prgm
- Dental Hygiene Prgm
- Medical Assistant Prgm
- Phlebotomy Prgm
- Radiography Prgm
- Surgical Technology Prgm

Rocky Mount

Nash Community College
William Carver II, MBA, President
522 N Old Carriage Rd
PO Box 7488
Rocky Mount, NC 27804-0488
919 443-4011
Type: Junior or Comm Coll
Control: State, County, or Local Govt
• Phlebotomy Prgm
• Physical Therapist Assistant Prgm

Salisbury

Catawba College
Robert Knott, PhD, President
2300 W Innes St
Salisbury, NC 28144
704 637-4414
Type: 4-year Coll or Univ
Control: Nonprofit (Private or Religious)
• Athletic Training Prgm

Rowan-Cabarrus Community College
Richard L Brownell, EdD, President
PO Box 1595
1333 Jake Alexander Blvd
Salisbury, NC 28145-1595
704 637-0760
Type: Junior or Comm Coll
Control: State, County, or Local Govt
• Dental Assisting Prgm
• Radiography Prgm

Sanford

Central Carolina Community College
Mathew Garrett, BS MA EdD, President
1105 Kelly Dr
Sanford, NC 27330
919 775-5401
Type: Junior or Comm Coll
Control: State, County, or Local Govt
• Medical Assistant Prgm (2)
• Veterinary Technology Prgm

Shelby

Cleveland Community College
L Steve Thornburg, EdD, President
137 S Post Rd
Shelby, NC 28150
704 484-4089
Type: Junior or Comm Coll
Control: State, County, or Local Govt
• Radiography Prgm
• Surgical Technology Prgm

Siler City

Body Therapy Institute
Rick Rosen, MA LMT, Codirector
300 Southwind Rd
Siler City, NC 27344
919 663-3111
Type: Vocational or Tech Sch
Control: For Profit
• Massage Therapy Prgm

Smithfield

Johnston Community College
Donald Reichard, President
PO Box 2350
Smithfield, NC 27577
919 209-2050
Type: Junior or Comm Coll
Control: State, County, or Local Govt
• Diagnostic Med Sonography Prgm
• Medical Assistant Prgm
• Radiography Prgm

Spruce Pine

Mayland Community College
Thomas Williams, EdD, President
PO Box 547
Spruce Pine, NC 28777
828 765-7351
Type: Junior or Comm Coll
Control: State, County, or Local Govt
• Medical Assistant Prgm

Statesville

Mitchell Community College
Douglas O Eason, PhD, President
West Broad St
Statesville, NC 28677
704 878-3200
Type: Junior or Comm Coll
Control: State, County, or Local Govt
• Medical Assistant Prgm

Supply

Brunswick Community College
Steven Greiner, EdD, President
PO Box 30
50 College Road
Supply, NC 28462
910 754-6900
Type: Junior or Comm Coll
Control: State, County, or Local Govt
• Health Information Tech Prgm
• Phlebotomy Prgm

Sylva

Southwestern Community College
Cecil Groves, PhD, President
447 College Dr
Sylva, NC 28779
800 586-4091
Type: Junior or Comm Coll
Control: State, County, or Local Govt
• Clin Lab Technician/Med Lab Technician Prgm
• Health Information Tech Prgm
• Phlebotomy Prgm
• Physical Therapist Assistant Prgm
• Radiography Prgm
• Respiratory Therapist (Advanced) Prgm

Tarboro

Edgecombe Community College
Deborah L Lamm, EdD, President
2009 W Wilson St
Tarboro, NC 27886
252 823-5166
Type: Junior or Comm Coll
Control: State, County, or Local Govt
• Health Information Tech Prgm
• Medical Assistant Prgm
• Radiography Prgm
• Respiratory Therapist (Advanced) Prgm
• Surgical Technology Prgm

Troy

Montgomery Community College
Mary Kirk, EdD, President
1011 Page St
Troy, NC 27371
910 576-6222
Type: Junior or Comm Coll
Control: State, County, or Local Govt
• Medical Assistant Prgm

Washington

Beaufort County Community College
David McLawhorn, EdD, President
PO Box 1069
Highway 264 East
Washington, NC 27889
252 946-6194
Type: Junior or Comm Coll
Control: State, County, or Local Govt
• Clin Lab Technician/Med Lab Technician Prgm

Weldon

Halifax Community College
Harold Mitchell, EdD, Interim President
PO Box 809
Weldon, NC 27890
252 536-4221
Type: Junior or Comm Coll
Control: State, County, or Local Govt
• Clin Lab Technician/Med Lab Technician Prgm
• Dental Hygiene Prgm
• Phlebotomy Prgm

Wentworth

Rockingham Community College
Robert C Keys, PhD, President
PO Box 38
Wentworth, NC 27375-0038
910 342-4261
Type: Junior or Comm Coll
Control: State, County, or Local Govt
• Phlebotomy Prgm
• Respiratory Therapist (Advanced) Prgm
• Surgical Technology Prgm

Whiteville

Southeastern Community College
Kathy Matlock, PhD, President
PO Box 151
Whiteville, NC 28472-0151
910 642-7141
Type: Junior or Comm Coll
Control: State, County, or Local Govt
• Clin Lab Technician/Med Lab Technician Prgm
• Phlebotomy Prgm

Wilkesboro

Wilkes Community College
Gordon Burns, PhD, President
1328 Collegiate Dr
PO Box 120
Wilkesboro, NC 28697-0120
336 838-6100
Type: Junior or Comm Coll
Control: State, County, or Local Govt
• Dental Assisting Prgm
• Medical Assistant Prgm

Williamston

Martin Commuity College
Ann R Britt, EdD, President
1161 Kehukee Park Rd
Williamston, NC 27892
919 792-1521
Type: Junior or Comm Coll
Control: State, County, or Local Govt
• Dental Assisting Prgm
• Medical Assistant Prgm
• Physical Therapist Assistant Prgm

Wilmington

Cape Fear Community College
Eric B McKeithan, EdD, President
411 N Front St
Wilmington, NC 28401-3993
910 362-7555
Type: Junior or Comm Coll
Control: State, County, or Local Govt
• Dental Assisting Prgm
• Dental Hygiene Prgm
• Diagnostic Med Sonography Prgm
• Occupational Therapy Asst Prgm
• Phlebotomy Prgm
• Radiography Prgm

Miller-Motte College
Ruth Hodge, BS, Executive Director
5000 Market St
Wilmington, NC 28405
910 392-4660
Type: 4-year Coll or Univ
Control: For Profit
• Medical Assistant Prgm (2)
• Surgical Technology Prgm (2)

Wilson

Barton College
Norval C Kneten, PhD, President
PO Box 5000
Wilson, NC 27893
252 399-6309
Type: 4-year Coll or Univ
Control: Nonprofit (Private or Religious)
• Athletic Training Prgm

Wilson Technical Community College
Frank L Eagles, EdD, President
904 Herring Ave
Wilson, NC 27893
252 291-1195
Type: Junior or Comm Coll
Control: State, County, or Local Govt
• Surgical Technology Prgm

Wingate

Wingate University
Jerry McGee, EdD, President
PO Box 3055
Wingate, NC 28714
704 233-8111
Type: 4-year Coll or Univ
Control: Nonprofit (Private or Religious)
• Athletic Training Prgm
• Pharmacy Prgm

Winston-Salem

Forsyth Technical Community College
Gary M Green, EdD, President
2100 Silas Creek Pky
Winston-Salem, NC 27103
336 734-7414
Type: Junior or Comm Coll
Control: State, County, or Local Govt
• Dental Assisting Prgm
• Dental Hygiene Prgm
• Diagnostic Med Sonography Prgm
• Medical Assistant Prgm
• Nuclear Medicine Technology Prgm
• Radiation Therapy Prgm
• Radiography Prgm
• Respiratory Therapist (Advanced) Prgm

Wake Forest University
Nathan Hatch, PhD, President
7622 Reynolda Station
Winston-Salem, NC 27109
910 759-5000
Type: 4-year Coll or Univ
Control: Nonprofit (Private or Religious)
• Counseling Prgm

Wake Forest University Baptist Medical Center
Medical Center Blvd
Winston-Salem, NC 27157-1072
Type: Acad Health Ctr/Med Sch
Control: Nonprofit (Private or Religious)
• Clin Lab Scientist/Med Technologist Prgm

Wake Forest University School of Medicine
William Applegate, MD MPH, Interim Pres, Dean
Medical Ctr Blvd
Winston-Salem, NC 27157
336 716-5026
Type: Acad Health Ctr/Med Sch
Control: Nonprofit (Private or Religious)
• Allopathic Medicine Prgm
• Physician Assistant Prgm

Winston-Salem State University
Michelle Howard-Vital, PhD, Interim Chancellor
601 Martin Luther King Jr Dr
Winston-Salem, NC 27110
336 750-2141
Type: 4-year Coll or Univ
Control: State, County, or Local Govt
• Clin Lab Scientist/Med Technologist Prgm
• Nursing Prgm
• Occupational Therapy Prgm
• Physical Therapy Prgm
• Rehabilitation Counseling Prgm
• Therapeutic Recreation Specialist Prgm

North Dakota

Bismarck

Bismarck State College
Larry Skogen, PhD, President
PO Box 5587
Bismarck, ND 58506-5587
701 224-5430
Type: Junior or Comm Coll
Control: State, County, or Local Govt
• Clin Lab Technician/Med Lab Technician Prgm
• Phlebotomy Prgm
• Surgical Technology Prgm

Medcenter One
James Cooper, President/CEO
300 N Seventh St
Bismarck, ND 58506-5525
701 323-6104
Type: Hosp or Med Ctr: 100-299 Beds
Control: Nonprofit (Private or Religious)
• Nursing Prgm
• Radiography Prgm

United Tribes Technical College
David M Gipp, PhD, President
3315 University Dr
Bismarck, ND 58504
701 255-3285
Type: Vocational or Tech Sch
Control: Nonprofit (Private or Religious)
• Health Information Tech Prgm

University of Mary
Sister Thomas Welder, OSB MM, President
7500 University Dr
Bismarck, ND 58504-9652
701 355-8100
Type: 4-year Coll or Univ
Control: Nonprofit (Private or Religious)
• Athletic Training Prgm
• Nursing Prgm
• Occupational Therapy Prgm
• Physical Therapy Prgm

North Dakota

University of Mary/St Alexius Medical Ctr
Richard A Tschider, MA, Administrator
PO Box 5510
Bismarck, ND 58506-5510
701 224-7600
Type: Hosp or Med Ctr: 100-299 Beds
Control: Nonprofit (Private or Religious)
• Emergency Med Tech-Paramedic Prgm
• Respiratory Therapist (Advanced) Prgm

Fargo

MeritCare Medical Center
Roger Gilbertson, MD, President
801 N Broadway
Fargo, ND 58122
701 234-6954
Type: Hosp or Med Ctr: 500> Beds
Control: Nonprofit (Private or Religious)
• Clin Lab Scientist/Med Technologist Prgm
• Radiography Prgm

NDSU/MeritCare Hospital Consortium
Gary Lee, BA RRT, CEO
MeritCare Hospital
PO Box MC
Fargo, ND 58122-0118
701 234-5190
Type: 4-year Coll or Univ
Control: State, County, or Local Govt
• Respiratory Therapist (Advanced) Prgm

North Dakota State University
Joseph Chapman, PhD, President
PO Box 5167
Fargo, ND 58105-5167
701 231-8011
Type: 4-year Coll or Univ
Control: State, County, or Local Govt
• Athletic Training Prgm
• Counseling Prgm
• Dietetics-Coordinated Prgm
• Dietetics-Didactic Prgm
• Exercise Science Prgm
• Nursing Prgm
• Pharmacy Prgm
• Veterinary Technology Prgm

Grand Forks

University of North Dakota
Charles Kupchella, PhD, President
Box 8193
Grand Forks, ND 58202-8193
701 777-2121
Type: Acad Health Ctr/Med Sch
Control: State, County, or Local Govt
• Allopathic Medicine Prgm
• Athletic Training Prgm
• Clin Lab Scientist/Med Technologist Prgm
• Cytotechnology Prgm
• Dietetics-Coordinated Prgm
• Histotechnician Prgm
• Music Therapy Prgm
• Nursing Prgm
• Occupational Therapy Prgm
• Physical Therapy Prgm
• Physician Assistant Prgm
• Psychology Prgm
• Speech-Language Pathology Prgm

Minot

Minot State University
David Fuller, President
500 University Ave W
Minot, ND 58707
701 858-3031
Type: 4-year Coll or Univ
Control: State, County, or Local Govt
• Speech-Language Pathology Prgm

Trinity Health
Terry G Hoff, FCHA, President
1 Burdick Expwy West
Minot, ND 58701
701 857-5000
Type: Hosp or Med Ctr: 100-299 Beds
Control: Nonprofit (Private or Religious)
• Radiography Prgm

Wahpeton

North Dakota State College of Science
John Richman, PhD, President
800 N Sixth St
Wahpeton, ND 58076-0002
701 671-2222
Type: Junior or Comm Coll
Control: State, County, or Local Govt
• Dental Assisting Prgm
• Dental Hygiene Prgm
• Health Information Tech Prgm
• Occupational Therapy Asst Prgm
• Pharmacy Technician Prgm

Williston

Williston State College
Joseph McCann, PhD, President
1410 University Ave
PO Box 1326
Williston, ND 58802-1326
701 774-4200
Type: Junior or Comm Coll
Control: State, County, or Local Govt
• Physical Therapist Assistant Prgm

Nova Scotia, Canada

Halifax

Dalhousie University
Tom Traves, President
Halifax, NS B3H 3J5
902 424-2511
Type: 4-year Coll or Univ
Control: State, County, or Local Govt
• Allopathic Medicine Prgm
• Medical Librarian Prgm

IWK Grace Health Centre
5850 University Ave
PO Box 3070
Halifax, NS B3J 3G9
Type: Hosp or Med Ctr: 500> Beds
Control: State, County, or Local Govt
• Orthoptist Prgm

Ohio

Ada

Ohio Northern University
Kendall Baker, PhD, President
525 S Main St
Ada, OH 45810
419 772-2031
Type: 4-year Coll or Univ
Control: Nonprofit (Private or Religious)
• Athletic Training Prgm
• Clin Lab Scientist/Med Technologist Prgm
• Pharmacy Prgm

Akron

Akron General Medical Center
Alan Bleyer, MHA, President
400 Wabash Ave
Akron, OH 44307
330 846-6548
Type: Hosp or Med Ctr: 500> Beds
Control: Nonprofit (Private or Religious)
• Cytotechnology Prgm
• Emergency Med Tech-Paramedic Prgm

Akron Institute
David LaRue, Campus President
1600 S Arlington Ste 100
Akron, OH 44306
330 724-1600
Type: Vocational or Tech Sch
Control: For Profit
• Medical Assistant Prgm

Children's Hospital Medical Ctr of Akron
William H Considine, MHA, President
One Perkins Square
Akron, OH 44308-1062
330 543-8293
Type: Hosp or Med Ctr: 100-299 Beds
Control: Nonprofit (Private or Religious)
• Clin Lab Scientist/Med Technologist Prgm
• Radiography Prgm

Summa Health System
Thomas Strauss, PhD, President and CEO
525 E Market St
PO Box 2090
Akron, OH 44309-2090
330 375-3000
Type: Hosp or Med Ctr: 500> Beds
Control: Nonprofit (Private or Religious)
• Emergency Med Tech-Paramedic Prgm

University of Akron
Luis M Proenza, PhD, President
Buchtel Hall 114
Akron, OH 44325-4702
330 972-7074
Type: 4-year Coll or Univ
Control: State, County, or Local Govt
• Athletic Training Prgm
• Audiologist Prgm
• Counseling Prgm
• Dietetics-Coordinated Prgm
• Dietetics-Didactic Prgm
• Medical Assistant Prgm
• Nursing Prgm
• Respiratory Therapist (Advanced) Prgm
• Speech-Language Pathology Prgm
• Surgical Technology Prgm

Alliance

Mount Union College
Richard F Giese, PhD, President
1972 Clark Ave
Alliance, OH 44601
330 823-6050
Type: 4-year Coll or Univ
Control: Nonprofit (Private or Religious)
• Athletic Training Prgm

Ashland

Ashland County - West Holmes Career Center
Michael McDaniel, BS MS, Superintendent
1783 State Rte 60
Ashland, OH 44805
419 289-3313
Type: Vocational or Tech Sch
Control: For Profit
• Medical Assistant Prgm

Ashland University
Fred Finks, DMin, President
205 Founders Hall
Ashland, OH 44805
419 289-5050
Type: 4-year Coll or Univ
Control: Nonprofit (Private or Religious)
• Athletic Training Prgm
• Nursing Prgm

Athens

Ohio University
Roderick McDavis, PhD, President
Cutler Hall 108
Athens, OH 45701
740 593-1804
Type: 4-year Coll or Univ
Control: State, County, or Local Govt
• Athletic Training Prgm
• Audiologist Prgm
• Counseling Prgm
• Dietetics-Didactic Prgm
• Medical Assistant Prgm
• Music Therapy Prgm
• Nursing Prgm
• Osteopathic Medicine Prgm
• Physical Therapy Prgm
• Psychology Prgm
• Rehabilitation Counseling Prgm
• Speech-Language Pathology Prgm

Batavia

Univ of Cincinnati - Clermont College
David H Devier, PhD, Dean
4200 Clermont College Dr
Batavia, OH 45103
513 732-5209
Type: Junior or Comm Coll
Control: State, County, or Local Govt
• Surgical Technology Prgm

Berea

Baldwin-Wallace College
Mark Collier, PhD, President
275 Eastland Rd
Berea, OH 44017
440 826-2424
Type: 4-year Coll or Univ
Control: Nonprofit (Private or Religious)
• Athletic Training Prgm
• Music Therapy Prgm

Bluffton

Bluffton College
Elmer Neufeld, President
280 W College Ave
Bluffton, OH 45817
419 358-3000
Type: 4-year Coll or Univ
Control: Nonprofit (Private or Religious)
• Dietetics-Didactic Prgm

Bowling Green

Bowling Green State University
Sidney A Ribeau, PhD, President
220 McFall Ctr
Bowling Green, OH 43403
419 372-2211
Type: 4-year Coll or Univ
Control: State, County, or Local Govt
• Athletic Training Prgm
• Clin Lab Scientist/Med Technologist Prgm
• Dietetic Internship Prgm
• Dietetics-Didactic Prgm
• Health Information Tech Prgm
• Psychology Prgm
• Rehabilitation Counseling Prgm
• Respiratory Therapist (Advanced) Prgm
• Speech-Language Pathology Prgm

Canfield

Mahoning County Career & Technical Center
Roan Craig, PhD, Superintendent
7300 N Palmyra Rd
Canfield, OH 44406-9710
330 729-4100
Type: Vocational or Tech Sch
Control: State, County, or Local Govt
• Medical Assistant Prgm

Canton

Aultman Hospital
Edward Roth, MBA, President
2600 Sixth St SW
Canton, OH 44710
330 438-6241
Type: Hosp or Med Ctr: 500> Beds
Control: Nonprofit (Private or Religious)
• Nuclear Medicine Technology Prgm
• Radiation Therapy Prgm
• Radiography Prgm

Canton City Schools
Dianne Talarico, Superintendent
617 McKinley Ave SW
Canton, OH 44707
330 438-2530
Type: Vocational or Tech Sch
Control: State, County, or Local Govt
• Medical Assistant Prgm

Malone College
Canton, OH 44709
Type: 4-year Coll or Univ
Control: Nonprofit (Private or Religious)
• Nursing Prgm

Mercy Medical Center
Thomas E Cecconi, President/CEO
1320 Mercy Dr NW
Canton, OH 44708
330 489-1001
Type: Hosp or Med Ctr: 500> Beds
Control: Nonprofit (Private or Religious)
• Diagnostic Med Sonography Prgm
• Radiography Prgm

Stark State College of Technology
John O'Donnell, EdD, President
6200 Frank Ave NW
Canton, OH 44720-7299
330 494-6170
Type: Vocational or Tech Sch
Control: State, County, or Local Govt
• Clin Lab Technician/Med Lab Technician Prgm
• Dental Hygiene Prgm
• Health Information Tech Prgm
• Medical Assistant Prgm
• Occupational Therapy Asst Prgm
• Physical Therapist Assistant Prgm
• Respiratory Therapist (Advanced) Prgm

Cedarville

Cedarville University
William Brown, PhD, President
251 N Main St
Cedarville, OH 45314
937 766-7900
Type: 4-year Coll or Univ
Control: Nonprofit (Private or Religious)
• Athletic Training Prgm
• Nursing Prgm

Centerville

RETS Tech Center
Duncan Anderson, President
555 East Alex-Bell Rd
Centerville, OH 45459
937 433-3410
Type: Vocational or Tech Sch
Control: For Profit
• Medical Assistant Prgm

Chesapeake

Collins Career Center
Steve Dodgion, BA MSEd, Superintendent
11627 St Rte 243
Chesapeake, OH 45619
740 867-6641
Type: Vocational or Tech Sch
Control: Nonprofit (Private or Religious)
• Pharmacy Technician Prgm
• Phlebotomy Prgm
• Radiography Prgm
• Respiratory Therapist (Advanced) Prgm
• Surgical Technology Prgm

Chillicothe

Pickaway Ross Joint Vocational School
Brett Smith, Superintendent
895 Crouse Chapel Rd
Chillicothe, OH 45601-9010
740 642-2111
Type: Vocational or Tech Sch
Control: Nonprofit (Private or Religious)
• Medical Assistant Prgm

Cincinnati

Brown Mackie College
Richard Thome, MS, President
2791 Mogadore Rd
Cincinnati, OH 45215
513 771-2424
Type: Junior or Comm Coll
Control: For Profit
• Medical Assistant Prgm (2)

Christ Hospital
Susan Croushore, Senior Executive Officer
2139 Auburn Ave
Cincinnati, OH 45219
513 585-1399
Type: Hosp or Med Ctr: 300-499 Beds
Control: Nonprofit (Private or Religious)
• Dietetic Internship Prgm
• Perfusion Prgm

Cincinnati Children's Hospital Medical Center
Nancy L Zimpher, President
3333 Burnet Ave
Cincinnati, OH 45229
513 556-2201
Type: Hosp or Med Ctr: 300-499 Beds
Control: Nonprofit (Private or Religious)
• Genetic Counseling Prgm

Cincinnati School of Medical Massage
111250 Cornell Park Dr, Ste 203
Cincinnati, OH 45242
Type: Vocational or Tech Sch
Control: For Profit
• Massage Therapy Prgm

Cincinnati State Tech & Comm College
Ronald D Wright, PhD, President
3520 Central Pkwy
Cincinnati, OH 45223
513 569-1511
Type: Junior or Comm Coll
Control: State, County, or Local Govt
• Clin Lab Technician/Med Lab Technician Prgm
• Diagnostic Med Sonography Prgm
• Dietetic Technician-AD Prgm
• Health Information Tech Prgm
• Medical Assistant Prgm
• Occupational Therapy Asst Prgm
• Respiratory Therapist (Advanced) Prgm
• Surgical Technology Prgm

Good Samaritan Hospital
375 Dixmyth Ave
Cincinnati, OH 45220-2489
513 872-1983
Control: Nonprofit (Private or Religious)
• Dietetic Internship Prgm

UC Raymond Walters College
Nancy Zimpher, PhD, President
PO Box 210063
Cincinnati, OH 45221-0063
513 745-5600
Type: Junior or Comm Coll
Control: State, County, or Local Govt
• Veterinary Technology Prgm

University of Cincinnati
Nancy L Zimpher, PhD, President
PO Box 210063
Cincinnati, OH 45221-0063
513 556-2201
Type: 4-year Coll or Univ
Control: State, County, or Local Govt
• Allopathic Medicine Prgm
• Athletic Training Prgm
• Audiologist Prgm
• Counseling Prgm
• Dental Hygiene Prgm
• Dietetics-Coordinated Prgm
• Dietetics-Didactic Prgm
• Emergency Med Tech-Paramedic Prgm
• Health Information Admin Prgm
• Medical Assistant Prgm
• Nuclear Medicine Technology Prgm
• Nursing Prgm
• Pharmacy Prgm
• Physical Therapist Assistant Prgm
• Physical Therapy Prgm
• Psychology Prgm
• Radiation Therapy Prgm
• Radiography Prgm
• Speech-Language Pathology Prgm

University of Cincinnati Medical Center
Nancy Zimpher, PhD, President
Admin Bldg
Cincinnati, OH 45221-0063
513 558-2201
Type: Acad Health Ctr/Med Sch
Control: State, County, or Local Govt
• Clin Lab Scientist/Med Technologist Prgm
• Specialist in BB Tech Prgm

Xavier University
Michael J Graham, SJ PhD, President
3800 Victory Pkwy
Cincinnati, OH 45207-4511
513 745-3501
Type: 4-year Coll or Univ
Control: Nonprofit (Private or Religious)
• Athletic Training Prgm
• Nursing Prgm
• Occupational Therapy Prgm
• Psychology Prgm
• Radiography Prgm

Clayton

Miami Valley Career Technology Center
John Boggess, PhD, Superintendent
6800 Hoke Rd
Clayton, OH 45315
937 854-6272
Type: Vocational or Tech Sch
Control: State, County, or Local Govt
• Medical Assistant Prgm

Cleveland

Case Western Reserve University
Edward Hundert, President
University Circle
Cleveland, OH 44106
216 368-2000
Type: Acad Health Ctr/Med Sch
Control: Nonprofit (Private or Religious)
• Allopathic Medicine Prgm
• Anesthesiologist Asst Prgm
• Dentistry Prgm
• Dietetic Internship Prgm
• Dietetics-Didactic Prgm
• Genetic Counseling Prgm
• Psychology Prgm
• Speech-Language Pathology Prgm

Cleveland Clinic Foundation
Delos M Cosgrove, MD, Chairman
9500 Euclid Ave H18
Cleveland, OH 44195-5108
216 444-2300
Type: Hosp or Med Ctr: 500> Beds
Control: Nonprofit (Private or Religious)
• Dietetic Internship Prgm
• Perfusion Prgm
• Radiation Therapy Prgm

Cleveland State University
Michael Schwartz, PhD, President
2121 Euclid Ave
Rhodes Tower 1201
Cleveland, OH 44115-2440
216 687-3544
Type: 4-year Coll or Univ
Control: State, County, or Local Govt
• Counseling Prgm
• Nursing Prgm
• Occupational Therapy Prgm
• Physical Therapy Prgm
• Speech-Language Pathology Prgm

Cuyahoga Community College
Jerry Sue Thornton, PhD, President, District
 Admin
700 Carnegie Ave
Cleveland, OH 44115
216 987-4850
Type: Junior or Comm Coll
Control: State, County, or Local Govt
• Clin Lab Technician/Med Lab Technician Prgm
• Dental Hygiene Prgm
• Diagnostic Med Sonography Prgm
• Dietetic Technician-AD Prgm
• Health Information Tech Prgm
• Medical Assistant Prgm
• Nuclear Medicine Technology Prgm
• Occupational Therapy Asst Prgm
• Pharmacy Technician Prgm
• Phlebotomy Prgm
• Physical Therapist Assistant Prgm
• Physician Assistant Prgm
• Radiography Prgm
• Respiratory Therapist (Advanced) Prgm
• Surgical Technology Prgm
• Veterinary Technology Prgm

John Carroll University
20700 N Park Blvd
Cleveland, OH 44118-4581
216 397-1886
Type: 4-year Coll or Univ
Control: Nonprofit (Private or Religious)
• Counseling Prgm

Louis Stokes Cleveland VA Med Ctr
10701 East Blvd
Cleveland, OH 44106-1702
216 421-3028
Control: Fed Govt
• Dietetic Internship Prgm

MetroHealth Medical Center
Terry R White, MBA, President/CEO
2500 Metro Health Dr
Cleveland, OH 44109-1998
216 459-5700
Type: Hosp or Med Ctr: 500> Beds
Control: State, County, or Local Govt
• Dietetic Internship Prgm

Ohio College of Podiatric Medicine
Thomas V Melitto, DPM
10515 Carnegie Ave
Cleveland, OH 44106
216 231-3300
Type: Acad Health Ctr/Med Sch
Control: Nonprofit (Private or Religious)
• Podiatric Medicine Prgm

University Hospitals Case Medical Center
Farah M Walters, MS, President/CEO
11100 Euclid Ave
Cleveland, OH 44106
216 844-7565
Type: Hosp or Med Ctr: 500> Beds
Control: Nonprofit (Private or Religious)
• Dietetic Internship Prgm

Columbus

A G James Cancer Hosp & Research Inst
Dennis Smith, BS, Assoc Exec Director
300 W 10th Ave 519 CHRI
Columbus, OH 43210-1228
614 293-3121
Type: Hosp or Med Ctr: 100-299 Beds
Control: State, County, or Local Govt
• Radiation Therapy Prgm

American School of Technology
Susan Stella, BS BA, Director
2100 Morse Rd
Columbus, OH 43229
614 436-4820
Type: Vocational or Tech Sch
Control: For Profit
• Medical Assistant Prgm

ARC Blood Svcs - Central Ohio Region
Ambrose Ng, MD, Chief Executive Officer
995 E Broad St
Columbus, OH 43205
614 253-2740
Type: Nonhosp HC Facil, BB, or Lab
Control: Nonprofit (Private or Religious)
• Specialist in BB Tech Prgm

Bradford School
Dennis Bartels, President
2469 Stelzer Rd
Columbus, OH 43219
614 416-6200
Type: Vocational or Tech Sch
Control: For Profit
• Medical Assistant Prgm
• Veterinary Technology Prgm

Capital University
Denvy Bowman, PhD, President
Yochum Hall
1 College & Main
Columbus, OH 43209
614 236-6908
Type: 4-year Coll or Univ
Control: Nonprofit (Private or Religious)
• Athletic Training Prgm
• Nursing Prgm

Chamberlain College of Nursing
Gail Baumlein, PhD, Chief Nurse Administrator
1350 Alum Creek Dr
Columbus, OH 43209
614 252-8890
Control: Nonprofit (Private or Religious)
• Nursing Prgm

Columbus State Community College
M Valeriana Moeller, PhD, President
550 E Spring St
PO Box 1609
Columbus, OH 43216-1609
614 287-2402
Type: Junior or Comm Coll
Control: State, County, or Local Govt
• Clin Lab Technician/Med Lab Technician Prgm
• Dental Hygiene Prgm
• Dietetic Technician-AD Prgm
• Emergency Med Tech-Paramedic Prgm
• Health Information Tech Prgm
• Histotechnician Prgm
• Medical Assistant Prgm
• Phlebotomy Prgm
• Radiography Prgm
• Respiratory Therapist (Advanced) Prgm
• Surgical Technology Prgm
• Veterinary Technology Prgm

Mt Carmel College of Nursing
Ann E Schiele, President
127 S Davis Ave
Columbus, OH 43222
614 234-5032
Type: 4-year Coll or Univ
Control: Nonprofit (Private or Religious)
• Dietetic Internship Prgm
• Surgical Technology Prgm

Ohio Institute of Health Careers
Angelique Walker, BS MBA, School Director
1880 E Dublin-Granville Rd
Suite 100
Columbus, OH 43229
614 891-5030
Type: Vocational or Tech Sch
Control: For Profit
• Medical Assistant Prgm (2)

Ohio State University
Gordon Gee, PhD, President
190 N Oval Mall
Columbus, OH 43210
614 292-2424
Type: 4-year Coll or Univ
Control: State, County, or Local Govt
• Allopathic Medicine Prgm
• Athletic Training Prgm
• Audiologist Prgm
• Clin Lab Scientist/Med Technologist Prgm
• Dental Hygiene Prgm
• Dentistry Prgm
• Dietetic Internship Prgm (2)
• Dietetics-Coordinated Prgm
• Dietetics-Didactic Prgm
• Health Information Admin Prgm
• Nursing Prgm
• Occupational Therapy Prgm
• Optometry Prgm
• Pathologists' Assistant Prgm
• Perfusion Prgm
• Pharmacy Prgm
• Physical Therapy Prgm
• Psychology Prgm
• Rehabilitation Counseling Prgm
• Respiratory Therapist (Advanced) Prgm
• Speech-Language Pathology Prgm
• Veterinary Medicine Prgm

Ohio State University Medical Center
Fred Sanfilippo, MD PhD, CEO
200 Meiling Hall
370 West 9th Ave
Columbus, OH 43210
614 292-1200
Type: Hosp or Med Ctr: 300-499 Beds
Control: State, County, or Local Govt
• Nuclear Medicine Technology Prgm

Sleep Care Inc
Craig Pickerill, RPSGT, President
7634 Rivers Edge Dr
Columbus, OH 43235
614 901-8989
Type: Nonhosp HC Facil, BB, or Lab
Control: For Profit
• Polysomnographic Technology Prgm

Dayton

Dayton School of Medical Message
4457 Far Hills Ave
Dayton, OH 45429
Type: Vocational or Tech Sch
Control: Nonprofit (Private or Religious)
• Massage Therapy Prgm (2)

Miami Valley Hospital
Karl R Tague, President/CEO
One Wyoming St
Dayton, OH 45409
513 223-6192
Type: Hosp or Med Ctr: 500> Beds
Control: Nonprofit (Private or Religious)
• Dietetic Internship Prgm

Miami-Jacobs Career College
Darlene Waite, MBA, President
110 N Patterson Ave
PO Box 1433
Dayton, OH 45402
937 461-5174
Type: Junior or Comm Coll
Control: For Profit
• Medical Assistant Prgm
• Surgical Technology Prgm

Ohio Institute of Photography & Technology
Robert A Martin, BS, Executive Director
2029 Edgefield Rd
Dayton, OH 45439
937 294-6155
Type: Vocational or Tech Sch
Control: For Profit
• Medical Assistant Prgm

Sinclair Community College
Steven Lee Johnson, PhD, President
444 W Third St
Dayton, OH 45402-1460
937 512-2525
Type: Junior or Comm Coll
Control: State, County, or Local Govt
• Dental Hygiene Prgm
• Dietetic Technician-AD Prgm
• Health Information Tech Prgm
• Medical Assistant Prgm
• Occupational Therapy Asst Prgm
• Physical Therapist Assistant Prgm
• Radiography Prgm
• Respiratory Therapist (Advanced) Prgm
• Surgical Technology Prgm

University of Dayton
Raymond Fitz, PhD SM, President
300 College Pk
Dayton, OH 45469-1624
937 229-1000
Type: 4-year Coll or Univ
Control: Nonprofit (Private or Religious)
• Dietetics-Didactic Prgm
• Music Therapy Prgm
• Physical Therapy Prgm

Wright State University
Dave Hopkins, PhD, President
3640 Colonel Glenn Hwy
Dayton, OH 45435
937 775-2312
Type: 4-year Coll or Univ
Control: State, County, or Local Govt
• Allopathic Medicine Prgm
• Athletic Training Prgm
• Clin Lab Scientist/Med Technologist Prgm
• Counseling Prgm
• Nursing Prgm
• Psychology Prgm
• Rehabilitation Counseling Prgm

Defiance

Defiance College
Gerald E Wood, EdD, President
701 N Clinton St
Defiance, OH 43512
419 783-2300
Type: 4-year Coll or Univ
Control: Nonprofit (Private or Religious)
• Athletic Training Prgm

East Liverpool

Ohio Valley College of Technology
Debra A Sanford, BS, President
16808 St Clair Ave
PO Box 7000
East Liverpool, OH 43920
330 385-1070
Type: Vocational or Tech Sch
Control: For Profit
• Medical Assistant Prgm

Elyria

Lorain County Community College
Roy A Church, EdD, President
1005 N Abbe Rd
Elyria, OH 44035
800 995-5222
Type: Junior or Comm Coll
Control: State, County, or Local Govt
• Clin Lab Technician/Med Lab Technician Prgm
• Dental Hygiene Prgm
• Diagnostic Med Sonography Prgm
• Medical Assistant Prgm
• Phlebotomy Prgm
• Physical Therapist Assistant Prgm
• Radiography Prgm
• Surgical Technology Prgm

Findlay

University of Findlay
Debow Freed, PhD, President
1000 North Main St
Findlay, OH 45840
419 434-4510
Type: 4-year Coll or Univ
Control: Nonprofit (Private or Religious)
• Athletic Training Prgm
• Nuclear Medicine Technology Prgm
• Occupational Therapy Prgm
• Pharmacy Prgm
• Physical Therapy Prgm
• Physician Assistant Prgm

Granville

Denison University
Dale T Knobel, PhD, President
Doane Hall
Granville, OH 43023
740 587-6281
Type: 4-year Coll or Univ
Control: Nonprofit (Private or Religious)
• Athletic Training Prgm

Green

Portage Lakes Career Center
Mark Lukens, MA, Superintendent
4401 Shriver Rd
PO Box 248
Green, OH 44232-0248
330 896-8200
Type: Vocational or Tech Sch
Control: State, County, or Local Govt
• Medical Assistant Prgm

Groveport

Fairfield Career Center (EVSD)
Mark Weedy, MEd, Superintendent
4465 S Hamilton Rd
Groveport, OH 43125
614 836-5725
Type: Vocational or Tech Sch
Control: State, County, or Local Govt
• Medical Assistant Prgm

Hillsboro

Southern State Community College
Lawrence N Dukes, EdD, President
100 Hobart Dr
Hillsboro, OH 45133
937 393-3431
Type: Junior or Comm Coll
Control: State, County, or Local Govt
• Medical Assistant Prgm

Kent

Kent State University
Lester Lefton, PhD, President
Office of the President
Kent, OH 44242-0001
330 672-2210
Type: 4-year Coll or Univ
Control: State, County, or Local Govt
- Athletic Training Prgm
- Counseling Prgm
- Dietetic Internship Prgm
- Dietetics-Didactic Prgm
- Medical Librarian Prgm
- Nuclear Medicine Technology Prgm
- Nursing Prgm
- Occupational Therapy Asst Prgm (2)
- Physical Therapist Assistant Prgm (2)
- Psychology Prgm
- Radiography Prgm
- Rehabilitation Counseling Prgm
- Speech-Language Pathology Prgm

Kettering

Kettering College of Medical Arts
Charles Scriven, PhD, President
3737 Southern Blvd
Kettering, OH 45429
937 298-3399
Type: 4-year Coll or Univ
Control: Nonprofit (Private or Religious)
- Diagnostic Med Sonography Prgm
- Physician Assistant Prgm
- Radiography Prgm
- Respiratory Therapist (Advanced) Prgm

Kirtland

Lakeland Community College
Morris Beverage, Jr, EdM, President
7700 Clocktower Dr
Kirtland, OH 44094
440 525-7177
Type: Junior or Comm Coll
Control: State, County, or Local Govt
- Clin Lab Technician/Med Lab Technician Prgm
- Dental Hygiene Prgm
- Medical Assistant Prgm
- Radiography Prgm
- Respiratory Therapist (Advanced) Prgm
- Surgical Technology Prgm

Lima

Apollo Career Center
J Chris Pfister, Superintendent
3325 Shawnee Rd
Lima, OH 45806
419 998-2911
Type: Vocational or Tech Sch
Control: State, County, or Local Govt
- Medical Assistant Prgm
- Surgical Technology Prgm

Rhodes State College
Debra McCurdy, PhD, President
4240 Campus Dr
Lima, OH 45804
419 995-8200
Type: Junior or Comm Coll
Control: State, County, or Local Govt
- Dental Hygiene Prgm
- Medical Assistant Prgm
- Occupational Therapy Asst Prgm
- Physical Therapist Assistant Prgm
- Radiography Prgm
- Respiratory Therapist (Advanced) Prgm

University of Northwestern Ohio
Loren R Jarvis, LLD, President
1441 N Cable Rd
Lima, OH 45805
419 227-3141
Type: 4-year Coll or Univ
Control: Nonprofit (Private or Religious)
- Medical Assistant Prgm

Lucasville

Scioto County Joint Vocational School
Stan Jennings, MS, Superintendent
951 Vern Riffe Dr
Lucasville, OH 45648
740 259-5526
Type: Vocational or Tech Sch
Control: State, County, or Local Govt
- Surgical Technology Prgm

Mansfield

Medcentral College
Mansfield, OH 44903
Type: 4-year Coll or Univ
Control: Nonprofit (Private or Religious)
- Nursing Prgm

North Central State College
Ronald E Abrams, PhD, President
2441 Kenwood Circle
PO Box 698
Mansfield, OH 44901
419 755-4800
Type: Junior or Comm Coll
Control: State, County, or Local Govt
- Physical Therapist Assistant Prgm
- Radiography Prgm
- Respiratory Therapist (Advanced) Prgm

Marietta

Marietta College
Jean Scott, PhD, President
215 Fifth St
Marietta, OH 45750
740 376-4699
Type: 4-year Coll or Univ
Control: Nonprofit (Private or Religious)
- Athletic Training Prgm
- Physician Assistant Prgm

Marietta Memorial Hospital
Larry J Unroe, MHA, President
401 Matthew St
Marietta, OH 45750
740 374-1411
Type: Hosp or Med Ctr: 100-299 Beds
Control: Nonprofit (Private or Religious)
- Radiography Prgm

Washington County Career Center
DeWayne O Poling, MA, Director
1750 Lancaster St
Marietta, OH 45750
740 373-6283
Type: Vocational or Tech Sch
Control: State, County, or Local Govt
- Medical Assistant Prgm

Washington State Community College
Charlotte Hatfield, PhD, President
710 Colegate Dr
Marietta, OH 45750
740 374-8716
Type: Junior or Comm Coll
Control: State, County, or Local Govt
- Clin Lab Technician/Med Lab Technician Prgm
- Physical Therapist Assistant Prgm
- Respiratory Therapist (Advanced) Prgm

Marion

Marion Technical College
J Richard Bryson, PhD, President
1467 Mt Vernon Ave
Marion, OH 43302-5694
740 389-4636
Type: Vocational or Tech Sch
Control: Nonprofit (Private or Religious)
- Clin Lab Technician/Med Lab Technician Prgm
- Medical Assistant Prgm
- Physical Therapist Assistant Prgm
- Radiography Prgm

Maumee

Stautzenberger College
George Simon, President
1796 Indian Wood Circle
Maumee, OH 43537
800 552-5099
Type: Vocational or Tech Sch
Control: For Profit
- Medical Assistant Prgm
- Veterinary Technology Prgm (2)

Mayfield Heights

Cleveland Clinic
Fred DeGrandis, CEO, Western Region
6803 Mayfield Rd
Ste 500, Bldg 1
Mayfield Heights, OH 44124
440 312-8720
Type: Hosp or Med Ctr: 300-499 Beds
Control: Nonprofit (Private or Religious)
- Radiography Prgm

Medina

Medina County Career Center
Thomas Horwedel, MEd, Superintendent
1101 W Liberty St
Medina, OH 44256-9969
216 725-8461
Type: Vocational or Tech Sch
Control: State, County, or Local Govt
• Medical Assistant Prgm

Middleburg Heights

Cleveland Institute of Medical Massage
18334-D E Bagley Rd
Middleburg Heights, OH 44130
Type: Vocational or Tech Sch
Control: Nonprofit (Private or Religious)
• Massage Therapy Prgm

Polaris Career Center
Bob Timmons, MA, Superintendent
7285 Old Oak Blvd
Middleburg Heights, OH 44130
440 891-7600
Type: Vocational or Tech Sch
Control: Nonprofit (Private or Religious)
• Dental Assisting Prgm
• Medical Assistant Prgm

Sanford-Brown Institute
Ken Gibson, Executive Director
17535 Rosbough Dr, Ste 100
Middleburg Heights, OH 44130
440 239-9640
Type: Vocational or Tech Sch
Control: For Profit
• Diagnostic Med Sonography Prgm

Southwest General Health Center
Gary Rowe, MA, Interim President, CEO
18697 Bagley Rd
Middleburg Heights, OH 44130
216 816-8051
Type: Hosp or Med Ctr: 300-499 Beds
Control: Nonprofit (Private or Religious)
• Clin Lab Scientist/Med Technologist Prgm

Milan

EHOVE Ghrist Adult Career Center
Sahron Mastroianni, Superintendent
316 W Mason Rd
Milan, OH 44846
419 499-4663
Type: Vocational or Tech Sch
Control: State, County, or Local Govt
• Medical Assistant Prgm
• Surgical Technology Prgm

Mt St Joseph

College of Mt St Joseph
Sr Francis M Thrailkill, PhD OSH, President
5701 Delhi Pike
Mt St Joseph, OH 45051
513 244-4232
Type: 4-year Coll or Univ
Control: Nonprofit (Private or Religious)
• Athletic Training Prgm
• Physical Therapy Prgm

Mt Vernon

Knox County Career Center
Ray Richardson, Superintendent
306 Martinsburg Rd
Mt Vernon, OH 43050
614 397-5820
Type: Vocational or Tech Sch
Control: State, County, or Local Govt
• Medical Assistant Prgm

Nelsonville

Hocking College
John J Light, PhD, President
3301 Hocking Pkwy
Nelsonville, OH 45764
740 753-3591
Type: Junior or Comm Coll
Control: Nonprofit (Private or Religious)
• Dietetic Technician-AD Prgm
• Health Information Tech Prgm
• Medical Assistant Prgm
• Physical Therapist Assistant Prgm

Newark

Central Ohio Technical College
Bonnie Coe, PhD, President
1179 University Dr
Newark, OH 43055-1767
740 364-9509
Type: Junior or Comm Coll
Control: State, County, or Local Govt
• Diagnostic Med Sonography Prgm
• Radiography Prgm
• Surgical Technology Prgm

North Canton

Walsh University
Richard Jusseaume, President
2020 E Maple St
North Canton, OH 44720-3396
330 490-7102
Type: 4-year Coll or Univ
Control: Nonprofit (Private or Religious)
• Physical Therapy Prgm

Oberlin

Lorain Cnty Joint Voc School - Adult Career
William B Randall, MS, Superintendent
15181 St Rte 58
Oberlin, OH 44074
440 774-1056
Type: Vocational or Tech Sch
Control: State, County, or Local Govt
• Medical Assistant Prgm

Oxford

Miami University
David Hodge, PhD, President
201 Roudebush
Oxford, OH 45056
513 529-2345
Type: 4-year Coll or Univ
Control: State, County, or Local Govt
• Athletic Training Prgm
• Dietetics-Didactic Prgm
• Psychology Prgm
• Speech-Language Pathology Prgm

Parma

Bryant & Stratton College - Parma
Lisa Mason, Campus Director
12955 Snow Rd
Parma, OH 44130
216 265-3151
Type: 4-year Coll or Univ
Control: For Profit
• Medical Assistant Prgm

Parma Community General Hospital
Thomas A Selden, Jr, President, CEO
7007 Powers Blvd
Parma, OH 44129-5495
440 888-1800
Type: Hosp or Med Ctr: 300-499 Beds
Control: Nonprofit (Private or Religious)
• Emergency Med Tech-Paramedic Prgm

Pepper Pike

Ursuline College
Anne Marie Diederich, President
2550 Lander Rd
Pepper Pike, OH 44124
216 449-4200
Type: 4-year Coll or Univ
Control: Nonprofit (Private or Religious)
• Art Therapy Prgm
• Nursing Prgm

Piqua

Edison Community College
Kenneth A Yowell, President
1973 Edison Dr
Piqua, OH 45356
800 922-3722
Type: Junior or Comm Coll
Control: State, County, or Local Govt
• Medical Assistant Prgm
• Phlebotomy Prgm

Portsmouth

Shawnee State University
Rita Rice Morris, PhD, President
940 Second St
Portsmouth, OH 45662-4303
740 351-3208
Type: 4-year Coll or Univ
Control: State, County, or Local Govt
• Athletic Training Prgm
• Clin Lab Technician/Med Lab Technician Prgm
• Dental Hygiene Prgm
• Occupational Therapy Asst Prgm
• Occupational Therapy Prgm
• Physical Therapist Assistant Prgm
• Radiography Prgm
• Respiratory Therapist (Advanced) Prgm

Rio Grande

Buckeye Hills Career Center
D Kent Lewis, BS MS, Superintendent
PO Box 157
Rio Grande, OH 45674
740 245-5334
Type: Vocational or Tech Sch
Control: State, County, or Local Govt
• Surgical Technology Prgm

University of Rio Grande
Barry M Dorsey, PhD, President
218 N College Ave
PO Box 500
Rio Grande, OH 45674-0500
740 245-7204
Type: 4-year Coll or Univ
Control: Nonprofit (Private or Religious)
• Clin Lab Technician/Med Lab Technician Prgm
• Diagnostic Med Sonography Prgm

Rootstown

Northeastern Ohio Univ College of Medicine
Lois Margaret Nora, MD JD, President
4209 St Rte 44
PO Box 95
Rootstown, OH 44272
Type: 4-year Coll or Univ
Control: State, County, or Local Govt
• Allopathic Medicine Prgm
• Pharmacy Prgm

Springfield

Clark State Community College
Karen Rafinski, PhD, President
570 E Leffel Ln
Springfield, OH 45505
937 328-6001
Type: Junior or Comm Coll
Control: State, County, or Local Govt
• Clin Lab Technician/Med Lab Technician Prgm
• Physical Therapist Assistant Prgm

St Clairsville

Belmont Technical College
Joseph Bukowski, EdD, President
120 Fox-Shannon Pl
St Clairsville, OH 43950
740 695-9500
Type: Vocational or Tech Sch
Control: State, County, or Local Govt
• Medical Assistant Prgm

Steubenville

Jefferson Community College
Laura M Meeks, PhD, President
4000 Sunset Blvd
Steubenville, OH 43952
740 264-5591
Type: Junior or Comm Coll
Control: Fed Govt
• Clin Lab Technician/Med Lab Technician Prgm
• Dental Assisting Prgm
• Medical Assistant Prgm
• Radiography Prgm
• Respiratory Therapist (Advanced) Prgm

Sylvania

Lourdes College
George Matthews, PhD, President
6832 Convent Blvd
Sylvania, OH 43560-2898
419 885-3211
Type: 4-year Coll or Univ
Control: Nonprofit (Private or Religious)
• Nursing Prgm

Toledo

Davis College
Diane Brunner, MEd, President/CEO
4747 Monroe St
Toledo, OH 43623
419 473-2700
Type: Junior or Comm Coll
Control: For Profit
• Medical Assistant Prgm

Mercy College of Northwest Ohio
Paul Kessler, EdD, President
2221 Madison Ave
Toledo, OH 43624-1133
419 259-1279
Type: 4-year Coll or Univ
Control: Nonprofit (Private or Religious)
• Health Information Tech Prgm
• Nursing Prgm
• Radiography Prgm

Owens Community College

Christa Adams, PhD, President
Oregon Rd, PO Box 10000
Toledo, OH 43699
567 661-7210
Type: Junior or Comm Coll
Control: State, County, or Local Govt
• Dental Hygiene Prgm
• Diagnostic Med Sonography Prgm
• Dietetic Technician-AD Prgm
• Health Information Tech Prgm
• Occupational Therapy Asst Prgm
• Physical Therapist Assistant Prgm
• Radiography Prgm
• Surgical Technology Prgm

Professional Skills Institute
Patricia A Finch, RN, President
20 Arco Dr
Toledo, OH 43607
419 531-9610
Type: Acad Health Ctr/Med Sch
Control: For Profit
• Health Information Tech Prgm
• Physical Therapist Assistant Prgm

St Vincent Mercy Medical Center
Steven C Mickus, President
2213 Cherry St
Toledo, OH 43608
419 251-4152
Type: Hosp or Med Ctr: 500> Beds
Control: Nonprofit (Private or Religious)
• Clin Lab Scientist/Med Technologist Prgm

University of Toledo
Lloyd Jacobs, MD, President
2801 W Bancroft St
Toledo, OH 43606-3390
419 530-2211
Type: 4-year Coll or Univ
Control: Nonprofit (Private or Religious)
• Allopathic Medicine Prgm
• Athletic Training Prgm
• Cardiovascular Technology Prgm
• Counseling Prgm
• Health Information Admin Prgm
• Kinesiotherapy Prgm
• Nursing Prgm
• Occupational Therapy Prgm
• Pharmacy Prgm
• Physical Therapy Prgm
• Physician Assistant Prgm
• Psychology Prgm
• Respiratory Therapist (Advanced) Prgm
• Respiratory Therapist (Entry-Level) Prgm
• Speech-Language Pathology Prgm
• Therapeutic Recreation Specialist Prgm

Urbana

Urbana University
Robert L Head, PhD, President
579 College Way
Urbana, OH 43078
937 484-1300
Type: 4-year Coll or Univ
Control: Nonprofit (Private or Religious)
• Athletic Training Prgm
• Nursing Prgm

INSTITUTIONS

Warren

Trumbull Career & Technical Center
Wayne McClain, PhD, Superintendent
528 Educational Hwy
Warren, OH 44483
330 847-0503
Type: Vocational or Tech Sch
Control: State, County, or Local Govt
• Medical Assistant Prgm

Trumbull Memorial Hospital
Kris Hoce, MBA, President and CEO
1350 E Market St
Warren, OH 44482
216 841-9117
Type: Hosp or Med Ctr: 300-499 Beds
Control: Nonprofit (Private or Religious)
• Phlebotomy Prgm

Westerville

Otterbein College
C Brent DeVore, PhD, President
Roush Hall 302
Westerville, OH 43081
614 823-1410
Type: 4-year Coll or Univ
Control: Nonprofit (Private or Religious)
• Athletic Training Prgm
• Nursing Prgm

Wilmington

Wilmington College
Daniel DiBiasio, PhD, President
1870 Quaker Way
Pyle Center Box 1246
Wilmington, OH 45177
937 382-6661
Type: 4-year Coll or Univ
Control: Nonprofit (Private or Religious)
• Athletic Training Prgm

Wooster

College of Wooster
R Stanton Hales, Director
1189 Beall Ave
Wooster, OH 44691
330 263-2311
Type: 4-year Coll or Univ
Control: State, County, or Local Govt
• Music Therapy Prgm

Youngstown

Choffin Career & Technical Center
Wendy Webb, PhD, Superintendent
20 W Wood St
Youngstown, OH 44501
330 744-6915
Type: Vocational or Tech Sch
Control: State, County, or Local Govt
• Dental Assisting Prgm
• Surgical Technology Prgm

St Elizabeth Health Center
Robert Shroder, MHA, President/CEO
1044 Belmont Ave
Youngstown, OH 44501-1790
330 746-7211
Type: Hosp or Med Ctr: 300-499 Beds
Control: Nonprofit (Private or Religious)
• Nuclear Medicine Technology Prgm

Youngstown State University
David C Sweet, PhD, President
One University Plaza
Youngstown, OH 44555
330 941-3101
Type: 4-year Coll or Univ
Control: State, County, or Local Govt
• Clin Lab Technician/Med Lab Technician Prgm
• Counseling Prgm
• Dental Hygiene Prgm
• Dietetic Technician-AD Prgm
• Dietetics-Coordinated Prgm
• Dietetics-Didactic Prgm
• Emergency Med Tech-Paramedic Prgm
• Histotechnician Prgm
• Medical Assistant Prgm
• Physical Therapy Prgm
• Respiratory Therapist (Advanced) Prgm

Zanesville

Zane State College
Paul Brown, EdD, President
1555 Newark Rd
Zanesville, OH 43701-2694
740 454-2501
Type: Junior or Comm Coll
Control: State, County, or Local Government
• Clin Lab Technician/Med Lab Technician Prgm
• Medical Assistant Prgm
• Occupational Therapy Asst Prgm
• Phlebotomy Prgm
• Physical Therapist Assistant Prgm
• Radiography Prgm

Oklahoma

Ada

East Central University
Richard Rafes, PhD JD, President
1100 E 14th St
Ada, OK 74820
405 332-8000
Type: 4-year Coll or Univ
Control: State, County, or Local Govt
• Athletic Training Prgm
• Health Information Admin Prgm
• Rehabilitation Counseling Prgm

Valley View Regional Hospital
Ron Webb, MHA, President
Health Administration
430 N Monta Vista
Ada, OK 74820
405 332-2323
Type: Hosp or Med Ctr: 100-299 Beds
Control: Nonprofit (Private or Religious)
• Clin Lab Scientist/Med Technologist Prgm

Altus

Western Oklahoma State College
Randy Cumby, MEd, President
2801 N Main
Altus, OK 73521-1397
580 477-2000
Type: Junior or Comm Coll
Control: State, County, or Local Govt
• Radiography Prgm

Ardmore

Southern Oklahoma Technology Center
David Powell, PhD, Superintendent
2610 Sam Noble Pkwy
Ardmore, OK 73401
580 223-2070
Type: Vocational or Tech Sch
Control: State, County, or Local Government
• Surgical Technology Prgm

Bartlesville

Oklahoma Wesleyan University
Bartlesville, OK 74006
Type: 4-year Coll or Univ
Control: Nonprofit (Private or Religious)
• Nursing Prgm

Bethany

Southern Nazarene University
Loren P Gresham, PhD, President
6729 NW 39th Expwy
Bethany, OK 73008
405 491-6300
Type: 4-year Coll or Univ
Control: Nonprofit (Private or Religious)
• Athletic Training Prgm
• Nursing Prgm

Drumright

Central Technology Center
Phil Waul, MA, Superintendent
3 CT Circle
Drumright, OK 74030
918 352-2551
Type: Vocational or Tech Sch
Control: Nonprofit (Private or Religious)
• Surgical Technology Prgm

Edmond

University of Central Oklahoma
W Roger Webb, President
100 N University Dr
Edmond, OK 73034
405 974-2000
Type: 4-year Coll or Univ
Control: State, County, or Local Govt
• Dietetic Internship Prgm
• Dietetics-Didactic Prgm
• Speech-Language Pathology Prgm

El Reno

Canadian Valley Technology Center
Earl Cowan, EdD, Superintendent
6505 E Hwy 66
El Reno, OK 73036
405 262-2629
Type: Vocational or Tech Sch
Control: State, County, or Local Govt
• Surgical Technology Prgm

Enid

Autry Technology Center
James Strate, EdD, Superintendent
1201 W Willow
Enid, OK 73703
405 242-2750
Type: Vocational or Tech Sch
Control: State, County, or Local Govt
• Radiography Prgm
• Surgical Technology Prgm

Fort Cobb

SW Oklahoma St Univ/Caddo Kiowa Tech Ctr
Jerry L Martin, MEd, Superintendent
PO Box 190
Fort Cobb, OK 73038
405 643-5511
Type: Vocational or Tech Sch
Control: Nonprofit (Private or Religious)
• Occupational Therapy Asst Prgm
• Physical Therapist Assistant Prgm

Langston

Langston University
Ernest L Holloway, President
Langston, OK 73050
405 466-2231
Type: 4-year Coll or Univ
Control: State, County, or Local Govt
• Dietetics-Didactic Prgm
• Physical Therapy Prgm
• Rehabilitation Counseling Prgm

Lawton

Comanche County Memorial Hospital
Randy Segler, MHA, Chief Executive Officer
3401 W Gore Blvd Box 129
Lawton, OK 73502
405 355-8620
Type: Hosp or Med Ctr: 100-299 Beds
Control: State, County, or Local Govt
• Clin Lab Scientist/Med Technologist Prgm

Great Plains Technology Center
James Nisbett, MSEd, Superintendent
4500 W Lee Blvd
Lawton, OK 73505
580 355-6371
Type: Vocational or Tech Sch
Control: State, County, or Local Govt
• Radiography Prgm
• Respiratory Therapist (Entry-Level) Prgm
• Surgical Technology Prgm

Miami

Northeastern Oklahoma A&M College
Glenn E Mayle, EdD, President
200 I St
PO Box 3841
Miami, OK 74354
918 542-8441
Type: Junior or Comm Coll
Control: State, County, or Local Govt
• Clin Lab Technician/Med Lab Technician Prgm
• Physical Therapist Assistant Prgm

Midwest City

Rose State College
Terry Britton, PhD, President
6420 SE 15th
Midwest City, OK 73110-2797
405 733-7300
Type: Junior or Comm Coll
Control: State, County, or Local Govt
• Clin Lab Technician/Med Lab Technician Prgm
• Dental Assisting Prgm
• Dental Hygiene Prgm
• Health Information Tech Prgm
• Radiography Prgm
• Respiratory Therapist (Advanced) Prgm

Moore

Oklahoma Health Academy
Mike Pugliese, President
1939 N Moore Ave
Moore, OK 73160
405 912-2777
Type: Vocational or Tech Sch
Control: State, County, or Local Government
• Surgical Technology Prgm

Muskogee

Bacone College
Robert Duncan, DMin, President
Office of the President
Muskogee, OK 74403-1568
888 682-5514
Type: 4-year Coll or Univ
Control: Nonprofit (Private or Religious)
• Radiography Prgm

Indian Capital Technology Center
Tom Stiles, Superintendent
2403 N 41st St East
Muskogee, OK 74403
918 687-7565
Type: Vocational or Tech Sch
Control: State, County, or Local Govt
• Radiography Prgm

Muskogee Regional Medical Center
Anthony Armstrong, CEO
300 Rockefeller Dr
Muskogee, OK 74401
918 682-5501
Type: Hosp or Med Ctr: 300-499 Beds
Control: State, County, or Local Govt
• Clin Lab Scientist/Med Technologist Prgm

Norman

Moore Norman Technology Center
John Hunter, MEd, Superintendant
4701 12th Ave NW
Norman, OK 73070-4701
405 364-5763
Type: Vocational or Tech Sch
Control: State, County, or Local Govt
• Dental Assisting Prgm
• Diagnostic Med Sonography Prgm
• Medical Assistant Prgm
• Surgical Technology Prgm

University of Oklahoma
David L Boren, President
660 Parrington Oval
Norman, OK 73019
405 325-3916
Type: 4-year Coll or Univ
Control: State, County, or Local Govt
• Allopathic Medicine Prgm
• Medical Librarian Prgm
• Pharmacy Prgm
• Physician Assistant Prgm

Oklahoma City

Francis Tuttle Technology Center
Kay Martin, PhD, Superintendent/CEO
12777 N Rockwell Ave
Oklahoma City, OK 73142
405 717-4266
Type: Vocational or Tech Sch
Control: State, County, or Local Govt
• Medical Assistant Prgm
• Respiratory Therapist (Advanced) Prgm

Metro Technology Centers
James Branscum, EdD, Superintendent
1900 Springlake Dr
Oklahoma City, OK 73111
405 605-4400
Type: Vocational or Tech Sch
Control: State, County, or Local Govt
• Dental Assisting Prgm
• Medical Assistant Prgm
• Radiography Prgm
• Surgical Technology Prgm

Oklahoma City Community College
Paul W Sechrist, PhD, President
7777 S May Ave
Oklahoma City, OK 73159-4444
405 682-7502
Type: Junior or Comm Coll
Control: State, County, or Local Govt
• Emergency Med Tech-Paramedic Prgm
• Occupational Therapy Asst Prgm
• Physical Therapist Assistant Prgm

Platt College
Micheal A Pugliese, President
309 S Ann Arbor
Oklahoma City, OK 73128
405 946-7799
Type: Vocational or Tech Sch
Control: For Profit
• Surgical Technology Prgm (2)

INSTITUTIONS

Univ of Oklahoma Health Sciences Center
Joseph J Ferretti, PhD, SVP/Provost
1000 Stanton L Young, Ste 221
Oklahoma City, OK 73117-1213
405 271-2332
Type: Acad Health Ctr/Med Sch
Control: State, County, or Local Govt
- Audiologist Prgm
- Dental Hygiene Prgm
- Diagnostic Med Sonography Prgm
- Dietetic Internship Prgm
- Dietetics-Coordinated Prgm
- Dietetics-Didactic Prgm
- Genetic Counseling Prgm
- Nuclear Medicine Technology Prgm
- Occupational Therapy Prgm (2)
- Physical Therapy Prgm
- Physician Assistant Prgm
- Radiation Therapy Prgm
- Radiography Prgm
- Speech-Language Pathology Prgm

University of Oklahoma Health Sciences Center
940 NE 13th St
Oklahoma City, OK 73104
Type: Hosp or Med Ctr: 300-499 Beds
Control: Nonprofit (Private or Religious)
- Dentistry Prgm

Poteau

Carl Albert State College
Joe E White, PhD, President
1507 S McKenna
Poteau, OK 74953-5208
918 647-1210
Type: Junior or Comm Coll
Control: Nonprofit (Private or Religious)
- Physical Therapist Assistant Prgm
- Radiography Prgm

Seminole

Seminole State College
James W Utterback, PhD, President
2701 Boren Blvd
PO Box 351
Seminole, OK 74818-0351
405 382-9950
Type: Junior or Comm Coll
Control: State, County, or Local Govt
- Clin Lab Technician/Med Lab Technician Prgm

Stillwater

Meridian Technology Center
Andrea Kelly, EdD, Superintendent
1312 S Sangre St
Stillwater, OK 74074
405 377-3333
Type: Vocational or Tech Sch
Control: State, County, or Local Govt
- Radiography Prgm

Oklahoma State University
Marlene Strathe, Interim President, CEO
Stillwater, OK 74078
405 744-5000
Type: 4-year Coll or Univ
Control: State, County, or Local Govt
- Athletic Training Prgm
- Counseling Prgm
- Dietetic Internship Prgm
- Dietetics-Didactic Prgm
- Osteopathic Medicine Prgm
- Psychology Prgm
- Speech-Language Pathology Prgm
- Therapeutic Recreation Specialist Prgm
- Veterinary Medicine Prgm
- Veterinary Technology Prgm

Tahlequah

Northeastern State University
W Roger Webb, President
Tahlequah, OK 74464
918 456-5511
Type: 4-year Coll or Univ
Control: State, County, or Local Govt
- Dietetics-Didactic Prgm
- Optometry Prgm
- Speech-Language Pathology Prgm

Tishomingo

Murray State College
William Pennington, PhD, President
One Murray Campus
NAH 116
Tishomingo, OK 73460
580 371-2371
Type: Junior or Comm Coll
Control: State, County, or Local Govt
- Physical Therapist Assistant Prgm
- Veterinary Technology Prgm

Tulsa

Community Care College
Teresa Knox, CEO
4242 S Sheridan
Tulsa, OK 74145
918 610-0027
Type: Vocational or Tech Sch
Control: For Profit
- Surgical Technology Prgm

Oral Roberts University
Tulsa, OK 74171
Control: Nonprofit (Private or Religious)
- Nursing Prgm

Orthoptic Teaching Program of Tulsa
6606 S Yale Ste 110
Tulsa, OK 74136
Type: Hosp or Med Ctr: 300-499 Beds
Control: Nonprofit (Private or Religious)
- Orthoptist Prgm

Saint Francis Hospital
Jake Henry, MD, CEO
6161 S Yale Ave
Tulsa, OK 74136
918 494-6342
Type: Hosp or Med Ctr: 500> Beds
Control: Nonprofit (Private or Religious)
- Clin Lab Scientist/Med Technologist Prgm

Tulsa Community College
Thomas McKeon, EdD, President, CEO
Central Office
6111 E Skelly Dr
Tulsa, OK 74135-6198
918 595-7868
Type: Junior or Comm Coll
Control: State, County, or Local Govt
- Clin Lab Technician/Med Lab Technician Prgm
- Dental Hygiene Prgm
- Health Information Tech Prgm
- Medical Assistant Prgm
- Occupational Therapy Asst Prgm
- Phlebotomy Prgm
- Physical Therapist Assistant Prgm
- Radiography Prgm
- Respiratory Therapist (Advanced) Prgm
- Veterinary Technology Prgm

Tulsa Technology Center
Gene Callahan, EdD, Superintendent
6111 E Skelly Dr
Tulsa, OK 74135-6100
918 828-5007
Type: Vocational or Tech Sch
Control: State, County, or Local Govt
- Radiography Prgm
- Surgical Technology Prgm

University of Tulsa
Steadman Upham, PhD, President
600 S College Ave
Tulsa, OK 74104
918 631-2000
Type: 4-year Coll or Univ
Control: Nonprofit (Private or Religious)
- Athletic Training Prgm
- Psychology Prgm
- Speech-Language Pathology Prgm

Weatherford

Southwestern Oklahoma State University
John Hays, EdD, President
100 Campus Dr
Weatherford, OK 73096
580 774-3766
Type: 4-year Coll or Univ
Control: State, County, or Local Govt
- Athletic Training Prgm
- Health Information Admin Prgm
- Music Therapy Prgm
- Pharmacy Prgm
- Radiography Prgm

Wetumka

Wes Watkins Technology Center District 25
James R Moore, MS, Superintendent
7892 Hwy 9
Wetumka, OK 74883
405 452-5500
Type: Vocational or Tech Sch
Control: State, County, or Local Govt
- Surgical Technology Prgm

Ontario, Canada

Brantford

Mohawk College
411 Elgin St
Brantford, ON N3T 5V2
Type: 4-year Coll or Univ
Control: State, County, or Local Govt
• Orientation and Mobility Specialist Prgm
• Vision Rehabilitation Therapy Prgm

Guelph

University of Guelph
Alastair Summerlee, President
50 Stone Rd E
Guelph, ON N1G 2W1
519 824-4120
Type: 4-year Coll or Univ
Control: State, County, or Local Government
• Veterinary Medicine Prgm
• Veterinary Technology Prgm

Hamiliton

McMaster University
1400 Main St W
IAHS - 403
Hamiliton, ON L8N 3Z5
905 525-9140
Type: 4-year Coll or Univ
Control: Nonprofit (Private or Religious)
• Allopathic Medicine Prgm

Kingston

Queen's University
Kingston, ON K7L 3N6
Type: Acad Health Ctr/Med Sch
Control: State, County, or Local Govt
• Allopathic Medicine Prgm

London

University of Western Ontario
London, ON N6G 1H1
Control: Nonprofit (Private or Religious)
• Allopathic Medicine Prgm
• Medical Librarian Prgm
• Physical Therapy Prgm

Ottawa

University of Ottawa
501 Smyth Rd
Ottawa, ON K1H 8M5
Control: Nonprofit (Private or Religious)
• Allopathic Medicine Prgm
• Ophthalmic Med Technologist Prgm
• Psychology Prgm

Thunder Bay, Sudbury

Northern Ontario Medical School
Thunder Bay, Sudbury, ON P7B 5E1
Type: Acad Health Ctr/Med Sch
Control: State, County, or Local Government
• Allopathic Medicine Prgm

Toronto

Hospital for Sick Children
Mary Jo Haddad
555 University Ave
Toronto, ON M5G 1X8
416 813-5798
Type: Hosp or Med Ctr: 100-299 Beds
Control: Nonprofit (Private or Religious)
• Orthoptist Prgm

ICT Kikkawa College
Shirley Desborough, Chief Executive Officer
2340 Dundas St W
Unit G-04
Toronto, ON M6P 4A9
416 762-4857
Type: Vocational or Tech Sch
Control: For Profit
• Massage Therapy Prgm

ICT Northumberland College
Shirley Desborough, RMT CST AT, Chief
   Executive Officer
2340 Dundas St W
Toronto, ON M6P 4A9
416 762-4857
Type: Vocational or Tech Sch
Control: For Profit
• Massage Therapy Prgm

University of Toronto
David Naylor, MD DPhil, President
Simcoe Hall, Room 206
27 King's College Circle
Toronto, ON M5S 1A1
416 978-2121
Type: 4-year Coll or Univ
Control: Nonprofit (Private or Religious)
• Allopathic Medicine Prgm
• Genetic Counseling Prgm
• Medical Illustrator Prgm
• Medical Librarian Prgm
• Physical Therapy Prgm

York University
Toronto, ON M3J 1P3
Type: 4-year Coll or Univ
Control: Nonprofit (Private or Religious)
• Psychology Prgm (2)

Waterloo

University of Waterloo
Thomas Freddo, OD PhD, Director
Waterloo, ON N2L 3G1
519 888-4567
Type: 4-year Coll or Univ
Control: Nonprofit (Private or Religious)
• Optometry Prgm
• Psychology Prgm

Windsor

University of Windsor
Windsor, ON N9B 3P4
519 253-3000
Type: 4-year Coll or Univ
Control: Nonprofit (Private or Religious)
• Music Therapy Prgm

Oregon

Albany

Linn-Benton Community College
Rita Cavin, PhD, President
6500 SW Pacific Blvd
Albany, OR 97321
541 917-4999
Type: Junior or Comm Coll
Control: State, County, or Local Govt
• Dental Assisting Prgm
• Medical Assistant Prgm

Beaverton

College of Emergency Services (CESWA)
Carl T Miller, MS EMT-P, CEO, Program Director
9735 SW Sunshine Ct #1000
Beaverton, OR 97005
503 644-9999
Type: Junior or Comm Coll
Control: Nonprofit (Private or Religious)
• Emergency Med Tech-Paramedic Prgm

Bend

Central Oregon Community College
James Middleton, EdD, President
2600 NW College Way
Bend, OR 97701
541 383-7201
Type: Junior or Comm Coll
Control: State, County, or Local Govt
• Dental Assisting Prgm
• Health Information Tech Prgm
• Medical Assistant Prgm

Corvallis

Oregon State University
Edward Ray, PhD, President
646 Kerr Administration Bldg
Corvallis, OR 97331
541 737-4133
Type: 4-year Coll or Univ
Control: State, County, or Local Govt
• Athletic Training Prgm
• Counseling Prgm
• Dietetics-Didactic Prgm
• Pharmacy Prgm
• Veterinary Medicine Prgm

Eugene

Lane Community College
Mary Spilde, PhD, President
4000 E 30th Ave
Eugene, OR 97405-0640
541 463-3000
Type: Junior or Comm Coll
Control: State, County, or Local Govt
• Dental Assisting Prgm
• Dental Hygiene Prgm
• Medical Assistant Prgm
• Respiratory Therapist (Advanced) Prgm

INSTITUTIONS

University of Oregon
David B Frohnmayer, President
Eugene, OR 97403
503 346-3111
Type: 4-year Coll or Univ
Control: State, County, or Local Govt
• Psychology Prgm
• Speech-Language Pathology Prgm

Forest Grove

Pacific University
Philip Creighton, PhD, President
2043 College Way
Forest Grove, OR 97116-1797
503 352-2214
Type: 4-year Coll or Univ
Control: Nonprofit (Private or Religious)
• Occupational Therapy Prgm
• Optometry Prgm
• Pharmacy Prgm
• Physical Therapy Prgm
• Physician Assistant Prgm
• Psychology Prgm

Gresham

Mt Hood Community College
Robert M Silverman, PhD, President
26000 SE Stark St
Gresham, OR 97030-3300
503 491-7212
Type: Junior or Comm Coll
Control: State, County, or Local Govt
• Dental Hygiene Prgm
• Medical Assistant Prgm
• Physical Therapist Assistant Prgm
• Respiratory Therapist (Advanced) Prgm
• Surgical Technology Prgm

Klamath Falls

Oregon Institute of Technology
Martha Anne Dow, PhD, President
3201 Campus Dr
Klamath Falls, OR 97601-8801
503 885-1101
Type: 4-year Coll or Univ
Control: State, County, or Local Govt
• Dental Hygiene Prgm
• Respiratory Therapist (Advanced) Prgm

Marylhurst

Marylhurst University
Nancy Wilgenbusch, PhD, President
17600 Pacific Hwy
Marylhurst, OR 97036-0261
503 636-8141
Type: 4-year Coll or Univ
Control: Nonprofit (Private or Religious)
• Art Therapy Prgm
• Music Therapy Prgm

McMinnville

Linfield College
Thomas Hellie, PhD, President
900 SE Baker St
McMinnville, OR 97128
503 434-2234
Type: 4-year Coll or Univ
Control: Nonprofit (Private or Religious)
• Athletic Training Prgm
• Nursing Prgm

Monmouth

Western Oregon University
John Minahan, PhD, President
345 N Monmouth Ave
Monmouth, OR 97361
503 838-8888
Type: 4-year Coll or Univ
Control: State, County, or Local Govt
• Rehabilitation Counseling Prgm

Newberg

George Fox University
David Brandt, PhD, President
414 N Meridian St #6305
Newberg, OR 97132
503 554-2102
Type: 4-year Coll or Univ
Control: Nonprofit (Private or Religious)
• Athletic Training Prgm
• Psychology Prgm

Oregon City

Clackamas Community College
Earl P Johnson, PhD, President
19600 S Molalla Ave
Oregon City, OR 97045
503 657-6958
Type: Hosp or Med Ctr <100 Beds
Control: State, County, or Local Govt
• Clinical Assisting Prgm
• Medical Assistant Prgm

Pendleton

Blue Mountain Community College
John Turner, President
2411 NW Carden
PO Box 100
Pendleton, OR 97801
541 278-5950
Type: Junior or Comm Coll
Control: State, County, or Local Govt
• Dental Assisting Prgm

Portland

Concorde Career Institute - Portland
Kevin Lambert, School Director
1425 NE Irving, Bldg 300
Portland, OR 97232
503 281-4181
Type: Vocational or Tech Sch
Control: For Profit
• Dental Assisting Prgm
• Medical Assistant Prgm
• Surgical Technology Prgm

East-West Coll of the Healing Arts
David Slawson
525 NE Oregon St
Portland, OR 97232
503 233-6500
Type: Vocational or Tech Sch
Control: For Profit
• Massage Therapy Prgm

Everest College
Mickey Sieracki, MA MT(ASCP), President
425 SW Washington St
Portland, OR 97204
503 222-3225
Type: Vocational or Tech Sch
Control: For Profit
• Medical Assistant Prgm

Heald College - Portland
Amy McCombs, BA MA, President
625 SW Broadway
Ste 200
Portland, OR 97205
415 808-1400
Type: Vocational or Tech Sch
Control: Nonprofit (Private or Religious)
• Medical Assistant Prgm

Oregon Health & Science University
Joseph E Robertson, MD MBA, President
3181 SW Sam Jackson Pk Rd, L101
Portland, OR 97239
503 494-8252
Type: Acad Health Ctr/Med Sch
Control: Nonprofit (Private or Religious)
• Allopathic Medicine Prgm
• Clin Lab Scientist/Med Technologist Prgm
• Dentistry Prgm
• Dietetic Internship Prgm
• Emergency Med Tech-Paramedic Prgm
• Nursing Prgm
• Physician Assistant Prgm
• Radiation Therapy Prgm

Portland Community College
Preston Pulliams, EdD, District President
PO Box 19000
Portland, OR 97280-0990
503 977-4365
Type: Junior or Comm Coll
Control: State, County, or Local Govt
• Clin Lab Technician/Med Lab Technician Prgm
• Dental Assisting Prgm
• Dental Hygiene Prgm
• Dental Lab Technician Prgm
• Health Information Tech Prgm
• Medical Assistant Prgm
• Ophthalmic Med Technician Prgm
• Radiography Prgm
• Veterinary Technology Prgm

Portland State University
Daniel Bernstine, President
Portland, OR 97207-0751
503 725-3000
Type: 4-year Coll or Univ
Control: State, County, or Local Govt
• Audiologist Prgm
• Counseling Prgm
• Rehabilitation Counseling Prgm
• Speech-Language Pathology Prgm

University of Portland
Portland, OR 97203
Type: 4-year Coll or Univ
Control: State, County, or Local Govt
• Nursing Prgm

Salem

Chemeketa Community College
Gretchen Schuette, PhD, President
4000 Lancaster Dr NE
PO Box 14007
Salem, OR 97309-7070
503 399-6591
Type: Junior or Comm Coll
Control: State, County, or Local Govt
• Dental Assisting Prgm
• Emergency Med Tech-Paramedic Prgm

Mid Willamette Valley Dietetic Internship
Capital Manor Retirement Community
1955 Dallas Hwy NW, Ste 1200
Salem, OR 97304
503 362-4101
Control: For Profit
• Dietetic Internship Prgm

Pennsylvania

Abington

Abington Memorial Hospital
Richard Jones, MS, President and CEO
1200 Old York Rd
Abington, PA 19001
215 576-2000
Type: Hosp or Med Ctr: 500> Beds
Control: Nonprofit (Private or Religious)
• Nuclear Medicine Technology Prgm
• Radiography Prgm

Allentown

Cedar Crest College
Jill L. Sherman, PhD, President
100 College Dr
Allentown, PA 18104-6196
610 437-4471
Type: 4-year Coll or Univ
Control: Nonprofit (Private or Religious)
• Dietetics-Didactic Prgm
• Nuclear Medicine Technology Prgm

Lehigh Valley Hospital
Elliot J Sussman, MD MBA, President/CEO
Cedar Crest and I-78
PO Box 689
Allentown, PA 18105-1556
610 402-2204
Type: Hosp or Med Ctr: 500> Beds
Control: Nonprofit (Private or Religious)
• Emergency Med Tech-Paramedic Prgm

Sodexho Health Care Services
Allentown, PA 18106
Control: For Profit
• Dietetic Internship Prgm
• Dietetics-Preprofessional Practice Prgm

Altoona

Altoona Regional Health System
James W Barner, MBA, President/CEO
620 Howard Ave
Altoona, PA 16601-4899
814 889-2223
Type: Hosp or Med Ctr: 500> Beds
Control: Nonprofit (Private or Religious)
• Clin Lab Scientist/Med Technologist Prgm

Greater Altoona Career & Technology Center
Lanny F Ross, DEd, Executive Director
1500 Fourth Ave
Altoona, PA 16602
814 946-8450
Type: Vocational or Tech Sch
Control: State, County, or Local Govt
• Medical Assistant Prgm

Annville

Lebanon Valley College
Stephen C MacDonald, President
Humanities 102
Annville, PA 17003-0501
717 867-6211
Type: Acad Health Ctr/Med Sch
Control: Nonprofit (Private or Religious)
• Physical Therapy Prgm

Aston

Neumann College
Rosalie Mirenda, DNSC, President
One Neumann Dr
Aston, PA 19014
610 558-5501
Type: 4-year Coll or Univ
Control: Nonprofit (Private or Religious)
• Athletic Training Prgm
• Clin Lab Scientist/Med Technologist Prgm
• Physical Therapy Prgm

Bethlehem

Moravian College
Bethlehem, PA 18018
Type: 4-year Coll or Univ
Control: Nonprofit (Private or Religious)
• Nursing Prgm

Northampton Community College
Arthur Scott, EdD, President
3835 Green Pond Rd
Bethlehem, PA 18020
610 861-5458
Type: Junior or Comm Coll
Control: State, County, or Local Govt
• Dental Hygiene Prgm
• Diagnostic Med Sonography Prgm
• Radiography Prgm
• Surgical Technology Prgm

St Luke's Hospital
Richard Anderson, President
801 Ostrum St
Bethlehem, PA 18015
610 954-4900
Type: Hosp or Med Ctr: 300-499 Beds
Control: Nonprofit (Private or Religious)
• Surgical Technology Prgm

Bloomsburg

Bloomsburg University
Jessica S Kozloff, PhD, President
Bloomsburg, PA 17815
570 389-4000
Type: 4-year Coll or Univ
Control: State, County, or Local Govt
• Audiologist Prgm
• Nursing Prgm
• Speech-Language Pathology Prgm

Blue Bell

Montgomery County Community College
Karen Stout, EdD, President
340 DeKalb Pike
East House
Blue Bell, PA 19422
215 641-6506
Type: Junior or Comm Coll
Control: State, County, or Local Govt
• Clin Lab Technician/Med Lab Technician Prgm
• Dental Hygiene Prgm
• Medical Assistant Prgm
• Phlebotomy Prgm
• Radiography Prgm
• Surgical Technology Prgm

Blue Ridge Summit

Synergy Healting Arts Center & Massage School
13593 Monterey Ln
Blue Ridge Summit, PA 17214
Type: Vocational or Tech Sch
Control: Nonprofit (Private or Religious)
• Massage Therapy Prgm

Bradford

Bradford Regional Medical Center
George E Leonhardt, President/CEO
116 Interstate Pkwy
PO Box 0218
Bradford, PA 16701-0218
814 368-4143
Type: Hosp or Med Ctr: 100-299 Beds
Control: Nonprofit (Private or Religious)
• Radiography Prgm

Bryn Mawr

Harcum College
Jon DeTemple, PhD, President
750 Montgomery Ave
Bryn Mawr, PA 19010
610 526-6024
Type: Junior or Comm Coll
Control: Nonprofit (Private or Religious)
• Clin Lab Technician/Med Lab Technician Prgm
• Dental Assisting Prgm
• Dental Hygiene Prgm
• Physical Therapist Assistant Prgm
• Radiography Prgm
• Veterinary Technology Prgm

Butler

Butler County Community College
Nicholas Neupauer, EdD, President
PO Box 1203
College Dr
Butler, PA 16003-1203
412 287-8711
Type: Junior or Comm Coll
Control: State, County, or Local Govt
• Medical Assistant Prgm
• Physical Therapist Assistant Prgm

California

California University of Pennsylvania
Angelo Armenti, Jr, PhD, President
250 University Ave
California, PA 15419
412 938-4400
Type: 4-year Coll or Univ
Control: State, County, or Local Govt
• Athletic Training Prgm
• Nursing Prgm
• Physical Therapist Assistant Prgm
• Speech-Language Pathology Prgm

Camp Hill

Holy Spirit Hospital
Romaine Niemeyer, MHA, President
503 N 21st St
Camp Hill, PA 17011-2288
717 763-2106
Type: Hosp or Med Ctr: 300-499 Beds
Control: Nonprofit (Private or Religious)
• Radiography Prgm

Center Valley

DeSales University
Bernard O'Connor, OSFS PhD, President
2755 Station Ave
Center Valley, PA 18034-9568
610 282-1100
Type: 4-year Coll or Univ
Control: Nonprofit (Private or Religious)
• Physician Assistant Prgm

Chambersburg

Wilson College
Lorna Duphiney Edmundson, President
1015 Philadelphia Ave
Chambersburg, PA 17204
717 264-3226
Type: Acad Health Ctr/Med Sch
Control: For Profit
• Veterinary Technology Prgm

Chester

Widener University
James T Harris, EdD, President
One University Pl
Chester, PA 19013
610 499-4102
Type: 4-year Coll or Univ
Control: Nonprofit (Private or Religious)
• Nursing Prgm
• Physical Therapy Prgm
• Psychology Prgm

Clarion

Clarion University of Pennsylvania
Joseph Grunenwald, President
Clarion, PA 16214
814 393-2000
Type: 4-year Coll or Univ
Control: State, County, or Local Govt
• Medical Librarian Prgm
• Speech-Language Pathology Prgm

Clearfield

Clearfield Hospital
David McConnell, CHE NHA, Acting
   President/CEO
PO Box 992
Clearfield, PA 16830
814 768-2497
Type: Hosp or Med Ctr <100 Beds
Control: Nonprofit (Private or Religious)
• Radiography Prgm

Cresson

Mount Aloysius College
Mary Ann Dillon, MD RSM
7373 Admiral Peary Hwy
Cresson, PA 16630
814 886-4131
Type: 4-year Coll or Univ
Control: Nonprofit (Private or Religious)
• Medical Assistant Prgm
• Occupational Therapy Asst Prgm
• Physical Therapist Assistant Prgm
• Surgical Technology Prgm

Dallas

Misericordia Unversity
Michael MacDowell, EdD, President
301 Lake St
Dallas, PA 18612-1098
570 674-6265
Type: 4-year Coll or Univ
Control: Nonprofit (Private or Religious)
• Diagnostic Med Sonography Prgm
• Nursing Prgm
• Occupational Therapy Prgm
• Physical Therapy Prgm
• Radiography Prgm

Danville

Geisinger Medical Center
Glenn Steele, MD, President
100 N Academy Ave
Danville, PA 17822-2201
570 271-5200
Type: Hosp or Med Ctr: 300-499 Beds
Control: Nonprofit (Private or Religious)
• Cardiovascular Technology Prgm
• Dietetic Internship Prgm
• Radiography Prgm

East Stroudsburg

East Stroudsburg University
Robert J Dillman, PhD, President
200 Prospect St
East Stroudsburg, PA 18301
717 422-3546
Type: 4-year Coll or Univ
Control: State, County, or Local Govt
• Athletic Training Prgm
• Exercise Physiology Prgm
• Exercise Science Prgm
• Speech-Language Pathology Prgm

Edinboro

Edinboro University of Pennsylvania
Jeremy D Brown, President
219 Meadville St
Edinboro, PA 16444
814 732-2711
Type: 4-year Coll or Univ
Control: State, County, or Local Govt
• Counseling Prgm
• Dietetics-Coordinated Prgm
• Nursing Prgm
• Rehabilitation Counseling Prgm
• Speech-Language Pathology Prgm

Elizabethtown

Elizabethtown College
Theodore E Long, PhD, President
One Alpha Dr
Elizabethtown, PA 17022-2298
717 361-1193
Type: 4-year Coll or Univ
Control: Nonprofit (Private or Religious)
• Music Therapy Prgm
• Occupational Therapy Prgm

Elkins Park

Pennsylvania College of Optometry
8360 Old York Rd
Elkins Park, PA 19027-1598
Type: Acad Health Ctr/Med Sch
Control: Nonprofit (Private or Religious)
• Low Vision Therapy Prgm
• Optometry Prgm
• Orientation and Mobility Specialist Prgm
• Physician Assistant Prgm
• Teacher of the Visually Impaired Prgm
• Vision Rehabilitation Therapy Prgm

Erie

Gannon University
Antoine M Garibaldi, PhD, President
109 University Square
Erie, PA 16541-0001
814 871-5800
Type: 4-year Coll or Univ
Control: Nonprofit (Private or Religious)
• Dietetics-Coordinated Prgm
• Nursing Prgm
• Occupational Therapy Prgm
• Physical Therapy Prgm
• Physician Assistant Prgm
• Radiography Prgm
• Respiratory Therapist (Advanced) Prgm

Great Lakes Institute of Technology
Tony Piccirillo, President/CEO
5100 Peach St
Erie, PA 16509
814 864-6666
Type: Vocational or Tech Sch
Control: For Profit
• Diagnostic Med Sonography Prgm
• Pharmacy Technician Prgm
• Surgical Technology Prgm

Lake Erie Coll of Osteopathic Medicine - Erie
1858 W Grandview Blvd
Erie, PA 16509
Type: Acad Health Ctr/Med Sch
Control: Nonprofit (Private or Religious)
• Osteopathic Medicine Prgm
• Pharmacy Prgm

Mercyhurst College
Thomas Gamble, PhD, President
501 E 38th St
Glenwood Hills
Erie, PA 16546
814 824-2000
Type: 4-year Coll or Univ
Control: Nonprofit (Private or Religious)
• Athletic Training Prgm
• Dietetics-Coordinated Prgm
• Physical Therapist Assistant Prgm

Saint Vincent Health Center
Sr Catherine Manning, MBA, President
232 W 25th St
Erie, PA 16544
814 452-5111
Type: Hosp or Med Ctr: 300-499 Beds
Control: Nonprofit (Private or Religious)
• Clin Lab Scientist/Med Technologist Prgm

Tri-State Business Institute
Guy Euliano, President
5757 W 26th St
Erie, PA 16506
814 838-7673
Type: Vocational or Tech Sch
Control: For Profit
• Dental Hygiene Prgm
• Medical Assistant Prgm

Glenside

Arcadia University
Jerry M Greiner, PhD, President
450 S Easton Rd
Glenside, PA 19038
215 572-2908
Type: 4-year Coll or Univ
Control: Nonprofit (Private or Religious)
• Genetic Counseling Prgm
• Physical Therapy Prgm
• Physician Assistant Prgm

Grantham

Messiah College
Kim Phipps, PhD, President
Grantham, PA 17027
717 766-2511
Type: 4-year Coll or Univ
Control: Nonprofit (Private or Religious)
• Athletic Training Prgm
• Dietetics-Didactic Prgm
• Nursing Prgm

Greensburg

Seton Hill University
JoAnne W Boyle, PhD, President
Box 231K
Greensburg, PA 15601
724 838-4211
Type: 4-year Coll or Univ
Control: Nonprofit (Private or Religious)
• Art Therapy Prgm
• Dietetics-Coordinated Prgm
• Physician Assistant Prgm

Gwynedd Valley

Gwynedd-Mercy College
Kathleen Cieplak Owens, PhD, President
1325 Sumneytown Pike
PO Box 901
Gwynedd Valley, PA 19437-0901
610 641-5560
Type: 4-year Coll or Univ
Control: Nonprofit (Private or Religious)
• Cardiovascular Technology Prgm
• Health Information Admin Prgm
• Health Information Tech Prgm
• Radiation Therapy Prgm
• Respiratory Therapist (Advanced) Prgm
• Respiratory Therapist (Entry-Level) Prgm

Harrisburg

Harrisburg Area Community College
Edna Baehre, PhD, President
One HACC Dr
Harrisburg, PA 17110-2999
717 780-2340
Type: Junior or Comm Coll
Control: State, County, or Local Govt
• Clin Lab Technician/Med Lab Technician Prgm
• Dental Assisting Prgm
• Dental Hygiene Prgm
• Diagnostic Med Sonography Prgm
• Emergency Med Tech-Paramedic Prgm
• Health Information Tech Prgm
• Medical Assistant Prgm
• Respiratory Therapist (Advanced) Prgm
• Respiratory Therapist (Entry-Level) Prgm
• Surgical Technology Prgm (2)

Immaculata

Immaculata University
Sr R Patricia Fadden, IHM EdD, President
1145 King Rd
Immaculata, PA 19345
610 647-4400
Type: 4-year Coll or Univ
Control: State, County, or Local Govt
• Dietetic Internship Prgm
• Dietetics-Didactic Prgm
• Music Therapy Prgm
• Nursing Prgm
• Psychology Prgm

Indiana

Indiana University of Pennsylvania
Tony Atwater, PhD, President
201 Sutton Hall
1011 South Dr
Indiana, PA 15705
724 357-2200
Type: 4-year Coll or Univ
Control: State, County, or Local Govt
• Athletic Training Prgm
• Dietetic Internship Prgm
• Dietetics-Didactic Prgm
• Nursing Prgm
• Psychology Prgm
• Respiratory Therapist (Advanced) Prgm
• Speech-Language Pathology Prgm

Jenkintown

Manor College
Sr Mary Cecilia Jurasinski, OSBM, President
700 Fox Chase Rd
Jenkintown, PA 19046
215 885-2360
Type: Junior or Comm Coll
Control: Nonprofit (Private or Religious)
• Dental Assisting Prgm
• Dental Hygiene Prgm
• Veterinary Technology Prgm

Johnstown

Commonwealth Tech Inst at Hiram G Andrews Ctr
Donald Rullman, BA, Director
727 Goucher St
Johnstown, PA 15905
814 255-8231
Type: Vocational or Tech Sch
Control: State, County, or Local Govt
• Dental Assisting Prgm

Conemaugh Memorial Medical Center
Scott Becker, MBA MPH, CEO
1086 Franklin St
Johnstown, PA 15905
814 534-9000
Type: Hosp or Med Ctr: 500> Beds
Control: Nonprofit (Private or Religious)
• Clin Lab Scientist/Med Technologist Prgm
• Histotechnician Prgm
• Radiography Prgm
• Surgical Technology Prgm

Kittanning

Armstrong County Memorial Hospital
Jack Hoard, President/CEO
One Nolte Dr
Kittanning, PA 16201
412 543-8404
Type: Hosp or Med Ctr: 100-299 Beds
Control: Nonprofit (Private or Religious)
• Radiography Prgm

Lancaster

Lancaster Gen Coll of Nursing & Hlth Sciences
Mary Grace Simcox, EdD, President
410 N Lime St
Lancaster, PA 17602
717 544-4787
Type: Junior or Comm Coll
Control: Nonprofit (Private or Religious)
- Cardiovascular Technology Prgm
- Clin Lab Scientist/Med Technologist Prgm
- Diagnostic Med Sonography Prgm
- Nuclear Medicine Technology Prgm
- Radiography Prgm
- Surgical Technology Prgm

Lock Haven

Lock Haven University
Keith Miller, PhD, President
Sullivan 202
Lock Haven, PA 17745
570 484-2000
Type: 4-year Coll or Univ
Control: State, County, or Local Govt
- Athletic Training Prgm
- Physician Assistant Prgm

Loretto

St Francis University
Rev Gabriel Zeis, TOR, President
PO Box 600
Loretto, PA 15940-0600
814 472-3001
Type: 4-year Coll or Univ
Control: Nonprofit (Private or Religious)
- Nursing Prgm
- Occupational Therapy Prgm
- Physical Therapy Prgm
- Physician Assistant Prgm

Mansfield

Mansfield University
Maravene Loeschke, PhD, President
500 North Hall
Mansfield, PA 16933
570 662-4046
Type: 4-year Coll or Univ
Control: State, County, or Local Govt
- Dietetics-Didactic Prgm
- Music Therapy Prgm
- Radiography Prgm
- Respiratory Therapist (Advanced) Prgm

McKees Rock

Ohio Valley General Hospital
William F Provenzano, FACHE, President
25 Heckel Rd
McKees Rock, PA 15136
Type: Hosp or Med Ctr: 100-299 Beds
Control: Nonprofit (Private or Religious)
- Radiography Prgm

Media

Delaware County Community College
Jerome Parker, PhD, President
901 S Media Line Rd
Media, PA 19603-1094
610 359-5100
Type: Junior or Comm Coll
Control: State, County, or Local Govt
- Medical Assistant Prgm
- Surgical Technology Prgm

Millersville

Millersville University of Pennsylvania
Francine McNairey, PhD, President
Biemesderfer Executive Ctr
Millersville, PA 17551
717 872-3592
Type: 4-year Coll or Univ
Control: State, County, or Local Govt
- Respiratory Therapist (Advanced) Prgm

Monaca

Community College of Beaver County
Joe D Forrester, EdD, President
One Campus Dr
Monaca, PA 15061
724 775-8561
Type: Junior or Comm Coll
Control: State, County, or Local Govt
- Phlebotomy Prgm

Monroeville

Western School of Health & Business
Kenneth Richards, MBA, President
1 Monroeville Center, Ste 250
Monroeville, PA 15146
412 373-6400
Type: Vocational or Tech Sch
Control: For Profit
- Diagnostic Med Sonography Prgm
- Pharmacy Technician Prgm
- Radiography Prgm
- Respiratory Therapist (Advanced) Prgm
- Surgical Technology Prgm
- Veterinary Technology Prgm

Moon Township

Robert Morris College/Allegheny Gen Hosp
Edward A Nicholson, PhD, President
Narrows Run Road
Moon Township, PA 1518
Type: Consortium
Control: Nonprofit (Private or Religious)
- Nursing Prgm
- Osteopathic Medicine Prgm

Nanticoke

Luzerne County Community College
Thomas Leary, MA, Interim President
1333 S Prospect St
Nanticoke, PA 18634-3899
570 740-0384
Type: Junior or Comm Coll
Control: State, County, or Local Govt
- Dental Assisting Prgm
- Dental Hygiene Prgm
- Respiratory Therapist (Advanced) Prgm
- Surgical Technology Prgm

New Castle

Jameson Health System
Thomas White, FACHE, President and CEO
1000 S Mercer St
South Campus
New Castle, PA 16101
724 658-9001
Type: Hosp or Med Ctr: 100-299 Beds
Control: Nonprofit (Private or Religious)
- Nuclear Medicine Technology Prgm

Jameson Hospital
Thomas White, FACHE, President/CEO
1211 Wilmington Ave
New Castle, PA 16105
412 658-3511
Type: Hosp or Med Ctr: 100-299 Beds
Control: Nonprofit (Private or Religious)
- Radiography Prgm

New Kensington

Career Training Academy
John M Reddy, BS, President
950 Fifth Ave
New Kensington, PA 15068
724 337-1000
Type: Vocational or Tech Sch
Control: For Profit
- Medical Assistant Prgm

Newton

Bucks County Community College
James J Linksz, EdD, President
275 Swamp Rd
Tyler Hall 220
Newton, PA 18940
215 968-8222
Type: Junior or Comm Coll
Control: State, County, or Local Govt
- Medical Assistant Prgm
- Radiography Prgm

Oaks

Cortiva Inst - Penn School of Muscle Therapy
Jeff Mann, PDMT NCBTMB, President
1173 Egypt Rd
PO Box 400
Oaks, PA 19456-0400
610 666-9060
Type: Vocational or Tech Sch
Control: For Profit
- Massage Therapy Prgm

Philadelphia

Albert Einstein Medical Center
Barry Freedman, MBA, President
5501 Old York Rd
Philadelphia, PA 19141-3098
215 456-7010
Type: Hosp or Med Ctr: 500> Beds
Control: Nonprofit (Private or Religious)
• Radiography Prgm

ARAMARK Healthcare
1717 Arch St, 42nd Fl
Philadelphia, PA 19103
Control: For Profit
• Dietetic Internship Prgm

Chestnut Hill College
Philadelphia, PA 19118
Type: 4-year Coll or Univ
Control: Nonprofit (Private or Religious)
• Psychology Prgm

Community College of Philadelphia
Stephen M Curtis, PhD, President
1700 Spring Garden St
Philadelphia, PA 19130
215 751-8028
Type: Junior or Comm Coll
Control: State, County, or Local Govt
• Clin Lab Technician/Med Lab Technician Prgm
• Dental Hygiene Prgm
• Health Information Tech Prgm
• Medical Assistant Prgm
• Phlebotomy Prgm
• Radiography Prgm
• Respiratory Therapist (Advanced) Prgm

Drexel University
Constantine N Papadakis, President
32nd and Chestnut Sts
Philadelphia, PA 19104
215 895-2000
Type: 4-year Coll or Univ
Control: Nonprofit (Private or Religious)
• Allopathic Medicine Prgm
• Art Therapy Prgm
• Dance/Movement Therapy Prgm
• Dietetics-Didactic Prgm
• Medical Librarian Prgm
• Music Therapy Prgm
• Nursing Prgm
• Pathologists' Assistant Prgm
• Perfusion Prgm
• Physical Therapy Prgm
• Physician Assistant Prgm
• Psychology Prgm
• Radiography Prgm

Holy Family University
Sr M Francesca Onley, PhD CSFN, President
Grant & Frankford Aves
Philadelphia, PA 19114
215 637-7700
Type: 4-year Coll or Univ
Control: Nonprofit (Private or Religious)
• Nursing Prgm
• Radiography Prgm

Hospital of the Univ of Pennsylvania
Wilbur B Pittinger, Exec Director
21 Penn Tower, 3400 Spruce St
Philadelphia, PA 19114
215 662-2992
Type: Hosp or Med Ctr: 500> Beds
Control: Nonprofit (Private or Religious)
• Allopathic Medicine Prgm

La Salle University
Michael McGinniss, President
1900 W Olney Ave
Philadelphia, PA 19141-1108
Type: 4-year Coll or Univ
Control: State, County, or Local Govt
• Dietetics-Coordinated Prgm
• Dietetics-Didactic Prgm
• Nursing Prgm
• Psychology Prgm
• Speech-Language Pathology Prgm

National Massage Therapy Insitute
Division of PSB
10050 Roosevelt Blvd
Philadelphia, PA 19116
Type: Acad Health Ctr/Med Sch
Control: For Profit
• Massage Therapy Prgm

Pennsylvania Hospital
Kathleen Kinslow, RN BSN MBA, CEO
800 Spruce St
Philadelphia, PA 19107
215 829-3312
Type: Hosp or Med Ctr: 300-499 Beds
Control: Nonprofit (Private or Religious)
• Clin Lab Scientist/Med Technologist Prgm

Philadelphia College of Osteopathic Medicine
Matthew Schure, PhD, President, CEO
4170 City Ave
Evans Hall - President's Office
Philadelphia, PA 19131-1694
215 871-6800
Type: Acad Health Ctr/Med Sch
Control: Nonprofit (Private or Religious)
• Osteopathic Medicine Prgm
• Physician Assistant Prgm
• Psychology Prgm

Philadelphia University
Stephen Spinelli, PhD, President
School House Ln and Henry Ave
Philadelphia, PA 19144
215 951-2970
Type: 4-year Coll or Univ
Control: Nonprofit (Private or Religious)
• Occupational Therapy Prgm
• Physician Assistant Prgm

St Christopher Hospital School of Rad Tech
Jill Tillman, MBA, Interim CEO
Erie Ave at Front
Philadelphia, PA 19134
215 427-5480
Type: Hosp or Med Ctr: 100-299 Beds
Control: For Profit
• Radiography Prgm

St Christopher's Hospital for Children
E Erie Ave at N Front St
Philadelphia, PA 19134
Type: Hosp or Med Ctr: 300-499 Beds
Control: For Profit
• Clin Lab Scientist/Med Technologist Prgm

Temple University
Ann Weaver Hart, PhD, President
President's Office
2nd Fl - Sullivan Hall
Philadelphia, PA 19122
215 204-7405
Type: 4-year Coll or Univ
Control: State, County, or Local Govt
• Allopathic Medicine Prgm
• Athletic Training Prgm
• Dentistry Prgm
• Health Information Admin Prgm
• Music Therapy Prgm
• Nursing Prgm
• Occupational Therapy Prgm
• Pharmacy Prgm
• Physical Therapy Prgm
• Podiatric Medicine Prgm
• Psychology Prgm
• Speech-Language Pathology Prgm
• Therapeutic Recreation Specialist Prgm

Thomas Jefferson University
Robert L Barchi, MD PhD, President
1020 Walnut St, 641 Scott Bldg
Philadelphia, PA 19107-5587
215 955-6617
Type: Acad Health Ctr/Med Sch
Control: Nonprofit (Private or Religious)
• Allopathic Medicine Prgm
• Clin Lab Scientist/Med Technologist Prgm
• Cytotechnology Prgm
• Diagnostic Med Sonography Prgm
• Magnetic Resonance Prgm
• Nursing Prgm
• Occupational Therapy Prgm
• Physical Therapy Prgm
• Radiation Therapy Prgm
• Radiography Prgm

Thompson Institute
Shawn Bartley, EdD, President
3010 Market St
Philadelphia, PA 19104
215 594-4000
Type: Vocational or Tech Sch
Control: For Profit
• Medical Assistant Prgm (2)

Univ of Penn MC/Hosp of the Univ of Penn
Ralph Muller
3400 Spruce St Silverstein One
21 Penn Tower
Philadelphia, PA 19104
215 662-2203
Type: Hosp or Med Ctr: 500> Beds
Control: Nonprofit (Private or Religious)
• Radiography Prgm

Univ of Penn School of Dental Medicine
Marjorie K Jeffcoat, DMD, Dean
240 S 40th St
Robert Shattner Center
Philadelphia, PA 19104
215 898-8961
Type: Acad Health Ctr/Med Sch
Control: Nonprofit (Private or Religious)
• Dentistry Prgm

University of Pennsylvania
Amy Gutmann, President
100 College Hall
Philadelphia, PA 19104
215 898-7221
Type: 4-year Coll or Univ
Control: Nonprofit (Private or Religious)
• Nursing Prgm
• Psychology Prgm
• Veterinary Medicine Prgm

University of the Sciences in Philadelphia
Philip P Gerbino, PhD, President
600 S 43rd St
Philadelphia, PA 19104-4495
215 596-8970
Type: 4-year Coll or Univ
Control: Nonprofit (Private or Religious)
• Occupational Therapy Prgm
• Pharmacy Prgm
• Physical Therapy Prgm

Pittsburgh

Adajio Health
960 Penn Ave, Ste 600
Pittsburgh, PA 15222
412 288-9039
Control: Nonprofit (Private or Religious)
• Dietetic Internship Prgm

Bidwell Training Center
William E Strickland, Jr, President and CEO
1815 Metropolitan St
Pittsburgh, PA 15233-2200
412 323-4000
Type: Vocational or Tech Sch
Control: Nonprofit (Private or Religious)
• Pharmacy Technician Prgm

Bradford School - Pittsburgh
Vincent Graziano, MBA, President
125 West Station Square Dr, Ste 129
Pittsburgh, PA 15219
412 391-6710
Type: Vocational or Tech Sch
Control: For Profit
• Dental Assisting Prgm
• Medical Assistant Prgm

Carlow University
Mary Hines, PhD, President
3333 Fifth Ave
Pittsburgh, PA 15213
Type: 4-year Coll or Univ
Control: Nonprofit (Private or Religious)
• Nursing Prgm

Chatham University
Esther L Barazzone, PhD, President
Woodland Rd
Pittsburgh, PA 15232-2826
412 365-1160
Type: 4-year Coll or Univ
Control: Nonprofit (Private or Religious)
• Occupational Therapy Prgm
• Physical Therapy Prgm
• Physician Assistant Prgm

Comm College of Allegheny County
Sutin Stewart, PhD, President
800 Allegheny Ave
Pittsburgh, PA 15233
412 323-2323
Type: Junior or Comm Coll
Control: State, County, or Local Govt
• Clin Lab Technician/Med Lab Technician Prgm
• Diagnostic Med Sonography Prgm
• Dietetic Technician-AD Prgm
• Health Information Tech Prgm
• Medical Assistant Prgm
• Nuclear Medicine Technology Prgm
• Occupational Therapy Asst Prgm
• Pharmacy Technician Prgm
• Physical Therapist Assistant Prgm
• Radiation Therapy Prgm
• Radiography Prgm
• Respiratory Therapist (Advanced) Prgm
• Surgical Technology Prgm

Connelley Technical Institute
Joseph Poerio, MS, Director of Adult Educ
1501 Bedford Ave
Pittsburgh, PA 15219
412 338-3703
Type: Vocational or Tech Sch
Control: State, County, or Local Govt
• Surgical Technology Prgm

Ctr for Emer Med of Western Pennsylvania
Douglas Garretson, BA NREMT-P, VP, COO
230 McKee Pl, Ste 500
Pittsburgh, PA 15213
412 647-5300
Type: Consortium
Control: Nonprofit (Private or Religious)
• Emergency Med Tech-Paramedic Prgm

Duquesne University
Charles Dougherty, PhD, President
600 Forbes Ave
Administration Bldg Rm 510
Pittsburgh, PA 15282
412 396-6060
Type: 4-year Coll or Univ
Control: Nonprofit (Private or Religious)
• Athletic Training Prgm
• Counseling Prgm
• Health Information Admin Prgm
• Music Therapy Prgm
• Nursing Prgm
• Occupational Therapy Prgm
• Pharmacy Prgm
• Physical Therapy Prgm
• Physician Assistant Prgm
• Psychology Prgm
• Speech-Language Pathology Prgm

Everest Institute
James Callahan, President
100 Forbes Ave, Ste 1200
Pittsburgh, PA 15222
412 261-4520
Type: Vocational or Tech Sch
Control: For Profit
• Medical Assistant Prgm

Kaplan Career Institute - ICM Campus
Richard A Gooding, President
10 Wood St
Pittsburgh, PA 15222-1977
412 261-4644
Type: Vocational or Tech Sch
Control: For Profit
• Medical Assistant Prgm
• Occupational Therapy Asst Prgm

Univ Health Center of Pittsburgh
Leslie Davis, MS, CEO
300 Halket St
Pittsburgh, PA 15213
412 641-4664
Type: Hosp or Med Ctr: 300-499 Beds
Control: Nonprofit (Private or Religious)
• Cytotechnology Prgm

University of Pittsburgh
Mark A Nordenberg, JD, Chancellor
Rm 107 Cathedral of Learning
Pittsburgh, PA 15260
412 624-4200
Type: 4-year Coll or Univ
Control: State, County, or Local Govt
• Allopathic Medicine Prgm
• Athletic Training Prgm (2)
• Audiologist Prgm
• Dental Hygiene Prgm
• Dentistry Prgm
• Dietetics-Coordinated Prgm
• Dietetics-Didactic Prgm
• Genetic Counseling Prgm
• Health Information Admin Prgm
• Medical Librarian Prgm
• Nursing Prgm
• Occupational Therapy Prgm
• Orientation and Mobility Specialist Prgm
• Pharmacy Prgm
• Physical Therapist Assistant Prgm
• Physical Therapy Prgm
• Psychology Prgm
• Rehabilitation Counseling Prgm
• Respiratory Therapist (Advanced) Prgm
• Speech-Language Pathology Prgm

UPMC Health System
Elizabeth Concordia, MAS, President and CEO
200 Lothrop St
Ste N739MUH
Pittsburgh, PA 15213-2582
412 647-8788
Type: Hosp or Med Ctr: 500> Beds
Control: Nonprofit (Private or Religious)
• Radiography Prgm

UPMC Presbyterian Shadyside
Liz Concordia, CEO
5230 Centre Ave
Pittsburgh, PA 15232
412 622-2010
Type: Hosp or Med Ctr: 500> Beds
Control: Nonprofit (Private or Religious)
• Dietetic Internship Prgm
• Perfusion Prgm

Vet Tech Institute
125 Seventh St
Pittsburgh, PA 15222
Type: Vocational or Tech Sch
Control: For Profit
• Veterinary Technology Prgm

Pottsville

McCann School of Business and Technology
Linda Walinsky, MPA
Regional Executive Director
2638 Woodglen Rd
Pottsville, PA 17901
570 622-3293
Type: Vocational or Tech Sch
Control: For Profit
• Surgical Technology Prgm

Reading

Alvernia College
Thomas F Flynn, PhD, President
400 Saint Bernardine St
Reading, PA 19607-1799
610 796-8324
Type: 4-year Coll or Univ
Control: Nonprofit (Private or Religious)
• Athletic Training Prgm
• Nursing Prgm
• Occupational Therapy Prgm

Reading Area Community College
Anna Weitz, EdD, President
10 S Second St
PO Box 1706
Reading, PA 19603
610 372-4721
Type: Junior or Comm Coll
Control: State, County, or Local Govt
• Clin Lab Technician/Med Lab Technician Prgm
• Respiratory Therapist (Advanced) Prgm
• Respiratory Therapist (Entry-Level) Prgm

Reading Hospital & Medical Center
Scott Wolfe, MS, CEO
PO Box 16052
Reading, PA 19612-6052
610 988-8258
Type: Hosp or Med Ctr: 500> Beds
Control: Nonprofit (Private or Religious)
• Clin Lab Scientist/Med Technologist Prgm
• Radiography Prgm
• Surgical Technology Prgm

St Joseph Medical Center
John Morahan, President/CEO
2500 Bernville Road
PO Box 316
Reading, PA 19605
610 378-2000
Type: Hosp or Med Ctr: 100-299 Beds
Control: Nonprofit (Private or Religious)
• Radiography Prgm

Sayre

Robert Packer Hospital
Mary N Mannix, MSHA, President and COO
Guthrie Square
Sayre, PA 18840
717 888-6666
Type: Hosp or Med Ctr: 300-499 Beds
Control: Nonprofit (Private or Religious)
• Clin Lab Scientist/Med Technologist Prgm

Schnecksville

Lehigh Carbon Community College
Donald W Snyder, MBA JD LLM, President
4525 Education Pk Dr
Schnecksville, PA 18078-2598
610 799-2121
Type: Junior or Comm Coll
Control: State, County, or Local Govt
• Health Information Tech Prgm
• Medical Assistant Prgm
• Occupational Therapy Asst Prgm
• Physical Therapist Assistant Prgm
• Veterinary Technology Prgm

Scranton

Johnson College
Ann L Pipinski, EdD, President and CEO
3427 N Main Ave
Scranton, PA 18508-1495
570 342-6404
Type: Vocational or Tech Sch
Control: Nonprofit (Private or Religious)
• Radiography Prgm
• Veterinary Technology Prgm

Lackawanna College
Raymond S Angeli, MS, President
501 Vine St
Scranton, PA 18509
570 961-7850
Type: Junior or Comm Coll
Control: Nonprofit (Private or Religious)
• Diagnostic Med Sonography Prgm

Marywood University
Sr Anne Munley, PhD, President
2300 Adams Ave
Scranton, PA 18509
570 348-6231
Type: 4-year Coll or Univ
Control: Nonprofit (Private or Religious)
• Art Therapy Prgm
• Athletic Training Prgm
• Counseling Prgm
• Dietetic Internship Prgm
• Dietetics-Coordinated Prgm
• Dietetics-Didactic Prgm
• Music Therapy Prgm
• Physician Assistant Prgm
• Psychology Prgm
• Speech-Language Pathology Prgm

University of Scranton
Rev Scott J Pilarz, SJ PhD, President
Scranton, PA 18510-4622
570 941-7500
Type: 4-year Coll or Univ
Control: Nonprofit (Private or Religious)
• Counseling Prgm
• Nursing Prgm
• Occupational Therapy Prgm
• Physical Therapy Prgm
• Rehabilitation Counseling Prgm

Seneca

UPMC Northwest
Neil E Todhunter, CHE NHA, President/CEO
100 Fairfield Dr
Seneca, PA 16346
814 676-7140
Type: Hosp or Med Ctr: 100-299 Beds
Control: Nonprofit (Private or Religious)
• Radiography Prgm

Sewickley

Sewickley Vlly Hosp/Heritage Valley Hlth Sys
Norman Mitry, President and CEO
720 Blackburn Rd
Sewickley, PA 15143
724 773-2024
Type: Hosp or Med Ctr: 300-499 Beds
Control: Nonprofit (Private or Religious)
• Radiography Prgm

Sharon

Sharon Regional Health System
John A Zidansek, MHA, President/CEO
740 E State St
Sharon, PA 16146
412 983-3911
Type: Hosp or Med Ctr: 100-299 Beds
Control: Nonprofit (Private or Religious)
• Radiography Prgm

Shippensburg

Shippensburg University
Shippensburg, PA 17257-2210
717 532-9121
Type: 4-year Coll or Univ
Control: State, County, or Local Govt
• Counseling Prgm

Slippery Rock

Slippery Rock University of Pennsylvania
G Warren Smith, PhD, President
300 Old Main
Slippery Rock, PA 16057
412 738-2000
Type: 4-year Coll or Univ
Control: State, County, or Local Govt
• Athletic Training Prgm
• Counseling Prgm
• Exercise Science Prgm
• Music Therapy Prgm
• Physical Therapy Prgm
• Therapeutic Recreation Specialist Prgm

Spring Mills

Central Pennsylvania Institute of Sci & Tech
Henry Yeagley, Chairman
198 Pennfield Lane
Spring Mills, PA 16875
814 422-8446
Type: Vocational or Tech Sch
Control: State, County, or Local Govt
• Medical Assistant Prgm

St David

Eastern University
David Black, President
1300 Eagle Rd
St David, PA 19087
Type: 4-year Coll or Univ
Control: State, County, or Local Govt
• Athletic Training Prgm
• Nursing Prgm

State College

Mount Nittany Medical Center
Thomas Murray
1800 E Park Ave
State College, PA 16803
814 231-7000
Type: Acad Health Ctr/Med Sch
Control: For Profit
• Clin Lab Scientist/Med Technologist Prgm

South Hills School of Business & Technology
S Paul Mazza, JD, President
480 Waupelani Dr
State College, PA 16801
814 234-7755
Type: Vocational or Tech Sch
Control: For Profit
• Health Information Tech Prgm

Summerdale

Central Pennsylvania College
Todd A Milano, BS, President
College Hill and Valley Rds
Summerdale, PA 17093-0309
800 759-2727
Type: 4-year Coll or Univ
Control: For Profit
• Medical Assistant Prgm
• Physical Therapist Assistant Prgm

University Park

Penn State University
Graham Spanier, President
201 Old Main
University Park, PA 16802
814 865-4700
Type: 4-year Coll or Univ
Control: State, County, or Local Govt
• Allopathic Medicine Prgm
• Athletic Training Prgm
• Audiologist Prgm
• Clin Lab Technician/Med Lab Technician Prgm
• Counseling Prgm
• Dietetic Internship Prgm
• Dietetic Technician-AD Prgm
• Dietetics-Didactic Prgm
• Nursing Prgm
• Occupational Therapy Asst Prgm (3)
• Physical Therapist Assistant Prgm (4)
• Psychology Prgm
• Radiography Prgm (2)
• Rehabilitation Counseling Prgm
• Speech-Language Pathology Prgm

Upland

Crozer-Keystone Medical Center
Joseph Saunders, President
One Medical Center Blvd
Upland, PA 19013
610 447-2766
Type: Hosp or Med Ctr: 300-499 Beds
Control: Nonprofit (Private or Religious)
• Diagnostic Med Sonography Prgm
• Electroneurodiagnostic Tech Prgm
• Radiography Prgm
• Respiratory Therapist (Advanced) Prgm

Villanova

Villanova University
Villanova, PA 19085
Type: 4-year Coll or Univ
Control: Nonprofit (Private or Religious)
• Nursing Prgm

Washington

Penn Commercial Inc
Robert S Bazant, BS, Director
242 Oak Spring Rd
Washington, PA 15301
724 222-5330
Type: Vocational or Tech Sch
Control: For Profit
• Medical Assistant Prgm

Washington Hospital
Telford W Thomas, MHA, President/CEO
155 Wilson Ave
Washington, PA 15301
724 223-3007
Type: Hosp or Med Ctr: 300-499 Beds
Control: Nonprofit (Private or Religious)
• Radiography Prgm

Waynesburg

Waynesburg College
Timothy R Thyreen, LHD, President
51 W College St
Waynesburg, PA 15370
412 852-3212
Type: 4-year Coll or Univ
Control: Nonprofit (Private or Religious)
• Athletic Training Prgm
• Nursing Prgm

West Chester

West Chester University
Madeleine Wing Adler, PhD, President
102 Phillips Hall
West Chester, PA 19383
610 436-2471
Type: 4-year Coll or Univ
Control: State, County, or Local Govt
• Athletic Training Prgm
• Dietetics-Didactic Prgm
• Nursing Prgm
• Respiratory Therapist (Advanced) Prgm
• Speech-Language Pathology Prgm

Wilkes-Barre

King's College
Rev Thomas J. O'Hara, CSC PhD, President
133 N River St
Wilkes-Barre, PA 18711
570 208-5899
Type: 4-year Coll or Univ
Control: Nonprofit (Private or Religious)
• Athletic Training Prgm
• Physician Assistant Prgm

Nesbitt Coll of Pharm & Nursing Sch of Pharm
Bernard Graham, PhD, Dean
Wilkes-Barre, PA 18766
570 408-4280
Type: Acad Health Ctr/Med Sch
Control: For Profit
• Perfusion Prgm

Wilkes University
Wilkes-Barre, PA 18766
Control: Nonprofit (Private or Religious)
• Nursing Prgm

Wilkes-Barre General Hospital
William Host, MD, CEO
575 N River St
Wilkes-Barre, PA 18764
570 552-3006
Type: Hosp or Med Ctr: 300-499 Beds
Control: Nonprofit (Private or Religious)
• Diagnostic Med Sonography Prgm
• Radiography Prgm

Wyoming Valley Health Care System
William Host, MD, President/CEO
575 N River St
Wilkes-Barre, PA 18764
570 552-3000
Type: Hosp or Med Ctr: 300-499 Beds
Control: Nonprofit (Private or Religious)
• Nuclear Medicine Technology Prgm

Williamsport

Pennsylvania College of Technology
Davie Jane Gilmour, PhD, President
One College Ave
Williamsport, PA 17701-5799
570 326-3761
Type: 4-year Coll or Univ
Control: State, County, or Local Govt
• Dental Hygiene Prgm
• Emergency Med Tech-Paramedic Prgm
• Health Information Tech Prgm
• Occupational Therapy Asst Prgm
• Physician Assistant Prgm
• Radiography Prgm
• Surgical Technology Prgm

Williamsport Hosp & Medical Center
Steve Johnson, President
777 Rural Ave
Williamsport, PA 17701
570 321-3170
Type: Hosp or Med Ctr: 100-299 Beds
Control: Nonprofit (Private or Religious)
• Clin Lab Scientist/Med Technologist Prgm

Wyomissing

Berks Technical Institute
Kenneth S Snyder, President
Four Park Plaza
Wyomissing, PA 19610
610 372-1722
Type: Vocational or Tech Sch
Control: For Profit
• Medical Assistant Prgm

York

Baltimore School of Massage
170 Red Rock Rd
York, PA 17402
Type: Acad Health Ctr/Med Sch
Control: For Profit
• Massage Therapy Prgm

York College of Pennsylvania
George W Waldner, PhD, President
Country Club Rd
York, PA 17405-7199
717 846-7788
Type: 4-year Coll or Univ
Control: Nonprofit (Private or Religious)
• Nursing Prgm
• Respiratory Therapist (Advanced) Prgm
• Respiratory Therapist (Entry-Level) Prgm

York Hospital/WellSpan Health
Richard L Seim, MBA, President
1001 S George St
York, PA 17405
717 851-2650
Type: Hosp or Med Ctr: 500> Beds
Control: Nonprofit (Private or Religious)
• Clin Lab Scientist/Med Technologist Prgm
• Radiography Prgm

YTI Career Institute
Timothy E Foster, BA, CEO
1405 Williams Rd
York, PA 17402
717 757-1100
Type: Vocational or Tech Sch
Control: Nonprofit (Private or Religious)
• Medical Assistant Prgm

Youngwood

Westmoreland County Community College
Steven C Ender, EdD, President
145 Pavilion Lane
Youngwood, PA 15697-1895
724 925-4000
Type: Junior or Comm Coll
Control: State, County, or Local Govt
• Dental Assisting Prgm
• Dental Hygiene Prgm
• Dietetic Technician-AD Prgm
• Medical Assistant Prgm
• Surgical Technology Prgm

Prince Edward Island, Canada

Charlottetown

University of Prince Edward Island
H. Wade MacLauchlan, President
550 University Ave
Charlottetown, PE C1A 4P3
Type: 4-year Coll or Univ
Control: State, County, or Local Government
• Veterinary Medicine Prgm

Puerto Rico

Bayamon

Universidad Central del Caribe
Jose Ginel Rodriguez, MD, Interim President
PO Box 60-327
Bayamon, PR 00960-6032
787 798-3001
Type: 4-year Coll or Univ
Control: Nonprofit (Private or Religious)
• Allopathic Medicine Prgm
• Radiography Prgm

Caguas

Huertas Junior College
Edwin Ramos, JD, President
PO Box 8429
Caguas, PR 00726
809 743-1242
Type: Junior or Comm Coll
Control: For Profit
• Health Information Tech Prgm

Carolina

Universidad del Este
Alberto Maldonado-Ruiz, Esq, Chancellor
PO Box 2010
Carolina, PR 00984-2010
787 257-7373
Type: 4-year Coll or Univ
Control: Nonprofit (Private or Religious)
• Health Information Tech Prgm
• Radiography Prgm

Gurabo

Universidad Del Turabo
Gurabo, PR 00778
Control: Nonprofit (Private or Religious)
• Dietetics-Coordinated Prgm
• Nursing Prgm

Humacao

University of Puerto Rico at Humacao
Hilda Colon Plumey, EdD, Chancellor
CUH Postal Station 100, Carr 908
Humacao, PR 00791-4300
787 850-9374
Type: 4-year Coll or Univ
Control: State, County, or Local Govt
• Occupational Therapy Asst Prgm
• Physical Therapist Assistant Prgm

Mayaguez

Universidad Adventista de las Antillas
Myrna Colon-Contreras, PhD, President
PO Box 118
Mayaguez, PR 00681
787 834-9595
Type: 4-year Coll or Univ
Control: Nonprofit (Private or Religious)
• Health Information Tech Prgm

Ponce

Ponce School of Medicine
Ponce, PR 00732
Type: Acad Health Ctr/Med Sch
Control: Nonprofit (Private or Religious)
• Allopathic Medicine Prgm
• Psychology Prgm

Ponce Technological University College
University of Puerto Rico
PO Box 7186
Ponce, PR 00732
Type: Vocational or Tech Sch
Control: Nonprofit (Private or Religious)
• Physical Therapist Assistant Prgm

Pontifical Catholic University
Marcelina Velez de Santiago, MS CHEM,
    President
2250 Las Americas Ave, Ste 564
Ponce, PR 00717-9997
787 841-2000
Type: 4-year Coll or Univ
Control: Nonprofit (Private or Religious)
• Clin Lab Scientist/Med Technologist Prgm

San German

Inter American University of Puerto Rico
Prof Agnes Mojica, MA, Chancellor
Call Box 5100
San German, PR 00683
787 892-5634
Type: 4-year Coll or Univ
Control: Nonprofit (Private or Religious)
• Clin Lab Scientist/Med Technologist Prgm (2)
• Health Information Tech Prgm
• Optometry Prgm
• Radiography Prgm

San Juan

Carlos Albizu University
San Juan, PR 00902
Control: Nonprofit (Private or Religious)
• Psychology Prgm (2)

Puerto Rico Department of Health
PO Box 70184
San Juan, PR 00936
787 274-6831
Control: State, County, or Local Govt
• Dietetic Internship Prgm

INSTITUTIONS

University of Puerto Rico
Marilyn Mendoza, PhD, Director
Medical Sciences Campus
PO Box 23345
San Juan, PR 00931
787 764-0000
Type: 4-year Coll or Univ
Control: State, County, or Local Govt
• Allopathic Medicine Prgm
• Clin Lab Scientist/Med Technologist Prgm
• Cytotechnology Prgm
• Dental Assisting Prgm
• Dentistry Prgm
• Dietetic Internship Prgm
• Dietetics-Didactic Prgm
• Health Information Admin Prgm
• Medical Librarian Prgm
• Nuclear Medicine Technology Prgm
• Nursing Prgm
• Occupational Therapy Prgm
• Ophthalmic Med Technician Prgm
• Pharmacy Prgm
• Physical Therapy Prgm
• Radiography Prgm
• Rehabilitation Counseling Prgm
• Veterinary Technology Prgm

VA Caribbean Healthcare System
10 Calle Casia
San Juan, PR 00921
Control: Fed Govt
• Dietetic Internship Prgm

Quebec, Canada

Montreal

McGill University
Jennifer Fitzpatrick, MS, Director, GC program
Human Genetics, Stewart Biology N5/13
1205 Dr Penfield Ave
Montreal, QC H3G 1Y5
514 398-3600
Type: Acad Health Ctr/Med Sch
Control: Nonprofit (Private or Religious)
• Allopathic Medicine Prgm
• Genetic Counseling Prgm
• Medical Librarian Prgm
• Psychology Prgm

University de Montreal
Pavillon Marguerite-D'Youville
CP 6128-Succ Centreville
Montreal, QC H3C 3J7
Control: Nonprofit (Private or Religious)
• Allopathic Medicine Prgm
• Medical Librarian Prgm
• Optometry Prgm
• Veterinary Medicine Prgm

Quebec City

University Laval
Pavillon Vandry
Quebec City, QC G1K 7P4
Control: Nonprofit (Private or Religious)
• Allopathic Medicine Prgm

Sherbrooke

University of Sherbrooke
Sherbrooke, QC J1K 2R1
Type: Acad Health Ctr/Med Sch
Control: State, County, or Local Government
• Allopathic Medicine Prgm

West Montreal

Concordia University
Frederick H Lowy, MD
1455 de Maisonneuve Blvd
West Montreal, QC H3G 1M8
514 848-4850
Type: 4-year Coll or Univ
Control: Nonprofit (Private or Religious)
• Art Therapy Prgm
• Psychology Prgm

Rhode Island

Kingston

University of Rhode Island
Robert L Carothers, PhD, President
35 Campus Ave
Kingston, RI 02881-1303
401 874-2444
Type: 4-year Coll or Univ
Control: State, County, or Local Govt
• Audiologist Prgm
• Cytotechnology Prgm
• Dietetic Internship Prgm
• Dietetics-Didactic Prgm
• Medical Librarian Prgm
• Nursing Prgm
• Pharmacy Prgm
• Physical Therapy Prgm
• Psychology Prgm
• Speech-Language Pathology Prgm

Newport

Salve Regina University
M Therese Antone, EdD RSM, President
100 Ochre Point Ave
Newport, RI 02840
Type: Acad Health Ctr/Med Sch
Control: Nonprofit (Private or Religious)
• Rehabilitation Counseling Prgm

North Providence

Our Lady of Fatima Hospital
H John Keimig, MHA, President
200 High Service Ave
North Providence, RI 02904
401 456-3000
Type: Hosp or Med Ctr: 100-299 Beds
Control: Nonprofit (Private or Religious)
• Clin Lab Scientist/Med Technologist Prgm

Providence

Brown Medical School
Providence, RI 02912
Type: Acad Health Ctr/Med Sch
Control: Nonprofit (Private or Religious)
• Allopathic Medicine Prgm

Johnson & Wales University
Morris J Gaebe, Chancellor
8 Abbott Park Palace
Providence, RI 02903-3703
401 598-1000
Type: 4-year Coll or Univ
Control: Nonprofit (Private or Religious)
• Dietetics-Didactic Prgm

Rhode Island Hospital
Joseph Amaral, MD, President/CEO
593 Eddy St
Providence, RI 02905
401 444-5123
Type: Hosp or Med Ctr: 500> Beds
Control: For Profit
• Clin Lab Scientist/Med Technologist Prgm
• Diagnostic Med Sonography Prgm
• Nuclear Medicine Technology Prgm
• Radiography Prgm

Warwick

Community College of Rhode Island
Ray M Di Pasquale, PhD, President
400 East Ave
Warwick, RI 02886
401 825-2188
Type: Junior or Comm Coll
Control: State, County, or Local Govt
• Clin Lab Technician/Med Lab Technician Prgm
• Dental Assisting Prgm
• Dental Hygiene Prgm
• Massage Therapy Prgm
• Occupational Therapy Asst Prgm
• Physical Therapist Assistant Prgm
• Radiography Prgm
• Respiratory Therapist (Advanced) Prgm

New England Institute of Technology
Richard I Gouse, BA, President
2500 Post Rd
Warwick, RI 02886-2251
401 467-7744
Type: 4-year Coll or Univ
Control: Nonprofit (Private or Religious)
• Occupational Therapy Asst Prgm
• Surgical Technology Prgm

Saskatchewan, Canada

Saskatoon

Orthoptic Clinic Eye Care Centre
Saskatoon, SK S7K 5T6
306 655-8058
Type: Hosp or Med Ctr: 100-299 Beds
Control: For Profit
• Orthoptist Prgm

Saskatoon SK

University of Saskatchewan
1121 College Dr
Saskatoon SK, SK S7N 0W3
Control: Nonprofit (Private or Religious)
• Allopathic Medicine Prgm
• Psychology Prgm
• Veterinary Medicine Prgm

South Carolina

Anderson

AnMed Health Medical Center
John Miller, MHA, President
800 N Fant St
Anderson, SC 29621
864 261-1109
Type: Hosp or Med Ctr: 500> Beds
Control: Nonprofit (Private or Religious)
• Radiography Prgm

Forrest Junior College
John Re, PhD, President
601 E River St
Anderson, SC 29624
864 225-7653
Type: Junior or Comm Coll
Control: For Profit
• Medical Assistant Prgm

Beaufort

Technical College of the Lowcountry
Anne McNutt, PhD, President
PO Box 1288
Beaufort, SC 29901
843 525-8211
Type: Vocational or Tech Sch
Control: For Profit
• Radiography Prgm
• Surgical Technology Prgm

Charleston

Charleston Southern University
Jairy C Hunter, PhD, President
PO Box 118087
Charleston, SC 29423-8087
803 863-7000
Type: 4-year Coll or Univ
Control: Nonprofit (Private or Religious)
• Athletic Training Prgm
• Music Therapy Prgm

College of Charleston
Leo I Higdon, Jr, President
66 George St
Charleston, SC 29424-0001
843 953-5500
Type: 4-year Coll or Univ
Control: State, County, or Local Govt
• Athletic Training Prgm

Medical University of South Carolina
Ray Greenberg, MD, President
135 Cannon St, PO Box d50001
Charleston, SC 29425-2701
803 792-2211
Type: 4-year Coll or Univ
Control: State, County, or Local Govt
• Allopathic Medicine Prgm
• Cytotechnology Prgm
• Dentistry Prgm
• Dietetic Internship Prgm
• Histotechnology Prgm
• Nursing Prgm
• Occupational Therapy Prgm
• Perfusion Prgm
• Pharmacy Prgm
• Physical Therapy Prgm
• Physician Assistant Prgm
• Speech-Language Pathology Prgm

Miller-Motte Technical College
Julie S Corner, MEd, Campus Director
8085 Rivers Ave
Charleston, SC 29406
843 574-0101
Type: Vocational or Tech Sch
Control: For Profit
• Medical Assistant Prgm
• Surgical Technology Prgm

South Carolina College of Pharmacy
Joseph T DiPiro, PharmD, Executive Dean
280 Calhoun St
Charleston, SC 29425
843 792-8450
Type: Acad Health Ctr/Med Sch
Control: Nonprofit (Private or Religious)
• Pharmacy Prgm

Trident Technical College
Mary D Thornley, EdD, President
PO Box 118067
Charleston, SC 29423-8067
843 574-6241
Type: Vocational or Tech Sch
Control: State, County, or Local Govt
• Clin Lab Technician/Med Lab Technician Prgm
• Dental Assisting Prgm
• Dental Hygiene Prgm
• Emergency Med Tech-Paramedic Prgm
• Medical Assistant Prgm
• Occupational Therapy Asst Prgm
• Pharmacy Technician Prgm
• Physical Therapist Assistant Prgm
• Radiography Prgm
• Respiratory Therapist (Advanced) Prgm
• Veterinary Technology Prgm

Clemson

Clemson University
Constantine W Curris, President
201 Sikes Hall
Clemson, SC 29634
803 656-3311
Type: 4-year Coll or Univ
Control: State, County, or Local Govt
• Counseling Prgm
• Dietetics-Didactic Prgm
• Nursing Prgm
• Therapeutic Recreation Specialist Prgm

Columbia

Midlands Technical College
Marshall (Sonny) White, PhD, President
PO Box 2408
Columbia, SC 29202-2408
803 738-7600
Type: Junior or Comm Coll
Control: State, County, or Local Govt
• Clin Lab Technician/Med Lab Technician Prgm
• Dental Assisting Prgm
• Dental Hygiene Prgm
• Health Information Tech Prgm
• Medical Assistant Prgm
• Nuclear Medicine Technology Prgm
• Pharmacy Technician Prgm
• Physical Therapist Assistant Prgm
• Radiography Prgm
• Respiratory Therapist (Advanced) Prgm
• Surgical Technology Prgm

Palmetto Health Baptist
Charles D Beaman, Jr, President
Taylor at Marion St
Columbia, SC 29220
803 771-5042
Type: Hosp or Med Ctr: 300-499 Beds
Control: Nonprofit (Private or Religious)
• Clin Lab Scientist/Med Technologist Prgm

SC Dept of Health & Environmental Control
Mills Complex, PO Box 101106
Columbia, SC 29211-0106
803 737-3954
Control: State, County, or Local Govt
• Dietetic Internship Prgm

Sister of Charity Providence Hospital
Stephen Purves, MHA, President
2435 Forest Dr
Columbia, SC 29204
803 256-5313
Type: Hosp or Med Ctr: 300-499 Beds
Control: Nonprofit (Private or Religious)
• Cardiovascular Technology Prgm

South University
Anne F Patton, BBA, President
3810 Main St
Columbia, SC 29203
803 799-9082
Type: Junior or Comm Coll
Control: For Profit
• Medical Assistant Prgm

University of South Carolina
Andrew Sorenson, PhD, President
Osborne 203
Columbia, SC 29208
803 777-2001
Type: 4-year Coll or Univ
Control: State, County, or Local Govt
• Allopathic Medicine Prgm
• Athletic Training Prgm
• Counseling Prgm
• Genetic Counseling Prgm
• Medical Librarian Prgm
• Nursing Prgm (2)
• Pharmacy Prgm
• Physical Therapy Prgm
• Psychology Prgm
• Rehabilitation Counseling Prgm
• Speech-Language Pathology Prgm

INSTITUTIONS

Conway

Horry - Georgetown Technical College
H Neyle Wilson, BS MEd, President
PO Box 261966
Conway, SC 29528
843 349-5201
Type: Junior or Comm Coll
Control: Nonprofit (Private or Religious)
- Dental Assisting Prgm
- Dental Hygiene Prgm
- Radiography Prgm
- Surgical Technology Prgm

Due West

Erskine College
Randy T Ruble, PhD, President
2 Washington St
Due West, SC 29639
864 379-8833
Type: 4-year Coll or Univ
Control: Nonprofit (Private or Religious)
- Athletic Training Prgm

Florence

Florence-Darlington Technical College
Charles W Gould, PhD, President
PO Box 100548
Florence, SC 29501-0548
843 661-8000
Type: Vocational or Tech Sch
Control: State, County, or Local Govt
- Clin Lab Technician/Med Lab Technician Prgm
- Dental Assisting Prgm
- Dental Hygiene Prgm
- Health Information Tech Prgm
- Radiography Prgm
- Respiratory Therapist (Advanced) Prgm
- Surgical Technology Prgm

McLeod Regional Medical Center
Robert Colones, MA, President and CEO
555 E Cheves St
PO Box 100551
Florence, SC 29506
843 777-2297
Type: Hosp or Med Ctr: 300-499 Beds
Control: Nonprofit (Private or Religious)
- Clin Lab Scientist/Med Technologist Prgm

Gaffney

Limestone College
Walt Griffin, PhD, President
1115 College Dr
Gaffney, SC 29340
864 488-4616
Type: 4-year Coll or Univ
Control: Nonprofit (Private or Religious)
- Athletic Training Prgm

Graniteville

Aiken Technical College
Susan Winsor, PhD, President
2276 Jefferson Davis Hwy
PO Box 400
Graniteville, SC 29829
803 593-9954
Type: Vocational or Tech Sch
Control: State, County, or Local Govt
- Dental Assisting Prgm
- Medical Assistant Prgm
- Radiography Prgm
- Surgical Technology Prgm

Greenville

Greenville Technical College
Thomas E Barton, Jr, EdD, President
PO Box 5616
Greenville, SC 29606-5616
864 250-8175
Type: Vocational or Tech Sch
Control: State, County, or Local Govt
- Clin Lab Technician/Med Lab Technician Prgm
- Dental Assisting Prgm
- Dental Hygiene Prgm
- Diagnostic Med Sonography Prgm
- Emergency Med Tech-Paramedic Prgm
- Health Information Tech Prgm
- Medical Assistant Prgm
- Occupational Therapy Asst Prgm
- Pharmacy Technician Prgm
- Physical Therapist Assistant Prgm
- Radiography Prgm
- Respiratory Therapist (Advanced) Prgm
- Surgical Technology Prgm

Greenwood

Lander University
Daniel W Ball, President
320 Stanley Ave
Greenwood, SC 29649
864 388-8300
Type: 4-year Coll or Univ
Control: State, County, or Local Govt
- Athletic Training Prgm

Piedmont Technical College
Lex D Walters, PhD, President
PO Box 1467
Emerald Rd
Greenwood, SC 29647-1467
864 941-8324
Type: Vocational or Tech Sch
Control: State, County, or Local Govt
- Medical Assistant Prgm
- Radiography Prgm
- Respiratory Therapist (Advanced) Prgm
- Surgical Technology Prgm

Newberry

Newberry College
Mitchell Zais, PhD, President
2100 College St
Holland Hall-101
Newberry, SC 29108
803 321-5102
Type: Acad Health Ctr/Med Sch
Control: For Profit
- Veterinary Technology Prgm

Orangeburg

Orangeburg Calhoun Technical College
Anne Crook, PhD, President
3250 St Matthews Rd
Orangeburg, SC 29118
803 535-1200
Type: Junior or Comm Coll
Control: State, County, or Local Govt
- Clin Lab Technician/Med Lab Technician Prgm
- Medical Assistant Prgm
- Radiography Prgm

South Carolina State University
Andrew Hugine, PhD, President
300 College St NE
Orangeburg, SC 29117
803 536-7014
Type: 4-year Coll or Univ
Control: State, County, or Local Govt
- Counseling Prgm
- Dietetics-Didactic Prgm
- Nursing Prgm
- Orientation and Mobility Specialist Prgm
- Rehabilitation Counseling Prgm
- Speech-Language Pathology Prgm

Pendleton

Tri-County Technical College
Ronnie L Booth, PhD, President
PO Box 587
Pendleton, SC 29670
864 646-8361
Type: Junior or Comm Coll
Control: State, County, or Local Govt
- Clin Lab Technician/Med Lab Technician Prgm
- Dental Assisting Prgm
- Medical Assistant Prgm
- Respiratory Therapist (Advanced) Prgm
- Surgical Technology Prgm
- Veterinary Technology Prgm

Rock Hill

Winthrop University
Anthony J Digiorgio, PhD, President
701 Oakland Ave
Rock Hill, SC 29733
803 323-2225
Type: 4-year Coll or Univ
Control: State, County, or Local Govt
- Athletic Training Prgm
- Counseling Prgm
- Dietetic Internship Prgm
- Dietetics-Didactic Prgm

York Technical College
Greg Rutherford, PhD, President
452 S Anderson Rd
Rock Hill, SC 29730
803 327-8050
Type: Junior or Comm Coll
Control: State, County, or Local Govt
- Clin Lab Technician/Med Lab Technician Prgm
- Dental Assisting Prgm
- Dental Hygiene Prgm
- Radiography Prgm
- Surgical Technology Prgm

Spartanburg

Spartanburg Community College
Dan L Terhune, EdD, President
PO Drawer 4386
Spartanburg, SC 29305-4386
864 592-4610
Type: Junior or Comm Coll
Control: State, County, or Local Govt
- Clin Lab Technician/Med Lab Technician Prgm
- Dental Assisting Prgm
- Medical Assistant Prgm
- Pharmacy Technician Prgm
- Radiation Therapy Prgm
- Radiography Prgm
- Respiratory Therapist (Advanced) Prgm
- Surgical Technology Prgm

Sumter

Central Carolina Technical College
Kay Raffield, President
506 N Guignard Dr
Sumter, SC 29150
803 778-1961
Type: Vocational or Tech Sch
Control: State, County, or Local Govt
- Medical Assistant Prgm
- Surgical Technology Prgm

West Columbia

Lexington Medical Center
Mike Biedeger, President
2720 Sunset Blvd
West Columbia, SC 29169
803 791-2000
Type: Hosp or Med Ctr: 300-499 Beds
Control: State, County, or Local Govt
- Clin Lab Scientist/Med Technologist Prgm

South Dakota

Aberdeen

Presentation College
Lorraine Hale, PhD, President
1500 N Main St
Aberdeen, SD 57401-1299
605 229-8404
Type: 4-year Coll or Univ
Control: Nonprofit (Private or Religious)
- Clin Lab Technician/Med Lab Technician Prgm
- Medical Assistant Prgm
- Radiography Prgm
- Surgical Technology Prgm

Brookings

South Dakota State University
Peggy Gordon Miller, EdD, President
Office of the President - AD 222
Brookings, SD 57007
605 688-4151
Type: 4-year Coll or Univ
Control: State, County, or Local Govt
- Athletic Training Prgm
- Counseling Prgm
- Dietetics-Didactic Prgm
- Nursing Prgm
- Pharmacy Prgm

Madison

Dakota State University
Douglas Knowlton, PhD, President
314 Heston Hall
Madison, SD 57042-1799
605 256-5112
Type: 4-year Coll or Univ
Control: State, County, or Local Govt
- Health Information Admin Prgm
- Health Information Tech Prgm
- Respiratory Therapist (Advanced) Prgm

Mitchell

Dakota Wesleyan University
Robert Duffet, PhD, President
1200 W University
Box 911
Mitchell, SD 57301
605 995-2601
Type: 4-year Coll or Univ
Control: Nonprofit (Private or Religious)
- Athletic Training Prgm

Mitchell Technical Institute
Chris Paustian, MA, Director
821 N Capital St
Mitchell, SD 57301
605 995-3022
Type: Vocational or Tech Sch
Control: State, County, or Local Govt
- Clin Lab Technician/Med Lab Technician Prgm
- Medical Assistant Prgm
- Radiography Prgm

Rapid City

National American University
Jerry L Gallentine, PhD, President
14 St Joseph St
Rapid City, SD 57709
605 394-4900
Type: 4-year Coll or Univ
Control: For Profit
- Athletic Training Prgm
- Medical Assistant Prgm
- Veterinary Technology Prgm

Rapid City Regional Hospital
Tim Sughrue, MBA, President/CEO
353 Fairmont Blvd
Rapid City, SD 57701
605 341-8100
Type: Hosp or Med Ctr: 300-499 Beds
Control: Nonprofit (Private or Religious)
- Clin Lab Scientist/Med Technologist Prgm
- Radiography Prgm

Western Dakota Technical Institute
Rich Gross, MEd PhD, Director
800 Mickelson Dr
Rapid City, SD 57703
605 394-4034
Type: Vocational or Tech Sch
Control: Nonprofit (Private or Religious)
- Pharmacy Technician Prgm
- Surgical Technology Prgm

Sioux Falls

Augustana College
Robert Oliver, PhD, President
2001 S Summit Ave
Sioux Falls, SD 57197
605 336-4111
Type: 4-year Coll or Univ
Control: State, County, or Local Govt
- Athletic Training Prgm
- Nursing Prgm

Avera McKennan Hospital
Fred Slunecka, MHA, President/CEO
800 E 21st St
PO Box 5045
Sioux Falls, SD 57117-5045
605 322-7808
Type: Hosp or Med Ctr: 300-499 Beds
Control: Nonprofit (Private or Religious)
- Emergency Med Tech-Paramedic Prgm
- Radiography Prgm

Colorado Technical University
Vicki Strunk, President
3901 W 59th St
Sioux Falls, SD 57108
605 361-0200
Type: 4-year Coll or Univ
Control: For Profit
- Medical Assistant Prgm

Sanford Medical Center
Kelby K Krabbenhoft, MBA, President
1305 W 18th St
Sioux Falls, SD 57117-5039
605 333-6574
Type: Hosp or Med Ctr: 300-499 Beds
Control: Nonprofit (Private or Religious)
- Clin Lab Scientist/Med Technologist Prgm
- Radiography Prgm

Southeast Technical Institute
Jeff Holcomb, MBA, Director and CEO
2320 N Career Ave
Sioux Falls, SD 57107
605 367-7485
Type: Vocational or Tech Sch
Control: Nonprofit (Private or Religious)
- Cardiovascular Technology Prgm
- Diagnostic Med Sonography Prgm
- Nuclear Medicine Technology Prgm
- Surgical Technology Prgm

INSTITUTIONS

Vermillion

University of South Dakota
Jim Abbott, JD, President
414 E Clark St
Vermillion, SD 57069-2390
605 677-5641
Type: 4-year Coll or Univ
Control: State, County, or Local Govt
• Allopathic Medicine Prgm
• Audiologist Prgm
• Counseling Prgm
• Dental Hygiene Prgm
• Dietetic Internship Prgm
• Occupational Therapy Prgm
• Physical Therapy Prgm
• Physician Assistant Prgm
• Psychology Prgm
• Speech-Language Pathology Prgm

Watertown

Lake Area Technical Institute
Deb Shehard, President
230 11th St NE
PO Box 730
Watertown, SD 57201-0730
605 882-5284
Type: Vocational or Tech Sch
Control: State, County, or Local Govt
• Clin Lab Technician/Med Lab Technician Prgm
• Dental Assisting Prgm
• Medical Assistant Prgm
• Occupational Therapy Asst Prgm
• Physical Therapist Assistant Prgm

Yankton

Avera Sacred Heart Hospital
Pamela J Rezac, PhD, CEO
501 Summit St
Yankton, SD 57078
605 668-8000
Type: Hosp or Med Ctr: 100-299 Beds
Control: Nonprofit (Private or Religious)
• Radiography Prgm

Mt Marty College
Sr Jacquelyn Ernster, PhD, President
Yankton, SD 57078
605 668-1514
Type: 4-year Coll or Univ
Control: Nonprofit (Private or Religious)
• Nursing Prgm

Tennessee

Blountville

Northeast State Technical Comm College
William W Locke, PhD, President
PO Box 246
2425 Hwy 75
Blountville, TN 37617-0246
423 323-3191
Type: Junior or Comm Coll
Control: State, County, or Local Govt
• Cardiovascular Technology Prgm
• Clin Lab Technician/Med Lab Technician Prgm
• Dental Assisting Prgm
• Emergency Med Tech-Paramedic Prgm
• Surgical Technology Prgm

Bristol

King College
Bristol, TN 37620
Type: 4-year Coll or Univ
Control: Nonprofit (Private or Religious)
• Nursing Prgm

National College of Business and Technology
Frank E Longaker, MBA, President
1328 Highway 11W
Bristol, TN 37620
540 986-1800
Type: Junior or Comm Coll
Control: For Profit
• Medical Assistant Prgm (3)

Chattanooga

Chattanooga State Technical Comm College
James L Catanzaro, PhD, President
4501 Amnicola Hwy
Chattanooga, TN 37406-1097
423 697-4455
Type: Junior or Comm Coll
Control: State, County, or Local Govt
• Dental Assisting Prgm
• Dental Hygiene Prgm
• Diagnostic Med Sonography Prgm
• Emergency Med Tech-Paramedic Prgm
• Health Information Tech Prgm
• Medical Assistant Prgm
• Nuclear Medicine Technology Prgm
• Pharmacy Technician Prgm
• Physical Therapist Assistant Prgm
• Radiation Therapy Prgm
• Radiography Prgm
• Respiratory Therapist (Advanced) Prgm
• Surgical Technology Prgm

Miller-Motte Technical College - Chattanooga
June Kearns, AAS, Campus Director
6020 Shallowford Rd
Chattanooga, TN 37421
423 510-9675
Type: Vocational or Tech Sch
Control: For Profit
• Medical Assistant Prgm
• Surgical Technology Prgm

University of Tennessee - Chattanooga
Roger G Brown, PhD, Chancellor
615 McCallie Ave
101 Founders Hall, Dept 5605
Chattanooga, TN 37403-2598
423 425-4141
Type: 4-year Coll or Univ
Control: State, County, or Local Govt
• Athletic Training Prgm
• Counseling Prgm
• Dietetics-Didactic Prgm
• Nursing Prgm
• Occupational Therapy Prgm
• Physical Therapy Prgm

Clarksville

Austin Peay State University
Sherry Hoppe, EdD, President
Office of the President
Clarksville, TN 37044
615 648-7566
Type: 4-year Coll or Univ
Control: State, County, or Local Govt
• Clin Lab Scientist/Med Technologist Prgm

Miller-Motte Technical College - Clarksville
Virginia Castleberry, BA MS, Campus Director
1820 Business Park Dr
Clarksville, TN 37040
931 553-0071
Type: Vocational or Tech Sch
Control: For Profit
• Medical Assistant Prgm
• Surgical Technology Prgm

Cleveland

Cleveland State Community College
Carl Hite, PhD, President
3535 Adkisson Dr
PO Box 3570
Cleveland, TN 37320-3570
423 472-7141
Type: Junior or Comm Coll
Control: State, County, or Local Govt
• Medical Assistant Prgm

Lee University
Carolyn Dirksen, PhD, VP Academic Affairs
1120 N Ocoee St
Cleveland, TN 37320-3450
423 614-8118
Type: 4-year Coll or Univ
Control: Nonprofit (Private or Religious)
• Athletic Training Prgm

Columbia

Columbia State Community College
O Rebecca Hawkins, PhD, President
Hwy 412 PO Box 1315
Columbia, TN 38401
615 540-2722
Type: Junior or Comm Coll
Control: State, County, or Local Govt
• Emergency Med Tech-Paramedic Prgm
• Radiography Prgm
• Respiratory Therapist (Advanced) Prgm
• Veterinary Technology Prgm

Cookeville

MedVance Institute
Deborah Schwarzberg, MA MT(ASCP), President
1025 Highway 111
Cookeville, TN 38501
615 586-3660
Type: Vocational or Tech Sch
Control: For Profit
• Clin Lab Technician/Med Lab Technician Prgm
• Radiography Prgm (2)
• Surgical Technology Prgm

Tennessee Technological University
Robert R Bell, President
1000 N Dixie Ave
Cookeville, TN 38505-0001
931 372-3101
Type: 4-year Coll or Univ
Control: State, County, or Local Govt
• Dietetics-Didactic Prgm
• Nursing Prgm

Crossville

Tennessee Technology Center - Crossville
James Purcell, Director
910 Miller Ave
PO Box 2959
Crossville, TN 38557
931 484-7502
Type: Vocational or Tech Sch
Control: State, County, or Local Govt
• Surgical Technology Prgm

Dayton

Bryan College
Stephen D Livesay, PhD, President
721 Bryan Dr
Box 7792
Dayton, TN 37321
423 775-7201
Type: 4-year Coll or Univ
Control: Nonprofit (Private or Religious)
• Athletic Training Prgm

Dickson

Tennessee Technology Center - Dickson
Bobby F Sullivan, MS, Director
740 Hwy 46 S
Dickson, TN 37055
615 441-6220
Type: Vocational or Tech Sch
Control: State, County, or Local Govt
• Dental Assisting Prgm
• Surgical Technology Prgm

Dyersburg

Dyersburg State Community College
Karen A Bowyer, PhD, President
1510 Lake Rd
Dyersburg, TN 38024
731 286-3301
Type: Junior or Comm Coll
Control: State, County, or Local Govt
• Health Information Tech Prgm
• Surgical Technology Prgm

Gallatin

Volunteer State Community College
Warren Nichols, EdD, President
1480 Nashville
Gallatin, TN 37066-3188
615 230-3500
Type: Junior or Comm Coll
Control: State, County, or Local Govt
• Clin Lab Technician/Med Lab Technician Prgm
• Dental Assisting Prgm
• Diagnostic Med Sonography Prgm
• Emergency Med Tech-Paramedic Prgm
• Health Information Tech Prgm
• Ophthalmic Med Technician Prgm
• Physical Therapist Assistant Prgm
• Polysomnographic Technology Prgm
• Radiography Prgm
• Respiratory Therapist (Advanced) Prgm
• Respiratory Therapist (Entry-Level) Prgm

Greenville

Tusculum College
Dolphus E Henry, PhD, President
106 McCormick
60 Old Shiloh Rd
Greenville, TN 37743
800 729-0256
Type: 4-year Coll or Univ
Control: Nonprofit (Private or Religious)
• Athletic Training Prgm

Harriman

Roane State Community College
Gary Goff, EdD, President
276 Patton Ln
Harriman, TN 37748-5011
865 882-4501
Type: Junior or Comm Coll
Control: State, County, or Local Govt
• Dental Hygiene Prgm
• Emergency Med Tech-Paramedic Prgm
• Health Information Tech Prgm
• Massage Therapy Prgm
• Occupational Therapy Asst Prgm
• Ophthalmic Dispensing Optician Prgm
• Physical Therapist Assistant Prgm
• Polysomnographic Technology Prgm
• Radiography Prgm
• Respiratory Therapist (Advanced) Prgm

Harrogate

Lincoln Memorial University
Nancy Moody, DSN, President
PO Box 2028
Cumberland Gap Pkwy
Harrogate, TN 37752
423 869-6391
Type: 4-year Coll or Univ
Control: Nonprofit (Private or Religious)
• Athletic Training Prgm
• Clin Lab Scientist/Med Technologist Prgm
• Osteopathic Medicine Prgm
• Veterinary Technology Prgm

Hohenwald

Tennessee Technology Center - Hohenwald
Rick C Brewer, MEd ED SPEC, Director
813 W Main St
Hohenwald, TN 38462
931 796-5351
Type: Vocational or Tech Sch
Control: Nonprofit (Private or Religious)
• Surgical Technology Prgm

Jackson

Jackson State Community College
Bruce Blanding, PhD, President
2046 N Parkway St
Jackson, TN 38301-3797
731 424-3520
Type: Junior or Comm Coll
Control: State, County, or Local Govt
• Clin Lab Technician/Med Lab Technician Prgm
• Emergency Med Tech-Paramedic Prgm
• Physical Therapist Assistant Prgm
• Radiography Prgm
• Respiratory Therapist (Advanced) Prgm

Tennessee Technology Center - Jackson
Don Williams, PhD, Director
2468 Technology Center Dr
Jackson, TN 38301
731 424-0691
Type: Vocational or Tech Sch
Control: State, County, or Local Govt
• Pharmacy Technician Prgm
• Surgical Technology Prgm

Union University
David S Dockery, PhD, President
1050 Union University Dr
Jackson, TN 38305
731 661-5180
Type: 4-year Coll or Univ
Control: Nonprofit (Private or Religious)
• Athletic Training Prgm
• Nursing Prgm

Jefferson City

Carson-Newman College
J Cordell Maddox, President
1646 Russell Ave
Jefferson City, TN 37760
615 471-4000
Type: 4-year Coll or Univ
Control: Nonprofit (Private or Religious)
• Athletic Training Prgm
• Dietetics-Didactic Prgm
• Nursing Prgm

Joelton

Meridian Institute of Surgical Assisting
Dennis A Stover, CST SA-C, President
PO Box 758
Joelton, TN 37080
615 298-1416
Type: Hosp or Med Ctr: 100-299 Beds
Control: For Profit
• Surgical Assistant Prgm

Johnson City

East Tennessee State University
Paul E Stanton, Jr, MD, President
College of Public and Allied Health
Box 70734
Johnson City, TN 37614
423 439-4211
Type: 4-year Coll or Univ
Control: State, County, or Local Govt
- Allopathic Medicine Prgm
- Audiologist Prgm
- Counseling Prgm
- Dental Hygiene Prgm
- Dietetic Internship Prgm
- Dietetics-Didactic Prgm
- Nursing Prgm
- Pharmacy Prgm
- Physical Therapy Prgm
- Radiography Prgm
- Respiratory Therapist (Advanced) Prgm
- Speech-Language Pathology Prgm

Knoxville

Fort Sanders Regional Medical Center
Jim Burkhart, MHA FACHE, Sr Vice President
9352 Park W Blvd
PO Box 22993
Knoxville, TN 37933-0993
865 541-1100
Type: Hosp or Med Ctr: 500> Beds
Control: Nonprofit (Private or Religious)
- Surgical Technology Prgm

South College
Stephen A South, BS, President
3904 Lonas Dr
Knoxville, TN 37909
865 251-1800
Type: 4-year Coll or Univ
Control: For Profit
- Medical Assistant Prgm
- Nuclear Medicine Technology Prgm
- Physical Therapist Assistant Prgm
- Physician Assistant Prgm
- Radiography Prgm

Tennessee Technology Center - Knoxville
David Esa, MSEd, Director
1100 Liberty St
Knoxville, TN 37919
615 546-5567
Type: Vocational or Tech Sch
Control: For Profit
- Dental Assisting Prgm
- Medical Assistant Prgm
- Surgical Technology Prgm

Tennessee Wesleyan College
Knoxville, TN 37932
Type: 4-year Coll or Univ
Control: Nonprofit (Private or Religious)
- Nursing Prgm

Univ of Tennessee Medical Ctr at Knoxville
Joseph Landsman, President and CEO
1924 Alcoa Hwy
Knoxville, TN 37920-6999
865 544-9430
Type: Hosp or Med Ctr: 500> Beds
Control: Nonprofit (Private or Religious)
- Clin Lab Scientist/Med Technologist Prgm
- Nuclear Medicine Technology Prgm
- Radiography Prgm
- Veterinary Medicine Prgm

University of Tennessee - Knoxville
Loren Crabtree, PhD, Chancellor
810 Andy Holt Tower
Knoxville, TN 37996
865 974-3265
Type: 4-year Coll or Univ
Control: State, County, or Local Govt
- Audiologist Prgm
- Counseling Prgm
- Dietetic Internship Prgm
- Dietetics-Didactic Prgm
- Medical Librarian Prgm
- Nursing Prgm
- Psychology Prgm
- Rehabilitation Counseling Prgm
- Speech-Language Pathology Prgm
- Therapeutic Recreation Specialist Prgm

Lebanon

Cumberland University
Harvill C Eaton, PhD, President
One Cumberland Square
Lebanon, TN 37087-3408
615 444-2562
Type: 4-year Coll or Univ
Control: Nonprofit (Private or Religious)
- Athletic Training Prgm

Martin

University of Tennessee - Martin
Tom Rakes, EdD, Chancellor
325 Adminstration Bldg
Martin, TN 38238
731 881-7500
Type: 4-year Coll or Univ
Control: State, County, or Local Govt
- Athletic Training Prgm
- Dietetic Internship Prgm
- Dietetics-Didactic Prgm

McMinnville

Tennessee Technology Center - McMinnville
Andy Forrester, MS, Director
241 Vo-Tech Dr
McMinnville, TN 37110
931 473-5587
Type: Vocational or Tech Sch
Control: State, County, or Local Govt
- Medical Assistant Prgm
- Surgical Technology Prgm

Memphis

Baptist College of Health Sciences
Betty Sue McGarvey, DSN, President
1003 Monroe Ave
Memphis, TN 38104-3199
901 572-2585
Type: 4-year Coll or Univ
Control: Nonprofit (Private or Religious)
- Diagnostic Med Sonography Prgm
- Nuclear Medicine Technology Prgm
- Nursing Prgm
- Radiation Therapy Prgm
- Radiography Prgm
- Respiratory Therapist (Advanced) Prgm

Concorde Career College - Memphis
Tommy Stewart, AAS, Director
5100 Poplar Ave, Ste 132
Memphis, TN 38137
901 761-9494
Type: Vocational or Tech Sch
Control: For Profit
- Dental Assisting Prgm
- Medical Assistant Prgm
- Pharmacy Technician Prgm
- Respiratory Therapist (Advanced) Prgm
- Surgical Technology Prgm

Methodist Le Bonheur Healthcare
Peggy Troy, RN MSN, CEO
Methodist Professional Bldg
1211 Union Ave, Ste 700
Memphis, TN 38104
901 516-0546
Type: Hosp or Med Ctr: 500> Beds
Control: Nonprofit (Private or Religious)
- Diagnostic Med Sonography Prgm

Methodist University Hospital
Cecelia Sawyer, CEO
1265 Union Ave
Memphis, TN 38104
901 516-0543
Type: Hosp or Med Ctr: 500> Beds
Control: Nonprofit (Private or Religious)
- Nuclear Medicine Technology Prgm
- Radiography Prgm

Southern College of Optometry
Richard W Phillips, OD FAAO, President
1245 Madison Ave
Memphis, TN 38104
901 722-3200
Type: Junior or Comm Coll
Control: Nonprofit (Private or Religious)
- Optometry Prgm

Southwest Tennessee Community College
Nathan L Essex, President
5983 Macon Cove
Memphis, TN 38134-7693
901 333-7822
Type: Junior or Comm Coll
Control: State, County, or Local Govt
- Clin Lab Technician/Med Lab Technician Prgm
- Dietetic Technician-AD Prgm
- Emergency Med Tech-Paramedic Prgm
- Phlebotomy Prgm
- Physical Therapist Assistant Prgm
- Radiography Prgm

Tennessee Technology Center - Memphis
Russell Shelton, Director
550 Alabama Ave
Memphis, TN 38105-3799
901 543-6156
Type: Vocational or Tech Sch
Control: State, County, or Local Govt
- Dental Assisting Prgm
- Medical Assistant Prgm
- Pharmacy Technician Prgm
- Surgical Technology Prgm

University of Memphis
Shirley C Raines, President
Memphis, TN 38152
901 678-2000
Type: 4-year Coll or Univ
Control: State, County, or Local Govt
- Audiologist Prgm
- Counseling Prgm
- Dietetic Internship Prgm
- Dietetics-Didactic Prgm
- Nursing Prgm
- Psychology Prgm
- Rehabilitation Counseling Prgm
- Speech-Language Pathology Prgm

University of Tennessee Health Science Ctr
Hershel P. Wall, MD, Interim Chancellor
62 S Dunlap
Hyman Admin Bldg, Ste 200
Memphis, TN 38163
901 448-4796
Type: Acad Health Ctr/Med Sch
Control: State, County, or Local Govt
- Allopathic Medicine Prgm
- Clin Lab Scientist/Med Technologist Prgm
- Cytotechnology Prgm
- Dental Hygiene Prgm
- Dentistry Prgm
- Health Information Admin Prgm
- Nursing Prgm
- Occupational Therapy Prgm
- Pharmacy Prgm
- Physical Therapy Prgm

Milligan College

Milligan College
Donald R Jeanes, DD, President
PO Box 1
Milligan College, TN 37682
423 461-8710
Type: 4-year Coll or Univ
Control: Nonprofit (Private or Religious)
- Nursing Prgm
- Occupational Therapy Prgm

Morristown

Walters State Community College
Wade B McCamey, EdD, President
500 S Davy Crockett Pkwy
Morristown, TN 37813-6899
423 585-2600
Type: Junior or Comm Coll
Control: State, County, or Local Govt
- Emergency Med Tech-Paramedic Prgm
- Health Information Tech Prgm
- Pharmacy Technician Prgm
- Physical Therapist Assistant Prgm
- Respiratory Therapist (Entry-Level) Prgm

Murfreesboro

Middle Tennessee State University
Sydney McPhee, PhD, President
Cope Administration Bldg 110
Murfreesboro, TN 37132
615 898-2622
Type: 4-year Coll or Univ
Control: State, County, or Local Govt
- Athletic Training Prgm
- Counseling Prgm
- Dietetics-Didactic Prgm
- Nursing Prgm

National HealthCare LP
PO Box 1398
Murfreesboro, TN 37133-1398
615 890-2020
Control: For Profit
- Dietetic Internship Prgm

Tennessee Technology Center - Murfreesboro
Carol Puryear, BS MS, Director
1303 Old Fort Pkwy
Murfreesboro, TN 37130
615 898-8010
Type: Vocational or Tech Sch
Control: State, County, or Local Govt
- Dental Assisting Prgm
- Pharmacy Technician Prgm
- Surgical Technology Prgm

Nashville

Belmont University
Robert C Fisher, PhD, President
1900 Belmont Blvd
Nashville, TN 37212
615 460-6793
Type: 4-year Coll or Univ
Control: Nonprofit (Private or Religious)
- Nursing Prgm
- Occupational Therapy Prgm
- Physical Therapy Prgm

Lipscomb University
L Randolph Lowry III, BA MPA JD, President
3901 Granny White Pike
Nashville, TN 37204
615 279-6194
Type: 4-year Coll or Univ
Control: Nonprofit (Private or Religious)
- Dietetic Internship Prgm
- Dietetics-Didactic Prgm

Meharry Medical College
1005 Dr D B Todd Jr Blvd
Nashville, TN 37208
615 327-6000
Type: Acad Health Ctr/Med Sch
Control: Nonprofit (Private or Religious)
- Allopathic Medicine Prgm
- Dentistry Prgm

Nashville General Hospital
Reginald Coopwood, MD, CEO
1818 Albion St
Nashville, TN 37208
615 341-4490
Type: Hosp or Med Ctr: 500> Beds
Control: State, County, or Local Govt
- Radiography Prgm

Nashville State Community College
George H Van Allen, EdD, President
120 White Bridge Rd
PO Box 90285
Nashville, TN 37209-4515
615 353-3236
Type: Junior or Comm Coll
Control: State, County, or Local Govt
- Occupational Therapy Asst Prgm
- Surgical Assistant Prgm
- Surgical Technology Prgm

Tennessee State University
Melvin Johnson, DBA, President
3500 John A Merritt Blvd
Nashville, TN 37209-1561
615 963-7406
Type: 4-year Coll or Univ
Control: State, County, or Local Govt
- Clin Lab Scientist/Med Technologist Prgm
- Dental Hygiene Prgm
- Dietetics-Didactic Prgm
- Health Information Admin Prgm
- Occupational Therapy Prgm
- Physical Therapy Prgm
- Respiratory Therapist (Advanced) Prgm
- Speech-Language Pathology Prgm

Tennessee Technology Center - Nashville
Charles F Malin, Director
100 White Bridge Rd
Nashville, TN 37209
Type: Vocational or Tech Sch
Control: For Profit
- Pharmacy Technician Prgm

Trevecca Nazarene University
Dan Boone, DMin, President
333 Murfreesboro Rd
Nashville, TN 37210
615 248-1251
Type: 4-year Coll or Univ
Control: Nonprofit (Private or Religious)
- Physician Assistant Prgm

Vanderbilt University
Nicholas S. Zeppos, Interim Chancellor
Nashville, TN 37240-0001
615 322-7311
Type: 4-year Coll or Univ
Control: Nonprofit (Private or Religious)
- Allopathic Medicine Prgm
- Counseling Prgm
- Psychology Prgm
- Teacher of the Visually Impaired Prgm

Vanderbilt University Medical Center
Harry R Jacobson, MD, Vice Chancellor, Hlth Aff
1161 21st Ave S
D-3300 MCN
Nashville, TN 37232
615 322-2151
Type: Acad Health Ctr/Med Sch
Control: Nonprofit (Private or Religious)
- Audiologist Prgm
- Clin Lab Scientist/Med Technologist Prgm
- Diagnostic Med Sonography Prgm
- Dietetic Internship Prgm
- Nuclear Medicine Technology Prgm
- Perfusion Prgm
- Radiation Therapy Prgm
- Speech-Language Pathology Prgm

Paris

Tennessee Technology Center - Paris
Bradley White, PhD, Interim Director
312 S Wilson St
Paris, TN 38242
731 644-7365
Type: Vocational or Tech Sch
Control: State, County, or Local Govt
• Surgical Technology Prgm

Texas

Abilene

Abilene Christian University
Royce L Money, PhD, President
ACU Box 29100
Abilene, TX 79699
325 674-2000
Type: 4-year Coll or Univ
Control: Nonprofit (Private or Religious)
• Dietetics-Didactic Prgm
• Speech-Language Pathology Prgm

Hardin-Simmons University
Craig Turner, PhD, President
2200 Hickory
HSU Box 16000
Abilene, TX 79698
325 670-1227
Type: 4-year Coll or Univ
Control: Nonprofit (Private or Religious)
• Athletic Training Prgm
• Physical Therapy Prgm

Hendrick Medical Center
Tim Lancaster, FACHE, President
1900 Pine
Abilene, TX 79601-2316
325 670-2364
Type: Hosp or Med Ctr: 300-499 Beds
Control: Nonprofit (Private or Religious)
• Radiography Prgm

Patty Hanks Shelton School of Nursing
Abilene, Tx 79601
Type: Acad Health Ctr/Med Sch
Control: Nonprofit (Private or Religious)
• Nursing Prgm

SWT/HMC Respiratory Care School Consortium
Jeff Lawrence, Program Director
1900 N Pine St
Abilene, TX 79601
915 670-2368
Type: Consortium
Control: Nonprofit (Private or Religious)
• Respiratory Therapist (Entry-Level) Prgm

Alpine

Sul Ross State University
R Vic Morgan, PhD, President
SR Box C-114
Alpine, TX 79830
432 837-8032
Type: 4-year Coll or Univ
Control: State, County, or Local Govt
• Veterinary Medicine Prgm

Alvin

Alvin Community College
A Rodney Allbright, JD, President
3110 Mustang Rd
Alvin, TX 77511
281 756-3598
Type: Junior or Comm Coll
Control: State, County, or Local Govt
• Diagnostic Med Sonography Prgm
• Respiratory Therapist (Advanced) Prgm

Amarillo

Amarillo College
Steven Jones, EdD, President
PO Box 447
Amarillo, TX 79178-0001
806 371-5123
Type: Junior or Comm Coll
Control: State, County, or Local Govt
• Clin Lab Technician/Med Lab Technician Prgm
• Dental Hygiene Prgm
• Nuclear Medicine Technology Prgm
• Occupational Therapy Asst Prgm
• Physical Therapist Assistant Prgm
• Radiation Therapy Prgm
• Radiography Prgm
• Respiratory Therapist (Advanced) Prgm
• Surgical Technology Prgm

Arlington

Concorde Career Institute - Arlington
Rebecca Zielinski, RN, Campus President
601 Ryan Plaza Dr, Ste 200
Arlington, TX 76011
817 267-1594
Type: Vocational or Tech Sch
Control: For Profit
• Surgical Technology Prgm

University of Texas at Arlington
James D Spaniolo, President
321 Davis Hall, Box 19125
Arlington, TX 76019-0125
817 272-2101
Type: Acad Health Ctr/Med Sch
Control: State, County, or Local Government
• Athletic Training Prgm
• Nursing Prgm

Athens

Trinity Valley Community College
Ronald C Baugh, MS, President
100 Cardinal Dr
Athens, TX 75751
903 675-6211
Type: Junior or Comm Coll
Control: State, County, or Local Govt
• Surgical Technology Prgm

Austin

Austin Community College
Stephen Kinslow, PhD, President
5930 Middle Fiskville Rd
Austin, TX 78752-4390
512 223-7598
Type: Junior or Comm Coll
Control: State, County, or Local Govt
• Clin Lab Technician/Med Lab Technician Prgm
• Dental Hygiene Prgm
• Diagnostic Med Sonography Prgm
• Emergency Med Tech-Paramedic Prgm
• Occupational Therapy Asst Prgm
• Pharmacy Technician Prgm
• Phlebotomy Prgm
• Physical Therapist Assistant Prgm
• Radiography Prgm
• Surgical Technology Prgm

Austin State Hospital
Carl Schock, Superintendent
4110 Guadalupe St
Austin, TX 78751
512 419-2041
Type: Hosp or Med Ctr: 500> Beds
Control: State, County, or Local Govt
• Clin Lab Scientist/Med Technologist Prgm

Texas WIC
1100 West 49th St
Austin, TX 78756
Control: State, County, or Local Govt
• Dietetic Internship Prgm

University of Texas at Austin
William Powers, PhD, President
1 University Station
Austin, TX 78712
512 471-3434
Type: 4-year Coll or Univ
Control: State, County, or Local Govt
• Athletic Training Prgm
• Audiologist Prgm
• Dietetics-Coordinated Prgm
• Dietetics-Didactic Prgm
• Medical Librarian Prgm
• Nursing Prgm
• Pharmacy Prgm
• Psychology Prgm
• Rehabilitation Counseling Prgm
• Speech-Language Pathology Prgm

Virginia College at Austin
Harvey Giblin, MEd, Campus President
6301 E Hwy 290
Austin, TX 78723
512 279-2802
Type: Vocational or Tech Sch
Control: For Profit
• Surgical Technology Prgm

Baytown

Lee College
Martha Ellis, PhD, President
PO Box 818
Baytown, TX 77520
281 425-6300
Type: Junior or Comm Coll
Control: Nonprofit (Private or Religious)
• Health Information Tech Prgm

Beaumont

CHRISTUS Hospital - St Elizabeth
Mario Murdano, MBA, Administrator
2830 Calder St
PO Box 5405
Beaumont, TX 77726-5405
409 892-7171
Type: Hosp or Med Ctr: 300-499 Beds
Control: Nonprofit (Private or Religious)
• Clin Lab Scientist/Med Technologist Prgm
• Phlebotomy Prgm

Lamar Institute of Technology
Paul J. Szuch, EdD, President
855 E Lavaca
PO Box 10043
Beaumont, TX 77705
409 880-8405
Type: Vocational or Tech Sch
Control: State, County, or Local Govt
• Dental Hygiene Prgm
• Diagnostic Med Sonography Prgm
• Health Information Tech Prgm
• Radiography Prgm
• Respiratory Therapist (Advanced) Prgm

Lamar University
James Simmons, President
PO Box 10001
Beaumont, TX 77710
409 880-8405
Type: 4-year Coll or Univ
Control: State, County, or Local Govt
• Audiologist Prgm
• Dietetic Internship Prgm
• Dietetics-Didactic Prgm
• Speech-Language Pathology Prgm

Memorial Hermann Baptist Hospital Beaumont
David Parmer, MS, President
Hospital Admin and Accounting
PO Drawer 1591
Beaumont, TX 77704
409 212-5012
Type: Hosp or Med Ctr: 300-499 Beds
Control: Nonprofit (Private or Religious)
• Radiography Prgm

Beeville

Coastal Bend College
Thomas Baynum, PhD, President
3800 Charco Rd
Beeville, TX 78102
361 354-2200
Type: Junior or Comm Coll
Control: State, County, or Local Govt
• Dental Hygiene Prgm

Belton

University of Mary Hardin-Baylor
Jerry Bawcom, PhD, President
900 Colllege St
Belton, TX 76502
254 295-8642
Type: 4-year Coll or Univ
Control: Nonprofit (Private or Religious)
• Athletic Training Prgm
• Nursing Prgm

Big Spring

Howard College
Cheryl T Sparks, EdD, President
1001 Birdwell Ln
Big Spring, TX 79720
432 264-5000
Type: Junior or Comm Coll
Control: State, County, or Local Govt
• Dental Hygiene Prgm
• Health Information Tech Prgm
• Surgical Technology Prgm

Brenham

Blinn College
Don E Voelter, PhD, President
902 College Ave
Brenham, TX 77833
979 830-4112
Type: Junior or Comm Coll
Control: State, County, or Local Govt
• Dental Hygiene Prgm
• Physical Therapist Assistant Prgm
• Radiography Prgm

Brownsville

Univ Tx at Brownsville/Tx Southmost Coll
Juliet Garcia, PhD, President
83 Ft Brown
Brownsville, TX 78520
956 544-8200
Type: 4-year Coll or Univ
Control: State, County, or Local Govt
• Clin Lab Technician/Med Lab Technician Prgm
• Diagnostic Med Sonography Prgm
• Radiography Prgm
• Respiratory Therapist (Advanced) Prgm
• Respiratory Therapist (Entry-Level) Prgm

Bryan

St Joseph Regional Health Center
John J Buckley, Jr, FACHE
2801 Franciscan Dr
Bryan, TX 77802-2544
979 776-3777
Type: Hosp or Med Ctr: 100-299 Beds
Control: Nonprofit (Private or Religious)
• Surgical Technology Prgm

Canyon

West Texas A&M University
J Patrick O'Brien, President/CEO
Office of the President, WTAMU Box 60247
Canyon, TX 79016
806 656-2000
Type: 4-year Coll or Univ
Control: State, County, or Local Govt
• Athletic Training Prgm
• Music Therapy Prgm
• Nursing Prgm
• Speech-Language Pathology Prgm

Carthage

Panola College
Gregory S Powell, EdD, President
1109 W Panola
Carthage, TX 75633-2397
903 693-2022
Type: Junior or Comm Coll
Control: State, County, or Local Govt
• Health Information Tech Prgm
• Occupational Therapy Asst Prgm

Cisco

Cisco Junior College
Colleen Smith, PhD, President
101 College Heights Drive
Cisco, TX 76437
254 442-2567
Type: Junior or Comm Coll
Control: State, County, or Local Govt
• Medical Assistant Prgm
• Surgical Technology Prgm

College Station

Baylor College of Dentistry, Texas A&M HSC
Nancy Dickey, MD, President
TAMU 1364
College Station, TX 77843-1364
979 458-7200
Type: 4-year Coll or Univ
Control: State, County, or Local Govt
• Dental Hygiene Prgm
• Dentistry Prgm

Texas A&M University
Robert Gates, President
College Station, TX 77843
409 845-3211
Type: 4-year Coll or Univ
Control: State, County, or Local Govt
• Allopathic Medicine Prgm
• Athletic Training Prgm
• Clin Lab Scientist/Med Technologist Prgm
• Counseling Prgm (2)
• Dietetic Internship Prgm (2)
• Dietetics-Didactic Prgm (2)
• Nursing Prgm (2)
• Pharmacy Prgm
• Psychology Prgm
• Speech-Language Pathology Prgm
• Veterinary Medicine Prgm

Conroe

Montgomery College
Thomas E Butler, EdD, President
3200 College Park Dr
Conroe, TX 77384
936 273-7222
Type: Junior or Comm Coll
Control: State, County, or Local Govt
• Physical Therapist Assistant Prgm
• Radiography Prgm

INSTITUTIONS

Corpus Christi

Del Mar College
Carlos A Garcia, PhD, President
101 Baldwin Blvd
Corpus Christi, TX 78404
361 698-1203
Type: Junior or Comm Coll
Control: State, County, or Local Govt
- Clin Lab Technician/Med Lab Technician Prgm
- Dental Assisting Prgm
- Dental Hygiene Prgm
- Diagnostic Med Sonography Prgm
- Health Information Tech Prgm
- Nuclear Medicine Technology Prgm
- Occupational Therapy Asst Prgm
- Physical Therapist Assistant Prgm
- Radiography Prgm
- Respiratory Therapist (Advanced) Prgm
- Surgical Technology Prgm

Corsicana

Navarro College
Richard Sanchez, EdD, President
3200 W 7th Ave
Corsicana, TX 75110-4818
903 875-7308
Type: Junior or Comm Coll
Control: State, County, or Local Govt
- Clin Lab Technician/Med Lab Technician Prgm
- Occupational Therapy Asst Prgm

Cypress

Cy-Fair College
Diane K Troyer, PhD, President
9191 Barker-Cypress Rd
Cypress, TX 77433
281 290-3940
Type: Junior or Comm Coll
Control: State, County, or Local Govt
- Diagnostic Med Sonography Prgm
- Medical Assistant Prgm
- Radiography Prgm

Dallas

ATI Health Education Centers
Joe Mehlmann, President
2777 Stemmons Freeway
Dallas, TX 75207
214 630-5651
Type: Vocational or Tech Sch
Control: For Profit
- Respiratory Therapist (Advanced) Prgm

ATI-Career Training
Gerald Parr, BS, Executive Director
10003 Technology Blvd W
Dallas, TX 75220
214 902-8191
Type: Vocational or Tech Sch
Control: For Profit
- Respiratory Therapist (Advanced) Prgm

Baylor University Med Center
John McWhorter, MHA, President/CEO
3500 Gaston Ave
3535 Worth St
Dallas, TX 75204
214 820-4642
Type: Hosp or Med Ctr: 500> Beds
Control: Nonprofit (Private or Religious)
- Dietetic Internship Prgm
- Nuclear Medicine Technology Prgm
- Radiography Prgm

Dallas County Community College
Sharon Blackman, EdD, Dean of Technical Educ
12800 Abrams Rd
Dallas, TX 75243-2199
972 238-6954
Type: Junior or Comm Coll
Control: State, County, or Local Govt
- Health Information Tech Prgm

El Centro College
Michael Jackson, PhD, Acting President
801 Main St
Dallas, TX 75202-3604
214 860-2011
Type: Junior or Comm Coll
Control: State, County, or Local Govt
- Cardiovascular Technology Prgm
- Clin Lab Technician/Med Lab Technician Prgm
- Diagnostic Med Sonography Prgm
- Medical Assistant Prgm
- Radiography Prgm
- Respiratory Therapist (Advanced) Prgm
- Surgical Technology Prgm

Presbyterian Hospital of Dallas
8200 Walnut Hill Ln
Dallas, TX 75231-4402
214 345-7558
Control: Nonprofit (Private or Religious)
- Dietetic Internship Prgm

Richland College
Stephen Mittelstet, PhD, President
12800 Abrams Rd
Dallas, TX 75243
214 238-6364
Type: Junior or Comm Coll
Control: State, County, or Local Govt
- Medical Assistant Prgm
- Pharmacy Technician Prgm

Sanford-Brown Institute - Dallas
Gary C Jack, BS MS, Executive Director
2998 N Stemmons Frwy
Dallas, TX 75247
214 638-6400
Type: Vocational or Tech Sch
Control: For Profit
- Diagnostic Med Sonography Prgm

Southern Methodist University
R Gerald Turner, President
6425 Boaz St
PO Box 296
Dallas, TX 75275
214 768-2000
Type: 4-year Coll or Univ
Control: Nonprofit (Private or Religious)
- Music Therapy Prgm

Univ of Texas Southwestern Med Ctr
Kern Wildenthal, MD PhD, President
5323 Harry Hines Blvd, B12.100
Dallas, TX 75390-9082
214 648-2508
Type: Junior or Comm Coll
Control: State, County, or Local Govt
- Allopathic Medicine Prgm
- Clin Lab Scientist/Med Technologist Prgm
- Dietetics-Coordinated Prgm
- Emergency Med Tech-Paramedic Prgm
- Medical Illustrator Prgm
- Orthotist/Prosthetist Prgm
- Physical Therapy Prgm
- Physician Assistant Prgm
- Psychology Prgm
- Rehabilitation Counseling Prgm
- Specialist in BB Tech Prgm

Westwood College
8390 LBJ Freeway, Ste 100
Dallas, TX 75243
214 570-0100
Type: Vocational or Tech Sch
Control: State, County, or Local Govt
- Medical Assistant Prgm

Denison

Grayson County College
Alan Scheibmeir, PhD, President
6101 Grayson Dr
Denison, TX 75020
903 465-6030
Type: Junior or Comm Coll
Control: State, County, or Local Govt
- Clin Lab Technician/Med Lab Technician Prgm
- Dental Assisting Prgm

Denton

Texas Woman's University
Ann Stuart, PhD, President and Chancellor
Box 425587
TWU Station (ACT-15)
Denton, TX 76204-3587
940 898-3201
Type: 4-year Coll or Univ
Control: State, County, or Local Govt
- Counseling Prgm
- Dental Hygiene Prgm
- Dietetic Internship Prgm (2)
- Dietetics-Didactic Prgm
- Medical Librarian Prgm
- Music Therapy Prgm
- Nursing Prgm
- Occupational Therapy Prgm (3)
- Physical Therapy Prgm
- Speech-Language Pathology Prgm

University of North Texas
Lee Jackson, Chancellor
Denton, TX 76203-5008
940 565-2000
Type: 4-year Coll or Univ
Control: State, County, or Local Govt
- Audiologist Prgm
- Counseling Prgm
- Medical Librarian Prgm
- Psychology Prgm (2)
- Rehabilitation Counseling Prgm
- Speech-Language Pathology Prgm

Edinburg

Univ of Texas - Pan American
Blandina Cardenas, PhD, President
1201 W University Dr
Edinburg, TX 78541-2999
956 381-2100
Type: 4-year Coll or Univ
Control: State, County, or Local Govt
• Clin Lab Scientist/Med Technologist Prgm
• Dietetics-Coordinated Prgm
• Nursing Prgm
• Occupational Therapy Prgm
• Physician Assistant Prgm
• Rehabilitation Counseling Prgm
• Speech-Language Pathology Prgm

El Paso

Career Centers of Texas
Sally Crickard, Executive Director
8360 Burnham Rd, Ste 100
El Paso, TX 79907
915 595-1935
Type: Vocational or Tech Sch
Control: For Profit
• Medical Assistant Prgm
• Surgical Technology Prgm

Computer Career Center
Lee Chayes, MA, President
6101 Montana
El Paso, TX 79925
915 779-8031
Type: Vocational or Tech Sch
Control: For Profit
• Medical Assistant Prgm

El Paso Community College
Richard M Rhodes, PhD, President
PO Box 20500
El Paso, TX 79998-0500
915 831-6511
Type: Junior or Comm Coll
Control: State, County, or Local Govt
• Clin Lab Technician/Med Lab Technician Prgm
• Dental Assisting Prgm
• Dental Hygiene Prgm
• Diagnostic Med Sonography Prgm
• Health Information Tech Prgm
• Medical Assistant Prgm
• Ophthalmic Dispensing Optician Prgm
• Pharmacy Technician Prgm
• Physical Therapist Assistant Prgm
• Radiography Prgm
• Surgical Technology Prgm

University of Texas at El Paso
Diana Natalicio, PhD, President
500 W University Ave
El Paso, TX 79968
915 747-5555
Type: 4-year Coll or Univ
Control: State, County, or Local Govt
• Clin Lab Scientist/Med Technologist Prgm
• Nursing Prgm
• Occupational Therapy Prgm
• Physical Therapy Prgm
• Speech-Language Pathology Prgm

Fort Sam Houston

Brooke Army Medical Center
William Fox, Jr, BG MC MD, Commanding
    General
Fort Sam Houston, TX 78234-6200
210 916-0499
Type: Dept of Defense
Control: Fed Govt
• Cytotechnology Prgm

Interservice
MCCS-HMT, Physical Therapy Branch
3151 Scott Rd
Fort Sam Houston, TX 78234-6138
Type: Dept of Defense
Control: Fed Govt
• Interservice Physician Assistant Prgm
• Physical Therapy Prgm

US Army Medical Dept Center & School
Russell Czerw, DC US Army, Major General
2250 Stanley Rd, Ste 301
Fort Sam Houston, TX 78234-6100
210 221-6325
Type: Dept of Defense
Control: Fed Govt
• Cardiovascular Technology Prgm
• Clin Lab Technician/Med Lab Technician Prgm
• Occupational Therapy Asst Prgm
• Optometric Technician Prgm
• Pharmacy Technician Prgm
• Radiography Prgm
• Respiratory Therapist (Entry-Level) Prgm

Fort Worth

Career Centers of Texas - Ft Worth Campus
Nancy Tedros, MBA, Executive Director
2001 Beach St, Ste 201
Fort Worth, TX 76103
Type: Hosp or Med Ctr: 500> Beds
Control: State, County, or Local Govt
• Radiography Prgm

Tarrant County Jr College - South
Jerry Mullen, Dean, Instruction
5301 Campus Dr
Fort Worth, TX 76119-5998
817 534-4861
Type: Junior or Comm Coll
Control: State, County, or Local Govt
• Dietetic Technician-AD Prgm

Texas Christian University
Victor Boschini, EdD, Chancellor
TCU 297080
Fort Worth, TX 76129
817 257-7783
Type: 4-year Coll or Univ
Control: Nonprofit (Private or Religious)
• Athletic Training Prgm
• Dietetics-Coordinated Prgm
• Dietetics-Didactic Prgm
• Nursing Prgm
• Speech-Language Pathology Prgm

Texas Wesleyan University
Harold G Jeffcoat, EdD, President
1201 Wesleyan St
Fort Worth, TX 76105
817 531-4401
Type: 4-year Coll or Univ
Control: State, County, or Local Govt
• Athletic Training Prgm

Univ of North Texas Hlth Sci Ctr at Ft Worth
Ronald Blanck, DO, President
3500 Camp Bowie Blvd
Fort Worth, TX 76107
817 735-2555
Type: Acad Health Ctr/Med Sch
Control: State, County, or Local Govt
• Osteopathic Medicine Prgm
• Physician Assistant Prgm

Friendswood

Texas School of Business
Kevin Green, JD, Executive Director
3208 FM 528
Friendswood, TX 77546
281 443-8900
Type: Vocational or Tech Sch
Control: For Profit
• Medical Assistant Prgm (4)

Gainesville

North Central Texas College
Eddie Hadlock, EdD, President
1525 W California St
Gainesville, TX 76240
940 668-7731
Type: Junior or Comm Coll
Control: State, County, or Local Govt
• Surgical Technology Prgm

Galveston

Galveston College
Myles Shelton, EdD, President
4015 Ave Q
Galveston, TX 77550-2782
409 944-1200
Type: Junior or Comm Coll
Control: State, County, or Local Govt
• Emergency Med Tech-Paramedic Prgm
• Nuclear Medicine Technology Prgm
• Radiation Therapy Prgm
• Radiography Prgm
• Surgical Technology Prgm

University of Texas Medical Branch
David Callender, PhD, President
301 University Blvd
Galveston, TX 77555
409 772-3055
Type: Acad Health Ctr/Med Sch
Control: State, County, or Local Govt
• Allopathic Medicine Prgm
• Clin Lab Scientist/Med Technologist Prgm
• Nursing Prgm
• Occupational Therapy Prgm
• Pharmacy Technician Prgm
• Physical Therapy Prgm
• Physician Assistant Prgm
• Respiratory Therapist (Advanced) Prgm
• Specialist in BB Tech Prgm

INSTITUTIONS

Georgetown

Southwestern University
Jake B Schrum, BA MDiv, President
1001 East University Ave
Georgetown, TX 78627-0770
512 863-1454
Type: 4-year Coll or Univ
Control: Nonprofit (Private or Religious)
• Athletic Training Prgm

Houston

Academy of Health Care Professions
A John Emerald, BA, CEO
1900 N Loop W, Ste 100
Houston, TX 77092
713 425-3100
Type: Vocational or Tech Sch
Control: For Profit
• Surgical Technology Prgm

Baylor College of Medicine
Peter Traber, MD, President/CEO
BCMC 143A, One Baylor Plaza
Houston, TX 77030
713 798-4433
Type: Acad Health Ctr/Med Sch
Control: Nonprofit (Private or Religious)
• Allopathic Medicine Prgm
• Physician Assistant Prgm

Bradford School
Robert Puig, MA, Dir/Chief Acad Officer
4669 SW Freeway, Ste 300
Houston, TX 77027
713 629-1500
Type: Vocational or Tech Sch
Control: For Profit
• Medical Assistant Prgm

Gulf Coast School of Blood Bank Technology
Bill T Teague, BS MT(ASCP)SBB, President/CEO
1400 La Concha Ln
Houston, TX 77054-1802
713 790-1200
Type: Nonhosp HC Facil, BB, or Lab
Control: Nonprofit (Private or Religious)
• Specialist in BB Tech Prgm

Harris County Hosp Dist/Ben Taub Gen Hosp
David Lopez, MS, CEO, President
2525 Holly Hall
Houston, TX 77266
713 566-6400
Type: Hosp or Med Ctr: 500> Beds
Control: State, County, or Local Govt
• Radiography Prgm

Houston Community College
Mary Spangler, EdD, Chancellor
3100 Main, Ste 12D
PO Box 667517
Houston, TX 77266
713 718-5059
Type: Junior or Comm Coll
Control: State, County, or Local Govt
• Clin Lab Technician/Med Lab Technician Prgm
• Dental Assisting Prgm
• Diagnostic Med Sonography Prgm
• Emergency Med Tech-Paramedic Prgm
• Health Information Tech Prgm
• Histotechnician Prgm
• Medical Assistant Prgm
• Nuclear Medicine Technology Prgm
• Occupational Therapy Asst Prgm
• Physical Therapist Assistant Prgm
• Radiography Prgm
• Respiratory Therapist (Advanced) Prgm
• Surgical Technology Prgm

MedVance Institute
Deborah Schwarzberg, PhD, President
6220 Westpark
Houston, TX 77057
Type: Vocational or Tech Sch
Control: For Profit
• Radiography Prgm
• Surgical Technology Prgm

Memorial Hermann Healthcare System
Dan Wolterman, CEO, President
7737 SW Freeway PB II
Houston, TX 77074
713 776-5484
Type: Hosp or Med Ctr: 500> Beds
Control: Nonprofit (Private or Religious)
• Radiography Prgm

Methodist Hospital
Ron Girotto, CEO, President
6565 Fannin, D 200
Houston, TX 77030
713 790-2481
Type: Hosp or Med Ctr: 500> Beds
Control: Nonprofit (Private or Religious)
• Clin Lab Scientist/Med Technologist Prgm

Michael E DeBakey VA Medical Center
Robert F Stott, MPH, Hospital Director
2002 Holcombe Blvd 00/580
Houston, TX 77030
713 794-7100
Type: Dept of Veterans Affairs
Control: Fed Govt
• Dietetic Internship Prgm

North Harris College
Stephen Head, PhD, President
2700 W W Thorne Dr
Houston, TX 77073-3499
281 618-5444
Type: Junior or Comm Coll
Control: Nonprofit (Private or Religious)
• Emergency Med Tech-Paramedic Prgm
• Health Information Tech Prgm
• Pharmacy Technician Prgm

San Jacinto College North
Charles Grant, PhD, President
5800 Uvalde Rd
Houston, TX 77049-4599
281 459-7100
Type: Junior or Comm Coll
Control: State, County, or Local Govt
• Emergency Med Tech-Paramedic Prgm
• Health Information Tech Prgm
• Medical Assistant Prgm
• Pharmacy Technician Prgm

San Jacinto College South
Linda Watkins, PhD, President
13735 Beamer Rd
Houston, TX 77089
281 922-3400
Type: Junior or Comm Coll
Control: State, County, or Local Govt
• Pharmacy Technician Prgm
• Physical Therapist Assistant Prgm

Sanford-Brown Institute - Houston
James Garrett, BS, Executive Director
10500 Forum Pl, Ste 200
Houston, TX 77036
713 779-1110
Type: Vocational or Tech Sch
Control: For Profit
• Diagnostic Med Sonography Prgm
• Surgical Technology Prgm

Texas Heart Institute
Denton A Cooley, MD, President
PO Box 20345, MC 1-224
Houston, TX 77225
832 355-4026
Type: Hosp or Med Ctr <100 Beds
Control: Nonprofit (Private or Religious)
• Perfusion Prgm

Texas Southern University
Priscilla Slade, PhD, President
3100 Cleburne St
Houston, TX 77004
713 313-7341
Type: 4-year Coll or Univ
Control: State, County, or Local Govt
• Clin Lab Scientist/Med Technologist Prgm
• Dietetics-Didactic Prgm
• Health Information Admin Prgm
• Pharmacy Prgm
• Respiratory Therapist (Advanced) Prgm

Univ of Texas Hlth Sci Ctr at Houston
James Willerson, MD, President
PO Box 20036
Houston, TX 77225-0708
713 500-3000
Type: Acad Health Ctr/Med Sch
Control: State, County, or Local Govt
• Dental Hygiene Prgm
• Dentistry Prgm
• Dietetic Internship Prgm
• Nursing Prgm

Univ of Texas M D Anderson Cancer Ctr
John Mendelsohn, MD, President
1515 Holcombe Blvd, Box 213
Houston, TX 77030
713 792-6000
Type: Hosp or Med Ctr: 500> Beds
Control: State, County, or Local Govt
• Clin Lab Scientist/Med Technologist Prgm
• Cytogenetic Technology Prgm
• Cytotechnology Prgm
• Diagnostic Molecular Scientist Prgm
• Histotechnician Prgm
• Medical Dosimetry Prgm
• Radiation Therapy Prgm

Univ of Texas Medical School at Houston
PO Box 20708
Houston, TX 77225
Type: Acad Health Ctr/Med Sch
Control: State, County, or Local Govt
• Allopathic Medicine Prgm
• Genetic Counseling Prgm

University of Houston
Thomas M Stauffer, PhD, President
2700 Bay Area Blvd
Houston, TX 77058-1098
713 488-9336
Type: 4-year Coll or Univ
Control: State, County, or Local Govt
• Dietetic Internship Prgm
• Dietetics-Didactic Prgm
• Optometry Prgm
• Pharmacy Prgm
• Psychology Prgm
• Speech-Language Pathology Prgm

Huntsville

Sam Houston State University
James Gaertner, PhD, President
Box 2026
Huntsville, TX 77341
936 294-1013
Type: 4-year Coll or Univ
Control: State, County, or Local Govt
• Dietetic Internship Prgm
• Dietetics-Didactic Prgm
• Music Therapy Prgm
• Psychology Prgm

Hurst

Tarrant County College
Larry Darlage, PhD, President, NE Campus
828 W Harwood Rd
Hurst, TX 76054-3219
817 515-6200
Type: Junior or Comm Coll
Control: Nonprofit (Private or Religious)
• Dental Hygiene Prgm
• Emergency Med Tech-Paramedic Prgm
• Health Information Tech Prgm
• Physical Therapist Assistant Prgm
• Radiography Prgm
• Respiratory Therapist (Advanced) Prgm
• Surgical Technology Prgm

Irving

DeVry University - Dallas
4800 Regent Blvd
Irving, TX 75063
Type: 4-year Coll or Univ
Control: State, County, or Local Govt
• Health Information Tech Prgm

Kilgore

Kilgore College
William M Holda, EdD, President
1100 Broadway
Kilgore, TX 75662
903 983-8100
Type: Junior or Comm Coll
Control: State, County, or Local Govt
• Medical Assistant Prgm
• Physical Therapist Assistant Prgm
• Surgical Technology Prgm

Killeen

Central Texas College
James R Anderson, PhD, Chancellor
US Hwy 190 W
Killeen, TX 76541-9990
817 526-1211
Type: Junior or Comm Coll
Control: State, County, or Local Govt
• Clin Lab Technician/Med Lab Technician Prgm

Kingwood

Kingwood College - NHMCCD
Linda Stegall, EdD, President
20000 Kingwood Dr
Kingwood, TX 77339
281 312-1640
Type: Junior or Comm Coll
Control: State, County, or Local Govt
• Dental Hygiene Prgm
• Occupational Therapy Asst Prgm
• Respiratory Therapist (Advanced) Prgm

Lackland AFB

US Military Dietetic Internship Consortium
Lackland AFB, TX 78236-5300
Type: Consortium
Control: Fed Govt
• Dietetic Internship Prgm

Lake Jackson

Brazosport College
Millicent Valek, PhD, President
500 College Dr
Lake Jackson, TX 77568
979 230-3200
Type: Junior or Comm Coll
Control: State, County, or Local Govt
• Emergency Med Tech-Paramedic Prgm

Lancaster

Cedar Valley College
Jennifer Wimbish, PhD, President
3030 N Dallas Ave
Lancaster, TX 75134
Type: Acad Health Ctr/Med Sch
Control: For Profit
• Veterinary Technology Prgm

Laredo

Laredo Community College
Juan L Maldonado, PhD, President
West End Washington St
Laredo, TX 78040-4395
956 721-5101
Type: Junior or Comm Coll
Control: State, County, or Local Govt
• Clin Lab Technician/Med Lab Technician Prgm
• Occupational Therapy Asst Prgm
• Physical Therapist Assistant Prgm
• Radiography Prgm

Levelland

South Plains College
Kelvin Sharp, EdD, President
1401 S College Ave
Levelland, TX 79336
806 894-9611
Type: Junior or Comm Coll
Control: State, County, or Local Govt
• Emergency Med Tech-Paramedic Prgm
• Health Information Tech Prgm
• Radiography Prgm
• Respiratory Therapist (Advanced) Prgm
• Surgical Assistant Prgm
• Surgical Technology Prgm

Lubbock

Covenant Medical Center
Charley Trimble, President, CEO
3615 19th St
PO Box 1201
Lubbock, TX 79408
806 725-0579
Type: Hosp or Med Ctr: 500> Beds
Control: Nonprofit (Private or Religious)
• Radiography Prgm

Texas Tech Univ Health Sciences Center
John Baldwin, MD, President
3601 4th St, Stop 6258
Lubbock, TX 79409-2013
806 743-2900
Type: Acad Health Ctr/Med Sch
Control: State, County, or Local Govt
• Allopathic Medicine Prgm
• Athletic Training Prgm
• Audiologist Prgm
• Clin Lab Scientist/Med Technologist Prgm
• Diagnostic Molecular Scientist Prgm
• Occupational Therapy Prgm
• Pharmacy Prgm
• Physical Therapy Prgm
• Physician Assistant Prgm
• Speech-Language Pathology Prgm

INSTITUTIONS

Texas Tech University
David Schmidly, PhD, President
PO Box 2005
Lubbock, TX 79409
806 742-2121
Type: 4-year Coll or Univ
Control: State, County, or Local Govt
- Counseling Prgm
- Dietetic Internship Prgm
- Dietetics-Didactic Prgm
- Nursing Prgm
- Orientation and Mobility Specialist Prgm
- Psychology Prgm
- Rehabilitation Counseling Prgm

Lufkin

Angelina College
Larry M Phillips, EdD, President
PO Box 1768
3500 South First
Lufkin, TX 75902-1768
936 639-1301
Type: Junior or Comm Coll
Control: State, County, or Local Govt
- Pharmacy Technician Prgm
- Radiography Prgm
- Respiratory Therapist (Advanced) Prgm

Marshall

East Texas Baptist University
Bob Riley, EdD, President
1209 N Grove
Marshall, TX 75670
903 923-2222
Type: 4-year Coll or Univ
Control: Nonprofit (Private or Religious)
- Athletic Training Prgm
- Nursing Prgm

McAllen

South Texas College
Shirley Reed, EdD, President
3201 W Pecan Blvd
PO Box 9701
McAllen, TX 78501-9701
956 872-8366
Type: Junior or Comm Coll
Control: State, County, or Local Govt
- Health Information Tech Prgm
- Occupational Therapy Asst Prgm
- Pharmacy Technician Prgm
- Physical Therapist Assistant Prgm

McKinney

Collin County Community College
Cary A Israel, JD, President
2200 W University Dr
McKinney, TX 75071
972 758-3801
Type: Junior or Comm Coll
Control: State, County, or Local Govt
- Dental Hygiene Prgm
- Respiratory Therapist (Advanced) Prgm

Midland

Midland College
David E Daniel, EdD, President
3600 N Garfield
Midland, TX 79705
432 685-4520
Type: Junior or Comm Coll
Control: State, County, or Local Govt
- Diagnostic Med Sonography Prgm
- Health Information Tech Prgm
- Radiography Prgm
- Respiratory Therapist (Advanced) Prgm
- Veterinary Technology Prgm

Nacogdoches

Stephen F Austin State University
Baker Patillo, PhD, President
1936 North St
Austin Bldg
Nacogdoches, TX 75962
936 468-2011
Type: 4-year Coll or Univ
Control: State, County, or Local Govt
- Athletic Training Prgm
- Counseling Prgm
- Dietetic Internship Prgm
- Dietetics-Didactic Prgm
- Orientation and Mobility Specialist Prgm
- Rehabilitation Counseling Prgm
- Speech-Language Pathology Prgm

Odessa

Odessa College
Greg Wilson, PhD, President
201 W University
Odessa, TX 79764-8299
915 335-6410
Type: Junior or Comm Coll
Control: State, County, or Local Govt
- Physical Therapist Assistant Prgm
- Radiography Prgm

Orange

Lamar State College - Orange
J Michael Shahan, PhD, President
410 Front St
Orange, TX 77630-5802
409 883-7750
Type: Junior or Comm Coll
Control: State, County, or Local Govt
- Clin Lab Technician/Med Lab Technician Prgm
- Dental Assisting Prgm
- Pharmacy Technician Prgm

Paris

Paris Junior College
Pamela Anglin, EdD, President
2400 Clarksville St
Paris, TX 75460
903 782-0330
Type: Junior or Comm Coll
Control: State, County, or Local Govt
- Surgical Technology Prgm

Pasadena

San Jacinto College Central
Monte Blue, EdD, President
8060 Spencer Hwy
PO Box 2007
Pasadena, TX 77501-2007
281 476-1501
Type: Junior or Comm Coll
Control: State, County, or Local Govt
- Clin Lab Technician/Med Lab Technician Prgm
- Dietetic Technician-AD Prgm
- Emergency Med Tech-Paramedic Prgm
- Radiography Prgm
- Respiratory Therapist (Advanced) Prgm
- Surgical Technology Prgm

Port Arthur

Lamar State College - Port Arthur
W Sam Monroe, LLD, President
PO Box 310
Port Arthur, TX 77641-0310
409 984-7101
Type: Junior or Comm Coll
Control: State, County, or Local Govt
- Surgical Technology Prgm

Prairie View

Prairie View A&M University
Charles A Hines, President
Prairie View, TX 77446
409 857-3311
Type: 4-year Coll or Univ
Control: State, County, or Local Govt
- Dietetic Internship Prgm
- Dietetics-Didactic Prgm
- Nursing Prgm

Richardson

University of Texas at Dallas
Franklyn G Jenifer, President
PO Box 8630688
Richardson, TX 75083
214 883-2111
Type: 4-year Coll or Univ
Control: State, County, or Local Govt
- Audiologist Prgm
- Speech-Language Pathology Prgm

San Angelo

Angelo State University
Joseph Rallo, PhD, President
2601 W Ave N
ASU Station #11007
San Angelo, TX 76909-0001
325 942-2555
Type: 4-year Coll or Univ
Control: State, County, or Local Govt
- Athletic Training Prgm
- Physical Therapy Prgm

San Antonio

Baptist Health System
Trip Pilgrim, MBA, President/CEO
215 E Quincy
San Antonio, TX 78215
210 297-1140
Type: Hosp or Med Ctr: 500> Beds
Control: For Profit
- Radiography Prgm
- Surgical Technology Prgm

Hallmark Institute of Technology
Ronald Usiewicz, PhD, Campus Director
10401 IH - 10 West
San Antonio, TX 78230
210 690-9000
Type: Vocational or Tech Sch
Control: For Profit
- Medical Assistant Prgm

Northwest Vista College
Jacqueline Claunch, President
3535 N Ellison Dr
San Antonio, TX 78251-4217
210 348-2001
Type: Junior or Comm Coll
Control: State, County, or Local Govt
- Pharmacy Technician Prgm

Our Lady of the Lake University
Elizabeth A Sueltenfuss, President
411 SW 24th St
San Antonio, TX 78207
210 434-6711
Type: 4-year Coll or Univ
Control: Nonprofit (Private or Religious)
- Speech-Language Pathology Prgm

Palo Alto College
Ana Cha Guzman, EdD, President
1400 W Villaret Blvd
San Antonio, TX 78224
210 921-5260
Type: Junior or Comm Coll
Control: State, County, or Local Govt
- Veterinary Technology Prgm

San Antonio College
Robert E Zeigler, PhD, President
1300 San Pedro Ave
San Antonio, TX 78212-4299
210 733-2190
Type: Junior or Comm Coll
Control: State, County, or Local Govt
- Dental Assisting Prgm
- Medical Assistant Prgm

San Antonio College of Med & Dental Assts
Esther P Jones, Executive Director
4205 San Pedro
San Antonio, TX 78212
210 733-0777
Type: Vocational or Tech Sch
Control: For Profit
- Medical Assistant Prgm

St Mary's University
One Camino Santa Maria
San Antonio, TX 78228
210 436-3011
Type: 4-year Coll or Univ
Control: Nonprofit (Private or Religious)
- Counseling Prgm

St Philip's College
Adena Loston, PhD, President
1801 Martin Luther King Dr
San Antonio, TX 78203-2098
210 531-3591
Type: Junior or Comm Coll
Control: State, County, or Local Govt
- Clin Lab Technician/Med Lab Technician Prgm
- Health Information Tech Prgm
- Histotechnician Prgm
- Occupational Therapy Asst Prgm
- Physical Therapist Assistant Prgm
- Radiography Prgm
- Surgical Technology Prgm

Univ of Texas Hlth Sci Ctr at San Antonio
Francisco Cigarroa, MD, President
7703 Floyd Curl Dr
San Antonio, TX 78229-3900
210 567-2050
Type: Acad Health Ctr/Med Sch
Control: State, County, or Local Govt
- Clin Lab Scientist/Med Technologist Prgm
- Cytogenetic Technology Prgm
- Dental Hygiene Prgm
- Dental Lab Technician Prgm
- Dentistry Prgm
- Emergency Med Tech-Paramedic Prgm
- Histotechnician Prgm
- Nursing Prgm
- Occupational Therapy Prgm
- Physical Therapy Prgm
- Physician Assistant Prgm
- Respiratory Therapist (Advanced) Prgm
- Specialist in BB Tech Prgm

University of Texas Health Science Center
Francisco Cigarroa, MD, President
7703 Floyd Curl Dr
San Antonio, TX 78229-3900
210 616-2000
Type: Acad Health Ctr/Med Sch
Control: State, County, or Local Govt
- Allopathic Medicine Prgm

University of the Incarnate Word
Louis J Agnese, Jr, PhD, President
4301 Broadway
San Antonio, TX 78209
210 829-3900
Type: 4-year Coll or Univ
Control: Nonprofit (Private or Religious)
- Athletic Training Prgm
- Dietetic Internship Prgm
- Dietetics-Didactic Prgm
- Music Therapy Prgm
- Nuclear Medicine Technology Prgm
- Nursing Prgm
- Pharmacy Prgm

US Military Consortium
San Antonio, TX 78236
Type: Nonhosp HC Facil, BB, or Lab
Control: Fed Govt
- Dietetic Internship Prgm

San Marcos

Texas State University - San Marcos
Denise M Trauth, PhD, President
601 University Dr
San Marcos, TX 78666
512 245-2121
Type: 4-year Coll or Univ
Control: State, County, or Local Govt
- Athletic Training Prgm
- Clin Lab Scientist/Med Technologist Prgm
- Counseling Prgm
- Dietetic Internship Prgm
- Dietetics-Didactic Prgm
- Health Information Admin Prgm
- Physical Therapy Prgm
- Radiation Therapy Prgm
- Respiratory Therapist (Advanced) Prgm
- Speech-Language Pathology Prgm
- Therapeutic Recreation Specialist Prgm

Seguin

Texas Lutheran University
Jon Moline, PhD, President
1000 W Court St
Seguin, TX 78155
830 372-8000
Type: 4-year Coll or Univ
Control: Nonprofit (Private or Religious)
- Athletic Training Prgm

Sheppard AFB

882d Training Group
Nancy Dezell, Col USAF, CEO
939 Missile Rd
Sheppard AFB, TX 76311-2245
940 676-2700
Type: Dept of Defense
Control: Fed Govt
- Clin Lab Technician/Med Lab Technician Prgm
- Dental Assisting Prgm

School of Health Care Sciences - Air Force
Sheppard AFB, TX 76311
Type: Dept of Defense
Control: Fed Govt
- Dental Lab Technician Prgm

US Air Force
Colonel K A Siniscalchi, Commander
882 TRG
939 Missile Rd, Ste 2
Sheppard AFB, TX 76311-2263
940 676-2700
Type: Dept of Defense
Control: Fed Govt
- Optometric Technician Prgm

USAF School of Health Care Sciences
Col Nancy Dezell, RN BAN MSN, Group
   Commander
882TRG/CC
939 Missile Rd
Sheppard AFB, TX 76311
940 676-2700
Type: Dept of Defense
Control: Fed Govt
- Pharmacy Technician Prgm
- Radiography Prgm
- Respiratory Therapist (Entry-Level) Prgm

INSTITUTIONS

Stephenville

Tarleton State University
Dennis P McCabe, PhD, President
Tarleton Station
Stephenville, TX 76402
817 968-9100
Type: 4-year Coll or Univ
Control: State, County, or Local Govt
• Clin Lab Scientist/Med Technologist Prgm
• Clin Lab Technician/Med Lab Technician Prgm
• Histotechnician Prgm
• Nursing Prgm

Temple

Scott & White Hospital
John Roberts, MD, President
2401 S 31st St
Temple, TX 76508
254 774-2111
Type: Hosp or Med Ctr: 500> Beds
Control: Nonprofit (Private or Religious)
• Clin Lab Scientist/Med Technologist Prgm

Temple College
Marc A Nigliazzo, PhD, President
2600 S First St
Temple, TX 76504
254 298-8600
Type: Junior or Comm Coll
Control: State, County, or Local Govt
• Dental Hygiene Prgm
• Respiratory Therapist (Advanced) Prgm
• Surgical Technology Prgm

Texas City

College of the Mainland
Homer Hayes, PhD, President
1200 Amburn Rd
Texas City, TX 77591
409 938-1211
Type: Junior or Comm Coll
Control: State, County, or Local Govt
• Emergency Med Tech-Paramedic Prgm

Tomball

Tomball College - NHMCCD
Raymond M Hawkins, PhD, President
30555 Tomball Pkwy
Tomball, TX 77375-4036
281 351-3333
Type: Junior or Comm Coll
Control: State, County, or Local Govt
• Occupational Therapy Asst Prgm
• Veterinary Technology Prgm

Tyler

Tyler Junior College
William R Crowe, PhD, President
PO Box 9020
Tyler, TX 75711
903 510-2380
Type: Junior or Comm Coll
Control: State, County, or Local Govt
• Clin Lab Technician/Med Lab Technician Prgm
• Dental Hygiene Prgm
• Diagnostic Med Sonography Prgm
• Health Information Tech Prgm
• Ophthalmic Dispensing Optician Prgm
• Radiography Prgm
• Respiratory Therapist (Advanced) Prgm
• Surgical Technology Prgm

University of Texas at Tyler
Rodney Maybry, PhD, President
3900 University Blvd
Tyler, TX 75799
903 566-7100
Type: 4-year Coll or Univ
Control: State, County, or Local Govt
• Nursing Prgm

Vernon

Vernon College
Steve Thomas, PhD, President
4400 College Dr
Vernon, TX 76384
940 552-6291
Type: Junior or Comm Coll
Control: State, County, or Local Govt
• Health Information Tech Prgm
• Pharmacy Technician Prgm
• Surgical Technology Prgm

Victoria

Citizens Medical Center
David Brown, FACHE, Administrator
2701 Hospital Dr
Victoria, TX 77901
512 573-9181
Type: Hosp or Med Ctr: 100-299 Beds
Control: State, County, or Local Govt
• Radiography Prgm

Victoria College
Jimmy Goodson, EdD, President
2200 E Red River
Victoria, TX 77901
361 573-3291
Type: Junior or Comm Coll
Control: State, County, or Local Govt
• Clin Lab Technician/Med Lab Technician Prgm
• Respiratory Therapist (Advanced) Prgm

Waco

Baylor University
John Lilley, PhD, President/CEO
1 Bear Pl #97096
Waco, TX 76798
254 710-3555
Type: 4-year Coll or Univ
Control: Nonprofit (Private or Religious)
• Athletic Training Prgm
• Dietetics-Didactic Prgm
• Nursing Prgm
• Psychology Prgm
• Speech-Language Pathology Prgm

Hillcrest Baptist Medical Center
Jim Gebhart, FACHE, COO
3000 Herring Ave
Waco, TX 76708
254 202-9400
Type: Hosp or Med Ctr: 300-499 Beds
Control: Nonprofit (Private or Religious)
• Clin Lab Scientist/Med Technologist Prgm

McLennan Community College
Dennis F Michaelis, PhD, President
1400 College Dr
Waco, TX 76708
254 299-8601
Type: Junior or Comm Coll
Control: State, County, or Local Govt
• Clin Lab Technician/Med Lab Technician Prgm
• Electroneurodiagnostic Tech Prgm
• Health Information Tech Prgm
• Physical Therapist Assistant Prgm
• Radiography Prgm
• Veterinary Technology Prgm

Texas State Technical College
Bill Segura, PhD, Chancellor
3801 Campus Dr
Waco, TX 76705
254 867-4836
Type: Junior or Comm Coll
Control: State, County, or Local Govt
• Dental Assisting Prgm (2)
• Dental Hygiene Prgm
• Health Information Tech Prgm (2)
• Medical Assistant Prgm
• Surgical Technology Prgm

Weatherford

Weatherford College
Joe Birmingham, EdD, President
225 College Park
Weatherford, TX 76086-5699
817 594-5471
Type: Junior or Comm Coll
Control: State, County, or Local Govt
• Pharmacy Technician Prgm
• Respiratory Therapist (Advanced) Prgm

Wharton

Wharton County Junior College
Betty McCrohan, MS, President
911 Boling Hwy
Wharton, TX 77488
979 532-6400
Type: Junior or Comm Coll
Control: State, County, or Local Govt
- Dental Hygiene Prgm
- Emergency Med Tech-Paramedic Prgm
- Health Information Tech Prgm
- Physical Therapist Assistant Prgm
- Radiography Prgm
- Surgical Technology Prgm

Wichita Falls

Midwestern State University
Jesse Rogers, PhD, President
3410 Taft Blvd
Wichita Falls, TX 76308-2099
940 397-4211
Type: 4-year Coll or Univ
Control: State, County, or Local Govt
- Athletic Training Prgm
- Dental Hygiene Prgm
- Nursing Prgm
- Radiography Prgm
- Respiratory Therapist (Advanced) Prgm

United Regional Health Care Systems
Phyllis Cowling, CEO
1600 10th St
Wichita Falls, TX 76301
940 764-3055
Type: Hosp or Med Ctr: 300-499 Beds
Control: State, County, or Local Govt
- Clin Lab Scientist/Med Technologist Prgm

United Kingdom

Garthdee Aberdeen

Robert Gordon University
William Stevely, Vice Chancellor/President
Garthdee Rd
Garthdee Aberdeen, UK AB107QG
Control: State, County, or Local Govt
- Physical Therapy Prgm

Utah

Cedar City

Southern Utah University
Steven D Bennion, PhD, President
351 W University Blvd
Cedar City, UT 84720
435 586-7702
Type: 4-year Coll or Univ
Control: State, County, or Local Govt
- Athletic Training Prgm
- Nursing Prgm

Kaysville

Davis Applied Technology College
Michael J Bouwhuis, MEd, Campus President
550 East 300 South
Kaysville, UT 84037
801 593-2500
Type: Vocational or Tech Sch
Control: State, County, or Local Govt
- Dental Assisting Prgm
- Medical Assistant Prgm
- Surgical Technology Prgm

Logan

Bridgerland Applied Technology College
Richard L Maughan, MS PhD, Campus President
1301 West 600 North
Logan, UT 84321
435 753-6780
Type: Vocational or Tech Sch
Control: State, County, or Local Govt
- Dental Assisting Prgm
- Medical Assistant Prgm

Utah State University
Stan Albrecht, President
Logan, UT 84322
435 797-1000
Type: 4-year Coll or Univ
Control: State, County, or Local Govt
- Audiologist Prgm
- Dietetic Internship Prgm
- Dietetics-Coordinated Prgm
- Dietetics-Didactic Prgm
- Music Therapy Prgm
- Rehabilitation Counseling Prgm
- Speech-Language Pathology Prgm

Ogden

Ogden-Weber Applied Technology College
Collette Mercier, MA, President
200 N Washington Blvd
Ogden, UT 84404
801 627-8304
Type: Vocational or Tech Sch
Control: State, County, or Local Govt
- Dental Assisting Prgm
- Medical Assistant Prgm

Stevens-Henager College
Vicky Dewsnup, President, Regional Dir
1890 South 1350 West
PO Box 9428
Ogden, UT 84409-0428
801 394-7791
Type: 4-year Coll or Univ
Control: For Profit
- Medical Assistant Prgm (2)
- Respiratory Therapist (Advanced) Prgm
- Surgical Technology Prgm

Weber State University
F Ann Milner, EdD, President
1001 University Circle
Ogden, UT 84408-1001
801 626-7071
Type: 4-year Coll or Univ
Control: State, County, or Local Govt
- Athletic Training Prgm
- Clin Lab Scientist/Med Technologist Prgm
- Clin Lab Technician/Med Lab Technician Prgm
- Dental Hygiene Prgm
- Emergency Med Tech-Paramedic Prgm
- Health Information Admin Prgm
- Health Information Tech Prgm
- Respiratory Therapist (Advanced) Prgm
- Respiratory Therapist (Entry-Level) Prgm

Orem

Careers Unlimited
575 E University Pkwy, Ste 1-163
Orem, UT 84097
Control: For Profit
- Dental Assisting Prgm

Utah Valley State College
William A Sederburg, PhD, President
800 W University Pkwy
Orem, UT 84058-5999
801 863-8550
Type: 4-year Coll or Univ
Control: State, County, or Local Govt
- Dental Hygiene Prgm
- Emergency Med Tech-Paramedic Prgm

Provo

AmeriTech College
Connie A Garland, BS CDA, CEO Administrator
1675 N Freedom Blvd, Ste 3B
Provo, UT 84604-6927
801 377-2900
Type: Vocational or Tech Sch
Control: For Profit
- Dental Assisting Prgm
- Medical Assistant Prgm
- Surgical Technology Prgm

Brigham Young University
Cecil O Samuelson, MD, President
D 346 ASB
Provo, UT 84602
801 422-2521
Type: 4-year Coll or Univ
Control: Nonprofit (Private or Religious)
- Athletic Training Prgm
- Clin Lab Scientist/Med Technologist Prgm
- Dietetic Internship Prgm
- Dietetics-Didactic Prgm
- Nursing Prgm
- Psychology Prgm
- Speech-Language Pathology Prgm
- Therapeutic Recreation Specialist Prgm

Provo College
Gordon C Peters, MBA, Campus President
1450 W North
Provo, UT 84601-1305
801 818-8912
Control: For Profit
- Dental Assisting Prgm
- Medical Assistant Prgm
- Physical Therapist Assistant Prgm

INSTITUTIONS

Salt Lake City

Intermountain Healthcare
Nancy Nowak, CPA MBA, Director
36 S State St
Salt Lake City, UT 84111
801 442-2805
Type: Hosp or Med Ctr: 300-499 Beds
Control: Nonprofit (Private or Religious)
• Surgical Technology Prgm

Latter Day Saints Business College
Steven K Woodhouse, MBA, President
411 E South Temple
Salt Lake City, UT 84111
801 524-8101
Type: Vocational or Tech Sch
Control: Nonprofit (Private or Religious)
• Medical Assistant Prgm

Salt Lake Community College
Cynthia Bioteau, PhD, President
4600 S Redwood Rd
PO Box 30808
Salt Lake City, UT 84130-0808
801 957-4226
Type: Junior or Comm Coll
Control: State, County, or Local Govt
• Clin Lab Technician/Med Lab Technician Prgm
• Dental Hygiene Prgm
• Medical Assistant Prgm
• Occupational Therapy Asst Prgm
• Physical Therapist Assistant Prgm
• Radiography Prgm
• Surgical Technology Prgm

Unified Fire Authority/Utah Valley State Coll
Don Berry, Fire Chief
3380 S 900 W
Salt Lake City, UT 84119
801 743-7200
Type: Junior or Comm Coll
Control: State, County, or Local Govt
• Emergency Med Tech-Paramedic Prgm

University of Phoenix - Utah
Brian Mueller, CEO
Salt Lake City, UT 84123
Type: 4-year Coll or Univ
Control: State, County, or Local Govt
• Counseling Prgm

University of Utah
Michael K Young, JD, President
201 S President Circle, Rm 203
Salt Lake City, UT 84112
801 581-5701
Type: 4-year Coll or Univ
Control: State, County, or Local Govt
• Allopathic Medicine Prgm
• Athletic Training Prgm
• Audiologist Prgm
• Dietetics-Coordinated Prgm
• Nursing Prgm
• Occupational Therapy Prgm
• Pharmacy Prgm
• Physical Therapy Prgm
• Psychology Prgm
• Therapeutic Recreation Specialist Prgm

University of Utah Health Science Center
Michael K Young, JD, President
203 Park Bldg
Salt Lake City, UT 84112
801 581-5701
Type: Acad Health Ctr/Med Sch
Control: State, County, or Local Govt
• Audiologist Prgm
• Clin Lab Scientist/Med Technologist Prgm
• Cytotechnology Prgm
• Genetic Counseling Prgm
• Nuclear Medicine Technology Prgm
• Physician Assistant Prgm
• Speech-Language Pathology Prgm

Westminster College
Salt Lake City, UT 84105
Type: 4-year Coll or Univ
Control: Nonprofit (Private or Religious)
• Nursing Prgm

St George

Dixie State College of Utah
Lee G Caldwell, PhD, President
225 South 700 East
St George, UT 84770-3876
435 652-7501
Type: Junior or Comm Coll
Control: State, County, or Local Govt
• Dental Hygiene Prgm
• Emergency Med Tech-Paramedic Prgm
• Radiography Prgm
• Surgical Technology Prgm

West Jordan

Utah Career College
Nate Herrmann, Regional Director
1902 West 7800 South
West Jordan, UT 84088
801 304-4224
Type: Vocational or Tech Sch
Control: For Profit
• Medical Assistant Prgm
• Veterinary Technology Prgm

West Valley City

Everest College
Larry Banks, President
3280 West 3500 South
West Valley City, UT 84119
801 840-4800
Type: Junior or Comm Coll
Control: For Profit
• Medical Assistant Prgm

Vermont

Burlington

Champlain College
David F Finney, PhD, President
163 S Willard St
PO Box 670
Burlington, VT 05402
802 865-2700
Type: 4-year Coll or Univ
Control: Nonprofit (Private or Religious)
• Radiography Prgm

Fletcher Allen Health Care
Melinda Estes, MD, CEO and President
111 Colchester Ave
Burlington, VT 05401-1429
802 847-5959
Type: Hosp or Med Ctr: 300-499 Beds
Control: Nonprofit (Private or Religious)
• Cytotechnology Prgm

University of Vermont
Daniel Fogel, PhD, President
349 Waterman Bldg
Burlington, VT 05405
802 656-3186
Type: 4-year Coll or Univ
Control: State, County, or Local Govt
• Allopathic Medicine Prgm
• Athletic Training Prgm
• Clin Lab Scientist/Med Technologist Prgm
• Counseling Prgm
• Dietetics-Coordinated Prgm
• Dietetics-Didactic Prgm
• Nuclear Medicine Technology Prgm
• Nursing Prgm
• Physical Therapy Prgm
• Psychology Prgm
• Speech-Language Pathology Prgm

Castleton

Castleton State College
David Wolk, MS, President
Woodruff Hall
Castleton, VT 05735
802 468-1201
Type: 4-year Coll or Univ
Control: State, County, or Local Govt
• Athletic Training Prgm

Essex Junction

Center for Technology - Essex
Kathy Finck, Director
Three Educational Dr
Essex Junction, VT 05452
802 879-5562
Type: Vocational or Tech Sch
Control: State, County, or Local Govt
• Dental Assisting Prgm

Northfield

Norwich University
Richard W Schneider, PhD, President
158 Harmon Dr
Northfield, VT 05663
802 485-2065
Type: 4-year Coll or Univ
Control: Nonprofit (Private or Religious)
• Athletic Training Prgm

Randolph Center

Vermont Technical College
Ty Handy, MBA, President
PO Box 500
Randolph Center, VT 05061
802 728-1258
Type: Junior or Comm Coll
Control: State, County, or Local Govt
• Dental Hygiene Prgm
• Respiratory Therapist (Advanced) Prgm
• Veterinary Technology Prgm

Virginia

Annandale

Northern Virginia Community College
Robert Templin, PhD, President
4001 Wakefield Chapel Rd
Annandale, VA 22003-3796
703 323-3101
Type: Junior or Comm Coll
Control: State, County, or Local Govt
• Clin Lab Technician/Med Lab Technician Prgm
• Dental Hygiene Prgm
• Emergency Med Tech-Paramedic Prgm
• Health Information Tech Prgm
• Physical Therapist Assistant Prgm
• Respiratory Therapist (Advanced) Prgm
• Veterinary Technology Prgm

Arlington

ACT College
Jeffrey Moore, MBA, President and CEO
1100 Wilson Blvd
Arlington, VA 22209
Type: 4-year Coll or Univ
Control: State, County, or Local Govt
• Radiography Prgm

Argosy University
Arlington, VA 22209
Type: 4-year Coll or Univ
Control: State, County, or Local Govt
• Psychology Prgm

Marymount University
James Bundschuh, President
2807 N Glebe Rd
Arlington, VA 22207-4299
703 522-5600
Type: 4-year Coll or Univ
Control: Nonprofit (Private or Religious)
• Counseling Prgm
• Nursing Prgm
• Physical Therapy Prgm

Big Stone Gap

Mountain Empire Community College
Terrance Suarez, PhD, President
3441 Mountain Empire Rd
Big Stone Gap, VA 24219
540 523-2400
Type: Junior or Comm Coll
Control: State, County, or Local Govt
• Respiratory Therapist (Advanced) Prgm

Blacksburg

Edward Via Virginia Coll of Opteopathic Med
2265 Kraft Dr
Blacksburg, VA 24060
Type: Acad Health Ctr/Med Sch
Control: Nonprofit (Private or Religious)
• Osteopathic Medicine Prgm

Virginia Polytechnic Inst & State Univ
Charles W Steger, President
Blacksburg, VA 24061
540 231-6000
Type: 4-year Coll or Univ
Control: State, County, or Local Govt
• Counseling Prgm
• Dietetic Internship Prgm
• Dietetics-Didactic Prgm
• Psychology Prgm
• Veterinary Medicine Prgm

Bridgewater

Bridgewater College
Phillip C Stone, JD, President
402 E College St
Bridgewater, VA 22812
540 828-5605
Type: 4-year Coll or Univ
Control: State, County, or Local Govt
• Athletic Training Prgm

Charlottesville

Piedmont Virginia Community College
Frank Friedman, PhD, President
501 College Dr
Charlottesville, VA 22902
434 961-5200
Type: Junior or Comm Coll
Control: State, County, or Local Govt
• Emergency Med Tech-Paramedic Prgm
• Surgical Technology Prgm

University of Virginia
John Casteen, President
PO Box 400224
Charlottesville, VA 22904-4224
434 924-3337
Type: 4-year Coll or Univ
Control: State, County, or Local Govt
• Allopathic Medicine Prgm
• Counseling Prgm
• Nursing Prgm (2)
• Psychology Prgm (2)
• Speech-Language Pathology Prgm

University of Virginia Health System
Edward R Howell, MS, VP and CEO, Hlth Systems
PO Box 800809
Charlottesville, VA 22908
434 243-9308
Type: Hosp or Med Ctr: 500> Beds
Control: State, County, or Local Govt
• Dietetic Internship Prgm
• Radiation Therapy Prgm
• Radiography Prgm

Virginia School of Massage
Charlottesville, VA 22903
Type: Acad Health Ctr/Med Sch
Control: For Profit
• Massage Therapy Prgm

Danville

Averett University
Richard A Pfau, PhD, President
420 W Main St
Danville, VA 24541
434 791-5670
Type: 4-year Coll or Univ
Control: Nonprofit (Private or Religious)
• Athletic Training Prgm

Danville Regional Medical Center
Warren E Callaway, FACHE, President
142 S Main St
Danville, VA 24541
804 799-3700
Type: Hosp or Med Ctr: 300-499 Beds
Control: Nonprofit (Private or Religious)
• Radiography Prgm

Emory

Emory & Henry College
Rosalind Reichard, PhD, President
PO Box 947
Emory, VA 24327-0947
276 944-6107
Type: 4-year Coll or Univ
Control: Nonprofit (Private or Religious)
• Athletic Training Prgm

Fairfax

George Mason University
Alan G Merten, PhD, President
4400 University Dr
Fairfax, VA 22030-4444
703 993-8700
Type: 4-year Coll or Univ
Control: State, County, or Local Govt
• Athletic Training Prgm
• Nursing Prgm
• Psychology Prgm
• Therapeutic Recreation Specialist Prgm

Falls Church

Inova Fairfax Hospital
Jolene Tournabeni, Administrator
3300 Gallows Rd
Falls Church, VA 22046
703 698-3371
Type: Hosp or Med Ctr: 500> Beds
Control: State, County, or Local Govt
• Clin Lab Scientist/Med Technologist Prgm

National Massage Therapy Institute
803 W Board St
Falls Church, VA 22046
Type: Acad Health Ctr/Med Sch
Control: For Profit
• Massage Therapy Prgm

Farmville

Longwood University
Patricia Cormier, PhD, President
201 High St
Farmville, VA 23909-1899
804 395-2000
Type: 4-year Coll or Univ
Control: State, County, or Local Govt
• Athletic Training Prgm
• Therapeutic Recreation Specialist Prgm

Fishersville

Augusta Medical Center
David Deering, MBA, COO
PO Box 1000
78 Medical Center Dr
Fishersville, VA 22939
540 332-4818
Type: Hosp or Med Ctr: 100-299 Beds
Control: Nonprofit (Private or Religious)
• Clin Lab Scientist/Med Technologist Prgm

Fredericksburg

Mary Washington Hospital
Fred M Rankin III, MPH, President/CEO
1001 Sam Perry Blvd
Fredericksburg, VA 22401
540 741-1414
Type: Hosp or Med Ctr: 300-499 Beds
Control: Nonprofit (Private or Religious)
• Radiography Prgm

Grundy

University of Appalachia College of Pharmacy
Eleanor Sue Cantrell, MD, President
PO Box 2858
Grundy, VA 24614
Type: Acad Health Ctr/Med Sch
Control: Nonprofit (Private or Religious)
• Pharmacy Prgm

Hampton

Hampton University
William R Harvey, President
Hampton, VA 23668
804 727-5000
Type: 4-year Coll or Univ
Control: Nonprofit (Private or Religious)
• Nursing Prgm
• Pharmacy Prgm
• Physical Therapy Prgm
• Speech-Language Pathology Prgm

Thomas Nelson Community College
Charles Taylor, EdD, President
PO Box 9407
Hampton, VA 23670
757 825-2711
Type: Junior or Comm Coll
Control: State, County, or Local Govt
• Clin Lab Technician/Med Lab Technician Prgm

Harrisonburg

Eastern Mennonite University
Loren E Swartzendruber, President
Harrisonburg, VA 22802
540 432-4000
Type: Acad Health Ctr/Med Sch
Control: For Profit
• Nursing Prgm

James Madison University
Linwood Rose, EdD, President
Office of the President, MSC 7608
Harrisonburg, VA 22807
540 568-6868
Type: 4-year Coll or Univ
Control: State, County, or Local Govt
• Athletic Training Prgm
• Audiologist Prgm
• Counseling Prgm
• Dietetic Internship Prgm
• Dietetics-Didactic Prgm
• Nursing Prgm
• Occupational Therapy Prgm
• Physician Assistant Prgm
• Speech-Language Pathology Prgm

Rockingham Memorial Hospital
T Carter Melton, Jr, MHA, President
235 Cantrell Ave
Harrisonburg, VA 22801
540 433-4101
Type: Hosp or Med Ctr: 100-299 Beds
Control: Nonprofit (Private or Religious)
• Clin Lab Scientist/Med Technologist Prgm
• Radiography Prgm

Leesburg

Loudoun County Dept of Fire-Rescue
Joseph Pozzo, MA, Chief
16600 Courage Court
Leesburg, VA 20175
703 777-0333
Type: Vocational or Tech Sch
Control: State, County, or Local Govt
• Emergency Med Tech-Paramedic Prgm

Lynchburg

Centra Health Systems of Lynchburg
George W Dawson, MHA, President/CEO
1920 Atherholt Rd
Lynchburg, VA 24501
804 947-4705
Type: Hosp or Med Ctr: 500> Beds
Control: Nonprofit (Private or Religious)
• Clin Lab Technician/Med Lab Technician Prgm

Central Virginia Community College
Darrel W Staat, DA, President
3506 Wards Rd
Lynchburg, VA 24502
804 832-7601
Type: Junior or Comm Coll
Control: State, County, or Local Govt
• Radiography Prgm
• Respiratory Therapist (Advanced) Prgm

Liberty University
Ronald Godwin, PhD, CEO
1971 University Blvd
Lynchburg, VA 24502
434 582-7600
Type: 4-year Coll or Univ
Control: Nonprofit (Private or Religious)
• Athletic Training Prgm
• Nursing Prgm

Lynchburg College
Kenneth R Garren, President
1501 Lakeside Dr
Lynchburg, VA 24501-3199
804 544-8100
Type: 4-year Coll or Univ
Control: Nonprofit (Private or Religious)
• Athletic Training Prgm
• Counseling Prgm
• Nursing Prgm

Miller-Motte Technical College
David Tipps, MA, Campus Director
1011 Creekside Lane
Lynchburg, VA 24502
434 239-5222
Type: Vocational or Tech Sch
Control: For Profit
• Medical Assistant Prgm
• Surgical Technology Prgm

Newport News

Medical Careers Institute
Barbara Larar, Director
1001 Omni Blvd, Ste 200
Newport News, VA 23606
757 873-2423
Type: Vocational or Tech Sch
Control: For Profit
• Medical Assistant Prgm
• Radiography Prgm

Riverside School of Health Careers
Tracee Carmean, VP Education
316 Main St
Newport News, VA 23601
757 240-2202
Type: Consortium
Control: Nonprofit (Private or Religious)
• Radiography Prgm
• Surgical Technology Prgm

Norfolk

Eastern Virginia Medical School
Harry T Lester, MD, President
PO Box 1980
Norfolk, VA 23507
757 446-5600
Type: Acad Health Ctr/Med Sch
Control: Nonprofit (Private or Religious)
• Allopathic Medicine Prgm
• Art Therapy Prgm
• Physician Assistant Prgm
• Surgical Assistant Prgm

Norfolk State University
Carolyn Meyers, PhD, President
700 Park Ave
Echols Hall Rm 165
Norfolk, VA 23504
757 823-8670
Type: 4-year Coll or Univ
Control: State, County, or Local Govt
• Clin Lab Scientist/Med Technologist Prgm
• Dietetics-Didactic Prgm
• Kinesiotherapy Prgm

Old Dominion University
Roseann Runte, PhD, President
Koch Hall
Norfolk, VA 23529-0001
757 683-3159
Type: 4-year Coll or Univ
Control: State, County, or Local Govt
• Clin Lab Scientist/Med Technologist Prgm
• Counseling Prgm
• Cytotechnology Prgm
• Dental Hygiene Prgm
• Exercise Science Prgm
• Nuclear Medicine Technology Prgm
• Nursing Prgm
• Ophthalmic Med Technologist Prgm
• Physical Therapy Prgm
• Speech-Language Pathology Prgm

Sentara Norfolk General Hospital
Rodney Hochman, MD, CEO
600 Gresham Dr
Norfolk, VA 23507
757 668-3361
Type: Hosp or Med Ctr: 500> Beds
Control: Nonprofit (Private or Religious)
• Cardiovascular Technology Prgm

Tidewater Community College
Deborah M DiCroce, EdD, President
121 College Place
Norfolk, VA 23510
757 822-1050
Type: Junior or Comm Coll
Control: State, County, or Local Govt
• Diagnostic Med Sonography Prgm
• Emergency Med Tech-Paramedic Prgm
• Health Information Tech Prgm
• Medical Assistant Prgm
• Occupational Therapy Asst Prgm
• Physical Therapist Assistant Prgm
• Radiography Prgm
• Respiratory Therapist (Advanced) Prgm

Tidewater Tech
Jerry Yagen
1760 E Little Creek Rd
Norfolk, VA 23518
757 588-2121
Type: Vocational or Tech Sch
Control: For Profit
• Dental Assisting Prgm

Petersburg

Southside Regional Medical Center
David S Dunham, MHA, Exec Director
801 S Adams St
Petersburg, VA 23803
804 862-5903
Type: Hosp or Med Ctr: 300-499 Beds
Control: State, County, or Local Govt
• Radiography Prgm

Virginia State University
Eddie N Moore, Jr, President
Petersburg, VA 23806
804 524-5000
Type: 4-year Coll or Univ
Control: State, County, or Local Govt
• Dietetic Internship Prgm
• Dietetics-Didactic Prgm

Portsmouth

Naval School of Health Sciences
Susan E Herron, CAPT NC USN, Commanding
  Officer
1001 Holcomb Rd
Portsmouth, VA 23708-5200
757 953-5040
Type: Dept of Defense
Control: Fed Govt
• Electroneurodiagnostic Tech Prgm
• Nuclear Medicine Technology Prgm
• Pharmacy Technician Prgm
• Radiography Prgm
• Surgical Technology Prgm

Radford

Radford University
Penelope Kyle, MBA JD, President
PO Box 6890
Martin Hall
Radford, VA 24142
540 831-5401
Type: 4-year Coll or Univ
Control: State, County, or Local Govt
• Athletic Training Prgm
• Counseling Prgm
• Dietetics-Didactic Prgm
• Music Therapy Prgm
• Nursing Prgm
• Speech-Language Pathology Prgm
• Therapeutic Recreation Specialist Prgm

Richlands

Southwest Virginia Community College
William Snydor, PhD, President
PO Box SVCC
Richlands, VA 24641-1101
276 964-7315
Type: Junior or Comm Coll
Control: State, County, or Local Govt
• Diagnostic Med Sonography Prgm
• Emergency Med Tech-Paramedic Prgm
• Occupational Therapy Asst Prgm
• Radiography Prgm
• Respiratory Therapist (Advanced) Prgm

Richmond

Bon Secours St Mary's Hospital
Joey S Battles, MA Ed RT(R), Association
  Directorr
8550 Magellan Pkwy - Ste 700
Richmond, VA 23227
Type: Hosp or Med Ctr: 300-499 Beds
Control: Nonprofit (Private or Religious)
• Radiography Prgm

Bryant & Stratton College - Richmond
John Staschak, President
8141 Hull St Road
Richmond, VA 23235
804 745-2444
Type: 4-year Coll or Univ
Control: For Profit
• Medical Assistant Prgm

J Sargeant Reynolds Community College
Gary Rhodes, EdD, President
PO Box 85622
Richmond, VA 23285-5622
804 523-5200
Type: Junior or Comm Coll
Control: State, County, or Local Govt
• Clin Lab Technician/Med Lab Technician Prgm
• Dental Assisting Prgm
• Dental Lab Technician Prgm
• Emergency Med Tech-Paramedic Prgm
• Ophthalmic Dispensing Optician Prgm
• Respiratory Therapist (Advanced) Prgm
• Respiratory Therapist (Entry-Level) Prgm
• Surgical Technology Prgm

Virginia Commonwealth Univ/Health System
Euguene P Trani, PhD, President
PO Box 842512
Richmond, VA 23284-2512
804 828-1200
Type: Acad Health Ctr/Med Sch
Control: State, County, or Local Govt
• Dentistry Prgm
• Dietetic Internship Prgm
• Emergency Med Tech-Paramedic Prgm
• Genetic Counseling Prgm
• Occupational Therapy Prgm
• Pharmacy Prgm
• Physical Therapy Prgm

Virginia Commonwealth University
Eugene P Trani, PhD, President
910 W Franklin St
Richmond, VA 23284-2512
804 828-1200
Type: 4-year Coll or Univ
Control: State, County, or Local Govt
• Allopathic Medicine Prgm
• Clin Lab Scientist/Med Technologist Prgm
• Dental Hygiene Prgm
• Nuclear Medicine Technology Prgm
• Radiation Therapy Prgm
• Radiography Prgm
• Rehabilitation Counseling Prgm

Virginia Department of Health
Div of Public Health Nutrition
1500 E Main St Rm 132
Richmond, VA 23219
804 786-5420
Control: State, County, or Local Govt
• Dietetic Internship Prgm

Roanoke

Carilion Medical Center
Nancy H Agee, RN MN
PO Box 13367
Belleview & Jefferson Sts
Roanoke, VA 24033-3367
540 981-8385
Type: Hosp or Med Ctr: 500> Beds
Control: Nonprofit (Private or Religious)
• Clin Lab Scientist/Med Technologist Prgm

Jefferson College of Health Sciences
Carol M Seavor, EdD, President
920 S Jefferson St
PO Box 13186
Roanoke, VA 24031-3186
888 985-8483
Type: 4-year Coll or Univ
Control: Nonprofit (Private or Religious)
• Emergency Med Tech-Paramedic Prgm
• Nursing Prgm
• Occupational Therapy Asst Prgm
• Occupational Therapy Prgm
• Physical Therapist Assistant Prgm
• Physician Assistant Prgm
• Respiratory Therapist (Advanced) Prgm

National College
Frank E Longaker, MBA, President
PO Box 6400
Roanoke, VA 24017
540 986-1800
Type: Junior or Comm Coll
Control: For Profit
• Health Information Tech Prgm
• Medical Assistant Prgm (7)
• Surgical Technology Prgm (2)

Virginia Western Community College
Robert Sandel, PhD, President
3095 Colonial Ave SW
PO Box 14045
Roanoke, VA 24015
540 857-7311
Type: Junior or Comm Coll
Control: State, County, or Local Govt
• Dental Hygiene Prgm
• Radiation Therapy Prgm
• Radiography Prgm

Salem

National College of Business and Technology
Frank Longake, MBA, President
1813 E Main St
Salem, VA 24153
540 986-1800
Type: Junior or Comm Coll
Control: For Profit
• Medical Assistant Prgm (2)

Roanoke College
Michael Maxey, PhD, President
221 College Lane
Salem, VA 24153
540 375-2200
Type: 4-year Coll or Univ
Control: Nonprofit (Private or Religious)
• Athletic Training Prgm

Virginia Beach

Bryant & Stratton College - Virginia Beach
Lee E Hicklin, Director
301 Centre Pointe Dr
Virginia Beach, VA 23462
757 499-7900
Type: Junior or Comm Coll
Control: For Profit
• Medical Assistant Prgm

Cayce/Reilly School of Massotherapy
215 67th St
Virginia Beach, VA 23451
Type: Acad Health Ctr/Med Sch
Control: For Profit
• Massage Therapy Prgm

Regent University
Rosemarie Hughes, PhD, Dean
School of Psychology and Counseling
1000 Regent University Dr, CRB 174
Virginia Beach, VA 23464-9800
757 226-4000
Control: Nonprofit (Private or Religious)
• Counseling Prgm
• Psychology Prgm

Virginia Consortium Program in Clinical Psych
Virginia Beach, VA 23453
Type: Acad Health Ctr/Med Sch
Control: For Profit
• Psychology Prgm

Weyers Cave

Blue Ridge Community College
James Perkins, PhD, President
PO Box 80
Weyers Cave, VA 24486
540 234-9261
Type: 4-year Coll or Univ
Control: State, County, or Local Govt
• Veterinary Technology Prgm

Williamsburg

College of William & Mary
Timothy J Sullivan, President
PO Box 8795
Williamsburg, VA 23187-8794
757 221-4000
Type: 4-year Coll or Univ
Control: State, County, or Local Govt
• Counseling Prgm

Winchester

Shenandoah University
James Davis, PhD, President
1460 University Dr
Winchester, VA 22601
540 665-4505
Type: 4-year Coll or Univ
Control: Nonprofit (Private or Religious)
• Athletic Training Prgm
• Music Therapy Prgm
• Nursing Prgm
• Occupational Therapy Prgm
• Pharmacy Prgm
• Physical Therapy Prgm
• Physician Assistant Prgm
• Respiratory Therapist (Advanced) Prgm

Winchester Medical Center Inc
1840 Amherst St
PO Box 3340
Winchester, VA 22601
Type: Hosp or Med Ctr: 300-499 Beds
Control: Nonprofit (Private or Religious)
• Radiography Prgm

Wytheville

Wytheville Community College
Charlie White, PhD, President
1000 E Main St
Wytheville, VA 24382
276 223-4700
Type: Junior or Comm Coll
Control: State, County, or Local Govt
• Clin Lab Technician/Med Lab Technician Prgm
• Dental Hygiene Prgm
• Physical Therapist Assistant Prgm

Yorktown

Tri-Service Optician School (TOPS)
CDR Lee Cornforth, USN OD MBA, Training
  Officer
Naval Ophthalmic Support & Trng Activity
160 Main Rd, Ste 360
Yorktown, VA 23691-9984
757 887-7329
Type: Dept of Defense
Control: Fed Govt
• Ophthalmic Dispensing Optician Prgm

Washington

Auburn

Green River Community College
Richard Rutkowski, MBA, President
12401 SE 320th St
Auburn, WA 98002-3622
253 833-9111
Type: Junior or Comm Coll
Control: State, County, or Local Govt
• Occupational Therapy Asst Prgm
• Physical Therapist Assistant Prgm

Bellevue

Bellevue Community College
B Jean Floten, MS, President
3000 Landerholm Circle SE
Bellevue, WA 98007-6484
425 564-2301
Type: Junior or Comm Coll
Control: State, County, or Local Govt
• Diagnostic Med Sonography Prgm
• Nuclear Medicine Technology Prgm
• Radiation Therapy Prgm

Bellingham

Bellingham Technical College
Gerald Pumphrey, EdD, President
3028 Lindbergh Ave
Bellingham, WA 98225
360 738-0221
Type: Junior or Comm Coll
Control: State, County, or Local Govt
• Dental Assisting Prgm
• Emergency Med Tech-Paramedic Prgm
• Surgical Technology Prgm

Western Washington University
Karen W Morse, PhD, President
516 High St
Old Main 450, MS 9000
Bellingham, WA 98225
360 650-3480
Type: 4-year Coll or Univ
Control: State, County, or Local Govt
• Counseling Prgm
• Rehabilitation Counseling Prgm
• Speech-Language Pathology Prgm

Whatcom Community College
Harold G Heiner, PhD, President
237 W Kellogg Rd
Bellingham, WA 98226
360 676-2170
Type: Junior or Comm Coll
Control: State, County, or Local Govt
• Medical Assistant Prgm
• Physical Therapist Assistant Prgm

Bremerton

Olympic College
David Mitchell, PhD, President
1600 Chester Ave
Bremerton, WA 98337-1699
360 792-6050
Type: Junior or Comm Coll
Control: State, County, or Local Govt
• Medical Assistant Prgm

Cheney

Eastern Washington University
Rodolfo Ar,valo, PhD, President
214 Showalter Hall
526 5th St
Cheney, WA 99004-2431
509 359-2371
Type: 4-year Coll or Univ
Control: State, County, or Local Govt
• Athletic Training Prgm
• Counseling Prgm
• Dental Hygiene Prgm
• Occupational Therapy Prgm
• Physical Therapy Prgm
• Speech-Language Pathology Prgm
• Therapeutic Recreation Specialist Prgm

Des Moines

Highline Community College
Jack Bermingham, Interim President
PO Box 98000
Des Moines, WA 98198-9800
206 878-3710
Type: Junior or Comm Coll
Control: State, County, or Local Govt
• Medical Assistant Prgm
• Respiratory Therapist (Advanced) Prgm

Ellensburg

Central Washington University
Jerilyn McIntyre, PhD, President
400 E University Way
Ellensburg, WA 98926-7501
509 963-2111
Type: 4-year Coll or Univ
Control: State, County, or Local Govt
• Dietetic Internship Prgm
• Dietetics-Didactic Prgm
• Emergency Med Tech-Paramedic Prgm

Everett

Everest College
Kimberly Lothyan, EdC, President
906 SE Everett Mall Way
Suite 600
Everett, WA 98251
425 789-7960
Type: Vocational or Tech Sch
Control: For Profit
• Medical Assistant Prgm (3)

Everett Community College
Charles Earl, President
2000 Tower St
Everett, WA 98201
425 388-9572
Type: Junior or Comm Coll
Control: State, County, or Local Govt
• Medical Assistant Prgm

Kirkland

Lake Washington Technical College
L Michael Metke, EdD, President
11605 132nd Ave NE
Kirkland, WA 98034
425 739-8100
Type: Vocational or Tech Sch
Control: State, County, or Local Govt
• Dental Assisting Prgm
• Dental Hygiene Prgm
• Medical Assistant Prgm

Northwest University
Kirkland, WA 98033
Type: 4-year Coll or Univ
Control: Nonprofit (Private or Religious)
• Nursing Prgm

Lakewood

Clover Park Technical College
John Walstrum, PhD, President
4500 Steilacoom Blvd SW
Lakewood, WA 98499-4098
253 589-5678
Type: Junior or Comm Coll
Control: State, County, or Local Govt
• Clin Lab Technician/Med Lab Technician Prgm
• Dental Assisting Prgm
• Medical Assistant Prgm
• Surgical Technology Prgm

Pierce College
Michele Johnson, PhD, President
9401 Farwest Dr SW
Lakewood, WA 98498-1999
253 964-6500
Type: Junior or Comm Coll
Control: State, County, or Local Govt
• Dental Hygiene Prgm
• Veterinary Technology Prgm

Longview

Lower Columbia College
James McLaughlin, PhD, President
1600 Maple St
Longview, WA 98632
360 577-2320
Type: Junior or Comm Coll
Control: State, County, or Local Govt
• Medical Assistant Prgm

Mt Vernon

Skagit Valley College
James M Ford, PhD, President
2405 E College Way
Mt Vernon, WA 98273
360 416-7997
Type: Junior or Comm Coll
Control: State, County, or Local Govt
• Medical Assistant Prgm

Olympia

South Puget Sound Community College
Gerald Pumphrey, PhD, President
2011 Mottman Rd SW
Olympia, WA 98512-6292
360 596-5206
Type: Junior or Comm Coll
Control: State, County, or Local Govt
• Dental Assisting Prgm
• Medical Assistant Prgm

Pasco

Columbia Basin College
Lee R Thornton, PhD, President
2600 N 20th Ave
Pasco, WA 99301
509 547-0511
Type: Junior or Comm Coll
Control: State, County, or Local Govt
• Dental Hygiene Prgm
• Emergency Med Tech-Paramedic Prgm

Pullman

Washington State University
Elson Floyd, PhD, President
422 French Administration
PO Box 641048
Pullman, WA 99164-1048
509 335-6666
Type: 4-year Coll or Univ
Control: State, County, or Local Govt
• Athletic Training Prgm
• Audiologist Prgm
• Dietetics-Coordinated Prgm (2)
• Dietetics-Didactic Prgm
• Nursing Prgm
• Pharmacy Prgm
• Psychology Prgm
• Speech-Language Pathology Prgm
• Veterinary Medicine Prgm

Renton

Renton Technical College
Donald E Bressler, PhD, President
4000 NE Fourth St
Renton, WA 98056
206 235-2235
Type: Vocational or Tech Sch
Control: State, County, or Local Govt
• Dental Assisting Prgm
• Medical Assistant Prgm
• Ophthalmic Assistant Prgm
• Pharmacy Technician Prgm
• Surgical Technology Prgm

Seattle

Antioch University - Seattle
Toni Murdock, President
2326 Sixth Ave
Seattle, WA 98121-1814
Type: 4-year Coll or Univ
Control: State, County, or Local Govt
• Art Therapy Prgm

Bastyr University
Joseph E Pizzorno, Jr, President
144 NE 54th St
Seattle, WA 98105
206 523-9585
Type: 4-year Coll or Univ
Control: Nonprofit (Private or Religious)
• Dietetic Internship Prgm
• Dietetics-Didactic Prgm

Cortiva Inst - Brian Utting School of Massage
Arlin Schmidt
900 Thomas St
Seattle, WA 98109
Type: Vocational or Tech Sch
Control: For Profit
• Massage Therapy Prgm

Cortiva Institute - Seattle
Dina Boon, LMP, President
425 Pontius Ave N, Ste 100
Seattle, WA 98109
206 282-1233
Type: Vocational or Tech Sch
Control: For Profit
• Massage Therapy Prgm

Harborview Med Ctr - Univ of Washington
David Jaffe, MPA, Admin/Executive Director
325 Ninth Ave
Seattle, WA 98104
206 731-3036
Type: Hosp or Med Ctr: 300-499 Beds
Control: State, County, or Local Govt
• Emergency Med Tech-Paramedic Prgm

North Seattle Community College
Ron LaFayette, PhD, President
9600 College Way N
Seattle, WA 98103
206 527-3602
Type: Junior or Comm Coll
Control: State, County, or Local Govt
• Medical Assistant Prgm

Pima Medical Institute - Seattle
Richard Luebke, Sr, BS, President
9709 Third Ave NE, #400
Seattle, WA 98115
206 322-6100
Type: Vocational or Tech Sch
Control: For Profit
• Radiography Prgm

Sea Mar Community Health Center
8720 14th Ave S
Seattle, WA 98108-4807
206 726-3730
Control: Nonprofit (Private or Religious)
• Dietetic Internship Prgm

Seattle Central Community College
Mildred Ollee, EdD, President
1701 Broadway, 2BE4180
Seattle, WA 98122
206 587-4144
Type: Junior or Comm Coll
Control: State, County, or Local Govt
• Dental Hygiene Prgm
• Ophthalmic Dispensing Optician Prgm
• Respiratory Therapist (Advanced) Prgm
• Surgical Technology Prgm

Seattle Pacific University
3307 Third Ave W
Seattle, WA 98119
206 281-2050
Type: 4-year Coll or Univ
Control: Nonprofit (Private or Religious)
• Dietetics-Didactic Prgm
• Nursing Prgm
• Psychology Prgm

Seattle University
Stephen Sundborg, SJ STD, President
901 12th Ave
PO Box 222000
Seattle, WA 98122-4460
206 296-5960
Type: 4-year Coll or Univ
Control: Nonprofit (Private or Religious)
• Diagnostic Med Sonography Prgm
• Nursing Prgm

Seattle Vocational Institute
Norward J Brooks, PhD, Director
2120 S Jackson
Seattle, WA 98144
206 587-4940
Type: Vocational or Tech Sch
Control: State, County, or Local Govt
• Dental Assisting Prgm
• Medical Assistant Prgm

University of Washington
Mark Emmert, PhD, President
301 Gerberding Hall
Box 351230
Seattle, WA 98195-1230
206 543-5010
Type: Acad Health Ctr/Med Sch
Control: State, County, or Local Govt
• Allopathic Medicine Prgm
• Audiologist Prgm
• Clin Lab Scientist/Med Technologist Prgm
• Dentistry Prgm
• Dietetic Internship Prgm
• Dietetics-Didactic Prgm
• Health Information Admin Prgm
• Medical Librarian Prgm
• Nursing Prgm
• Occupational Therapy Prgm
• Orthotist/Prosthetist Prgm
• Pharmacy Prgm
• Physical Therapy Prgm
• Physician Assistant Prgm
• Psychology Prgm
• Speech-Language Pathology Prgm

Shoreline

Shoreline Community College
Lee Lambert, JD, Interim President
16101 Greenwood Ave N
Shoreline, WA 98133
206 546-4551
Type: Junior or Comm Coll
Control: State, County, or Local Govt
• Clin Lab Technician/Med Lab Technician Prgm
• Dental Hygiene Prgm
• Dietetic Technician-AD Prgm
• Health Information Tech Prgm

Spokane

Apollo College
George Montgomery, BA, President and CEO
10102 E Knox Ste 200
Spokane, WA 99206
509 532-8888
Type: Junior or Comm Coll
Control: For Profit
• Radiography Prgm

Gonzaga University
Spokane, WA 99258
Type: 4-year Coll or Univ
Control: Nonprofit (Private or Religious)
• Nursing Prgm

Sacred Heart Medical Center
Michael Wilson, MA, President/CEO
W 101 Eighth Ave
PO Box 2555
Spokane, WA 99220-2555
509 455-3040
Type: Hosp or Med Ctr: 500> Beds
Control: Nonprofit (Private or Religious)
• Clin Lab Scientist/Med Technologist Prgm

Spokane Community College
Joe Dunlap, EdD, President
N 1810 Greene St MS 2150
Spokane, WA 99217
509 533-7042
Type: Junior or Comm Coll
Control: State, County, or Local Govt
• Cardiovascular Technology Prgm
• Dental Assisting Prgm
• Emergency Med Tech-Paramedic Prgm
• Health Information Tech Prgm
• Medical Assistant Prgm
• Optometric Technician Prgm
• Pharmacy Technician Prgm
• Radiography Prgm
• Respiratory Therapist (Advanced) Prgm
• Surgical Technology Prgm

Spokane Falls Community College
Mark Palek, President
3410 W Fort George Wright Dr, MS3160
Spokane, Wa 99224-5288
509 533-3535
Type: Junior or Comm Coll
Control: State, County, or Local Govt
• Physical Therapist Assistant Prgm

Whitworth College
William P Robinson, PhD, President
300 W Hawthorne Rd
Spokane, WA 99251
509 777-1000
Type: 4-year Coll or Univ
Control: Nonprofit (Private or Religious)
• Athletic Training Prgm

Tacoma

Bates Technical College
David Borofsky, EdD, President
1101 S Yakima Ave
Tacoma, WA 98405
253 680-7100
Type: Vocational or Tech Sch
Control: State, County, or Local Govt
• Dental Assisting Prgm
• Dental Lab Technician Prgm

Pacific Lutheran University
Tacoma, WA 98447
Type: 4-year Coll or Univ
Control: Nonprofit (Private or Religious)
• Nursing Prgm

St Joseph Medical Center
Joseph W Wilezek, President and CEO
1717 South J St
Tacoma, WA 98401-2197
Type: Acad Health Ctr/Med Sch
Control: For Profit
• Pharmacy Technician Prgm

Tacoma Community College
Pamela Transue, PhD, President
6501 S 19th St
Tacoma, WA 98466
253 566-5100
Type: Junior or Comm Coll
Control: State, County, or Local Govt
• Emergency Med Tech-Paramedic Prgm
• Health Information Tech Prgm
• Radiography Prgm
• Respiratory Therapist (Advanced) Prgm

Tacoma Fire Department
Ron Stephens, Fire Chief
901 Fawcett Ave
Tacoma, WA 98402
253 591-5737
Type: Consortium
Control: State, County, or Local Govt
• Emergency Med Tech-Paramedic Prgm

University of Puget Sound
Ronald R Thomas, PhD, President
1500 N Warner St, CMB 1094
Tacoma, WA 98416-0510
253 879-3201
Type: 4-year Coll or Univ
Control: Nonprofit (Private or Religious)
• Occupational Therapy Prgm
• Physical Therapy Prgm

Vancouver

Clark College
Robert Knight, MA, President
1933 Fort Vancouver Way
Vancouver, WA 98663-3598
360 992-2000
Type: Junior or Comm Coll
Control: State, County, or Local Govt
• Dental Hygiene Prgm
• Medical Assistant Prgm

Everest College
Edward Yakimchick, BA, President
120 NE 136th Ave, Ste 130
Vancouver, WA 98684
360 254-3282
Type: Vocational or Tech Sch
Control: For Profit
• Medical Assistant Prgm

Northwest Regional Training Center
Marty James, Administrator
11606 NE 66th St, Ste 103
Vancouver, WA 98662
360 759-4404
Type: Vocational or Tech Sch
Control: State, County, or Local Govt
• Emergency Med Tech-Paramedic Prgm

Wenatchee

Wenatchee Valley College
James Richardson, MSEd, President
1300 Fifth St
Wenatchee, WA 98801
509 682-6668
Type: Junior or Comm Coll
Control: State, County, or Local Govt
• Clin Lab Technician/Med Lab Technician Prgm
• Medical Assistant Prgm

Yakima

Yakima Regional CLS Program
Rick Garnier, CEO
1120 W Spruce St
Yakima, WA 98902
Type: 4-year Coll or Univ
Control: Nonprofit (Private or Religious)
• Clin Lab Scientist/Med Technologist Prgm

Yakima Valley Community College
Linda J Kaminski, EdD, President
PO Box 22520
Yakima, WA 98907
509 574-4635
Type: Junior or Comm Coll
Control: State, County, or Local Govt
• Dental Hygiene Prgm
• Medical Assistant Prgm
• Surgical Technology Prgm
• Veterinary Technology Prgm

West Indies

Trinidad West Indies

Trinidad & Tobago Coll of Therapeutic Massage
68 Market St
Gopaul Lands, Marabella
Trinidad West Indies, WN
Type: Vocational or Tech Sch
Control: Nonprofit (Private or Religious)
• Massage Therapy Prgm

West Virginia

Athens

Concord University
Jerry Beasley, PhD, President
PO Box 1000
Campus Box Wall
Athens, WV 24712
304 384-9188
Type: 4-year Coll or Univ
Control: State, County, or Local Govt
• Athletic Training Prgm

Beckley

Mountain State University
Charles H Polk, EdD, President
PO Box 9003
Beckley, WV 25802
304 253-7351
Type: 4-year Coll or Univ
Control: Nonprofit (Private or Religious)
• Diagnostic Med Sonography Prgm
• Medical Assistant Prgm
• Occupational Therapy Asst Prgm
• Physical Therapist Assistant Prgm
• Physician Assistant Prgm
• Radiography Prgm

Bluefield

Bluefield Regional Medical Center
Lynn Whitaker, MBA, CEO
500 Cherry St
Bluefield, WV 24701
304 327-1701
Type: Hosp or Med Ctr: 100-299 Beds
Control: Nonprofit (Private or Religious)
• Clin Lab Technician/Med Lab Technician Prgm

Bluefield State College
Albert Walker, EdD, President
219 Rock St
Bluefield, WV 24701
304 327-4030
Type: 4-year Coll or Univ
Control: State, County, or Local Govt
• Nursing Prgm
• Radiography Prgm

Buckhannon

West Virginia Wesleyan College
Pamela Balch, MA, President
59 College Ave
Buckhannon, WV 26201-2995
304 473-8181
Type: 4-year Coll or Univ
Control: Nonprofit (Private or Religious)
• Athletic Training Prgm

Charleston

CAMC Health Education & Research Institute
Sharon A Hall, President
3200 MacCorkle Ave SE
Charleston, WV 25304
304 388-9900
Type: Hosp or Med Ctr: 500> Beds
Control: Nonprofit (Private or Religious)
• Cytotechnology Prgm

Carver Career Center
Jim Casdorph, MA, Principal
4799 Midland Dr
Charleston, WV 25306
304 348-1965
Type: Vocational or Tech Sch
Control: State, County, or Local Govt
• Pharmacy Technician Prgm
• Respiratory Therapist (Advanced) Prgm
• Surgical Technology Prgm

Mountain State School of Massage
Robert Rogers, LMTNCTMB, Executive Director
601 50th St
Charleston, WV 25304
304 926-8822
Type: Vocational or Tech Sch
Control: For Profit
• Massage Therapy Prgm

University of Charleston
Edwin H Welch, PhD, President
2300 McCorkle Ave SE
Charleston, WV 25304
304 357-4713
Type: 4-year Coll or Univ
Control: Nonprofit (Private or Religious)
• Athletic Training Prgm
• Pharmacy Prgm
• Radiography Prgm

Clarksburg

United Hospital Center
Bruce C Carter, MS, President
Three Hospital Plaza
Clarksburg, WV 26301
304 624-2332
Type: Hosp or Med Ctr: 300-499 Beds
Control: Nonprofit (Private or Religious)
• Radiography Prgm

Dunbar

Benjamin Franklin Career & Technical Ed Ctr
Alvin L Brown, BA MA MS, Principal
500 28th St
Dunbar, WV 25064
304 766-0369
Type: Vocational or Tech Sch
Control: State, County, or Local Govt
• Medical Assistant Prgm

Fairmont

Fairmont State Univ
Blair Montgomery, MS, President
230 Hardway Building
1201 Locust Ave
Fairmont, WV 26554
304 367-4692
Type: Junior or Comm Coll
Control: State, County, or Local Govt
• Clin Lab Technician/Med Lab Technician Prgm
• Health Information Tech Prgm
• Nursing Prgm
• Physical Therapist Assistant Prgm
• Veterinary Technology Prgm

Huntington

Cabell Huntington Hospital
Brent Marstellar, BS, President
1340 Hal Greer Blvd
Huntington, WV 25701
304 526-2111
Type: Hosp or Med Ctr: 300-499 Beds
Control: Nonprofit (Private or Religious)
• Cytotechnology Prgm

Huntington Junior College
Carolyn Smith, BA, President
900 Fifth Ave
Huntington, WV 25701
304 697-7550
Type: Junior or Comm Coll
Control: For Profit
• Medical Assistant Prgm

Marshall Community & Technical College
Dan D Angel, President
One John Marshall Dr
Huntington, WV 25755
304 696-2300
Type: Vocational or Tech Sch
Control: State, County, or Local Govt
• Health Information Tech Prgm
• Medical Assistant Prgm
• Physical Therapist Assistant Prgm

Marshall University
Stephen Kopp, PhD, President
One John Marshall Dr
Huntington, WV 25755
304 696-2300
Type: 4-year Coll or Univ
Control: State, County, or Local Govt
• Allopathic Medicine Prgm
• Athletic Training Prgm
• Clin Lab Scientist/Med Technologist Prgm
• Clin Lab Technician/Med Lab Technician Prgm
• Dietetic Internship Prgm
• Dietetics-Didactic Prgm
• Health Information Tech Prgm
• Psychology Prgm
• Speech-Language Pathology Prgm

St Mary's Medical Center
Michael Sellards, BS MHA, Exec Director/CEO
2900 First Ave
Huntington, WV 25702
304 526-1270
Type: Hosp or Med Ctr: 300-499 Beds
Control: Nonprofit (Private or Religious)
• Radiography Prgm

Institute

West Virginia State Comm & Tech College
Ervin V Griffin, PhD, President
PO Box 1000
105 Cole Complex
Institute, WV 25112
304 766-3111
Type: Junior or Comm Coll
Control: State, County, or Local Govt
• Nuclear Medicine Technology Prgm

Lewisburg

West Virginia of Osteopathic Medicine
400 N Lee St
Lewisburg, WV 24901
Type: Acad Health Ctr/Med Sch
Control: Nonprofit (Private or Religious)
• Osteopathic Medicine Prgm

Montgomery

Community & Technical College at WVU Tech
Beverly Jo Harris, EdD, President
208 Davis Hall
Montgomery, WV 25136
304 442-3149
Type: Junior or Comm Coll
Control: State, County, or Local Govt
• Dental Hygiene Prgm

Morgantown

Monongalia County Tech Education Center
John George, MA, Director/Principal
1000 Mississippi St
Morgantown, WV 26505
304 291-9240
Type: Vocational or Tech Sch
Control: State, County, or Local Govt
• Surgical Technology Prgm

West Virginia University
David C Hardesty, Jr, JD, President
102A Stewart Hall, PO Box 6201
Morgantown, WV 26506-6201
304 293-5531
Type: 4-year Coll or Univ
Control: State, County, or Local Govt
• Allopathic Medicine Prgm
• Athletic Training Prgm
• Audiologist Prgm
• Clin Lab Scientist/Med Technologist Prgm
• Counseling Prgm
• Dental Hygiene Prgm
• Dentistry Prgm
• Dietetic Internship Prgm
• Dietetics-Didactic Prgm
• Nursing Prgm
• Occupational Therapy Prgm
• Pharmacy Prgm
• Physical Therapy Prgm
• Psychology Prgm
• Rehabilitation Counseling Prgm
• Speech-Language Pathology Prgm

West Virginia University Hospitals
Bruce McClymonds, President
Rudy Memorial Hospital
PO Box 8136
Morgantown, WV 26505
304 598-4355
Type: Hosp or Med Ctr: 300-499 Beds
Control: Nonprofit (Private or Religious)
• Diagnostic Med Sonography Prgm
• Dietetic Internship Prgm
• Nuclear Medicine Technology Prgm
• Radiation Therapy Prgm
• Radiography Prgm

Mt Gay

Southern West Virginia Comm & Tech College
Joanne C Tomblin, MA, President
PO Box 2900
Mt Gay, WV 25637
304 792-7160
Type: Junior or Comm Coll
Control: State, County, or Local Govt
• Clin Lab Technician/Med Lab Technician Prgm
• Dental Hygiene Prgm
• Radiography Prgm
• Surgical Technology Prgm

Parkersburg

West Virginia University - Parkersburg
Marie Foster Gnage, PhD, President
300 Campus Dr
Parkersburg, WV 26104
304 424-8200
Type: Junior or Comm Coll
Control: State, County, or Local Govt
• Surgical Technology Prgm

Philippi

Alderson-Broaddus College
Stephen E Markwood, PhD, President
Box 2065
101 College Hill Rd
Philippi, WV 26416
304 457-6201
Type: 4-year Coll or Univ
Control: Nonprofit (Private or Religious)
• Athletic Training Prgm
• Physician Assistant Prgm

Princeton

Mercer County Technical Education Center
1397 Stafford Dr
Princeton, WV 24720
Type: Vocational or Tech Sch
Control: Nonprofit (Private or Religious)
• Dental Assisting Prgm

West Liberty

West Liberty State College
John McCollough, PhD, Interim President
Main Hall
West Liberty, WV 26074
304 336-8000
Type: 4-year Coll or Univ
Control: State, County, or Local Govt
• Clin Lab Scientist/Med Technologist Prgm
• Dental Hygiene Prgm
• Nursing Prgm

Wheeling

Ohio Valley Medical Center
Brian Felici, MS, President
2000 Eoff St
Wheeling, WV 26003
304 234-8294
Type: Hosp or Med Ctr: 100-299 Beds
Control: Nonprofit (Private or Religious)
• Radiography Prgm

West Virginia Northern Community College
Martin Olshinsky, PhD, President
1704 Market St
Wheeling, WV 26003
304 233-5900
Type: Junior or Comm Coll
Control: State, County, or Local Govt
• Health Information Tech Prgm
• Respiratory Therapist (Advanced) Prgm
• Surgical Technology Prgm

Wheeling Hospital
Donald H Hofreuter, MD, Administrator
Medical Park
Wheeling, WV 26003
304 243-3000
Type: Hosp or Med Ctr: 100-299 Beds
Control: Nonprofit (Private or Religious)
• Radiography Prgm

Wheeling Jesuit University
Rev Julio Giuletti, SJ, President
316 Washington Ave
Wheeling, WV 26003
304 243-2233
Type: 4-year Coll or Univ
Control: Nonprofit (Private or Religious)
• Nuclear Medicine Technology Prgm
• Nursing Prgm
• Physical Therapy Prgm
• Respiratory Therapist (Advanced) Prgm

Wisconsin

Appleton

Affinity Health System
Robert Turner, MS, COO
St Elizabeth Hospital
1506 S Oneida St
Appleton, WI 54915
920 831-8912
Type: Hosp or Med Ctr: 100-299 Beds
Control: Nonprofit (Private or Religious)
• Clin Lab Scientist/Med Technologist Prgm

Fox Valley Technical College
David Buettner, PhD, President
1825 N Bluemound Dr
PO Box 2277
Appleton, WI 54913-2277
920 735-5731
Type: Vocational or Tech Sch
Control: State, County, or Local Govt
• Dental Assisting Prgm
• Dental Hygiene Prgm
• Medical Assistant Prgm
• Occupational Therapy Asst Prgm

Cleveland

Lakeshore Technical College
Michael Lanser, EdD, Director
1290 North Ave
Cleveland, WI 53015
920 693-1123
Type: Vocational or Tech Sch
Control: State, County, or Local Govt
• Radiography Prgm

Eau Claire

Chippewa Valley Technical College
William A Ihlenfeldt, PhD, President
620 W Clairemont Ave
Eau Claire, WI 54701
715 833-6211
Type: Vocational or Tech Sch
Control: State, County, or Local Govt
• Clin Lab Technician/Med Lab Technician Prgm
• Diagnostic Med Sonography Prgm
• Health Information Tech Prgm
• Medical Assistant Prgm
• Radiography Prgm
• Respiratory Therapist (Advanced) Prgm
• Surgical Technology Prgm

INSTITUTIONS

Sacred Heart Hospital
Steve Ronstrom, MHA, Administrator
900 W Clairemont Ave
Eau Claire, WI 54701
715 839-4131
Type: Hosp or Med Ctr: 300-499 Beds
Control: Nonprofit (Private or Religious)
• Clin Lab Scientist/Med Technologist Prgm

University of Wisconsin - Eau Claire
Brian Levin-Stankevich, PhD, Chancellor
Schofield 204
105 Garfield Ave
Eau Claire, WI 54702-4004
715 836-2327
Type: 4-year Coll or Univ
Control: State, County, or Local Govt
• Athletic Training Prgm
• Music Therapy Prgm
• Nursing Prgm
• Speech-Language Pathology Prgm

Fennimore

Southwest Wisconsin Technical College
Karen Knox, EdD, President
1800 Bronson Blvd
Fennimore, WI 53809
608 288-3262
Type: Vocational or Tech Sch
Control: State, County, or Local Govt
• Medical Assistant Prgm

Fond du Lac

Marian College
Fond du Lac, WI 54935
Type: 4-year Coll or Univ
Control: State, County, or Local Govt
• Nursing Prgm

Moraine Park Technical College
Gayle Hytrek, PhD, President
235 N National Ave
PO Box 1940
Fond du Lac, WI 54936-1940
414 922-8611
Type: Vocational or Tech Sch
Control: State, County, or Local Govt
• Clin Lab Technician/Med Lab Technician Prgm
• Health Information Tech Prgm
• Medical Assistant Prgm
• Radiation Therapy Prgm

Grafton

Blue Sky School of Professional Massage
Karen Lewis, Dean, Co-Founder
220 Oak St
Manchester Mall
Grafton, WI 53024
262 376-1011
Type: Vocational or Tech Sch
Control: Nonprofit (Private or Religious)
• Massage Therapy Prgm (3)

Green Bay

Bellin Health Hosp/Bellin Health Systems Inc
George Kerwin, MBA, President and CEO
744 S Webster Ave
PO Box 23400
Green Bay, WI 54305-3400
414 433-7898
Type: Hosp or Med Ctr: 100-299 Beds
Control: Nonprofit (Private or Religious)
• Nursing Prgm
• Radiography Prgm

Northeast Wisconsin Technical College
H Jeffrey Rafn, PhD, President
2740 W Mason St, PO Box 19042
Green Bay, WI 54307-9042
920 498-5411
Type: Vocational or Tech Sch
Control: State, County, or Local Govt
• Clin Lab Technician/Med Lab Technician Prgm
• Dental Assisting Prgm
• Dental Hygiene Prgm
• Diagnostic Med Sonography Prgm
• Health Information Tech Prgm
• Medical Assistant Prgm
• Physical Therapist Assistant Prgm
• Respiratory Therapist (Advanced) Prgm
• Surgical Technology Prgm

University of Wisconsin - Green Bay
Mark L Perkins, Chancellor
Green Bay, WI 54311
414 465-2000
Type: 4-year Coll or Univ
Control: State, County, or Local Govt
• Dietetic Internship Prgm
• Dietetics-Didactic Prgm
• Nursing Prgm

Hayward

Lac Courte Oreills Ojibwa Community College
Danielle Hornett, PhD, President
13466 Trepania Rd
Hayward, WI 54843
715 634-4790
Type: Junior or Comm Coll
Control: State, County, or Local Govt
• Medical Assistant Prgm

Janesville

Blackhawk Technical College
Eric Larson, EdD, President
6004 Prairie Rd
PO Box 5009
Janesville, WI 53547-5009
608 756-4121
Type: Vocational or Tech Sch
Control: State, County, or Local Govt
• Dental Assisting Prgm
• Medical Assistant Prgm
• Physical Therapist Assistant Prgm
• Radiography Prgm

Kenosha

Carthage College
F Gregory Campbell, President
2001 Alford Park Dr
Kenosha, WI 53140-1994
262 551-5858
Type: 4-year Coll or Univ
Control: State, County, or Local Govt
• Athletic Training Prgm

Gateway Technical College
Bryan Albrecht, PhD, President
3520 30th Ave
Kenosha, WI 53144
262 564-2200
Type: Vocational or Tech Sch
Control: State, County, or Local Govt
• Dental Assisting Prgm
• Health Information Tech Prgm
• Medical Assistant Prgm (2)
• Physical Therapist Assistant Prgm
• Surgical Technology Prgm

La Crosse

Gundersen Lutheran Medical Foundation
Jeffrey Thompson, PhD, CEO
1900 South Ave
La Crosse, WI 54601
608 782-7300
Type: Hosp or Med Ctr: 300-499 Beds
Control: Nonprofit (Private or Religious)
• Nuclear Medicine Technology Prgm

University of Wisconsin - La Crosse
Joe Gow, PhD, Chancellor
1725 State St
135 Main Hall
La Crosse, WI 54601
608 785-8004
Type: 4-year Coll or Univ
Control: State, County, or Local Govt
• Athletic Training Prgm
• Medical Dosimetry Prgm
• Occupational Therapy Prgm
• Physical Therapy Prgm
• Physician Assistant Prgm
• Radiation Therapy Prgm
• Therapeutic Recreation Specialist Prgm

Viterbo College
Robert E Gibbons, PhD, President
818 S 9th St
La Crosse, WI 54601
608 784-0040
Type: 4-year Coll or Univ
Control: State, County, or Local Govt
• Dietetic Internship Prgm
• Dietetics-Coordinated Prgm
• Nursing Prgm

Western Technical College
J Lee Rasch, EdD, President/District Dir
304 N Sixth St
PO Box C-0908
La Crosse, WI 54602-0908
608 785-9210
Type: Vocational or Tech Sch
Control: State, County, or Local Govt
- Clin Lab Technician/Med Lab Technician Prgm
- Dental Assisting Prgm
- Electroneurodiagnostic Tech Prgm
- Health Information Tech Prgm
- Medical Assistant Prgm
- Occupational Therapy Asst Prgm
- Physical Therapist Assistant Prgm
- Radiography Prgm
- Respiratory Therapist (Advanced) Prgm
- Surgical Technology Prgm

Madison

Edgewood College
Daniel J Carey, PhD, President
1000 Edgewood College Dr
Madison, WI 53711
Type: 4-year Coll or Univ
Control: Nonprofit (Private or Religious)
- Nursing Prgm

Madison Area Technical College
Bettsey Barhorst, PhD, President
3550 Anderson St
Madison, WI 53704-2599
608 246-6676
Type: Vocational or Tech Sch
Control: State, County, or Local Govt
- Clin Lab Technician/Med Lab Technician Prgm
- Dental Hygiene Prgm
- Dietetic Technician-AD Prgm
- Medical Assistant Prgm
- Occupational Therapy Asst Prgm
- Optometric Technician Prgm
- Radiography Prgm
- Respiratory Therapist (Advanced) Prgm
- Surgical Technology Prgm
- Veterinary Technology Prgm

State Laboratory of Hygiene
Charles Brokopp, DPh, Director
Center for Health Studies - UW Madison
465 Henry Hall
Madison, WI 53706
608 262-1293
Type: Nonhosp HC Facil, BB, or Lab
Control: State, County, or Local Govt
- Cytotechnology Prgm

University of Wisconsin - Madison
John Wiley, PhD, Chancellor
500 Lincoln Dr
161 Bascom Hall
Madison, WI 53706-1380
608 262-9946
Type: 4-year Coll or Univ
Control: State, County, or Local Govt
- Allopathic Medicine Prgm
- Athletic Training Prgm
- Audiologist Prgm
- Clin Lab Scientist/Med Technologist Prgm
- Dietetics-Coordinated Prgm
- Dietetics-Didactic Prgm
- Genetic Counseling Prgm
- Medical Librarian Prgm
- Nursing Prgm
- Occupational Therapy Prgm
- Pharmacy Prgm
- Physical Therapy Prgm
- Physician Assistant Prgm
- Psychology Prgm
- Rehabilitation Counseling Prgm
- Speech-Language Pathology Prgm
- Veterinary Medicine Prgm

University of Wisconsin Hospital and Clinics
Carl Getto, MD, Interim President and CEO
600 Highland Ave
Dept of Administration
Madison, WI 53792-8310
608 263-8025
Type: Hosp or Med Ctr: 500> Beds
Control: State, County, or Local Govt
- Diagnostic Med Sonography Prgm
- Dietetic Internship Prgm
- Orthoptist Prgm
- Radiography Prgm

Marshfield

Marshfield Clinic
Reed Hall, MS JD, Executive Director
1000 N Oak Ave
Marshfield, WI 54449
715 387-5123
Type: Nonhosp HC Facil, BB, or Lab
Control: Nonprofit (Private or Religious)
- Cytotechnology Prgm

St Joseph's Hospital
Michael A Schmidt, CPA, CEO
611 St Joseph Ave
Marshfield, WI 54449
715 387-1713
Type: Hosp or Med Ctr: 500> Beds
Control: Nonprofit (Private or Religious)
- Clin Lab Scientist/Med Technologist Prgm
- Histotechnician Prgm
- Nuclear Medicine Technology Prgm
- Radiography Prgm

Menasha

Mercy Medical Center/Affinity Health System
Daniel Neufelder, MS, President
1570 Midway Place
Menasha, WI 54952
920 720-1713
Type: Hosp or Med Ctr: 100-299 Beds
Control: Nonprofit (Private or Religious)
- Radiography Prgm

Menomonie

University of Wisconsin - Stout
Charles W Sorensen, Chancellor
Menomonie, WI 54751
715 232-1123
Type: 4-year Coll or Univ
Control: State, County, or Local Govt
- Dietetic Internship Prgm
- Dietetics-Didactic Prgm
- Rehabilitation Counseling Prgm

Mequon

Concordia University Wisconsin
Patrick Ferry, PhD, President
12800 N Lake Shore Dr
Mequon, WI 53097
262 243-4368
Type: 4-year Coll or Univ
Control: Nonprofit (Private or Religious)
- Athletic Training Prgm
- Medical Assistant Prgm
- Nursing Prgm
- Occupational Therapy Prgm
- Physical Therapy Prgm

Milwaukee

Alverno College
Mary Meehan, President
3401 S 39th St, Box 343922
Milwaukee, WI 53234-3922
414 382-6000
Type: 4-year Coll or Univ
Control: Nonprofit (Private or Religious)
- Music Therapy Prgm
- Nursing Prgm

Aurora St Luke's Medical Center
Nick Turkal, MD, President
2900 W Oklahoma Ave
PO Box 2901
Milwaukee, WI 53201-2901
414 649-7500
Type: Hosp or Med Ctr: 500> Beds
Control: Nonprofit (Private or Religious)
- Diagnostic Med Sonography Prgm
- Nuclear Medicine Technology Prgm
- Radiography Prgm

Blood Center of Southeast Wisconsin
William V Miller, MD, President
PO Box 2178
Milwaukee, WI 53201-2178
414 937-6338
Type: Nonhosp HC Facil, BB, or Lab
Control: Nonprofit (Private or Religious)
- Specialist in BB Tech Prgm

Bryant & Stratton College - Milwaukee
Peter Pavone, MS, Dir, Milwaukee Colleges
310 W Wisconsin Ave, Ste 500 E
Milwaukee, WI 53203
414 276-5200
Type: 4-year Coll or Univ
Control: For Profit
- Medical Assistant Prgm

INSTITUTIONS

Cardinal Stritch University
Sister Mary Lea Schneider, President
6801 N Yates Rd
Milwaukee, WI 53217
414 410-4001
Type: 4-year Coll or Univ
Control: Nonprofit (Private or Religious)
• Nursing Prgm

Clement J Zablocki VA Medical Center
Glen Grippen, Director
5000 W National Ave
Milwaukee, WI 53295
414 384-2000
Type: Dept of Veterans Affairs
Control: Fed Govt
• Clin Lab Scientist/Med Technologist Prgm

Columbia St Mary's Hospitals
Leo Brideau, President, CEO
2025 E Newport Ave
Milwaukee, WI 53211
414 961-3638
Type: Hosp or Med Ctr: 300-499 Beds
Control: Nonprofit (Private or Religious)
• Diagnostic Med Sonography Prgm
• Radiography Prgm

Froedtert Memorial Lutheran Hospital
William D Petasnick, MHA, President
9200 W Wisconsin Ave
PO Box 26099
Milwaukee, WI 53226
414 805-3000
Type: Hosp or Med Ctr: 300-499 Beds
Control: Nonprofit (Private or Religious)
• Nuclear Medicine Technology Prgm
• Radiography Prgm

Lakeside School of Massage Therapy
Carole Ostendorf, PhD PT, Chief Executive
  Officer
1726 N 1st St, Ste 200
Milwaukee, WI 53212
414 372-4345
Type: Vocational or Tech Sch
Control: Nonprofit (Private or Religious)
• Massage Therapy Prgm (2)

Marquette University
Robert A Wild, SJ, President
O'Hara Hall
Milwaukee, WI 53201-1881
414 288-7223
Type: 4-year Coll or Univ
Control: Nonprofit (Private or Religious)
• Athletic Training Prgm
• Clin Lab Scientist/Med Technologist Prgm
• Dentistry Prgm
• Nursing Prgm
• Physical Therapy Prgm
• Physician Assistant Prgm
• Psychology Prgm
• Speech-Language Pathology Prgm

Medical College of Wisconsin
T Michael Bolger, JD, President
8701 Watetown Plank Rd
Milwaukee, WI 53226
414 257-8225
Type: Acad Health Ctr/Med Sch
Control: Nonprofit (Private or Religious)
• Allopathic Medicine Prgm

Milwaukee Area Technical College
Darnell Cole, PhD, President
700 W State St
Milwaukee, WI 53233-1443
414 297-6320
Type: Vocational or Tech Sch
Control: State, County, or Local Govt
• Cardiovascular Technology Prgm
• Clin Lab Technician/Med Lab Technician Prgm
• Dental Hygiene Prgm
• Dietetic Technician-AD Prgm
• Medical Assistant Prgm
• Occupational Therapy Asst Prgm
• Ophthalmic Dispensing Optician Prgm
• Phlebotomy Prgm
• Physical Therapist Assistant Prgm
• Radiography Prgm
• Respiratory Therapist (Advanced) Prgm
• Surgical Technology Prgm

Milwaukee School of Engineering
Hermann Viets, PhD, President
1025 N Broadway
Milwaukee, WI 53202-3109
414 277-7100
Type: 4-year Coll or Univ
Control: Nonprofit (Private or Religious)
• Nursing Prgm
• Perfusion Prgm

Mount Mary College
Patricia D O'Donoghue, President
2900 N Menomonee River Pkwy
Milwaukee, WI 53222-4597
414 258-4810
Type: 4-year Coll or Univ
Control: Nonprofit (Private or Religious)
• Art Therapy Prgm
• Dietetic Internship Prgm
• Dietetics-Coordinated Prgm
• Occupational Therapy Prgm

University of Wisconsin - Milwaukee
Carlos Santiago, PhD, Chancellor
PO Box 413
Milwaukee, WI 53201
414 229-4331
Type: 4-year Coll or Univ
Control: State, County, or Local Govt
• Athletic Training Prgm
• Clin Lab Scientist/Med Technologist Prgm
• Cytotechnology Prgm
• Medical Librarian Prgm
• Nursing Prgm
• Occupational Therapy Prgm
• Psychology Prgm
• Speech-Language Pathology Prgm

Wheaton Franciscan Healthcare - St Francis
Debra Standridge, MBA, President
3237 S 16th St
Milwaukee, WI 53215
414 647-5106
Type: Hosp or Med Ctr: 100-299 Beds
Control: Nonprofit (Private or Religious)
• Diagnostic Med Sonography Prgm

Wheaton Franciscan Healthcare - St Joseph
Ronald Groepper, RN MBA FACHE,
  President/CEO
5000 West Chambers St
Milwaukee, WI 53210
414 447-2847
Type: Hosp or Med Ctr: 300-499 Beds
Control: Nonprofit (Private or Religious)
• Radiography Prgm

Neenah

Theda Clark Regional Medical Center
John Toiusant, MD, President
130 Second St
PO Box 2021
Neenah, WI 54957-2021
920 729-3100
Type: Hosp or Med Ctr: 300-499 Beds
Control: Nonprofit (Private or Religious)
• Radiography Prgm

Oshkosh

University of Wisconsin - Oshkosh
Richard Wells, Chancellor
800 Algoma Blvd
Oshkosh, WI 54901
920 424-0200
Type: 4-year Coll or Univ
Control: State, County, or Local Govt
• Athletic Training Prgm
• Counseling Prgm
• Nursing Prgm

Pewaukee

Waukesha County Technical College
Barbara Prindiville, PhD, President
800 Main St
Pewaukee, WI 53072
414 691-5435
Type: Vocational or Tech Sch
Control: State, County, or Local Govt
• Dental Hygiene Prgm
• Medical Assistant Prgm
• Surgical Technology Prgm

Racine

Wheaton Franciscan Healthcare - All Saints
Kenneth R Buser, FACHE, President and CEO
3801 Spring St
Racine, WI 53405
262 687-4285
Type: Hosp or Med Ctr: 300-499 Beds
Control: Nonprofit (Private or Religious)
• Radiography Prgm

Rhinelander

Nicolet Area Technical College
Adrian Lorbetske, JD, President
PO Box 518
Rhinelander, WI 54501
715 365-4410
Type: Vocational or Tech Sch
Control: State, County, or Local Govt
• Medical Assistant Prgm

River Falls

University of Wisconsin - River Falls
Gary A Thibodeau, Chancellor
River Falls, WI 54022
715 425-3911
Type: 4-year Coll or Univ
Control: State, County, or Local Govt
• Speech-Language Pathology Prgm

Shell Lake

Wisconsin Indianhead Technical College
Charles Levine, PhD, Interim President
505 Pine Ridge Dr
Shell Lake, WI 54871-9300
715 468-2815
Type: Vocational or Tech Sch
Control: State, County, or Local Govt
• Medical Assistant Prgm (3)
• Occupational Therapy Asst Prgm
• Radiography Prgm

Stevens Point

University of Wisconsin - Stevens Point
Linda Bunnell, PhD, Chancellor
213 Main
Stevens Point, WI 54481
715 346-2123
Type: 4-year Coll or Univ
Control: State, County, or Local Govt
• Athletic Training Prgm
• Audiologist Prgm
• Clin Lab Scientist/Med Technologist Prgm
• Dietetics-Didactic Prgm
• Speech-Language Pathology Prgm

Superior

University of Wisconsin - Superior
Julius E Erlenbach, Chancellor
1800 Grand Ave
Superior, WI 54880-2898
715 394-8101
Type: 4-year Coll or Univ
Control: State, County, or Local Govt
• Counseling Prgm

Waukesha

Carroll College
Douglas N Hastad, DEd, President
100 N East Ave
Waukesha, WI 53186-5593
414 547-1211
Type: 4-year Coll or Univ
Control: Nonprofit (Private or Religious)
• Athletic Training Prgm
• Nursing Prgm
• Physical Therapy Prgm

Wausau

Aspirus Wausau Hospital
Diane Postler-Slattery, PhD, President and COO
333 Pine Ridge Blvd
Wausau, WI 54401
715 847-2988
Type: Hosp or Med Ctr: 300-499 Beds
Control: Nonprofit (Private or Religious)
• Clin Lab Scientist/Med Technologist Prgm

Northcentral Technical College
Lori A Weyers, PhD, President
1000 Campus Dr
Wausau, WI 54401-1899
715 675-3331
Type: Vocational or Tech Sch
Control: State, County, or Local Govt
• Dental Hygiene Prgm
• Medical Assistant Prgm
• Phlebotomy Prgm
• Radiography Prgm
• Surgical Technology Prgm

Whitewater

University of Wisconsin - Whitewater
Richard Telfer, Interim Chancellor
800 W Main
Hyer 421
Whitewater, WI 53190-1791
262 472-1918
Type: 4-year Coll or Univ
Control: State, County, or Local Govt
• Counseling Prgm
• Speech-Language Pathology Prgm

Wisconsin Rapids

Mid-State Technical College
John Clark, PhD, President
500 32nd St N
Wisconsin Rapids, WI 54494
715 423-5650
Type: Vocational or Tech Sch
Control: State, County, or Local Govt
• Medical Assistant Prgm (2)
• Phlebotomy Prgm
• Respiratory Therapist (Advanced) Prgm
• Surgical Technology Prgm

Wyoming

Casper

Casper College
Walter Nolte, PhD, President
125 College Dr
Casper, WY 82601
307 268-2547
Type: Junior or Comm Coll
Control: State, County, or Local Govt
• Occupational Therapy Asst Prgm
• Radiography Prgm

University of North Dakota at Casper College
Walter Nolte, President
125 College Dr
Casper, WY 82601-9958
Type: 4-year Coll or Univ
Control: State, County, or Local Govt
• Occupational Therapy Prgm

Cheyenne

Laramie County Community College
Darrel L Hammon, PhD, President
1400 E College Dr
Cheyenne, WY 82007
307 778-5222
Type: Junior or Comm Coll
Control: State, County, or Local Govt
• Dental Hygiene Prgm
• Radiography Prgm
• Surgical Technology Prgm

Laramie

University of Wyoming
Thomas Buchanan, PhD, President
Dept 3434
1000 E University Ave
Laramie, WY 82071
307 766-4121
Type: 4-year Coll or Univ
Control: State, County, or Local Govt
• Athletic Training Prgm
• Counseling Prgm
• Dietetics-Didactic Prgm
• Nursing Prgm
• Pharmacy Prgm
• Psychology Prgm
• Speech-Language Pathology Prgm

Sheridan

Sheridan College
Kevin Drumm, EdD, President
3059 Coffeen Ave
Box 1500
Sheridan, WY 82801
307 674-6446
Type: Junior or Comm Coll
Control: State, County, or Local Govt
• Dental Hygiene Prgm

Torrington

Eastern Wyoming College
Jack Bottenfield, PhD, President
3200 West C St
Torrington, WY 82240
307 532-8202
Type: Junior or Comm Coll
Control: State, County, or Local Govt
• Veterinary Technology Prgm

INSTITUTIONS

Section III

Additional Health Care Careers Information

Resources for Information on Health Care Careers

Web Sites

Alabama Health Careers
Alabama Hospital Association
www.AlabamaHealthCareers.com

Career Voyages
US Departments of Labor and Education
www.careervoyages.gov/healthcare-alliedhealth.cfm

CareerZone, California
Carl Perkins funding from the California Department of Education
www.cacareerzone.org

CareerZone, New York
New York State Department of Labor with a grant from the United States Department of Labor
www.nycareerzone.org

Colorado Health Career Guide
Central Colorado AHEC and Workforce Boulder County
www.coloradohealthcareers.org/index.htm

Diagnostic Detectives
Michigan Department of Community Health
www.medlabcareers.msu.edu

ExploreHealthCareers.org
American Dental Education Association, with funding by the Josiah Macy Jr. Foundation
www.explorehealthcareers.org

Health Care Career Advisor
Cookeville Regional Medical Center Education Department, Tennessee Hospital Association, and Putnam County Schools.
www.healthcareadvisortn.org

Health Care Careers Report
Labor Market Information Division, State of California
www.labormarketinfo.edd.ca.gov/cgi/career/
    ?PAGEID=3&SUBID=169

Health Careers Center, Mississippi Hospital Association
www.mshealthcareers.com

healthinformationcareers.com
American Health Information Management Association
www.healthinformationcareers.com

Health Occupations for Today and Tomorrow
Michigan Health Council
www.mihott.com

Health Occupations for Today and Tomorrow
South Dakota Department of Health/Office of Rural Health
www.sdjobs.org/sdhott

H.O.T. Jobs: Health Opportunities in Texas
East Texas Area Health Education Center
West Texas Area Health Education Center
Center for South Texas Programs
www.texashotjobs.org

Iowa Health Careers Information Center
Iowa Department of Public Health
www.idph.state.ia.us/healthcareers

Kids Into Health Careers
http://bhpr.hrsa.gov/kidscareers

Labs are Vital
Abbott Diagnostics Division
www.labsarevital.com

LifeWorks
Office of Science Education, National Institutes of Health
http://science.education.nih.gov/lifeworks.nsf

Louisiana Health Careers Directory
The Governor's Office of the Workforce Commission and the four Louisiana Area Health Education Centers (AHECs):
- North Louisiana AHEC
- Central Louisiana AHEC
- Southwest Louisiana AHEC
- Southeast Lousiana AHEC
www.lahealthcareers.com

My First Day
Minnesota Hospital Association and Virginia Hospital Association
www.myfirstday.org

My Health Career
Northern Area Health Education Center
www.myhealthcareer.org

New York Health Careers
www.healthcareersinfo.net

Vermont Health Care Careers Portal
University of Vermont College of Medicine AHEC Program
www.vthealthcareers.org

Scholarship Information

Health Career Opportunity Program
Health Resources and Services Administration, Bureau of Health Professions
301 443-2100
http://bhpr.hrsa.gov/diversity/hcop/default.htm

Federal Student Aid
US Department of Education
800 443-3243
http://tinyurl.com/4tfej

College is Possible
American Council on Education
202 939-9300
www.collegeispossible.org

National Organizations

Association of Academic Health Centers
1400 16th Street NW, Suite 720
Washington, DC 20036-2401
202 265-9600
202 265-7514 Fax
www.ahcnet.org

Founded in 1958, the Association of Academic Health Centers (AHC) is a national, nonprofit organization that consists of over 100 institutional members throughout the United States that are the health complexes of the major universities. Generally, academic health centers consist of an allopathic or osteopathic school of medicine, at least one other health professions school or program, and one or more teaching hospitals. These institutions are the nation's primary resources for education in the health professions, biomedical and health services research, and many aspects of patient care.

The AHC is dedicated to improving the health of the people by advancing the leadership of academic health centers in health professions' education, biomedical and health services research, and health care delivery.

Association of Schools of Allied Health Professions
1730 M Street NW, Suite 500
Washington, DC 20036
202 293-4848
202 293-4852 Fax
www.asahp.org

The Association of Schools of Allied Health Professions (ASAHP) works to promote collaboration and partnerships across allied health education and practice, influence health care policy, promote and strengthen research and scholarship, promote and support academic leadership, and promote high quality and innovation in education. ASAHP publishes the *Journal of Allied Health* and holds an annual conference and other meetings.

Health Occupations Students of America
6021 Morriss Road, Suite 111
Flower Mound, TX 75028
800 321-HOSA
972 874-0063 Fax
www.hosa.org

Health Occupations Students of America (HOSA) is a national student organization in secondary and postsecondary schools, with members in 2,086 chapters and 40 state associations. As part of the public school system, HOSA offers health career information on a daily basis to over 2,000,000 high school students. Its Career Awareness Campaign is designed to promote health career opportunities in grades K-12 and to mobilize thousands of HOSA members in spreading the word about the value of a career in health care.

The HOSA Web site features a "Career Center" to help its nearly 70,000 members obtain information about potential career choices in health care. It includes information about successful HOSA members who are now practicing health professionals, workforce links, and career information with links to professional association's Web sites.

Health Professions Network
1850 Samuel Morse Drive
Reston, VA 20190-5316
703 708-9000
703 708-9015 Fax
www.healthpronet.org

The Health Professions Network is a group of volunteers representing allied health professional associations interested in interdisciplinary communication, discussion, and collaboration. Participants meet at least annually to engage in discussion of issues relating to health care and to serve as a conduit for interdisciplinary problem solving and preparation for future health care delivery. The Network also sponsors Allied Health Professions Week, an annual event held in November that honors health care providers working in the allied health professions and promotes these fields to students considering a career in health care.

National Association of Advisors for the Health Professions
PO Box 1518
Champaign, IL 61824-1518
217 355-0063
217 355-1287 Fax
E-mail: naahpja@aol.com
www.naahp.org

Established in 1974, the National Association of Advisors for the Health Professions (NAAHP) is an organization of over 800 pre-health professions advisors at colleges and universities throughout the US, including schools of allied health, allopathic medicine, chiropractic, dentistry, nursing, optometry, osteopathic medicine, pharmacy, podiatric medicine, and veterinary medicine. The NAAHP coordinates the activities and efforts of four independent regional associations—Central (CAAHP), Northeast (NEAAHP), Southeast (SAAHP) and West (WAAHP)—to help health professions' advisors across the nation function together and speak with one voice.

National Commission for Certifying Agencies
2025 M Street NW, Suite 800
Washington, DC 20036
202 857-1165
202 367-2165 Fax
http://www.noca.org/Resources/NCCAAccreditation/tabid/82/Default.aspx

The National Commission for Certifying Agencies (NCCA), the accreditation body of the National Organization for Competency Assurance (NOCA), is the only national accreditation body for private certification organizations in all disciplines. The NCCA works to ensure the health, welfare, and safety of the public through the accreditation of a variety of certification programs/organizations that assess professional competency. The NCCA uses a peer review process to establish accreditation standards, evaluate compliance with the standards, recognize organizations/programs that demonstrate compliance, and serve as a resource on quality certification.

National Network of Health Career Programs in Two-Year Colleges

Cullen Johnson, Executive Director
714 Harsh Road
Marblehead, OH 43440
800 592-1299 code 50
419 798-5490 Fax
E-mail: texascj@bright.net
www.nn2.org

The National Network of Health Career Programs in Two-Year Colleges is an organization of health education leaders from 2-year colleges across the nation dedicated to:
- promoting and encouraging innovation, collaboration, cooperation, and communication with 2-year colleges sponsoring health career programs;
- developing new leaders in health career education; and
- expressing and advocating the interests of health career programs in 2-year colleges (ie, accreditation issues, practice issues, federal policy issues, etc).

National Society of Allied Health

2139 Georgia Avenue NW, Suite 1C
Washington, DC 20001
202 806-4960
www.nsah.org

Formed in 1978, this nonprofit professional organization draws its members from historically and predominantly black colleges and universities that offer allied health programs. Included are individuals who work as educators, clinicians, and researchers; allied health students become members through induction into the National Society of Allied Health Honor Society.

The organization's major goal is to improve the health care status of African Americans and other at-risk populations through education, employment, community service, and research.

Publications

Occupational Outlook Handbook
US Department of Labor, Bureau of Labor Statistics
www.bls.gov/oco

Diversity: Allied Health Careers
Quarterly magazine
www.diversityalliedhealth.com

Health Workforce Research Organizations

The Bureau of Health Professions, Health Resources and Services Administration, recognizes six federally designated regional workforce analysis centers throughout the US:
- California Center for Health Workforce Studies,
  University of California at San Francisco
  http://futurehealth.ucsf.edu/cchws.html
- Center for Health Workforce Studies,
  State University of New York at Albany
  http://chws.albany.edu
- Illinois Regional Health Workforce Center,
  University of Illinois at Chicago
  www.uic.edu/sph/ichws/
- Regional Center for Health Workforce Studies, Center for Health Economics and Policy, The University of Texas Health Science Center at San Antonio
  www.uthscsa.edu/rchws/index.asp
- Southeast Regional Center for Health Workforce Studies
  www.healthworkforce.unc.edu/data.html

- WWAMI Center for Health Workforce Studies,
  University of Washington
  http://depts.washington.edu/uwchws/

In addition to these federally designated centers, some states have centers that focus on state-specific health workforce concerns:
- Michigan Center for Health Professions,
  Michigan Health Council
  www.mhc.org
- Center for Health Workforce Planning,
  Iowa Department of Public Health
  www.idph.state.ia.us/hpcdp/workforce_planning.asp
- North Carolina Health Professions Data System (HPDS)
  Cecil G. Sheps Center for Health Services Research at the University of North Carolina at Chapel Hill
  www.shepscenter.unc.edu/hp

Other Sources of Health Professions' Data

Enrollment Snapshot of Radiography, Radiation Therapy and Nuclear Medicine Programs, Fall 2006
www.asrt.org/media/pdf/research/enrollmentsurvey06.pdf
American Society of Radiologic Technologists
800 444-2778
www.asrt.org

2000-01 Demographic Survey of Undergraduate and Graduate Programs in Communication Sciences and Disorders
www.capcsd.org/survey/2002/2000-01DemographicsSurvey.pdf

These data cover audiology and speech-language pathology educational programs.

Council of Academic Programs in Communication Sciences and Disorders
952 920-0966
925 920-6098 Fax
E-mail: cap@incnet.com
www.capcsd.org

22nd Annual Report on Physician Assistant Educational Programs in the United States, 2005-2006
www.paeaonline.org/publications.html

Physician Assistant Education Association
Attn: Geraldene Darden
703 548-5538, ext 306
703 548-5539 Fax
E-mail: gdarden@paeaonline.org
www.paeaonline.org

Trends in Dietetics Education: 2006-2007
www.eatright.org/ada/files/2007_Annual_Report.pdf
Data collected by the Commission on Accreditation for Dietetics Education for dietitian and dietetic technician programs are published annually in the *CADE Annual Report*.

Commission on Accreditation for Dietetics Education
American Dietetic Association
800 877-1600, ext 4872
312 899-0040
312 899-4817 Fax
E-mail: cade@eatright.org

ADDITIONAL INFORMATION

Descriptions of Other Health Professions

The American Medical Association (AMA) receives frequent requests for information on health professions that are not listed in the *Directory*. The following organizations and resources may be able to provide more information and/or listings of educational programs in these professions. Please note that these organizations are not affiliated with the AMA and that the organizations and professions listed are not in any sense "recognized" or "approved" by the AMA.

Anesthesia Technologist/Technician

Anesthesia technicians and technologists are integral members of the anesthesia patient care team. Their role is to assist anesthesiologist and anesthetists in acquiring, preparing, and using the equipment and supplies required to administer anesthesia. In this role, they contribute to safe, efficient, and cost-effective anesthesia care.

Depending on individual expertise and training, the tasks of the anesthesia technician and technologist may include equipment maintenance and servicing such as cleaning and sterilizing, assembling, calibrating and testing, troubleshooting, requisitioning and recording of inspections and maintenance, and operating a variety of mechanical, pneumatic, and electronic equipment used to monitor the patient undergoing anesthesia.

Anesthesia technologists with the appropriate training may perform inspection, maintenance, and on-site repairs.

The anesthesia technician or technologist may also be responsible for purchasing and distributing supplies and equipment and maintaining inventories and service records. Individuals functioning as anesthesia technicians or technologists should be capable of a level of self-direction and supervision commensurate with their training.

American Society of Anesthesia Technologists and Technicians
55 Harristown Road, 2nd Floor
Glen Rock, NJ 07452
201 652-6622
201 447-3831 Fax
E-mail: customercare@asatt.org
www.asatt.org

Cancer Registrar

Cancer registrars are data management experts who report cancer statistics for various health care agencies. Registrars work closely with physicians, administrators, researchers, and health care planners to provide support for cancer program development, ensure compliance of reporting standards, and serve as a valuable resource for cancer information with the ultimate goal of preventing and controlling cancer. The cancer registrar is involved in managing and analyzing clinical cancer information for the purpose of education, research, and outcome measurement.

The cancer registrar's primary responsibility is to ensure that timely, accurate, and complete data are incorporated and maintained on all types of cancer diagnosed and/or treated within an institution or other defined population. Information is entered into the database manually and through database linkage and computer interfaces.

Cancer registrars bridge the information gap by capturing a complete summary of the patient's disease from diagnosis through their lifetime. The information is not limited to the episodic information contained in the health care facility record. The summary or abstract is an ongoing account of the cancer patient's history, diagnosis, treatment, and current status.

In addition to managing and reporting cancer data, registrars serve in multiple other professional activities. Cancer registrars participate in cancer program, institution, and community benefit activities as part of the active leadership structure. Registrars provide benchmarking services, monitor quality of care and clinical practice guidelines, assess patterns of care and referrals, and monitor adverse outcomes including mortality and co-morbidity. Cancer registrars can provide consultative services on many issues including registry management and program standards.

National Cancer Registrars Association
1340 Braddock Place, Suite 203
Alexandria, VA 22314
703 299-6640
703 299-6620 Fax
E-mail: mhechter@ncra-usa.org
www.ncra-usa.org

Chaplain

Chaplains are specialized ministers with advanced training who serve in a variety of institutional settings, such as hospitals, correctional institutions, long term care facilities, rehabilitation centers, hospice programs, the military, and other specialized settings. They are considered members of the treatment team and provide pastoral/spiritual care to patients, family members, and staff.

They respond to crisis situations related to codes, traumas, deaths, grieving, and end of life care. They also attend rounds, accept referrals, are available for consults, and visit patients in their assigned areas. Chaplains work as religious specialists in the institution, with training in spiritual screening and spiritual assessments, and utilize those skills in working with patients on spiritual issues and needs, while being careful to keep professional boundaries clear. Chaplains may also have other skills in medical ethics, clinical quality improvement, patient rights, and hospital accreditation.

Four units of Clinical Pastoral Education (approved by the Association for Clinical Pastoral Education, or ACPE), a graduate theological degree, endorsement by a faith group, and appearance before a Certification Committee are standard requirements for certification as a chaplain by the Association of Professional Chaplains (APC).

The APC serves chaplains in all types of health and human service settings. Almost 4,000 of its members are chaplains involved in pastoral care and represent more than 150 faith groups. As a national, not-for-profit professional association, the APC advocates for quality spiritual care of all persons in institutional settings. The ACPE accredits institutions, sets standards, certifies supervisors, and trains ministers for specialized work as institutional chaplains.

Association for Professional Chaplains
1701 E Woodfield Road, Suite 400
Schaumburg, IL 60173
847 240-1014
847 240-1015 Fax
E-mail: info@professionalchaplains.org
www.professionalchaplains.org

Association for Clinical Pastoral Education
1549 Clairmont Road, Suite 103
Decatur, GA 30033-4611
404 320-1472
404 320-0849 Fax
www.acpe.edu

Health Advocate

The health advocate promotes patients' rights in the increasingly complex health care system of the US. Currently, Sarah Lawrence University in New York offers the nation's only master's degree program in health advocacy. Graduates of this program work in diverse professional capacities in health care: as patient representatives and administrators, on ethics committees and medical policy boards, and at hospitals and consumer health agencies. Salaries range from $35,000 to $45,000 for entry level to $65,000 to $75,000 for managers.

The health advocacy program at Sarah Lawrence is a 52-credit program. The curriculum includes core courses, discipline-based courses (eg, health law, economics, history, bioethics, evaluation and assessment, psychology, health care delivery and policy, and topics in physiology), and fieldwork.

Sarah Lawrence College
Health Advocacy Program
One Mead Way
Bronxville, NY 10708
914 395-2371
914 395-2664 Fax
E-mail: grad@slc.edu
www.slc.edu/grad_healthadvocacy.php

Horticultural Therapist

Horticultural therapy is a complementary therapy profession using gardening and horticultural activities to improve the social, educational, psychological, and physical adjustment of persons. The professional horticultural therapist uses a treatment plan in working with persons who are mentally and physically disabled and others with special needs, including people who are developmentally disabled, the elderly, substance abusers, public offenders, and socially disadvantaged. Horticultural therapists practice in diverse locations, including hospitals and institutions, vocational training facilities, nursing homes and halfway houses, rehabilitation facilities, older adult centers, correctional facilities, schools, arboreta and botanical gardens, parks and recreational settings, farms and horticultural businesses, and community gardens.

Nearly 20 schools in the US offer educational programs or curricula in horticultural therapy.

American Horticultural Therapy Association
3570 E 12th Avenue, Suite 206
Denver, CO 80206
800 634-1603
303 322-2485 Fax
E-mail: info@ahta.org
www.ahta.org

Medical Coder

A medical coder, a member of the health information service team, uses a classification system to assign code numbers and letters to each symptom, diagnosis, disease, procedure, and operation that appears in the patient's chart. These codes are used for insurance reimbursement, research, health planning analysis, and to make clinical decisions. A high degree of accuracy and a working knowledge of medical terminology, anatomy, and physiology are important skills for these professionals.

Career opportunities include:
- Inpatient Hospital Coder
- Reimbursement Specialist
- Outpatient Coder
- Coding Abstracting Analyst
- Insurance Claim Analyst
- Managed Care Organization Coder
- Procedural Coder
- Physician's Office/Clinic Coder

American Health Information Management Association (AHIMA)
233 N Michigan Avenue, Suite 2150
Chicago, IL 60601-5800
312 233-1100
312 233-1500 Fax
E-mail: info@ahima.org
www.ahima.org/careers

Medical Transcriptionist

Medical transcriptionists are specialists in medical language and healthcare documentation who interpret and transcribe dictation by physicians and other health professionals regarding patient assessment, workup, therapeutic procedures, clinical course, diagnosis, prognosis, and so on, editing dictated material for grammar and clarity as necessary and appropriate.

American Association for Medical Transcription
4230 Kiernan Avenue
Suite 130
Modesto, CA 95356
800 982-2182
209 527-9620
209 527-9633 Fax
E-mail: ahdi@ahdionline.org
www.ahdionline.org

ADDITIONAL INFORMATION

Section IV

Health Professions Education Data

Health Professions Education Data

Every year, the American Medical Association (AMA) surveys health professions' educational programs accredited by the following organizations:

- Accreditation Council for Occupational Therapy Education
- Accreditation Review Commission on Education for the Physician Assistant
- American Art Therapy Association
- American Board of Genetic Counseling
- American Dance Therapy Association
- American Orthoptic Council
- American Society of Health-System Pharmacists
- Association for Education and Rehabilitation of the Blind and Visually Impaired
- Commission on Accreditation for Health Informatics and Information Management Education
- Commission on Accreditation of Allied Health Education Programs
- Commission on Accreditation of Athletic Training Education
- Commission on Accreditation of Ophthalmic Medical Programs
- Commission on Dental Accreditation of the American Dental Association
- Commission on Massage Therapy Accreditation
- Commission on Opticianry Accreditation
- Council for Accreditation of Counseling and Related Educational Programs
- Council on Academic Accreditation in Audiology and Speech-Language Pathology
- Council on Accreditation of the National Recreation and Park Association
- Council on Rehabilitation Education
- Joint Review Committee on Education in Radiologic Technology
- Joint Review Committee on Educational Programs in Nuclear Medicine Technology
- National Accrediting Agency for Clinical Laboratory Sciences
- National Association of Schools of Music

The program population is established from periodic accreditation data and updates provided by each agency throughout the year. Accrediting agencies also forwarded to the AMA administrative changes received from educational programs and sponsoring institutions.

The AMA recognizes and thanks the accrediting agencies for their work in ensuring an accurate population and an up-to-date *Directory*. Specifically, the agencies helped AMA staff develop and test the survey instrument and ensured a high survey response rate by contacting programs that had not yet responded by the initial survey deadline of October 31, 2007.

Annual Survey of Health Professions Education Programs

In 2002, for the first time, the AMA used an online survey instrument to collect data on health professions education programs. This process was also used for the 2007 survey cycle, beginning in May and extending through November 2007. The online survey, available at www.ama-assn.org/go/hpsurvey, helps reduce survey mailing costs and allows for the collection of racial/ethnic program data, which had been discontinued in 1996 due to the financial burden and the difficulty of obtaining accurate data. Program directors received the survey via e-mail, which directs them to the survey site and provides institution ID, program ID, and login password. Those program directors without a valid e-mail address on file received this information via US mail.

To ensure a high response rate and data quality, nonrespondents received reminder e-mails/mailings/phone calls/faxes after the original surveys were sent, both from the AMA and from the accrediting agencies. Telephone, fax, and e-mail inquiries of program personnel helped clarify questionable responses.

Data collected were for the 2006-2007 academic year, generally September 1, 2006, through August 31, 2007.

Data Collected
The survey collected the following data:

Student data
- data on program enrollments, attrition, and graduates by gender and race/ethnicity

Program data
- Tuition cost (in-state and out-of-state)
- Class capacity per start date or session
- Availability of evening/weekend classes
- Program length(s)
- Program start date(s)
- Degree/credential(s) awarded
- Program stipend offered
- Data on employment/additional education of recent program graduates
- Name, address, telephone/fax numbers, and e-mail address of program official(s)
- Program Web site
- Availability of education/courses in medical/health care terms in non-English languages
- Availability of education in cultural competence or patient communication

Health Professions Education Data Book
Data collected on the survey, which had in the past been published in this section of the *Directory*, are now available in the *Health Professions Education Data Book*.

The 2007-2008 edition of the Data Book, published in May 2007, included the following tables, for academic year 2005-2006:

Section A: Data on Enrollments, Attrition, and Graduates, Programs, and Sponsoring Institutions
- Accredited or Approved Programs by Occupation, 1985, 1990, 1995, and 2006
- Number of Programs and Enrollments, Attrition, and Graduates by Occupation
- Enrollments by Occupation and Degree/Award
- Graduates by Occupation and Degree/Award
- Accredited Programs by Type of Sponsoring Institution
- Institutions Sponsoring Accredited Programs by Ownership Type
- Accredited Programs by Occupation and Type of Sponsoring Institution
- Enrollments, Graduates, and Number of Programs by State/Province and Occupation

Section B: Data on Enrollments, Attrition, and Graduates by Occupation, Gender, and Race-Ethnic Origin
- Enrollments, Attrition, and Graduates by Occupation and Gender
- Enrollments by Occupation and Gender/Race-Ethnic Origin
- Attrition by Occupation and Gender/Race-Ethnic Origin
- Graduates by Occupation and Gender/Race-Ethnic Origin
- Enrollments, Attrition, and Graduates by Race/Ethnic Origin and Gender
- Enrollments, Attrition, and Graduates by Gender and Type of Sponsoring Institution
- Enrollments, Attrition, and Graduates by Gender and Type of Sponsoring Institution for Whites
- Enrollments, Attrition, and Graduates by Gender and Type of Sponsoring Institution for Blacks
- Enrollments, Attrition, and Graduates by Gender and Type of Sponsoring Institution for Hispanics
- Enrollments, Attrition, and Graduates by Gender and Type of Sponsoring Institution for Native Americans/Alaskan Natives
- Enrollments, Attrition, and Graduates by Gender and Type of Sponsoring Institution for Asians/Pacific Islanders
- Enrollments, Attrition, and Graduates by Gender and Institutional Control Type
- Enrollments, Attrition, and Graduates by Gender and Institutional Control Type for Whites
- Enrollments, Attrition, and Graduates by Gender and Institutional Control Type for Blacks
- Enrollments, Attrition, and Graduates by Gender and Institutional Control Type for Hispanics
- Enrollments, Attrition, and Graduates by Gender and Institutional Control Type for Native Americans/Alaskan Natives
- Enrollments, Attrition, and Graduates by Gender and Institutional Control Type for Asians/Pacific Islanders

Section C: Data on Employment, Cultural Competence/Patient Communication Curricula, Tuition, Program Length, and Salary
- Percentage of Graduates Finding Employment Within 6 Months and/or Seeking Additional Education, by Occupation
- Number of Programs Offering Cultural Competence/Patient Communication Curricula, by Occupation
- Average First-Year Tuition, by Occupation
- Average Program Length, by Occupation
- Health Professions Salary Ranges

For more information or to order, call 312 464-5333 or e-mail enza.perrone@ama-assn.org.

The AMA's Role in Health Professions Education Data Collection

Since the early seventies, the AMA has annually collected program enrollment and graduate data for the allied health professions. Since 1989, enrollment, attrition, and graduate data have been compiled by gender. Collection of data on race/ethnic origin was discontinued after the 1995 survey; starting in 2002, these data are now available in the *Health Professions Education Data Book* (see above).

In addition, a wide variety of data collected on the survey are available through the AMA's Health Professions Data Service. For example, data on such variables as enrollment, attrition, and graduates, as well as program size, length, and tuition, can be broken out by state, profession, and/or accrediting agency. For more information, contact

American Medical Association
Medical Education Products
515 N State St
Chicago, IL 60610
312 464-5333
312 464-5830 Fax
E-mail: fred.lenhoff@ama-assn.org

Table 1. Accredited or Approved Programs by Occupation, 1985, 1990, 1995, 2000, 2005, and 2007

Occupation	1985	1990	1995	2000	2005	2007
Anesthesiologist Assistant	0	2	2	2	3	4
Art Therapist	—	—	—	28	31	33
Athletic Trainer	0	0	29	122	285	354
Audiologist	149	111	120	109	95	85
Cardiovascular Technologist	0	2	14	24	28	30
Clinical Assistant	0	0	0	2	2	2
Clinical Laboratory Scientist/Medical Technologist	584	420	357	255	228	223
Clin Lab Tech/Med Lab Tech	225	215	223	242	201	203
Counselor	43	146	239	334	190	187
Cytogenetic Technologist	0	0	6	6	5	6
Cytotechnologist	58	46	67	48	48	44
Dance Therapist	7	7	6	5	5	6
Dental Assistant	290	244	229	256	269	266
Dental Hygienist	198	202	212	255	279	279
Dental Laboratory Technician	58	49	37	30	21	21
Dentist	—	—	—	—	—	56
Diagnostic Medical Sonographer	24	43	77	76	130	149
Diagnostic Molecular Scientist	0	0	0	0	3	4
Dietetic Technician	80	62	70	67	66	52
Dietitian/Nutritionist	444	439	529	544	545	532
Electroneurodiagnostic Technologist	20	14	14	11	12	14
Emergency Medical Technician-Paramedic	20	72	96	122	201	213
Exercise Physiologist	0	0	0	0	0	2
Exercise Science Professional	0	0	0	0	0	8
Genetic Counselor	10	14	20	23	31	30
Health Information Administrator	54	55	53	51	46	46
Health Information Technician	85	108	142	175	179	194
Histotechnician	*	*	*	24	25	27
Histotechnologist	43*	37*	31*	2	2	3
Kinesiotherapist	0	0	0	5	7	6
Low Vision Therapist	—	—	—	—	1	1
Magnetic Resonance Technologist	—	—	—	—	—	2
Massage Therapist	—	—	—	63	63	82
Medical Assistant	168	185	221	475	511	557
Medical Dosimetrist	—	—	—	—	—	4
Medical Illustrator	5	6	5	5	5	5
Medical Librarian	69	63	57	56	56	55
Music Therapist	65	65	67	61	62	70
Nuclear Medicine Technologist	141	107	120	88	98	99
Nurse	—	—	—	—	—	463
Occupational Therapist	61	69	98	142	157	151
Occupational Therapy Assistant	60	69	108	185	134	137
Ophthalmic Assistant	—	—	—	—	—	5
Ophthalmic Dispensing Optician	17	17	24	24	23	21
Ophthalmic Medical Technician/Technologist	9	10	10	16	15	16
Optometric Technician	—	—	—	—	—	5
Optometrist	—	—	—	—	—	19
Orientation and Mobility Specialist	—	—	—	—	—	17
Orthoptist	—	—	—	16	18	15
Orthotist/Prosthetist	0	0	1	7	8	8
Pathologists' Assistant	0	0	0	5	7	8
Perfusionist	19	26	33	23	21	20
Pharmacist	—	—	—	—	—	101
Pharmacy Technician	8	29	56	96	96	90
Phlebotomist	0	39	68	66	54	55
Physical Therapist	109	122	145	196	209	202
Physical Therapist Assistant	69	107	179	286	238	222
Physician (allopathic)	—	—	—	—	—	142
Physician (osteopathic)	—	—	—	—	—	28
Physician Assistant	52	48	64	126	136	139
Podiatrist	—	—	—	—	—	8
Polysomnographic Technologist	0	0	0	0	0	7
Psychologist	—	—	—	—	—	229

DATA

Table 1. Accredited or Approved Programs by Occupation, 1985, 1990, 1995, 2000, 2005, and 2007 *(cont'd)*

Occupation	1985	1990	1995	2000	2005	2007
Radiation Therapist	101	104	120	72	77	80
Radiographer	744	672	677	583	601	616
Rehabilitation Counselor	—	—	—	83	98	99
Respiratory Therapist (Advanced)	232	259	286	310	315	323
Respiratory Therapist (Entry-Level)	182	159	174	105	43	40
Specialist in Blood Bank Technology	59	29	24	15	13	14
Speech-Language Pathologist	†	194	222	224	238	237
Surgical Assistant	3	3	‡	‡	5	7
Surgical Technologist	102	113	143	257	394	418
Teacher of the Visually Impaired	—	—	—	—	—	8
Therapeutic Recreation Specialist	—	—	—	43	40	40
Veterinarian	—	—	—	—	—	32
Veterinary Technologist	—	—	—	—	—	135
Vision Rehabilitation Therapist	—	—	—	9	9	7
Total	**4,338**	**4,370**	**5,012**	**6,417**	**6,651**	**8,118**

—These occupations were not part of the accreditation systems reflected in this Directory, or did not have accredited programs at the time.

* Before 1996, numbers for HT and HTL were not broken out.

† The number of speech-language pathologist programs for 1985 is included in the number of audiologist programs.

‡ Surgeon assistant programs were listed with physician assistant programs.

Table 2. Percentage of Graduates Finding Employment Within 6 Months and/or Seeking Additional Education, by Occupation, Academic Year 2006-2007

Occupation	# of responding prgms	Found Job (%)	Additional Education (%)	Both (%)
Anesthesiologist Assistant	2	100.0	2.5	0.0
Art Therapist	12	89.6	5.3	7.7
Athletic Trainer	207	48.1	42.8	18.0
Audiologist	33	72.7	0.3	1.2
Cardiovascular Technologist	18	89.5	5.3	7.2
Clinical Assistant	1	75.0	0.0	0.0
Clinical Laboratory Scientist/Medical Technologist	199	96.6	3.8	5.5
Clinical Laboratory Technician/Medical Laboratory Technician	153	91.8	10.1	13.2
Counselor	47	86.7	8.5	3.6
Cytogenetic Technologist	3	97.2	2.8	4.2
Cytotechnologist	32	91.1	7.4	2.2
Dance/Movement Therapist	3	88.0	0.0	3.0
Dental Assistant	158	83.6	11.0	8.6
Dental Hygienist	180	92.0	2.4	6.0
Dental Laboratory Technician	7	82.7	17.9	4.0
Diagnostic Medical Sonographer	77	93.1	4.5	4.3
Diagnostic Molecular Scientist	2	94.5	0.0	5.5
Electroneurodiagnostic Technologist	9	98.1	5.6	11.1
Emergency Medical Technician-Paramedic	74	91.0	13.0	15.1
Exercise Physiologist	1	100.0	0.0	0.0
Exercise Science Professional	2	90.0	10.0	0.0
Genetic Counselor	18	86.9	0.9	0.1
Health Information Administrator	24	81.3	10.7	7.0
Health Information Technician	86	84.9	5.0	8.5
Histotechnician	20	88.7	8.3	7.8
Histotechnologist	3	100.0	3.3	3.3
Kinesiotherapist	4	65.0	25.3	26.8
Massage Therapist	17	58.5	18.7	27.1
Medical Assistant	299	82.9	8.9	10.4
Medical Illustrator	4	86.5	4.0	1.3
Music Therapist	27	80.0	7.8	10.3
Nuclear Medicine Technologist	90	94.9	1.5	2.8
Occupational Therapist	102	93.8	1.8	3.7
Occupational Therapy Assistant	81	88.6	3.5	3.1
Ophthalmic Dispensing Optician	5	88.4	27.0	4.2
Ophthalmic Medical Technician/Technologist	8	86.5	1.0	0.0
Orientation and Mobility Specialist	5	71.0	3.0	6.0
Orthoptist	11	81.9	0.0	0.0
Orthotist/Prosthetist	5	79.6	24.0	22.0
Pathologists' Assistant	7	98.6	1.4	0.0
Perfusionist	10	94.7	3.3	0.0
Pharmacy Technician	35	77.5	9.0	10.5
Phlebotomist	41	60.5	20.5	15.0
Physician Assistant	93	92.6	1.3	2.8
Polysomnographic Technologist	5	77.6	0.8	1.4
Radiation Therapist	46	94.0	3.0	5.6
Radiographer	436	92.6	11.6	18.0
Rehabilitation Counselor	32	93.2	5.5	5.3
Respiratory Therapist (Advanced)	188	97.9	7.5	11.1
Respiratory Therapist (Entry-Level)	17	92.2	34.3	27.1
Specialist in Blood Bank Technology	11	90.9	2.3	18.2
Speech-Language Pathologist	89	93.2	1.4	3.8
Surgical Assistant	4	70.0	0.0	2.5
Surgical Technologist	189	82.8	6.2	9.9
Therapeutic Recreation Specialist	14	71.6	10.6	3.7
Vision Rehabilitation Therapist	3	100.0	0.0	0.0

Table 3. Average First-Year Tuition, by Occupation, Academic Year 2006-2007

Occupation	Tuition
Anesthesiologist Assistant	$27,450
Art Therapist	$17,125
Athletic Trainer	$12,054
Audiologist	$8,865
Cardiovascular Technologist	$9,578
Clinical Assistant	$1,408
Clinical Laboratory Scientist/Medical Technologist	$6,206
Clinical Laboratory Technician/Medical Laboratory	$3,392
Counselor	$22,771
Cytogenetic Technologist	$6,067
Cytotechnologist	$8,200
Dance/Movement Therapist	$16,980
Dental Assistant	$4,397
Dental Hygienist	$5,037
Dental Laboratory Technician	$3,228
Diagnostic Medical Sonographer	$6,281
Diagnostic Molecular Scientist	$5,061
Electroneurodiagnostic Technologist	$3,436
Emergency Medical Technician-Paramedic	$4,022
Genetic Counselor	$12,313
Health Information Administrator	$8,034
Health Information Technician	$3,188
Histotechnician	$3,870
Histotechnologist	$10,900
Kinesiotherapist	$4,445
Massage Therapist	$8,172
Medical Assistant	$6,294
Medical Illustrator	$5,910
Music Therapist	$10,093
Nuclear Medicine Technologist	$7,422
Occupational Therapist	$13,120
Occupational Therapy Assistant	$3,941
Ophthalmic Dispensing Optician	$2,781
Ophthalmic Medical Technician/Technologist	$6,131
Orientation and Mobility Specialist	$3,138
Orthoptist	$1,913
Orthotist/Prosthetist	$8,355
Pathologists' Assistant	$14,108
Perfusionist	$16,669
Pharmacy Technician	$4,627
Phlebotomist	$1,481
Physician Assistant	$20,573
Polysomnographic Technologist	$6,509
Radiation Therapist	$5,600
Radiographer	$4,675
Rehabilitation Counselor	$6,746
Respiratory Therapist (Advanced)	$5,209
Respiratory Therapist (Entry-Level)	$4,520
Specialist in Blood Bank Technology	$5,036
Speech-Language Pathologist	$7,985
Surgical Assistant	$4,154
Surgical Technologist	$6,304
Therapeutic Recreation Specialist	$3,796
Vision Rehabilitation Therapist	$1,757

Table 4. Average Program Length, by Occupation, Academic Year 2006-2007

Occupation	# of Months
Anesthesiologist Assistant	26.0
Art Therapist	25.9
Athletic Trainer	33.1
Audiologist	44.0
Cardiovascular Technologist	20.4
Clinical Assistant	9.0
Clinical Laboratory Scientist/Medical Technologist	16.1
Clinical Laboratory Technician/Medical Laboratory	21.0
Counselor	32.9
Cytogenetic Technologist	14.2
Cytotechnologist	13.3
Dance/Movement Therapist	24.3
Dental Assistant	12.0
Dental Hygienist	22.2
Dental Laboratory Technician	20.9
Diagnostic Medical Sonographer	19.0
Diagnostic Molecular Scientist	18.0
Electroneurodiagnostic Technologist	20.6
Emergency Medical Technician-Paramedic	16.2
Exercise Physiologist	12.0
Exercise Science Professional	48.0
Genetic Counselor	20.5
Health Information Administrator	30.8
Health Information Technician	22.0
Histotechnician	16.1
Histotechnologist	15.0
Kinesiotherapist	34.3
Massage Therapist	13.1
Medical Assistant	15.9
Medical Illustrator	22.5
Music Therapist	46.8
Nuclear Medicine Technologist	19.3
Occupational Therapist	32.4
Occupational Therapy Assistant	22.3
Ophthalmic Dispensing Optician	16.6
Ophthalmic Medical Technician/Technologist	21.4
Orientation and Mobility Specialist	15.0
Orthoptist	23.5
Orthotist/Prosthetist	19.6
Pathologists' Assistant	21.6
Perfusionist	20.1
Pharmacy Technician	11.4
Phlebotomist	4.6
Physician Assistant	27.8
Polysomnographic Technologist	13.8
Radiation Therapist	20.6
Radiographer	23.8
Rehabilitation Counselor	25.2
Respiratory Therapist (Advanced)	22.5
Respiratory Therapist (Entry-Level)	20.4
Specialist in Blood Bank Technology	15.7
Speech-Language Pathologist	26.1
Surgical Assistant	13.0
Surgical Technologist	14.9
Therapeutic Recreation Specialist	36.9
Vision Rehabilitation Therapist	19.0

DATA

Table 5. Health Professions Salary Ranges

Occupation	Starting Salary	Overall Average	Upper Ranges	Year of Data
Anesthesiologist assistant	$95,000-$120,000		$160,000-$180,000	2006
Art therapist	$32,000	$38,000-$48,000	$50,000-$80,000	2006
Athletic trainer	$35,000	$45,000	$55,000-$75,000	2005
Audiologist	$52,000	$65,000	$78,000 (management)	2006
Cardiovascular technologist	$36,000-$45,000	$50,000-$65,000	$75,000 plus	2006
Clinical lab scientist/med technologist		$44,500-$52,000		2005
CLS/MT manager		$69,500-$72,000		2005
Clinical lab technician/medical lab technician		$37,100-$41,000		2005
Counselor	$23,560	$42,110	$67,170	2004
Cytotechnologist	$46,000	$68,645	$105,600	2005
Cytotech supervisor	$48,000	$70,646	$100,000	2002
Dental assistant		$15.48/hr		2004
Dental hygienist		$30.30/hr		2004
Dental lab technician		$15.40/hr		2003
Dentist		$114,000	$315,000	2004
Diagnostic medical sonographer		$61,984	$67,253	2005
Diagnostic molecular scientist	$35,000-$47,000		$45,000-$82,000 (management)	2002
Dietetic technician	$30,000-$40,000*		$38,000-$53,000	2007
Dietitian/nutritionist	$42,000-$55,000*		$60,000-$91,000	2007
Electroneurodiagnostic technologist	$35,610	$44,621	$49,192-$52,187	2006
Emergency medical technician-paramedic	$16,090	$25,310	$43,240	2004
Genetic counselor	$40,900	$59,000	$150,000	2006
Health information administrator	$40,000	$54,700	$85,000	2003
Health information technician	$30,000	$39,100	$50,000	2003
Histologic technician		$40,500		2005
Histotechnologist		$44,970-$49,360		2005
Kinesiotherapist	$32,500-$38,000	$48,000	$60,000	2006
Low vision therapist		$44,777		2002
Magnetic resonance technologist	$44,410	$66,861	$78,210	2004
Marriage and family counselor/therapist		$57,119		1997
Massage therapist		$20,000- $49,000		2005
Medical assistant	$22,650	$27,951	$30,000	2004
Medical illustrator	$40,000-$45,000	$45,000-$75,000	$90,000-$130,000	2002
Medical librarian	$41,000	$58,000	$158,000	2005
Music therapist		$42,364		2004
Nuclear med technologist	$56,400	$69,083	$83,505	2007
Nurse	$37,300	$52,330	$74,760	2004
Occupational therapist	$46,334	$58,080	$80,000	2006
Occupational therapy assistant	$33,000	$39,728	$55,100	2006
Ophthalmic assistant	$21,500	$40,040	$44,833	2005
Ophthalmic dispensing optician	$27,000			1997
Ophthalmic laboratory technician	$15,100		$25,000	2000
Ophthalmic medical technologist	$45,000	$58,481	$70,400- $125,000	2005
Ophthalmic technician	$39,000	$47,438	$56,643	2005
Optometrist		$105,000		2006
Orientation and mobility specialist		$46,564		2002
Orthoptist	$35,000-$42,000	$45,000-$50,000	$80,000	2000
Orthotist and prosthetist	$22,000-$35,000	$42,000-$60,000		2003
Pathologists' assistant	$55,000-$75,000		$75,000-$100,000	2005
Perfusionist	$60,000-$75,000	$70,000-$90,000	$100,000 (manager)	2006
Pharmacy technician	$19,000	$27,000	$35,000	2002
Pharmacist		$94,927		2006
Phlebotomist		$24,315-$29,120		2005
Physical therapist	$54,000	$70,000	$100,000	2006
Physical therapist assistant	$30,000	$37,000		2005

Table 5. Health Professions Salary Ranges *(cont'd)*

Occupation	Starting Salary	Overall Average	Upper Ranges	Year of Data
Physician assistant	$71,004	$84,396	$111,000-$200,000	2006
Psychologist	$32,380	$54,950	$92,250	2004
Radiographer	$36,918	$59,735	$64,580	2004
Radiation therapist	$65,381	$72,300	$80,067	2004
Rehabilitation counselor	$27,500-$51,700	$34,300-$55,000	$55,000-$75,000+	2006
Vision rehabilitation Therapist		$37,055		2002
Respiratory therapist	$41,537	$56,222	$74,880	2005
Specialist in blood bank technology	$45,000 (bench techs)	$54,000 (supervisors)	$66,000 (managers)	2006
Speech-language pathologist (schools)	$40,041	$52,131-$57,000	$80,000 (management)	2006
Speech-language pathologist (health care)	$52,694	$60,000	$72,985 (management)	2005
Surgical technologist		$34,010		2004
Teacher of the visually impaired	$47,086			2002
Therapeutic recreation specialist (CTRS)	$30,000	$39,000	$60,000-$70,000	2004
Veterinarian	$39,020	$66, 590	$118,430	2004
Veterinary technologist and technician	$8.51/hr	$11.99.hr	$17.12/hr	2004

*Data valid for those employed full time in their current primary position for 5 years or less.

DATA